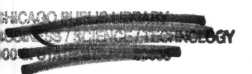

Pathology of Environmental and Occupational Disease

PATHOLOGY OF ENVIRONMENTAL AND OCCUPATIONAL DISEASE

John E. Craighead, MD
Professor
Department of Pathology
University of Vermont Medical School
Colchester Research Facility
Colchester, Vermont

with 324 illustrations, 7 in color

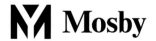 Mosby

St. Louis   Baltimore   Berlin   Boston   Carlsbad   Chicago   London   Madrid
Naples   New York   Philadelphia   Sydney   Tokyo   Toronto

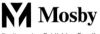
Mosby

Dedicated to Publishing Excellence

Executive Editor: Susan M. Gay
Senior Managing Editor: Lynne Gery
Project Manager: Linda Clarke
Senior Production Editor: Patricia C. Walter
Interior Design: Sheilah Barrett
Cover Design: Ellen Dawson
Manufacturing Supervisor: Karen Lewis

Printed in the United States of America.
Composition by The Clarinda Company.
Printing/binding by Maple-Vail, York.

Mosby–Year Book, Inc.
11830 Westline Industrial Drive
St. Louis, Missouri 63146

Library of Congress-in-Publication Data

Craighead, John E.
    Pathology of environmental and occupational disease / John E.
Craighead.
       p.   cm.
    Includes bibliographical references and index.
    ISBN 0-8016-7776-9
    1. Environmentally induced diseases. 2. Occupational diseases.
I. Title.
    [DNLM: 1. Environmental Health. 2. Environmental Pollutants-
-adverse effects. 3. Occupational Diseases. WA 30 C886p 1995]
RB152.C76 1995
616.9′8--dc20
DNLM/DLC
for Library of Congress
                                         94-31205
                                            CIP

95 96 97 98 99 / 9 8 7 6 5 4 3 2 1

Contributors

Richard Albertini, MD, PhD

Professor of Medicine and Director, Vermont Cancer Center, University of Vermont, Burlington, Vermont

19 DNA Damage and Repair

H. Clarke Anderson, MD

Professor of Pathology and Harrington Professor of Orthopedic Research, University of Kansas Medical Center; Attending in Pathology, University Hospital, Kansas City, Kansas

31 Skeletal System

**David V. Bates,
MD, FRCP, FRCPC, FACP, FRSC**

Professor Emeritus of Medicine, University of British Columbia, Vancouver, British Columbia, Canada

2 Outdoor Air Quality and Pollution

Carl G. Becker, MD

Professor and Chair of Pathology, Medical College of Wisconsin; Director of Clinical Laboratories and Pathology, United Regional Medical Services, Milwaukee, Wisconsin

13 Tobacco Abuse

Richard F. Branda, MD

Professor of Medicine, University of Vermont College of Medicine, Burlington, Vermont

9 Alimentary and Nutritional Excesses and Deficiencies

Kenneth P. Cantor, PhD, MPH

Epidemiologist, National Cancer Institute, Bethesda, Maryland

16 Water Quality and Pollution

Stephen F. Cleary, PhD

Professor of Physiology and Biophysics, Medical College of Virginia/Virginia Commonwealth University, Richmond, Virginia

12 Electromagnetic Energy

John E. Craighead, MD

Professor of Pathology, University of Vermont Colchester Research Facility, Colchester, Vermont

3 Indoor Air Quality and Pollution
6 Inorganic and Organic Dust Pollutants
9 Alimentary and Nutritional Excesses and Deficiencies
26 Carcinogenesis
28 Airways and Lung
33 Reproductive System

Gunther F. Craun

President, Global Consulting for Environmental Health, Radford, Virginia

16 Water Quality and Pollution

Gary Curhan, MD

Instructor in Medicine, Harvard Medical School, Boston; Chief of Clinical Nephrology, Brockton/West Roxbury VA Medical Center, West Roxbury, and Associate Physician, Brigham and Women's Hospital, Boston, Massachusetts

9 Alimentary and Nutritional Excesses and Deficiencies

Elizabeth D. Dolci, PhD

Assistant Professor, Department of Environmental Health Sciences, Johnson State College, Johnson, Vermont

18 Cell Membranes

Kevin Driscoll, PhD

Section Head, Human Safety Department, The Procter & Gamble Company, Cincinnati, Ohio

24 Mediators of Inflammation

Harriet P. Dustan, MD

Emeritus Professor of Medicine, University of Alabama School of Medicine, Birmingham, Alabama

9 Alimentary and Nutritional Excesses and Deficiencies

John L. Farber, MD

Professor of Pathology and Pharmacology, Jefferson Medical College, Thomas Jefferson University, Philadelphia, Pennsylvania

17 Mechanisms of Cell Injury

Vincent F. Garry, MD

Associate Professor of Laboratory Medicine and Pathology, University of Minnesota Medical School, Minneapolis, Minnesota

8 Agricultural Pesticides

Doyle G. Graham, MD, PhD

Professor of Pathology, Director of Neuropathology, and Director, Integrated Toxicology Program, Duke University Medical Center, Durham, North Carolina

30 Central and Peripheral Nervous Systems

Jack Griffith, PhD

Adjunct Professor of Epidemiology, Department of Epidemiology, School of Public Health, University of North Carolina at Chapel Hill, Chapel Hill, North Carolina

8 Agricultural Pesticides

J.W. Grisham, MD

Kenan Professor and Chair of Pathology and Professor of Medicine, University of North Carolina at Chapel Hill; Chair, Department of Pathology, UNC Hospitals, Chapel Hill, North Carolina

29 Liver

Miles P. Hacker, PhD

Professor, Department of Pharmacology, University of Vermont College of Medicine, Burlington, Vermont

22 Nitric Oxide

Michael G. Hitchcock, MBChB

Assistant Professor of Pathology, Duke University Medical Center, Durham, North Carolina

37 The Eye

Sally A. Huber, PhD

Associate Professor of Pathology, University of Vermont College of Medicine, Burlington, Vermont

25 Immunopathology

Anne E. Huot, PhD

Associate Professor, Department of Medical Technology, University of Vermont, Burlington, Vermont

22 Nitric Oxide

Yvonne M.W. Janssen, PhD

Postdoctoral Fellow, Department of Pathology, University of Vermont College of Medicine, Burlington, Vermont

21 Active Oxygen Species

Michael Kashgarian, MD

Professor of Pathology and Biology, Yale University School of Medicine; Director, Diagnostic Electron Microscopy and Renal Pathology, Yale New Haven Hospital, New Haven, Connecticut

32 Urinary System

Gordon K. Klintworth, MD, PhD

Professor of Pathology, Joseph A.C. Wadsworth Research Professor of Ophthalmology, and Director of Research, Duke University Eye Center, Durham, North Carolina

37 The Eye

Steven L. Kunkel, MS, PhD

Professor of Pathology, The University of Michigan Medical School, Ann Arbor, Michigan

24 Mediators of Inflammation

Robert W. Leader, DVM

Professor Emeritus, Department of Pathology, Michigan State University, East Lansing, Michigan

9 Alimentary and Nutritional Excesses and Deficiencies

Orville A. Levander, PhD

USDA/ARS, Beltsville Human Nutrition Research Center, Nutrient Requirements and Functions Laboratory, Beltsville, Maryland

9 Alimentary and Nutritional Excesses and Deficiencies

Michael M. Lipsky, PhD

Professor of Pathology, University of Maryland School of Medicine, Baltimore, Maryland

5 Chemical Toxicity

George Lumb, MD

Emeritus Professor of Pathology, Hahnemann University School of Medicine, Philadelphia, Pennsylvania; Scholar in Residence, Department of Pathology, Duke University Medical Center, Durham, North Carolina

4 Metal Toxicity

Laura H. McArthur, PhD, RD

Assistant Professor of Environmental Studies and Nutrition, University of Vermont, Burlington, Vermont

9 Alimentary and Nutritional Excesses and Deficiencies

Donald R. Mattison, MD

Professor of Environmental and Occupational Health, and Dean, University of Pittsburgh Graduate School of Public Health; Professor of Obstetrics and Gynecology, University of Pittsburgh School of Medicine, Pittsburgh, Pennsylvania

33 Reproductive System

Thomas J. Montine, MD, PhD

Department of Pathology, Duke University Medical Center, Durham, North Carolina

30 Central and Peripheral Nervous Systems

Brooke Taylor Mossman, PhD

Professor of Pathology, University of Vermont College of Medicine, Burlington, Vermont

21 Active Oxygen Species

George F. Murphy, MD

Herman Beerman Professor of Dermatology, Professor of Pathology, and Director of Dermatopathology Research and Training, University of Pennsylvania, Philadelphia, Pennsylvania

27 Skin

Brian J. Nickoloff, MD, PhD

Associate Professor of Pathology and Dermatology, University of Michigan Medical School, Ann Arbor, Michigan

24 Mediators of Inflammation

R. Julian Preston, PhD

Adjunct Professor, Integrated Toxicology Program, Duke University, and Toxicology Department, North Carolina State University, Durham, North Carolina

20 Genetic Injury

Timothy Quinlan, MS

Research Fellow, Department of Pathology, University of Vermont, Burlington, Vermont

21 Active Oxygen Species

John T. Reeves, MD

Professor of Medicine and Pediatrics, University of Colorado Health Sciences Center, Denver, Colorado

7 High Altitude and Human Disease

Cheryl F. Rosen, MD, FRCPC

Assistant Professor of Medicine, University of Toronto Faculty of Medicine, Women's College Hospital, Toronto, Ontario, Canada

10 Ultraviolet Radiation

Emanuel Rubin, MD

Gonzalo E. Aponte Professor of Pathology and Chair of Pathology and Cell Biology, Jefferson Medical College of Thomas Jefferson University; Attending Physician-in-Chief (Pathology), Thomas Jefferson University Hospital, Philadelphia, Pennsylvania

14 Alcohol Abuse

Joseph Sataloff, MD

Professor of Otolaryngology, Jefferson Medical College, Thomas Jefferson University, Philadelphia, Pennsylvania

36 Auditory Function

Robert Thayer Sataloff, MD, DMA

Professor of Otolaryngology, Jefferson Medical College, Thomas Jefferson University, Philadelphia, Pennsylvania; Adjunct Professor of Otolaryngology, Georgetown University, Washington, DC

35 Phonation
36 Auditory Function

Stephen H. Schneider, PhD

Professor of Biological Science and Senior Fellow, Institute for International Studies, Stanford University, Stanford, California

1 Climatic Change

Anthony R. Scialli, MD

Director, Residency Traning Program, Department of Obstetrics and Gynecology, Georgetown University Medical Center; Director, Reproductive Toxicology Center, Columbia Hospital for Women Medical Center, Washington, DC

34 Teratology

Robert M. Strieter, MD

Associate Professor of Medicine, The University of Michigan Medical School, Ann Arbor, Michigan

24 Mediators of Inflammation

Russell P. Tracy, PhD

Associate Professor of Pathology and Biochemistry, University of Vermont College of Medicine, Burlington, Vermont

9 Alimentary and Nutritional Excesses and Deficiencies

Thomas R. Tritton, PhD

Professor of Pharmacology, University of Vermont College of Medicine, Burlington, Vermont

18 Cell Membranes

Benjamin F. Trump, MD

Professor and Chair of Pathology, University of Maryland School of Medicine, Baltimore, Maryland

5 Chemical Toxicity

Arthur C. Upton, MD

Clinical Professor of Pathology and Radiology, University of New Mexico School of Medicine, Albuquerque, New Mexico; Professor Emeritus of Environmental Medicine, New York University School of Medicine, New York, New York

11 Ionizing Radiation

William M. Valentine, PhD, DVM

Assistant Research Professor of Pathology, Duke
University Medical Center, Durham, North Carolina

30   Central and Peripheral Nervous Systems

Bennett Van Houten, PhD

Senior Scientist and Associate Professor of Human
Biological Chemistry and Genetics, University of Texas
Medical Branch at Galveston, Galveston, Texas

19   DNA Damage and Repair

Bernard M. Wagner, MD

Research Professor of Pathology, New York University
School of Medicine, New York, New York

9   Alimentary and Nutritional Excesses and Deficiencies

Peter A. Ward, MD

Godfrey D. Stobbe Professor and Chair of Pathology,
The University of Michigan Medical School and
Hospitals, Ann Arbor, Michigan

24   Mediators of Inflammation

Charles V. Wetli, MD

Deputy Chief Medical Examiner of Dade County; Clinical
Associate Professor of Pathology, University of Miami
School of Medicine, Miami, Florida

15   Illicit Drug Abuse

Robert C. Woodworth, PhD

Professor and Vice Chair of Biochemistry, University of
Vermont College of Medicine, Burlington, Vermont

9   Alimentary and Nutritional Excesses and Deficiencies
23   Energy-Producing Metabolic Pathways

Chung S. Yang, PhD

Professor II and Associate Chair, Robert Wood Johnson
Medical School, Piscataway, New Jersey

9   Alimentary and Nutritional Excesses and Deficiencies

Wei-Cheng You, MD

Beijing Institute for Cancer Research, Beijing Medical
University, Beijing, China

9   Alimentary and Nutritional Excesses and Deficiencies

To those physicians and scientists who have gone before us,

and to those in the future who will follow in their footsteps

To what extent is human disease attributable to environmental factors? Various estimates have been made, but the question invariably focuses on how, in fact, we define environment. This text addresses environmental disease broadly; occupational diseases are considered to be the result of specific types of exposure experienced in the workplace. Thus, it too is environmental disease. Simply stated, environmental disease results from our interactions with the world around us (in contrast to genetic, immunologic, metabolic, transmissible, and iatrogenic disease). This book integrates concepts of causation and pathogenesis in the context of the resulting disease and the tissue changes (i.e., pathology) that accompany it. However, this is not a traditional pathology text replete with descriptions and illustrations of gross and microscopic lesions. For detailed morphological information on a specific disease, the reader should turn to references that describe the clinical conditions and the associated tissue alterations.

An understanding of environmental disease invariably reflects an appreciation of the etiological factors that are responsible. Thus, in Part I entitled Causes of Environmental and Occupational Diseases, the reader can garner a sense of the geographical, ecological, cultural, economic, and technical aspects of an exposure that proves to be a causative or contributing factor in disease. By their nature, these complex factors are exceedingly diverse. The editor has refrained from developing this text into an exhaustive, encyclopedic presentation of factual material. But the detail provided is important if we are to understand the subtle influences that determine the outcome of an environmental exposure. In Part I, considerable space is devoted to nutrition and alimentary toxicology within the perspectives of their important role in the development of many diseases. Infectious diseases pose a difficult problem for the editor because so many common conditions are a result of exposure to a microorganism in our environment, rather than a result of transmission from one person to another. The writers of the chapters concerned with the various organ systems in Part III have brought to our attention specific human infectious diseases, but inevitably, the presentation is incomplete, considering the vast variety of organisms in our environment to which we are exposed.

Part II, Pathogenic Mechanisms of Environmental and Occupational Disease, is a comprehensive examination of comtemporary pathogenic concepts concerned with the mechanisms involved in the generation of disease. Our understanding is ever-changing, paced by the explosive growth in our fundamental knowledge of cell and molecular biology. Although based on concepts of general pathology, it is evident that the environmental experiences of humans invariably invoke specific and often unique mechanistic processes related to exposures to toxic substances in the workplace and the world around us (for example, mesothelioma, hepatic angiosarcoma, and chloroacne). As our modern world becomes increasingly complex, so do the diseases that seemingly are inevitable outcomes.

Finally, Part III, entitled Organ Pathology of Environmental and Occupational Disease approaches these diseases specifically from the perspective of the human experience. Although an enormous body of experimental information invariably has accumulated, the appropriate study of disease in man is based on an understanding of the conditions as they occur in human populations worldwide. Thus, epidemiological study is required to formulate cause-and-effect relationships. Although animal models of disease are critical considerations, in this presentation we have not stressed models as surrogates unless correlates with human disease exist. It is paradoxical, for example, that hepatocarcinomas occur infrequently in developed countries, whereas so many commonly used modern chemicals readily produce these tumors in standard animal toxicity studies. Does this imply that the animal studies are misleading, or does it suggest that unrecognized cofactors contribute to hepatotoxicity and carcinogenicity in areas of the world undergoing rapid industrialization?

Because environmental exposures of a great diversity of types are now an everyday experience, establishing a cause-and-effect relationship between a specific exposure and an illness in an individual case is a difficult, if not impossible, challenge. Epidemiological studies often can demonstrate a "risk" resulting from a hypothetical exposure, but they cannot predict and rationalize a diversity of technical considerations in individual situations that influence the outcome. The inevitable biological differences between one individual and another is a variable that, as yet, has not been addressed satisfactorily. Laboratory studies and animal models provide concrete evidence of the potential toxicity of a substance in our environment, but the information is often of limited use when the exposure is relatively small or transient and by a route not easily duplicated or tested in animals. The clinical scientist and pathologist face a difficult task in determining whether or not an illness or a specific lesion is related to a potentially toxic substance in the environment. Deciphering these riddles will continue to be a challenge for biomedical scientists.

The approach in this book permits the reader to bridge from causation to mechanism, to human disease (or the inverse) without undue repetition and redundancy in the text. Because of the diversity of the subject matter and the great variability in our knowledge, chapters differ in emphasis and depth. The science of some environmental topics is relatively mature (for example, air pollution), whereas other sciences are in their infancy (for example, electromagnetic energy). Rather than constrain the contributing authors, the editor has permitted substantial liberty in the scope and focus of the individual presentations.

John E. Craighead

Contents

Part I

CAUSES OF ENVIRONMENTAL AND OCCUPATIONAL DISEASE

Chapter 1

CLIMATIC CHANGE

Stephen H. Schneider

THE MEDIA DEBATE

To provide a perspective as to whether there are any significant public health implications over the prospect that human activities may alter the climate, it is first necessary to
review that debate, including its physical, biological, and
social scientific interactions. Several years after "global
warming" hit the headlines in North America in the wake
of the heat wave and fires of 1988, so much misinforma-
tion about the greenhouse effect had been circulated that
public understanding was often confused and public policy
making paralyzed since that time. The airwaves and printed
pages have been clogged by opposing advocates offering
assertions and counterassertions about the alleged serious-
ness or triviality of global warming.

As a climatologist identified with this subject, I am constantly asked to explain what is actually happening and its
importance. The experience since those hotter-than-usual
summers of 1987 and 1988 has confirmed for me at least
two crucial points: (1) The extent of public concern *should
be shaped* by the best scientific and economic knowledge
available about possible long-term climate change and its
effects on, for example, farms, floods, sea levels, forest

fires, ecosystems, and cardiovascular or tropical diseases;
(2) the extent of public concern *is being shaped* by the blurring of scientific and economic knowledge under the impact of political opinion, media miscommunication, and a
polarized debate among battling scientists.

Scientists too often share responsibility with the media
for not communicating complex scientific issues clearly to
the public. Most members of the general public as well as
many officials in government do not recognize that many
scientists spend the bulk of their time arguing about what
they do not know. We simply must spend more time making clear the distinctions among (1) what is well-known and
accepted by most knowledgeable scientists, (2) what is
known with some degree of reliability, and (3) what is
highly speculative.

The public debate on global warming rarely separates
those components, thereby leaving the false impression that
the scientific community is in overall intellectual disarray
on every aspect of the issue. In fact, the 15-year-old, often-
reaffirmed U.S. National Academy of Sciences consensus
estimate (1.5° C to 4.5° C global average warming if the
atmospheric concentration of carbon dioxide [CO_2] were to
double) still reflects the best approximation derivable from
a wide range of current climate models[20] and ancient climatic eras.[17,27] The earth has not been more than 1° C to
2° C warmer now than during the 1×10^4 year era over
which human civilization developed. The previous ice age,
in which mile-high ice sheets stretched from New York to
Chicago to the Arctic or across northern Europe, was "only"
5° C colder on a global average than the current 1×10^4
year interglacial epoch. This estimate of 1.5° C to 4.5° C
warming from CO_2 doubling still includes those studies that
halved the "best guess" on warming from over 4° C to 2.5°
C. Perhaps some new discovery next week will push it back
up again, but even if not, that enduring 1.5° C to 4.5° C

3

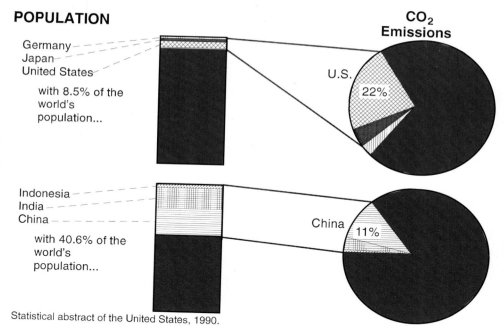

Fig. 1-1. Global inequities in carbon dioxide (CO_2) generation by developed and developing countries in relation to percentage of world population.

Statistical abstract of the United States, 1990.

warming consensus estimate is still widely believed by knowledgeable experts.

Changes of this magnitude on a global scale could dramatically alter climatic patterns, affecting agriculture, water supplies, disease patterns, ecosystems, endangered species, storms, sea level, and coastal flooding. All aspects, however, must be stated in terms of probabilities because few scientists state unequivocally that they believe the future climate will be in or out of the 1.5° C to 4.5° C warming range. Rather, most believe this range to be reasonably probable.[19] Therefore, if scientific opinion is to be communicated accurately, it must be by conveying issues in probabilistic terms—even if those probabilities are heuristically, rather than objectively, determinable.[50] What counts is the nature of the evidence and the spectrum of opinions of a broadly representative group of experts.[20,33] The media should focus on providing perspective on the range of views, not pitting one extreme against another.

The following global warming–related points are accepted, I believe, by a large fraction of the relevant expert communities. One good source for discussions on the following points is the National Academy of Sciences study on global warming and its implications.[33] (The parentheses after each of these statements indicate my own estimate of the likelihood of the statement being valid.)

1. Greenhouse gases, such as water vapor (H_2O), carbon dioxide (CO_2), methane (CH_4), nitrous oxide (N_2O), and chlorofluorocarbons (CFCs), trap infrared radiative energy in the lower atmosphere. (Certain)

2. The natural greenhouse effect from clouds, water vapor, CO_2, and methane is responsible for some 33° C of natural surface temperature warming. (Certain)

3. Since the Industrial Revolution, humans have altered the natural greenhouse effect by adding 25% more CO_2 (Fig. 1-1), 100% more methane, and a host of other greenhouse gases, such as N_2O and CFCs. (Certain)

4. Greenhouse gas accumulations from human activities since preindustrial times should have added some 1 to 2 watts of infrared radiative energy over every square meter of earth. This is well established, based on our considerable knowledge of the structure of the atmosphere and extensive validation from satellites and other measurements—even though the extra 1 to 2 watts cannot be directly measured yet. (Very likely)

5. The earth has, in fits and starts, warmed up by about 0.5° C over the past century; the 1980s is the warmest decade on record and 1990, 1991, and 1988 were (in order) the warmest years in the thermometer records. (Very likely)

6. Although no highly significant correlations between the observed warming and the buildup of human-induced greenhouse gases can be claimed for at least another decade or two, the likelihood that the 0.5° C twentieth-century warming trend is wholly a natural phenomenon is small (I would estimate perhaps a 10% to 20% chance).[49] (Likely)

7. Most climatic models project a warming of several degrees or so in the next 50 years (Fig. 1-2), given standard greenhouse gas emission scenarios, and

they portend a potential long-term (i.e., A.D. 2100 to 2200) warming of as high as 5° C to 10° C.[20] (Good chance, at least an even bet)

8. The natural, sustained, globally averaged rate of surface air temperature change (from the breakup of the last ice age 1.5×10^4 years ago to the full establishment of our current interglacial age some 5 to 8 $\times 10^3$ years ago) is about 1° C per 1×10^3 years. Even the minimum projected human-induced rates of global climate change are on the order of 1° C per 100 years up to a potentially catastrophic rate of 5° C per 100 years (Fig. 1-2). This is some 10 to 100 times faster than the typical sustained, global averaged rates of climate change in which human civilization evolved and the current distribution of species and ecosystems emerged. (Very likely)

9. Different species (e.g., specific kinds of trees, insects, birds, mammals) would all respond differently to projected climatic changes. For example, birds can migrate rapidly, but the vegetation some birds need for survival habitat would respond only very slowly perhaps over centuries. This implies a rending of the structures of communities of plants, insects, and animals[41] at rates that exceed most clear prehistoric or geological metaphors.[15] (Very likely)

10. Most forest species migrate at rates of some 1 km/year, and many would not be able to "keep up" with temperature changes at the rate of several degrees centimeter per century[11] without human intervention to transplant them (i.e., ecological engineering). (Likely)

11. Current engineering and economic practices in terms of building standards, automobile mileage, power production, or manufacturing are retarded relative to the energy efficiency of best-available technologies or techniques. From 10% to 40% reductions in current CO_2 emissions in the United States could result if current inefficient practices and infrastructures were replaced by state-of-the-art, proven efficient practices and equipment.[33,36] (Very likely)

12. Despite the slowness (approximately 1° C per 1000 years) of the sustained globally averaged natural rate of climatic change over most of the past 1.6×10^5 years, there are a few examples of rapid changes in pollen records in Europe[59] and ice cores in Greenland.[16] The possibilities of such "surprise" scenarios arising from greenhouse gas emissions, although currently difficult to assess, are sufficiently dramatic to require both scientific and policy assessments. (Speculative, but urgent)

The uncertainties in temperature projections over the next century range over a factor of 10 (Fig. 1-2). This is an attempt to include uncertainty from human behavioral

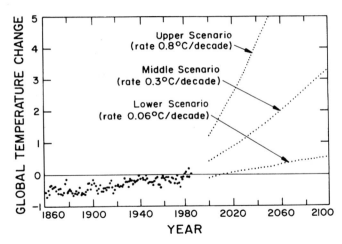

Fig. 1-2. Three scenarios for global temperature change to 2100 derived from combining uncertainties in future trace greenhouse gas projections with those of modeling the climatic response to those projections. The dots represent global surface temperature up to the mid 1980s. Sustained global temperature changes beyond 2° C (3.6° F) would be unprecedented during the era of human civilization. The middle-to-upper range represents climatic change at a 10 to 100 times faster pace than sustained natural global average rates of change. (From Jager J: *Developing policies for responding to climatic change.* Summary of the discussions and recommendations of the workshops held in Villach, 1987, Publication No. WMO/TO-No.225. Geneva, 1988, World Meteorological Organization; with permission.)

activities that create greenhouse gas emissions, biological factors that influence the carbon cycle (and thus CO_2 and CH_4 concentrations), and physical factors such as the "feedback effects" of clouds or ice (all of which, taken together, lead to the wide differences seen in Fig. 1-2).[22]

WHAT IS KNOWN WITH SOME RELIABILITY

A major criticism of the concept of global warming is the imperfect match between the erratic warming of the earth and the relatively gradual increase in greenhouse gases over the past hundred years (Fig. 1-3). It has been alleged that the temperature trends in the twentieth century cannot be attributed to greenhouse gas buildup because most of the warming in the twentieth century took place between 1915 and the 1940s, followed by northern hemisphere cooling at the time the global greenhouse gases began to build up rapidly. Then, from the mid-1970s to 1992, there was a dramatic warming, with the last 12 of those years containing over six of the warmest years on record.

This problem of cause and effect is akin to a criminal investigation in which the whereabouts of one principal suspect is fairly well-known, but the whereabouts of other possible secondary suspects have not been carefully observed. In this case, of course, the "crime" is the 0.5° C warming trend of the twentieth century, and the known principal "suspect" is greenhouse gases. Unfortunately, some possible role for the unwatched "suspects" cannot be ruled out because there are no quantitatively accurate ways of mea-

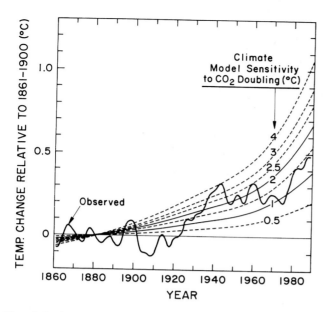

Fig. 1-3. Observed global mean temperature changes (1861-1989) compared with predicted values. The observed changes are given in Section 7 of reference 19. The data have been smoothed to show the decadal and longer time-scale trends more clearly. Predictions are based on observed concentration changes and concentration/forcing relationships as provided in Section 2 of reference 19 and have been calculated using an upwelling-diffusion climate model. (From Wigley TML, Raper SCB: *Detection of the enhanced greenhouse effect on climate.* In Jager J, Ferguson HL, editors: *Climate change: Science, impacts and policy.* Proc. Second World Climate Conference, Cambridge, UK, 1991, Cambridge University Press; with permission.)

suring precisely what these suspects did (other potential climatic influences or "forcings" as they are called). These suspects include sunspot activity, atmospheric particles from volcanic eruptions, industry, automobiles, and agriculture. It has long been known that most of these particles, for example, tend to cool the planet, counteracting some of the greenhouse effect, at least regionally.

Charlson and colleagues[1] picked up on the old debate[1,45,52] by focusing on the cooling potential of human emissions of sulfur dioxide (SO_2) (largely from burning of sulfur-contaminated oil or coal) and added some quantitative insights. They concluded that sulfuric acid or other sulfate aerosol particles (a form of smog) could both directly and indirectly (by brightening clouds) reflect enough sunlight away so as to nearly compensate for the extra human-caused greenhouse effect (attributable to surface-layer heating from CO_2, CH_4, and CFCs) over most of the northern hemisphere land masses since the 1960s. Because this reflection of sunlight is a daytime phenomenon, but the addition of greenhouse gases occurs both during the day and at night, some scientists have begun to suspect that the SO_2 effect combined with the anticipated global warming from greenhouse gas emissions would, at least over land in the northern hemisphere, result in a nighttime warming trend.[25]

Karl and colleagues[24] noted that over the United States, the former U.S.S.R., and China (precisely those places most affected by SO_2 emissions), warming trends over the past 30 years indeed largely occurred at night. Thirty years, however, is too short to lead to any statistically confident conclusions. Furthermore, estimating radiative effects on the day-night temperature cycle from regionally patchy aerosols requires sophisticated calculations that are yet to be made. Nevertheless, these latest results add (not subtract as some critics have contended) to the confidence that greenhouse gas buildups would eventually warm the earth by some 1.5° C to 4.5° C[20] in the twenty-first century.

One final aspect needs mentioning. We should not take comfort in the possibility that sulfuric acid particles will "save us" from global warming for two reasons. First, such chemicals are a principal ingredient of acid rain and health-threatening smog. Second, aerosols are, as many scientists have noted for decades, a regional phenomenon,[51] whereas "greenhouse" heat-trapping effects are spread uniformly over the globe. Thus, even if, on a hemispheric average, sulfur aerosols were to reject exactly as much extra solar heat into space as greenhouse gases trapped in the infrared wavelengths near the surface, this situation would not be a cancellation of climatic effects. This is because cooling would be in patterned, half-continental–sized patches, whereas the heating would be more globally distributed. The likely result would be a distortion of normal heating patterns, such as the land/ocean thermal contrast. Such distortions would likely lead to regional climatic anomalies (unanticipated local/regional climatic events) even if the net hemisphere temperature changes were small as a result of the hemisphere-scale heating/cooling compensations.[49] In short, we cannot "cure" global warming with SO_2 emissions and escape risk-free.

The updated interim report of the Intergovernmental Panel on Climate Change (IPCC)[20] acknowledged these uncertainties. It concluded once again that 1.5° C to 4.5° C warming is likely to be the actual long-term temperature response to CO_2 doubling over the next 50 years or so (the time frame in which a greenhouse gas buildup equivalent to a CO_2 doubling is typically forecast to occur).

Most scientists still agree, however, that without 10 to 20 more years of observations, it will be difficult to pin anything down to 99% certainty. In fact, such seemingly objective probabilities are, in essence, heuristic in any case.[49]

Of course, the assignment of an intuitive probability should not be viewed as pejorative because most nonintuitive probabilities, such as the significance level to which a global climate signal can be attributed to human activities,[54] are not objective (despite pretensions to the contrary by some statisticians). The assignment of formal statistical significance requires two fundamentally intuitive assumptions: (1) What is the long-term (i.e., low-frequency) natural climatic variability, and (2) what have been the time histories of both natural and anthropogenic "forcings" (such as greenhouse gas buildups or changes in solar output or aerosols). Thus, rather than delude ourselves into a false sense of analytic security based on some arbitrary statistical confidence limit, it is better to recognize that most probabilities assigned to the likelihood of specific environmental consequences in the global change area are intuition-dependent, based on the plausibility of underlying assumptions.

In this context of uncertainty, but not implausibility, a strategic approach would seem prudent.[32] Accordingly, even relatively low probability or unassignable probability events are analyzed for their potential consequences. Where does the moderate degree of certainty for significant climatic change projection (i.e., point 7 alone) come from? I believe this substantial consensus arises largely from the established knowledge of heat trapping and from validation exercises for models that test features of the present and past climate. Many aspects of these models have already been validated to a considerable degree, although not to the full satisfaction of responsible scientists. For example, it is known from observations that the last ice age, which was about 5° C colder on a global average than the present era, was associated with CO_2 concentrations about 25% less than our current interglacial time (at least before the Industrial Revolution). Methane, another potent greenhouse gas, also was lower by about half during the ice age, relative to interglacial preindustrial levels.

Ice in Antarctica contains gas bubbles that serve as records of atmospheric composition going back over 1.6×10^5 years. Cores drilled into the ice sheets show that in the previous interglacial warm age (some 1.2 to 1.4×10^5 years ago), temperatures were comparable to (or perhaps up to 2° C warmer than) those in the present interglacial period, as were levels of atmospheric CO_2 and methane.

The well-correlated change in these greenhouse gases and in planetary temperature over geological epochs allows an empirical way to estimate the sensitivity of climate to change in greenhouse gas concentrations. Such studies find geological-scale temperature changes from greenhouse gas variations roughly of the magnitude that would be expected, based on projections from today's computer models.[17,27] We still cannot assert, however, that this greenhouse gas/geological temperature coincidence is proof that our models are quantitatively correct because other factors were operating during the ice age–interglacial cycles. The best we can say is that the evidence is strong but circumstantial.

One related point may be useful. It typically takes tens of thousands of years for ice age glaciers to build up but only about 1×10^4 years to deglaciate. Each warm "interglacial epoch" also typically lasts 1×10^4 years. Because our current interglacial period is now about 1×10^4 years old, some have suggested that global warming could be a "good thing" as it will hold back the next ice age. What this view ignores is that the time frame for natural interglacial-to-glacial transitions (including major ice build-ups) is tens of thousands of years, whereas the potential for global warming of 1° C to 10° C is only a century or two—a radical rate of climatic change relative to most sustained, natural global climate changes in geological history. Another difficulty is the recent discovery of rapid climate oscillations evidenced in Greenland ice from the 2° C warmer climate of the previous interglacial era some 120 to 140 thousand years age.[16] This has led to speculation that a warmer world (by a few degrees), resulting from a few more decades of greenhouse gas buildup, might lead to a nasty surprise: a loss of current climatic stability. This is not yet a well-documented finding, however; it awaits confirmation.

WHAT IS HIGHLY SPECULATIVE?

Any prediction of what climatologists call the detailed regional distribution of climatic anomalies is speculative. That is, it is still difficult to be confident in projecting where and when it will be wetter and drier, how many floods might occur in the spring in California, or how many forest fires might occur in Wyoming in August—although some plausible scenarios can be given. How much the sea level will change is also speculative,[47] with most estimates ranging from a 0 to 1-m rise by the year 2100. Perhaps the best way to think about sea level rise is by a probability distribution, such as that shown in Fig. 1-4.[55]

ECOLOGICAL IMPACTS: THE POTENTIALLY MOST SERIOUS CONSEQUENCE

Because the projection of time-evolving, regional climatic changes is still speculative, so too is any confident assessment of the agricultural, hydrological, ecological, or health consequences of global warming. We can construct, however, a variety of plausible specific scenarios of climatic changes over space and time and then ask: "So what?"[38,53] Indeed, such exercises have led to conflicting assessments of the agricultural consequences,[33] greater concern for the hydrological consequences,[56] and serious concern for the ecological implications of most global warming scenarios.[33,39] This last issue is examined in more detail next.

A new assessment paradigm: interactions and surprises

The assumptions associated with the standard paradigm of global climate change impact assessment, although recognizing a wide range of uncertainty, are essentially surprise free. One approach is to postulate low (or uncertain) probability cases in which little climate change, on the one hand, or catastrophic surprises, on the other hand, might occur and multiply the lower probability times the much larger potential costs or benefits. Analysts, however, customarily use a few standard general circulation climate model (GCM) CO_2-doubling scenarios to "bracket the uncertainty," rather than to assume extremely serious or rela-

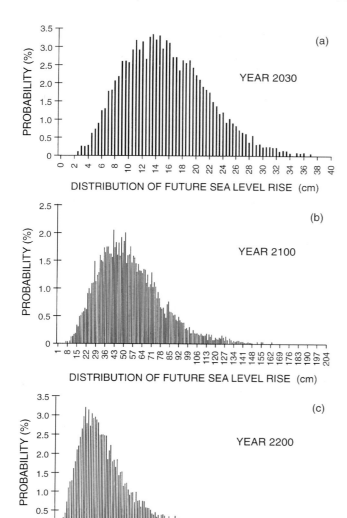

Fig. 1-4. Probability of a given sea level rise at three future times based on the Monte Carlo estimation technique of Titus and Narayanan. (From Titus J, Narayaman V: Probability distribution of future sea level rise [submitted].)

tively negligible cases of climatic change. I believe that a strategic approach—i.e., one that considers a wide range of probabilities and consequences—is more appropriate (as in Fig. 1-4), given the high plausibility of surprises, even if we have but little capacity to anticipate specific details right now. For example, two critical assumptions of the standard assessment paradigm are that climate extremes— drought, floods, superhurricanes—either remain unchanged or will change with the mean change in climate according to unchanged variability distributions. As Mearns and co-workers[30] have shown, however, changes in the daily temperature variance or the autocorrelation of daily weather extremes can either significantly reduce or dramatically enhance the vulnerability of agriculture, ecosystems,

or other climate extreme–sensitive components of the environment to global warming. How such variability measures might change as the climatic mean changes is as yet highly uncertain.[31,40] Nevertheless, the possibility that variability will change with climate change is not at all remote, even though it is not possible to ascertain credibly with current techniques how that might occur.

Another assumption in cost-to-benefit calculations of the standard assessment paradigm is that "nature" is either constant or irrelevant.[9] For example, ecological services such as pest control or waste recycling are assumed as constants, or of no value in most assessment calculations. Yet, as argued shortly, should climatic change occur in the middle to upper range of that typically projected (Fig. 1-2), it is highly likely that communities of species will be disassembled, and the probability of significant alterations to existing patterns of pests and weeds seems virtually certain. Some argue that pests, should their patterns be altered, can simply be controlled by pesticides and herbicides or medicines. The side effects of such controls are well-known to many. What is not considered in the standard paradigm,— but I believe should be— is the consideration of a "surprise" scenario such as a change in public consciousness regarding the value of nature that would reject pesticide/herbicide application as a response to global changes. A related potential "surprise" is the suggestion that halogenated compounds are causing damage to the endocrine systems of humans and animals, leading to a twenty-first century human and animal health crisis.[6]

Although it has long been known that understanding and projection of the impact of human activities on climate and the converse involve detailed interactive studies of social, physical, biological, and chemical systems, the multidisciplinary nature of the analysis is exceedingly difficult to undertake in practice.[3,46] There have been a number of attempts to develop multidisciplinary assessments, which spawned the movement toward an international geosphere/biosphere program[21] and the Global Change program.[28] These efforts certainly suggest a major recognition of the need to integrate physical, biological, and social factors, putting us in a better position to make a heuristic judgment on appropriate mitigation or adaptation policies.

Fig. 1-5 is a simplified system diagram that stresses physical, biological, and social interactions as they might affect food security. I can choose several examples at various points in this simple picture (simple only in the sense that it is much simpler than reality, although still complex to analyze) that provide an opportunity to identify plausible surprises and interactions. Indeed, interactions among physical, biological, and social systems may well prove to be the biggest surprise of all for adaptability of human systems to climate change. In our context, climatic influences on food security could, in turn, have major public health implications.

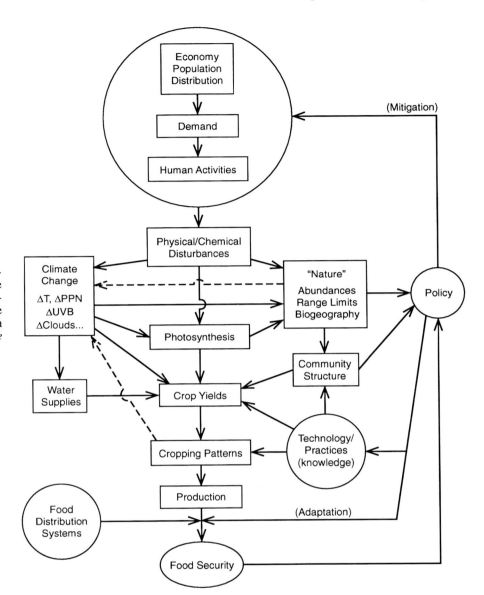

Fig. 1-5. System flow chart for diagnosing interactions between climatic change factors and food security. (Adapted and redrawn by author from Schneider SH: The future of climate: potential for interaction and surprises, *Global Environ Change* [submitted].)

Fig. 1-5 is my suggested economic-environment-food security assessment flow chart. It is designed to approximate the way one might model the food security system as affected by climate change, rather than a description of full reality. In addition, although interconnected systems in reality do not flow linearly from the social sphere to food security as this flow chart suggests, if small enough "time steps" are taken and the process is repeated many times, the practical necessity of proceeding linearly eventually will cause smaller errors.

In Fig. 1-5, the upper circle represents, in essence, the "demand side," which leads to human activities that are responsible for the global change, i.e., greenhouse gas increases, increase in sulfur oxide emissions, and habitat fragmentation. Population, technology, and affluence are multiplicative factors that combine on a global scale to provide

scenarios for future potential physical and chemical disturbances. Based on these human behavioral assumptions, physical and chemical disturbances then can be applied to the next level of analysis, such as models of climate change—typically in the form of general circulation models—to determine changes in temperature (ΔT), precipitation (ΔPPN), ultraviolet light (ΔUVB) (if ozone depletion is involved), and clouds. In reality, an intermediate step is needed to determine the way the naturally disturbed and human-disturbed carbon cycle operates. This is because the CO_2 and methane introduced into the system do not just sit but are actively transformed by atmospheric, oceanic, and biospheric chemical processes as well as by direct disturbances to physical and biological sources and sinks (e.g., deforestation or agriculture). Changes in decomposition rates of soil organic matter arising from the effects of in creases in temperature on soil microbial activity are good candidates for "surprise," as is potential photosynthetic enhancement of crops, forests, and other biota. The latter already has been postulated by a wide range of people as a "positive surprise."[18,43] That is why there is a direct arrow in Fig. 1-5 from the disturbances to photosynthesis. Notice also a direct arrow from photosynthesis to "nature," because the effect of CO_2 enhancement of photosynthesis is not likely to have equal effects on all vegetative species (agricultural or natural).

It seems virtually certain that natural biological systems primarily will respond to CO_2 enhancement by conferring competitive advantage on some species at the expense of others. The phrase "winners and losers" has no traditional economic meaning in this context because the conservation of nature is difficult to define in human value terms if dollars are the sole measure of worth. The only statement that can be made with some assurance is that the larger and more rapid the change in the environmental system, the more communities of species will be altered by differential CO_2 photosynthetic enhancement within natural systems. This likely will lead to "surprises," which currently are neither calculated nor valued, positively or negatively, in any of the current assessments of climate change, but rather debated philosophically in the typical dichotomy of "economists versus environmentalists."[7-9]

It is already clear that changes in climate would change the abundances and range limits of many species.[5,10,29] As Root and Schneider[42] have noted, however, this combination of differential photosynthetic enhancement (along with the differential responses of various species to climatic changes) will undoubtedly lead to reorganizations of biological communities with potential implications for evapotranspiration (which might, in turn, affect soil moisture and runoff) as well as have implications for pest management, biodiversity preservation, and conservation of nature. For

example, as Fig. 1-6 shows (using the standard assessment paradigm of three CO_2-doubled, equilibrium general circulation model runs to drive an ecological model), a change in climate would dramatically alter the distribution patterns of ticks in North America, substantially reducing the populations in hot southern zones and dramatically increasing the population in northern zones.[53] Not only does this have implications for human health, but also for natural communities because insects are food for birds, which, in turn, depend on vegetation for nesting and serve as prey for animals such as foxes, all of which taken together are part of the community structure of ecosystems.

It is typically assumed that individual species may respond to climate change by shifting their range limit or abundances. Most studies, however, concentrated on individual species at the scale of a field plot the size of a tennis court.[23] "Scaling up" such studies to larger geographical and biological community levels is not yet based on validated general theory and has been attempted in only a few studies.[14,26,42] It is inferred from such studies that the migration rates for specific species of vegetation, mammals, insects, reptiles, and birds are all different, yet the interactions among these species may have unique properties—i.e., biological communities—which suggests that climate change could disrupt the community structure.

The climate-health connection

The case of ticks (because they have implications for the health of humans and animals) suggests another category of "surprises" for which there already has been considerable analysis: human health (Fig. 1-6). Several studies have suggested that increased environmental heat stress could lead to increased mortality rates for those with cardiovascular disease (Fig. 1-7A).[57] It is usually noted, however, that adaptations, ranging from simple acclimatization to proper choice of clothing, nutrition, diet, and housing, can

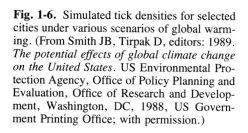

Fig. 1-6. Simulated tick densities for selected cities under various scenarios of global warming. (From Smith JB, Tirpak D, editors: 1989. *The potential effects of global climate change on the United States.* US Environmental Protection Agency, Office of Policy Planning and Evaluation, Office of Research and Development, Washington, DC, 1988, US Government Printing Office; with permission.)

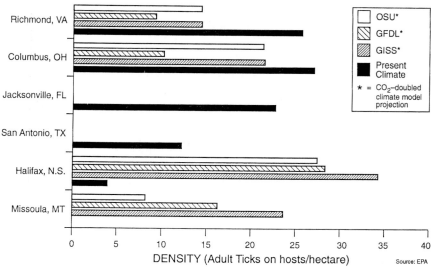

substantially mitigate vulnerability to each stress (Fig. 1-7*B*). There is potential for surprise impact on human health if adaptations are not properly anticipated. More important is the potential for the redistribution of much more serious disease factors that are climate-associated.[57] Table 1-1 provides an example of serious concern for expanding the range of malaria or altering the habitats of other potential disease vectors. Dobson and Carper[12] have also suggested that significant redistribution of tsetse fly zones could spare some currently infested areas while affecting vast other tracts not currently threatened. The potential of surprise to human and animal health with a combination of

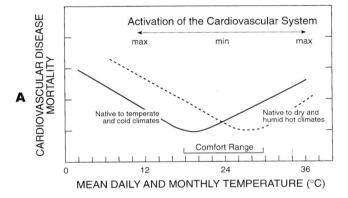

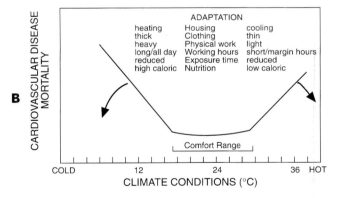

Fig. 1-7. A, Relationship between cardiovascular disease mortality rate and adaptation to local climates. The cardiovascular system is activated and strained under both heat and cold conditions with a minimum of strain at comfort temperatures. People native to temperate and cold climates prefer and tolerate lower comfort temperatures, whereas those native to dry and humid hot climates prefer and tolerate higher comfort temperatures. On the global scale, comfort temperatures range from about 17° C to 30° C. Cold-native people show a higher vulnerability to heat and heat-native people to cold. **B,** The physiological strain in cold and hot climates can be mitigated or prevented by a variety of single or combined behaviors, which are different or opposite in cold and hot climates. (From Weihe WH, Mertens R: *Human well-being, diseases and climate.* In Jager J, Ferguson HL, editors: *Climate change: science, impacts and policy.* Proc. Second World Climate Conference, Cambridge, UK, 1991, Cambridge University Press; with permission.)

heat stress, altered disease patterns, and the interactions of these factors with malnourishment is a synergism that must not be neglected in future impact assessments.

Referring again to Fig. 1-5, the food security oval appears just below the box labeled crop yields. It is affected by photosynthesis and water supplies as determined by climate and human adaptations, such as fertilization or groundwater pumping. Yields also are subject to influence from changes to biological community structure, such as those shown in the "nature" side of the box in Fig. 1-5 (pests, soil organic matter, or soil microbes) that should be included in the analysis. It is useful here to focus on climate change/food security impact assessment studies.[44,50]

Crop yields then are translated to cropping patterns, based on land use, technology, and knowledge, which leads to overall production. Then, depending on economic and political factors that influence food distribution systems, food security can be ascertained. Currently, it is estimated that perhaps half- a billion to a billion people are "food insecure" owing to dietary restrictions, political strife, poverty, maldistribution, and the normal variability of the weather that results in droughts, floods, or weather-related pest attacks.[4] The possibility that a world of doubled current population by the mid-twenty-first century could not easily become food secure is debated.[7,8]

It is already a formidable scientific challenge to try to explain the range limits and abundances of most species today, even though they have had thousands of years of stable climate in which to adapt. Therefore, to predict the highly transient response of biological communities faced with sustained global climatic changes at 10 to 100 times faster rates than natural, sustained average rates of global climatic change over the past 1×10^4 years is speculative at best. We do have some knowledge, however, as previously indicated, of what factors can affect individual species and roughly how rapidly they can respond to various disturbances. Therefore, statements such as "disruptions of ecosystems," "tearing apart of communities of species," and even "ecological chaos" are plausible "forecasts," should global warming materialize at the mid or high end of projected rates of 1° C to 5° C over the next 100 years. Should such disruptions affect natural ecosystems, there could be significant implications for human health, as noted earlier.

IS IT TOO EXPENSIVE TO ACT NOW?

Other aspects of the global warming issue that are highly speculative are the overall social and economic consequences of typical warming scenarios; the costs of actions to mitigate CO_2, CH_4, N_2O, or CFC emissions; and whether to use technological schemes to offset warming (so-called geoengineering).[33] Should such costs slow development, some have argued, that too could have an impact on human health.

Table 1-1. Examples of major vector-borne tropical diseases

Disease	Causative agent	Vector	Population at risk* (millions)	Prevalence of infection (millions)	Present distribution	Likelihood of spreading owing to climatic change
Malaria	*Plasmodium* spp. (protozoa)	*Anopheles* mosquitos	2100	270	Tropics/subtropics	+++
Lymphatic filariasis	Nematode worms: family filaridae	Various mosquito species	900	90	Tropics/subtropics	++
Onchocerciasis (river blindness)	*Onchocerca volvulus* (filaridae)	*Simulium* blackflies	90	17.6	Africa/Latin America	+
Schistosomiasis (bilharziasis)	*Schistosoma* flatworms	Water snails	600	200	Tropics/subtropics	++
African trypanosomiasis (sleeping sickness)	*Trypanosoma* spp. (protozoa)	Tsetse flies	50	25,000 new cases/year	Tropical Africa	+
Leishmaniases	*Leishmania* spp. (protozoa)	Sandflies	350	12	Asia/S. Europe/Africa/S. America	?
Arboviral diseases						
Dengue fever	Dengue virus	*Aedes* mosquitos		30-60 million infections per year	Tropics/subtropics	++
Yellow fever	Yellow fever virus	Various mosquito species		>3000 deaths in 1986-1988	Africa/The Americas	+
Japanese encephalitis	Japenese encephalitis virus	Various mosquito species			Asia/Pacific Islands	+
Other arboviral diseases	90+ other viruses	Anthropods, mainly mosquitos and ticks			Cosmopolitan	+

+ + +, Highly likely; + +, very likely; +, likely; *?*, unknown.
From Weihe WH, Mertens R: Human well-being, diseases, and climate. In Jager J, Ferguson HL, editors: *Climate change: science, impacts and policy,* proceedings of the Second World Climate Conference. Cambridge, UK, 1991, Cambridge University Press.
*Based on a world population estimated at 4.8 million (1989).

The final, and perhaps most difficult, criticism made against those proposing action to slow global warming is that immediate policy steps to cut CO_2 emissions are too expensive. For example, some newspaper articles by greenhouse critics suggest that if CO_2 emissions are cut, the United States will be bankrupt and the Third World even more impoverished. There is substantial Third World opposition to the prospect that developing countries may not be allowed to have their own industrial revolutions, and development certainly will influence public health status.

Some developing Eastern countries, notably India and China, have abundant coal supplies. They would like to repeat Western history and use these resources as low-cost routes to industrialization. Of course, these countries in the 1990s have between them 2 billion people, whereas the entire world population did not total 2 billion people in Victorian times. So the magnitude of the global impact of developing countries using coal would be greater than that of developing Western nations in the past. Needless to say, such arguments are not greeted sympathetically in China or India, where the large discrepancy in per capita consumption between developed and developing countries is correctly noted.

CAN CARBON DIOXIDE BE CUT BY TWENTY PERCENT?

It is sensible, I believe, to argue that currently developing countries need not repeat the experience of Victorian industrialization with smog-choked cities, acid rain, and inefficient power production, given that modern technology has many better solutions. For example, electrical power generation efficiency today is near 50%, whereas it was half that at the turn of the century. Unfortunately, developing countries typically respond that efficient high-technology power production initially is more expensive than the traditional options that are cheaper and more available to them. This dilemma sets up the obvious need for a bargain by which developed countries with technology and capital help to provide those resources to developing countries, which, in turn, develop their industries with the least-polluting, most efficient technologies, even if they cost more initially.

Critics of emissions reductions cite the supposed annual cost of a 20% CO_2 emissions reduction at tens of billions of dollars annually. Some studies have suggested that carbon taxes to promote switching to energy systems that pollute less could cost the United States "$800 billion, under optimistic scenarios of available fuel substitutes and increasing energy efficiency, to $3.6 trillion under pessimistic scenarios...to [the year] 2100." This statement, quoted from the February 1990 "Economic Report of the President" to Congress, was based on the initial results of the first wave of economic model simulations.

Let us pursue the economic modeling issue a bit further. When only the supposed costs to the economy (typically measured as gross national product [GNP] loss from a hypothetical carbon tax) are shown, seemingly staggering figures emerge.[34] The costs can be seen to run into the trillions by the year 2105 (as a result of a 20% reduction in CO_2 emissions in one economic model[34]). The benefit of this "20% cut" is a 30% reduction in global warming by the year 2105, only considered to be "worth" one percent or less of the GNP loss because the model assumes the primary negative economic consequence of warming to be an agricultural-water supply loss of up to 1% of GNP in the United States (about $40 billion per year in 1990).[34] No value is placed on the potential for catastrophic effects on ecosystems or public health concerns or the security implications of long-term, large climatic changes (perhaps up to 10° C in the twenty-second century). Effects such as the tearing apart of communities of species or the impacts of increases in tropical cyclone intensities on the political stability of South Asia are not explicitly considered. The underlying economic growth assumptions that drive the conclusions of this analysis are revealing. The underlying scenario for economic development projects that there will be more than a 450% growth in per capita consumption from 1965 to 2105 in all scenarios; the untaxed "business as usual" scenario implies 460% growth, whereas even the "draconian" 20% reduction in CO_2 resulting from the carbon tax scenarios still allows 450% world per capita consumption growth over this time period.[34] In my value system, it is unconscionable to risk unabated, unprecedentedly rapid rates of climate change with potentially serious risks to public health, agricultural, hydrological, and (especially)

ecological systems of the earth merely because it will reduce our per capita growth in consumption from some 460% to "only" 450%. To avoid carbon taxes because they might cost trillions of dollars without also looking at the negligible effect these taxes would have on overall projected consumption, and the major effect they would have on lowering CO_2 emissions, is to have no balanced perspective on the economics and ethics of measures that could mitigate CO_2 emissions.

In any event, although it is possible to use analytic methods and simulation models to investigate costs and benefits of different specific climate change or emission scenarios, these tools are even less well validated for long-term studies than climatic models and also do not include many significant factors.[13,35,37,48] It is my opinion that the primary value of physical, biological, or economic analytical methods is to help a decision-maker—personal, corporate, or governmental—obtain more complete knowledge of the potential benefits or risks of various alternative actions. This will aid in formulating a heuristic judgment that incorporates what is quantifiable with those aspects that are not (e.g., the "value" of a species facing extinction or the likelihood of altered disease vectors). It is a gross misunderstanding of analytic methods, be they climatic, ecological, or economic, to believe they provide the sole bases for arriving at "the answer" for policy choices.

CLIMATIC INSURANCE

The global warming debate then is both scientific and political. It is essential for the public to understand, however, that there are vastly greater disagreements over what to do about the prospect of global warming (a political value issue) than over the probability that significant change will occur in the twenty-first century (a scientific debate). Estimates of climatic effects range from mildly beneficial (i.e., longer growing seasons) to catastrophic (i.e., more super-hurricanes or expanded disease patterns or mass extinctions). These uncertain impacts reflect the wide range of plausible climate futures forecast by most assessment groups (Fig. 1-2). Although accelerated research will undoubtedly bring more reliable answers sooner, this analyst does not believe it likely that any feasible level of research effort will identify the detailed consequences of our continuing greenhouse gas emissions in less than a few decades (the time it will take the climate system itself to begin to answer the questions).

Slowing the rate of buildup of the greenhouse gases that threaten unprecedented global warming neither requires economically catastrophic measures nor will it bankrupt industrial nations or doom poor countries to increasing poverty as is often asserted. Rather, prudent investments in energy-efficient equipment, buildings, and power plants, combined with sensible reforestation, population control, and consumption reduction programs, can both reduce the rate of buildup of greenhouse gases and pay their own way.

It is ludicrous simply to claim that reductions in greenhouse gas emission are too costly without weighing the overall, systemwide economic, environmental, health, and strategic benefits of such investments.

The prospect of "surprises" for events of low probability or currently unassessable probability suggests the obvious need for flexibility in managing all systems that depend on environmental factors that are influenced by human activities. More attention needs to be given to the emerging climatic impact paradigm of strategic analysis for a spectrum of probabilities and outcomes. Typically, impact assessments, as mentioned earlier, tend to focus on "best guesses." I certainly understand, even applaud, such analyses as important early steps in the attempt to incorporate uncertainty into physical, biological, and social components of environmental impact assessment. The alternative paradigm, however, needs to begin to creep into analytic activities. Meanwhile, it will remain a gamble whether benign or catastrophic outcomes will unfold, and it will require many decades to resolve the uncertainties.

REFERENCES

1. Charlson RJ, Pilat MJ: Climate: the influence of aerosols, *J Appl Meteorol* 8:1001, 1969.
2. Charlson RJ et al: Perturbation of the northern hemisphere radiative balance by backscattering from anthropogenic sulfate aerosols, *Tellus* 43ab:152, 1991.
3. Chen RS: Interdisciplinary research and integration: the case of CO_2 and climate, *Climatic Change* 3:429, 1981.
4. Chen RS, Kates RW: Climate change and world food security, *Global Environ Change* March 1994, Vol 4, No 1.
5. COHMAP Members: Climatic change of the last 18,000 years: observations and model simulations, *Science* 241:1043, 1988.
6. Colborn T, Clement C, editors: *Chemically induced alterations in sexual and functional development: the wildlife/human connection,* Princeton, NJ, 1992, Princeton Scientific Publishing.
7. Crosson P, Anderson JR: *Resources and global food prospects, supply and demand for cereals to 2030,* World Bank Technical Paper No. 184. Washington, DC, 1992, The World Bank.
8. Daily G, Ehrlich P: Population sustainability and earth carrying capacity, *BioScience* 42:761, 1992.
9. Daly HE: *Ecological economics and sustainable development.* In Rossi C, Tiezzi E, editors: *Ecological physical chemistry, proceedings of an international workshop,* Amsterdam, 1991, Elsevier.
10. Davis MB: *Ecological systems and dynamics.* In *Toward an understanding of global change,* Washington, DC, 1988, National Academy Press.
11. Davis MB: *Climatic change and the survival of forest species.* In Woodwell GM, editor: *The earth in transition: patterns and processes of biotic impoverishment,* Cambridge, Mass, 1990, Cambridge University Press.
12. Dobson A, Carper R: *Global warming and potential changes in host-parasite and disease-vector relationships.* In Peters R, Lovejoy T, editors: *Global warming and biological diversity,* New Haven, Conn, 1992, Yale University Press.
13. Dowlatabadi H, Lave L: Letters, *Science* 259:1381, 1993.
14. Ehleringer JP, Field CB, editors: *Scaling physiological processes: leaf to globe.* New York, 1993, Academic Press.
15. Graham RW, Grimm EC: Effects of global climate change on the patterns of terrestrial biological communities, *Trends in Ecology and Evolution* 5:289, 1990.
16. Greenland Ice Core Project (GRIP) Members: Climate instability during the last interglacial period recorded in the GRIP ice core, *Nature* 364:203, 1993.
17. Hoffert MI, Covey C: Deriving global climate sensitivity from palaeoclimate reconstructions, *Nature* 360:573, 1992.
18. Idso SB: The aerial fertillization effect of CO_2 and its implications for global carbon cycling and maximum greenhouse warming, *Bull Am Meteorol Soc* 72:962, 1991.
19. Intergovernmental Panel on Climate Change, Houghton JT, Jenkins GJ, Ephraums JJ, editors: *Climate change: the IPCC scientific assessment,* Cambridge, Mass, 1990, Cambridge University Press.
20. Intergovernmental Panel on Climate Change, Houghton JT, Jenkins GJ, Ephraums JJ, editors: *Climate change 1992: the supplementary report to the IPCC scientific assessment,* Cambridge, Mass, 1992, Cambridge University Press.
21. International Geosphere-Biosphere Programme: *A study of global change,* Stockholm, 1991, IGBP Press.
22. Jager J: *Developing policies for responding to climatic change.* Summary of the discussions and recommendations of the workshops held in Villach, 1987, Publication No. WMO/TD-No. 225. Geneva, 1988, World Meteorological Organization.
23. Kareiva P, Andersen M: *Spatial aspects of species interactions.* In Hastings A, editor: *Community ecology,* workshop held at Davis, California, April 1986, New York, 1988, Springer.
24. Karl TR et al: Global warming: evidence for asymmetric diurnal temperature change, *Geophys Res Lett* 18:2253, 1992.
25. Kerr RA: 1992: Pollutant haze cools the greenhouse, *Science* 255:682, 1992.
26. Levin SA: The problem of pattern and scale in ecology, *Ecology* 73:1943, 1992.
27. Lorius C et al: The ice-core record: Climate sensitivity and future greenhouse warming, *Nature* 347:139, 1990.
28. Malone TF, Roederer JG, editors: *Global change,* New York, 1984, ICSU Press.
29. McDonald KA, Brown JH: Using montane mammals to model extinctions due to global change, *Conservation Biol* 6:409, 1992.
30. Mearns LO, Katz RW, Schneider SH: Changes in the probabilities of extreme high temperature events with changes in global mean temperature, *J Climate Appl Meteorol* 23:1601, 1984.
31. Mearns LO et al: Analysis of climate variability in general circulation models: comparison with observations and changes in variability in $2\times CO_2$ experiments, *J Geophys Res* 95:20469-20490, 1990.
32. Morgan MG: Risk analysis and management, *Scientific American,* July, 32-41, 1993.
33. National Academy of Sciences: *Policy implications of greenhouse warming,* Washington, DC, 1991, National Academy Press.
34. Nordhaus W: *Rolling the "dice": an optimal transition path for controlling greenhouse gases.* Paper presented at the Annual Meeting of the American Association for the Advancement of Science, 1992, Chicago.
35. Nordhaus W: Letters—response, *Science* 259:1383, 1993.
36. Office of Technology Assessment: *Changing by degrees, steps to reduce greenhouse gases,* Washington, DC, 1991, US Government Printing Office.
37. Oppenheimer M: Letters, *Science* 259:1382, 1993.
38. Pearman GI, editor: *Greenhouse: planning for climate change,* Melbourne, Australia, 1988, CSIRO.
39. Peters R, Lovejoy T, editors: *Global warming and biological diversity,* New Haven, Conn, 1992, Yale University Press.
40. Rind DR, Goldberg R, Ruedy R: Change in climate variability in the 21st century, *Climatic Change* 14:5, 1989.
41. Root TL: *Effects of global climate change on North American birds and their communites.* In Kingsolver J, Kareiva P, Huey R, editors: *Biotic interactions and global change,* Sunderland, Mass, 1992, Sinauer Associates.
42. Root TL, Schneider SH: Can large-scale climatic models be linked with multiscale ecological studies? *Conservation Biol* 7:256, 1993.

43. Rosenberg NJ: Implications of policies to prevent climate change for future food security, *Global Environ Change,* March, 1994, Vol 4, No 1.
44. Rosenzweig C et al: Climate change and world food supply, *Global Environ Change* March, 1994, Vol 4, No 1.
45. Schneider SH: A comment on "climate: the influence of aerosols," *J Appl Meteorol* 10:840, 1971.
46. Schneider SH: The whole earth dialogue, *Iss Sci Technol* 4:93, 1988.
47. Schneider SH: Will sea levels rise or fall? *Nature* 356:11, 1992.
48. Schneider SH: Pondering greenhouse policy, *Science* 259:1381, 1993.
49. Schneider SH: Detecting climatic change signals: are there any fingerprints? *Science* 263:341-347.
50. Schneider SH: The future of climate: potential for interaction and surprises, *Global Environ Change* (submitted).
51. Schneider SH, Mesirow LE: *The Genesis strategy: climate and global survival,* New York, 1973, Plenum Publishing.
52. SMIC Report: *Study of man's impact on climate,* Cambridge, Mass, 1971, MIT Press.
53. Smith JB, Tirpak D, editors: 1989. *The potential effects of global climate change on the United States.* US Environmental Protection Agency, Office of Policy Planning and Evaluation, Office of Research and Development, Washington, DC, 1988, US Government Printing Office.
54. Solow AR, Broadus JM: On the detection of greenhouse warming, *Climatic Change* 15:449, 1989.
55. Titus J, Narayanan V: Probability distribution of future sea level rise, (submitted).
56. Waggoner PE, editor: *Climate change and US water resources,* New York, 1990, John Wiley & Sons.
57. Weihe WH, Mertens R: *Human well-being, diseases and climate.* In Jager J, Ferguson HL, editors: *Climate change: science, impacts and policy.* Proc. Second World Climate Conference, Cambridge, UK, 1991, Cambridge University Press.
58. Wigley TML, Raper SCB: *Detection of the enhanced greenhouse effect on climate.* In Jager J, Ferguson HL, editors: *Climate change: science impacts and policy.* Proc Second World Climate Conference, Cambridge, UK, 1991, Cambridge University Press.
59. Woillard GM, Mook WG: Carbon 14 dates at Grande Pile: correlation of land and sea chronologies, *Science* 215:159, 1982.

Chapter 2

OUTDOOR AIR QUALITY
AND POLLUTION

David V. Bates

The study of the effect of air pollution on people has been complicated by a number of factors:

The dominance of cigarette smoking in the genesis of lung disease

The difficulty of drawing conclusions about causation from demonstrated associations

The difficulty of comparisons between populations living in different pollution environments but with many other differences between them, such as climate, living conditions, and methods of heating and cooking

The uncertainty of the importance of some outcome measurements, such as small transient declines in lung function

The difficulty of separating the effects of different pollutants, when they commonly rise together

After the obvious associations between acute mortality and discrete air pollution episodes in the 1950s and 1960s in the West were lessened by control methods, there was a temptation to dismiss continuing evidence of adverse health effects as essentially unimportant. In the developing world, immediate economic objectives have taken precedence over long-term concerns about the impact of pollution.

During the past two decades, however, there have been substantial advances in environmental epidemiology, and other lines of evidence have become available, such as that deducible from controlled human exposures to pollutant mixtures. It is remarkable that it took 28 years after the 1952 London pollution episode before the increased sensitivity of asthmatics to sulfur dioxide (SO_2) was discovered.

In this chapter, the evidence for adverse health effects from air pollutants is summarized. The references are those that document the effect in question and are taken from studies in which care was taken to exclude the effect of other variables, or in which the exposure data was more detailed. There is an inevitable choice between studying a small sample of individuals with precise exposure monitoring or studying a large population and inferring their exposure by reference to area monitoring. Both types of study are needed for a full understanding.

There are many different patterns of air pollution, and these vary by region and by season of the year. Individuals may encounter high levels of pollutants simultaneously (as in the London fog of December 1952,[54] in which particulates from coal burning, sulfur dioxide, and sulfuric acid aerosol were all present in the fog) or sequentially, as in the contemporary Northeast of North America, where a high ozone level may be encountered one afternoon and a peak of sulfuric acid aerosol may occur on the next day.

PROBLEMS IN ASSESSMENT

As in all areas of environmental epidemiology, there are two main problems in such studies: the assessment of exposure and the measurement of outcome.

Exposure assessment

Over the past 5 years, a great deal of attention has been given to the problem of exposure assessment.[55] In studies involving millions of subjects, area monitoring is necessarily used as a measure of exposure, although the actual exposures within a large population must vary considerably. Because more time is spent indoors than outdoors, outdoor ambient monitoring may bear little relationship to actual exposure in the majority of people. Several strategies have been adopted to overcome this difficulty. In the case of oxides of nitrogen, which have both outdoor and indoor sources, measurements of indoor concentrations together with ambient levels may be used in the study. When schoolchildren are being studied, air monitoring can be conducted in the school yard. Activity patterns and complex computer models can be used to calculate individual exposures in panel studies.[57] In studies of children at summer camps, air monitoring equipment can be established at the camp.

In time-series studies, such as those relating particulate

levels of air pollution to mortality, although there may be no knowledge of the actual exposure of the victims, the constancy of the relationship indicates that in such instances area monitoring provides an adequate differentiation between pollutant exposure on different days. The same is true of studies of hospital admissions in relation to ambient pollution.

Measurements of effect

Measurements of significant health outcomes present difficulties no less serious than those of exposure measurement. Changes in daily mortality are the least controversial of outcomes, but ill health induced by air pollution has many outcomes other than this. The epidemiological literature dealing with air pollution in the past presents a distorted view of the reality, in that it would suggest that chronic lung disease is due to cigarettes; and air pollution is primarily important in causing transient increases in mortality. Such a perspective minimizes the role of air pollution in leading to the chronic lung disease in the first place. The 1965 study, from which Fig. 2-1 is taken, is important because it shows that living in a more polluted environment at that time caused a lowering in forced expiratory volume in one second (FEV$_1$) in men with similar smoking histories.

The box on p. 19 shows different outcomes of pollution exposure, ranked in an arbitrary order of significance. The interpretation of transient declines in pulmonary function is

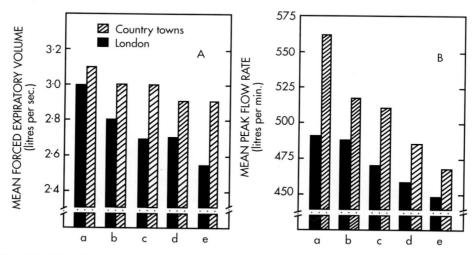

Fig. 2-1. Mean forced expiratory volume (1.0 sec) **(A)** and mean peak flow rate **(B)**, both standardized to age 40, in *(a)* nonsmokers; *(b)* ex-smokers; *(c)* smokers, 1 to 14 g/day; *(d)* smokers, 15 to 24 g/day; *(e)* smokers ≥25 g/day. The data show significantly lower lung function in nonsmokers and smokers in those residing in London, compared with those in country towns. The levels of SO$_2$ and particulate pollution in the country towns were less than half those in London at this time. Mean value and number of subjects: **A,** *(a)* 3·1 (30) and 3·0 (13); *(b)* 3·0 (77) and 2·8 (36); *(c)* 3·0 (142) and 2·7 (74); *(d)* 2·9 (134) and 2·7 (98); *(e)* 2·9 (40) and 2·5 (29). **B,** *(a)* 562 (31) and 491 (13); *(b)* 517 (77) and 488 (36); *(c)* 510 (142) and 470 (74); *(d)* 485 (134) and 458 (98); *(e)* 468 (41) and 448 (29). (From Holland WW, Reid DD: The urban factor in chronic bronchitis, *Lancet* 1:445, 1965, with permission.)

Relative significance of adverse health indicators of effects of air pollution

Least

Changes in general indices of ill health

Small episodic FEV_1 declines

Increased symptoms in populations in more polluted regions

Cross-sectional FEV_1 differences

Increased prevalence of respiratory diseases

Increased hospital admission rates for respiratory disease in more polluted regions

Cross-sectional respiratory mortality differences not related to episodes

Increased hospital emergency visits in association with episodic increases in pollution

Increased hospital admissions in episodes

Increased respiratory or total mortality in most episodes of increased pollution

Most

FEV_1, Forced expiratory volume in one second.

open to question. Comparisons of populations that show an increased incidence of respiratory symptoms in one compared with the other may also be difficult to interpret if the difference is small. Major advances have been made in the application of lung function studies in the field,[7] and these have been used both to detect transient changes when a pollution episode occurs[9] and to note systematic differences.[68]

Comparisons of differential changes in such indices as the overall rate of hospital admissions are complicated by the many factors that may influence such numbers. For this reason, the demonstration of a systematic relationship between pollution levels and emergency visits or admissions to hospital on a daily basis may be more sensitive and reliable. When mortality is being studied, examination of causes of death that change when pollution is higher, gives insight into the effects that are occurring and significantly supports a causal inference from such associations.[63] Because all diseases that are likely to be adversely affected by air pollution are multifactorial, there is necessarily considerable difficulty in determining how important exposure to air pollutants may be (for instance) in influencing an apparent increase in the prevalence of a disease such as asthma. As noted subsequently, mortality from cardiovascular disease seems to be an invariable feature of time-series analyses of mortality and pollutants. Undoubtedly, cardiovascular disease is multifactorial; but the mechanism for this effect is as yet unknown.

Difficulties are also caused by the definition of such common diseases as asthma. If the question asked is "Have you had doctor-diagnosed asthma?", about 5% of a population replies in the affirmative. If the question is whether the child or individual experiences chest wheezing on oc-

casion, three times more people will reply affirmatively. Hence difficulties in definition make comparisons between populations uncertain. Detecting significant increases in acute respiratory infections in young children, which may indeed be related to pollutants,[18] is difficult because such infections are common.

More general questions, such as possible impacts on the normal aging process of the lung, are even more complex to study and evaluate, although there may be theoretical reasons why such effects might be expected.

OUTDOOR AIR POLLUTION
Sulfur dioxide and particulates (see Chapter 6)

This is the oldest form of pollution, attributable in large part to open burning of sulfur-containing coal. Claude Monet spent the winter of 1901 in London, and his paintings of the Thames, with Waterloo and Charing Cross bridges, and of the Houses of Parliament provide a remarkable record of the interplay of fog, sunshine, and air pollutants in causing shifting colors and images.[64]

The ordinance in Pittsburgh against air pollution in 1946 represented the first effort to deal with this problem.[70] It was the London episode in December 1952,[54] however, with the excess mortality of about 4000, that forced a reluctant government to take the problem seriously. Such episodes provided incontrovertible evidence that extreme levels of air pollution were a hazard to elderly people, probably most of whom had preexisting lung or heart disease. Nevertherless, the mortality in children under age 5 was also increased in this episode.

The research resulting from this episode led to the cross-sectional study by Holland and Reid, published in 1965.[35] This landmark study was important because cigarette smoking was taken into account, all the men studied were of the same socioeconomic group, and climatic factors were uniform. At that time, levels of air pollution in London were at least twice as high as in the country towns the researchers studied. The difference in FEV_1 they found between these populations (Fig. 2-1) indicated that the effect of living in such a polluted city as London was not only to influence acute mortality, but also to lead to long-term decrements in lung function. It is now known that the FEV_1 is a powerful indicator of survival.[3] Hence living and working in London must have influenced longevity at this time. It is also realized now that growing up in such pollution may have limited the maximal FEV_1 achieved. Not only may the rate of decline of this index (which occurs in populations unexposed to pollutants) be increased by the air pollution, but also the initial value achieved may have been lower if one grew up in this atmosphere.

There has been much discussion of whether it is the SO_2 directly, the levels of particulate, or the concomitant presence of sulfuric acid aerosol that produces these effects. Models may be devised that indicate the importance of one

Table 2-1. Respiratory disease in Polish army inductees: adverse health outcomes associated with air pollution levels, arranged in an arbitrary descending order of severity*

Sample: 574,878 19-year-old inductees into the Polish army			
Annual mean ambient SO_2 (ppm)	Number of centers	Chronic bronchitis (Rate per 1000)	Asthma (Rate per 1000)
<0.005	7	1.18	1.19
0.005-0.010	37	1.22	2.55
0.010-0.012	61	1.86	2.64
0.012-0.020	66	1.92	2.96
0.020-0.028	34	3.09	4.46
>0.028	36	3.83	6.23

Data collected in Poland by Dr. Clyde Hertzman for the World Bank.[30]
*No smoking data. Diagnostic criteria not precisely stated. Although smoking history was not recorded, at the age of 19 this is unlikely to have had a major effect on chronic bronchitis, nor would it have affected asthma. Inductees came from all social classes and were required to complete a questionnaire from which these data are drawn.

of these factors over the others; the reality must surely be that they are at least additive in their effects.

This form of air pollution influences symptoms of chronic respiratory disease in children, as shown by cross-sectional[16] and panel studies.[26] It is still of great importance in Eastern Europe, where little attempt was made to control this type of pollution,[19] and in Third World countries such as the People's Republic of China. A study conducted of nonsmoking women in Beijing[80] confirmed the decrement in FEV_1 that results from exposure to smoke from coal burning. Relatively little reliable health data have come out of Eastern Europe. Table 2-1 shows some incomplete information from Poland,[30] of interest because of the large size of the sample. It confirms a dose-response relationship between increasing levels of SO_2 (and probably concomitant) particulate pollution and the incidence of asthma and chronic bronchitis.

Although gross particulate pollution has been largely controlled in the West, associations are still found between SO_2 (at low levels) and such indices as acute emergency hospital visits for respiratory disease, both in the general population[5,49] and in patients with chronic obstructive lung disease.[69] Indices of mortality also show relationships.[15,28,38] Although asthmatic subjects are much more sensitive to SO_2 than others, the levels at which these effects occur are much lower than the level of 0.5 ppm, which may have an adverse impact on a significant percentage of asthmatics.[74] In all these studies, the role of fine particulate pollution, rather than that of SO_2, may well be dominant. Levels of SO_2 may be acting as a surrogate for PM10 (particulates less than 10 microns in size) pollution, as noted in the next section.

Fine particulates

When gross particulate pollution from coal burning was controlled, either directly or by fuel substitution, it was commonly assumed that fine particulate pollution was of little consequence; a proposed level of 150 $\mu g/m^3$ for a 1-hour standard for PM10 was thought by some to be overzealous.[36]

In a modern city, automobiles are responsible for much of the fine particulate pollution, but aerosol sulfates, formed from the neutralization of sulfuric acid aerosol by ammonia, are important in many regions in the summer, and particulates from wood smoke or agricultural burning may be important during fall and winter.[45] In areas of high vehicle density and strong sunlight, such as Los Angeles or Mexico City, the composition of fine particles is extremely complex. Basic elements, such as elemental and organic carbon, aluminum, silicon, calcium, titanium, and many others, can be detected; nitrates, sulfates, and ammonium ions are also present.[12]

Data have indicated that PM10 is associated with daily mortality in a variety of different environments. These include Detroit; St. Louis; Steubenville, Ohio; Santa Clara County, California; Los Angeles; Provo, Utah; and Philadelphia.[63] In Philadelphia it has been shown that both cardiovascular and respiratory mortality are affected. Furthermore, asthma emergency visits are related to PM10 levels (which never exceeded the U.S. standard) in Seattle.[44] A strong relationship of sulfates to hospital admissions in the summer in southern Ontario has been demonstrated.[6] In Provo, Utah, where a local steel mill is responsible for a considerable fraction of the PM10 pollution, respiratory function in children and medication use in asthmatics[60] and hospital admissions for respiratory disease in children[59] are related to changes in levels of PM10.

All of this evidence, taken together, indicates that whenever a temperature inversion occurs and levels of PM10, SO_2, and nitrogen dioxide (NO_2) rise together, it is probable that PM10 is the most important component from the point of view of adverse health effects. The technology to record daily levels of PM10 has only recently become available; further epidemiological studies in a variety of different climates are needed to confirm the importance of PM10 in mixtures of air pollutants.

In the Third World, where biomass fuels may be used indoors with inadequate ventilation, particulate pollution is responsible for major respiratory effects. This problem is noted later in Chapter 3.

Photochemical oxidants

In 1952, the same year as the infamous London fog, Haagen-Smit,[27] a chemist working in Los Angeles, first clarified the basic process of ground-level ozone formation. In its simplest terms, nitric oxide *(NO)* emitted from cars is quickly oxidized to NO_2. Then in the presence

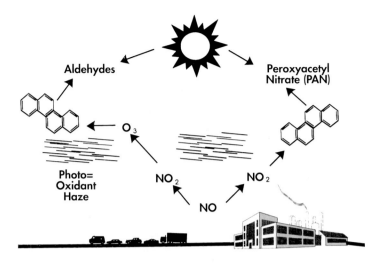

Aldehydes

Peroxyacetyl Nitrate (PAN)

O₃

Photo= Oxidant Haze

NO₂

NO₂

NO

Fig. 2-2. Chemical events in nitric oxide *(NO)* polluted air. Sunlight catalyzes the formation of nitrogen dioxide (NO_2), and ozone *(O_3)* and peroxyacetyl nitrite *(PAN)* are generated. These and other complex reactions in the atmosphere result in photooxidant production.

of sunlight of sufficient intensity and hydrocarbons, ozone *(O_3)* is formed, together with other compounds, some of which exist only for a few minutes (Fig. 2-2). Ozone, however, at low concentrations can travel hundreds of miles. Hence rural areas with ozone-sensitive crops or forested regions are exposed to levels of ozone 10 or 15 times higher than the normal background concentration of about 20 ppb. One of the transient compounds, peroxyacetyl nitrite (PAN), causes smarting of the eyes in this type of air pollution. Ozone does not affect the eyes but is an irritant of the respiratory tract at low concentrations.

Over the past 20 years, controlled-exposure experiments with ozone have illuminated the effects of this gas. In young normal subjects with intermittent exercise, lung function as judged by a simple test of maximal expiratory flow rate (FEV_1) is affected after 2 hours of exposure to 80 ppb and continues to decline if the exposure continues for another 4 hours.[37] Ozone causes inflammation in the lung[47] and nasal mucosa[11] (Fig. 2-3). The first adverse effect is to reduce the subject's maximal inspiration,[29] probably by stimulation of irritant receptors. Although the effects are not greater in asthmatics, the facts that their respiratory flow rates are already reduced and their airway responsiveness is already abnormal mean that in them the consequences of exposure may be more serious.[48]

Because for years many people have lived in areas with high oxidant levels, such as the Los Angeles suburbs, it might be expected that the effects on a normal population would be precisely defined by now. This is not the case. There is evidence that ozone worsens asthma[77] and that respiratory symptoms may be higher in regions of higher oxidant pollution.[32] A comparison of two populations of children living in areas with different ozone concentrations[81] found no differences in spirometry, or respiratory symptoms, but did find differences in lymphocyte populations and in airway responsiveness. The mean serum immuno-

globulin E (IgE) levels were not different between the two populations. Hospital data indicate that summer pollution with ozone, probably accompanied by peaks of acid aerosol, is accompanied by higher rates of hospital admission for acute respiratory diseases. This data has come from southern Ontario;[6] metropolitan Toronto:[72] upper New York state;[71] New Jersey;[13] and Atlanta, Georgia.[75] Fig. 2-4 shows the data from the study of metropolitan Toronto. A short-term study in Los Angeles found no relationship between ozone levels and hospital emergency visits in children,[61] but the period of observation may have been too short.

We have little idea of the possible long-term effects of living in an oxidant atmosphere. In a paper read to a meeting of the Air and Waste Management Association in Los Angeles, however, Russell Sherwin from the University of California, Los Angeles,[65] reviewed evidence that he had collected from 107 young adults aged 14 to 25 years who died of nonrespiratory traumatic causes in Los Angeles County (Fig. 2-5). The lungs of 29 of the 107 showed severe respiratory bronchiolitis, of the kind first described by Niewohner and others [56] in young smokers. Moderate changes were present in an additional 51 of the young adults. When fully analyzed by quantitative morphometry,[79] and when control comparisons have been made with populations in low oxidant regions,[1] these data may be the first to show that current ozone exposures are causing the same lesions that have been observed in primates exposed to ozone.[23] Calculations from theoretical dosimetric studies indicate that the terminal respiratory bronchiole is the region of the lung that receives the highest concentration of ozone.[51]

In marked contrast to the case of SO_2, therefore, ozone is known to be intensely biologically active. There is no safety margin between current levels and the minimal-effect level for this pollutant. In many locations, ozone travels with acid aerosols (which is not surprising because it en-

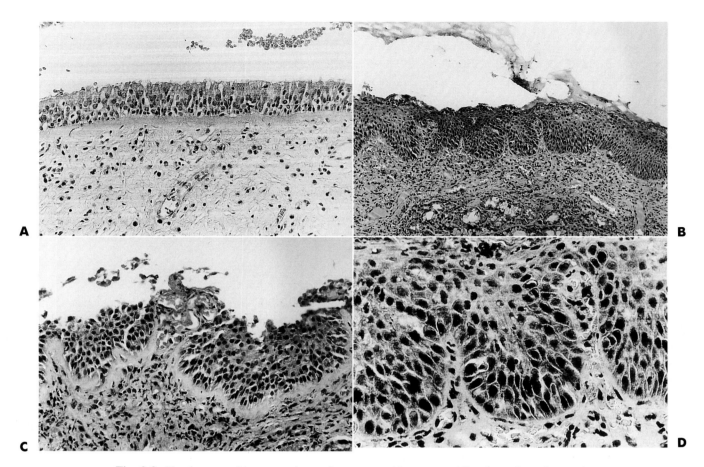

Fig. 2-3. Nasal mucosa biopsy specimens from nonsmoking men residing for at least 5 years in Vera Cruz, Mexico (low atmospheric ozone) (**A**) or in southwest metropolitan Mexico City for varying periods of time (high atmospheric ozone) (**B-D**). In Mexico City, atmospheric ozone concentrations range from approximately 0.1 to 0.2 ppm. **A,** Normal nasal mucosa. (Ca ×50.) **B,** Nasal mucosa with a moderate chronic inflammatory infiltrate and evidence of both mucous hypersecretion and superficial squamous metaplasia. (×62.) **C,** Nasal mucosa exhibiting epithelial projections and a disarray of mucosa cells and sloughing of superficial cells. (×100.) **D,** Nasal mucosa showing atypicalities and variation in cell size and orientation. (From Calderon-Garciduenas L, et al: Histopathologic changes of the nasal mucosa in southwest metropolitan Mexico City inhabitants. *Am J Pathol* 140:225, 1992, with permission).

hances the formation of sulfurous acid [H_2SO_3] from SO_2). Studies of FEV_1 in children at summer camp in Canada and the United States have indicated that the summer mix of pollutants, including ozone, is associated with measurable declines in function.[43] The same is true in adults jogging during their lunch hour,[66] many of whom were found to have ventilation levels in excess of 60 L/min (they had selected their own exercise level).

The significance of a transient fall in FEV_1 is unclear, but if it indicates that inflammation has been induced, the question that must be addressed is whether repetitive inflammation has long-term consequences.

Ozone may aggravate asthma by facilitating the entry of allergens or by inducing inflammation. This phenomenon has been known from animal studies, and Boushey[8] has pointed to its possible importance. The preliminary data of Molfino et al[52] are the first direct indication that this mechanism may be important in humans. Koenig et al[46] showed that preexposure to ozone caused an enhanced response to SO_2 in asthmatics. Thus, there are grounds for suspecting that ozone exposure might worsen the asthmatic state, but it would be premature to ascribe the increased prevalence of this multifactorial disease to ozone alone.

Ozone and acid aerosols

As noted in the previous paragraph, ozone in combination with acid aerosols (mostly sulfates) has been shown to be important in some studies of morbidity in the northeastern United States and Canada. In 1986, the first direct measurements of sulfuric acid aerosol were made in this re-

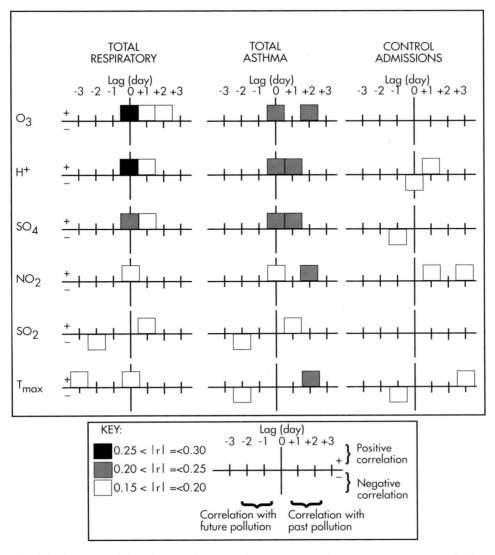

Fig. 2-4. Cross-correlations between hospital admissions and environmental measurements in Toronto, Ontario: 1986, 1987, and 1988 summers combined (after detrending and day-of-week control). O_3, Ozone; SO_4, sulfates; NO_2, nitrogen dioxide; SO_2, sulfur dioxide; T_{max}, maximum temperature. (From Thurston GD, Ito K, Lippmann M, Bates DV: Respiratory hospital admissions and summertime haze air pollution in Toronto, Ontario: consideration of the role of acid aerosols, *Environ Res,* 1994, in press; with permission.)

gion.[39] It became apparent that ozone, sulfates, and sulfuric acid aerosol commonly rose together when a summer episode occurred in this region. Furthermore, the acid aerosol could travel across the countryside before being neutralized by ammonia. A remarkable concordance between peaks of sulfuric acid aerosol has been shown to occur in the summer in Buffalo and in Toronto[73] (and presumably across the countryside in between, exposing working agricultural populations to much higher levels of pollution than formerly existed).

It is not yet clear whether the morbidity effects from this mixture are to be attributed primarily to ozone or to the acidity. It has been pointed out that the acid loading in a child exercising outdoors in this atmosphere may approximate levels that have been shown to affect asthmatic children.[67] The concomitant ozone is often above the minimal-effect level. More observations from different regions are required to throw light on this question.

In view of the large populations being exposed to this summer mixture at present, it is a matter of considerable importance that this risk should be more precisely defined. It is of interest that in Holland, where there are many thousands of pigs and cattle, atmospheric ammonia is so high that peaks of acid aerosol are not found in association with

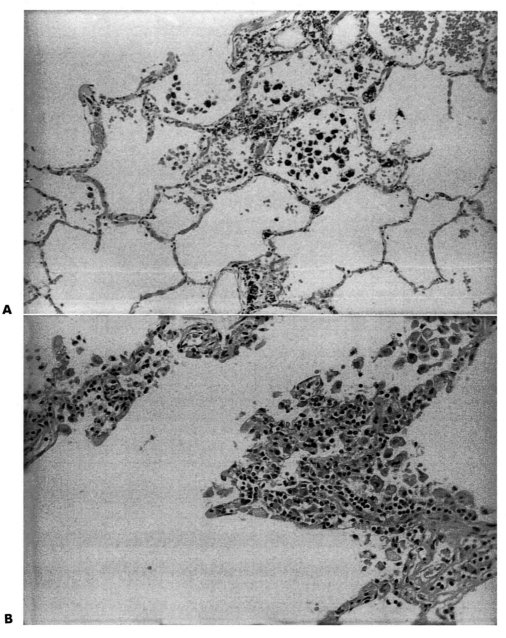

Fig. 2-5. Lung histological features of nonsmoking 21-year-old (**A**) and 23-year-old (**B**) Los Angeles County white male residents who died unexpectedly. **A,** Pigmented histiocytes are exhibited in air spaces accompanied by marked edematous changes in air space walls. (×183.) **B,** The walls of air spaces show infiltrates of lymphocytes, and prominent numbers of histiocytes are found. (×457.) These centriacinar region lesions are believed to reflect the effects of air pollution in the Los Angeles basin. (Courtesy Dr. Russell P. Sherwin, University of Southern California.)

ozone, although ammonium sulfate levels do rise together with it.[33,34]

Hydrogen sulfide, ammonia, chlorine

Individuals may be exposed to these gases either as a result of industrial accidents or if they live downwind from a processing plant. Communities have been exposed to hydrogen sulfide from acid gas plants in Alberta, both chronically and intermittently to exposures of about 1.0 ppm. Although these exposures may cause subjective symptoms, such as nausea, eye irritation, headache, and fatigue,[21,25] there is no evidence that the incidence of lung cancer or chronic respiratory disease is affected.[14] Ammonia exposure results from accidental spills or escapes of the gas. Acute adverse effects (sometimes with chronic consequences) have been documented following such exposures.

Exposures to chlorine occur in many industries, of which the pulp and paper industry is a principal one. Kennedy et al[41] have shown that such intermittent exposures to this gas may be associated with a chronically reduced level of lung function.

SENSITIVE SUBGROUPS

Depending on how the term *asthma* is defined, between 4% and 7% of the population might be considered to be asthmatic (see Chapter 28). A higher percentage give a history of "wheezy illnesses," and if tests of airway reactivity are used, about a quarter of the normal population appear to have levels of response that fall out of the normal range, although many of these do not have any respiratory history. Subjects with undoubted clinical asthma requiring medication have been shown to be much more sensitive to SO_2 than are others; as noted previously, the effects of ozone, by lowering an already abnormally low ventilatory capability and increasing an already elevated airway responsiveness, are more of a hazard to such subjects than to others. In addition, ozone is known to affect lung permeability,[40] and this may lead to a facilitated penetration of allergens.[52] Exacerbations of asthma are now known to be accompanied by evidence of inflammation in the lung, and this is another effect of ozone. These effects indicate that asthmatics should be regarded as a sensitive group in the population, but they do not prove that air pollution exposure leads to an increased prevalence of the disease.

Elderly patients with chronic obstructive lung disease, whose lung function is compromised by this, also constitute a sensitive group. As noted previously, studies of mortality in Philadelphia found that with elevations in the particulate pollution (PM10), the risk of death increased in these subjects. Furthermore, it has been shown that such patients, with mild air flow obstruction, have a greater response to NO_2 than do normal subjects of the same age.[53] It is of interest that a significant association was found in Vancouver between winter levels of NO_2 and emergency treatments for respiratory disease in patients older than 61 years.[5]

It should be noted that all patients with asthma and emphysema have nonuniform ventilation distribution in the lung. This has the effect of causing a higher dose of inhaled pollutants to be delivered into the well-ventilated regions than would occur if ventilation were normal and uniform.[2] This means that patients with nonuniform ventilation distribution within the lung would be at higher risk from inhaled pollutants than those with uniform ventilation distribution.

In acute air pollution episodes, such as occurred in London in 1952, cardiovascular mortality is invariably elevated. It has also been found to be elevated when fine particulate pollution increases, as in time-series studies in Philadelphia. The mechanism of such an effect is unclear. Incorrect diagnoses are always a possibility, but it is conceivable that in someone on the edge of heart failure, some minor change in the lung might be important.

That children might be sensitive to air pollution, by reason of their lung growth pattern being interfered with, has long been suspected. Lower FEV_1 levels have been noted in some heavily polluted regions, and there are data suggesting that lower respiratory infections in the first 2 years of life might be influenced by ambient pollution.[18] These early studies, however, did not necessarily take into account such domestic factors as gas cooking or passive cigarette smoke inhalation because their importance was not known at that time. Cross-sectional comparisons are always difficult to interpret because these circumstances, together with socioeconomic factors, undoubtedly play a major role in determining the frequency of such infections, particularly in children.

With photochemical pollution, the peak in ozone concentrations often occurs just after midday and in the early afternoon. Children coming home from school or exercising during recess periods, for example, may encounter higher ozone concentrations than office personnel. In the case of ozone, not only does exercise increase the delivered dose of the gas, but also the changed pattern of breathing has been shown, by dosimetric modeling studies, to lead to a major increase in the ozone concentration at the wall of the terminal bronchiole.[51] As noted earlier, it is this region of the lung that has been found to be first affected in primates exposed to near ambient levels of ozone.[23] Anyone exercising heavily outdoors, whether recreational or occupational, is at greater risk of adverse effects from inhaled pollutants.

INFERENCES OF CAUSALITY

Sir Austin Bradford Hill,[31] a distinguished British biostatistician, considered in 1965 the criteria that were of assistance in concluding that a causal relationship existed when a statistical association had been found. This question has been the subject of an instructive volume of essays.[62] Most air pollution studies demonstrate the presence of associations between pollutant levels and some health outcome. The question of a causal attribution is therefore central to this area of study. Whittemore[76] in 1980 noted that air pollution studies did not lead to any dose-response conclusion, and usually there are too few replicate studies in different regions to permit conclusions to be drawn that would be comparable to those that are sometimes possible in occupational exposure settings.

Four of Bradford Hill's nine criteria are particularly important in relation to studies of air pollution. "Biological plausibility" is one of these, and Bradford Hill noted that this was a criterion that could not be demanded before a causal inference was made. With air pollutants, there are no known mechanisms whereby extremely low concentrations of SO_2 might lead to long-term outcomes or to increased hospital emergency visits for respiratory disease except for the sensitivity of asthmatics to this gas (but this is to higher concentrations as a rule). In the case of ozone, this gas is extremely reactive, and current data indicate that any respiratory outcome might be thought to be biologically plausible. The data on adverse outcomes in relation to PM10 levels, including increased cardiovascular mortality, lack a convincing biological basis at the low levels at which effects occur.

A second important feature is that the associations between pollutants and outcomes should be demonstrable in different regions and in different populations. The observation that the association between PM10 level and daily mortality is present in different places with different populations and climates reinforces the causal hypothesis.

A third important criterion is that of "coherence." It is unlikely that raised levels of air pollutants would result in increased mortality and *not* lead to such outcomes as increased hospital admissions or attendances at physician's offices. The London episode in 1952 led to increased demand for hospital admissions and increased attendances for respiratory conditions at a family practice on the outskirts of London.[54] An air pollution episode in Germany led to a significant increase in ambulance use.[78] The effect of PM10 pollution has been shown to be not only on mortality, but also on lung function of children, on worsening of asthma, and on hospital admissions. This internal "coherence" provides supporting evidence for a causal inference.[4] The biological plausibility criterion is supported if there is some concordance between animal data and human observations. In the case of ozone, there is some "coherence" between controlled human studies and animal exposure data[58] but, with the exception of Sherwin's observations noted earlier,[65] no strong "coherence" with epidemiological data.

Another of Hill's criteria was the strength of the demonstrated association. It is important to recognize that associations may be weakened (and often are) by imprecision of the exposure assessment or by the fact that the health outcome is a multifactorial disease, such as asthma. Statistical techniques have improved the possibility of excluding factors that may be correlated with pollutant levels; the fact that ozone levels and ambient temperature usually are significantly correlated means that if daily mortality is being studied, careful consideration must be given to the roles of temperature and oxidants.[42] Long-term trends in disease levels and in pollutants might lead to a false association, and for this reason studies may be limited to a summer period and the regression calculated only from divergence of some health outcome from a baseline level only within the same year.[6]

These concerns are of major importance when, as is presently the case, phenomena other than catastrophic mortality in the presence of a severe pollution episode are being considered.

CONCLUDING REMARKS

The control of major industrial and domestic pollutant emissions, which has been a feature of industrialized nations since 1960, has led some observers to conclude that present levels of air pollution do not constitute any significant threat to health.[17,20] It is unlikely that catastrophic episodes will occur in the Western world in the future. Nevertheless, it would be premature to conclude that all problems had been solved. In addition to the formidable problems in the Third World of lead dissemination from gasoline and gross particulate pollution, the following aspects of pollution in the industrialized world suggest that the problems are far from being solved:

1. The continuing evidence that ozone and acidic air pollution in Canada and the United States are associated with increased hospital admissions for asthma and respiratory disease (Fig. 2-2).
2. The fact that in Los Angeles and Mexico City, and in many other regions, children are growing up in levels of oxidant pollution higher than those that cause morphometric changes in controlled animal exposures. Until it has been shown that such repetitive exposures are without serious long-term consequences in humans, there is no reason to dismiss contemporary pollutant levels as unimportant.
3. The occurrence in London, England, in December 1991, of levels of NO_2 (from automobiles) of 400 ppb for periods of several hours on 2 consecutive days.[22] This level is well above the minimal-effect level in controlled human exposures; it is not yet known if there were any measurable health outcomes.
4. The unexplained increase in the prevalence of asthma.[10,24,50] It would be premature to ascribe this to air pollution levels and equally unwise to dismiss these contaminants as unimportant factors in relation to this multifactorial disease, given our knowledge of the biological potency of ozone and the levels to which millions of people are now exposed.

REFERENCES

1. Adesina AM et al: Bronchiolar inflammation and fibrosis associated with smoking, *Am Rev Respir Dis* 143:144, 1991.
2. Bates DV: *Overview on characterizing study groups and their responses.* In Utell MJ, Frank R, editors: *Susceptibility to inhaled pollutants,* ASTM STP 1024, Philadelphia, 1989, American Society for Testing and Materials.
3. Bates DV: *Respiratory function in disease,* ed 3, Philadelphia, 1989, WB Saunders.
4. Bates DV: Health indices of the adverse effects of air pollution: the question of coherence, *Environ Res,* 59:336, 1992.
5. Bates DV, Baker-Anderson M, Sizto R: Asthma attack periodicity: a study of hospital emergency visits in Vancouver, *Environ Res* 51:51, 1990.
6. Bates DV, Sizto R: Hospital admissions and air pollutants in south-

ern Ontario: the acid summer haze effect, *Environ Res* 43:317, 1987.

7. Becklake MR: *Uses of pulmonary function tests in epidemiology.* In Bates DV: *Respiratory function in disease,* Philadelphia, 1989, WB Saunders.
8. Boushey HA: *Ozone and asthma.* In Utell MJ, Frank R, editors: *Susceptibility to inhaled pollutants,* ASTM STP 1024, Philadelphia, 1989, American Society for Testing and Materials.
9. Brunekreef B: Pulmonary function changes associated with an air pollution episode in January 1987, *J Air Poll Control Assoc* 39:1444, 1989.
10. Burney PGJ, Chinn S, Rona RJ: Has the prevalence of asthma increased in children? Evidence from the National Study of Health and Growth 1973-1986, *Br Med J* 300:1306, 1990.
11. Calderon-Garciduenas L et al: Histopathologic changes of the nasal mucosa in southwest metropolitan Mexico City inhabitants. *Am J Pathol* 140:225, 1992.
12. Chow JC et al: A neighbourhood-scale study of PM10 source contributions in Rubidoux, California, *Atmos Environ* 26A:693, 1992.
13. Cody RP et al: The effect of ozone associated with summertime photochemical smog and the frequency of asthma visits to hospital emergency departments, *Environ Res* 58:184, 1992.
14. Dales RE et al: Respiratory health of a population living downwind from natural gas refineries, *Am Rev Respir Dis* 139:595, 1989.
15. Derriennic F et al: Short-term effects of sulphur dioxide pollution on mortality in two French cities, *Int J Epidemiol* 18:186, 1989.
16. Dockery DW et al: Effects of inhalable particles on respiratory health of children, *Am Rev Respir Dis* 139:587, 1989.
17. Doll R: Prospects for prevention, *Br Med J* 286:445, 1983.
18. Douglas JWB, Waller RW: Air pollution and respiratory infections in children, *Br J Prevent Soc Med* 20:1, 1966.
19. East Europe's dark dawn, *National Geographic* 179:36, 1991.
20. Eisenbud M: *An environmental odyssey: people, pollution, and politics in the life of a practical scientist,* Seattle, WA, 1990, University of Washington Press.
21. Energy Resources Conservation Board: *Lodgepole blowout report.* Report to the Lieutenant Governor in council with respect to an inquiry held into the blowout of the well, Amoco Dome Brazeau River 13-12-48-12, Calgary, Alberta, Canada, 1984, Energy Resources Conservation Board.
22. Environmental Technology Executive Agency of the Department of Trade and Industry: Initial analysis of NO₂ pollution episode, December 1991, England, 1992, Warren Spring Laboratory.
23. Eustis SL et al: Chronic bronchiolitis in nonhuman primates after prolonged ozone exposure, *Am J Pathol* 105:121, 1981.
24. Gergen PJ, Mullally DI, Evans R III: National survey of prevalence of asthma among children in the United States, 1976 to 1980, *Pediatrics* 81:1, 1988.
25. Glass DC: A review of the health effects of hydrogen sulphide exposure, *Ann Occup Hyg* 34:323, 1990.
26. Goren AI, Hellman S: Prevalence of respiratory symptoms and diseases in schoolchildren living in a polluted and in a low polluted area in Israel, *Environ Res* 45:28, 1988.
27. Haagen-Smit AJ: Chemistry and physiology of Los Angeles smog, *Ind Eng Chem* 44:1342, 1952.
28. Hatzakis A: Short-term effects of air pollution on mortality in Athens, *Int J Epidemiol* 15:73, 1986.
29. Hazucha M, Bates DV, Bromberg P: Mechanism of action of ozone on the human lung, *J Appl Physiol* 67:1535, 1989.
30. Hertzman C: *Poland: health and environment in the context of socioeconomic decline,* Discussion paper HPRU 90, 2D, Vancouver, BC, 1990, Health Policy Research Unit, University of British Columbia.
31. Hill AB: The environment and disease: association or causation? *Proc Roy Soc Med* 58:295, 1965.
32. Hodgkin JE et al: COPD prevalence in nonsmokers in high and low photochemical air pollution areas, *Chest* 86:830, 1984.

33. Hoek G, Brunekreef B: *Effects of low level winter air pollution concentrations on respiratory health of Dutch children.* In Hoek G: *Acute effects of ambient air pollution episodes on respiratory health of children,* thesis, Holland, 1992, Landbouwuniversiteit te Wageningen.
34. Hoek G et al: Acute effects of ambient ozone on pulmonary function of children in the Netherlands. *Am Rev Respir Dis* 147:111, 1993.
35. Holland WW, Reid DD: The urban factor in chronic bronchitis, *Lancet* 1:445, 1965.
36. Holland WW et al: Health effects of particulate pollution: reappraising the evidence, *Am J Epidemiol* 110:527, 1979.
37. Horstman DH et al: Ozone concentration and pulmonary response relationships for 6.6-hour exposures with five hours of moderate exercise to 0.08, 0.10, and 0.12 ppm, *Am Rev Respir Dis* 142:1158, 1990.
38. Imai M, Yoshida K, Kitabatake M: Mortality from asthma and chronic bronchitis associated with changes in sulfur oxides air pollution, *Arch Environ Health* 41:29, 1986.
39. Keeler GJ et al: Transported acid aerosols measured in southern Ontario, *Atmos Environ* 24A:2935, 1990.
40. Kehrl HR et al: Ozone exposure increases human respiratory epithelial permeability in humans, *Am Rev Respir Dis* 135:1124, 1987.
41. Kennedy SM et al: Lung health consequences of reported accidental chlorine gas exposures among pulpmill workers, *Am Rev Respir Dis* 143:74, 1991.
42. Kinney PL, Ozkaynak H: Associations of daily mortality and air pollution in Los Angeles County, *Environ Res* 54:99, 1991.
43. Kinney PL, Ware JH, Spengler JD: A critical evaluation of acute ozone epidemiology results, *Arch Environ Health* 43:168, 1988.
44. Reference deleted in proofs. See Ref. 63a.
45. Koenig JQ et al: Wood smoke: health effects and legislation, *Northw Environ J* 4:41, 1988.
46. Koenig JQ et al: Prior exposure to ozone potentiates subsequent response to sulfur dioxide in adolescent asthmatic subjects, *Am Rev Respir Dis* 141:377, 1990.
47. Koren HS et al: Ozone-induced inflammation in the lower airways of human subjects, *Am Rev Respir Dis* 139:407, 1989.
48. Kreit JW et al: Ozone-induced changes in pulmonary function and bronchial responsiveness in asthmatics, *J Appl Physiol* 66:217, 1989.
49. Levy D, Gent M, Newhouse MT: Relationship between acute respiratory illness and air pollution levels in an industrial city, *Am Rev Respir Dis* 116:167, 1977.
50. Mao Y et al: Increased rates of illness and death from asthma in Canada, *Can Med Assoc J* 137:620, 1987.
51. Miller FJ, McDonnell WF, Gerrity TR: *Exercise and regional dosimetry: an overview.* In Utell MJ, Frank R, editors: *Susceptibility to inhaled pollutants,* ASTM STP 1024, Philadelphia, 1989, American Society for Testing and Materials.
52. Molfino NA et al: Effect of low concentrations of ozone on inhaled allergen responses in asthmatic subjects, *Lancet* 338:199, 1991.
53. Morrow PE et al: Pulmonary performance of elderly normal subjects and subjects with chronic obstructive pulmonary disease exposed to 0.3 ppm nitrogen dioxide, *Am Rev Respir Dis* 145:291, 1992.
54. *Mortality and morbidity during the London fog of December 1952 London:* Her Majesty's Stationery Office; Report No. 95 on Public Health and Medical Subjects, 1954.
55. National Academy of Sciences: *Human exposure assessment for airborne pollutants. Advances and opportunities,* Washington, DC, 1991, National Academy Press.
56. Niewohner DE, Kleinerman J, Rice DB: Pathologic changes in the peripheral airways of young cigarette smokers, *N Engl J Med* 291:755, 1974.
57. Ostro BD et al: Asthmatic responses to airborne acid aerosols, *Am J Public Health* 81:694, 1991.
58. Pinkerton KE et al: Differentiated bronchiolar epithelium in alveolar

ducts of rats exposed to ozone for 20 months. *Am J Pathol* 142:947, 1993.

59. Pope CA: Respiratory hospital admissions associated with PM10 pollution in Utah, Salt Lake, and Cache valleys, *Arch Environ Health* 46:90, 1991.

60. Pope CA et al: Respiratory health and PM10 pollution: a daily time series analysis, *Am Rev Respir Dis* 144:668, 1991.

61. Richards W et al: Los Angeles air pollution and asthma in children, *Ann Allergy* 47:348, 1981.

62. Rothman KJ, editor: *Causal inference,* Chestnut Hill, MA, 1988, Epidemiology Resources.

63. Schwartz J, Dockery DW: Increased mortality in Philadelphia associated with daily air pollution concentrations, *Am Rev Respir Dis* 145:600, 1992.

63a. Schwartz J, et al: Particulate air pollution and hospital emergency room visits for asthma in Seattle, *Am Rev Respir Dis,* 147:826, 1993.

64. Seiberling G: *Monet in London,* High Museum of Art, Atlanta Georgia, Seattle, London, 1988, University of Washington Press.

65. Sherwin RP, Richters V: Centriacinar region (CAR) disease in the lungs of young adults. A preliminary report. In Berglund RL, Lawrson DR, McKee DJ, editors: *Tropospheric ozone and the environment,* Pittsburgh, 1991, Air and Waste Management Association.

66. Spektor DM et al: Effects of ambient ozone on respiratory function in healthy adults exercising outdoors, *Am Rev Respir Dis* 138:821, 1988.

67. Spengler JD et al: Exposures to acid aerosols, *Environ Health Perspect* 79:43, 1989.

68. Stern B et al: Respiratory health effects associated with ambient sulfates and ozone in two rural Canadian communities, *Environ Res* 49:20, 1989.

69. Sunyer J et al: Effects of urban air pollution on emergency room admissions for chronic obstructive pulmonary disease, *Am J Epidemiol* 134:277, 1991.

70. Tarr JA: Changing fuel use behavior and energy transitions: the Pittsburgh smoke control movement 1940-1950, *J Social History* 14:561, 1981.

71. Thurston GD et al: A multi-year study of air pollution and respiratory hospital admissions in three New York state metropolitan areas: results for 1988 and 1989 summers, *J Expos Anal Environ Epidemiol,* 2:429, 1992.

72. Thurston GD et al: Respiratory hospital admissions and summertime haze air pollution in Toronto, Ontario: consideration of the role of acid aerosols, *Environ Res,* 1994, in press.

73. Thurston GD et al: The nature and origins of acid aerosol pollution measured in metropolitan Toronto, Ontario, *Environ Res,* 1994, in press.

74. U.S. Environmental Protection Agency: *Review of the national ambient air quality standards for sulfur oxides: updated assessment of scientific and technical information.* Draft addendum to the 1982 Office of Air Quality Protection Staff Paper, Washington, DC, 1986, U.S. Environmental Protection Agency.

75. White MC et al: Childhood asthma and ozone pollution in Atlanta (pilot study), *Environ Res,* 1994, in press.

76. Whittemore AS: Air pollution and respiratory disease, *Annu Rev Public Health* 2:397, 1981.

77. Whittemore AS, Korn EL: Asthma and air pollution in the Los Angeles area, *Am J Public Health* 70:687, 1980.

78. Wichmann HE et al: Health effects during a smog episode in West Germany in 1985, *Environ Health Perspect* 79:89, 1989.

79. Wright JL: Small airways disease: its role in chronic airflow obstruction, *Semin Respir Med* 13:72, 1992.

80. Xu X, Dockery DW, Wang L: Effects of air pollution on adult pulmonary function, *Arch Environ Health* 46:198, 1991.

81. Zwick H et al: Effects of ozone on the respiratory health, allergic sensitization, and cellular immune system in children, *Am Rev Respir Dis* 144:1075, 1991.

Chapter 3

INDOOR AIR QUALITY
AND POLLUTION

John E. Craighead

Sick building syndrome
Biologicals
Volatile organic compounds
Combustion products
Radon
Lead
Asbestos

Table 3-1. Approximate proportion of day spent at various sites by adults in urban United States

Location	Percent
Home	60
Work	25
Transit (auto, bus, train)	6
Other structures (stores, restaurants)	7
Outside	2

Modified from Letz GA: Sick building syndrome: acute illness among office workers—the role of building ventilation, airborne contaminants and work stress, *Allergy Proc* 11:109, 1990.

Most residents of developed countries spend a substantial proportion of their time indoors (Table 3-1). The indoor air is a microenvironment that only partially reflects outdoor air conditions (see Chapter 2). This is particularly the case in modern, mechanically ventilated buildings in which, for economic reasons, attempts are increasingly being made to reduce the exchange of outdoor air with indoor air. After the energy crisis in the early 1970s, ventilatory standards were reduced, and, as a result, the turnover of indoor-generated pollutants increased substantially. Approximately half of the workforce in developed countries are employed in offices. The remainder work in countless occupations in which potentially unique types of air pollutant exposures occur. Indoor employment accounts for roughly 25% of the modern worker's day. The average adult spends roughly 60% of his or her time in the home environment; homemakers and children under school age generally spend much of their time in the house on a daily basis (Table 3-1). This chapter considers the nature of the environmental exposures that occur indoors, at work, and at home, and the illness

related to them. In general, the long-term health effects (if any) of the exposures discussed here are unknown. Specific respiratory disease processes occurring in the workplace are considered in Chapter 28.

SICK BUILDING SYNDROME

Since the 1970s, outbreaks of acute, nonspecific minor illnesses, primarily of the upper aerodigestive tract, the external eye, and central nervous system (see box on next page), have been reported among indoor workers, particularly those employed in offices.* In many of these episodes, the relationship of the syndrome to the indoor environment appears to have been established because the symptoms seem to disappear when affected persons leave the building. Moreover, studies that attempt to simulate the polluted indoor environment have shown that illness can be induced experimentally by manipulating the environment. The spe-

*References 19, 23, 24, 29, 30, 44, 47, 51, 54.

Dr. David Bates provided a critique and brought to the author's attention information incorporated into this chapter.

**Symptoms commonly reported
in building-related illness**

Irritation of mucus membranes and respiratory tract
  Itching or burning eyes
  Dry or irritated throat
  Rhinitis, sinus congestion, sneezing
  Cough, chest tightness
Skin irritation, including rashes
Central nervous system/systemic effects
  Headaches
  Drowsiness, fatigue, malaise
  Confusion, irritability, difficulty concentrating
  Dizziness

Table 3-2. Presumptive causation of outbreaks of sick building syndrome

Cause	Percent
Inadequate ventilation	50
Inside contaminants	19
Outside contaminants	11
Biologicals	5
Building materials	4

Modified from Samet JM, Marbury C, Spangler JD: Health effects and sources of indoor air pollution. Part II, *Am Rev Respir Dis* 137:221, 1988.

cific cause of most outbreaks, however, is not established, although the primary problems in a substantial number of cases are believed to be inadequate ventilation and inadequate air turnover (Table 3-2). Even this conclusion has been questioned by the results of experimental studies. For example, Menzies and colleagues[31] showed that symptom patterns and the numbers of building inhabitants affected did not change when air turnover was experimentally increased. Chronicity of symptoms among office workers has been claimed, and in several studies, 50% to 80% of building inhabitants are affected at one time or another. This would suggest that some of us chronically exhibit a variety of nonspecific symptoms or are subjects of suggestion or mass hysteria. Regardless of the vagueness of the sick building syndrome and its causation, a number of indoor air pollutants have been identified in homes and offices in low concentrations and to a variable extent have been appropriately or incorrectly implicated.

Although little research has been focused on pathogenetic mechanisms in humans, it might be speculated that the various pollutants act as irritants and, in so doing, trigger the generation of a variety of cytokines (Chapter 24), which affect multiple organ systems. Evidence supporting such speculation is lacking at present. Invariably the nonspecific symptoms of the sick building syndrome overlap those of preexisting respiratory infections and allergic reactions of varying degrees of severity.

Potential disease-causing indoor air pollutants can be classified into (1) biologicals, (2) volatile organic compounds, and (3) products of combustion (see box on next page).

BIOLOGICALS

Most, if not all, homes and occupational settings are contaminated with a multiplicity of obscure organisms that give rise to potentially irritating or allergenic (or both) biological products. Rug mites are an inevitable inhabitant of buildings, where they feed on spilled food and animal products (hair and dander).[34,41] Cockroaches and other vermin

and microorganisms (including their spores) inhabit the nooks and crannies of most buildings, and pets are kept in more than half of U.S. homes. These diverse biota, their feces and urine proteins, carcasses and body parts, hair, and sloughed skin are the potential triggers of acute allergic reactions (asthma) in susceptible hosts. It is likely that they give rise to more minor allergic complaints in many people, but specific documentation is lacking, and the mechanisms are not clearly defined.

VOLATILE ORGANIC COMPOUNDS

Volatile organic compounds of presumptive relevance and their sources are listed in the box on page 31. These compounds are the constituents of insulation materials, carpets, draperies and other furnishings, paints, waxes, solvents, soaps, perfumes, detergents, and countless other consumer items found in the home and workplace. A research group in Aarhus, Denmark,[27,32] carried out carefully controlled experimental exposures to mixtures of hydrocarbons that they had found were most commonly present when the occupants complained of symptoms. The reproducibility of the experiments provided strong evidence of the reality of the complaints. In their studies, one substance was not found to be the cause of the syndrome, but the "cocktail" of eight hydrocarbons was often considered to be responsible. Of the many volatile indoor air pollutants, formaldehyde is one of the most ubiquitous (and well-studied) because of its wide use in the synthetic chemical industry and more specifically in the manufacturing of insulation materials and various types of plywood, particle boards, and so forth.[3] Table 3-3 summarizes information on the range of concentrations of formaldehyde that have been found in surveys of various types of dwellings; the symptoms recognized to be associated with formaldehyde over a range of concentrations are listed in Table 3-4. It is apparent that in some closed environments, formaldehyde alone might be expected to contribute to the development of symptoms consistent with the sick building syndrome. Because of its almost universal presence in a variety of construction materials and consumer items, formaldehyde has been the subject of restrictive regulation in some jurisdictions.

Indoor air pollutants possibly contributing to sick building syndrome

Biologicals	*Sources*
Rug mites	Fecal material, body parts
Cats and dogs	Saliva and dander
Wild and pet rodents and birds	Urine proteins
Fungi and bacteria	Mycelia and spores

Combustion products

Tobacco smoke
Automobile exhaust
Energy generation (space and water heating; cooling; fireplaces)
Particulates, carbon monoxide, nitrogen oxides, polycyclic aromatic hydrocarbons

*Volatile and semivolatile organic compounds**	*Sources*
Formaldehyde	Particle board, plywood, furniture, urea formaldehyde for insulation
Benzene	Smoking, auto exhaust
Tetrachloroethylene	Passive smoking, driving, pumping gas, wearing or storing dry-cleaned clothes, visiting dry cleaners
p-Dichlorobenzene	Room deodorizers, moth cakes
Chloroform	Tap water
Methylene chloride	Paint strippers, solvents
1,1,1-Trichloroethane	Dry-cleaned clothes, aerosol sprays, fabric protectors
Carbon tetrachloride	Industrial-strength cleansers
Aromatic hydrocarbons	Paints, adhesives, gasoline, combustion sources (toluene, xylenes, ethylbenzene, trimethylbenzenes)
Aliphatic hydrocarbons	Paints, adhesives, gasoline, combustion sources (octane, decane, undecane)
Terpenes (limonene, pinene)	Scented deodorizers, polishes, fabrics, fabric softeners, cigarettes, food, beverages
Insecticides	(See Chapter 8)
Polychlorobiphenyls *(PCBs)*	Transformers, fluorescent ballasts, ceiling tiles

*Modified from Samet J: Environmental controls and lung disease, Report of the ATS Workshop on Environmental Controls and Lung Disease, Santa Fe, 1988, *Am Rev Respir Dis* 142:915, 1990.

Table 3-3. Formaldehyde concentrations in indoor air

Location	Concentration (ppm)
Mobile homes	0.01-3.68
Apartments and public buildings	0.03-0.2
Detached housing	0-0.3

Modified from Letz GA: Sick building syndrome: acute illness among office workers—the role of building ventilation, airborne contaminants and work stress, *Allergy Proc* 11:109, 1990.

Table 3-4. Symptoms pattern in relation to formaldehyde air concentration

ppm*	Symptoms
<0.5	None
0.05-1.5	Neurological complaints
0.01-2.0	Eye irritation
0.1-25	Upper airway irritation

*Indoor concentrations generally range from 0-0.3 ppm in U.S. detached homes and 0-2 ppm in manufactured housing.

COMBUSTION PRODUCTS

The relative importance of gaseous and particulate pollutants in the home and workplace is determined by architectural design and the potential for circulation of outside air (either relatively clean or polluted). The type of indoor heat-generating equipment and its maintenance also are critical. Table 3-5 provides information on the concentrations of products of combustion from various forms of hydrocarbon fuels. The increasingly popular use of woodstoves as a primary or supplementary source of heat has resulted in gas and particle accumulations not heretofore observed with the traditional home heating fuels, gas and oil. This is accompanied by the generation of substantial amounts of the potentially carcinogenic polycyclic aromatic hydrocarbons.[7]

Table 3-5. Comparison of emissions from selected residential space heating and transportation sources

Source	Carbon monoxide	Nitrous oxide	Sulfur dioxide	Benzo(a)pyrene	Particulates
Residential space heating	lb/10^6 BTU	lb/10^6 BTU	lb/10^6 BTU	μg/10^6 BTU	lb/10^6 BTU
Gas	0.02	0.08	0.0006	8×10^2	0.02
Oil	0.04	0.09	0.3-7	9×10^3	0.07
Coal	3.5	0.1	0.5-7	2.5×10^7	0.6
Wood (fireplace)	3.0	0.25		4.5×10^3	1.3
Wood (stove)	22	0.07	0.03	1.4×10	1.2
Transportation	lb/50 mi	lb/50 mi	lb/50 mi	μg/50 mi	lb/50 mi
Highway vehicles	2.4	0.34	0.02	50	0.06

Modified from Cooper JA: Environmental impact of residential wood combustion emissions and its implications, *J Air Pollut Cont Assoc* 30:855, 1980.

The efficiency of combustion, the effective convection of effluents to the outside air, and the maintenance and function of the heat-generating equipment are critical determinants influencing the concentrations of combustion products that find their way into the living space.

Oxides of nitrogen are given off by unvented gas stoves. Homes with these appliances have higher concentrations of the gas indoors than homes with electric stoves. In a study of 1567 white children by Neas and his colleagues,[36] a 15-ppb increase in annual mean nitrogen oxide (NO_2) concentration in the home was associated with an increased cumulative incidence of lower respiratory symptoms in girls, with a slightly lower incidence in boys. Pulmonary function was unaffected by this potentially irritating cytotoxic gas, but it is impossible to know what other nonspecific symptoms might be attributed to it. The use of kerosene heaters indoors gives rise to highly acidic aerosol atmospheres, with the production of nitric acid.[53] No specific adverse health effects have been described as a consequence of this exposure.

In energy-conscious countries of the developed world, households are increasingly turning to wood as fuel for space heating. In developing countries, the use of biomass fuels, such as cow dung, in poorly ventilated cooking areas is the source of high concentrations of fine particulates and carbon monoxide (CO) in the home.[40] Some of the most striking accumulations of carbon in lung tissue that I, as a pathologist, have noted were among peasants residing in primitive grass and wood dwellings in Africa. In these circumstances, chimneys to remove smoke are either inadequate or nonexistent, and ventilation is poor. A vivid illustration of the effects of such conditions is given by a study of women in a village at 11,200 feet altitude near the river Indus.[39] Chronic cough was common in both men and women. In the women, the timed forced expiratory volume was significantly reduced during winter compared with summer, and the CO in their blood tripled during winter. It is hardly surprising that respiratory diseases are the sec-

ond most common cause of death among children under age 5 in the Third World;[28] gross indoor particulate pollution no doubt plays a contributory, but at present undefined, role. Of all the indoor combustion products, tobacco smoke is the most common and pervasive. The health effects of sidestream tobacco smoke and the apparent high concentrations of particulates and hydrocarbons found within it are of particular importance (see Chapters 3 and 13).[22,26,48,55]

Homes and office complexes with attached or basement garages exhibit special problems with regard to the potential for automotive exhaust to enter buildings directly or through air intake vents.

RADON

In 1879, workers in a pitchblende (uranium ore) mine in Schneeburg, Germany, were found to experience a substantial risk of lung cancer.[20] This observation was made at least a half-century before the major epidemic of cigarette smoking began in developed countries and almost 20 years before the discovery of radium by the Curies in 1898. Autopsy studies of workers from another central European uranium mine (Joschimstal, Czechoslovakia) in the 1930s showed that 50% died of bronchogenic carcinoma. Subsequent work established the association of lung cancer with high concentrations of radon in the air of these mines. This public health tragedy was played out again on the Colorado plateau of North America among miners of uranium ores during and after World War II.[5] Although in the Colorado outbreak cancer developed among radon-exposed nonsmokers,[46] the major impact was reflected in the apparent interaction of the alpha emitters of radon daughter products with the carcinogens and promoters in cigarette smoke and their effects on the respiratory mucosa.

Awareness of the potential significant negative impact on health of radon in residential buildings first developed in Sweden in the 1970s. In the United States, the significance of indoor radon pollution was abruptly brought into

Table 3-6. Sources of global atmospheric radon

Source	Input to atmosphere (million Ci/yr)
Emanation from soil	2000
Groundwater (potential)	500
Emanation from oceans	30
Phosphate residues	3
Uranium mill tailings	2
Coal residues	0.02
Natural gas	0.01
Coal combustion	0.001

Modified from National Council on Radiation Protection and Measurement: *Exposures from the uranium series with emphasis on radon and its daughters,* Report No. 77, Bethesda, MD, 1984, National Council on Radiation Protection and Measurements.

Table 3-7. Mean uranium and radium content of common geological deposits

Deposit	Uranium (ppm)	Radium (pCi/g)
Igneous rock, acid	3	—
Igneous rock, neutral	1.5	—
Igneous rock, basic	0.6	—
Igneous rock, ultrabasic	0.03	—
Granite	4	1
Sedimentary rocks	1.3	0.3
Phosphate deposits (Florida)	120	—
Phosphate deposits (Algeria)	25	—
Bituminous shale (Tennessee)	65	—
Sand and gravel	—	0.4

Modified from Eisenbud M: *Environmental radioactivity (from natural, industrial, and military sources),* ed 3, Orlando, 1987, Academic Press.

focus by the discovery of a substantial concentration of radon daughters in the body of an employee of a nuclear power plant who triggered radiation detectors when entering the plant. Further investigation yielded the imposing finding that the basement of this worker's home contained 2700 picocuries per liter of air. The level was almost 700-fold greater than the U.S. Environmental Protection Agency (EPA) current action level of 4 pCi/L.

Radium-226 is the major radioactive decay product of uranium-238, a ubiquitous element in rock and soil (Table 3-6). It in turn decays to odor-free, colorless radon-222 gas, which further breaks down (half-life, 3.8 days) into several nongaseous daughters having half-lives ranging from less than 1 second to 27 minutes (polonium-218, lead-214, and polonium-210). Alpha particles, the major radioactive product of radon decay, are emitted by lead-214 and polonium-218. Inhaled high-energy, high-mass particles of these solid isotopes are believed to interact with the respiratory mucosa in a distribution pattern favoring deposition at bifurcations of intermediate-size bronchi in the lungs. Presumptively the isotopes diffuse to, or in proximity to, the progenitor cells of the bronchial epithelium. As a result, carcinogenic mutations occur consequent to alpha particle release. This is a hypothetical construct, however, unproven by experimentation. Bronchogenic carcinoma appears to be the only adverse health effect of radon exposure in homes, in the workplace, and in public buildings.[5,11]

Radium is a basic constituent of igneous rock, such as basalt and granite. Over eons of geological time, however, it has accumulated by erosion in relatively high concentrations in sedimentary deposits and certain soils.[16] Thus the geological sources of radon gas are complex (Table 3-7). Radon accounts for more than half of the natural and anthrophogenic radiation to which humans are exposed (Fig. 3-1).[6] When buildings are situated in proximity to deposits, radon seeps through cracks in foundations, in sumps,

and around piping to accumulate in basements. Radon also is found in potable groundwater and some deposits of natural gas that are piped into the home. The concentrations, of course, are quite variable because they indirectly reflect the radon leached from the rock in which the water (i.e., aquifer) and gas are located. Some building materials also contain radon sources. Because of the geological complexities and the peculiarities of individual buildings, the radon concentrations in any one structure can only be determined by analytical means.

Determination of risks to building inhabitants is a complex issue in which universal agreement doubtlessly never will be obtained. Data on which calculations are based is almost exclusively derived from studies of uranium miners exposed to high concentrations of radon in the mines.[5] In addition to being exposed to radon, these workers commonly smoke and potentially experience other risk factors for lung cancer (i.e., exposure to silicas, asbestos, heavy metals, and combustion products)[13] (see Chapters 3 and 4). Systematic studies of uranium miners on the Colorado plateau have consistently demonstrated a relative risk of three to four times, with a shortened latency period (Fig. 3-2). At the exceedingly high concentrations of radon found in some mines, the risk probably is increased tenfold to twentyfold. Although modern studies are controlled for cigarette use, the cocarcinogenic effects of radon and smoke are more difficult to analyze. An increase in lung cancer, however, also occurs in nonsmokers, as has been shown in studies of uranium miners who are Navajo Native Americans.[46] It is currently unclear whether the combined carcinogenic effects of smoking and radon are additive or synergistic and thus multiplicative.

Data on indoor air concentrations of radon in homes, offices, and public buildings are limited despite extensive, ongoing studies.[2] Figure 3-3 summarizes information from

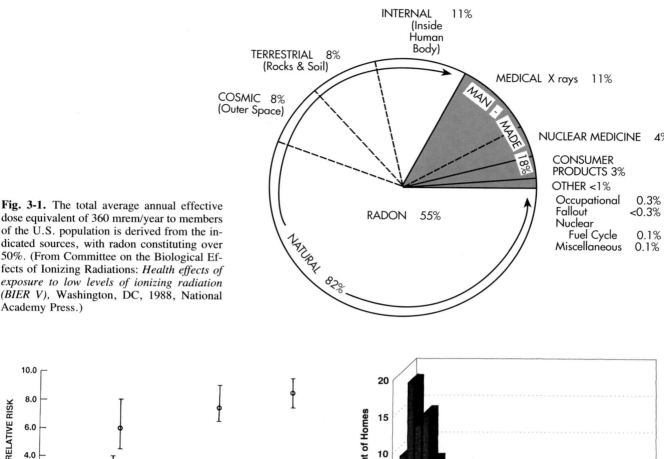

Fig. 3-1. The total average annual effective dose equivalent of 360 mrem/year to members of the U.S. population is derived from the indicated sources, with radon constituting over 50%. (From Committee on the Biological Effects of Ionizing Radiations: *Health effects of exposure to low levels of ionizing radiation (BIER V),* Washington, DC, 1988, National Academy Press.)

Fig. 3-2. Risk of bronchogenic carcinoma related to radon exposure. Note the dose-response relationship with a plateau. (Modified from Committee on the Biological Effects of Ionizing Radiations: *Health risks of radon and other internally deposited alpha-emitters (BIER IV),* Washington, DC, 1988, National Academy Press.)

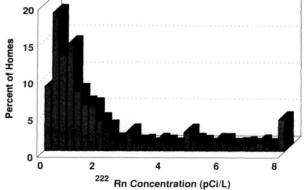

Fig. 3-3. Percentage of single-family houses with indicated detectable radon-222 (^{222}Rn) concentrations. The sample includes 552 homes from 19 studies. (Adapted from Needleman HL, editor: *Lead toxicity,* Washington, DC, 1990, U.S. Department of Health and Human Services, Public Health Service, Agency for Toxic Substances and Disease Registry.)

several surveys of homes throughout the United States indicating the relative concentrations of radon in air.[38] It illustrates the enormous range in the exposures experienced by average Americans. Table 3-8 provides data on indoor radon concentrations by location as documented in five different studies. The enormous variability between structures in various geographical sites (Fig. 3-4), and even in the local setting, reflects the complexities of geological accumulations of radon in rock, soil, and water. Although detailed studies of naturally occurring radon radiation have largely been conducted in developed countries (particularly the

United States), outdoor terrestrial background radiation has also been found to exceed the normal range (0.2 to 0.6 mGy/yr) in several regions of the world (Brazil, India, People's Republic of China, Italy, France, Iran, Madagascar, and Nigeria).[6] For example, in the village of Guarapari, Brazil, the monazite sand in the local soils contains high concentrations of thorium, a source of both gamma and alpha radiation. On the Kerala Coast of India, an estimated 70,000 residents are exposed to roughly fourfold increases in the radiation products of thorium owing to the presence of this substance in the monazite sands in the soil. In a re-

Chapter 3 Indoor air quality and pollution   **35**

Table 3-8. Comparisons of indoor radon concentrations in different parts of houses (geometrical means)

Characterization of houses studied	Radon concentration (pCi/L)		
	Basement	First floor	Second floor
New York–New Jersey	1.7	0.83	0.7
Central Maine	2.46	1.40	1.12
Houston		0.39	
Eastern Pennsylvania			
Summer	3.40	1.22	
Winter	5.90	4.40	
Northeastern United States			
Nonefficient	1.3	0.3	
Energy efficient	3.57	1.60	2.01

Modified from Bodansky D, Robkin M, Stadler D, editors: *Indoor radon and its hazards,* Seattle, 1987, University of Washington Press.

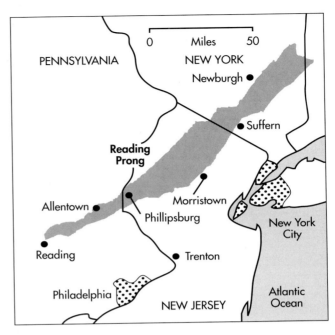

Fig. 3-4. "The Reading Prong" copyright 1993 by Consumers Union of U.S., Inc., Yonkers, NY 10703-1057. Reprinted by permission from *Consumer Reports,* October 1993.

gion of Guangding Province, People's Republic of China, the naturally occurring soil thorium, uranium, and radium are responsible for an exposure of 3 to 5 mSv (300 to 400 mrem) (see Chapter 11).[6,57]

Based on these findings, we must ask what information serves as the basis for the widespread concern regarding the effects of radon in the home. Unfortunately, important data are lacking, and the few epidemiological studies to assess health risk thus far conducted on those exposed to low-level concentrations have been inconclusive. As a result, estimates of risk are based on straight-line mathematical extrapolations (assuming no threshold) from mortality data accumulated in animal models and radiation workers exposed to substantially greater concentrations of radon.

The accuracy of the risk assessments for members of the general population are fraught with unresolvable problems. They are compounded by enormous differences in concentrations of radon in individual residences, by architectural considerations, by the locations of sleeping and recreational quarters, and by the age and smoking habits as well as the relative susceptibility of each individual.

Based on a variety of considerations, the EPA has established the "action level" for radon to be 4 pCi/L of inhalable air. The number of homes exceeding this concentration ranges from 4% in the Northeast to 55% in the so-called Reading Prong region of northeastern Pennsylvania and west central New Jersey (a geographically defined region in which naturally occurring radon sources are found in unusually high concentrations). Overall, 11% of American homes are believed by the EPA to exceed the action level. Based on these considerations, the EPA has estimated a relative risk of 0.3% (i.e., one lung cancer death per 300 members of a population) for the average American owing to environmental exposure to radon.[45] For a life-time exposure to radon at 4 pCi/L, the EPA has esti-

mated that the risk for developing lung cancer is 1% to 5%, whereas the National Research Council (BEIR IV)[5] concluded the risk is 0.8% to 1.4%. Regardless of the incalculable variables, it is evident that radon in the home poses a significant public health problem, particularly among smokers. It seems likely that a proportion of the bronchogenic carcinomas occurring in older, nonsmoking members of the population (approximately 15% of men and 25% of women) over 50 years of age may be due to radon exposure in the home or workplace (see Chapter 28).[43]

LEAD

Concern regarding the unique susceptibility of children and the widespread presence of lead in the indoor environment has mushroomed in recent years. Concomitantly, evidence has accumulated to indicate that neurobehavioral dysfunction is demonstrable in children of both high and low socioeconomic status with blood lead concentrations of 10 µg/dl or more, manyfold lower than was believed just a few years ago.[1,37,42] Although the overt toxicity of industrial lead exposure has long been recognized (see Chapter 4) (Table 3-9), the potential hazard of lead paint in the home has been less widely appreciated. In the 1950s, public health surveys of homes were first initiated in the United States. These surveys consistently demonstrated a relative increase in the blood concentrations of lead among a substantial proportion of the children surveyed. It was particularly the case in children of lower socioeconomic status

Table 3-9. Summary of lowest observed effect level for lead-induced health effects in adults and children

Blood lead concentration (μg/dl)	Health effect
>100	Adults: Encephalopathic signs and symptoms
>80	Adults: Anemia
	Children: Encephalopathic signs and symptoms
	Chronic nephropathy (e.g., aminoaciduria)
>70	Adults: Clinically evident peripheral neuropathy
	Children: Colic and other gastrointestinal symptoms
>60	Adults: Female reproductive effects
	Central nervous system symptoms (i.e., sleep disturbances, mood changes, memory and concentration problems, headaches)
>50	Adults: Decreased hemoglobin production
	Decreased performance on neurobehavioral tests
	Altered testicular function
	Gastrointestinal symptoms (i.e., abdominal pain, constipation, diarrhea, nausea, anorexia)
	Children: Reduced hemoglobin synthesis
>25	Adults: Elevated erythrocyte protoporphyrin levels in men
15-25	Adults: Elevated erythrocyte protoporphyrin levels in women
	Children: Decreased intelligence and growth
>10	Fetus: Preterm delivery
	Impaired learning
	Reduced birth weight
	Impaired mental ability

From *MMWR* 41(17), May 1, 1992.

Table 3-10. Estimated rates of white children (ages 0.5 to 5 years) with blood lead concentrations greater than 10 μg/dl

Family income ($)	Prevalence (%)
≥15,000	32
6000-14,999 (× 10³)	50
<6000	68
Total	40

Modified from Sayre JW, Ernhart CB: Control of lead exposure in childhood. Are we doing it correctly? *Am J Dis Child* 146:1275, 1992 (editorial).

Table 3-11. Lead in paints from residential houses in Oakland, California, 1987-1990

Paint concentration greater than 5000 ppm	Percent
Exterior	72
Interior	37

Modified from *MMWR* 46(17), May 1, 1982.

residing in older homes (Table 3-10). The use of lead in paints for residential dwellings was regulated in 1977, shortly after its potential health implications were first appreciated. Both the exteriors and interiors of a substantial proportion (more than 80%) of buildings constructed before that time were painted with compounds containing lead (Table 3-11), because the metal instilled durability to the paint while serving as a dryer and pigment. Now, this aging paint on older buildings is chipping and breaking down into dust that accumulates in and around buildings. As a result, the soils on the exteriors and the dust in the interiors of these buildings are contaminated (Table 3-12).

Until recently, aerosolized lead in the exhaust of internal combustion engines was considered a widespread but

Table 3-12. Geometrical mean lead concentrations in dust in and surface garden soils within 5 cm surrounding houses of various age in Brighton, England

House age	n	Lead concentration μg/g	
		House dust	Soil
Pre-1870	20	982	1146
1870-1919	38	1874	1014
1920-1939	31	619	368
1940-1959	22	433	292
1960-1986	28	241	131

Modified from Thornton I et al: Lead exposure in young children from dust and soil in the United Kingdom, *Environ Health Perspect* 89:55, 1990.

Table 3-13. Airborne concentrations of asbestos fibers (5 μ or longer) in the ambient air of buildings of various types

Building type	No. of buildings	Mean	90th Percentile	Maximum
School	48	0.00051	0.0016	0.0080
Residence	96	0.00019	0.0005	0.0025
Public and commercial	54	0.00020	0.0004	0.0065
All buildings	198	0.00027	0.0007	0.0080

Modified from Health Effects Institute: *Asbestos research: asbestos in public and commercial buildings: a literature review and synthesis of current knowledge,* Washington, DC, 1991, Health Effects Institute.

unquantitated potential health hazard for urban residents. Although old chipping paint containing lead in homes may be a significant hazard for many children who ingest it (a practice called pica), absorption of the lead from the digestive tract is much less efficient than its uptake from the lungs. Thus the contribution of airborne lead originating in automotive exhaust and household dust most probably is a more significant factor for the youthful urban resident than ingested lead paint fragments. The movement to eliminate tetraethyl lead from gasoline in the United States has been followed by a reduction in blood lead concentrations in the populations of several heavily polluted urban areas.[50] This observation suggests that aerosolized lead in automotive exhaust may be a more important source of pollution than was previously appreciated.

ASBESTOS

Few environmental subjects have stirred more controversy and litigation than those related to the health effects of asbestos. Among the many unresolved issues is the concern that asbestos in the insulation and flooring of homes, businesses, and public buildings poses a subtle, long-term health risk for the inhabitants. During the middle decades of this century, asbestos in various formulations was incorporated into materials that were sprayed on structural components of buildings; incorporated into acoustical tile, wallboard, and floor tile; and used in spackling compounds and paints. With only a few exceptions, this asbestos was the chrysotile type, a mineral that differs structurally and chemically from the commercial and highly pathogenic amphibole asbestos types, crocidolite and amosite (see Chapter 6).

Concerns regarding the possible health risks of asbestos in public buildings are founded on the epidemic of asbestos-related disease that developed in Europe and America after World War II. They were fanned by the supposition among some members of the scientific community that airborne asbestos poses a risk for the development of mesothelioma in those who inhale it, regardless of the concentration in the ambient air (see Chapters 6 and 28). Thus, if 15% to 20% of workers heavily exposed in the industrial setting ultimately develop malignant mesotheliomas (see Chapter 28) as a result of their occupational exposure to airborne as-

bestos, a calculable risk, however small, exists for the occupants of public buildings, even though only negligible amounts of airborne asbestos are found in the ambient environment.[15]

Based on these considerations, the EPA initiated a national program dictating routine inspections of school buildings to detect sources of the presumptively hazardous release of asbestos from construction materials.[17] With this action, as well as the exceptionally intense media coverage and publicity by advocates and public health officials, many schools, public buildings, and business places were extensively renovated to eliminate asbestos-containing material, regardless of its conditions. These well-intentioned but often needless and expensive actions finally provoked a public and scientific outcry[10,33,52] that precipitated a temporizing response by the EPA.[18] Furthermore, justifiable concerns have arisen regarding the hazards for workers involved in asbestos abatement and the contamination of buildings by residual asbestos debris if the abatement is poorly conducted.

As can be seen in Table 3-13, the concentrations of respirable asbestos in the air of households and public buildings is exceedingly low and far beneath the ambient air concentrations permitted by current regulations of the U.S. Occupational Safety and Health Administration (OSHA) (i.e., 0.2 fibers/ml^3 of air time-weighted average [8 hr/day, 5 days/wk, year round]). The argument championed by several regulatory agencies of the U.S. government ignores several important concepts. The first is that asbestos dust concentrations in the ambient indoor air do not differ from the amounts detected in the outdoor air surrounding the buildings.[4,9,14,21] This, of course, is because asbestos (usually in low concentrations) in the building insulation and flooring is encased in binding materials and thus is not released to be respirable. The second concept relates to the type of asbestos involved because it is universally agreed that chrysotile is substantially less pathogenic than the amphiboles.[8] Moreover, it is doubtful that chrysotile exposure in low concentrations causes mesothelioma, as has been found by numerous epidemiological studies.[12] The basic notion that risk is proportional to the ambient fiber concentration in the air is highly suspect and an unrealistic basis for establishing public policy. Regardless, when the hypo

Table 3-14. Estimates of risk from asbestos exposure in schools in comparison to other risks in U.S. society

Cause	Annual rate (deaths per million)
Asbestos exposure in schools	0.005 to 0.093
Whooping cough vaccination (1970-1980)	1 to 6
Aircraft accidents (1979)	6
High school football (1970-1980)	10
Drowning (ages 5-14)	27
Motor vehicle accident, pedestrian (ages 5-14)	32
Home accidents (ages 1-14)	60
Long-term smoking	1200

Data derived from Hughes JM, Weill H: Asbestos exposure—quantitative assessment of risk, *Am Rev Respir Dis* 133:5, 1986.

thetical risk based on linear dose-response mathematical extrapolations is determined, it becomes evident that the calculated risk of developing a mesothelioma later in life owing to schoolroom exposure is substantially less than the health risks of any one of a number of everyday activities that characterize modern life (Table 3-14).[21,25] Because air concentrations of asbestos in public buildings are almost invariably equivalent to those in outside air, one wonders what standards for airborne asbestos would be acceptable to those who argue that asbestos should be removed from public buildings.

Justifiable concerns of a different type, however, exist in homes and public buildings with heating systems insulated by asbestos. Many buildings house equipment insulated decades in the past when amphibole asbestos as well as chrysotile was used. As these heating systems age, insulation deteriorates and breaks down. Thus the potential exists for exposure of household residents, custodians, and repairmen during routine maintenance or renovations. This possibility warrants caution by those who are required to remove or repair heating systems in older buildings. The EPA and OSHA have promulgated demanding regulations that dictate practices for asbestos removal from buildings.

In past decades, households contaminated with asbestos from the work clothes of insulators and shipyard workers resulted in the subtle exposure of family members to inordinate amounts of pathogenic amphibole asbestos. As a result, mesotheliomas have tragically occurred in an occasional household resident and family member inadvertently exposed many years in the past. This experience has led to the implementation of OSHA regulations limiting the wearing of work clothes home from the occupational setting.

REFERENCES

1. Baghurst PA, et al: Environmental exposure to lead and children's intelligence at the age of seven years. The Port Pirie cohort study, *N Engl J Med* 327:1279, 1992.
2. Bodansky D, Robkin M, Stadler D, editors: *Indoor radon and its hazards,* Seattle, 1987, University of Washington Press.
3. Broder I et al: Formaldehyde exposure and health status in households, *Environ Health Perspect* 95:101, 1991.
4. Burdett GJ, Jaffrey SAMT: Airborne asbestos concentrations in buildings, *Ann Occup Hyg* 30:185, 1986.
5. Committee on the Biological Effects of Ionizing Radiations: *Health risks of radon and other internally deposited alpha-emitters (BIER IV),* Washington, DC, 1988, National Academy Press.
6. Committee on the Biological Effects of Ionizing Radiations: *Health effects of exposure to low levels of ionizing radiation (BIER V),* Washington, DC, 1988, National Academy Press.
7. Cooper JA: Environmental impact of residential wood combustion emissions and its implications, *J Air Pollut Cont Assoc* 30:855, 1980.
8. Cordier S et al: Epidemiologic investigation of respiratory effects related to environmental exposure to asbestos inside insulated buildings, *Arch Environ Health* 42:303, 1987.
9. Corn M et al: Airborne concentrations of asbestos in 71 school buildings, *Reg Toxicol Pharmacol* 13:99, 1991.
10. Council on Scientific Affairs (American Medical Association): Asbestos removal, health hazards, and the EPA, *JAMA* 266:696, 1991.
11. Council on Scientific Affairs (American Medical Association): Radon in homes, *JAMA* 258:668, 1987.
12. Craighead JE: Current pathogenetic concepts of diffuse malignant mesothelioma, *Hum Pathol* 18:544, 1987.
13. Craighead JE: Do silica and asbestos cause lung cancer? *Arch Pathol Lab Med* 116:16, 1992.
14. Crump KS, Farrar DB: Statistical analysis of data on airborne asbestos levels collected in an EPA survey of public buildings, *Reg Toxicol Pharmacol* 10:51, 1989.
15. Department of Labor, Occupational Safety and Health Administration [regulations]: Occupational exposure to asbestos, tremolite, anthophyllite, and actinolite, *Fed Reg* 51:22612, 1986.
16. Eisenbud M: *Environmental radioactivity (from natural, industrial, and military sources),* ed 3, Orlando, 1987, Academic Press.
17. Environmental Protection Agency [regulations]: Asbestos-containing materials in schools, *Fed Reg* 52:41826, 1987.
18. Environmental Protection Agency: *Communicating about risk: EPA and asbestos in schools,* Washington, DC, 1992, US Environmental Protection Agency.
19. Finnegan MJ, Pickering CAC, Burge PS: The sick building syndrome: prevalence studies, *Br Med J* 289:1573, 1984.
20. Greenberg M, Selikoff IJ: Lung cancer in the Schneeberg mines: a reappraisal of the data reported by Harting and Hesse in 1879, *Ann Occup Hyg* 37:5, 1993.
21. Health Effects Institute: *Asbestos research: asbestos in public and commercial buildings: a literature review and synthesis of current knowledge,* Washington, DC, 1991, Health Effects Institute.
22. Hein H et al: Indoor dust exposure: an unnoticed aspect of involuntary smoking, *Arch Environ Health* 46:98, 1991.
23. Hodgson MJ et al: Symptoms and microenvironmental measures in nonproblem buildings, *J Occup Med* 33:527, 1991.
24. Hoffman RE, Wood RC, Kreiss K: Building-related asthma in Denver office workers, *Am J Public Health* 83:89, 1993.
25. Hughes JM, Weill H: Asbestos exposure—quantitative assessment of risk, *Am Rev Respir Dis* 133:5, 1986.
26. Janerich DT et al: Lung cancer and exposure to tobacco smoke in the household, *N Engl J Med* 323:632, 1990.
27. Kjaergaard S, Molhave L, Pedersen OF: Human reactions to indoor air pollutants: n-decane, *Environ Int* 15:473, 1989.
28. Leowski J: Mortality from acute respiratory infections in children under 5 years of age; global estimates, *World Health Stat Q* 39:138, 1986.
29. Letz GA: Sick building syndrome: acute illness among office workers—the role of building ventilation, airborne contaminants and work stress, *Allergy Proc* 11:109, 1990.
30. Mendell MJ, Smith AH: Consistent pattern of elevated symptoms in

air-conditioned office buildings: a reanalysis of epidemiologic studies, *Am J Public Health* 80:1193, 1990.

31. Menzies R et al: The effect of varying levels of outdoor-air supply on the symptoms of sick building syndrome, *N Engl J Med* 328:821, 1993.

32. Molhave L: Volatile organic compounds as indoor air pollutants. In Gammasge RB, Kaye SV, editors: *Indoor air and human health,* Chelsea, MI, 1985, Lewis Publishers.

33. Mossman BT et al: Asbestos: scientific developments and implications for public policy, *Science* 247:294, 1990.

34. Murray AB, Ferguson AC, Morrison BJ: Sensitization to house dust mites in different climatic areas, *J Allergy Clin Immunol* 76:108, 1985.

35. National Council on Radiation Protection and Measurement: *Exposures from the uranium series with emphasis on radon and its daughters,* Report No. 77, Bethesda, MD, 1984, National Council on Radiation Protection and Measurements.

36. Neas LM et al: Association of indoor nitrogen dioxide with respiratory symptoms and pulmonary function in children, *Am J Epidemiol* 134:204, 1991.

37. Needleman HL, editor: *Lead toxicity,* Washington, DC, 1990, US Department of Health and Human Services, Public Health Service, Agency for Toxic Substances and Disease Registry.

38. Nero AV et al: *Distribution of airborne ^{222}radon concentrations in U.S. homes,* Publication No. LBL-19346, Berkeley, CA, 1984, Lawrence Berkeley Laboratory.

39. Norboo T et al: Domestic pollution and respiratory illness in a Himalayan village, *Int J Epidemiol* 20:749, 1991.

40. Pandey MR et al: Indoor air pollution in developing countries and acute respiratory infection in children, *Lancet* 1:427, 1989.

41. Platts-Mills TAE, de Weck AL: Dust mites, allergens and asthma: a worldwide problem, *J Allergy Clin Immunol* 83:416, 1989.

42. Rosen JF: Health effects of lead at low exposure levels, *Am J Dis Child* 146:1278, 1992 (editorial).

43. Rosenow EC, Carr DT: Bronchogenic carcinoma, *Cancer* 29:232, 1979.

44. Samet J: Environmental controls and lung disease, Report of the ATS Workshop on Environmental Controls and Lung Disease, Santa Fe, 1988, *Am Rev Respir Dis* 142:915, 1990.

45. Samet J, editor: *Radon toxicity,* Washington, DC, 1990, US Department of Health and Human Services, Public Health Service Agency for Toxic Substances and Disease Registry.

46. Samet JM: Uranium mining and lung cancer in Navajo men, *N Engl J Med* 310:1451, 1983.

47. Samet JM, Marbury MC, Spengler JD: Health effects and sources of indoor air pollution. Part II, *Am Rev Respir Dis* 137:221, 1988.

48. Saracci R, Riboli E: Passive smoking and lung cancer: current evidence and ongoing studies at the International Agency for Research on Cancer, *Mutat Res* 222:117, 1989.

49. Sayre JW, Ernhart CB: Control of lead exposure in childhood. Are we doing it correctly? *Am J Dis Child* 146:1275, 1992 (editorial).

50. Sebastian I: *Issues in urban air pollution: Mexico City diagnostic study. Environment working paper,* 1990, The World Bank.

51. Skov P, Valbjorn O, Pedersen BV: Influence of indoor climate on the sick building syndrome in an office environment, *Scand J Work Environ Health* 16:363, 1990.

52. Spengler JD: *Harvard's Energy and Environmental Policy Center finds fear of asbestos in buildings out of proportion to public health risk* (press release, August 9, 1989), Cambridge, MA, Harvard University.

53. Spengler JD et al: Exposures to acid aerosols, *Environ Health Perspect* 79:43, 1989.

54. Stolwijk JAJ: Sick-building syndrome, *Environ Health Perspect* 95:99, 1991.

55. Surgeon General of the United States: *The health consequences of involuntary smoking.* Rockville, MD, 1986, Office on Smoking and Health, Centers for Disease Control, US Department of Health and Human Services.

56. Thornton I et al: Lead exposure in young children from dust and soil in the United Kingdom, *Environ Health Perspect* 89:55, 1990.

57. United Nations Scientific Committee on the Effects of Atomic Radiations (UNSCEAR): *Ionizing radiation: sources and biological effects,* United Nations publication no. 93.IX.8 06300p, New York, 1982, United Nations.

Chapter 4

METAL TOXICITY

George Lumb

Metals are important from the environmental point of view because of their toxic potential for humans. Increasing technological use of metals is one manifestation of human progress after the stone age. Beautiful metal and pottery *objets d'art* were produced as early as the ninth century, B.C., largely because iron had just been discovered in Central Italy. Hippocrates, who is responsible for so many "first" observations, described a man with abdominal colic who had been extracting metals. This may well be the first description of colic related to lead poisoning. In modern times, particularly during this century, the use of metals in a large variety of sophisticated products has increased rapidly, along with increases in world population. This large group of products is related, in turn, to scientific research materials required in their development and themselves dangerous; generation of waste products in vast quantities that are dangerous, and use of fossil fuels clearly dangerous to produce the energy required in manufacture both for usage and for disposal. All of these facets of this interwoven pattern, in addition to any advantages that may result, also lead to direct toxic effects on humans as well as indirect toxic results owing to air, water, and soil pollution. This results in a wide ecological involvement not only of humans, but also of fish, mammals, and plants, including crops, on all of which humans depend.

Metals have been shown to have cycles of their distribution as a result of many natural phenomena. One is the occurrence of volcanic eruptions, the most famous of which occurred on the island of Krakatoa in August 1833. This eruption converted the island into a rocky wasteland in a few days, and the distribution of pollutants, including many particulate metal-containing materials, was noted throughout the world. At about this time in England, the famous painter Turner was producing his oil paintings of strange sky patterns and colors, which at the time caused him to be considered a lunatic. His perceptions were partly due to the volcanic eruption but of course were principally due to the man-made environmental pollution that was occurring at the beginning of the industrial age in England. Changes in concentration of metals can occur therefore as a result of violent natural phenomena such as volcanos or simple phenomena such as rainwater dissolution of rock and ores that occurs over long periods and transports material into adjacent streams and rivers to be distributed widely. One of the most important of the man-made distributions of metals results from the use of fossil fuels, causing gaseous effluents to be released into the atmosphere. Along with other pollutants, this produces the acid rain that increases the dissolution of rocks by rainwater. One of the most significant metal-polluting problems caused by human activities occurred when lead was added to gasoline in the 1920s. Enormous increases of lead in air, water, and soil in many parts of the world resulted.[116] The realization of the problem of lead in gasoline is leading to control.

Metals are sometimes defined as "heavy" and "light," based on the metal's atomic number and position in the periodic table. Examples of heavy metals are nickel, chromium, and cadmium; "light" metals include beryllium and aluminum. In this chapter it is impossible to discuss in detail the wide variety of both groups of metals, therefore, a selection was made based largely on the metal's important potential for harmful effects to humans.

GENERAL PRINCIPLES AND PROBLEMS

It is difficult to give many specific general principles that apply to all the heavy and light metals because they have such diverse activities, different origins, and different metabolic processes. A few, however, can be identified. Metals rarely interface with biological systems in their elemental form. An exception to this is mercury, which can do so. Most metals, however, affect humans in the form of one of their salts. Some metals are essential in low concentrations but dangerous at high doses. Examples of these are chromium, selenium, and iron.

Many metals accumulate in the body, such as nickel, chromium, and beryllium. Fortunately, chelating agents are available, which are useful in the treatment of many toxic results of exposure to metals. These chelating agents are most useful in the acute stages of toxic exposure, particularly when the exposure and the results of it are obvious. "Chelation" is taken from the Greek word meaning "to grab." The effect of such substances is to change and remove the offending metal substance or salt from the body through excretion. One of the most successful of these is the chelating agent developed for nickel. This is discussed further in the section on nickel. Another widely used chelating agent is British anti-Lewisite (BAL). This substance was developed in World War I in relation to gas attacks but has been used widely in the treatment of exposure to many metallic substances and is a useful form of treatment, particularly in the acute stages.

Establishment of "acceptable" levels for metals in the air or water and of similar levels for human tissues or "body load" is difficult because of the great variations in potential exposure. Workers in the same factory may be exposed to metals in other settings as well. For instance, they may live in urban or rural areas, in or near a manufacturing plant,

near a smelting works, or near a polluted landfill, which may or may not be recognized as such. Thus, workers in the same factory may have markedly different additional exposures outside the factory. An interesting example of the sort of problem that is faced may be quoted in relation to nickel and its presence in cigarette smoke. This is mentioned again in the section on nickel.

Another problem always difficult to resolve, particularly when lung cancers occur in the presence of industrial exposures to carcinogens, is the fact that many workers also smoke cigarettes. The relationship between smoking and metal exposure in causing cancer is not always clear. When workers die of cancer, however, the asssumption is frequently made that cigarette smoking has been the cause, and the exposure to other carcinogens is discounted.

It is easy, but unfortunately ineffective, to be dogmatic. For instance, although smoking is dangerous, it is not possible to prohibit tobacco growing. Although nickel and chromium are dangerous, it may not be possible to reduce them to zero levels in workplaces or find alternative "safe" substances to replace them. An alternative can sometimes be found as with the development of new safer insulating materials to replace asbestos or the substitution of hexachlor for chlordane in termite control. Such improvements, however, have usually followed major tragedies and public outcry, which demanded intensive search for alternative methods.

Experience with the development of new therapeutic agents indicates the opportunities and also the difficulties of this problem. A therapeutic drug is designed to benefit humans, and if during animal safety studies for preliminary clinical trials potential dangers are encountered, chemists must try to find possible "safe" analogues, or abandon the substance and start again.

Such approaches are not applied in general industry. Metals such as nickel and chromium have been in use for a century or more, and the cost of attempting their replacement by safer substances seems impossible to manufacturers, lawmakers, and politicians. As a result, therefore, strict control of the workplace, and routine frequent testing of workers are essential.

In some industries, workers are exposed to more than one metal. Although it would seem reasonable to assume that an additive effect might result, no effective epidemiological studies have been performed to analyze this question. An example of the problem is found where sintering and roasting of nickel ores produces lesser quantities of chromium and arsenic, which are mixed with the potent nickel subsulfide (Ni_3S_2), nickel oxide (NiO), and nickel dust. All three metals are carcinogens[144] (see Chapter 2 on Carcinogenesis).

Despite all these difficulties, however, the Environmental Protection Agency (EPA) and many other similar agencies have accumulated and published valuable material to help in planning safety procedures. The Public Health Service Agency for Toxic Substances and Disease Registry (ATSDR) of the Department of Health and Human Services has published "Profiles" of many substances that include most of the information available, not only in the United States, but also from sources all over the world. Included in these profiles are "regulations and advisories," in which recommendations are made based on the current information available. This information includes MRL and chronic oral reference doses (RFD). RFDs are usually based on "no observed adverse effect levels" (NoAL) in animal studies. When such information is published, it is updated at reasonable intervals. Details of current knowledge are included in the discussions of the various metals in this chapter.[6-11] There are some general problems associated with the collection of such material from humans. The principal one is contamination. Particularly with metals, this may involve the method of collecting specimens, especially when these are taken from tissues in the human body. It is obvious that if a specimen is being removed, a stainless steel scalpel will have to be used, and therefore careful consideration must be given in the assessment of the results obtained. The main contaminants from stainless steel are chromium and nickel, but these are buried in the substance of the metal, beneath the highly polished surface. Containers and solutions may also contain metals that could contaminate the specimen. The same problem of contamination applies when one attempts to measure water pollution, air pollution, and particularly soil and earth pollution. When the frequent updates of the profiles are made, the allowable levels and MRLs tend to fall. This trend is due principally to increasing knowledge of long-term exposure to low levels of potentially dangerous substances.

Chromium

Sources of exposure and mechanisms of effect. Direct exposure to significant excess of chromium is most likely to occur in or near manufacturing plants where the important chrome ore (chromite) or chromates are used. The principal uses for chromium and its salts are in steel production, chromium plating, paint and pigment manufacture, and leather tanning. Cement production is also important because cement contains chromium, and there is frequently considerable air pollution in areas where it is manufactured. Combustion of natural gas, oil, and coal produces significant chromium in air pollution. Wastewaters from any of these sources must be carefully monitored, and improper disposal of solid waste into landfills and other sites, such as building projects where "fill" is used, is also potentially dangerous.

Chromium occurs in several different valency states, but only chromium III and VI have been shown to have demonstrable relationships to bodily function. Chromium III is essential for effective glucose and lipid metabolism, and it has been shown that dietary supplements of chromium III can improve glucose utilization and tolerance in diabet-

ics and malnourished patients, particularly children and the elderly. It has been suggested that chromium III deficiency may be a factor in atherogenesis.[103]

Although chromium is present in many foods, particularly unrefined sugar and butter, no human or animal toxicity has been recorded as being due to consuming food containing chromium.[134]

Chromium VI is universally considered to be a "dangerous" substance when humans are exposed to its chromite ore or the salts (oxides, chromates, and sulfides). It is recognized worldwide as a carcinogenic agent, specifically leading to lung cancer.[9] Most of the recognized histological types have been reported[69] (see Chapter 28).

Chromium carcinogenesis in experimental animals has been extensively reviewed in two publications.[72,142] These experiments have been performed with a variety of chromium salts, including chromium powder, introduced directly into the bone or into the muscle or by injection subcutaneously, intrapleurally, and intraperitoneally. These experiments have all used hexavalent chromium compounds, and the resulting tumors have been local sarcomas. Laskin and co-workers,[82,85] have managed to produce squamous cell carcinoma and adenocarcinoma in the lungs of rats but only after intrabronchial implantation of pellets of calcium chromate. The rat is notoriously resistant to induction of malignant lung tumors. These tumors seldom arise spontaneously in normal rats, and the experiments with tobacco smoke and nicotine have also demonstrated the difficulty of inducing cancer of the lung in rats. The fact that malignant lung tumors can be produced at all therefore increases the significance of the carcinogenic effect of chromium.

In vitro studies of potential chromium carcinogenicity have included investigation of chromates in strains of *Escherichia coli* (Ames test). The results of these tests showed that hexavalent chromium was mutagenic in many of the strains of *E. coli*, and the mutagenicity was not modified by any absence of the pathways for repair of DNA of a genetic nature.[153] These researchers came to the conclusion that the chromates exerted their effects by direct modification of DNA bases so that base-pair errors arose at subsequent cell divisions. Although this is indirect evidence, it does seem to be of some importance, and it may point, at least, to research into the mechanism of chromium carcinogenesis in humans. Other important experimental observations were findings by Fradkin and others.[45] These workers were able to show that tissue culture cells of BHK21 would show in vitro transformation when grown in the presence of calcium chromate. These alterations in growth properties were irreversible and persisted after the cells had been removed from the artificial medium containing the calcium salt. In the experiments both with *E. coli* and with the tissue cultures of BHK21, no evidence of mutagenic changes or transformation of cells was found in the presence of chromium III salts.

Regulations and advisories. A low minimum risk level (MRL) has been established by ATSDR for inhalation exposure to chromium VI. It is 2×10^{-5} mg of Cr VI/m^3. There is no satisfactory MRL for ingestion because insufficient information is available. Because the exposure to most people at risk is by inhalation in or near factories, however, this is a useful measure and indicates that even slightly higher levels than this must be taken seriously, particularly when the exposure is long-standing. As stated previously, deficiencies of chromium III can be deleterious. The Committee on Dietary Allowances of the National Research Council has recommended a daily intake for adults of 50 to 200 μg/day of all types of chromium, most of which should be chromium III. This recommendation is based on the absence of any signs of chromium deficiency.[9]

Pathogenesis and specific lesions. Chromium is a generalized respiratory tract irritant when inhaled and characteristically causes nasal septal irritation followed by perforation and less frequently by nasal and palatal bone erosions, all of which have been described.[98,99] Changes of a general irritative nature leading to nonspecific inflammatory changes have been described throughout the upper respiratory tract.[25,90] Dental caries and alveolar disease are common in chromate poisoning.[37,41]

An interesting finding in exposed workers followed with serial x-ray films is increased lung markings and hilar lymph node enlargement, which can be demonstrated before pulmonary carcinoma is manifested. These diffuse lung changes have been designated as a form of pneumoconiosis (chromitosis). Chromium has been demonstrated in the interstitial tissue and in the septa of the lung as well as in the enlarged hilar lymph nodes.[2,88,89,93,98]

It is considered that the lung acts as a reservoir from which the metal can be released for months or years after exposure has ceased.[99] This would account probably for the long latent period between exposure and lung cancer development, which is so frequently seen. Although no experimental work has been performed in animals to address this mechanism, I would suggest a strong possibility that a similar process may be at work to that which has been investigated in rats using nickel, a closely related chemical[94-96] (see the section on nickel below).

The question of carcinogenicity with chromium III remains in some doubt, although Norseth[119] believes that soluble chromium III and chromium III bound to ligands can produce carcinoma in certain animals, and the positive results relate to their biological availability.

The long-term follow-up of workers in a chromate plant[98,99] is the best available epidemiological and pathological study. It identifies the cumulative nature of chromium in the body, the likelihood of storage particularly in the lung, the chemical and pathological features already discussed, and the importance of renal damage with pyelonephritis and excretion of chromium. Analysis of chromium at autopsy shows the largest concentrations in the lung but with high levels in thyroid, liver, adrenal, and even positive evidence in spinal bone.[99]

Nickel

Sources of exposure and mechanisms of effect. Nickel occurs naturally as an ore in combination with iron, copper, or both. From these, it is separated by the process of smelting, which involves raising the ore to high temperatures followed by processes of separation, which need not concern us here. The smelting process itself involves potentially dangerous air pollution, including emission of sulfur dioxide and nickel compounds, including nickel carbonyl, the extremely potent toxin and carcinogen. The latter is principally carcinogenic in the respiratory tract and the lung in particular. Fortunately a metal-binding agent (a form of chelation) diethyl dithio-carbamatetrihydrate (dithiocarb) developed by Sunderman[149,155] is used successfully in the treatment of acute poisoning. Nickel is a constituent of the air in cities, mostly as a result of fossil fuel combustion and gasoline engine exhaust. It is also present in cigarette smoke. The principal uses of nickel are in stainless steel and steel alloys, batteries, many electronic devices, and coins.

In contrast to other metals, such as chromium, selenium, or arsenic, which, in addition to toxic or even carcinogenic effects, may have certain values at specific dose levels, nickel has no human physiological role; it is important from the environmental point of view only because of its potential for toxicity and malignant tumor development.

Regulations and advisories. No MRL has been established for nickel. Other agencies, however, have provided some figures. The Occupational Safety and Health Administration (OSHA) has issued a permissible exposure limit for nickel and soluble nickel compounds of 1 mg/m^3.[120] Federal law requires that the National Response Center be notified when there is a release of a hazardous substance of any nature in excess of what they call the reportable quantity (RQ). The RQ for nickel metal, nickel carbonyl, and nickel cyanide is 1 pound per industrial site.

Pathogenesis and specific lesions. Skin irritation and skin rashes sometimes associated with asthmalike attacks have been reported in industrial close contact, either from nickel compounds or from gaseous effluent. It has even been reported that skin changes can occur when wearing nickel-containing jewelry.[142] The first significant review of a large number of cases of lung cancer in nickel workers came from the nickel refineries of Wales in 1937, where nasal cavity and lung carcinomas were identified.[11] Corroborative reports soon followed,[18,32,33,107] and Doll and co-workers[33] recorded 10.5 times the expected risk in nickel workers. Reports from Norway,[122] Canada,[101,146,154] and Russia[131-133] expressed essentially similar findings.

Sintering and roasting are considered the most dangerous exposures of nickel subsulfide and nickel oxide together with nickel dust and metallic particles of nickel. This group

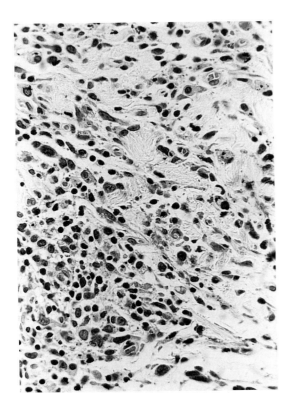

Fig. 4-1. Bizarre cells highly suspicious for malignancy found in a biopsy. (Hematoxylin and eosin × 500.) (From Lumb GD, Sunderman FW, The mechanism of malignant tumor induction by nickel subsulfide. *Ann Clin Lab Sci* 18:353-366, 1988. Copyright 1988 by the Institute for Clinical Science.)

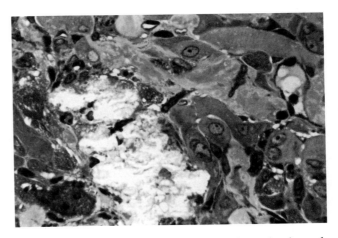

Fig. 4-2. Necrotizing and abnormal regenerating striated muscle cells in an area of (intramuscular) tumor development. (Hematoxylin and eosin × 400.) (From Lumb GD, Sunderman FW, The mechanism of malignant tumor induction by nickel subsulfide. *Ann Clin Lab Sci* 18:353-366, 1988. Copyright 1988 by the Institute for Clinical Science.)

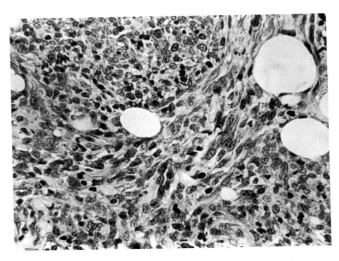

Fig. 4-3. Tumors arising following subcutaneous innoculation 10 months previously. The storiform pattern of malignant fibrous histiocytoma is seen. (Hematoxylin and eosin × 400.) (From Lumb GD, Sunderman FW, The mechanism of malignant tumor induction by nickel subsulfide. *Ann Clin Lab Sci* 18:353-366, 1988. Copyright 1988 by the Institute for Clinical Science.)

of nickel-containing substances is generally agreed to include the most significant carcinogenic forms.[101,143]

The cancers of the respiratory tract are claimed to be primarily of the squamous cell type, but an association of this morphological type with nickle exposure is doubtful (see Chapter 28). Increased risk of gastric carcinoma and soft tissue sarcomas has been reported in the Russian literature.[131,132] The principal compounds of nickel occurring in dusts in industrial surroundings are those that are insoluble and therefore of greatest potential for remaining as contaminants. The most important in this category are nickel subsulfide and nickel oxide.[101,143]

Lung cancer, however, is the most important environmentally related problem. It has a long latency period between exposure and the appearance of the tumor. The following experiments suggest a mechanism by which this occurs.[94,96] Experimental work using nickel subsulfide implanted into muscle and into subcutaneous tissue in the axilla as a pellet in rats has shown that when serial biopsies were performed, the first demonstrable changes at the site of implantation were degenerating muscle or connective tissue fibers with necrosis associated with nonspecific inflammatory cell proliferation of histiocytic type (Fig. 4-1). Later, atypicalities were seen in both regenerating muscle fibers and fibroblasts (Fig. 4-2). These atypicalities were striking. Finally, frank malignancy with invasiveness and metastases was demonstrated (10 months) (Fig. 4-3). These malignant tumors closely resembled the malignant fibrous histiocytoma of humans.[94,96] These tumors could be transplanted with resulting fomation of malignant tumors identical to the primary tumors. These arose quite rapidly (5 to 8 weeks). Tissue cultures were prepared from the original malignant tumors and transplants up to the F3 generation (Fig. 4-4). Cells from these cultures, when innoculated subcutaneously, produced invasive malignancy even more rapidly (3 to 4 weeks) than the transplanted tumors (Fig.

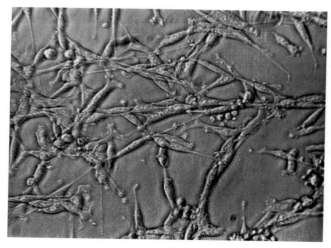

Fig. 4-4. Cells from tissue culture of tumor material from F2 gereration transplant from a subcutaneously induced tumor. (× 400.) (From Lumb GD, Sunderman FW, The mechanism of malignant tumor induction by nickel subsulfide. *Ann Clin Lab Sci* 18:353-366, 1988. Copyright 1988 by the Institute for Clinical Science.)

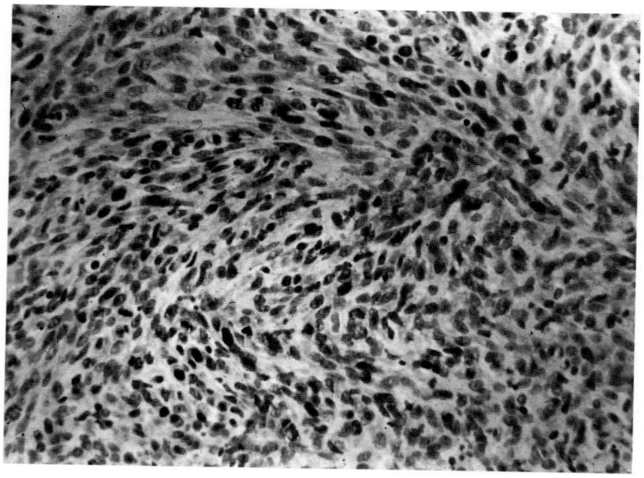

Fig. 4-5. Typical storiform pattern of malignant fibrous histiocytoma. (Hematoxylin and eosin × 400.) (From Lumb GD, Sunderman FW, The mechanism of malignant tumor induction by nickel subsulfide. *Ann Clin Lab Sci* 18:353-366, 1988. Copyright 1988 by the Institute for Clinical Science.)

4-5). They showed the typical pattern of malignant fibrous histiocytoma.

This sequence of events of long latency to malignancy following subcutaneous inoculation of nickel subsulfide with intervening cell damage with necrosis and cell repair leading first to completely atypical cell formation and then later to malignancy was quite remarkable. It represents the development pattern of so-called epigenetic carcinogenesis of cytotoxic variety.*

These experiments indicate a reason for the latent period of tumor development in the rat (10 months in an estimated 40-month life span or 25% of its life). If this is equated with the 75-year life span in humans, the result is a projected latent period of 19 years.

Although no animal experiments of a similar nature have been performed with chromium, certain features noted in epidemiological studies in humans[98,99] seem to suggest a similar sequence of events in malignant development with this metal. (See the previous comments on chromium.)

The presence of nickel in tobacco smoke deserves further mention. It was pointed out as long ago as 1961,[145,150] as a result of experiments to show lung carcinogenecity in rats exposed to nickel carbonyl, that the rats developed lung cancer after inhaling nickel carbonyl three times weekly for a year. The estimated total dosage was 1930 µg of nickel. The amount of nickel contained in the mainstream smoke of a cigarette was shown to be 0.37 µg of nickel. Thus the authors pointed out that the amount of nickel inhaled by the experimental

rats was comparable to that contained in the mainstream smoke of 260 packs of cigarettes; that is, less than one pack a day, or roughly 12 to 13 cigarettes a day. It would seem that, in addition to concentrating on nicotine as the carcinogenic agent in cigarettes, some attention should also be paid to nickel, particularly in the smoke, both inhaled and in the adjacent polluted air.

Studies of the mechanisms by which nickel can enter target cells are important. Nickel carbonyl is soluble in lipids and can pass across cell membranes without metabolic change. This fact may account for its high toxic and malignant potential.[147,148]

The insoluble forms such as nickel subsulfide are more difficult to explain. In the experiments discussed earlier with personal observations by the author, we were certainly able to convince ourselves that nickel particles could be demonstrated not only adjacent to, but also inside atypical regenerating cells within the developing tumors.[94,96]

A number of authors have described different mechanisms whereby insoluble nickel salts and particles may become solubilized by body fluids or otherwise altered to make cell entry possible. For a full account of these experiments and theories, the reader is referred to a review by Sunderman.[144]

Nickel production and usage involve a dangerous group of substances. Workplaces must be carefully and frequently monitored. The workforce must be carefully protected, not only by clothing, masks, and gloves, but also by weekly urine testing. This is the best and easiest test for human monitoring. All waste material must be classified as hazardous and dealt with according to well-defined EPA and National Institute for Occupational Safety and Health

*References 3, 22, 94-96, 114, 115.

(NIOSH) regulations. Such precautions are observed by most major organizations.

Arsenic

Forms of chemical structure and sources of exposure. Arsenic has a complex chemistry and is manifested as many different compounds. Trivalent and pentavalent forms exist, and both forms are common in nature. Inorganic compounds include a pentoxide, arsenic acid, and various salts, such as an arsenate of lead and also of calcium. These are pentavalent. Inorganic trivalent compounds most commonly found are the trioxide, the trichloride, and sodium arsenite. Organic forms also occur in both trivalent and pentavalent forms and may be methylated by organisms in soil as well as freshwater and saltwater.[159]

The main occupational risk from exposure to arsenic is in facilities in which herbicides and insecticides are manufactured. The base substance used for the preparation of these products is arsenic trioxide (As_2O_3), which, in turn, is obtained by roasting arsenic-containing ores in which arsenic is combined, usually with iron ($FeAsS$, As_2S_3, and As_2S_2). Other important areas in which arsenic can be dangerous to workers and to those outside are zinc-, copper-, and lead-smelting industries, which release arsenic into the air and frequently contaminate not only the smelting operation, but also the surrounding areas. It has been suggested that the increased incidence of lung cancer discovered in populations living near smelting industries is due to the pollution by arsenic in its trivalent form, arising as an effluent from the industrial source.[21]

Arsenic is widespread in nature and finds its way mostly in its pentavalent form into food. It is found in water, principally as a result of air effluents from industry and also partly from herbicides and pesticides that contaminate groundwater. Many of these substances contain phosphate fertilizers, which frequently contain arsenic.

Ubiquitous arsenic in nature is usually pentavalent, whereas arsenic that contaminates the environment by its being added to it is trivalent. The trivalent form is more toxic and is recognized as a carcinogen, particularly of the skin and the lung. More recently, the evidence of lung cancer has been shown epidemiologically to be increased in workers who inhale arsenic compounds.[80,86,104]

The principal uses of arsenic in industry depend on its toxicity, which makes its compounds effective as the aforementioned herbicides and insecticides, and it is also used for the preservation of wood. It is, however, used in the manufacture of a variety of chemicals and is also one of the added substances in the manufacture of glass.

Pathogenesis and specific lesions. Arsenic is excreted from the body principally in the urine, but it also appears in sweat, desquamated skin, and hair. The hair can be a convenient tool for investigating arsenic contamination in humans. Arsenic can cross the placental barrier and can be demonstrated in human milk and in the tissue of fetuses and newborn infants. Similar levels have been demonstrated in maternal and umbilical cord blood.[76]

In the past arsenic was used for medicinal purposes, particularly on skin rashes and even as a possible treatment for skin cancer. This is remarkable because by using this form of treatment it was first recognized that arsenic was, in fact, a specific factor in the causation of skin cancers. This was determined as long ago as the end of the nineteenth century.[70,156]

Medicinal use of arsenic has largely been abandoned in human medicine, in favor of more specific and precise therapies, with greater margins of safety and less risk of abuse. Parasitic diseases were effectively treated by arsenic until more widespread preventive methods and specific antiparasitic chemicals were developed. Veterinarians still use arsenicals, which is a potential source of danger particularly for children whose pets are treated.

Most of the research into the dangers of arsenic has centered on its potential as a carcinogen. The first studies were mostly in relation to the association between arsenic poisoning and skin cancer, and there are numerous well-recorded examples of this in the literature.* The first good investigation into the mortality of arsenical workers, and thus into the relationship of arsenic to cancers of the respiratory tract and skin, came in 1948 as a result of experience with arsenical production in Great Britain.[68] Since this time there have been numerous investigations, and at present there is no doubt that a direct relationship exists between arsenic poisoning and, principally, squamous cell carcinomas of the respiratory tract, mostly affecting the lung. An interesting paper related to lung cancer dealt with French vineyard workers who had been chronically exposed to arsenic insecticides (see Chapters 26 and 28).[50,51]

Iatrogenic exposure to arsenicals has led to a well-documented incidence of skin and lung cancer, but also cases of malignancy of other organs, such as the liver and the reticuloendothelial tissues, have been reported.[56,106,139] The liver tumor best documented is hemangioendothelial sarcoma.[83,127,129]

Mention must be made also of *arsine*. This is a gas resulting from the combination of arsenic with hydrogen. It is formed during refinement of nonferrous metals. It is a hemolytic agent, and exposed humans first suffer dyspnea, vomiting and nausea, and blood hemolysis. Death may occur with renal failure and hemoglobinuria. In nonfatal cases, persistent anemia and jaundice have been reported.[43,44]

Although numerous studies have been performed, there is little evidence that arsenic compounds are carcinogenic in experimental animals.[47] One final word may be added relating to the use of arsenic in homicides: the relatively

---

*References 31, 34, 45, 133, 162, 163.

easy access to arsenical-containing substances used as pesticides makes this possible.

Mercury

Sources of exposure and mechanisms of effect. Mercury plays no role whatsoever in human physiology compared with several of the other metals discussed in this chapter.[38,61,111,113] The largest proportion of the environmental contamination of air, water, and land occurs by natural processes, for the metal is released from the earth's crust by a process known as degassing (approximately 2.5×10^4 to 1.5×10^5 tons per year).[118,160] Mercury can be readily transmitted in the air over vast areas. Thus, mercury released from the earth's crust in one part of the world can cover enormous areas as shown by measurements of the arctic ice mass both at the North and the South poles.

Mining, smelting, and other industrial discharge were factors in environmental pollution in the past, but these sources have been reduced considerably by regulation. A problem that remains, however, is the presence of mercury in fossil fuels (approximately 1 ppm). Burning coal, natural gas, or petroleum products releases mercury into the atmosphere. The major industrial uses of inorganic mercury are in chloralkali production[92] and the preparation of chlorine and caustic soda, in the manufacturing of plastics, fungicides, and germicides. The use of mercury in plastics is particularly important in relation to the preparation of both indoor and outdoor vinyl paints. The potential for mercury entering the atmosphere from this source during application and during fire has only been recognized in recent years. Other major uses for mercury in the United States include the manufacturing of electrical wiring and switches, fluorescent lights, and dry cell batteries. In municipal waste, dry cell batteries and electrical wiring equipment are likely to be major sources of pollution. It has been claimed that mercury has potential health effects as a result of its use and subsequent release as a vapor from dental amalgam. Currently, this is a controversial issue.[40]

Several sources of mercury when considered together are of particular concern to humans. Mercury vapor in the air and mercury released from the earth's crust by natural processes have the potential for traveling widely in the atmosphere. The combustion of fossil fuels (e.g., automotive exhausts, coal-burning incinerators, trash-to-steam incinerators) also serves as a significant atmospheric source of the element. This mercury in the air is frequently mixed with the other gases contributing to acid rain, which pollutes surface water.* The other potential sources of widespread effects in humans are where mercury is in herbicides and germicides. In this way, it contaminates soil and groundwater and is metabolized by certain grains. Alarming poisoning has resulted from this source in many countries, including the United States. Fish ingest the poisonous material from

aquatic biota and later may be eaten by humans. Surveys conducted in the United States by the National Academy of Science and the Food and Drug Administration indicate that the consumption of fish is the most important source of exposure for the general population.[111]

Mercury exists in three chemical forms: elemental (Hg_0), organic, and inorganic (Hg_1,Hg_2). Mercury is one of the few metals that is a toxicant to humans in its elemental form. It is principally important when inhaled as a vapor (as commonly occurs). It has the ability to pass directly through the respiratory tract and across the alveolar bed into the blood stream.[75,105] It is lipid soluble and therefore can attack red cells. It is particularly toxic in the central nervous system. Metallic mercury is only slightly soluble in water, but it readily dissolves in organic solvents. Inorganic mercury occurs as a result of two forms of oxidation. Hg_2 is the more reactive and is capable of forming complexes with organic substances. Hg_1 is less toxic; both are soluble in water. Organic mercury compounds occur in many forms. The most important from the perspective of human toxicity are methyl and ethyl mercury and the family of alkoxyalkyl, which are used therapeutically in diuretics.[78] These organic forms are also lipid soluble and can readily pass through cell membranes.

Pathogenesis and specific lesions. The elemental forms of mercury form covalent bonds with sulfur. It would appear that this property accounts for most of the biological effects and properties of the metal. When the sulfur is in the form of sulfhydryl groups, divalent mercury replaces the hydrogen atom to form mercaptides. Inorganic and organic mercurial forms produce mercaptides of different chemical structure but apparently similar biological properties. Even at low concentrations, mercurials are capable of inactivating sulfhydryl enzymes and thus interfering with cellular metabolism and function. The affinity of mercury for thiols is the basis for using penicillamine for the treatment of mercury poisoning.[138]

All three forms of mercury are highly toxic. They have the ability to change from one form to another in tissues. Chronic mercury poisoning in humans owing to gastrointestinal uptake of Hg^{2+} primarily affects the kidneys (see Chapter 32 on the Urinary System), whereas chronic mercury poisoning owing to inhalation affects the central nervous system in particular (see Chapter 30).[41] This seemingly strange differential effect of the same element appears to be due to the fact that the lipid-soluble Hg_0 is readily transferred from the blood to the brain; its subsequent oxidation in the brain causes it to remain at that site on a chronic basis. Organic mercury compounds seem to express their toxicity in a different manner. Methyl mercury, which is an important organic toxic agent, specifically damages the brain, so the manifestations are largely neurologic.[39,102]

Systemic effects have been described in many organs. There is evidence to suggest that metallic mercury can affect the cardiovascular system in humans, and gastrointes-

*References 54, 79, 108, 126, 137, 158.

tinal effects have been described in the form of cramps, diarrhea, and other more minor symptoms. Hematological and hepatic effects have also been recorded. Mercury is transported readily across the placenta.[48,49] Regardless of the chemical form, fetal tissues attain high concentrations, at least equal to or in excess of the amounts in the mother's tissues. Measurements of mercury in the body of humans remain limited from the point of view of developing information regarding toxicity.*

Metallic mercury, in elemental form, is oxidized to divalent mercury after it has been absorbed into the tissues. Methylmercury, probably the most dangerous of all forms in terms of human toxicity, is converted to divalent mercury by removal of the carbon–mercury bond. It is transformed in the liver and secreted in bile, then reabsorbed from the gastrointestinal tract and mostly excreted through the kidneys. Within cells, binding can occur to a variety of enzyme systems in the microsomes and mitochondria, which may result in cell death.[5,128]

Although a wide variety of organs and systems are affected by mercury in all its forms, the chief target areas are the central and peripheral nervous systems and the kidney. Various forms of behavioral and other symptoms have been described in the involvement of the brain, particularly tremors, irritability, forgetfulness, and rather "difficult to define" symptoms, many of which have been immortalized by the author, Austin Dobson, better known as Lewis Carroll, in his description of the Mad Hatter in *Alice in Wonderland*. The Mad Hatter is typical of one of the forms of mercury poisoning, which was quite characteristic of the fur and hat trade, when mercury was used in the processing of felt. This practice has, of course, been abandoned. Pathological findings in the brain have shown selective involvement of neurons with necrosis and lysis and replacement with glial cells in the cerebral cortex and cerebellum. Cerebral atrophy can result.[151]

Mercury, or quicksilver, as it was originally called, has always had an element of magic about it: the name of the planet, the name of a Greek god, the nature of the appearance of the quicksilver itself, and its use by alchemists in their search for a way to make gold. It was used as a medication by ancient Hebrews and Egyptians, long before the Christian era, and its use has continued over the centuries. It is only recently, in the twentieth century, that its real dangers have become apparent, particularly in terms of central nervous system disorders. A rather amusing quote recorded by Goldwater in 1972[57] is from a journal called *The Surgeons Mate: Military and Domestic Surgery:* "The hottest, the coldest, a true healer, a wicked murderer, a precious medicine and a deadly poison, a friend that can flatter and lie." In 1639, they knew it was poisonous, but it took us until the twentieth century to do anything about it.

*References 12, 14, 17, 16, 26, 97, 161.

Lead

Sources of exposure and mechanisms of effect. Lead is widespread in the environment. Its main sources of origin are from mining and smelting. The latter involves the generation of fumes and dust containing lead oxide in large quantities. Similar contamination with the oxide occurs in factories where storage batteries are manufactured. The air and water pollution that occurs as a result of these activities means that inevitably groundwater, crops, and food contain lead. Lead is an important component of most paints and is used in gasoline manufacture. The principal problems in the workplace are for those employed as smelters or engaged in the manufacture of storage batteries. Here the contaminant is particulate and is mostly inhaled, although inevitably some enters the digestive tract.[35]

Lead in paint presents a real hazard, both at the time of manufacture and particularly in old buildings, where cracking and flaking occur. In recent years, lead in pipes as well as cooking and eating utensils has largely been eliminated. Old buildings, however, along with modern human desire to use "antiques" can be hazardous (see Chapter 6).

For the general population, the main source of lead is food. There is, however, some indication that the human load is decreasing somewhat since the 1970s. EPA reported levels under 100 μg/day in 1986 compared with 400 to 500 μg per day levels reported in 1940.[61] The body load is not entirely dependent on food and varies considerably according to the surroundings. Municipal water supplies in most areas contain lead, but with regulation in recent years it is not considered to be a hazard. However, lead in water supplies must continue to be monitored carefully. Ten micrograms to a maxium of 20 μg may be ingested by humans, of which about 10% is absorbed and less than 5% is retained.[61]

It is most important to be aware that infants, in particular, and children in general, are significantly more susceptible than adults to the hazards of lead. Studies have shown absorption of greater than 40% in children, with retention of 30% to 32% compared with the 5% retention in adults.[61] Because of this fact, children's tendency to suck on colored objects and flaking paint is particularly dangerous (see Chapter 3). Children also have a tendency to eat dirt and soil. Therefore, families living near paint, smelting, or battery manufacturing works should be cautioned on soil and groundwater contamination. The industries themselves must be carefully controlled against air and water effluent. Lead contamination is, however, not uncommon around such facilities. In addition to the major contaminating industries already mentioned, all fossil fuel incinerators, including trash to steam plants generate lead in their effluents.

Regulations and advisories. ATSDR has not developed an MRL. Neither do reference concentrations (RFC) nor reference doses (RFD) exist. This is because ATSDR does not believe that any threshold has been demonstrated for the most sensitive effects that might affect humans. The EPA[35] has determined that the critical effect is on the central nervous system and has described what it calls an "action" level in water of 0.015 mg/L. In an effort to protect human health by trying to achieve a level as close to zero as possible at consumers' taps, a series of regulations has been issued for the construction of pipes and outlets in buildings of all descriptions.[10]

Lead from lead-containing gasoline exhaust has been controlled considerably in the United States.[4] In many parts of Europe and in developing countries, it is still a major problem.

Pathogenesis and specific lesions. Lead in the body is found mainly in the bones, where it has a long half-life of 20 years or more.[61] In children, it tends to concentrate around the epiphyses. It is slowly turned over from bones and released, which means that blood levels may remain high for years after exposure[24] (see Chapter 31).

Lead is excreted mainly through the kidneys by glomerular filtration and some tubular resorption. In tubular lining cells, characteristic nuclear inclusion bodies are found at an early stage of lead intoxication. These are best seen by electron microscopy. The significance of these bodies and other aspects of lead nephropathy have been studied extensively by Goyer.[58-60,63,64]

In contradistinction to the long half-life of lead in bones, the half-life in soft tissues is short; only 20 to 30 days.[61] An important feature of lead transport in the body is its ready passage across the placenta and thus into the fetus and infant. The implication of this in the light of the above-mentioned susceptibility of infants is obvious. In addition, therefore, to the hazards for children from paint and soil ingestion, great care must be taken to monitor milk, both human and raw milk from cows.[62]

The toxicological manifestations of lead absorption in humans include gastrointestinal, hematological, central and peripheral nervous system manifestations, and renal damage. Other recorded effects of lead poisoning are sterility, abortions, and neonatal deaths (see Chapters 33 and 34).

Acute toxicity is not common in the general population, but chronic effects can be insidious. Several of the varieties of changes mentioned previously may occur simultaneously, and symptoms and signs may mimic other well-known syndromes. Thus lead colic is a common early symptom of lead poisoning, but unless the physician is alerted to the possibility of lead exposure, this condition can easily be missed.

Anemias may be severe because lead interferes with the hemoglobin development and heme synthesis. The red cells in patients with lead anemia are hypochromic and microcitic, which a physician may confuse with iron deficiency anemia. A characteristic finding, however, is an increased number of reticulocytes and red cells with basophilic stippling.

Blue gums (Burton's lines) are seen in children with lead encephalopathy but can also be observed in adults. I saw this gingival phenomenon clearly, when being shown a cloisonné factory near Tokyo, in those employed painting the chinaware by hand; they frequently licked the small brushes to keep a fine tip.

Central nervous system neuropathies are most severe in children, as might be expected. They are manifested by a variety of symptoms, including dizziness, ataxia, and, in the most severe cases in which there has been high exposure, coma and death. When there is recovery, epilepsy may occur. Follow-up of these children has shown various forms of speech defects and mental retardation. The severity of these defects is dose dependent.[15,115,130]

Peripheral neuropathies are seen mostly in patients with excessive exposure in paint manufacture. Wrist and foot drop were frequently seen in the past, particularly in house painters, but now that precautions are taken, lead levels are low, and the condition is uncommon (see Chapter 30).

It is inappropriate herein to attempt a comprehensive account of all of the numerous varieties of clinical and pathological changes in lead poisoning. The reader is referred to standard textbooks on the subject or, for a brief and easily read review, to an account by Landrigan.[84]

An important role of patient care is to institute suitable testing for pregnant women who may have been exposed to lead. This is necessary to prevent transplacental transfer to the fetus by eliminating the "source of poisoning." Chelating agents such as ethylene diaminetetra-acetic acid (EDTA) and BAL can be administered to prevent both mortality and morbidity. They must, however, be used with great care and constant observation.[91]

In experimental animals (rats and mice), renal carcinomas have been produced, but no convincing evidence indicates that lead is carcinogenic in humans.[74]

Once again however, it must be pointed out that our knowledge of long-term, low-dose effect is minimal. Vigilance must be pursued and every effort exerted to minimize lead levels in the environment, particularly in view of its widespread distribution.

Beryllium

Sources of exposure and mechanisms of effect. Coal combustion provides the majority of beryllium in the environment. It is estimated that five times the beryllium in the atmosphere comes from coal and oil combustion when compared with other industrial sources. The industrial processes involved in preparing beryllium products include extraction, ceramic manufacture, and beryllium alloy manufacture. Beryllium has been used widely in ceramic manufacture for many years, but the advent of the space age has increased the use of its alloys in nuclear reactors, x-ray windows, missile fuels, spacecraft of all types, and space optics. Human exposure comes mainly in industrial facilities, and in common with most environmental problems, particularly those related to metals, much more needs to be learned in terms of long-term, low-level exposures. This is important because beryllium is cumulative and is probably stored in fibrotic nodules resulting from tissue damage.

Regulations and advisories. No standards as to safe levels for beryllium have been issued either by the World Health Organization or ATSDR, but the EPA[36] has given figures known as "ambient water quality criteria" (AWQC), and these are from 0.68 to 68 ng/L for consumption of 2 L of ambient water. This is obviously a considerable difference, and much further work needs to be done to narrow the range.

Pathogenesis and specific lesions. Numerous experiments have been performed in rats, leading to valuable data on body disposal.[61] Fifty percent of inhaled beryllium is cleared from the body in about 2 weeks, but the remainder is removed slowly as it becomes fixed in fibrotic granulomatous nodules, particularly in the lungs but also in other tissues. Ingested beryllium is absorbed only in an acid medium such as the stomach. It is deposited in most organs, with colloidal portions in the liver, spleen, and bone marrow,[135] but ultimately the majority ends up in the bones with the exception of the fibrotic granulomatous nodules in the lungs referred to previously. The half-life is short except in the lung, and it is excreted in the urine, where measurements can be made to estimate and monitor body load. The effects in humans are principally on the skin and in the lungs. A contact dermatitis is common, mostly from exposure to soluble products. Contact with an insoluble product causes chronic granulomatous lesions with ulceration and tissue necrosis. If the insoluble material becomes embedded, the resulting lesions will not heal until it is removed.[141] Lung lesions include acute effects, chronic granulomatous lesions (berylliosis), and possible carcinoma, but this association has not been established (see later) (see Chapter 28). The acute effects are those of a violent inflammatory process involving all levels of the respiratory tract from the nasal region to the alveoli. It occurs rapidly, following inhalation of soluble compounds. The compound most commonly involved in berylliosis is the fluoride produced during the industrial process of extraction. Severity is dose related, and some deaths have occurred, although if the exposure is recognized immediately and the patient is removed from the area of danger, recovery occurs within several weeks.

Berylliosis was first recognized in workers exposed to insoluble beryllium compounds and in particular to beryllium oxide, which is used in the manufacture of fluorescent bulbs and lamps. Dyspnea and cyanosis are typical symptoms, and chest films reveal diffuse small nodules throughout the lungs with a histological picture resembling sarcoidosis. These are the lesions that progress to fibrous nodules, within which the beryllium is retained.

Beryllium is interesting in that it is the only metal in which lung malignancy was recognized in experimental animals before being suspected in humans. This might give some encouragement to those who have become somewhat skeptical of the value of animal toxicology testing in the safety assessment of new drugs. There is growing epidemiological evidence of increased numbers of lung cancers in beryllium workers,[81] but the numbers are not yet sufficient for complete certainty, and both the International Agency for Research on Cancer (IARC)[74] and EPA[36] acknowledge "sufficient evidence" for carcinogenicity in animals but only "limited evidence" in humans. In vitro studies by DiPaolo and Casto[30] have shown morphological transformation both in mammalian and in Syrian hamster cells. This is suggestive of malignant potential in humans. They have also shown that beryllium decreases the fidelity of DNA synthesis, but when it is tested as a mutagen in a bacterial system (Ames test), the results are negative. For all these reasons, therefore, suspicion of malignancy in humans is considerable, but a definitive decision is not available. The current information is certainly sufficient to demand careful monitoring of levels in industrial facilities and of the workers. Frequent urine testing is the best method for human surveillance.

In common with other metals, notably nickel and chromium, there is a long latency period between exposure and pathological manifestations. This has varied from 10 years to as long as 20 years.[66]

Care must be taken to monitor industrial facilities, as there are occasions when contamination of rivers and groundwater, in particular, results from escape of contaminated material from these factories.

Aluminum

Sources of exposure and mechanisms of effect. Aluminum is widespread in nature. It is the third most abundant element and accounts for 8% of the earth's crust. It occurs naturally in the form of ores mixed with many other substances and is extremely reactive but is never found in its elemental state. The largest source of particle-borne aluminum is escape of dust from ores and rock materials in the earth's surface.[87,140] A significant amount of dust occurs as a result of volcanic eruptions, a subject that has only recently been recognized as being of importance. The principal source of aluminum in the environment is from the ore bauxite. It is from bauxite ($Al_2O_3 \cdot H_2O$) that aluminum metal is produced. Production is the result of three major steps: refining, followed by electrolytic reduction, and casting the aluminum into ingots.[23,29,73]

Aluminum is a constituent of acid rain, which is now a well-known phenomenon. It is largely the product of combustion of many fuels, including fossil fuels, but also of the gaseous effluents of trash-to-steam plants and industrial smelting of a large number of metals, including aluminum itself, nickel, and chromium.[121]

Another important source of air pollution by aluminum comes from the exhausts of gasoline-driven automobiles.[121]

Acid rain was originally thought to be composed principally of sulfur and nitrogen oxides capable of being converted to acids and then deposited on land and into both freshwater and saltwater (hence its name). Further analyses have exposed many other particulate materials, among them, aluminum. An important feature of acid rain is the ability of the gaseous materials to travel long distances from their site of origin before the rain is precipitated. The importance of the association of aluminum with acid rain and with other acid substances, such as the weathering of sulfide ores exposed to the atmosphere or of inactive mines and tailing dumps where large quantities of sulfuric acid and metals such as aluminum are released, is the fact that lowering pH increases the mobility of monometric forms of aluminum.[55]

According to the Toxics Release Inventory (TRI), an estimated total of 869.3 million pounds of aluminum and aluminum compounds were released to the environment from manufacturing and processing facilities in the United States in 1987 alone. Of this total, an estimated 47.2 million pounds of aluminum and aluminum compound were released into the air from the same sources.[152]

The Public Health Service cautions that these figures represent first-time and somewhat incomplete estimation of releases. They are well aware of the fact that not all of the sources of chemical wastes were included; therefore it seems inevitable that this amount of toxic release, large though it is, will be considerably larger when continuing estimations are made over the next several years. It is difficult to collect information regarding, on the one hand, how much toxic substance is released and, on the other hand, how much is required to do damage or produce toxic effects on the human organism. Accuracy can occur only with long-term research. It is inevitable, therefore, that the amounts released will appear to increase as more accurate methods are used, and the allowable amounts suggested for contamination in air, water, or total body storage will decrease.

Human exposure is inevitable because aluminum is so widespread. It is present in the air, water, and soil as well as in food. Further contribution to human exposure occurs because aluminum is used in packaging, processing, and preserving foods and also in the treatment of drinking water.

It is a component of antiperspirants and cosmetics and is widely used as an antacid. It is used for the manufacture of many containers, including food containers and cooking utensils. There is ample evidence that the amount of aluminum released into the food from cooking utensils increases with the number of times the container is used.[65,77,109]

Studies related to ecological factors but that also affect human exposure have included milk and uptake into beef tissue[13] and a number of fish, including brook trout, rainbow trout, and smallmouth bass.[27] These few examples show how widespread the distribution can be into all areas

of food production, and all of these, in turn, affect humans.

Regulations and advisories. It is perhaps a surprising fact that no international regulations relating to aluminum or its compounds have been found by the ATSDR. Clearly much work is required in this area. Aluminum has not been recognized as a potential toxic substance in humans or animals until recently. This recognition of its availability for toxicity has largely been due to two major factors. One is the analysis of the constituents of so-called acid rain, and the other is the establishment of the TRI by the EPA.

Pathogenesis and specific lesions. At present, information seems to indicate that intakes of aluminum have to be considerable in the human to produce harmful effects, but much more research is required to understand fully long-term, low-level exposure. Aluminum accumulates principally in bones and in the lungs, and blood concentrations never seem to reach high levels.[52] Aluminum, by forming a complex with pectin in the gastrointestinal tract, seems to be able to affect absorption of other substances. A positive effect is a diminution of cholesterol absorption, but this, if significant, is offset by some negative features, such as binding with phosphorus, which may lead to osteomalacia by causing lowering of phosphate levels. Calcium ion and folate absorption can also be affected.[110] Aluminum compounds, which are frequently used as antacids, tend to cause constipation and some other problems, which are discussed later.

Toxicology studies in animals, particularly in cats and rabbits, have shown interesting neurological effects, including tremors, ataxia, and behavioral changes. These have not been reproduced in rats, and it is necessary to expose monkeys for more than a year before any changes can be detected. Neurofibrillary tangles (NFTs) have been described in many areas of the brain, which have interest for correlation with human experience, but at the present state of knowledge, much more information is required before positive relationships can be established.[19,20,136]

Human studies of various forms of dementia and related neurological disorders and their possible association with elevated levels of aluminum in various organs and tissues are of great interest. One of these problems that was among the first to be studied is known as "dialysis dementia," which was reported in patients on long-term dialysis for chronic renal disease.[1] This can be a progressive series of changes arising after several years of dialysis. It is manifested by speech disorders progressing to dementia, convulsions, and death. Increased aluminum levels have been found in the muscles, bones, and brain.

The problem can be avoided if aluminum hydroxide, which has been used in these patients for the treatment of indigestion, which is common in people suffering from chronic renal diseases, is avoided and careful attention is paid to monitoring aluminum in the dialysate fluid. Progression of the dementia can be slowed or arrested by the use of aluminum chelating agents.[157] The relation of the cause of the dementia to aluminum has provided an important therapeutic lesson for the treatment of stomach upsets in patients with renal disease who do not require dialysis. It is recognized that increased aluminum absorption occurs in the presence of impaired renal function; therefore aluminum hydroxide, although an effective antacid, should be avoided.

A second group of possibly aluminum-related conditions with neurological changes resembling Alzheimer's disease has been described in the native populations of certain Pacific Islands, particularly the islands of Guam and Rota. This condition has been named "amyotrophic lateral sclerosis and parkinsonism-dementia syndrome of Guam" (Guam ALS-PD syndrome). The volcanic soil of these islands contains high levels of aluminum and manganese, with low levels of calcium and magnesium, a combination that could lead to increased tissue levels of aluminum if ingested.[53] These islanders have shown degenerative nerve diseases with cell loss and neurofibrillary degeneration of the Alzheimer's type. It has been suggested that the typical diet on Guam may be the source of the aluminum, perhaps partially by inhalation as well as ingestion.[28] It has been suggested that the pathway of inhaled aluminum may be via the olfactory pathways.[124]

The third relationship of aluminum to disease, and perhaps the most interesting, is Alzheimer's disease itself. At the present stage of investigation, no definitive statement can be made, but increased levels of aluminum have been found in the brains of patients with Alzheimer's disease. These levels vary considerably, and interest centers as much on how the aluminum reaches the brain as on the actual levels. The resolution of this particular question should give good indication of the mechanisms and cause of the aluminum-Alzheimer relationship.[100]

NFTs are found in this disease, but they are different both morphologically and chemically from those found in "dialysis dementia." Using x-ray spectrometry, Perl and Brody[123] demonstrated aluminum in the nuclei of NFT-containing neurons but no aluminum in normal neurons in human tissues. Suggestions have been made that the aluminum accumulations may result from a genetically related defect in the blood-brain barrier, but as yet little is known of the bioavailability of aluminum.[123]

Reviews and epidemiological studies have appeared from England,[67,71,125] but much ongoing research is needed before definitive information can result that, it is hoped, may lead to effective treatment of this most unusual disease.

CONCLUSIONS

Beneficial or harmful effects in humans may result from exposure to many heavy and light metals. Dose relationship is the cause of this paradox; low doses can be essential, whereas high doses can cause toxicity or malignancy.

Latency in the development of tumors, following exposure to a number of metals, is a problem in accurate diagnosis of cause and also in establishing precautions at the site of origin of the carcinogen. Epidemiological studies are difficult to perform, as industrial workers frequently leave to work and live at considerable distances from the source of contamination. When 10 to 20 years later, illness develops, possibly ending in death from malignancy, neither the patient nor the family may associate the cause with an exposure to metals at a previous place of employment.

These problems provide fruitful opportunities for research into all aspects of the toxicology and carcinogenesis of metals. Epidemiology studies are particularly important.

REFERENCES

1. Alfrey AC et al: Syndrome of dyspraxia and multifocal seizures associated with chronic hemodialysis, *Trans Am Soc Artif Intern Organs* 18:257, 1972.
2. Alwens W, Jonas W: Der Chromat-Lungenkrebe, *Acta Union Internat contro cancer* 3:108, 1988.
3. Andersen M: Mechanistic considerations in chemical carcinogenesis: pharmacokinetics, *Proc Tox Forum* 68, 1986.
4. Annest JL et al: Chronological trend in blood lead levels between 1976 and 1980, *N Engl J Med* 308:1373, 1983.
5. Anwar WA, Gabal MS: Cytogenetic study in workers occupationally exposed to mercury fulminate, *Mutagenesis* 6:189, 1992.
6. Association for Toxic Substances and Disease Registry: *Toxicological profile for aluminum and compounds*. U.S. Public Health Service, TP-91-01, revised July, 1992.
7. Association for Toxic Substances and Disease Registry: *Toxicological profile for arsenic*. U.S. Public Health Service, TP-92/02 published 3/89 and revised 4/93.
8. Association for Toxic Substances and Disease Registry: *Toxicological profile for beryllium*. U.S. Public Health Service, TP-92/04 published 12/88 and revised 4/93.
9. Association for Toxic Substances and Disease Registry: *Toxicological profile for chromium*. U.S. Public Health Service, TP-92/08 published 7/89 and revised 4/93.
10. Association for Toxic Substances and Disease Registry: *Toxicological profile for lead*. U.S. Public Health Service, TP-92/12 published 6/90 and revised 4/93.
11. Association for Toxic Substances and Disease Registry: *Toxicological profile for nickel*. U.S. Public Health Service, TP-92/14 published 12/89 and revised 4/93.
12. Baader EW: Berufkrebs, *New Ergeh Geb Krebskrunkh* 1:104, 1937.
13. Baes CF et al: *A review and analysis of parameters for assessing transport of environmentally-released radionuclides through agriculture*, US Department of Energy, ORNL-5786, 1984.
14. Bakig F: Methylmercury poisoning in Iraq. An interuniversity report, *Science* 181:230, 1973.
15. Bellinger D et al: A follow-up study of the academic attainment and classroom behavior of children with elevated dentine lead levels, *Biol Trace Elem Res* 6:207, 1986.
16. Bencko V, Wagner V, Wagnerova M: Immunological profiles in workers occupationally exposed to inorganic mercury, *J Hyg Epidemiol Microbiol Immunol* 34:9, 1990.
17. Berlin M: *Mercury*. In Friberg L, Nordberg GF, Vouk VB, editors: *Handbook on the toxicology of metals*, Vol II, *specific metals*, 2nd ed, Amsterdam, 1986, Elsevier Scientific Publishers.
18. Bidstrup PL: Cancer of the lung in nickel, arsenic and chromate workers, *Arch Belg Med Soc* 8:500, 1950.
19. Birchall J, Chappell J: The chemistry of aluminum and silicon in relation to Alzheimer's disease, *Clin Chem* 34:265, 1988.

20. Bizzi A, Gambetti P: Phosphorylation of neurofilaments is altered in aluminum intoxication, *Acta Neuropathol* 71:154, 1986.

21. Blot WJ, Fraumeni JR Jr: Arsenical air pollution and lung cancer, *Lancet* 2:142, 1975.

22. Bosan WS et al: Methylation of DNA guanine during the course of induction of liver cancer in hamsters by hydrazine or dimethylnitrosamine, *Carcinogenesis* 8:439, 1987.

23. Browning E: *Toxicity of industrial metals,* 2nd ed, New York, 1969, Appleton-Century-Crofts.

24. Bushnell PJ, Jaeger RJ: Hazards to health from environmental lead exposure. A review of recent literature, *Vet Hum Toxicol* 28:255, 1986.

25. Carter WW: The effect of chromium poisoning on the nose and throat: the report of a case, *Medical Journal and Record* 130:125, 1929.

26. Clarkson TW, Small H, Norseth T: Excretion and absorption of methylmercury after polythiol resin treatment, *Arch Environ Health* 26:173, 1973.

27. Cleveland L et al: *Chronic no-observed-effect concentrations of aluminum for brook trout exposed in low-calcium, dilute acidic water.* In Lewis TE (ed): *Environmental chemistry and toxicology of aluminum,* Chelsea, Mich, 1989, Lewis Publishers.

28. Crapper DR et al: Aluminum and calcium in soil and food from Guam, Palau and Jamaica: implications for amyotrophic lateral sclerosis and parkinsonism-dementia syndromes of Guam, *Environ Geochem Health* 11:47, 1989.

29. Dinman BD: *Aluminum, alloys and compounds.* In *Encyclopedia of occupational health and safety,* Vol I, 1983.

30. DiPaolo JA, Casto BC: Quantitative studies of in vitro morphologic transformation of Syrian hamster cells by inorganic metal salts, *Cancer Res* 39:1008, 1979.

31. Dobson RL, Pinto JS: *Arsenical carcinogenesis.* In Montagna E, Dobson RL, editors: *Advances in biology of skin,* Vol VIII, New York, 1955, Pergamon Press.

32. Doll R: Cancer of the lung and nose in nickel workers, *Br J Ind Med* 15:217, 1958.

33. Doll R, Morgan LG, Speizer FE: Cancers of the lung and nasal sinuses in nickel workers, *Br J Cancer* 24:623, 1970.

34. Ehlers G: Klinische und histologische Untersuchungen zur Frage armeimttelbedingter Arsentumoren, *Z Hauf-Geschlkr* 43:763, 1974.

35. Environmental Protection Agency: *Air quality criteria for lead,* Vols. I-IV, EPA/600/8-83/02aF, Washington, DC, 1987, US Environmental Protection Agency.

36. Environmental Protection Agency: *Health assessment document for beryllium,* EPA/600/8-84/026F, Washington, DC, 1987, US Environmental Protection Agency.

37. Environmental Protection Agency: *Health assessment document for chromium,* Final Report EPA 600/8 83 014F, August 1984.

38. Environmental Protection Agency: *Mercury health effects update: Health issue assessment.* Final Report, Document No. EPA 600 8-84-019F, Washington, DC, 1984, US Environmental Protection Agency, Office of Health and Environmental Assessment.

39. Falk SA, Klein R, Haseman J: Acute methylmercury intoxication and ototoxicity in guinea pigs, *Arch Pathol Lab Med* 97:297, 1974.

40. Fan PL: Safety of amalgam, *CDA J* 53:34, 1987.

41. Fawer RF, et al: Measurement of hand tremor induced by industrial exposure to metallic mercury, *Br J Ind Med* 40:204, 1983.

42. Federal Security Agency, Public Health Service: *Health of workers in chromate producing industry, a study,* Division of Occupational Health of the Bureaus of State Services, 1952.

43. Fowler BA, Vouk V: *Bismuth.* In Friberg L, Nordberg GF, Vouck VB, editors: *Handbook on the toxicology of metals, Vol II,* specific metals, 2nd ed, Amsterdam, 1986, Elsevier Scientific Publications.

44. Fowler BA, Weissberg JB: Arsine poisoning, *N Engl J Med* 291:1171, 1974.

45. Fradkin A et al: In vitro transformation of BHK21 cells grown in the presence of calcium chromate, *Cancer Res* 35:1058, 1975.

46. Friedrich EG Jr: Vulvar carcinoma in situ in identical twins—an occupational hazard, *Obstet Gynecol* 39:837, 1972.

47. Frost DV: Arsenicals in biology—retrospect and prospect, *Fed Proc* 26:194, 1967.

48. Gale TF: Embryopathic effects of different routes of administration of mercuric acetate on the hamster, *Environ Res* 8:207, 1974.

49. Gale T, Ferm V: Embryopathic effects of mercuric salts, *Life Sci* 10:1341, 1971.

50. Galy P et al: Les cancers broncho-pulmonaires de l'intoxication arsenicale chronique chez les vitleulteurs du Beaujolais, *Lyon Med* 210:735, 1963.

51. Galy P et al: Le cancer pulmonaire d'orgine arsenicale des vignerons du Beaujolais, *J Franc Med Chir Thorac* 17:303, 1963.

52. Ganrot PO: Metabolism and possible health effects of aluminum, *Env Health Perspect* 65:363, 1986.

53. Garruto RM et al: Imaging of calcium and aluminum in neurofibrillary tangle-bearing neurons in parkinsonism-dementia of Guam. *Proc Natl Acad Sci USA* 81:1875, 1984.

54. Glass GE, Sorensen JA, Schmidt KW: New source identification of mercury contamination in the Great Lakes, *Environ Sci Technol* 24:1059, 1990.

55. Goenaga X, Williams DJA: Aluminum speciation in surface waters from a Welsh upland area, *Env Pollut* 52:131, 1988.

56. Goldman AL: Lung cancer in Bowen's disease, *Am Rev Respir Dis* 108:1205, 1973.

57. Goldwater LJ: *Mercury: a history of quicksilver,* Baltimore, 1972, York Press.

58. Goyer RA: Lead and the kidney, *Curr Top Pathol* 55:147, 1971.

59. Goyer RA: Lead toxicity: a problem in environmental pathology, *Am J Pathol* 64:176, 1971.

60. Goyer RA: *The nephrotoxic effects of lead.* In Bach P et al, editors: *Nephrotoxicity, assessment and pathogenesis,* Chichester, UK, 1982, John Wiley & Sons.

61. Goyer RA: *Toxic effects of metals.* In Amdur MO, Doull J, Klaassen CD, editors: *Casarett and Doull's toxicology,* 4th ed, New York, 1991, Pergamon Press.

62. Goyer RA: Transplacental transport of lead, *Env Health Perspect* 1994, in press.

63. Goyer RA, Wilson MH: Lead-induced inclusion bodies: results of EDTA treatment, *Lab Invest* 32:149, 1975.

64. Goyer RA et al: *Lead induced nephrotoxicity: kidney calcium as an indicator of tubular injury.* In Bach PH, Lock EA, editors: *Nephrotoxicity,* 1989, Plenum Publishing.

65. Greger JL, Goetz W, Sullivan D: Aluminum levels in foods cooked and stored in aluminum pans, trays and foil, *J Food Prot* 48:772, 1985.

66. Hammond PB, Beliles RP: *Metals.* In Doull J, Klaassen CD, Amdur MO, editors: *Casarett and Doull's toxicology,* 2nd ed. New York, 1980, MacMillan Press.

67. Henderson AS: The epidemiology of Alzheimer's disease, *Br Med Bull* 42:3, 1986.

68. Hill AB, Faning EL: Studies in the incidence of cancer in a factory handling inorganic compounds of arsenic. I. Mortality experience in the factory, *Br J Ind Med* 5:2, 1948.

69. Hueper WC: *Occupational and environmental cancers of the respiratory system,* New York, 1966, Springer-Verlag.

70. Hutchinson J: On some examples of arsenic-keratoses of the skin and of arsenic cancer, *Trans Path Soc Lond* 39:352, 1988.

71. Ineichen B: Measuring the rising tide. How many dementia cases will there be by 2001? *Br J Psychol* 11:26, 1987.

72. International Agency for Research on Cancer: *Evaluation of carcinogenic risk of chemical to man, vol II, some inorganic and orga-*

nometallic compounds, Lyon, France, 1973, World Health Organization, International Agency for Research on Cancer.

73. International Agency for Research on Cancer: *Polynuclear aromatic compounds. Part 3. Industrial exposures in aluminum production, coal gasification, coke production and iron and steel founding,* vol 34, Lyon, France, 1984, World Health Organization, International Agency for Research on Cancer.

74. International Agency for Research on Cancer: *Monograph on the evaluations of carcinogenicity: an update of IARC monographs,* vol 1-42, suppl 7, Lyon, France, 1987, World Health Organization, International Agency for Research on Cancer.

75. Jaffe KM, Shurtleff DB, Robertson WO: Survival after acute mercury vapor poisoning—role of intensive supportive care, *Am J Dis Child* 137:749, 1983.

76. Kagey BT, Bumgarner JE, Creason JP: *Arsenic levels in maternal-fetal tissue sets.* In Hemphill OD, editor: *Trace substances in environmental health XI,* Columbia, Mo, 1977, University of Missouri Press.

77. King SW, Savory J, Wills MR: Clinical biochemistry of aluminum, *Crit Rev Clin Lab Sci* 14:1, 1981.

78. Klaassen CD: In Gilman AG, et al, editors: The *pharmacological basis of therapeutics,* 7th ed, New York, 1985, Macmillan.

79. Kohler CC, Heidinger RC, Call T: *Levels of PCBs and trace metals in crab orchard lake sediment, benthos, zooplankton and fish,* Report No. HWRICRR-043, Carbondale, Ill, 1990, Fishery Research Laboratory, University of So. Illinois.

80. Kuratsune M et al: Occupational lung cancer among copper smelters, *Int J Cancer* 13:552, 1974.

81. Kuschner M: The carcinogenicity of beryllium, *Env Health Perspect* 40:101, 1981.

82. Kuschner M, Laskin S: Experimental models in environmental carcinogenesis, *Am J Pathol* 64:183, 1971.

83. Lander JJ et al: Angiosarcoma of the liver associated with Fowler's solution (potassium arsenite), *Gastroenterology* 68:1582, 1975.

84. Landrigan PJ: Toxicity of lead at low dose, *Br J Ind Med* 46:593, 1989 (editorial).

85. Laskin S, Kuschner M, Drew RT: *Studies in pulmonary carcinogenesis.* In Hanna MG Jr, Nettesheim P, Gilbert JR, editors: *Inhalation carcinogenesis,* Washington, DC, 1970, US Atomic Energy Commission.

86. Lee AM, Fraumeni JF Jr: Arsenic and respiratory cancer in man: an occupational study, *J Natl Cancer Inst* 42:1045, 1969.

87. Lee RE Jr, Von Lehmden DJ: Trace metal pollution in the environment. *J Air Pollut Control Assoc* 23:853, 1973.

88. Letterer E: Examination of a chromium-silicotic lung, *Arch Gawerbepath* 9:486; abstracted in *J Ind Hyg Toxicol* 21:815, 1939.

89. Letterer E, Neidhardt K, Kiett H: Chromat-lungendreba and chromatatu-blunge, *Arch f Gewerbepath u Gawerbehyg* 12:3, 1944.

90. Lieberman H: Chrome ulcerations of the nose and throat, *N Engl J Med* 225:132, 1941.

91. Lilis R, Fischbein A: Chelation therapy in workers exposed to lead—a critical review, *JAMA* 235:2823, 1976.

92. Lindstedt G, Gottberg I, Holmgren B: Individual mercury exposure of chloralkali workers and its relation to blood and urinary mercury levels, *Scand J Work Environ Health* 5:59, 1979.

93. Lukanin WP: Zur pathologie der chromat-pneumokoniose, *Arch f Hyg* 104:188, 1980.

94. Lumb G, Sunderman FW Sr: *Mechanism of malignant tumor induction by nickel subsulfide.* In Nieboer E, Nriagu JO, editors: *Nickel and human health: current perspectives,* New York, 1992, John Wiley & Sons.

95. Lumb G, Sunderman FW Sr: The problem of latency in the development of tumors following exposure to nickel compounds, *Sci Total Environ* 1994, in press.

96. Lumb G et al: Histogenesis of subcutaneous malignant tumors resulting from nickel subsulfide implantation, *Ann Clin Lab Sci* 17:286, 1987.

97. Lundgren K-D, Swensson A, Ulfvarson U: Studies in humans on the distribution of mercury in the blood and the excretion in urine after exposure to different mercury compounds, *Scand J Clin Lab Invest* 20:164, 1967.

98. Mancuso TF: Occupational cancer and other health hazards in a chromate plant: a medical appraisal. II. Clinical and toxicologic aspects, *Ind Med Surg* 20:393, 1951.

99. Mancuso TF, Hueper WC: Occupational cancer and other health hazards in a chromate plant: a medical appraisal. I. Lung cancers in chromate workers, *Ind Med Surg* 20:359, 1951.

100. Martyn CM et al: Geographical relation between Alzheimer's disease and aluminum in drinking water, *Lancet* 1:59, 1989.

101. Mastromatteo E: Nickel: a review of its occupational health aspects, *J Occup Med* 9:127, 1967.

102. McKeown-Eyssen GE, Ruedy J, Neims A: Methylmercury exposure in northern Quebec: II. Neurologic findings in children, *Am J Epidemiol* 118:470, 1983.

103. Mertz W: Chromium occurrence and function in biological systems, *Physiol Rev* 49:163, 1969.

104. Milham S Jr, Strong T: Human arsenic exposure in relation to a copper smelter, *Environ Res* 7:176, 1974.

105. Milne J, Christophers A, DeSilva P: Acute mercurial pneumonitis, *Br J Ind Med* 27:334, 1970.

106. Minkowitz S: Multiple carcinomata following ingestion of medicinal arsenic, *Ann Intern Med* 61:296, 1964.

107. Morgan JG: Some observations on the incidence of respiratory cancer in nickel workers, *Br J Ind Med* 15:224, 1958.

108. Murdock A, Hill K: Distribution of mercury in Lake St. Clair and the St. Clair River sediments, *Water Pollution Research Journal of Canada* 24:1, 1989.

109. Nagy S, Nikdel S: Tin, iron and aluminum contents of commercially canned single-strength grapefruit juice stored at varying temperatures, *J Agric Food Chem* 34:588, 1986.

110. Nagyvary J, вradbury EL: Hypocholesterolemic effects of Al^{3+} complexes, *Biochem Res Commun* 2:592, 1977.

111. National Academy of Science: *An assessment of mercury in the environment: scientific and technical assessments of environmental pollutants,* Washington, DC, 1977, National Academy Press.

112. National Research Council of Canada: *Effects of mercury in the Canadian environment,* Ottawa, Canada, 1979, National Research Council of Canada. Publication No. 16739.

113. National Toxicology Program: *NTP technical report on the toxicology and carcinogenesis studies of mercuric chloride (CAS No. 7487-94-7) in F344/N rats and B6C3F1 mice (gavage studies) as modified based on peer review),* Research Triangle Park, NC, 1992, NTP TR 408. NIH Publication No. 91-3139, National Toxicology Program, US Department of Health and Human Services, Public Health Service, National Institutes of Health.

114. Needleman HL et al: Deficits in psychologic and classroom performance of children with elevated blood lead levels, *N Engl J Med* 300:689, 1979.

115. Needleman HL et al: Long-term effects of childhood exposure to lead at low dose: an eleven year follow-up report, *N Engl J Med* 322:83, 1990.

116. Newberne PM et al: *Nongenotoxic mouse liver carcinogens. Banbury Report 25: nongenotoxic mechanisms in carcinogenesis,* Cold Spring Harbor Laboratory, 1987.

117. Newberne PM et al: The role of necrosis in hepatocellular proliferation and liver tumors. Mouse liver tumors, *Arch Toxicol* Suppl 10:54, 1987.

118. Ng A, Patterson C: Natural concentrations of lead in ancient arctic and antarctic ice, *Geochim Cosmochin Acta* 45:2109, 1981.

119. Norseth T: The carcinogenicity of chromium and its salts, *Br J Ind Med* 43:649, 1986.

120. Occupational Safety and Health Administration: *OSHA permissable exposure limits,* 29CFR1910.1000, 1985.

121. Ondov JM, Zoller WH, Gordon GE: Trace element emissions on aerosols from motor vehicles, *Environ Sci Technol* 16:318, 1982.

122. Pederson E, Hogetveit AC, Cancerson A: Cancer of respiratory organs among workers at a nickel refinery in Norway, *Int J Cancer* 12:32, 1973.

123. Perl DP, Brody AR: Detection of aluminum by SEM X-ray spectrometry within neurofibrillary tangle-bearing neurons of Alzheimer's disease, *Neurotoxicology* 1:133, 1980.

124. Perl DP, Good PF: Uptake of aluminum in central nervous system along nasal olfactory pathways, *Lancet* 1:1087, 1987.

125. Perl DP, Good PF: Aluminum, environment and central nervous system disease, *Environ Technol Lett* 9:901, 1988.

126. Rada RG, Wiener JG, Winfrey MR: Recent increases in atmospheric deposition of mercury to north-central Wisconsin lakes inferred from sediment analyses, *Arch Environ Contam Toxicol* 18:175, 1989.

127. Regelson W et al: Hemangioendothelial sarcoma of liver from chronic arsenic intoxication by Fowler's solution, *Cancer* 21:514, 1968.

128. Rosenman KD, Valciukas JA, Glickman L: Sensitive indicators of inorganic mercury toxicity, *Arch Environ Health* 41:208, 1986.

129. Roth F: Arsen-leber-tumoren (Hemongioendotheliom), *Z Krebsforsch* 61:468, 1957.

130. Rutter M, Jones RR, editors: *Lead versus health. Sources and effects of low level lead exposure,* New York, 1983, John Wiley & Sons.

131. Saknyn AV, Shabynina NK: Some statistical data on carcinogenesis hazards for workers engaged in the production of nickel from oxidized ores, *Gig Trud Prof Zabol* 14:10, 1970.

132. Saknyn AV, Shabynina NK: Epidemiology of malignant neoplasms in nickel plants, *Gig Trud Prof Zabol* 17:25, 1973.

133. Sanderson KV: Arsenic and skin cancer, *Trans St John's Hosp Dermatol Soc* 49:115, 1963.

134. Schroeder HA, Mitchener M: Scandium, chromium (VI), gallium, yttrium, rhodium, palladium, indium in mice: effects on growth and life span, *J Nutr* 101:1431, 1971.

135. Scott JK, Hodge HC: *Nonabsorbable dusts.* In DiPalma JR, editor: *Drill's pharmacology in medicine,* 4th ed, New York, 1971, McGraw-Hill.

136. Siegel N, Huag A: Aluminum interaction with calmodulin. Evidence for altered structure and function from optical enzymatic studies, *Biochim Biophys Acta* 14:36, 1981.

137. Skerfving S: Methylmercury exposure, mercury levels in blood and hair, and health status in Swedes consuming contaminated fish, *Toxicology* 2:3, 1974.

138. Snodgrass W, Sullivan JB, Rumack BH: Mercury poisoning from home gold ore processing: use of penicillamine and dimercaprol, *JAMA* 246:1929, 1981.

139. Sommers SS, McManus RG: Multiple arsenical cancers of skin and internal organs, *Cancer* 6:347, 1953.

140. Sorenson JRJ et al: Aluminum in the environment and human health, *Environ Health Perspect* 8:3, 1974.

141. Stokinger HE, editor: *Beryllium: its industrial hygiene aspects,* New York, 1966, Academic Press.

142. Sunderman FW Jr: Metal carcinogenesis in experimental animals, *Food Cosmet Tox* 9:105, 1971.

143. Sunderman FW Jr: The current status of nickel carcinogenesis, *Ann Clin Lab Sci* 3:156, 1973.

144. Sunderman FW Jr: A review of the carcinogenecities of nickel, chromium and arsenic compounds in man and animals, *Prev Med* 5:279, 1976.

145. Sunderman FW, Donnelly AJ: Studies of nickel carcinogenesis metastasizing pulmonary tumors in rats induced by the inhalation of nickel carbonyl, *Am J Pathol* 46:1027, 1965.

146. Sunderman FW Jr, Mastromatteo E: *Nickel carcinogenesis.* In Sunderman FW Jr et al, editors: *Nickel,* Washington, DC, 1975, National Academy of Sciences.

147. Sunderman FW Jr, Roszel NO, Clark RJ: Gas chromatography of nickel carbonyl in blood and breath, *Arch Environ Health* 16:836, 1968.

148. Sunderman FW Jr, Selin CE: The metabolism of nickel-63 carbonyl, *Toxicol Appl Pharmacol* 12:207, 1968.

149. Sunderman FW, Sunderman FW Jr: Nickel poisoning. VIII. Dithiocarb: a new therapeutic agent for persons exposed to nickel carbonyl, *Am J Med Sci* 236:26, 1958.

150. Sunderman FW, Sunderman FW Jr: Nickel poisoning. XI. Implication of nickel as a pulmonary carcinogen in tobacco smoke, *Am J Clin Pathol* 35:203, 1961.

151. Takeuchi T: *Neuropathology of Minimata disease in Kumamoto: especially at the chronic stage.* In Roizin L, Shiraki H, Grcevic N, editors: *Neurotoxicology,* vol I, New York, 1977, Raven Press.

152. *Toxics release inventory,* Washington, DC, 1989, US Environmental Protection Agency, Office of Toxic Substances.

153. Venitt S, Levy LS: Mutagenicity of chromates in bacteria and its relevance to chromate carcinogenesis, *Nature* 250:493, 1974.

154. Virtue JA: The relationship between the refining of nickel and cancer of the nasal cavity, *Can J Otolaryngol* 1:37, 1972.

155. West B, Sunderman FW: Nickel poisoning. VII. The therapeutic effectiveness of alkyl dithiocarbamates in experimental animals exposed to nickel carbonyl, *Am J Med Sci* 236:15, 1958.

156. White JC: Psoriasis, verruca, epithelioma: a sequence, *Am J Med Sci* 89:163, 1985.

157. Wills MR, Savory J: Aluminum poisoning dialysis encephalopathy, osteomalacia and anemia, *Lancet* 2:29, 1983.

158. Wilson BL, Mitchell DL: Trace metal study of sediment samples near electrical generating facility, *J Environ Sci Health* A26:493, 1991.

159. World Health Organization *Environmental health criteria 19. Arsenic.* Geneva, 1981, World Health Organization.

160. World Health Organization *Environmental health criteria 1. Mercury.* Geneva, 1976, World Health Organization.

161. Wulf HC, Kromann N, Kousgaard N: Sister chromatid exchange (SCE) in Greenlandic Eskimos: dose response relationship between SCE and seal diet, smoking, and blood cadmium and mercury concentrations, *Sci Total Environ* 48:81, 1986.

162. Yeh S: Skin cancer in chronic arsenicalism, *Human Pathol* 4:469, 1973.

163. Zachariae H: Arsenik og cancerrisko, *Ugeskr Laeg* 134:2720, 1972.

Chapter 5

CHEMICAL TOXICITY

Michael M. Lipsky
Benjamin F. Trump

Polycyclic aromatic hydrocarbons
  Benz[a]anthracene and benzo[a]pyrene
Vinyl chloride
Benzene
Benzidine
Formaldehyde
Carbon disulfide
Bis(chloromethyl) ether and chloromethyl methyl ether
Halogenated hydrocarbons
  Tetrachloroethylene (perchloroethylene)
  Carbon tetrachloride
  Chloroform
2,3,7,8-tetrachlorodibenzo-p-dioxin
Aflatoxin B_1
Nitrosamines
  N-Nitrosodiethylamine and N-nitrosodimethylamine

It is well recognized that occupational and environmental exposure to toxic agents can significantly impact human health. An important focus has been on cancer. The development of many human malignancies has been attributed to environmental influences.* A subset of these cancers can be attributed to direct occupational exposures. There has been considerable variability in the quantitative estimates of cancer attributable to occupation, with the range being from 1% to 10% of total cancers.[92,236,339,390] It has been suggested that this large variability in the published estimates is due to inaccurate measures of the proportion of exposed subjects, levels of exposure, and/or carcinogenic risk. These estimates can also be viewed in a different perspective. Tomatis[339] pointed out that the percentages of

cancer attributable to occupational risk are based on the general population. However, only 12% to 20% of the general population are actually at risk for occupational exposure. Then, for example, 4% of the cancer cases in the general population translates into 20% to 30% of the subgroup actually at risk.[339]

Regardless of the estimates, it is clear that occupational exposure to chemical carcinogens poses a real health hazard to the exposed workers. In addition to cancer, environmental and occupational exposures of humans to chemical toxins are responsible for inducing a variety of acute and chronic pathological alterations and deaths.

Environmental influences (nonoccupational) are here considered in a broad context as any influence arising external to the body. Many of these influences are life-style factors and include factors defined by our culture and personal habits, such as diet and smoking. However, a large proportion of these environmental factors are, in fact, chemicals, both synthetic and naturally occurring. In recent years the impact of nonoccupational exposures to synthetic chemical pollutants in the environment on human health and cancer risk has been debated.* Because of the wide distribution and persistence of many synthetic chemicals in the environment and their ability to induce cancers in laboratory animals, they would appear to be important.[265,339] It should be noted that of those chemicals that have been demonstrated to be carcinogenic in humans, all induce neoplasia in laboratory animals.[175,265] It should also be kept in mind that there are often significant variations in responses among different animal species that may modify the toxicological and carcinogenic profile observed after acute and chronic exposures to environmental toxicants. This fact

*References 92, 154, 155, 236, 265, 339, 390.

*References 15, 16, 161, 265, 339.

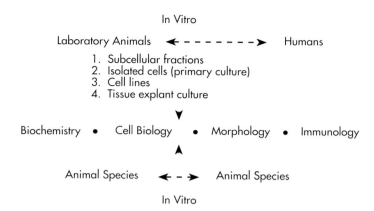

Fig. 5-1. Model for interspecies extrapolation research. (Adapted from Harris CC, Trump BF: Human tissues and cells in biomedical research, *Surv Synth Path Res* 1:165, 1983; Trump BF, Harris CC: Human tissues in biomedical research, *Hum Pathol* 10:245, 1979; Weston, et al: Genotoxicity of chemical and physical agents in cultured human tissues and cells, *Food Chem Toxicol* 24:675, 1986.)

does not invalidate interspecies extrapolations but should provide the impetus to perform mechanistic studies to identify the action of toxic and carcinogenic chemicals to gain a better understanding of the potential impact on human health.

Research strategies have been designed to provide a firmer basis for interspecies extrapolation and determination of toxic and carcinogenic mechanisms of action with the ultimate goal to understand and determine human risk from exposure to chemical toxicants. One approach that has been successfully utilized by Harris and colleagues [140,141,143,144] and the authors of this chapter[204,340] is a correlated in vivo–in vitro strategy involving both laboratory animals and human tissues and cells (Fig. 5-1). In this scheme, direct comparisons can be made with any number of parameters between human and laboratory animal tissues and cells in vitro. For example, distinct species differences are evident for the hepatocarcinogenicity of aflatoxin B_1, with the rat being sensitive and the mouse generally being resistant. In vitro experiments using primary liver cells from rats, mice, and humans demonstrated that the sensitive species (rats) produced a higher level of metabolic activation, binding of metabolites to DNA, DNA damage, mutagenicity, and ultrastructural alterations in nucleoli than did the resistant species (mouse).[66,67,158,204] The human tissue displayed responses similar to that of the rat but usually required a higher dose of the aflatoxin to be effective. The in vitro responses for each species correlated well with the in vivo potential for toxicity and carcinogenicity. A wide variety of experiments have demonstrated the metabolic activation and toxic potential of a number of important chemical carcinogens directly in human target tissues.[140-143,371]

It is our intent in this chapter to review important classes of chemicals that have been implicated as potential causes of human disease from environmental exposures in nonoc-

cupational and occupational settings and to provide some basic information on the mechanisms of action and responses to these agents. The reader is referred to Chapter 26 for a detailed discussion of chemical carcinogenesis.

POLYCYCLIC AROMATIC HYDROCARBONS

Polycyclic aromatic hydrocarbons (PAHs) are a group of chemicals that are ubiquitous in the environment and can be naturally occurring as well as man-made. They generally occur as colorless to yellow to golden solids that are insoluble in water and only slightly soluble in ethanol. They have no industrial uses but are produced primary for research purposes.[8,169,247] There are more than 100 different PAHs.[8] Fifteen of the more recognized PAHs are listed in the box on the next page. They are commonly formed during the combustion of organic materials such as wood, coal, gasolines, and other fuels and are present in industrial materials such as mineral oils, coal tar, coke tars, petroleum waxes, asphalt, crude oils, and creosote.[8,169,247] Industrial activity is a major source of PAH release into the environment.[8,70] Sources include incineration, power generation, the production of coal tar, coke, and asphalt, and the catalytic cracking of petroleum. Transportation sources of PAH emissions such as gasoline and diesel fuel exhausts can compromise up to 50% of urban resident exposures.[8,317] Moreover, PAH emissions occur from a variety of individual or consumer-related activities (in addition to fuel combustion) such as cigarette smoking, use of outdoor grills, and the burning of wood in fireplaces. The types of PAHs that are present in different areas varies widely and is dependent upon the mix of substances or processes giving rise to their emissions.

Exposure to PAHs occurs in the general population at low levels.[8,235] It is primarily by inhalation of tobacco and wood smoke and polluted air and by ingestion of contami-

Polycyclic aromatic hydrocarbons

Benz[a]anthracene
Benza[b]fluoranthene
Benzo[j]fluoranthene
Benzo[k]fluroanthene
Benzo[a]pyrene
Dibenz[a,h]acridine
Dibenz[a,j]acridine
Dibenz[a,h]anthracene
Dibenzo[c,g]carbazole
Dibenzo[a,e]pyrene
Dibenzo[a,h]pyrene
Dibenzo[a,i]pyrene
Dibenzo[a,l]pyrene
Chrysene
Indeno[1,2,3-cd]pyrene

nated food and of PAHs that naturally occur in food. Some foods shown to contain PAHs are smoked, barbecued, and charcoal-broiled foods, processed foods, seafood, meats, vegetables and vegetable oils, and roasted coffee.[8,70,169] Ingestion of food containing PAHs is most likely the primary source for nonsmokers in the general population.[8,70] Menzie and colleagues[235] estimated a mean daily exposure for adult males at 3 μg/day (maximum 15 μg/day). Low-level exposure may also take place via drinking water or by dermal exposure to PAH-containing products. Smoking cigarettes may result in an exposure level that is double that level.[235]

Occupational exposure to PAHs occurs in coal tar production plants, foundries, coke ovens, road and roof tarring operations, smoke houses, asphalt production plants, and wherever there is combustion of carbonaceous materials.[8] The highest level of human exposure is found among these occupational groups.

An association appears to exist between human cancer and exposure to mixtures of PAHs.[8] Epidemiological studies of relevant occupational groups, such as roofers and coke oven workers, have demonstrated increased cancer risk. However, identification of specific PAHs as the causative agents for cancer in these occupational groups is still not definitive.[8]

Benz[a]anthracene and Benzo[a]pyrene

Benz[a]anthracene (BaA) and benzo[a]pyrene (BaP) are two of the most common and most frequently studied of the PAHs. As with the other members of this chemical group, they are highly lipophilic and readily penetrate cell membranes.[8,90] They are also readily metabolized by cellular enzyme systems. Because it has been extensively studied, benzo[a]pyrene is used here to describe general patterns of metabolic transformation. Detailed and comprehensive discussions of this metabolism are readily

available. The initial metabolic activity centers on cytochrome P-450–dependent mixed-function oxidases. For PAHs these are called *aryl hydroxide hydroxylases* (AHH) (see Chapters 17 and 26).[8,90,121] This may result in the formation of arene oxides, which can undergo a variety of metabolic fates. They may covalently react with glutathione to form a water-soluble conjugate, either in a glutathione-s-transferase–catalyzed reaction or spontaneously. They may also spontaneously rearrange to phenols. Phenols act as intermediates in the oxidative formation of quinones.[260] Some of these products may undergo further oxidative reactions. For example, 9-o-benzo[a]pyrene may be oxidized to the K-region 4,5-oxide and then hydrated to the corresponding 4,5-dihydrodiol (4,5,9-triol). The arene oxides may also undergo epoxide hydrolase–catalyzed reactions (hydrations) to *trans*-dihydrodiols. The phenols and dihydrodiols can be conjugated by glucuronides and sulfate esters; the quinones may undergo these conjugations as well as form glutathione conjugates (see Fig. 26-3).[3,8,169]

The primary toxicological concern with PAH exposures is the carcinogenic and mutagenic potential of many of the members of this class of chemicals. Both BaA and BaP are considered to be chemical carcinogens and mutagens, and BaP has demonstrated a wide range of genotoxic and mutagenic capabilities in prokaryotic, eukaryotic, and mammalian cells in vitro and in vivo.* The genotoxicity and mutagenicity of BaP is keyed to its metabolic activation. The 7,8-diol-9,10-epoxide is considered to be the ultimate mutagenic metabolite of BAP. This can form when the epoxide metabolite of BaP is activated by the action of epoxide hydralase to form a dihydrodiol. Additional mixed-function oxidase activity can then result in the formation of the diol-epoxide. It is capable of covalently binding to nucleophilic sites in cellular macromolecules, including DNA. Although there is some evidence to suggest that enzymatic systems other than AHH may convert BaP to a genotoxin,[206] the primary route of metabolic activation is cytochrome P-450–dependent mixed-function oxidation. This is also true for many of the PAHs, including BaA. The genotoxic and carcinogenic potential of many of these PAHS appears linked to the formation of diol-epoxides in the bay region of the molecule.

Of major concern is the carcinogenic potential of many PAHs: BaP, BaA, and a number of the other PAHs are carcinogenic in experimental animals.[8,61,247] The PAHs have been shown to induce a wide spectrum of neoplasms in multiple organ systems, dependent upon the specific PAH and route of administration. These are summarized in a number of reviews and resports.[8,169,247] Both BaP and BaA have been demonstrated to be carcinogenic in experimental animals when administered by a variety of exposure routes. When painted on the backs of mice, BaP and BaA induce

*References 8, 160, 206, 253, 376.

skin neoplasia.* Exposure to BaP also induced skin neoplasms in rats, guinea pigs, and rabbits.

In addition, BaA has been demonstrated to induce papillomas in the forestomach, bladder carcinomas, sarcomas, and lung adenomas in adult mice.[8,169] When administered to newborn mice, BaA resulted in the induction of pulmonary adenomas and adenocarcinomas.[8,247] Of the PAH carcinogens, BaP is one of the most potent and most studied. In addition to skin neoplasms, it induced forestomach and mammary carcinomas in rats and sarcomas and fibrosarcomas in rats, hamsters, guinea pigs, newts, mice, and subhuman primates.[8,247] Intratracheal administration induced tracheal papillomas and carcinomas in hamsters and rats, Hepatocellular carcinomas were induced by BaP exposure in newborn mice and rainbow trout.[8,247] The wide variety of target tissues at risk after different routes of administration and the number of species affected demonstrate the carcinogenic hazards posed by PAH exposure. Although definitive studies on the causation of human cancers by individual PAHs are lacking, the cancer risk associated with certain occupational groups exposed to PAH mixtures demonstrates their carcinogenic potential in humans.† This carcinogenic potential for humans is further strengthened by numerous studies demonstrating metabolism, DNA binding, and mutagenesis of PAHs in human cells and tissues.‡

The potential for other types of toxicity in humans can only be inferred from studies in experimental animals. Other potential noncarcinogenic effects of PAH exposure include respiratory, immunological, reproductive, and developmental effects. These effects have been demonstrated in experimental animals and have not been directly reported in humans. In experimental animals BaP exposure can be immunosuppressive.[44,213,345,346] Studies have demonstrated effects on both cell-mediated[346,380] and humoral[43,213,372] immune function. Other PAHs have also demonstrated immunosuppressive activity. The degree of this activity seems to correlate with carcinogenic potential.[345] When studied in in vitro, BaP has also been shown to affect a number of enzymes and hormonal activities of human placenta[28,31,133] and to inhibit fecundity and fetal development in mice (see Chapter 33).[199,214]

VINYL CHLORIDE

Vinyl chloride (C_2H_3Cl) is a colorless vapor with a mild, sweet odor.[317] A synthetic compound, it is an important industrial chemical with a wide variety of uses. One principal use is for making polyvinyl chloride (PVC), which is commonly used in the production of numerous plastic products such as piping, coatings for cable and wires, automobile parts, furniture, and packaging materials.[6,75] In addition, vinyl chloride is used in vinyl chloride–vinyl acetate

copolymer products, including films and resins.[6] Vinyl chloride is soluble in a wide variety of liquids including alcohol, oil, chlorinated solvents, and most organic liquids.

Potential human exposures to vinyl chloride are primarily occupational, although it has been detected in the air around hazardous waste sites and landfills and near plastics production facilities.[6] The primary route of exposure is by inhalation, although for plastics workers the potential for dermal exposure exists. Inhalation exposure results in rapid absorption of vinyl chloride with widespread distribution throughout the body (as determined in animal experiments).[45,53,94,362,363]

Vinyl chloride is metabolized in mammalian tissues. A number of alternative pathways for metabolism have been postulated.[151] The primary pathway appears to be oxidative, involving cytochrome P-450–dependent mixed-function oxidases.[46,131,163] The initial interactions in this pathway result in the formation of the highly reactive intermedite metabolite, 2-chloroethylene oxide.[130,131] This metabolite has been demonstrated to bind covalently to cellular macromolecules, including DNA and RNA.* 2-Chloroethylene oxide and 2-chloroacetaldehyde (which can form from sponateous rearrangement of the ethylene oxide reactant) are detoxified primarily by glutathione-s-transferase–catalyzed conjugation with glutathione.[47,151] N-acetyl-s-(2-hydroxyethyl)cysteine and thioglycolic acid are two of the substituted cysteine derivatives that were identified in urine of rats.

Vinyl chloride exposure can result in a vareity of pathologic alterations in mammals.[344] Of prime interest is the induction of malignancies in multiple organ sites. Clinical observations that workers chronically exposed to vinyl chloride had an unusually high incidence of hepatic angiosarcoma, a rare form of cancer in the United States, provided the initial evidence that it was carcinogenic.† Subsequent studies have verified the increased incidence of hepatic angiosarcoma following chronic occupational exposures, particularly in those workers exposed to the highest concentrations of vinly chloride.‡

There are conflicting studies on the significance of neoplasm induction at other tissue sites in humans. Statistically significant increases in mortality due to lung or respiratory tract neoplasia, lymphoma, and other hematopoietic neoplasia and brain and other central nervous system (CNS) neoplasia have been reported.§ However, other investigations failed to demonstrate a statistically significant association between vinyl chloride exposure and CNS neoplasia or neoplasia in other organs.‖

Studies in experimental animals have also demonstrated

---

*References 8, 11, 40, 61, 169, 247, 309.
†References 137, 205, 215, 228, 283.
‡References 3, 26, 27, 143, 144.

*References 130, 131, 182, 363, 365.
†References 52, 77, 116, 167, 239, 366.
‡References 91, 179, 288, 333, 368, 389.
§References 37, 72, 239, 288, 366, 368.
‖References 91, 116, 167, 179, 389.

the carcinogenic potential of vinyl chloride. In many experiments chronic exposure has led to the development of hepatic angiosarcomas, indicating a similar target tissue in many mammalian species. Angiosarcomas were observed in rats, mice, and hamsters after inhalation exposure to vinyl chloride (52 weeks) at concentrations from 50 ppm and up.* A statistically significant increase in angiosarcomas was noted in female rats at the 50 ppm dose level and in male rats at the 200 ppm dose level.[221] In another study, male rats exposed to 100 ppm for 12 months (inhalation 6 hr/day for 6 days) had a statistically significant increase in angiosarcomas at sacrifice 6 months after the final dose (18 months).[38] Increased incidences of neoplasms at other organ sites was also noted in some studies. Maltoni and colleagues[221] reported increases in mammary neoplasms in female rats at a dose level as low as 5 ppm. Zymbal gland carcinomas and nephroblastomas were also increased in male and female rats.

BENZENE

Benzene (C_6H_6) is an industrial chemical produced in large quantities in the United States. It can also be given off naturally in a number of processes, including incomplete combustion of many organic substances, such as smoldering wood.[367] Benzene is also a natural component of materials derived from petroleum.[367] Most benzene is made from petroleum sources. It is a clear, colorless, volatile, and highly flammable liquid with a distinctive odor.[247,317] It is an additive in gasolines, is a solvent for inks, oils, and paints, and is used in the manufacturing of some types of rubber, lubricants, dyes, detergents, drugs, and pesticides.[4,247,317] It is a major component in the synthesis of many chemical compounds, including ethylbenzene, a prime raw material for the production of styrene in the plastics industry.[4,317]

Human exposure to benzene occurs in both occupational and nonoccupational settings. Essentially all of the benzene that is emitted into the environment is in the air.[4,357] Therefore, most human exposure to benzene is by inhalation.[147] In fact, most of the U.S. population are probably exposed to benzene from gasoline, and about 50% are exposed from industrial sources.[4] About 20% of the national exposure to benzene is from outdoor sources such as auto exhaust and industrial emissions.[357-359,361] The smoking of cigarettes is also an important source of benzene exposure for a large number of individuals in that benzene release accompanies tobacco combustion.[358,359] This accounts for about 50% of the national exposure (including secondhand smoke exposure).[360] Smokers had an average breath concentration of benzene that is approximately 10 times the amount of a nonsmoker.[359,360]

It was demonstrated by Sammett and colleagues[300] that benzene toxicity was dependent upon hepatic metabolism.

*References 157, 196, 197, 220, 221.

Patrial hepatectomy of rats decreased both the metabolism and the toxicity. There are several activation and/or detoxification pathways available for benzene.[152,298] It is metabolized by the cytochrome P-450–dependent mixed-function oxidase system. The specific cytochrome P-450 utilized for benzene metabolism is P450IIE, which also metabolizes alcohol and aniline.[4] The intial oxidative metabolism results in the formation of an epoxide, benzene oxide.[177] The epoxide ring can be hydroxylated, opened, and/or conjugated with glutathione.[152] The first two options lead to toxic metabolites; glutathione conjugation leads to detoxification. Ring hydroxylation is accomplished by acid-catalyzed opening of the benzene oxide and aromatization leading to the formation of a phenol.[152] The phenol can be converted to hydroquinone, which is oxidized to benzoquinone. The second type of ring opening can lead to the development of muconic acid from muconaldehyde.[152,377] In mouse liver microsomes, this is preceded by an NADPH-dependent ring opening leading to muconic dialydehyde,[377] which can be further metabolized to muconaldehyde and other toxic benzene metabolites. Glutathione conjugation of benzene oxide leads to the formation of mercapturic acid, which can be further metabolized to prephenyl and phenyl mercapturic acid and eliminated by biliary excretion.[152,298] Glucuronide and sulfate conjugates of benzene metabolites can also be formed and result in detoxificiation via water-soluble metabolite excretion into the urine. These detoxification pathways act upon the phenol metabolites of benzene after they are converted to catechol and trihydroxy benzene.[4,152]

Benzene metabolites can form covalent bonds with DNA, RNA, and proteins in rats and mice.* Kalf and colleagues[181] have shown a correlation between the covalent binding of benzene metabolites to DNA and inhibition of RNA synthesis in liver and bone marrow mitochondria.

Occupational benzene exposure has long been associated with toxic damage to the hematopoietic system and the development of leukemia.† Both aplastic anemia and pancytopenia have been associated with benzene exposure.[24,186] A causal relationship has been noted between benzene exposure and aplastic anemia, a disorder in which all cellular elements of the blood and bone marrow are depleted.[24] Investigations of occupational exposures have established a causal relationship between benzene exposure and acute myeloid leukemia.[4,247] Associations between other hematological neoplasms and benzene exposure have not been consistent. Askoy[22] has documented hematopoietic toxicity and increased incidence of leukemia in workers from Turkey exposed to benzene. Infante and colleagues[168] and Rinsky and associates[287,288] demonstrated an excess risk of leukemia and multiple myeloma in workers at two plants that manufacture rubber hydrochloride. They demonstrated

*References 207, 208, 212, 254, 297, 330.
†References 4, 21-23, 25, 168, 258, 287, 381.

a qualitative dose-response relationship between the leukemia and benzene exposure. Data from the human cases of benzene exposure and from animal studies indicate an association between hypocellularity of bone marrow and leukemia.

Chronic bioassays in animals also demonstrated the carcinogenic potential of benzene. Administration of benzene by gavage resulted in increased incidences of Zymbal glands carcinomas and oral cavity carcinomas in male and female rats and skin carcinomas in male rats.[247] In male and female mice, chronic gavage administration of benzene induced an increase in Zymbal gland carcinomas, alveolar and bronchial adenomas, and malignant lymphomas.[162,247] In male mice, carcinomas of the preputial gland were also evident, as were mammary gland carcinomas and carcinosarcomas in female mice.[162,247]

Benzene has been shown to be a genotoxin in human and animal studies. It causes primarily chromosomal aberrations in humans, with peripheral lymphocytes and bone marrow cells being the primary targets.* Numerous studies have reported the genotoxic effects of benzene in in vivo and in vitro systems derived from animals and bacteria.[4] Some of the assays that were positive for benzene genotoxicity included detection of chromosomal alterations in lymphocytes and bone marrow cells of rats and mice, sister chromatid exchange, RNA synthesis inhibition, Ames bacterial mutagenesis, and unscheduled DNA synthesis. Correlation between chromosomal aberrations and the mechanism of leukemia induction still have not been unequivocally demonstrated.[4,115,301]

BENZIDINE

Benzidine ($NH_2C_6H_4C_6H_4NH_2$) is a crystalline solid but with a significant vapor pressure.[317] It is a major raw material in the production of azo dyes[317]; however, it is also a potent chemical carcinogen.[174,247] There are more than 250 benzidine-based dyes and approximately 550 uses for the dyes. Benzidine-based dyes have been used in paper, textiles, and leather products, as a hardener in the rubber industry, and as a laboratory reagent. Because of the carcinogenic potential of many azo dyes, their use has been discontinued,[247,317] and the use of benzidine has fallen dramatically. Benzidine production and use are limited to closed systems with stringent environmental controls.[247]

Exposure of the general population to benzidine via exposure to the different azo dyes appears limited. The primary release of dyes from industrial sources is by wastewater discharges, sludges, and solid wastes generated by their use.[247] Potential health risks are basically limited to those who work with benzidine or the benzidine-based dyes.[60] It has been estimated that the carcinogenicity risk factor was 14 times higher for those workers than for the general population.[247]

The carcinogenicity of benzidine is related to its metabolism and patterns of binding to DNA.[35,184,224,225] Benzidine and most aromatic amines can be metabolically activated to hydroxylated and N-hydroxylated intermediates. They can be further acetylated and undergo conjugation with sulfates and glucuronides. The N-hydroxylated metabolite may also be esterified as a further activation step.[35,136] It has been reported that the monoacetylation product (N-acetyl benzidine) has a greater relative binding to DNA than benzidine, which has a greater relative binding than the N,N'-diacetyl benzidine. This was interpreted as monoacetylation being part of the activation sequence of the chemical and the second acetyl group insertion acting toward the detoxification of the chemical.[35]

Benzidine is a carcinogen in humans and experimental animals.[174,274] In humans it has been recognized as a potential urinary bladder carcinogen since the 1890s.[226] There is a strong association between benzidine exposure and the development of bladder cancer in humans.* This association was strengthened by the fact that the incidence of bladder cancer in workers decreased after efforts were made to decrease and/or eliminate occupational sources of exposure.[107,234,247]

Benzidine is also a carcinogen in animals. Experimental studies have demonstrated the induction of bladder cancer in dogs; cholangiocarcinomas and hepatocellular carcinomas in hamsters, rats, and mice; and Zymbal gland carcinomas, sarcomas, and mammary carcinomas in rats.†

FORMALDEHYDE

Formaldehyde is a colorless, flammable gas primarily sold as an aqueous solution (30% to 56%) containing methanol (0.5% to 15%) as a polymerization inhibitor.[247,317] It has a pungent odor and is also marketed in solid forms as trioxane (its cyclic trimer) and paraformaldehyde.[317] Formaldehyde is used in a variety of industrial processes. It is used in the production of urea-formaldehyde resins and phenol-formaldehyde resins. These are commonly used as adhesives in assembling different wood products such as particle board and plywood, as insulating foams, and as treatments and coatings for textiles and papers.[247,317] Formaldehyde has a large number of other miscellaneous uses, including disinfectants, fumigants, room deodorizers, seed treatments, preservatives, and tissue hardener and corrosion inhibitor in metal industries.[247] It has also been used in human and veterinary medicine.

The primary risk of exposures is for those who use formaldehyde in the production of other products or in different processes, for example, laboratory technicians who are involved in different histological procedures, pathologists,

---

*References 4, 113-115, 301, 306.

*References 32, 39, 60, 136, 222, 234, 341, 393, 394.
†References 136, 174, 247, 251, 321, 355.

and workers in the garment, printing, and publishing industries. Because of its widespread use in building materials and other sources, indoor air contamination with formaldehyde is widespread, although the levels present in the air vary widely.[383] A major source of formaldehyde, contributing to its ubiquitous presence in ambient air, is automobile exhaust.[247] Formaldehyde fumes may also be emitted from construction materials such as plywood and particle board, urea-formaldehyde foam insulation, and home furnishings in which fabrics have been treated with formaldehyde.[247]

Formaldehyde is rapidly metabolized by humans after exposure. It may be oxidized to formic acid in reactions that can be catalyzed by several enzyme systems.[71,328] The most important of these is NAD-dependent formaldehyde dehydrogenase, an enzyme that requires reduced glutathione as a cofactor.[383] The ultimate endpoint for this pathway is the production of CO_2. Formaldehyde may also react with proteins and nucleic acids, although it apparently reacts only with single-strand DNA.[69,106,145,201] Formaldehyde is also formed endogenously after metabolism of a variety of xenobiotics.[164] It is rapidly metabolized to formate.[219]

Formaldehyde exposure can produce irritation in the eye and skin.[383] It is also a sensitizing agent.[17] Acute toxic changes noted in some species following exposure have included squamous metaplasia of respiratory epithelium.[240,375,384]

In general, formaldehyde was mutagenic in a number of in vitro assay systems,[383] although there are a number of conflicting studies in the literature. Mammalian cell-mediated mutagenicity and cell transformation assays were the strongest indicators of the mutagenic potential of formaldehyde.[383] There has been no definitive evidence that formaldehyde is mutagenic in in vivo assay systems.[383] Formaldehyde induces DNA-protein cross-linking and DNA single-strand breaks in human cells in vitro.[126]

Inhalation exposure of rats to formaldehyde gas resulted in the development of squamous carcinomas in the nasal cavitites.[10,185,305,337] This was accompanied by irritation of the nasal cavities, regenerative hyperplasia, and metaplasia. There is limited evidence that formaldehyde is a human carcinogen.[175] Despite some suggestive studies on human cancers at a number of different tissue sites, including leukemias and nasopharyngeal and upper respiratory cancers, none of the data is conclusive.[383] In most of these studies, the numbers of cases were too small to achieve adequate power to determine a statistically significant cancer excess from formaldehyde exposure. Additional studies with adequate power did not demonstrate an excess of respiratory cancer.[383] The World Health Organization[383] concluded that formaldehyde is at most a weak human carcinogen, but the carcinogenic potential dictates that exposure to high levels of formaldehyde should be minimized.

CARBON DISULFIDE

Carbon disulfide (CS_2) is a highly refractive, flammable liquid that has a sweet (pure) or foul (commerical grade) odor. It is highly soluble in organic solvents but only slightly soluble in water.[317] Carbon disulfide was used in the vulcanization of rubber in the nineteenth century; in this century it has been used primarily in the viscose rayon industry in the production of cellulose, including cellophane and rayon.[34,331] It may also be used as a raw material in the production of carbon tetrachloride, pesticides, and a variety of other chemicals and industrial processes.[34,317] Exposure to carbon disulfide is primarily occupational. However, at least one recent study measured levels of carbon disulfide in the breath of normal volunteers working in New York City as well as in indoor and outdoor air samples.[266] The mean levels of carbon disulfide detected were 3.92 pmol/L (outdoor air), 8.26 pmol/L (indoor air), and 5.25 pmol/L (breath). Carbon disulfide has been detected in rural and urban air samples. In addition to industrial sources, carbon disulfide can originate from biogenic sources, including volcanic eruption. Schilling[303] suggested that because the air of industrialized countries was polluted with sulfur-containing compounds, then air pollution should be investigated as a source of potential causes of cardiovascular diseases.

The primary route of human exposure to carbon disulfide is by inhalation.[34] Percutaneous absorption is also a potential route of occupational exposure.[34,95] Regardless of the route or exposure, the major route of excretion of unmetabolized carbon disulfide is exhalation by the lung.[34] Additional (although minor) amounts of unmetabolized carbon disulfide are excreted by the kidneys into the urine. Two primary and distinctly different pathways have been described for the metabolism of carbon disulfide. These are (1) the formation of dithiocarbamates and glutathione conjugates and (2) mixed-function, oxidase-mediated generation of reactive sulfur, which can covalently bind to macromolecules.*

Dithiocarbamates may form after the carbon disulfide is metabolized to acid-labile carbon disulfides. These can be directly eliminated, can interact with amino acids to form the dithiocarbamates, or under some conditions can be metabolized back to carbon disulfide.[34] Similarly, carbon disulfide can form a water-soluble glutathione conjugate and be eliminated. Carbon disulfide can also be metabolized by cytochrome P-450.[80,86] This oxidative metabolism can result in the formation of an unstable oxygen intermediate that may spontaneously degrade to atomic sulfur and carbonyl sulfide.[34,86] Alternatively, the oxygen intermediate can react with water to give atomic sulfur and monothiocarbamate.[34]

Cardiovascular toxicity has long been associated with occupational exposure to carbon disulfide. In addition, there

---

*References 34, 48, 80, 86, 233.

have been reports of neurological, gastrointestinal, renal, hepatic, reproductive, and opthalmological toxicity in humans.[34] The cardiovascular toxicity was initially highlighted by Tiller and colleagues,[336] who demonstrated increased mortality from coronary heart disease in workers chronically exposed to carbon disulfide in viscose rayon factories. In a cohort study of men employed for more than 10 years in the rayon industry, they noted that death rates from coronary heart disease in workers exposed to carbon disulfide were more than twice that of nonexposed rayon workers. The Tiller group observations [336] have been supported in subsequent studies* that demonstrated similar associations between coronary heart disease and exposure to carbon disulfide in viscose rayon workers from different countries. Sweetnam and colleagues[331] studied a cohor of the workers described by Tiller and associates[336] which were followed for an additional 18 years. The patterns for mortality among workers aged 45 to 64 were similar to those described in the original study, with ischemic heart disease playing a major role. However, when the analysis was performed on men over the age of 65, there was a tendency for mortality to decline. They demonstrated that mortality was more closely related to recent exposure than to total exposure, indicating that the effects of carbon disulfide may be reversible.[331] This result was similar to that reported on a Finnish cohort of rayon workers. The initial studies demonstrated a fivefold excess in mortality from ischemical heart disease. However, after a preventive program was established that lowered the exposure levels to below 10 ppm, the mortality rates for the exposed and control groups were similar.[256] It was hypothesized that carbon disulfide acted as a cardiotoxin and that its effects were reversible after cessation of exposure. Recent studies have demonstrated carbon disulfide effects on specific cardiovascular parameters. Egeland and colleagues[96] demonstrated a positive linear trend between elevated levels of low-density lipoprotein cholesterol (LDL) concentration and diastolic blood pressure with increasing levels of carbon disulfide exposure. VanHoorne and colleagues[354] observed an increase in both diastolic and systolic blood pressure, LDL cholesterol concentration, and apolipoprotein A_1 and B with increasing exposure to carbon disulfide. They also observed a decrease in high-density lipoprotein cholesterol levels with increases in carbon disulfide exposure.

Studies of carbon disulfide toxicity in animals produced a variety of responses. In general, these studies reported cardiovascular alterations similar to those seen in humans.[34] They included morphological alterations similar to ischemia-induced lesions, right ventricular thickening with increased heart weight, thickening of the aortic wall, increased cholesterol content in the aorta, and elevation of serum cholesterol, phospholipid, and triglycerides.[19,34,385-388] Carbon disulfide was shown to enhance the effects of other cardiovascular toxins. It enhanced

cholesterol-induced atherogenesis in rabbits[387] and norepinephrine-induced myocardial necrosis in rats pretreated with phenobarbital.[63]

There have been a number of conflicting reports on the ophthalmological toxicity of carbon disulfide. There were apparent differences between studies on Japanese workers and Finnish workers.[34,329] In Japenese viscose rayon workers, a distinct retinopathy composed of microvascular alterations including microanuerysms and hemorrhages was clearly linked to carbon disulfide exposure.[329] The retinal capillary defects were similar to those seen in diabetes. However, no microvascular effects were induced by carbon disulfide in Finnish workers.[34] Other findings by a number of groups can typically be characterized as minor vascular changes, often atherosclerotic in origin (see Chapter 37).[122,338]

Carbon disulfide exposure can result in neurological effects, in particular, peripheral neuropathy of the central-peripheral distal axonal type.[1,73,178] Initial and follow-up studies by Ruijten and colleagues[295,296] demonstrated decreases in co-induction velocity of fast and slow motor nerve fibers of the peroneal nerve. In addition, the sensory refractory period of the sural nerve increased, and sensory conduction velocities were reduced. They also found exposure-related effects in the autonomic nervous system. There was a decrease in the heart frequency response to isometric muscle contraction and a decrease in maximal forced respiration.[295,296] These changes were noted with low-level occupational exposures. The authors interpreted the nature of the alterations and their relation to cumulative exposure to indicate that the effects on the peripheral nerves were not reversible after cessation of exposure. Behavioral abnormalities have also been associated with acute carbon disulfide exposure, including extreme irritability, uncontrolled anger, and a toxic manic-depressive psychosis (see Chapter 30).[307]

Carbon disulfide exposure has also been associated with toxic alterations in other organ systems in experimental animals. However, for the most part these data are conflicting or equivocal. The primary concern continues to be cardiovascular toxicity, especially after chronic exposures.

BIS(CHLOROMETHYL) ETHER AND CHLOROMETHYL METHYL ETHER

Bis(chloromethyl) ether (BCME; $ClCH_2OCH_2Cl$) is a colorless, volatile liquid with a suffocating odor.[317] It is water soluble; however, it rapidly decomposes in water to hydrogen chloride and formaldehyde.[247,317] Chloromethyl methyl ether (CME; $ClCH_2OCH_3$) is a volatile, corrosive liquid that usually contains 1% to 10% BCME as a contaminant.[68,317,351] These compounds are strong alkylating agents and are used in the synthesis of plastics and manufacture of ion exchange resins. Because of the acute toxicity of BCME, it is not used in industrial processes, but it is present by virtue of its presence as a contaminant in CME.

---

*References 96, 153, 216, 256, 303, 331, 373.

In the United States, BCME is not produced as a commercial product.[247,351]

Exposure to BCME and CME is primarily by inhalation and dermal contact in the workplace.[247] Potential exposure of the general population from environmental contamination is unlikely because both chemicals are rapidly degraded and/or decompose in water.[247] Because CME and BCME are reactive alkylating agents, they are not activated by metabolism but directly interact with cellular macromolecules.*

Pure CME is a weak carcinogen in laboratory animals.[350-352] It can act as an initiator for mouse skin carcinogenesis.[352] Subcutaneous injection of CME resulted in the development of fibrosarcomas in mice.[352] Inhalation exposure of rats and hamsters resulted in an increased (but low) incidence of respiratory tract neoplasms.[247] In experimental animals BCME is a potent carcinogen.[351] It is a strong initiator of mouse skin carcinogenesis.[352,353] When administered by subcutaneous injection, BCME induced fibrosarcomas in female rats and fibrosarcomas and pulmonary neoplasms in male and female mice.[119,352,353] Both squamous cell carcinoma of the lung cancer and esthesioneuroepithelioma of the nasal cavity were induced in rats by inhalation exposure to BCME.[193,200]

There are numerous reports of increased cancer risk in workers exposed to CME and BCME.† Because BCME is a contaminant in most CME preparations, it has been impossible to determine in humans if both chemicals are carcinogenic or if it is the BCME that is responsible for neoplasm induction. Therefore, CME is classified as a human carcinogen.[247] Occupational exposure to CME-BCME is associated with an increased risk of lung cancer, especially oat cell carcinoma (see Chapter 28).[108,299,334] Although dose-response studies have been difficult, heavily exposed workers have a relative risk tenfold or more above unexposed populations.[218,229,350] The risk of developing lung cancer increased with the duration and with cumulative exposure. In addition, the latency period for development of lung cancer in CME-BCME exposed workers was unusually short.[350]

HALOGENATED HYDROCARBONS

Halogenated hydrocarbons are, in large part, products of industrialization that do not occur in the natural environment. They were widely used in industrial and agricultural settings and are now ubiquitous contaminants of the environment. Some of the chemicals in this class continue to be extensively used in the workplace. Many are resistant to degradation and therefore steadily accumulate and pose persistent environmental problems. They are commonly present in "Superfund" hazardous waste sites. These chemicals display a diversity of toxic actions, including carcino-

genicity in laboratory rodents.[170,175,247,369] In many instances the mechanisms of toxic action are unknown, although the kidney and liver seem to be consistent target organs for acute and chronic toxicity. The carcinogenic potential of many (but not all) of the chemicals in this class appear to be mediated by nongenotoxic mechanisms, some of which are related to the extent of tissue injury and compensatory cell regeneration (repair) subsequent to the toxic injury.

TETRACHLOROETHYLENE (PERCHLOROETHYLENE)

Tetrachloroethylene (C_2Cl_4) is a lipid-soluble, colorless liquid extensively used in the dry-cleaning and textile-processing industries.[9,317] It is also used as an industrial solvent, an intermediate in the production of some fluorocarbons, an insulating fluid and cooling gas in electrical transformers, and a metal degreasing agent. Loss into the atmosphere has been estimated at 85% of the tetrachloroethylene used annually. Because of its widespread use, it has been detected in ambient air, primarily in urban areas but also in rural areas, and it has also been detected in ground, surface, and drinking water.[99]

There is significant human exposure to tetrachloroethylene in the workplace. The dry-cleaning industry accounts for over half, and the production of fluorocarbons accounts for another quarter of the total tetrachloroethylene used in the United States. Therefore, workers employed in these industries have the greatest potential for exposure. Nonoccupational environmental exposure may also occur to the general public in coin-operated laundromats adjacent to dry-cleaning establishments and from freshly dry-cleaned clothes.[247] The primary route of exposure of humans to tetrachloroethylene is by inhalation and dermal contact; however, absorption through the skin is minimal.[247] It can also be absorbed after ingestion. Tetrachloroethylene is readily absorbed by the lungs, and blood vessels rapidly (within a few hours) reach an equilibrium after exposure.[135]

Tetrachloroethylene undergoes oxidative metabolism via the cytochrome P-450 in mammals, with a major urinary metabolite being trichloroacetic acid.* Other metabolites that were identified included trichloroethanol, oxalic acid, and ethylene glycol. Controlled exposure experiments in rats, mice, and humans indicated that metabolism of tetrachloroethylene is a saturable process. The primary route of excretion is the lungs (for nonmetabolized compound), with metabolites being excreted in the urine and feces.[117,262] A second metabolic pathway for tetrachloroethylene that has been identified involves the conjugation of the parent compound to glutathione in the liver with further modification to N-acetyl-s-(1,2,2-trichlorovinyl)-L-cysteine, a compound that can be activated by renal β-lyase to a nephrotoxic intermediate with the capability of covalently binding to DNA

*References 119, 349, 350, 352, 353.
†References 68, 82, 108, 159, 218, 229, 261, 299, 334, 370.

*References 74, 135, 165, 244, 245, 262, 323, 391.

and other cellular macromolecules.[84,127,257] Glutathione conjugation of tetrachloroethylene increases at higher levels of exposure following saturation of the cytochrome P-450 pathway.[128]

In general, most studies to determine the genotoxic potential of tetrachloroethylene have been negative. Most of the metabolites formed from the oxidative metabolism of tetrachloroethylene are also not considered mutagenic.[9] These investigations included both in vitro and in vivo assays, such as the Ames test,[33,148] mammalian cell transformation assays,[342] unscheduled DNA synthesis in hepatocytes,[9,74] and sister chromatid exchanges.[248] However, when tetrachloroethylene was preincubated with glutathione and glutathione-s-transferases and assayed in an Ames test in the presence of a rat kidney S-9 fraction, it produced mutations in the target *Salmonella typhimurium*.[347] This assay system allowed for the formation of the glutathione conjugate [*S*-(1,2,2-trichlorovinyl)glutathione] of tetrachloroethylene, which would not have formed in most other mutagenesis systems.

Chronic exposure to tetrachloroethylene resulted in an increased incidence of hepatocellular carcinomas in male and female mice.[246-248] Liver neoplasms were not, however, induced in rats. The species difference in hepatocellular carcinogenesis appears to be due to differences in metabolism. Mice produce higher blood levels of trichloroacetic acid, which is known to induce proliferation of peroxisomes in mouse hepatocytes but not in rat hepatocytes.[123] Other liver alterations in mice were hepatocellular degeneration and necrosis and hepatic nuclear inclusions.[248] Subchronic alterations (13-week exposures) included centrilobular necrosis and bile stasis in the livers of mice. Tetrachloroethylene exposure also resulted in renal tubular cell carcinomas in male rats.[124,128,246] Additional renal alterations observed were karyomegaly and hyperplasia of proximal tubule epithelial cells and hyaline droplet accumulation karyomegaly of renal proximal tubule epithelial cells in rats and mice.[128,248]

A few epidemiologic studies have suggested a potential association between increased malignancies in humans and chronic tetrachloroethylene exposure.[41,42,64,93] However, the evidence is generally regarded as inconclusive because most occupational exposures are accompanied by exposure to other dry-cleaning agents or petroleum solvents.[9]

Carbon tetrachloride

Carbon tetrachloride (CCl_4) is a highly volatile, colorless liquid with a strong ethereal odor.[317] Although nonflammable, it produces highly toxic phosgene fumes when heated by flame (oxidative decomposition).[317] The primary use for carbon tetrachloride is in the production of chlorofluorocarbons.[7,317] It is also used as a degreasing agent and as a solvent for fats, lacquers, and varnishes.[7] The Food and Drug Administration (FDA) banned the use of carbon tetrachloride in consumer products used in the home, and

the Environmental Protection Agency (EPA) banned its use as a grain fumigant in 1985.[7,247]

There are no known natural sources of carbon tetrachloride. Its presence in the environment is due to its stability and slow rate of degradation.[250,312-314] The primary source of carbon tetrachloride in the environment is direct release into the air during its production, use, and disposal.[7] The majority of carbon tetrachloride in the environment is in the atmosphere, and it has been estimated to be increasing in concentration at a rate of about 25 ppb per year.[149,311] Exposure to carbon tetrachloride is possible for workers involved in flurorcarbon production and other workers in industrial areas where it is used. Because of its stability in the environment, there is potential for exposure of the general population.

In mammals, the metabolism of carbon tetrachloride is mediated by cytochrome P-450. The initial step is a one-electron reduction (reductive dehalogenation) and homolytic cleavage, which yields the trichloromethyl radical and chloride ion.[194,273,286,316] A variety of metabolic interactions may then occur. With respect to carbon tetrachloride toxicity, the homolytic cleavage may be followed by hydrogen abstraction of the trichloromethyl radical to form organic free radicals. These can react with molecular oxygen to form organic peroxy free radicals and ultimately organic peroxides.[276,281,282] These compounds can cleave homolytically to form free radicals, which interact with cellular macromolecules and cause lipid peroxidation.[276]

Carbon tetrachloride is generally considered to be nonmutagenic. There was no increased unscheduled DNA synthesis in rats exposed to a single dose of carbon tetrachloride in vivo or in hepatocytes exposed in vitro or in vivo.[76,237,238] However, it did induce S-phase DNA synthesis in adult mouse liver.[237] Most assays for genotoxicity were negative.* Although DNA strand breaks were induced in cultured cells by carbon tetrachloride, it was done only by concentrations that produced more than 50% lethal cytotoxicity. Binding of carbon tetrachloride metabolites to DNA and protein was reported by Diaz-Gomez and Castro[88] and Rocchi and colleagues.[289]

Acute toxic effects from carbon tetrachloride have been observed in human kidney and liver. Acute exposure induces a severe nephropathy (nephritis) in humans that is characterized by swelling, degeneration, and necrosis in proximal tubule epithelial cells and signs of renal dysfunction such as oliguria, anuria, proteinuria, edema, and hypertension.† Hepatotoxicity in humans includes elevated levels of hepatic enzymes in the serum, liver enlargement, fatty liver, degeneration, and necrosis.[146,223,252]

Both renal and hepatic toxicity have been noted in laboratory animals exposed to carbon tetrachloride. The renal toxicity is generally much less severe than the hepatotoxic-

---

*References 29, 81, 120, 209, 230, 291, 310, 343.
†References 132, 176, 223, 232, 252, 255, 327.

ity in most rodent species.[7] Renal pathologic alterations noted were proximal tubule cell swelling and some degeneration.[210] There is also wide variability in the renal response among rat strains, with some exhibiting no toxicity.[263,285,327] The hepatic toxicity of carbon tetrachloride has long been studied in laboratory animals. It is characterized by fat accumulation, inhibition of protein synthesis, lipid peroxidation resulting in destruction of the endoplasmic reticulum, hydropic vacuolation, and necrosis of centrilobular hepatocytes.*

Chronic administration of carbon tetrachloride to laboratory rodents is associated with an increased incidence of hepatocellular neoplasia. This was seen in studies using rats, mice, and hamsters† and often occurred in animals of both sexes. When it was administered by subcutaneous injection, an increase in mammary carcinomas was also observed in female rats.[247]

Chloroform

Chloroform ($CHCl_3$) is a clear, colorless, volatile liquid. It is nonflammable, but upon contact with a flame it can decompose to form hydrochloric acid, phosgene, and chlorine.[317] The primary use for chloroform is in the production of fluorocarbons.[5,317] It is also widely used as a solvent for many products and compounds, some of which are lacquers, resins, adhesives, and waxes, and in other industrial and manufacturing processes such as in the manufacture of artificial silk and as a solvent for extraction of some antibiotics.[5,317] Chloroform was initially used as an anesthetic, but that use has been discontinued. Chloroform is also an unwanted by-product that is formed during the chlorination of water and is often present at low levels in municipal water supplies.[36,56,192,292]

Exposure to chloroform occurs in both occupational and nonoccupational settings. Workers in a variety of industries in which chloroform is used as an intermediate or a solvent or occurs as a by-product can be exposed to it by inhalation, dermal absorption, or ingestion.[5,247,317] The general population may be exposed through drinking water or by inhalation of contaminated air.‡ Chloroform has been detected in the atmosphere and in indoor air.

Chloroform is enzymatically metabolized in mammals by cytochrome P-450–dependent mixed-function oxidases.§ Induction of hepatic mixed-function oxidase activity by phenobarbital and other inducers enhanced the toxicity of chloroform in rats.[231] Phenobarbital pretreatment of C57 Black mice also enhanced the binding of chloroform metabolites to microsomal lipids, whereas pretreatment with the mixed-function oxidase inhibitor piperonyl butoxide decreased the amount of binding.[166,189] The initial oxidative hydroxylation of chloroform leads to the production

of trichloromethanol, which is unstable and spontaneously dechlorinates to produce $COCl_2$.[269,316] This metabolite is electrophilic and readily forms covalent bonds with cellular macromolecules.

Chloroform is a hepatic and renal toxin in rats and mice.[5] Acute toxicity is manifested in both organs as cell degeneration and necrosis.* In the rat kidney there is also a strong regenerative response, resulting in large increases in DNA synthesis and mitosis in the renal epithelial cells lining the proximal tubules.[203] Chloroform also causes liver enlargement, hepatotoxicity, and kidney damage in humans, with alcoholics affected sooner and more severely than nonalcoholics.[267,304,326] Altered liver function was reported by Smith and colleagues[319] in patients anesthetized with chloroform. Case reports of fatal chloroform exposures demonstrate severe liver and kidney damage.[211,267,294]

The ability of chloroform metabolites to bind covalently to DNA and/or induce mutations is not completely resolved.[65,89,264,293] However, it is generally considered to be a weak mutagen at most. It does not induce mutations in bacterial mutagenesis tests, unscheduled DNA synthesis, or cell-mediated mutagenesis assays.† There is some evidence, however, that chloroform induces chromosomal aberrations in vivo in rat bone marrow cells[118] and sister chromatid exchanges in human lymphocytes in vitro.[242]

Chronic animal bioassays have demonstrated the carcinogenic potential of chloroform in rat kidney and mouse liver. Renal carcinomas were induced in male rats when chloroform was administered by gavage or in the drinking water.[180,284,369] Liver neoplasms were also induced in mice by gavage exposure but not when chloroform was administered in the drinking water.[180,369] Renal neoplasms were also induced in male mice after administration of chloroform in a toothpaste, but only in one of four strains tested.[290] The data are inadequate regarding the carcinogenicity of chloroform in humans.[247] Although some reports have suggested an association between chloroform exposure (via drinking water) and human cancer, a variety of confounding factors render these data inconclusive.[13,57,392]

2,3,7,8-TETRACHLORODIBENZO-*p*-DIOXIN

The chemical 2,3,7,8-tetrachlorodibenzo-*p*-dioxin (TCDD; $C_{12}H_4Cl_4O_2$) is a colorless, odorless, crystalline solid. It is insoluble in water, slightly soluble in methanol, and soluble in benzene, chloroform, dichlorobenzene, and chlororbenzene.[171,317] It has no known use and is primarily a research chemical.[247,317] It is not commerically produced in the United States. Polychlorinated dibenzo-*p*-dioxins are formed during the manufacture of all dichlorophenols, depending upon the temperatures reached;[317] TCDD is a concern because it is formed as an unwanted contaminant during the production of some organic sol-

---

*References 104, 173, 249, 280-282, 286, 318.
†References 7, 18, 85, 100, 102, 104, 173, 247, 369.
‡References 30, 36, 192, 312, 314, 359.
§References 188, 231, 316, 343.

*References 54, 79, 103, 166, 203, 242, 259, 335.
†References 87, 187, 238, 291, 343, 348.

vents, herbicide precursors and herbicides, and chlorine-bleached paper products.[14,110,277] It may also be present in emissions from coal-burning power plants, diesel engine exhaust, and the incomplete incineration of chlorine-containing wastes (such as PVC plastics).[55,62,97,98] It may also be produced in small amounts from natural sources such as forest fires. It can bioaccumulate in the food chain and is readily sequestered in fatty tissues.[278,322]

The herbicide 2,4,5-T was banned by the EPA in the later 1970s, as was the use of polychlorinated biphenyls (PCBs) in electrical transformers and heat exchangers, thus limiting two important sources of TCDD contamination. Current human exposures to TCDD are primarily from sources of environmental contamination and some occupational situations. Workers involved in the manufacture of some herbicides and organic solvents, as well as municipal and industrial incinerator and hazardous waste site workers, have the potential for exposure to TCDD.[55,62,97,202] Those involved in fighting fires and cleaning up transformer or capacitor fires and hazardous waste accidents are also at risk from TCDD exposure.[247] Because low levels of TCDD are virtually ubiquitous in industrialized countries and TCDD can bioaccumulate in the food chain, there is potential in certain areas for exposure of the general population.

Exposure to TCDD can occur by inhalation, dermal absorption, and ingestion. Metabolism of TCDD in mammals is slow,[356] and it is therefore distributed throughout the body and accumulates in tissues. Some reports imply that no metabolism occurs in mammalian systems.[202] However, TCDD accumulates in adipose tissue, and it readily accumulates in breast milk.[202,278,279] It can have a half-life of over 7 years in human adipose tissue. It induces the activity of aryl hydrocarbon hydroxylase, and its toxicity is mediated through binding to a cytosolic receptor and translocation to the nucleus.[202,270] Major metabolites are methoxylated and hydroxylated TCDD derivatives that can be conjugated to glucuronides and sulfates.

Although TCDD is a potent toxin and a carcinogen, there is a wide degree of variability among species in their sensitivity to toxicity and carcinogenicity. When administered by gavage, TCDD caused an increase in the incidence of hepatocellular carcinomas in male and female mice.[171,175,247] It induced hepatocellular carcinomas and squamous cell carcinomas of the hard palate nasal turbinates in female rats and squamous carcinomas of the tongue and hard palate nasal turbinates in male rats after dietary exposure.[190,191] Female mice developed fibrosarcomas after topical administration.[190,191] Liver tumors and thymic lymphomas were induced in infant mice exposed by subcutaneous injection.[247] It also induced cholangiocarcinomas and neoplasms of the lung, tongue, skin, and thyroid.[271,275] It is also an effective promoter of diethylnitrosamine-initiated hepatocellular carcinomas in rats and skin neoplasia in mice.[111,112,268,272]

No conclusive epidemiological studies link TCDD to cancer in humans. Most studies have focused on phenoxy herbicide exposures, probably reflecting contamination of the herbicides with TCDD. A few studies point to an association between soft tissue sarcoma and non-Hodgkin's lymphoma and TCDD.* However, there are other studies in which no excess deaths due to cancer were found after TCDD exposure.[109,129]

The most consistent pathologic condition in humans linked to TCDD exposure is chloracne.[28,227,243,270] It has developed in workers exposed by inhalation, ingestion, and dermal contact. The lesions generally resolve within 1 to 3 years.[243] After acute exposures related to industrial accidents, workers and other exposed populations have developed a number of acute health problems, including liver enlargement, peripheral neuropathy, and diarrhea. Most conditions did not persist.

In laboratory animals, TCDD is an acute poison; however, sensitivity to the toxicity varies greatly. Guinea pigs are some 5000 to 10,000 times more sensitive than hamsters to the lethal toxicity of TCDD.[202] In general, males are more sensitive than females. Acute toxicity in laboratory animals is characterized by hepatotoxicity, weight loss, thymic atrophy, thrombocytopenia, immunosuppression, and chloracne.[202,270]

AFLATOXIN B_1

Aflatoxin B_1 ($C_{17}H_{12}O_6$) is a pale yellow, crystalline mycotoxin that is fluorescent under ultraviolet light.[317] It is slightly soluble in water, insoluble in nonpolar solvents, and highly soluble in moderately polar solvents, especially dimethylsulfoxide. Aflatoxins are a product of the fungus *Aspergillus flavus* and *A. parasiticus* that has no commercial use or production. It is produced in small quantities for laboratory use. The fungal strains that produce aflatoxin B_1 are widespread in warmer climates and potential contaminants in a wide variety of foodstuffs.[12,308,325] Although this is controlled in many countries by harvest methods and storage of crops at low-moisture conditions, aflatoxin contamination persists in many areas of the world. The presence of aflatoxin in food has been epidemiologically linked to the development of hepatocellular carcinoma in Asian and African populations.[12,175,308]

Aflatoxin B_1 is metabolized by the cytochrome P-450–dependent mixed-function oxidase enzymes, ultimately resulting in AFB_1-2,3-epoxide.[332,379] This reactive metabolite covalently binds to RNA, protein, and DNA, particularly the N^7 atom of guanine, forming the AFB_1-N^7-guanyl adduct.[105,379] It is the AFB_1-DNA adduct that is thought to mediate the toxic and carcinogenic effects of aflatoxin B_1. Detoxification of aflatoxin B_1 can occur by conjugation with glutathione, as well as active repair of the AFB-DNA adducts.[83,105,379] There are species differences in the level of metabolism, glutathione conjugation, and repair of the

---

*References 101, 138, 139, 156, 382.

DNA adducts, which correlated with the hepatocarcinogenic response.

Aflatoxin B_1 is a potent hepatocarcinogen in some laboratory animals. There are, however, striking differences among species in the carcinogenic response. The mouse is relatively resistant to the hepatocarcinogenic effects.[78,105,324] The rat is relatively sensitive to aflatoxin B_1–induced carcinogenesis. Male rats fed as little aflatoxin B_1 as 1 g/kg of diet developed liver neoplasms, including hepatocellular carcinoma in excess of the control animals.[379] A linear dose-response relationship was also noted in rats for liver cancer.[379] A number of other studies demonstrated the hepatocarcinogenic potential of this chemical.[175] In addition, aflatoxin B_1 induced carcinomas in other organs in rats, including the kidney, colon, and glandular stomach.[175,247] Several other animal species, including salmonid fishes,[315] guppies,[302] ducks,[59] and some nonhuman primates,[2] developed hepatocellular carcinomas following aflatoxin B_1 exposure. Strong associations have been made between exposure to aflatoxin B_1 and human liver cancer.[175,247]

NITROSAMINES

Nitrosamines are among the most potent chemical carcinogens that have been tested in laboratory animals. As a chemical class, they induce neoplasia in a wide spectrum of both animal species and target organs.[175,247] For the most part, they are not currently produced commerically in the United States and are not in general industrial use. Their major use is as research chemicals. However, many of the nitrosamines have been detected in a wide variety of products and/or are formed during industrial processes.[247] Nitrosamines can be formed under the right set of conditions by interactions between nitrosating agents and primary and secondary amines. A number of nitrosamines are produced during rubber processing and may be present in the completed product.[247] Nitrosamines have also been detected in foods, including smoked and cured meats and fish, cheeses, some alcoholic beverages, spices, and soybean oil.[175,247] They are also components of tobacco products and tobacco smoke (see Chapters 13 and 26).[49-51,150]

Exposure to nitrosamines can occur by ingestion, dermal contact, and inhalation. Exposure to a variety of nitrosamines occurs during cigarette smoking. Consumers can be exposed to N-nitrosodiethanolamine in some facial cosmetics, lotions, and shampoos.[247] Workers in machine shops and manufacturing firms can be exposed to nitrosamines from the use of synthetic and semisynthetic cutting oils.[247]

Many nitrosamines are biochemically activated in target cells by oxidation via mixed-function oxidases to reactive electrophilic metabolites.[20,26,217] For example, N-nitrosodimethylamine (DMNA) is metabolically activated to alkylcarbonium ions that are capable of alkylating DNA at specific sites.[26] For DMNA, major DNA adducts include the O^6-methylguanine and 7-methylguanine. For longer-chain or cyclic nitrosamines, a hydroxylation is the critical activation reaction.[150,198,374] A few nitrosamines such as N-nitroso-N-methylurea are direct-acting alkylating agents.[374] For the discussion on toxic and carcinogenic potential, DMNA and N-nitrosodiethylamine (DENA) will serve as model compounds.

N-nitrosodiethylamine and N-Nitrosodimethylamine

Two of the most widespread nitrosamines are DENA and DMNA. Both DENA $(C_2H_5)_2$ NNO) and DMNA $[(CH_3)_2NNO]$ are volatile, yellow oils that are soluble in lipids, ether, organic solvents, alcohol, and water.[317] They both rapidly photodegrade when exposed to light, especially ultraviolet light. Most species studied to date appear to have some capability of metabolically activating these carcinogens. Human cells in vitro are capable of activating DMNA to metabolites that bind to DNA and are mutagenic.[26,142,144] However, adequate data do not exist to evaluate the carcinogenicity of DENA or DMNA directly in humans.[172,175,247]

Both DENA and DMNA are potent carcinogens in laboratory animals. Chronic exposure to either chemical results in the induction of multiple tumor types in a variety of animal species.[175,247] Hepatocellular neoplasms were induced in many species including rats, mice, fish, gerbils, guinea pigs, hamsters, hedgehogs, newts, and monkeys by either DMNA or DENA.[247] Tumors of the trachea and lung were induced in mice, hamsters, gerbils, and rats. Other neoplasms induced by these nitrosamines include forestomach and esophageal neoplasms in mice, rats, and hamsters; nasal cavity neoplasms in mice, hamsters, and gerbils; kidney neoplasms in rats and mice; hemangiosarcomas of the liver in mice and ducks, and cholangiocarcinomas in rats, hamsters, and mastomys (see Table 26-5).[175,247]

REFERENCES

1. Aaserud O, et al: Neurological examination, compuerized tomography, cerebral blood flow and neuropsychological examination in workers with long-term exposure to carbon disulfide, *Toxicology* 49:277, 1988.
2. Adamson RH, Correa P, Dalgard DW: Occurrence of a primary liver carcinoma in a rhesus monkey fed aflatoxin B_1, *J Natl Cancer Inst* 50:549, 1973.
3. Agarwal ID, Kleisch U, Keifer F: Metabolism of benzo[(a)]pyrene by human melanocytes in culture, *Carcinogenesis* 12:1963, 1991.
4. Agency for Toxic Substances and Disease Registry (ATSDR): *Toxicological profile for benzene*, TP-92/03, Atlanta, 1993, ATSDR.
5. Agency for Toxic Substances and Disease Registry (ATSDR): *Toxicological profile for chloroform*, Atlanta, 1993, ATSDR.
6. Agency for Toxic Substances and Disease Registry (ATSDR): *Toxicological profile for vinyl chloride*, TP-92/20, Atlanta, 1993, ATSDR.
7. Agency for Toxic Substances and Disease Registry (ATSDR): *Toxicological profile for carbon tetrachloride*, draft for public comment, Atlanta, 1993, ATSDR.
8. Agency for Toxic Substances and Disease Registry (ATSDR): *Toxicological profile for polycyclic aromatic hydrocarbons (PAH's)*, draft for public comment, Atlanta, 1993, ATSDR.

9. Agency for Toxic Substances and Disease Registry (ATSDR): *Toxicological profile for tetrachloroethylene*, Atlanta, 1993, ATSDR.

10. Albert RE, et al: Gaseous formaldehyde and hydrogen chloride induction of nasal cancer in the rat, *J Natl Cancer Inst* 68:597, 1982.

11. Albert RE, et al: Benzo(*a*)pyrene-induced skin damage and tumor promotion in the mouse, *Carcinogenesis* 12:1273, 1991.

12. Alpert ME, et al: Association between aflatoxin content of food and hepatoma frequency in Uganda, *Cancer* 28:253, 1971.

13. Alvanja M, Goldstein I, Susser M: *A case control study of gastrointestinal and urinary tract cancer mortality and drinking water chlorination.* In Jolley RJ, Gorchen H, Hamilton DH Jr, editors: *Water chlorination: environmental impact and health effects*, Ann Arbor, Mich, 1978, Ann Arbor Science Publications.

14. Amendola G, et al: The occurrence and fate of PCDDs and PCDFs in five bleached kraft pulp and paper mills, *Chemosphere* 18:1181, 1989.

15. Ames BN, Gold LS: Too many rodent carcinogens: mitogenesis increases mutagenesis, *Science* 249:970, 1990.

16. Ames BN, Shigenaga MK, Gold LS: DNA lesions, inducible DNA repair, and cell division: three key factors in mutagenesis and carcinogenesis, *Environ Health Perspect* 101(suppl 5):35, 1993.

17. Anderson J, et al: Induction of formaldehyde contact sensitivity: dose-response relationship in the guinea pig maximization test, *Acta Derm Venereol (Stockh)* 65;472, 1985.

18. Andervont HB: Induction of hepatomas in strain C3H mice with 4-0 tolylaxo-*o*-toluidine and carbon tetrachloride, *J Natl Cancer Inst* 20:431, 1958.

19. Antove G, et al: Effect of carbon disulphide on the cardiovascular system, *J Hyg Epidemiol Microbiol Immunol* 29:329, 1985.

20. Argus, et al: Dimethylnitrosamine-demethylase: absence of increased enzyme catabolism and multiplicity of effector sites in repression: hemoprotein involvement, *Chem Biol Interact* 13:127, 1976.

21. Askoy M: Benzene and leukemia, *Lancet* 1:441, 1978.

22. Askoy M: Different types of malignancies due to occupational exposure to benzene: a review of recent observations in Turkey, *Environ Res* 23:181, 1980.

23. Askoy M: Malignancies due to occupational exposure to benzene, *Am J Ind Med* 7:395, 1985.

24. Askoy M: Hematotoxicity and carcinogenicity of benzene, *Environ Health Perspect* 82:193, 1989.

25. Askoy M, Erdem S: Follow-up study on the mortality and the development of leukemia in 44 pancytopenic patients with chronic benzene exposure, *Blood* 52:285, 1978.

26. Autrup H, Harris CC: *Metabolism of chemical carcinogens by human tissues.* In Harris CC, Autrup HN, editors: *Human carcinogenesisi*, New York, 1983, Academic Press.

27. Autrup H, et al: Metabolism of (³H) benzo[*a*]pyrene by cultured human bronchus and cultured human pulmonary alveolar macrophages, *Lab Invest* 38:217, 1978.

28. Avigdor S, Zakheim D, Barnea ER: Quinone reductase activity in first trimester placenta: effect of cigarette smoking and polycyclic aromatic hydrocarbons, *Reprod Toxicol* 6:336, 1992.

29. Barber Ed, Donish WH, Mueller KR: A procedure for the quantitative measurement of the mutagenicity of volatile liquids in the Ames salmonella/microsome assay. *Mutat Res* 90:31, 1981.

30. Barkley J, et al: Gas chromatography mass spectrometry computer analysis of volatile halogenated hydrocarbons in man and his environment: a multimedia environmental study, *Biomed Mass Spectrom* 7:130, 1980.

31. Barnea ER, Shurtz-Swirski R: Modification of pulsatile human chorionic gonadotrophin secretion in first trimester placental explants induced by polycyclic aromatic hydrocarbons, *Hum Reprod* 7:305, 1988.

32. Barsotti M, Vigliani EC: Bladder lesions from aromatic amines, *Med Lav* 40:129, 1949.

33. Bartsch H, et al: Mutagenic and alkylating metabolites of haloethylenes, chlorobutadienes, and dichlorobutenes produced by rodent or human liver tissues, *Arch Toxicol* 41:249, 1979.

34. Beauchamp RO, et al: A critical review of the literature on carbon disulphide toxicity, *Crit Rev Toxicol* 11:169, 1983.

35. Beland FA, Kadlubar FF: Formation and persistence of arylamine DNA adducts in vivo, *Environ Health Perspect* 62:19, 1985.

36. Bellar TA, Lichtenberg JJ, Kroner RC: The occurrence of organohalides in chlorinated drinking water, *J AWWA* 66:703, 706, 1974.

37. Belli S, et al: A cohort study on vinyl chloride manufacturers in Italy: study design and preliminary results, *Cancer Lett* 35:253, 1987.

38. Bi W, et al: Effect of vinyl chloride on testes in rats, *Ecotoxicol Environ Safety* 10:281, 1985.

39. Bi W, et al: Mortality and incidence of bladder cancer in benzidine-exposed workers in China, *Am J Ind Med* 231:481, 1992.

40. Bingham E, Falk HL: Environmental carcinogens: the modifying effect of carcinogens on the threshold response, *Arch Environ Health* 19:779, 1969.

41. Blair A, Decoufle P, Grauman D: Causes of death among laundry and dry cleaning workers, *Am J Public Health* 69:508, 1979.

42. Blair A, et al: Cancer and other causes of death among a cohort of dry cleaners, *Br J Ind Med* 47;162, 1990.

43. Blanton RH: Modulation of immunocompetent cell populations by benzo(*a*)pyrene, *Toxicol Appl Pharmacol* 93:267, 1988.

44. Blanton RH, et al: Immunomodulation of polyaromatic hydrocarbons in mice and murine cells, *Cancer Res* 46:2735, 1986.

45. Bolt HM, et al: Disposition of (1,2,¹⁴C) vinyl chloride in the rat, *Arch Toxicol* 35:153, 1976.

46. Bolt HM, et al: Pharmacokinetics of vinyl chloride in the rat, *Toxicology* 7:179, 1977.

47. Bolt HM, et al: Binding kinetics of vinyl chloride and vinyl bromide at very low doses, in. quantitative aspects of risk assessment in chemical carcinogenesis, *Arch Toxicol Suppl* 3:129, 1980.

48. Bond EJ, DeMatteis F: Biochemical changes in rat liver after administration of carbon disulphide with particular reference to microsomal changes, *Biochem Pharmacol* 18:2531, 1969.

49. Brunneman KD, Hoffman D: *Chemical studies in tobacco smoke: analysis of volatile nitrosamines in tobacco smoke and polluted indoor environments. In: Environmental aspects of n-nitroso compounds*, IARC Scientific Publication 19, Lyon, 1978, International Agency for Research on Cancer.

50. Brunnemann KD, Hoffman D: Assessment of carcinogenic *n*-nitrosodiethanolamine in tobacco products and tobacco smoke, *Carcinogenesis* 2:1123, 1981.

51. Brunnemann KD, Yu L, Hoffman D: Assessment of carcinogenic volatile nitrosamines in snuff tobacco, *Carcinogenesis* 3;693, 1982.

52. Bryen D, et al: Mortality and cancer morbidity in a group of Swedish VCM and PCM production workers, *Environ Health Perspect* 17:167, 1976.

53. Buchter A, et al: Pharmacokinetics of vinyl chloride in the rhesus monkey, *Toxicol Lett* 6:33, 1980.

54. Bull RJ, et al: Enhancement of hepatotoxicity of chloroform in B6C3F$_1$ mice by corn oil: implications for chloroform carcinogenesis, *Environ Health Perspect* 69:1645, 1986.

55. Buser HR, Bosshart HP, Rappe C: Identification of polychlorinated dibenzo-*para*-dioxin isomers in fly-ash, *Chemosphere* 7:165, 1978.

56. Bush B, Narang RS, Syrotynski S: Screening for haloorganics in New York state drinking water, *Bull Environ Contam Toxicol* 18:436, 1977.

57. Cantor KP, et al: Associations of cancer mortality with halomethanes in drinking water, *J Natl Cancer Inst* 61:979, 1978.

58. Caputo R, et al: Cutaneous manifestations of tetrachlorodibenzo-*p*-

dioxin in children and adolescents: follow-up 10 years after the Sevaso, Italy, accident, *J Am Acad Dermatol* 19:812, 1988.

59. Carnaghan RS: Hepatic tumors in ducks fed a low level of toxic ground nut meal, *Nature* 208:308, 1965.

60. Case RA: Tumours of the urinary bladder in workmen engaged in the manufacture and use of certain dyestuff intermediates in the British chemical industry, *Br J Ind Med* 11:75, 1954.

61. Cavalieri EL, et al: Tumorigenicity of 6-halogenated derivatives of benzo[a]pyrene in mouse skin and rat mammary gland, *J Cancer Res Clin Oncol* 114:10, 1988.

62. Cavallaro A, et al: Sampling, occurence and evaluation of PCDDs and PCDFs from incinerated solid urban waste, *Chemosphere* 9:611, 1980.

63. Chandra SV, Butler WH, Neal RA: The effect of carbon disulphide on the myocardium of the rat, *Exp Mol Pathol* 17:249, 1972.

64. Chapman JAW, Connolly JG, Rosenbaum L: *Occupational bladder: a case controlled study.* In Connolly JE, editor: *Carcinoma of the bladder,* New York, 1981, Raven Press.

65. Colacci AS, et al: Chloroform bioactivation leading to nucleic acid binding, *Tumori* 77:285, 1991.

66. Cole KE, et al: In vitro binding of aflatoxin B_1 and 2-acetylaminofluorene to rat, mouse and human hepatocyte DNA: the relationship of DNA binding to carcinogenicity, *Carcinogenesis* 9:711, 1988.

67. Cole KE, et al: Comparative effects of three carcinogens on human, rat and mouse hepatocytes, *Carcinogenesis* 10:139, 1989.

68. Collingwood KW, Pasternack BS, Shore RE: An industry-wide study of respiratory cancer in chemical workers exposed to chloromethyl ethers, *J Natl Cancer Inst* 78:1127, 1978.

69. Collins CJ, Guild WR: Irreversible effects of formaldehyde on DNA, *Biochim Biophys Acta* 157:107, 1968.

70. Cooke M, Dennis AJ: *Polynuclear aromtic hydrocarbons: a decade of progress,* Columbus, 1988, Batelle.

71. Cooper JR, Kini MM: Editorial: biochemical aspects of methanol poisoning, *Biochem Pharmacol* 11:405, 1962.

72. Cooper WC: Epidemiological study of vinyl chloride workers: mortality through December 31, 1972, *Environ Health Perspect* 41:101, 1981.

73. Corsi G, et al: Chronic peripheral neuropathy in workers with previous exposure to carbon disulphide, *Br J Ind Med* 40:209, 1980.

74. Costa AK, Ivanetich KM: Tetrachloroethylene metabolism by the hepatic microsomal cytochrome *p*-450 system, *Biochem Pharmacol* 29:2863, 1980.

75. Cowfer JA, Magistro AJ: *Vinyl chloride.* In: *Kirk-Othmer encyclopedia of chemical technology,* vol 23, New York, 1983, John Wiley.

76. Craddock VM, Henderson AR: De novo and repair replication of DNA in liver of carcinogen-treated animals, *Cancer Res* 38:2135, 1978.

77. Creech JL, Johnson MN: Angiosarcoma of liver in the manufacture of polyvinyl chloride, *J Occup Med* 16:150, 1974.

78. Croy RG, Essigman JM, Wogan GN: Aflatoxin B_1: correlation of patterns of metabolism and DNA modification with biological effects, *Basic Life Sci* 24:49, 1983.

79. Culliford D, Hewitt HB: The influence of sex hormone status on the susceptibility of mice to chloroform-induced necrosis of the renal tubules, *J Endocrinol* 14:381, 1957.

80. Dalvi RR, Hunter AL, Neal RA: Toxicological implications of the mixed-function oxidase catalyzed metabolism of carbon disulphide, *Chem Biol Interact* 10:349, 1975.

81. Dean BJ, Hodson-Walker G: An *in vitro* chromosome assay using cultured rat liver cells, *Mutat Res* 64:329, 1979.

82. DeFonso LR, Kelton SC: Lung cancer following exposure to chloromethyl methyl ether, *Arch Environ Health* 31:125, 1976.

83. Degan GH, Neumann HG: Differences in aflatoxin B_1 susceptibility of rat and mouse are correlated with the capability *in vitro* to inactivate aflatoxin B_1 epoxide, *Carcinogenesis* 2:299, 1981.

84. Dekant W, Metzler M, Henschler D: Identification of S-1,2,2-trichlorovinyl-*n*-acetylcysteine as a urinary metabolite of tetrachloroethylene: bioactivation through glutathione conjugation as a possible explanation of its nephrocarcinogenicity, *J Biochem Toxicol* 1:57, 1986.

85. Della Porta GD, Terracine B, Shubik P: Induction with carbon tetrachloride of liver cell carcinomas in hamsters, *J Natl Cancer Inst* 26:855-863, 1961.

86. DeMatteis F, Seawright AA: Oxidative metabolism of carbon disulphide by the rat: effect of treatments which modify the liver toxicity of carbon disulphide, *Chem Biol Interact* 7:375, 1973.

87. DeSerres FJ, Ashby J: *Evaluation of short-term tests for carcinogens.* In: *Progress in mutation research,* Amsterdam, 1981, Elsevier.

88. Diaz-Gomez MI, Castro JA: Covalent binding of carbon tetrachloride metabolites to liver nuclear DNA, proteins and lipids, *Toxicol Appl Pharmacol* 56:199, 1980.

89. Diaz-Gomez MI, Castro JA: Covalent binding of chloroform metabolites to nuclear proteins: no evidence for binding to nucleic acids, *Cancer Lett* 9:213-218, 1980.

90. Dipple A: *Polynuclear aromatic hydrocarbons:* In Searle CE, editor: *Chemical carcinogens,* American Cancer Society monograph 173, Washington, DC, 1976, ACS.

91. Doll R: Effects of exposure to vinyl chloride, *Scand J. Work Environ Health* 14:61-78, 1988.

92. Doll R, Peto R: The causes of cancer: quantitative estimates of avoidable risks of cancer in the United States today, *J Natl Cancer Inst* 66:1191, 1981.

93. Duh RW, Asal NR: Mortality among laundry and dry-cleaning workers in Oklahoma, *Am J Public Health* 74:1278, 1984.

94. Duprat P, et al: Metabolic approach to industrial poisoning: blood kinetics and distribution of ^{14}C-vinyl chloride (VCM), *Acta Pharmacol Toxicol (Supp)* 41:142, 1977.

95. Dutkiewicz T, Baranowska R: *The significance of absorption of carbon disulphide through the skin in the evaluation of exposure.* In Brieger H, editor: *Toxicology of carbon disulphide,* Amsterdam, 1967, Excerpta Medical Foundation.

96. Egeland GM, et al: Effects of exposure to carbon disulphide on low density lipoprotein cholesterol concentration and diastolic blood pressure, *Br J Ind Med* 49:287, 1992.

97. Eiceman GA, Clement RE, Karasek FW: Analysis of fly-ash from municipal incinerators for trace organic compounds, *Anal Chem* 51:2343, 1979.

98. Environmental Protection Agency (EPA): *Health assessment document or polychlorinated dibenzo-p-dioxins,* Washington, DC, 1985, EPA.

99. Environmental Protection Agency (EPA): *Health assessment document for tetrachloroethylene (perchloroethylene),* Washington, DC, 1985, EPA.

100. Environmental Protection Agency (EPA). *Evaluation of the potential carcinogenicity of carbon tetrachloride (56-23-5): final report,* Washington, DC, 1988, EPA.

101. Eriksson M, et al: Soft tissue sarcomas and exposure to chemical substances: a case referent study, *Br J Ind Med* 38:27, 1981.

102. Eschenbrenner AB, Miller E: Studies on hepatomas: size and spacing of multiple doses in the induction of carbon tetrachloride hepatomas, *J Natl Cancer Inst* 4:385, 1944.

103. Eschenbrenner AB, Miller E: Sex diferences in kidney morphology and chloroform necrosis, *Science* 103:302, 1945.

104. Eschenbrenner AB, Miller E: Liver necrosis and the induction of carbon tetrachloride hepatomas in strain A mice, *J Natl Cancer Inst* 6:325, 1946.

105. Essigman JM, et al: Metabolic activation of aflatoxin B_1: patterns of

DNA adduct formation, removal and excretion in relation to carcinogenesis, *Drug Metab Rev* 13:581, 1982.

106. Feldman MY: Reactions of nucleic acids and nucleoproteins with formaldehyde. *Prog Nucleic Acid Res Mol Biol* 13:1, 1973.

107. Ferber KH, Hill WJ, Cobb DA: An assessment of the effect of improved working conditions on bladder tumor incidence in a benzidine manufacturing facility, *Am Ind Hyg Assoc J* 37:61, 1976.

108. Figueroa WG, Raszkowski R, Weiss W: Lung cancer in chloromethylmethyl ether workers, *N Eng J Med* 288:1096, 1973.

109. Fingerhut MA, et al: An evaluation of reports of dioxin exposure and soft tissue sarcoma pathology among chemical workers in the United States, *Scand J Work Environ Health* 10:299, 1984.

110. Firestone D: Etiology of chick edema disease, *Environ Health Perspect* 5:59, 1973.

111. Flodstrom S, Ahlborg UG: Tumor promoting effects of 2,3,7,8-tetrachlorodibenzo-p-dioxin (TCDD): effects of exposure duration, administration schedule and type of diet, *Chemosphere* 19:779, 1989.

112. Flodstrom S, et al: Modulation of 2,3,7,8-tetrachlorodibenzo-p-dioxin and phenobarbital-induced promotion of hepatocarcinogenesis in rats by the type of diet and vitamin A deficiency, *Fundam Appl Toxicol* 16:375, 1991.

113. Forni A: Chromosome changes and benzene exposure: a review, *Rev Environ Health* 3:5, 1979.

114. Forni A, Moreo L: Cytogenetic studies in a case of benzene leukemia, *Eur J Cancer* 3:251, 1967.

115. Forni A, Moreo L: Chromosome studies in a case of benzene-induced erythroleukemia, *Eur J Cancer* 5:459, 1969.

116. Fox AJ, Collier PF: Mortality experience of workers exposed to vinylchloride monomer in the manufacture of polyvinylchloride in Great Britian, *Br J Ind Med* 34:1, 1977.

117. Frantz SW, Watanabe PG: Tetrachlorethylene: balance and tissue distribution in male sprague dawly rats by drinking water administration, *Toxicol Appl Pharmacol* 69:66, 1983.

118. Fujie K, Aoki T, Wada M: Acute cytogenetic effects of trihalomethanes on rat bone marrow cells *in vivo, Mutat Res* 242:111, 1990.

119. Gargus JL, Reese WH, Rutter HA: Induction of lung adenomas in newborn mice by bis(chloromethyl)ether, *Toxicol Appl Pharmacol* 15:92, 1969.

120. Garry VF, et al: Preparation for human study of pesticide applicators: sister chromatid exchanges and chromosome aberrations in cultured human lymphocytes exposed to selected fumigants, *Teratogenesis Carcinog Mutagen* 10:21, 1990.

121. Gelboin HV: Benzo[a]pyrene metabolism, activation, and carcinogenesis: role and regulation of mixed-function oxidases and related enzymes, *Physiol Rev* 60:1107, 1980.

122. Gilioli R, et al: Study of neurological and neurophysiological impairment of carbon disulfide workers, *Med Lav* 69:120, 1978.

123. Goldsworthy TL, Popp JA: Chlorinated hydrocarbon-induced peroxisomal enzyme activity in relation to species and organ carcinogenicity, *Toxicol Appl Pharmacol* 88:225, 1987.

124. Goldsworthy TL, et al: Potential role of α-2u-globulinm, protein droplet accumulation and cell replication in the renal carcinogenicity of rats exposed to trichloroethylene, perchloroethylene and pentachloroethane, *Toxicol Appl Pharmacol* 88:367, 1988.

125. Gordon SJ, Meeks SA: A study of gaseous pollutants in the Houston, Texas area, *AICHE Symp Ser* 73:84, 1977.

126. Grafstrom RC, Fornace A, Harris CC: Repair of DNA damage caused by formaldehyde in human cells, *Cancer Res* 44:4323, 1984.

127. Green T, Odum J: Structure/activity studies of the nephrotoxic and mutagenic action of cysteine conjugates of chloro and fluoroalkenes, *Chem Biol Interact* 54:15, 1985.

128. Green T, et al: Perchloroethylene-induced rat kidney tumors: an investigation of the mechanisms involved and their relevance to humans, *Toxicol Appl Pharmacol* 103:77, 1990.

129. Greenwald P, et al: Sarcomas of soft tissue after Vietnam service, *J Natl Cancer Inst* 73:1107, 1984.

130. Guengerich FP, Crawford WM, Watanabe PG: Activation of vinyl chloride to covalently bound metabolites; role of 2-chloroethylene oxide and 2-chloroacetaldehyde, *Biochemistry* 18:517, 1979.

131. Guengerich FP, Watanabe PG: Metabolism of (^{14}C−) and (^{36}Cl)−labelled vinyl chloride *in vivo* and *in vitro, Biochem Pharmacol* 28:589, 1979.

132. Guild WR, Young JV, Merril JP: Anuria due to carbon tetrachloride intoxication, *Ann Intern Med* 48:1221, 1958.

133. Guyda DF: Metabolic effects of growth factors and polycyclic aromatic hydrocarbons on cultured human placental cells of early and late gestation, *J Clin Endocrinol Metab* 72:718, 1991.

134. Hahon N, Booth JA: Coinhibition of viral interferon induction by benzo(a)pyrene and chrysotile asbestos, *Environ Res* 40:102, 1986.

135. Hake CL, Stewart RD: Human exposure to tetrachloroethylene: inhalation and skin contact, *Environ Health Perspect* 21:231, 1977.

136. Haley TJ: Benzidine revisited: a review of the literature and problems associated with the use of benzidine and its cogeners, *Clin Toxicol* 8:13, 1975.

137. Hammond ED, et al: Inhalation of B[a]P and cancer in man, *Ann N Y Acad Sci* 271:116, 1976.

138. Hardell L: Malignant mesenchymal tumors and exposure to phenoxyacetic acids of chlorophenols, *Br J Cancers* 39:711, 1977.

139. Hardell L, Bengston NO: Epidemiological study of socioeconomic factors and clinical findings in Hodgkin's disease, and reanalysis of previous data regarding chemical exposure, *Br J Cancer* 48:217, 1984.

140. Harris CC, Autrup H: *Human carcinogenesis*, New York, 1984, Academic Press.

141. Harris CC, Trump BF: Human tissues and cells in biomedical research, *Surv Synth Path Res* 1:165, 1983.

142. Harris CC, et al: Metabolism of B(a)P, n-nitrosodimethylamine, and n-nitrosopyrrolidine and identification of the major carcinogen-DNA adducts formed in cultured human esophagus, *Cancer Res* 39:4401, 1979.

143. Harris CC, et al: *Carcinogen metabolism and carcinogen-DNA adducts in human tissues and cells*. In Greim H, et al, editors: *Biochemical basis of chemical carcinogenesis*, New York, 1982, Raven Press.

144. Harris CC, et al: *Carcinogen metabolism and carcinogenic DNA adducts in human tissues and cells*. In Marquardt H, Oesch F, editors: *Biochemical basis of chemical carcinogenesis* New York, 1984, Raven Press.

145. Haselkorn R, Doty P: The reaction of formaldehyde with polynucleotides, *J Biol Chem* 36:2738, 1961.

146. Hashimoto S, Glende EA, Recknagle RO: Hepatic lipid peroxidation in acute fatal human carbon tetrachloride poisoning, *N Engl J Med* 279:1082, 1968.

147. Hattemer-Frey HA, Travis CC, Land ML: Benzene: environmental partitioning and human exposure, *Environ Res* 53:221, 1990.

148. Haworth S, et al: *Salmonella* mutagenicity test results for 250 chemicals, *Environ Mutagen* 1(suppl):3, 1983.

149. Hazardous Substances Data Bank, *National toxicology information program*, Bethesda, Md, 1992, National Library of Medicine.

150. Hecht SS, Hoffman D: Tobacco-specific nitrosamines, an important group of carcinogens on tobacco and tobacco smoke, *Carcinogenesis* 9:875, 1988.

151. Hefner RE, Watanabe PG, Gehring PJ: Preliminary studies of the fate of inhaled vinyl chloride monomer in rats, *Ann N Y Acad Sci* 246:135, 1975.

152. Henderson RF, et al: The effect of dose, dose rate, route of administration and species on tissue and blood levels of benzene metabolites, *Environ Health Perspect* 82:9, 1989.

153. Hernberg S, et al: Coronary heart disease among workers exposed to carbon disulphide, *Br J Ind Med* 27:313, 1970.

154. Higginson J: Present trends in cancer epidemiology, *Can Cancer Res Conf* 8:40, 1979.

155. Higginson J, Muir CS: The role of epidemiology in elucidating the importance of environmental factor in human cancer, *Cancer Detect Prev* 1:79, 1976.

156. Hoar SK, et al: Agricultural herbicide use and risk of lymphoma and soft tissue sarcoma *JAMA* 256:1141, 1986.

157. Hong CB, et al: Follow-up study on the carcinogenicity of vinyl chloride and vinylidene chloride in rats and mice: tumor incidence and mortality subsequent to exposure, *J Toxicol Environ Health* 7:909, 1981.

158. Hsu, et al: Cell and species differences in metabolic activation of chemical carcinogens, *Mutat Res* 177:1, 1987.

159. Hsueth SZ, et al: Lung cancer exposure to chloromethyl methyl ether: an occupational survey, *Environ Sci* 31:841, 1984.

160. Huberman E, et al: Identification of mutagenic metabolites of benzo[a]pyrene in mammalian cells, *Proc Natl Acad Sci U S A*, 73:607, 1976.

161. Huff J: Absence of morphological correlation between chemical toxicity and chemical carcinogenesis, *Environ Health Perspect* 101(Suppl 5):45, 1993.

162. Huff JE, et al: Carcinogenesis studies of benzene, methyl benzene and dimethylbenzene, *Ann N Y Acad Sci* 534:427, 1988.

163. Hultmark D, et al: Ethanol inhibition of vinyl chloride metabolism in isolated rat hepatocytes, *Chem Biol Interact* 25:1, 1979.

164. Hutson DH: *Mechanisms of biotransformation.* In Hathaway DE, editor, *Foreign compound metabolism in mammals,* London, 1970, The Chemical Society.

165. Ikeda M, Imamura T: Biological half-life of trichloroethylene and tetrachloroethylene in human subjects, *Int Arch Arbeirtsmed* 31:209, 1973.

166. Ilett KF, et al: Chloroform toxicity in mice: correlation of renal and hepatic necrosis with covalent binding of metabolites to tissue macromolecules, *Exp Mol Pathol* 19:215, 1973.

167. Infante PF, Wagoner JK, Waxweiler RJ: Carcinogenic, mutagenic, and teratogenic risks associated with vinyl chloride, *Mutat Res* 41:131, 1976.

168. Infante PF, et al: Leukemia in benzene workers, *Lancet* 2:76, 1977.

169. International Agency for Research on Cancer: *IARC monographs on the evaluation of the carcinogenic risk of chemicals to man: certain polycyclic aromatic hydrocarbons and heterocyclic compounds,* vol 3, Lyon, 1973, IARC.

170. International Agency for Research on Cancer: *IARC monographs on the evaluation of the carcinogenic risk of chemicals to humans: some organochlorine pesticides,* vol 5, Lyon, 1974, IARC.

171. International Agency for Research on Cancer: *IARC monographs on the evaluation of the carcinogenic risk of chemicals to humans: some fumigants, the herbicides 2,4,-D and 2,4,5-T, chlorinated dibenzodioxins and miscellaneous industrial chemicals,* vol 15, Lyon, 1977, IARC.

172. International Agency for Research on Cancer: *IARC monographs on the evaluation of the carcinogenic risk of chemicals to humans: some n-nitroso compounds,* vol 17, Lyon, 1978, IARC.

173. International Agency for Research on Cancer: *IARC monographs on the evaluation of the carcinogenic risk of chemicals to humans: some halogenated hydrocarbons,* vol 20, Lyon, 1979, IARC.

174. International Agency for Research on Cancer: *IARC monographs on the evaluation of the carcinogenic risk of chemicals to man: some industrial chemicals and dyestuffs,* vol 29, Lyon, 1982, IARC.

175. International Agency for Research on Cancer: *IARC monographs on the evaluation of the carcinogenic risk of chemicals to humans: overall evaluations of carcinogenicity,* supplement 7, Lyon, 1987, IARC.

176. Jennings RB: Fatal fulminant acute carbon tetrachloride poisoning, *Arch Pathol* 59:269, 1955.

177. Jerina D: Role of arene oxide-oxepin system in the metabolism of aromatic substances, *Arch Biochem Biophys* 128:176, 1968.

178. Johnson BL, et al: Effects on the peripheral nervous system of workers' exposure to carbon disulfide, *Neurotoxicology* 4:53, 1983.

179. Jones RD, et al: A mortality study of vinyl chloride monomer workers employed in the United Kingdom in 1940–1974, *Scand J Environ Health* 14:153, 1988.

180. Jorgenson TA, et al: Carcinogenicity of chloroform in drinking water in male osborne-mendel rats and female B6C3F$_1$ mice, *Fundam Appl Toxicol* 5:760, 1985.

181. Kalf GF, Rushmore T, Snyder R: Benzene inhibits RNA synthesis in mitochondria from liver and bone marrow, *Chem Biol Interact* 42:353, 1982.

182. Kappus H, et al: Liver microsomal uptake of [^{14}C] vinyl chloride and transformation to protein alkylating metabolites *in vitro, Toxicol Appl Pharmacol* 37:461, 1976.

183. Keen P, Martin P: Is aflatoxin carcinogenic in man? The evidence in Swaziland. *Trop Geogr Med* 23:44, 1971.

184. Kennelly JC, et al: Binding of N-acetylbenzidine and N,N' diacetylbenzidine to hepatic DNA of rat and hamster in vivo and in vitro, *Carcinogenesis* 5:407, 1984.

185. Kerns WD, et al: Carcinogenicity of formaldehyde in rats and mice after long-term inhalation exposure, *Cancer Res* 43:4382, 1983.

186. Kipen HM, Cody FP, Goldstein BD: Use of longitudinal analysis of peripheral blood counts to validate historical reconstructions of benzene exposure, *Environ Health Perspect* 82:199, 1989.

187. Kirkland DJ, Smith KL, Van Abbe NJ: Failure of chloroform to induce chromosome damage or sister chromatid exchanges in cultured human lymphocytes and failure to induce reversion in *Escherichia coli, Food Cosmet Toxicol* 19:699, 1981.

188. Kluwe WM: *Mechanisms of acute nephrotoxicity: halogenated aliphatic hydrocarbons.* In Porter GA, editor: *Nephrotoxic mechanisms of drugs and experimental toxins,* New York, 1982, Plenum Press.

189. Kluwe WM, Hook JB: Metabolic activation of nephrotoxic haloalkanes, *Fed Proc* 39:3129, 1980.

190. Kociba RJ, et al: Results of a two-year chronic toxicity and oncogenicity study of 2,3,7,8-tetrachloro-p-dioxin in rats, *Toxicol Appl Pharmacol* 46:279, 1978.

191. Kociba RJ, et al: Toxicological studies of 2,3,7,8-tetrachloro-p-dioxin (TCDD) in rats, *Toxicol Occup Med* 4:281, 1978.

192. Krasner SW, et al: The occurrence of disinfection byproducts in the US drinking water, *J AWWA* 81:41, 1989.

193. Kuschner M, et al: Inhalation carcinogenicity of alpha-chloroethers. III, Lifetime and limited period inhalation studies with bis(chloromethyl)ether at 0.1 ppm, *Arch Environ Health* 30:73, 1975.

194. Lai EK, et al: *In vivo* spin-trapping of trichloromethyl radicals formed from carbon tetrachloride, *Biochem Pharmacol* 28:2231, 1979.

195. Lawrence CE, et al: Mortality patterns of New York state Vietman veterans, *Am J Public Health* 75:277, 1985.

196. Lee CC, et al: Inhalation toxicity of vinyl chloride and vinylidene chloride, *Environ Health Perspect* 21:25, 1977.

197. Lee CC, et al: Carcinogenicity of vinyl chloride and vinylidene chloride, *J Toxicol Environ Health* 4:15, 1978.

198. Lee M, et al: Substrate specificity and alkyl group selectivity in the metabolism of n-nitrosodialkylamines, *Cancer Res* 49:1470, 1989.

199. Leggraverend C, Guenther TM, Nebert DW: Importance of the route of administration for genetic differences in benzo(a)pyrene-induced in utero toxicity and teratogenicity, *Teratology* 29:35, 1984.

200. Leong BKJ, Kociba RJ, Jersey GC: A lifetime study of rats and mice exposed to vapors of bis(chloromethyl)ether, *Toxicol Appl Pharmacol* 58:269, 1981.

201. Lewin S: Reaction of salmon sperm deoxyribonucleic acid with formaldehye, *Arch Biochem Biophys* 113:584, 1966.

202. Lilienfeld DE, Gallo MA: 2,4-D, 2,4,5-T and 2,3,7,8-TCDD: an overview, *Epidemiol Rev* 11:28, 1989.

203. Lipsky MM, Skinner M, O'Connell C: Effects of chloroform and bromodichloromethane and DNA synthesis in male fischer 344 rat kidney, *Environ Health Perspect* 101:249, 1993.

204. Lipsky MM, et al: Interspecies comparisons of in vitro hepatocarcinogenesis, *Prog Clin Biol Res* 331:395, 1990.

205. Lloyd JW: Long-term mortality study of steelworkers. V, Respiratory cancer in coke plant workers, *J Occup Med* 13:53, 1971.

206. LoJacona F, Stecca C, Duverger M: Mutagenic activation of benzo[a]pyrene by human red blood cells, *Mutat Res* 268:21, 1992.

207. Longacre S, Kocsis J, Snyder R: Influence of strain differences in mice on the metabolism and toxicity of benzene, *Toxicol Appl Pharmacol* 60:398, 1981a.

208. Longacre S, et al: Toxicological and biochemical effects of repeated administration of benzene in mice, *J Toxicol Environ Health* 7:223, 1981.

209. Loveday KS, et al: Chromosome aberration and sister chromatid exchange tests in Chinese hamster ovary cells *in vitro* v. results with 46 chemicals, *Environ Mol Mutagen* 16:272,

210. Lundh HAB: Sequence comparison between kidney and liver lesions in the rat following carbon tetrachloride poisoning, *J Occup Med* 6:123, 1964.

211. Lunt RL: Delayed chloroform poisoning in obstetric practice, *Br Med J* 1:489, 1953.

212. Lutz WK, Schlatter CH: Mechanism of the carcinogenic action of benzene: irreversible binding to rat liver DNA, *Chem Biol Interact* 18:241, 1977.

213. Lyte M, Bick PH: Differential immunotoxic effects of the environmental chemical benzo(a)pyrene in young and aged mice, *Mech Ageing Dev* 30:333, 1985.

214. Mackenzie KM, Angevine DM: Infertility in mice exposed in utero to benzo[a]pyrene, *Biol Reprod* 24:183, 1981.

215. Maclure KM, MacMahon B: An epidemiological perspective of environmental carcinogensis, *Epidemiol Rev* 2:19, 1980.

216. MacMahon B, Monson RR: Mortality in the US rayon industry, *J Occup Med* 30:698, 1988.

217. Magee PM, Barnes JM: Carcinogenic nitroso compounds, *Adv Cancer Res* 10:163, 1967.

218. Maher KV, DeFonso LR: Respiratory cancer among chloromethyl ether workers, *J Natl Cancer Inst* 78:839, 1978.

219. Malorny G: Metabolism tests with sodium formate and formic acid in man, *Z Ernahrungswiss* 9:340, 1969.

220. Maltoni C, Cotti G: Carcinogenicity of vinyl chloride in spraguedawley rats after prenatal and postnatal exposure, *Ann N Y Acad Sci* 534:145, 1988.

221. Maltoni C, et al: Carcinogenicity bioassays of vinyl chloride monomer: a model of risk assessment on an experimental basis, *Environ Health Perspect* 41:329, 1981.

222. Mancuso TF, El-Attar AA: Cohort study of workers exposed to betanapthylamine and benzidine, *J Occup Med* 9:277, 1967.

223. Markham TN: Renal failure due to carbon tetrachloride *J Occup Med* 9:16, 1967.

224. Martin CN, Ekers SF: Studies on macromolecular binding of benzidine, *Carcinogenesis* 1:101, 1980.

225. Martin CN, et al: Binding of benzidine, N-acetylbenzidine, N,N'-diacetylbenzidine and direct blue 6 to rat liver DNA, *Environ Health Perspect* 49:101, 1983.

226. Matonski GM, Elliot EA: Bladder cancer epidemiology, *Epidemiol Rev* 3:203, 1981.

227. May G: Chloracne from the accidental production of tetrachlorobenzodioxin, *Br J Ind Med* 39:128, 1982.

228. Mazumdar S, et al: An epidemiological study of exposure to coal tar pitch volatiles among coke oven workers, *JAPCA* 25:382, 1975.

229. McCallum RI, Woolley V, Petrie A: Lung cancer associated with chloromethylmethyl ether manufacture: an investigation at two factories in the United Kindgom, *Br J Ind Med* 40:384, 1983.

230. McCann J, et al: Detection of carcinogens as mutagens in the salmonella/microsome test: assay of 300 chemicals. *Proc Natl Acad Sci USA* 72:5135, 1975.

231. McClean AEM: The effect of protein deficiency and microsomal enzyme induction by DDT and phenobarbitone on the acute toxicity of chloroform and a pyrrolizidine alkaloid, retrorsine, *Res Commun Chem Pathol Pharmacol* 31:99, 1970.

232. McGuire LW: Carbon tetrachloride poisoning, *JAMA* 99:989, 1932.

233. McKenna MJ, DiStephano V: Carbon disulphide. I, The metabolism of inhaled carbon disulphide in the rat, *J Pharmacol Exp Ther* 202:245, 1977.

234. Meigs JW, et al: Bladder tumor incidence among workers exposed to benzidine: a thirty year follow-up, *J Natl Cancer Inst* 76:1, 1986.

235. Menzie CA, Potocki BB, Santadonato J: Ambient concentrations and exposure to carcinogenic pahs in the environment, *Environ Sci Technol* 26:1278, 1992.

236. Merletti F, et al: Target organs for carcinogenicity of chemicals and industrial exposures in humans: a review of results in the IARC monographs on the evaluation of the carcinogenic risk of chemicals to humans, *Cancer Res* 44:2244, 1984.

237. Mirsalis JC, Butterworth BE: *The role of hyperplasia in liver carcinogenesis*. In Stevenson DE, et al, editors: *Mouse liver carcinogenesis mechanisms and species comparisions*, New York, 1990, Wiley-Liss.

238. Mirsalis JC, et al: Measurement of unscheduled DNA synthesis and s-phase synthesis in rodent hepatocytes following in vivo treatment: testing of 24 compounds, *Environ Mol Mutagen* 14:155, 1989.

239. Monson RR, Peters JM, Johnson MN: Proportional mortality among vinyl chloride workers, *Environ Health Perspect* 11:75, 1975.

240. Monticello TM, et al: Effect of formaldehyde gas on the respiratory tract of rhesus monkeys: pathology and cell proliferation, *Am J Pathol* 13:515, 1989.

241. Moore DH, et al: The effect of dose and vehicle on early tissue damage and regenerative activity after chloroform administration to mice, *Food Cosmet Toxicol* 20:951, 1982.

242. Morimoto K, Koizumi A: Trihalomethanes induce sister chromatid exchanges in human lymphocytes in vitro and mouse bone marrow cells *in vivo, Environ Res* 32:72, 1983.

243. Moses M, Prioleau PG: Cutaneous histological findings in chemical workers with and without chloracne with past exposure to 2,3,7,8-tetrachlorodibenzo-p-dioxin, *J Am Acad Dermatol* 12:497, 1985.

244. Moslen MT, Reynolds ES, Szabo S: Enhancement of the metabolism and hepatotoxicity of trichloroethylene and perchloroethylene, *Biochem Pharmacol* 26:369, 1977.

245. Monster AC, et al: Kinetics of tetrachloroethylene in volunteers: influence of exposure concentration and work load, *Int Arch Occup Environ Health* 42:303, 1979.

246. National Cancer Institute: *Biosassy of tetrachloroethylene for possible carcinogenicity*, DHEW Publ (NIH) 77-813, Washington, DC, National Cancer Institute.

247. National Toxicology Program: *Sixth annual report on carcinogens*, Rockville, MD, 1991, U S Dept Health and Human Services.

248. National Toxicology Program: *Technical report series. toxicology and carcinogenesis studies of tetrachloroethylene (perchloroethylene) (CAS no 127-18-4) in F344/N rats and B6C3F1 mice (inhalation studies)*, USPHS Publ (NIH) 86-2567, Research Triangle Park, NC, 1986, U S Dept Health and Human Services.

249. Nayak NC, et al: Diverse mechanisms of hepatocellular injuries due to chemicals: evidence in rats administered carbon tetrachloride, *Br J Exp Path* 56:103, 1975.

250. Neeley BW: Material balance analysis of trichlorofluoromethane and carbon tetrachloride in the atmosphere, *Sci Total Environ* 8:267, 1977.

251. Nelson CJ, et al: The influence of sex, dose, time and cross on neoplasia in mice given benzidine dihydrochloride, *Toxicol Appl Pharmacol* 64:171, 1982.

252. New PS, et al: Acute renal failure associated with carbon tetrachloride intoxication, *JAMA* 181:903, 1962.

253. Newbold RF, Brookes P: Exceptional mutagenicity of a benzo[a]pyrene diol epoxide in cultured mammalian cells, analysis of *Nature* 261:52, 1976.

254. Norpoth K, et al: Biomonitoring of benzene exposure by trace analysis of phenylguanine, *Int Arch Occup Environ Health* 60:163, 1988.

255. Norwood WD, Fuqua PA, Scudder BC: Carbon tetrachloride poisoning, *Arch Ind Hyg Occup Med* 1:90, 1950.

256. Nurminen M, Hernberg S: Effects of intervention on the cardiovascular mortality of workers exposed to carbon disulphide: a 15 year follow-up *Br Med J* 42:32, 1985.

257. Odum J, Green T: Perchloroethylene metabolism by the glutathione conjugation pathway, *Toxicologist* 7:1077, 1987.

258. Ott MG, et al: Mortality among workers occupationally exposed to benzene, *Arch Environ Health* 33:3, 1978.

259. Palmer AK, et al: Safety evaluation of toothpaste containing chloroform, II, Long-term studies in rats, *J Environ Pathol Toxicol* 2:821, 1979.

260. Panthanickal A, Marnett LJ: Arachadonic acid–dependent metabolism of a (+/−)-7,8-dihydroxy-dihydrobenzo[a]pyrene to polyguanylic acid-binding derivatives, *Chem Biol Inter* 33:239, 1981.

261. Pasternack BS, Shore RE, Albert RE: Occupational exposure to chloromethyl ethers, *J Occup Med* 19:741, 1977.

262. Pegg DG, et al: Disposition of (^{14}C) tetrachloroethylene following oral and inhalation exposure in rats, *Toxicol Appl Pharmacol* 51:465, 1979.

263. Perassi R, Martin A: Urinary protein of the rat during carbon tetrachloride poisoning, *Pathol Biol (Paris)* 21:569, 1973.

264. Pereira MNA, et al: Trihalomethanes as initiators and promoters of carcinogenesis, *Environ Health Perspect* 46:151, 1982.

265. Perera FP, Boffeta P, Nisbet IC: *What are the major carcinogens in the etiology of human cancer? Industrial carcinogens 14b.* In DeVita V, editor: *Important advances in oncology, 1989. p 249.*

266. Phillips M: Detection of carbon disulphide in breath and air: a possible new risk factor for coronary heart disease, *Occup Environ Health* 64:119, 1992.

267. Piersol GM, Tumen HJ, Kau LS: Fatal poisoning following the ingestion of chloroform, *Med Clin North Am* 17:587, 1933.

268. Pitot HC, et al: Quantitative evaluation of the promotion by 2,3,7,8-tetrachlorodibenzo-p-dioxin of hepatocarcinogenesis by diethylnitrosamine, *Cancer Res* 40:3616, 1980.

269. Pohl LR, et al: Phosgene: a metabolite of chloroform, *Biochem Biophys Res Commun* 79:684, 1977.

270. Poland A, Greenlee WF, Kende AS: Studies on the mechanism of action of the chlorinated dibenzo-p-dioxins and related compounds, *Ann N Y Acad Sci* 320:214, 1979.

271. Poland A, Knutson JC: 2,3,7,8-tetrachlorodibenzo-p-dioxin and related halogenated aromatic hydrocarbons: examination of the mechanism of toxicity, *Annu Rev Pharmacol Toxicol* 22:517, 1982.

272. Poland A, Palen D, Glover E: Tumor production by TCDD in skin of HRS/J hairless mice, *Nature* 300:271, 1982.

273. Poyer JL, et al: Spin-trapping of the trichloromethyl radical produced during enzymatic NADPH oxidation in the presence of carbon tetrachloride or bromotrichloromethane, *Biochem Biophys Acta* 539:402, 1978.

274. Price JM: *Etiology of bladder cancer.* In Maltry E, editor: *Benign and malignant tumors of the urinary bladder,* Boca Raton, Fla, 1971, Medical Examination Publishing Co.

275. Rao MS, et al: Carcinogenicity of 2,3,7,8-tetrachlorodibenzo-p-dioxin in the Syrian golden hamster, *Carcinogenesis* 9:1677, 1988.

276. Rao SB, Recknagle RO: Early incorporation of carbon labelled carbon tetrachloride into rat liver particulate lipids and proteins, *Exp Mol Pathol* 10:219, 1969.

277. Rappe C, Buser HR, Bosshardt HP: Dioxins, dibenzofurans, and other polyhalogenated aromatics: production, use, formation, and destruction, *Ann N Y Acad Sci* 320:295, 1979.

278. Rappe C, et al: *Chemistry and analysis of polychlorinated dioxins and dibenzofurans in biological samples.* In Poland A, Kimbrough R, editors: *Biological mechanisms of dioxin action,* Banbury report 18, Cold Spring Harbor, Maine, 1984, Cold Spring Harbor Laboratory.

279. Rappe C, et al: Dioxins and dibenzofurans in human tissues and milk of European origin, *Chemosphere* 15:1635, 1986.

280. Recknagle RO: Carbon tetrachloride hepatotoxicity, *Pharamcol Rev* 19:145, 1967.

281. Recknagle RO, Glende EA: Carbon tetrachloride hepatotoxicity: an example of lethal cleavage, *Crit Rev Toxicol* 2:263, 1973.

282. Recknagle RO, Goshal AK: Lipoperoxidation as a vector in carbon tetrachloride hepatotoxicity, *Lab Invest* 15:132, 1966.

283. Redmond C, et al: Long-term mortality study of steelworkers. VI, Mortality from malignant neoplasms among coke oven workers, *J Occup Med* 14:621, 1977.

284. Reuber MD: Carcinogenicity of chloroform, *Environ Health Perspect* 31:171, 1979.

285. Reuber MD, Glover EL: Cirrhosis and carcinoma of the liver in male rats given subcutaneous carbon tetrachloride, *J Natl Cancer Inst* 44:419, 1970.

286. Reynolds ES, Yee AG: Liver parenchymal cell injury. Part IV, Significance of early glucose-6-phosphatase expression and transient calcium influx following poisoning, *Lab Invest* 19:273, 1968.

287. Rinsky RA, et al: Benzene and leukemia: an epidemiological risk assessment, *N Engl J Med* 316:1044, 1987.

288. Rinsky RA, et al: Study of mortality among chemical workers in the Kanawha Valley of West Virginia, *Am J Ind Med* 13:429, 1988.

289. Rocchi P, et al: *In vivo* and *in vitro* binding of carbon tetrachloride with nucleic acids proteins in rat and mouse liver, *Int J Cancer* 11:419, 1973.

290. Roe FJC, Palmer AK, Worden AN: Safety evaluation of toothpaste containing chloroform. I, Long-term studies in mice, *J Environ Pathol Toxicol* 2:799, 1979.

291. Roldan-Aronja T, et al: An association between mutagenicity of the ara test of *Salmonella typhimuriam* and carcinogenicity in rodents for 16 halogenated aliphatic hydrocarbons, *Mutagenesis* 6:199, 1991.

292. Rook JJ: Formation of haloforms during chlorination of natural waters, *Water Treat Examin* 23:234, 1974.

293. Rosenthal SL: A review of the mutagenicity of chloroform, *Environ Mol Mutagen* 10:211, 1987.

294. Royston GD: Delayed chloroform poisoning following delivery, *Am J Obstet Gynecol* 10:808, 1924.

295. Ruijten MWM, Salle HJ, Verberk MM, Verification of effects on the nervous system of low level occupational exposure to CS$_2$, *Br J Ind Med* 50:301, 1993.

296. Ruijten MWM, et al: Special nerve functions and colour discrimination in workers with long-term low level exposure to carbon disulphide, *Br J Ind Med* 47:589, 1990.

297. Rushmore T, Snyder R, Kalf G: Covalent binding of benzene and its metabolites to DNA in rabbit bone marrow mitochondria *in vitro,* *Chem Biol Interact* 49:133, 1984.

298. Sabourin OPJ, et al: Differences in the metabolism and disposition of inhaled (3H) benzene by Fischer 344/N rats and B6C3F$_1$ mice. *Toxicol Appl Pharmacol* 94:128, 1988.

299. Sakabe H: Lung cancer due to exposure to bis(chloromethyl)ether, *Ind Health* 11:145, 1973.

300. Sammett D, et al: Partial hepatectomy reduces both the metabolism and toxicity of benzene, *J Toxicol Environ Health* 5:785, 1979.

301. Sasiadek M, Jagielski J, Smolik R: Localization of breakpoints in the karyotype of workers professionally exposed to benzene, *Mutat Res* 224:235, 1989.

302. Sato S, et al: Hepatic tumors in the guppy *(Lebistes reticulatus)* induced by aflatoxin B$_1$, dimethylnitrosamine, and 2-acetylamino-fluorene, *J Natl Cancer Inst* 50:765, 1973.

303. Schilling RSF: Coronary heart disease in viscose rayon workers, *Am Heart J* 80:1, 1970.

304. Schroeder HG: Acute and delayed chloroform poisoning, *Br J Anaesth* 37:972, 1966.

305. Sellakumar AR, et al: Carcinogenicity of formaldehyde and hydrogen chloride in rats, *Toxicol Appl Pharmacol* 81:401, 1985.

306. Sellyei M, Kelemem E: Chromosome study in a case of granulocytic leukemia with "pelgerisation" seven years after benzene pancytopenia, *Eur J Cancer* 7:83, 1971.

307. Seppäläinen AM, Haltia M: *Carbon disulfide.* In Spencer PS, Schaumburg HH, editors: *Experimental and clinical neurotoxicology,* Baltimore, 1980, Williams & Wilkins.

308. Shank RC, et al: Dietary aflatoxins and human liver cancer. II, Aflatoxins in market foods and foodstuffs in Thailand and Hong Kong, *Food Cosmet Toxicol* 10:61, 1972.

309. Shubik P, Porta GD: Carcinogenesis and acute intoxication with large doses of polycyclic hydrocarbons, *Am Med Assoc Arch Pathol* 64:691, 1957.

310. Simmon VF, Kavhanen K, Tardiff RG: *Mutagenic activity of chemicals identified in drinking water.* In Scott D, Bridges BA, Sobesl FH, editors: *Progress in genetic toxicology,* New York, 1977, Elsevier.

311. Simmonds PG, et al: Carbon tetrachloride lifetimes and emmissions determined from daily global measurements during 1975–1985, *J Atmospheric Chem* 7:35, 1988.

312. Singh HB, Salas LJ, Cavanaugh LA: Distribution, sources and sinks of atmospheric halogenated compounds, *Air Poll Cont* 27:332, 1977.

313. Singh HB, Salas LJ, Stiles RE: Distribution of selected gaseous organic mutagens and suspect carcinogens in ambient air, *Environ Sci Technol* 16:872, 1982.

314. Singh HB, et al: Measurements of some potentially hazardous chemicals in urban environments, *Atmos Environ* 15:601, 1981.

315. Sinnhuber RO, et al: Dietary factors and hepatoma in rainbow trout *(Salmo gairdneri)*. I, Aflatoxins in vegetable protein feedstuffs, *J Natl Cancer Inst* 41:711, 1968.

316. Sipes IG, Krishna G, Gillette JR, Bioactivation of carbon tetrachloride, chloroform and bromotrichloromethane: role of cytochrome p-450, *Life Sci* 20:1541, 1977.

317. Sittig M: *Handbook of toxic and hazardous chemicals,* Park Ridge, New Jersey, 1981, Noyes Publications.

318. Slater TF: Necrogenic action of carbon tetrachloride in the rat: a speculative mechanism based on activation, *Nature* 209:36, 1966.

319. Smith AA, et al: Chloroform, halothane, and regional anesthesia: a comparative study, *Anesth Analg* 52:1, 1973.

320. Smith JH, Hook JB: Mechanism of chloroform nephrotoxicity. III, Renal and hepatic microsomal metabolism of chloroform in mice, *Toxicol Appl Pharmacol* 73:511, 1984.

321. Spitz S, Maguigan WH, Dobriner K: The carcinogenic action of benzidine, *Cancer* 3:789, 1950.

322. Stalling DL, et al: Pattern of PCDD, PCDF, and PCB contamination in Great Lakes fish and birds and their characterization by principal component analysis, *Chemosphere* 14:627, 1985.

323. Stewart RD, et al: Human exposure to tetrachloroethylene vapor: relationship of expired air and blood concentrations to exposure and toxicity, *Arch Environ Health* 2:40, 1961.

324. Steyn M, Pitout MJ, Purchase IFH: A comparative study on aflatoxin B$_1$ metabolism in rats and mice, *Br J Cancer* 25:291, 1971.

325. Stoloff L: *Aflatoxins: an overview.* In Rodericks J, Hesseltine CW, Mehlman MA, editors: *Mycotoxins in human and animal health,* Park Forest South, Illinois, 1977, Pathtox Publishers.

326. Storms WW: Chloroform parties, *JAMA* 225:160, 1973.

327. Striker GE, et al: Structural and functional alterations in rat kidney during carbon tetrachloride intoxication, *Am J Pathol* 53:769, 1968.

328. Strittmatter P, Ball EG: Formaldehyde dehydrogenase, a glutathione-dependent enzyme system, *J Biol Chem* 213:445, 1955.

329. Sugimoto K, Goto S, Taniguchi H: Ocular fundus photography of workers exposed to carbon disulfide: a comparative epidemiological study between Japan and Finland, *Int Arch Occup Environ Health* 39:97, 1977.

330. Sun JD, et al: Benzene hemoglobin adducts in mice and rats: characterization of formation and physiological modeling, *Fundam Appl Toxicol* 15:468, 1990.

331. Sweetnam PM, Taylor SW, Elwood PC: Exposure to carbon disulphide and ischaemic heart disease in a viscose rayon factory, *Br J Ind Med* 44:220, 1987.

332. Swenson DH, Miller EC, Miller JA: Aflatoxin B$_1$-2,3-oxide; evidence for its formation in rat liver *in vivo* and by human liver microsomes *in vitro, Biochem Biophys Res Commun* 60:1036, 1974.

333. Teta MJ, et al: Mortality surveillance in a large chemical company: the Union Carbide Corporation experience, *Am J Ind Med* 17:435, 1990.

334. Theiss AM, Hey W, Zeller H: Zur toxikologie von dichlorodimethylather. Verdach auf kanzerogene wirkung auch beim mensch, *Arbeitsmed Arbeitsschutz* 23:97, 1973.

335. Thompson DJ, Warner SD, Robinson VB: Teratology studies on orally administered chloroform in the rat and rabbit, *Toxicol Appl Pharmacol* 29:379, 1980.

336. Tiller JR, Schilling RSF, Morris JN: Occupational toxic factor in mortality from coronary heart disease, *Br Med J* 4:407, 1968.

337. Tobe M, Naito K, Kurokawa Y: Chronic toxicity study on formaldehyde administered orally to rats, *Toxicology* 56:79, 1989.

338. Tolonen M, Nurminen M, Hernberg S: Ten-year coronary mortality of workers exposed to carbon disulfide, *Scand J Work Environ Health* 5:109, 1979.

339. Tomatis L: The contribution of the IARC monographs program to the identification of cancer risk factors, *Ann N Y Acad Sci* 534:31, 1988.

340. Trump BF, Harris CC: Human tissues in biomedical research, *Hum Pathol* 10:245, 1979.

341. Tsuchiya K, Okubo T, Ishizu S: An epidemiological study of occupational bladder tumors in the dye industry of Japan, *Br J Ind Med* 32:203, 1975.

342. Tu AS, et al: *In vitro* transformation of Balb/C 3T3 cell by chlorinated ethanes and ethylenes, *Cancer Lett* 28:85, 1985.

343. Uehleke H, et al: Metabolic activation of holoalkanes and tests *in vitro* for mutagenicity, *Xenobiotica* 7:393, 1977.

344. United States Environmental Protection Agency: *Scientific and technical assessment report on vinyl chloride and polyvinyl chloride,* Washington, DC, 1975, Office of Research and Development.

345. Urso P, Gengozian N: Depressed humoral immunity and increased tumor incidence in mice following *in utero* exposure to benzo[a]pyrene, *J Toxicol Environ Health* 6:569, 1980.

346. Urso P, et al: Suppression of humoral and cell-mediated immune responses *in vitro* by benzo(a)pyrene, *J Immunopharmacol* 8:223, 1986.

347. Vamvakas S, et al: Mutagenicity of tetrachloroethylene in the Ames test: metabolic activation by conjugation with glutathione, *J Biochem Toxicol* 4:21, 1989.

348. Van Abbe NJ, et al: Bacterial mutagenicity studies on chloroform, *in vitro, Food Cosmet Toxicol* 20:557, 1982.

349. Van Duuren BL: Prediction of carcinogenicity based on structure, chemical reactivity and possible metabolic pathways, *J Environ Pathol Toxicol* 3:11, 1980.

350. Van Duuren BL: Comparison of potency of human carcinogens: vinylchloride, chloromethylmethyl ether and bis(chloromethyl)ether, *Environ Res* 49:143, 1989.

351. Van Duuren BL, VanDuuren SB: *Chemistry, reactivity and carcinogenicity of chloroethers*. In Politzer P, Roberts L, editors: *Chemical carcinogens*, Amsterdam, 1988, Elsevier.

352. Van Duuren BL, et al: Alpha-haloethers: a new type of alkylating carcinogen, *Arch Environ Health* 19:472, 1968.

353. Van Duuren BL, et al: Carcinogenicity of halo-ethers, *J Natl Cancer Inst* 43:481, 1969.

354. VanHoorne M, De Bacquer D, De Backer G: Epidemiological study of the cardiovascular effects of carbon disulphide, *Int J Epidemiol* 21:745, 1992.

355. Vesselinovitch SD, Rao KVN, Mihailovich N: Factors modulating benzidine carcinogenicity bioassay, *Cancer Res* 35:2814, 1975.

356. Vinopal JH, Casida JE: Metabolic stability of 2,3,7,8 tetrachlorodibenzo-p-dioxin in mammalian liver microsomal systems and in living mice, *Arch Environ Contam Toxicol* 1:122, 1973.

357. Wallace LA: Major sources of benzene exposure, *Environ Health Perspect* 82:165, 1989.

358. Wallace LA: The exposure of the general population to benzene, *Cell Biol Toxicol* 297:314, 1989.

359. Wallace LA, Pellizzare ED: Personal air exposure and breath concentrations of benzene and other volatile hydrocarbons for smokers and nonsmokers, *Toxicol Lett* 35:113, 1986.

360. Wallace LA, et al: Concentrations of 20 volatile organic compounds in the air and drinking water of 350 residents of New Jersey compared with concentrations in their exhaled breath, *J Occup Med* 28:603, 1986.

361. Wallace LA, et al: The team study: personal exposures to toxic substances in air, drinking water, and breath of 400 residents of New Jersey, North Carolina, and North Dakota, *Environ Res* 43:290, 1987.

362. Watanabe PG, McGowan GR, Gehring PJ: Fate of ^{14}C-vinyl chloride after single oral administration in rats, *Toxicol Appl Pharmacol* 36:339, 1976.

363. Watanabe PG, Zempel JA, Gehring PG: Comparison of the fate of vinyl chloride following single and repeated exposure in rats, *Toxicol Appl Pharmacol* 44:391, 1978.

364. Watanabe PG, et al: Fate of ^{14}C-vinyl chloride following inhalation exposure in rats, *Toxicol Appl Pharmacol* 37:49, 1976.

365. Watanabe PG, et al: Hepatic macromolecular binding following exposure to vinyl chloride, *Toxicol Appl Pharmacol* 44:571, 1978.

366. Waxweiller RJ, et al: Neoplastic risk among workers exposed to vinyl chloride, *Ann N Y Acad Sci* 271:40, 1976.

367. Weaver NK, Gibson RL, Smith CE: *Occupational exposure to benzene in the petroleum and petrochemical industries*. In Mehlman MA, editor: *Advances in modern environmental toxicology, vol 4, Carcinogenicity and toxicity of benzene*, Princeton, 1983.

368. Weber H, Reinl W, Greiser E: German investigations on morbidity and mortality of workers exposed to vinyl chloride, *Environ Health Perspect* 41:91, 1981.

369. Weisberger EK: Carcinogenicity studies on halogenated hydrocarbons, *Environ Health Perspect* 21:7, 1977.

370. Weiss W: Epidemic curve of respiratory cancer due to chloromethyl ethers, *J Natl Cancer Inst* 69:1265, 1969.

371. Weston A, et al: Genotoxicity of chemical and physical agents in cultured human tissues and cells, *Food Chem Toxicol* 24:675, 1986.

372. White KJ, Holsapple MP: Direct suppression *in vitro* antibody production by mouse spleen cells by the carcinogen benzo(a)pyrene but not by the cogener benzo(e)pyrene, *Cancer Res* 44:3388, 1984.

373. Wilcosky TC: Mortality from heart disease among workers exposed to solvents, *J Occup Med* 25:879, 1983.

374. Williams GM, Weisburger JH: *Chemical carcinogenesis*. In Amdur MO, Doull J, Klaassen CD, editors: *Casarett and Doull's toxicology, the basic science of poisons*, New york, 1991, Pergamon Press.

375. Wilmer JWGM, et al: Subacute (4-week) inhalation toxicity study of formaldehyde in male rats: 8-hour intermittent versus 8-h continuous exposures, *J Appl Toxicol* 7:15, 1987.

376. Wislocki PG, et al: Mutagenicity and cytotoxicity of benzo[a]pyrene arene oxides, phenols, quinones, and dihydrodiols in bacterial and mammalian cells, *Cancer Res* 36:3350, 1976.

377. Witz G, et al: Comparative metabolism of benzene and trans, trans-muconic acid in DBA/2N and C57BL/6 mice, *Biochem Pharmacol* 40:1275, 1990.

378. Wogan GN: Markers of exposure to carcinogens: methods for human biomonitoring, *J Am Coll Toxicol* 8:871, 1989.

379. Wogan GN, Paglialunga S, Newberne PM: Carcinogenic effects of low dietary levels of aflatoxin B$_1$ in rats, *Food Cosmet Toxicol* 12:681, 1974.

380. Wojdani A, Alfred LJ: Alternations in cell mediated immune functions induced in mouse splenic lymphocytes by polycyclic aromatic hydrocarbons, *Cancer Res* 44:942, 1984.

381. Wong O: An industry wide mortality study of chemical workers occupationally exposed to benzene: I, general results, *Br J Ind Med* 44:365, 1987.

382. Woods JS, et al: Soft tissue sarcomas and military service in Vietnam: a case comparison group analysis of hospital patients, *J Natl Cancer Inst* 78:899, 1987.

383. World Health Organization: *Environmental health criteria 89 formaldehyde*, Geneva, 1989, WHO.

384. Woustersen PA, et al: Subchronic (13-week) inhalation toxicity study of formaldehyde in rats, *J Appl Toxicol* 7:43, 1987.

385. Wronska-Nofer T: Effect of carbon disulphide intoxication on fecal excretion of end products of cholesterol metabolism, *Int Arch Occup Environ Health* 40:261, 1977.

386. Wronska-Nofer T, Parke M: Influence of carbon disulphide on metabolic processes in the aorta wall: study of the rate of cholesterol synthesis and the rate of influx of ^{14}C cholesterol from serum into the aorta wall, *Int Arch Occup Environ Health* 42:63, 1978.

387. Wronska-Nofer T, Szendikowski S, Laurman W: The effect of carbon disulphide and atherogenic diet on the development of atherosclerotic changes in rabbits, *Atherosclerosis* 31:33, 1978.

388. Wronska-Nofer T, Szendzikowski S, Obrebska-Parke M: Influence of chronic carbon disulphide intoxication on the development of experimental atherosclerosis in rats, *Br J Ind Med* 37:387, 1980.

389. Wu W, et al: Cohort and case-control analyses of workers exposed to vinyl chloride: an update, *J Occup Med* 31:518, 1989.

390. Wynder E, Gori G: Contribution of the environment to cancer incidence: an epidemiologic exercise, *J Natl Cancer Inst* 58:825, 1977.

391. Yllner S: Urinary metabolites of ^{14}C tetrachloroethylene in mice, *Nature* 191:820, 1961.

392. Young TB, Kanarek MSD, Tsiatis AA: Epidemiological study of drinking water chlorination and Wisconsin female cancer mortality, *J Natl Cancer Inst* 67:1191, 1981.

393. Yun YX, Ji-Gang C, Yong-Ning H: Studies on the relation between bladder cancer and benzidine or its derived dyes in Shanghai, *Br J Ind Med* 47:544, 1990.

394. Zavon MR, Hoegg U, Bingham E: Benzidine exposure as a cause of bladder tumors, *Arch Environ Health* 27:1, 1973.

Chapter 6

INORGANIC AND ORGANIC DUST POLLUTANTS

John E. Craighead

The human respiratory tract is exposed on a continuous basis to a variety of inorganic and organic particulates in the air. These particles vary enormously in size (Fig. 6-1) and type and differ in pathogenic potential. Their capacity to cause disease depends, in part, on the site of deposition in the airway as well as the dosage and durability. Key to the occurrence of respiratory disease, however, are the factors and diseases that influence particulate clearance (such as preexisting pulmonary disease and smoking) and host susceptibility that permits an immune-mediated, ultimately pathogenic response to occur in some individuals (see Chapters 24 and 25). Exposures to suspended silicates, a diversity of plant and animal materials, and products of combustion are ubiquitous and a universal experience of humans. Many of these small respirable particulates are maintained in the ambient air indefinitely by brownian motion and are inhaled and cleared from the airways without adverse consequence.

This chapter provides an overview of the many types of particulates found in the ambient air we breathe and in the work environment. Because of enormous diversity of particulates in the air and the variability from one geographical location to another, only examples of the most important dusts from a health perspective are considered. Under unusual circumstances, inorganic dust exposures relating to meteorological (dust storms) or cataclysmic geological (volcanic) events (Fig. 6-2) can produce exposures of such magnitude as to overcome host clearance mechanisms, resulting in the accumulation of dust in the lungs. On a geographical scale, these geological events contribute to the background particle load of the ambient air. Thus, fine particulate dusts in the atmosphere over North America in recent years have reflected volcanic activity in the Pacific basin. During the 1930s, when drought and windstorms were turning the high plains states of North America into a "dust bowl," clouds of dust occasionally blanketed the sky of the eastern seaboard. Similarly, mariners far off the coast of sizable land masses have observed, on occasion, the accumulation of dust on decks of ships, an event described by Darwin while anchored in the Cape Verde Islands in 1846.[24] Studies of pulmonary tissue from California ranchers by Sherwin and coworkers[81] attest to the burden of silicates that accumulate in the lungs of those who spend their lifetime in the parched lands of the barren U.S. West. Additionally, atmospheric dust is derived from cosmic sources (i.e., the breakdown of meteorites as they enter earth's atmosphere), sea salt, and fires in both urban and rural settings.[74]

Common particulate causes of occupational asthma and a number of the recognized causes for hypersensitivity pneumonitis in specific settings are recorded in Tables 28-2 and 28-6. Occupational dust exposure poses a major health

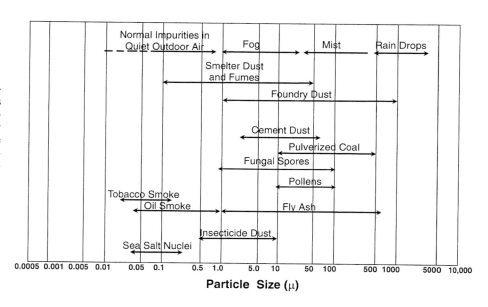

Fig. 6-1. Particle size by type of commonly encountered aerosols. Those less than 5 μ in diameter are highly respirable, whereas the remainder usually deposit in the upper airways and are eliminated by the nasal and tracheobronchial mucociliary escalator systems. (Adapted from Bates DV et al: Deposition and retention models for internal dosimetry of human respiratory tract, *Health Phys* 12:173, 1966.)

problem for workers in countless industries. The nature of the job and the materials used as well as the existence of, and adherence to, regulations is intrinsic to the ultimate outcome. Diseases consistent with silicosis and asbestosis among artesians were described by physicians before and in the early centuries of the Christian era. Although disease related to dust exposure in major industries was a health problem in the past, increasingly, dusty work conditions more frequently pose a threat to individuals or small groups of workers in specialized industries.* The imposing influence of regulatory bodies has yet to affect the expo-

*References 7, 12, 16, 19, 21, 27, 46, 54, 59, 62, 69, 85, 87-89, 92.

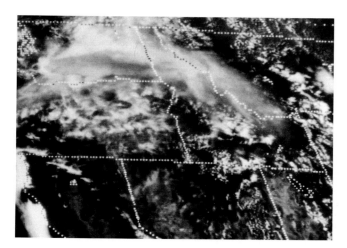

Fig. 6-2. Atmospheric dust cloud over northwest United States shortly after the eruption of Mount St. Helens in southwest Washington state. (Courtesy of NASA.)

sures sustained in many cottage industries. An outbreak of mesotheliomas among Native American silversmiths attests to the ubiquitous hazard of asbestos in the home workplace.[35] In the experience of the author, isolated cases of pneumoconiosis related to unique circumstances of dust exposure present the diagnostician and the public health official with imposing challenges. Frequently, histopathological evaluation of the lung tissue, supplemented by analytical studies, provides important clues for diagnosis and the identification of hazards.

As noted previously, the air we breathe invariably contains finely suspended dust particles that are unrelated to human sources (Fig. 6-3). Human activities, however, have resulted in the pollution of the air we breathe, even before the industrial revolution. Particles of carbon, fly ash, i.e., mullite,[47] and condensation nuclei of sulfur dioxide (SO_2) and nitrous oxides (NO_x) are products of modern industry and the generation of energy from petroleum products and coal. Tobacco smoke adds complex liquid and lipid, submicron particulates to the ambient air. Ash may serve as condensation nuclei. Fig. 6-4 graphically illustrates the relative but changing patterns of ambient particulate pollution in Beijing, People's Republic of China, and in selected cities in the United States where ongoing studies are currently being conducted.[28,95] Geographical considerations reflecting the distribution of industries, patterns of automotive transportation, sources of fuel for energy generation, heating systems for buildings, topography, and complex meteorological considerations ultimately influence the types and concentrations of dust in the air we breathe. Compelling, epidemiological evidence now implicates these particulates as major factors influencing respiratory dysfunction in urban residents, as a result of both indoor and outdoor pollution (see Chapters 2 and 3).

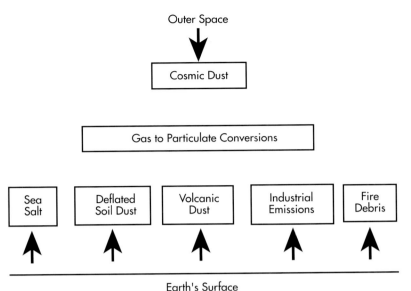

Fig. 6-3. Sources of airborne particulates reflected in ambient air. (From Pye K: *Aeolian dust and dust deposits,* New York, 1977, Academic Press; with permission.)

GEOLOGICAL CONSIDERATIONS

The earth's crust is a complex montage of geological formations representing the diverse internal forces and meteorological influences that have molded it. Deposits of a diversity of minerals in solid or particulate form and accumulations of complex mixtures of organic materials compose the elements of the earth's crust. A mineral is defined by Parkes[71] as an inorganic homogeneous substance that occurs naturally and has distinct crystal structure (prismatic, acicular, asbestiform, platy), chemical composition, and

physical properties. The structure, however, may be variable in a single mineral deposit or between different deposits. Igneous materials are fusion products of superheated magma in or on the surface of the earth's crust. In various combinations, the bulk of this material is comprised of free silica (i.e., crystalline silicon dioxide [SiO_2]) and combined silica (i.e., silicates), which are made up of cationic substituted SiO_2. Sedimentary geological deposits either are annealed into rocks of various degrees of hardness (sandstone, limestone, slate, and shale) or consist of deposits

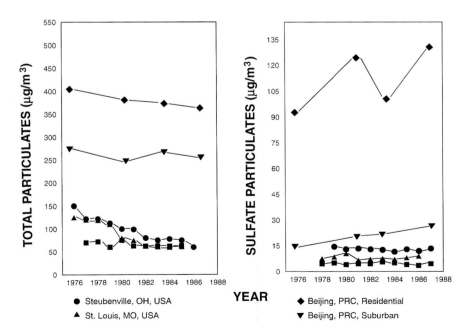

Fig. 6-4. Airborne particulates and, specifically, sulfate particulates in various selected urban environments in the United States and in two general locations in Beijing, People's Republic of China (PRC). Noteworthy is the gradual reduction in particulate concentrations in Steubenville, OH, and St. Louis, MO. In the former city, the concentrations of dust particulates are associated with respiratory symptoms. The high concentrations of dust in Beijing, PRC, reflect the use of coal as a major source of energy. (Adapted from references 28 and 95.)

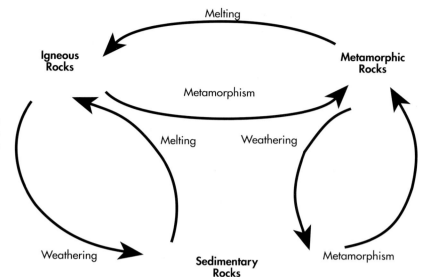

Fig. 6-5. Interrelationships of the three major types of rock. (From *Crystalline silica primer*, Washington DC, 1988, US Department of Interior, US Bureau of Mines.)

lacking structure and form (clays, coal). They can represent secondary accumulations of volcanic debris or the products of the erosive forces of water or wind. Alternatively, sedimentary deposits of organic origin are of three fundamental types: those composed predominantly of (1) carbon (coal, graphite, lignite, peat); (2) silicon (diatomaceous earth), and (3) Ca^{++} or Ca^{++}/Mg^{++} (limestone). Metamorphic rocks develop as a result of changes in preexisting sedimentary or igneous deposits through the impact of temperature or physical and hydrothermal forces. As a result, the crystalline structure or chemical makeup changes. Forms of metamorphic rocks of health importance are those that are asbestiform (asbestos), platy (talc), and crystalline (quartzite or metamorphic sandstone) (Fig. 6-5).

MINERALS DERIVED FROM INORGANIC SOURCES
Silica

The term silicon refers to the element Si; silicone to amorphous man-made polymers of SiO_2; and silica to the naturally occurring, amorphous or crystalline, SiO_2 (Fig.

6-6).[23] Free silica is found as crystals (Fig. 6-7) that develop in volcanic magma to form igneous rock. It is composed of silicon and oxygen and assumes several polymorphic forms, the most common of which is alpha quartz (Fig. 6-8).[2] Although alpha quartz is of igneous origin, humans frequently are exposed to it in pure form when working with the sedimentary rock—sandstone, for example, when sand blasting.[78] Tridymite (Fig. 6-8) and cristobalite are infrequently found as natural deposits but develop more commonly under conditions of high temperatures greater than 1000° C (Fig. 6-9). Thus, these polymorphs of SiO_2 pose a hazard for workers in foundries and those handling used fire bricks such as in open hearth furnaces of steel mills.[5,62] They are generally believed to be more pathogenic than alpha quartz, but the mineralogical and biological basis for differences is obscure. Amorphous SiO_2 is much less pathogenic than crystalline silica. It is found in volcanic tuff and man-made plate and fiberglass. Obsidian is one such glass, whereas perlite is a hydrated glass that finds application as a soil conditioner and in construction as an insulation material. Silicon carbide (carborundum) is a fusion product of

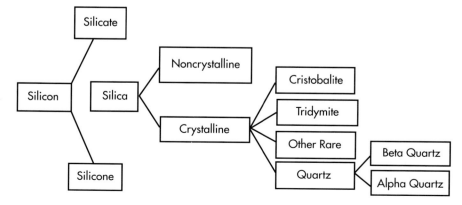

Fig. 6-6. Overall relationships of the noncrystalline and crystalline forms of silicon oxide. (From *Crystalline silica primer*, Washington, DC, 1988, US Department of Interior, US Bureau of Mines.)

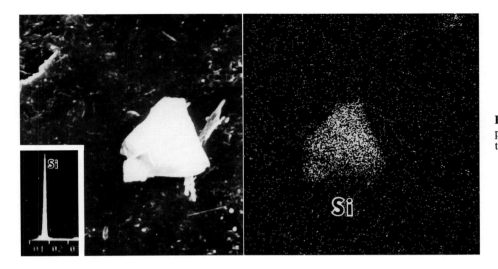

Fig. 6-7. Crystalline particle of alpha quartz with backscatter imaging to demonstrate the silicon atoms.

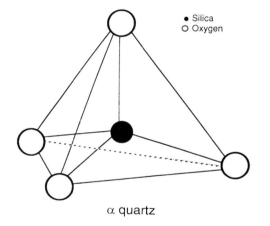

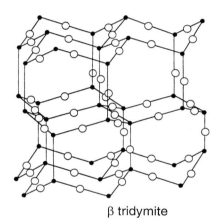

Fig. 6-8. Comparison of the crystalline structure of alpha quartz and beta tridymite. (Adapted from *Crystalline silica primer,* Washington, DC, 1988, US Department of Interior, US Bureau of Mines.)

• Silica
O Oxygen

α quartz

β tridymite

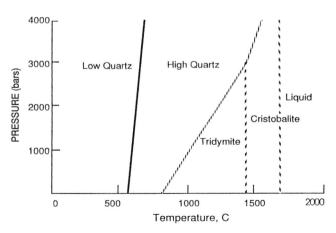

Fig. 6-9. Stability fields of the different forms of silica in glass, ceramic and fine china manufacturing. (From *Crystalline silica primer,* Washington, DC, 1988, US Department of Interior, US Bureau of Mines.)

SiO_2 and carbon. It is an exceedingly durable, heat-resistant particulate material used as an abrasive and in refractories.[42] In studies of the dust from Mount St. Helens, irregular particles of glass were frequently observed (see later) (Fig. 6-10).[22] Diatomaceous earth, which forms from diatome deposits (diatomite) and plant debris (such as from reeds and sugarcane), contains amorphous silica. It can undergo metamorphic transitions to crystalline tridymite and cristobalite under unique conditions of temperature and pressure. Because of the ubiquity of silica in rock of all types, it poses an ever-present hazard for workers in the extraction industries as well as those using earth products in a diversity of secondary and tertiary industries (Fig. 6-11; Table 6-1).

Silicates

Mineralogically, silicate particles are comprised of silicon dioxide into which one or more common cations (alu-

Table 6-1. Common sources of exposure to pathogenic mineral dusts in industrialized countries

Nature of exposure	Asbestos	Silica	Coal	Talc
Primary	Miners and millers of primary product	Miners of other minerals; quarriers of granite	Miners and millers	Miners and millers
Secondary	Shipbuilders, insulation workers, friction products and textile manufacturers	Sandblasters, stone masons, potters, abrasive manufacturers	Firemen, steam plant operators	Pharmaceutical and cosmetic manufacturers
Tertiary users	Electricians, carpenters, plumbers, roofers, auto mechanics, firefighters, refinery workers, welders	Welders, potters, users of abrasives, foundry and steel mill workers	Coke oven workers	Users of cosmetics; intravenous drug users

minum, magnesium, sodium, calcium, potassium [Al, Mg, Na, Ca, K]) have been substituted (Fig. 6-12).[23,67] The crystal structure of silicates is diverse because of the array of chemical materials and the geological mechanisms involved in their formation. As a result, the silicate particles are granular, platy, or fibrous in pure form and vary in their water of hydration. More commonly, they are found as mixtures of these forms. Silicate minerals are derived primarily as a result of volcanic or igneous activity but secondarily often occur as the result of sedimentation and, to variable degrees, as a consequence of metamorphosis of rock. The complexities of these processes result in variability between deposits having the same elemental composition and ultimately influence the commercial value of the deposit. Although asbestiform minerals, kaolin, and micaceous deposits are commonly found in the earth's crust, accumulations of relatively pure minerals having mercantile properties are rare. These considerations are further compounded by the presence of variable amounts of mineral contaminants such as silica and asbestos in deposit of silicates. For example, China clay (kaolinite) can contain particulate silica (known as China stone). Both talc and vermiculite are often contaminated with variable amounts of asbestos and a host of chemicals.[9,60,61] Contaminants of this type can have potential health effects among workers in the extraction industries and users of the end products (Table 6-1).

The earth's crust is comprised, to a large extent, of silicates of diverse origin. Vast areas of its surface represent volcanic and sedimentary deposits that, to a varying extent, are composed of potentially aerosolizable particulate materials. The complexities of soil development are reflected in mixtures of silica and silicates with variable amounts and types of organic material. The aerosolizability of these dusts reflects the physical form and size of the particle as well as wind current (Fig. 6-13; Table 6-2). Prevailing winds can result in almost worldwide distribution of fine particles

Table 6-2. Reported mineral composition of some windblown dusts by geographical location

Qu	Fe	Mi	Ch	Ka	Sm	Pa	Ca	Do	Gy	Ha	Other	Location
X	x	x	x	x	x		x					Arctic
X	x	x	x	x	x		x	x	x			South Israel
X	x	x		x	x							North Nigeria
X	x	X		x		x	X	x				England
X	x	x	x	x		x	x	x			H	Netherlands
X	x	X	x	x	x		x				H	Equatorial Atlantic
X	x	X	x	x	x							East Equatorial Pacific
X	x	X	x	x								North Atlantic
X	X	x					x				Gl	Ashkabad, Turkmenstan
X	x		x				x			x		New Mexico
X	x	X	x				x				A	Beijing, People's Republic of China

Qu, Quartz; *Fe*, feldspars; *Mi*, mica/illite; *Ch*, chlorite; *Ka*, kaolinite; *Sm*, smectite/mixed layer; *Pa*, palygorskite; *Ca*, calcite; *Do*, dolomite; *Gy*, Gypsum; *Ha*, halite.
Other: *H*, Hematite; *Gl*, glauconite; *A*, amphibole.
X, Dominant constituent; *x*, important constituent.
Adapted from Pye K: *Aeolian dust and dust deposits,* New York, 1987, Academic Press.

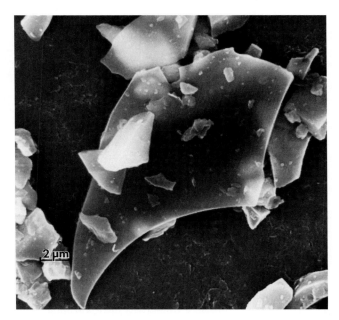

Fig. 6-10. A glass shard demonstrated by scanning electron microscopy among silicate dust particles from Mount St. Helens, Washington.

(Fig. 6-14). To a variable extent, we all imperceptibly breathe a diversity of silicate dust particles from our everyday atmospheric environment, which, to a large extent, are cleansed from the respiratory tract. Granular and platy silicates result in disease only when dust concentrations exceed the clearance threshold of the airways and the exposure occurs over long periods of time. To a large extent, only workers in the mineral extraction industries and dusty trades develop symptomatic pulmonary disease as a result of the inhalation of granular and platy silicates (Table 6-1).

Asbestiform particles are a special case that are considered in more detail later.

Thresholds have been defined largely by pragmatic legal and regulatory decisions and are often based on demonstrable radiological or functional changes in the lungs, rather than from pathological studies. Because dust accumulation in the lungs is undetectable except by autopsy study or the examination of bronchoalveolar washing cell sediments, little information has been systematically accumulated on subtle pathological effects of exposure. Substantial accumulations of talc[44,86] (Fig. 6-15), hematite,[49,58] slate,[45,86] and shale,[56,79,80] (Fig. 6-16) dusts and asbestos[75] can be found during postmortem studies of the lungs of workers dying of accidents or unrelated natural disease. It is only when the exposure is heavy and prolonged that respiratory insufficiency develops as a result of silicate dust exposure.

Clay minerals are a diverse, complex group of hydrated aluminum silicate minerals characterized by a particle size of less than 2 μ in diameter. The particle configuration is variable, but many are classified as phyllosilicates, i.e., silicate particulates that are composed of laminate sheets of base-substituted SiO_2 (Fig. 6-15). As noted previously, phyllosilicate mineral (platy) particulates[9] (Fig. 6-17) composed of magnesium silicates (talc) and aluminum silicates (kaolinite and mica) (Fig. 6-18) have potential health importance when exposure is heavy and prolonged.[25,55,66,91] A variety of less well-known silicates have diverse commercial uses, but their health importance is most probably limited (Table 6-3). Thus, disease caused by exposure to the relatively pure mineral has been largely restricted to miners and millers in the extraction industries. To a variable extent, these minerals are distributed worldwide and are found in igneous (granite), sedimentary (China clay), and metamorphic deposits (slate and shale) over a wide

Pottery and related products

Paving and roofing materials

Flat glass

Concrete, gypsum, plaster products

Masonry, stonework, tile setting
    and plastering

Medical and dental laboratories

Misc. chemical products

Roofing and sheet metal work

Combination electric and gas,
    and other utilities services

Abrasive, asbestos and misc.
    nonmetallic mineral products

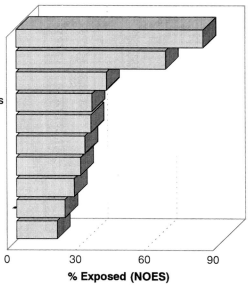

0   30   60   90

% Exposed (NOES)

Fig. 6-11. Sources and relative importance of different forms of silica dust exposure by industry. (Courtesy National Institute for Occupational Safety and Health.)

range of concentrations. The fibers of chrysotile asbestos (a magnesium silicate) have a basic platelike structure but are configured into a scroll-like asbestiform particle. Chrysotile contaminates some talc deposits. It is a metamorphic platy silicate of identical chemical composition. These structural differences reflect the unique forces of geological molding of the mineral deposits (a subject beyond the scope of this chapter).

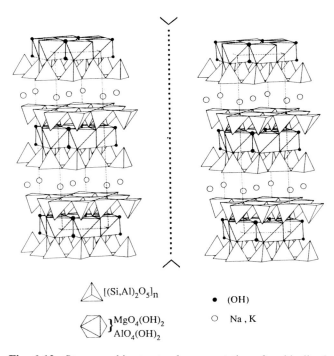

Fig. 6-12. Stereographic structural representation of an idealized platy silicate particle, mica. The structure is composed of continuous layers containing two tetrahedral aluminum silicate sheets that enclose octahedral coordinated cations, Al^{3+} or Mg^{2+} This layer or "sandwich" is held together by K^{1+} or Na^{1+} ions. (From Skinner HCW, Ross M, Frondel C: *Asbestos and other fibrous minerals. Mineralogy, crystal chemistry and health effects*, New York, 1988, Oxford University Press; with permission.)

Asbestiform minerals

The term asbestiform applies to fibrous material 5 μm or longer with a length-to-breadth ratio (aspect ratio) of at least 3.[20,75,93] This is a regulatory definition; almost invariably the ratio is much higher. Asbestos is a commercial term referring to a family of fibrous minerals that are fire and heat resistant and, to a variable extent, are insoluble in strong acid and alkali. These properties account for the unique usefulness of these minerals in insulation materials of all types and in countless other industrial applications (Table 6-1; Fig. 6-19). Although use of asbestos in developed countries has been substantially reduced by regulation, many millions of tons of the material are in place in buildings and manufactured products. These materials continue to be a subject of public health concern because they could pose a hazard for those who remove it or are involved in building renovation or remodeling.

The asbestos minerals are composed of two mineralogically distinct subfamilies: the amphiboles and serpentines (Fig. 6-20). The amphibole fibers are made up of replete, "loglike" crystalline subfibrils composed of hydrated mag-

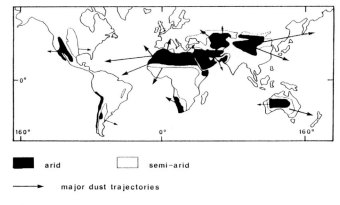

Fig. 6-13. Major dust trajectories from arid regions of the earth, resulting in significant air pollution by particulates. (From Pye K: *Aeolian dust and dust deposits*, New York, 1987, Academic Press; with permission.)

Table 6-3. Commercial applications of classes of clay minerals (with interchangeable mineralogical terms) having limited health importance

Kaolin (Kaolinite)	Bentonite (Montmorillonite, Smectite)	Fuller's Earth (Montmorillonite, Attapulgite [polygorsite])	Feldspar (K silicate [orthoclase], NaCa Silicate [plagioclase])
Cement and bricks	Foundry sand	Absorbents	Fluxes
Coated paper	Well-drilling mud	Carriers for pesticides	Ceramics
Ceramics	Iron-ore pelletizing	Paints/fillers	Paints/fillers
	Catalysts	Joint sealing compounds	Glass
	Filters	Well-drilling mud	
	Paints/fillers		

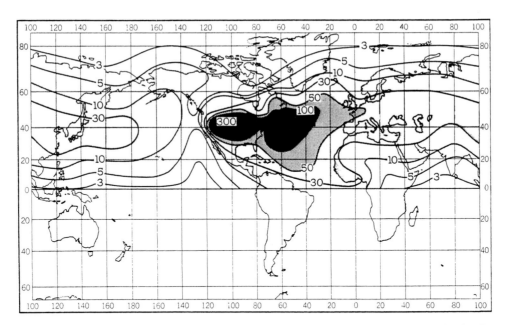

Fig. 6-14. Worldwide fallout of radioactive dust particulates after nuclear weapons testing in Nevada in 1953. Ground level explosion introduced dust into the troposphere. (From Machta L, List JR, Hubert LF: World-wide travel of atomic debris, *Science* 124:474, 1956; with permission.)

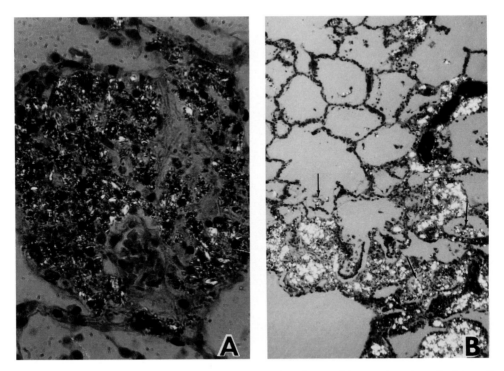

Fig. 6-15. A, Dust macule containing particulates of carbon and lancet-shaped particulates of highly birefringent talc. **B,** Accumulations of talc within the interstitium of lung. These photomicrographs were prepared from lung tissue of a long-term worker in a Vermont talc mine. (From Vallyathan NV, Craighead JE: Pulmonary pathology of workers exposed to nonasbestiform talc, *Hum Pathol* 12:28, 1981; with permission.)

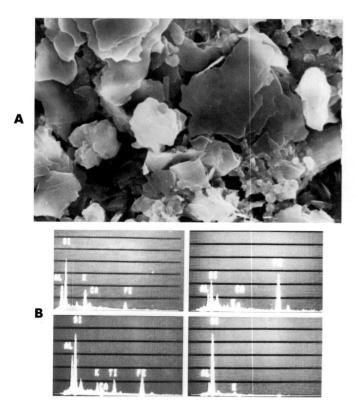

Fig. 6-16. **A,** Scanning electron micrograph of particulates extracted from the lung of a Vermont slateworker. **B,** The x-ray spectrographs illustrate different "fingerprints" of silicate particles in this mass of fine particulates.

nesium silicates into which are substituted specific cations (Fig. 6-21, *A*). Amphibole fibers are annealed together by tight chemical or electrostatic bonds to make a rigid, relatively indestructible particle (Fig. 6-22). In contrast, the serpentine chrysotile fibers are composed of numerous sub-

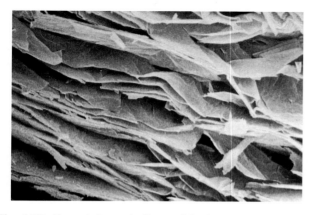

Fig. 6-17. Expanded vermiculite used for horticultural and insulation purposes. The platelike layers of silicates expand with heat owing to the vaporization of the water of hydration of the particle. The term "vermis" refers to worm, which characterizes the vermiculite firecracker that expands with heat to form a "worm."

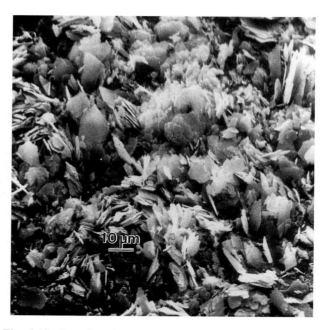

Fig. 6-18. Scanning electron micrograph of mica particulates extracted from the lungs of a worker who was exposed to mica occupationally. (From the American Medical Association.)

fibrils individually structured into rolled scrolls of platy magnesium silicate (Fig. 6-21, *B*). The subunit fibrils are loosely bound by electrostatic forces (Figs. 6-21 and 6-22). As a result, the fibers tend to be flexible and pliable and lack durability. In the environment and in human tissues, the magnesium ion, which serves as an electrostatic "glue" between the subfibrils, is readily dissolved. As a result, the fibers break down into the subunit fibrils (Figs. 6-23 and 6-24). It should be apparent from this brief description that the amphibole asbestos and chrysotile asbestos types are distinctly different from a mineralogical perspective. These differences are reflected in their respective capacities to cause disease.

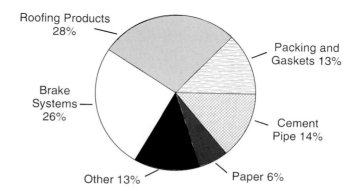

Fig. 6-19. Industrial utilization of asbestos in the United States, 1988. This pattern is rapidly changing because of federal efforts to restrict the use of asbestos in manufactured products. (From Asbestos Information Association of North America, with permission.)

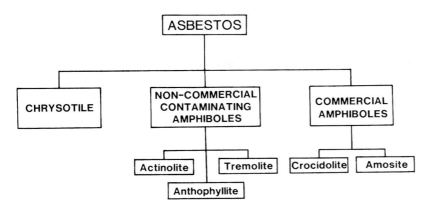

Fig. 6-20. Asbestos is a commercial term referring to two major classes of industrial asbestos, i.e., the amphiboles (crocidolite and amosite) and the serpentine (chrysotile). The noncommercial types of asbestos are often sporadic contaminants of other mineral products or other forms of chrysotile asbestos. (From Craighead JE: Current pathogenic concepts on diffuse malignant mesothelioma, *Hum Pathol* 18:554, 1987; with permission.)

The asbestos minerals form by the geological process of metamorphosis and are distributed widely in the earth's crust (Fig. 6-25). They are located in four types of rocks: (1) banded ironstone (amosite and crocidolite), (2) alpine-type ultramafic rocks (anthophyllite, tremolite and chrysotile), (3) stratiform ultramafic intrusions (tremolite and chrysotile), and (4) serpentinized limestone (chrysotile) (Fig. 6-23).[76] The ubiquity of asbestiform minerals in rock outcrops is exemplified by the common finding of both amphibole and chrysotile fibers in high concentrations in potable water, irrigation systems, and lakes (Tables 6-4, 6-5).* (There is no epidemiological evidence to suggest that the asbestiform particles in public water systems have health effects.) The serpentine rocks in which commercial fibrous chrysotile forms compose major strata over the earth's crust, although deposits of contemporary commercial importance are located in only a relatively small number of places worldwide. In the past, mines were established at many scattered sites. Currently, active chrysotile quarries and mines are located in Australia, Canada, China, Japan, Korea, Russia, South Africa, United States, and Zimbabwe. Amphiboles are presently extracted in South Africa and Bolivia (crocidolite), although major mines were formerly active in both Australia (crocidolite) and Finland (anthophyllite).

The length and breadth of the fibers of both amphiboles and chrysotile in ore bodies and commercial products is variable (Fig. 6-26). Although the majority of fibers in com-

*References 14, 17, 18, 64, 65.

mercial preparations are relatively short, asbestos products containing a relatively high proportion of long fibers and are used preferentially in some industries (such as textiles). Although products with relatively high concentrations of the longer fibers have considerable commercial value, the long fibers of amphibole have been found to be highly pathogenic. For example, the Western Australia Wittenoom mine yielded a crocidolite product that contained many unusually long fibers; as a result, the health risks to workers was so great that the mine was ultimately closed.[26]

The pathogenic properties of the relatively long, thin fibers (greater than 5 μm in length and less than 0.5 μm in breadth) has been established in numerous experimental studies.* Durable, long fibers of amphibole appear to establish an intense inflammatory response in tissue with the generation of oxygen radicals and cytokine by-products of the macrophage. This response probably accounts, in whole or in part, for its exceptional pathogenicity (see Chapter 28).

An abundant literature has accumulated on the airborne concentrations of asbestos in various occupational settings, in the outdoor environment and the community, and in public buildings (see Chapter 3).[15,51] These data are exceed-

*References 1, 29, 48, 83, 84.

Table 6-5. Asbestiform fibers in two major west coast United States water bodies

	California (bay area)	Washington (Puget Sound)
N, fibers	7375	6977
Mean length, μm	1.35	0.6
Standard deviation	1.99	0.52
Median length, μm	1.0	0.5
Range, μm	0.1-59.0	0.1-9.5
Distribution		
90% <	2.2 μm	1.1 μm
75% <	1.5 μm	0.7 μm
25% <	0.6 μm	0.3 μm
Percentage ≥ 5 μm	2.3%	0.2%

Table 6-4. Results of surveys in United States for asbestiform particles in potable water sources

Highest concentration, 10⁶ fibers/L	Number of cities
Below detectable limits	61
<1	27
1-10	7
>10	5

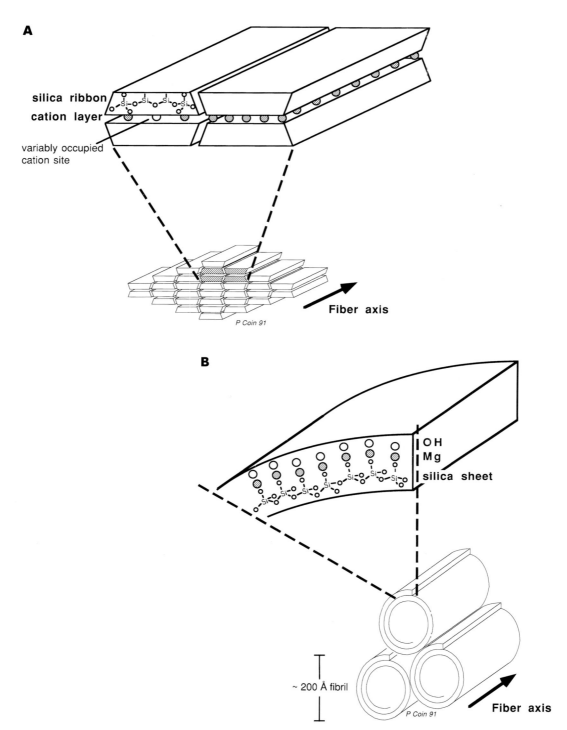

Fig. 6-21. A, Diagrammatic representation of the structure of an amphibole fiber demonstrating the platelike rods that form the subunits of the major fiber. **B,** Structure of chrysotile asbestos fibers. The layers of chrysotile are bound by magnesium, which can dissolve in lung tissue, resulting in the dissolution of the chrysotile fibers into the subunit fibrils. (From Roggli VL, Greenberg SD, Pratt PC: *Pathology of the asbestos-associated diseases,* Boston, 1992, Little, Brown, Figs. 1-5, 1-7; with permission.)

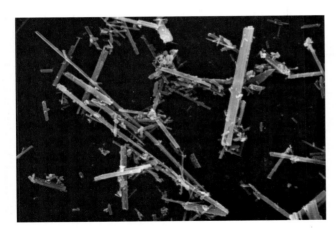

Fig. 6-22. Scanning electron micrograph of amphibole asbestos of the amosite type. Note the variability in fiber length and breadth. The majority of the fibers are relatively short and often blunt. These smaller particulates are not believed to be pathogenic.

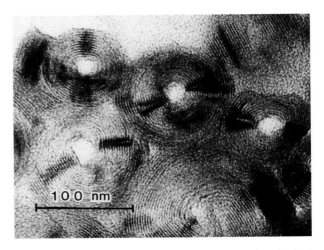

Fig. 6-24. Transmission electron micrograph showing the lattice image of the layered chrysotile fibers. (From Skinner HCW, Ross M, Frondel C: *Asbestos and other fibrous minerals. Mineralogy, crystal chemistry and health effects,* New York, 1988, Oxford University Press; with permission.)

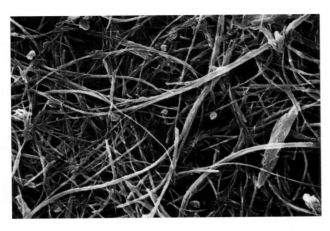

Fig. 6-23. Scanning electron micrograph of chrysotile asbestos. Note the variability in fiber length and width. The fibers are "splaying out" to release the fibrils that compose them.

ingly difficult for the uninitiated to interpret because the environmental assessment tools used over the past several decades have differed from laboratory to laboratory worldwide. In early decades of the twentieth century, environmental dust concentrations were quantitated based on millions of particles per cubic foot (mppcf), and various calculations were used to account for the proportion of the whole, believed to be asbestos. More recently, exposure has been quantitated by electron microscopy based on fibers per cubic centimeter, although some laboratories have developed gravimetric criteria for this purpose. The latter approach has many shortcomings. From an historical perspective, fibers in the environmental air initially were assessed by phase microscopy, but in recent years, scanning and transmission electron microscopic techniques have been employed. The latter approach was incorporated into the so-called AHERA (Asbestos Hazard Emergency Response

Act) protocols developed by the EPA to quantify asbestiform minerals in ambient air in public buildings.[39] These protocols standardize the techniques, something that was largely lacking in previous approaches. Fiber length is a variable that receives all too little attention in these assessments, particularly because it is now widely recognized that the majority of fibers in environmental dust samples are substantially shorter than 5 μ in length. As noted previously, long, thin fibers can be accorded the major credit for the causation of asbestos-related disease.

Asbestos bodies are a product of biological activity and thus are found in the lung tissues of exposed humans. They usually are composed of a core of amphibole fiber on which is layered a protein-iron–containing coagulum (Fig. 6-27). The bodies have a distinctive morphological feature but must be distinguished from other minerals and organic particulates that also attract this coated layer of biological product when deposited in the lung—the generic term ferruginous bodies is used to describe these structures.[20] Asbestos bodies are believed to develop in macrophages, but the fundamental mechanism leading to the deposit of the surface material is not known. The ratio of asbestos bodies to fibers in lung tissue digests from different individuals is, for unknown reasons, quite variable, ranging from 1:1 to 1:3000. Host factors may be an important contributor to the development of asbestos bodies because experimental animals differ in their capacity to produce asbestos bodies after experimental inoculation.

Manufactured vitreous and crystalline fibers

With the blossoming concern regarding the health risks of asbestos exposure, industry has increasingly used synthetic, inorganic fibers as asbestos substitutes. Simply de-

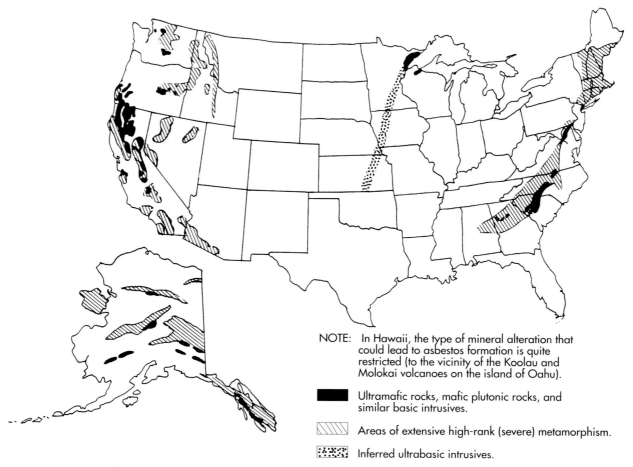

NOTE: In Hawaii, the type of mineral alteration that could lead to asbestos formation is quite restricted (to the vicinity of the Koolau and Molokai volcanoes on the island of Oahu).

███ Ultramafic rocks, mafic plutonic rocks, and similar basic intrusives.

▨ Areas of extensive high-rank (severe) metamorphism.

▒ Inferred ultrabasic intrusives.

Fig. 6-25. Distribution of ultra-basic and metamorphic rock formations in the United States. (From *Asbestos: An Information Resource*, Washington, DC, 1978, US Department of Health, Education, and Welfare, based on US Geological Survey: Tectonic map of North America.)

fined, these are fibers that can withstand temperatures of 1000° C without fragmentation or distortion.[41] They are made up of various amalgams of SiO_2 or aluminum silicates and contain a diversity of additives that instill specific properties: for example, aluminum oxide (Al_2O_3), titanium dioxide ($TiO)_3$, zinc oxide (ZnO), magnesium oxide (MgO), lithium oxide (Li_2O), barium oxide (BaO), calcium oxide (CaO), sodium oxide (Na_2O), potassium oxide (K_2O). To a large extent, the fibers are manufactured by an extrusion process. Thus they can be exceedingly long. Various binder, antistatic compounds and wetting agents provide additional surface properties. As a result, the end products do not create an excessively dusty work environment.[43] Manufactured fibers known as rock wool, slag wool, glass wool, and refractory ceramic fibers are used in yarns, paper, insulation and construction material of all types, blankets, and felts as well as composite materials of various kinds.[40]

Compelling epidemiological and experimental information associates malignant mesothelioma with exposure to long (i.e., > 5 μ) amphibole asbestos (see Chapter 28). Accordingly, concern has arisen regarding the potential pathogenetic effects of man-made inorganic fibers, particularly because fiberglass has been found to induce mesotheliomas in rats after intrathoracic inoculations. Indeed, the International Agency for Research in Cancer (IARC) has categorized fiberglass as a possible human carcinogen (an exceedingly controversial decision). Although epidemiological studies have failed to demonstrate an association between the occurrence of this unique tumor with employment in the fiberglass manufacturing industry,[38] concern is justified because the disease develops infrequently, even in workers exposed to high concentrations of amphibole asbestos. Moreover, the long latency period of the cancer precludes early detection of an increased risk.

Dosage and durability in tissue and fiber diameter are

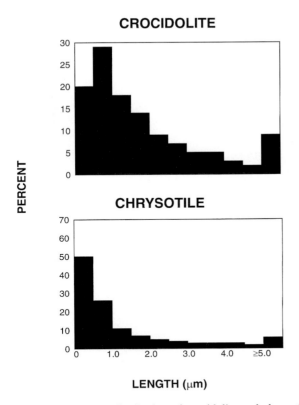

CROCIDOLITE

CHRYSOTILE

PERCENT

LENGTH (μm)

Fig. 6-26. Typical size distribution of crocidolite and chrysotile fibers after industrial purification. Note the majority of the fibers are relatively short and less than 5 μ in length. It is the longer fibers greater than 5 μ that are considered to be pathogenic. (Adapted from Hwang C-Y: Size and shape of airborne asbestos fibres in mines and mills, *Br J Ind Med* 40:273, 1983.)

Table 6-6. Some typical exposures to personnel during manufacture and use of ceramic fibers

Process description or job	Fiber/ml^3
Manufacturers	
Baling raw fiber	0.4
Bagging/chopping raw fiber	1.2
Mixing during product formation	0.4
Packing of products	0.02
Users	
Wrapping ceramic fiber blanket around pipe weld	0.8
Stripping and relining furnace panel	1.2
Kiln building	1.75
Handling blanket ceramic fiber	1.0
Machining and ventilation control of ceramic fire-board	0.6
Insulation work using blanket	1.0

Adapted from Friar JJ, Phillips AM: *Exposure to ceramic man-made mineral fibers.* In *Non-occupational exposure to mineral fibers,* Lyon, France, 1990, IARC.

additional considerations that influence the potential health effects of these materials. As shown in Table 6-6, exposures of manufacturers and users to refractory ceramic fibers are low, most probably because of the physical characteristics and length of the fibers and industrial controls that reduce the release of fibers into the working environment. Similar data have accumulated in environmental studies of other synthetic fibers. Manufactured vitreous fibers do not seem to persist in tissues once inhaled, in contrast to amphibole asbestos, which is retained indefinitely in the lungs of those who are exposed.

Volcanic tuff

As one reads this page, roughly 3000 active sites of volcanic activity are contributing to the dust burden of the atmosphere and, to a lesser extent, the stratosphere.[10,22] An estimated 4 to 25 · 10^6 tons of volcanic debris accumulate worldwide each year.[74] Fine dust remains suspended for indefinite periods, depending on particle size, and can be transported in the atmosphere for long distances (Figs. 6-2, 6-28). The density of these particulates and their broad dis-

tribution are believed to account for climatic changes over wide geographical regions. The bulk of the mass of cataclysmic eruptions is composed of large boulders and rocks, whereas the great majority of the particles are in the respirable range, i.e., less than 5 μ. Lava is a viscous product of a nonexplosive eruption that contains a relatively high concentration of crystalline and noncrystalline SiO$_2$. Its contribution of dust to the atmosphere is derived from aged igneous extrusions that ultimately erode and are aerosolized by wind. Vast areas of the earth's surface, such as in the American Northwest, are covered by these extensively eroded deposits of lava, which reflect volcanic activity in the geological past.

Magma, the core material of the volcano, wells up through the lithosphere from deep in the earth, usually, but not invariably, at the juncture of geological plates formed beneath the earth's crust. Magma consists of gas-laden superheated liquid material composed of variable amounts of silicate and silica. The dust in North America's most recent eruption at Mount St. Helens was composed of over 95% plagiclase, a complex aluminum silicate, with the remainder of the material being SiO$_2$, much of which was found as shards of glass (Fig. 6-10). Because silicates and noncrystalline glass shards have relatively little or no adverse effects on the lungs after inhalation, the risk of respiratory disease owing to volcanic dust has been largely limited to those experiencing extremely heavy exposure in close proximity to the explosive event (Fig. 6-29). In a few geographically circumscribed regions, however, deposits of lava have crystallized to form fibrous silicates. Thus, in the Anatollan region of southern Turkey, a fibrous aluminum silicate, classified as a zeolite (eronite), is found in depos-

Fig. 6-27. Asbestos fibers and bodies in lung tissue of industrial dust-exposed individuals. **A,** A hematoxylin and eosin–stained tissue section revealing the patterns of several asbestos bodies as observed by light microscopy. **B,** Scanning electron micrograph of the cut surface of a slice of lung exhibiting asbestos bodies embedded in lung tissue. **C,** Amphibole asbestos fibers in lung tissue demonstrated by scanning electron microscopy. **D,** Scanning electron micrograph of two asbestos bodies demonstrating the range in size of the particles. Note the beaded accumulations of the iron/protein coagulum, which form at the tips and around the shafts of the fibers. **E,** A higher magnification of an asbestos body by scanning electron microscopy. **F,** A backscatter x-ray spectrometry image of the fiber demonstrating iron within the coagulum, which surrounds the fiber. **G,** Scanning electron micrographic x-ray spectrographic of fibers of asbestos. Cation peaks characteristic of amphibole asbestos are not designated and are obscured by the "iron/protein coagulum" of the asbestos body. (From Corn M, editor: *Handbook of toxic substances,* New York, 1993, Academic Press; with permission.)

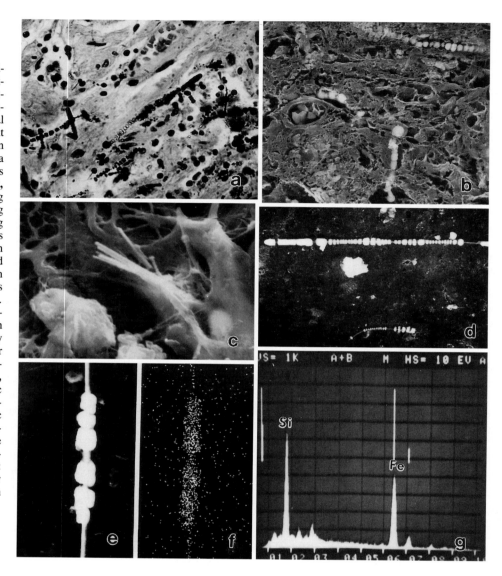

Fig. 6-28. Patterns of volcanic dust transport into the atmosphere. El Chichon, a Mexican volcano, erupted in a vertical axis from the core in the 1980s. Dust entered the stratosphere resulting in an exceptionally wide geographical dispersion. In contrast, Mount Saint Helens erupted on the northern escarpment. Dust dispersed in the troposphere and tropopause. Heavy deposits accumulated on the earth's surface in western Washington and in Idaho. (See Figure 6-2.)

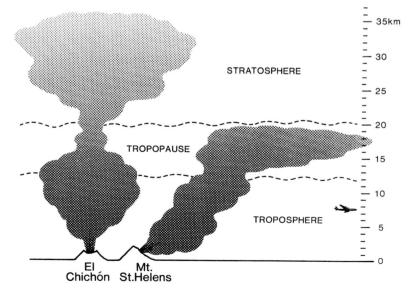

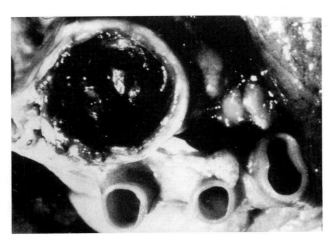

Fig. 6-29. Trachea at autopsy of an observer of the Mount St. Helens eruption who was suffocated by the volcanic dust. Note the obstruction of the trachea on cross section. (Adapted from Eisele JW et al: Deaths during the May 18, 1980, eruption of Mount St. Helens, *N Engl J Med* 305:931, 1981; with permission.)

its of volcanic tuff.[4,6] Similarly, lava deposits in central Turkey contain fibrous tremolite.[96] Malignant mesotheliomas have occurred among the indigenous populations of these regions, presumably as a result of lifelong exposure to these asbestiform dusts. Zeolites, some of which are fibrous and of volcanic origin, are widely distributed in the Great Basin and northwestern United States.

MINERALS DERIVED FROM ORGANIC SOURCES
Noncarbonaceous minerals

Limestone consists of the sedimentary deposits of the skeletal remains of a wide variety of mollusks, corals, crustaceans, and other lesser water-inhabiting species having a cytoskeleton containing calcium and magnesium salts. It is composed primarily of calcium carbonate and variable amounts of magnesium carbonate, with dolomite limestone being largely made up of the latter. Marble is the metamorphic expression of limestone. Its chemical impurities and the preserved skeletal remains of the zoata that formed it are reflected in the uniqueness of commercial deposits and their value. Limestone and marble dusts are not known to cause lung disease, presumably because the particulates dissolve readily in tissue. Some deposits contain impurities such as silica, but the concentrations are generally low and of little health relevance. Limestone and marble are used extensively in the building trades and for a variety of lesser purposes. Ground limestone is primarily used for soil conditioning. Wallastonite ($CaSiO_2$) is metamorphasized limestone that has been altered by the interaction of the sedimental deposits with igneous intrusions. It has a variety of uses as a substitute for silica and silicates.

Carbonaceous minerals

Coal is a general term referring to a complex group of minerals that are rich in carbon. Coal contains a wide variety of organic compounds (benzenes, phenols, napthalenes, and polynuclear aromatic hydrocarbons) in addition to carbon. The major inorganic mineral components of coal are clays, such as kaolinite, muscovite, and illite, and various salts, such as sulfides and chlorides.

The formation of coal has occurred through the continuous transformation of a diversity of plant materials over the past several hundred million years. Deposits increase in hardness and carbon content based on time and pressure considerations. The oldest coal (anthracite) has the highest content of carbon (approximately 92% to 95%), the greatest calorific value, and the lowest percentage of quartz, ash, and volatile matter. The youngest coal (lignite) has the lowest carbon content (approximately 65% to 75%), the least calorific value, the highest percentage of quartz and ash, and greater than 30% volatile matter. Bituminous coal is intermediate in age between anthracite and lignite. In the

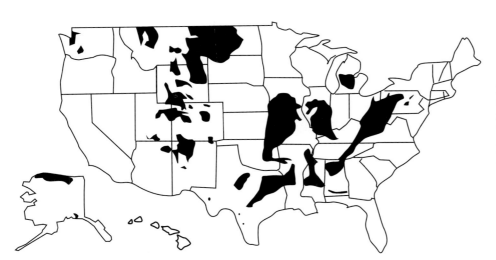

Fig. 6-30. Geographical distribution of major deposits of coal of various ranks in the United States. (Adapted from Merchant JA, editor: *Occupational respiratory diseases,* Washington, DC, 1986, U.S. Department of Health and Human Services, based on US Geological Survey, 1975.)

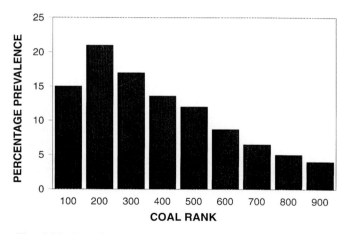

Fig. 6-31. Prevalence of coal worker's pneumoconiosis in British coal mine workers by rank of coal. (Adapted from Bennett JG et al: The relationship between coal rank and the prevalence of pneumoconiosis, *Br J Ind Med* 46:206, 1979.)

industry, coals are classified by "rank." Anthracite coal is accorded a high rank, whereas lignite has a low rank. Commercial deposits of coal are distributed at scattered sites in all seven continents, with major geological resources being found in the Russian Federation, the People's Republic of China, and the United States (Table 6-7; Fig. 6-30). Although coal consumption in the United States has been decreasing over the past several decades, it is still a major source of energy (and consequently pollution) in the People's Republic of China, the Russian Federation, and the central European countries. About 60% of the coal in the United States is used in electrical power generation with a substantial proportion of the remainder consumed in steel fabrication.

The profusion of small radiological opacities in simple coal worker's pneumoconiosis (CWP) correlates with the cumulative lifetime exposure to respirable coal dust (see Chapter 28). The density of opacities, in turn, correlates with the concentration of dust retained within the lung tissues. For reasons that are unclear, the risk of developing simple CWP varies from mine to mine even though the workers are believed to have been exposed to similar concentrations of dust. The risk of developing CWP is greatest in collieries mining high-rank coals (Fig. 6-31).[8] In this regard, it is interesting to note that the in vitro cytotoxicity of dusts has been shown to increase with the geological age and rank of the coal.

Underground mining practices dictate the concentrations of dust in the working environment. There has been a continuous improvement in underground conditions during this century (Table 6-8). Open-pit "strip" mining produces relatively little dust and is not associated with the development of CWP. Although quartz may be found within coal deposits to a variable extent, most silica dust exposures ex-

Table 6-7. Estimated recoverable world coal by major coal-producing countries (10^6 metric ton coal equivalent)

Australia	32,800
Canada	4,242
People's Republic of China	98,883
Federal Republic of Germany	34,419
India	12,427
Poland	59,600
Republic of South Africa	43,000
United Kingdom	45,000
United States	166,950
Soviet Union	109,900
Other countries	55,711
Total world	662,932

From *Coal—bridge to the future,* Cambridge, Mass, 1980, Ballinger Publishing.

perienced by miners are consequent to the removal of adjacent seams of rock, usually shale and slate, or in the digging of tunnels. Sand has been used on underground tracks to provide friction for mine locomotives, and the dust generated results in a pure silica respiratory exposure. As a result, underground coal miners often develop anthrosilicosis rather than a pure form of pneumoconiosis, attributable exclusively to coal dust exposure. There is some evidence to suggest that the silica dusts in the coal miner's environment influences the development of progressive massive fibrosis (see Chapter 28).

Natural graphite (plumbago) is composed of elemental crystalline carbon amalgamated with variable amounts of quartz and a variety of trace impurities, particularly silicates. Synthetic graphite is a high-temperature fusion product of coal. It is used in blast furnaces and in crucibles and ladels for highly reactive chemicals and molten metals. Exposure to particulate graphite can result in a pneumoconiosis.[46,50] Carbon black is hard crystalline carbon with many uses. It is reactive with cells and may have the capacity to injure pulmonary tissue.[68]

Table 6-8. Respirable dust concentrations (mg/m^3) in high-risk and selected occupations in the United States coal mining industry, by year

	Year	
Occupation	**1968**	**1977**
Continuous miner operator	6.5	1.3
Roofbolter	3.9	1.2
Cutter operator	5.9	1.1
Loader operator	6.0	1.3

Adapted from Merchant JA: *Coal worker's pneumoconiosis and exposures to other carbonaceous dust.* In Merchant JA, editor: *Occupational respiratory diseases,* Washington, DC, 1986, US Department of Health and Human Services.

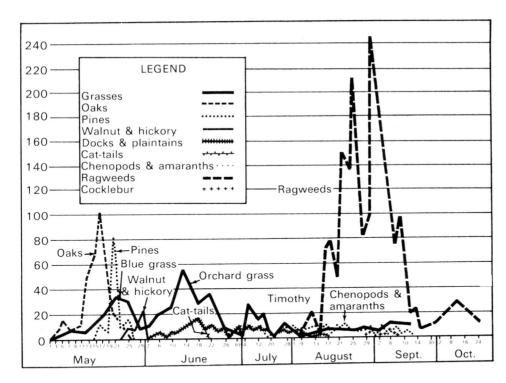

Fig. 6-32. Counts of pollen of common vegetation by months in Michigan. Tree pollen predominates in the spring; grasses during the summer; ragweed in early autumn. (From Wolbat GL: *Health effects of environmental pollutants,* St Louis, 1973, CV Mosby, Fig. 15-4; with permission.)

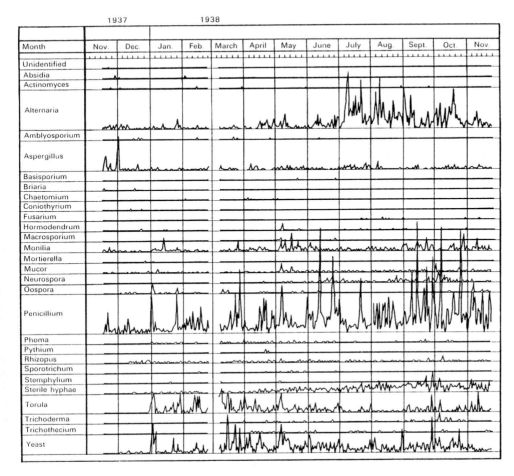

Fig. 6-33. Mold spores in the air of urban and rural Michigan during 2 years. Spore counts from the highest building in Detroit were averaged; spore counts were obtained on the third floor of a second Detroit building and averaged with data from a field 60 miles northwest of Detroit. Each count represents the results on an individual mold type during a year. Other studies have shown great variability from year to year, most probably reflecting meteorological conditions. (From Wolbat GL: *Health effects of environmental pollutants,* St Louis, 1973, CV Mosby; Fig. 15-5; with permission.)

Table 6-9. Infectious agents characteristically acquired from environmental sources

Infectious agent	Characteristic pathological lesion	Common environmental source
Bacteria		
Legionella pneumophila	Acute inflammation	Air coolers and conditioners, plumbing
Pseudomonas aeruginosa	Acute inflammation	Plumbing; hospital equipment
Bacillus anthracis	Acute inflammation and pulmonary edema	Animal products and carcasses; biological warfare
Yersinia pestis	Acute inflammation and pulmonary edema	Rodent carcasses
Rickettsia		
Coxiella burnetii	Acute inflammation and pulmonary edema	Animal products and carcasses; biological warfare
Fungus		
Monophasic fungus		
Aspergillus sp.		
Lung airways	Intra-airway fungus "ball"	Ubiquitous saprophyte
Lung parenchyma	Acute inflammation and abscesses	Ubiquitous saprophyte
Biphasic fungus imperfecti		
Histoplasma capsulatum	Granulomatous inflammation	Avian and bat guano
Histoplasma duboisii	Granulomatous inflammation	Soil
Coccidioides immitis	Acute granulomatous inflammation	Soil
Blastomyces dermatitidis	Acute granulomatous inflammation with abscesses	Soil
Paracoccidioides brasiliensis		Soil
Yeast		
Cryptococcus neoformans	Abscesses	Avian guano
Virus		
Hantavirus group	Hemorrhagic pulmonary edema	Rodent feces
Arenavirus	Hemorrhagic fever	Rodent feces

Table 6-10. Examples of organic dusts of agricultural importance

Organic particulates	Hay handling	Grain harvest	Commodity storage	Animal confinement	Mushroom production
Microorganisms					
Bacteria	X	X	X	X	X
Gram-negative	X	X	X	X	
Gram-positive			X	X	
Thermophilic					
Actinomycetes			X	X	X
Anaerobic microbes	?	?	?	?	?
Fungi	X	X	X	X	X
Microbial metabolites					
Endotoxins	X	X	X	X	?
Mycotoxins		?	X	X	
Proteases			?	X	
Macroorganisms					
Grain		X	X	X	
Insects (mites)			X	X	
Pollen	?			X	
Animal dander, hair				X	
Other plant parts	X		X	X	

?, Suspected but uncertain.
From Popendorf W: Report on agents, *Am J Ind Med* 10:251, 1986.

ORGANIC DUSTS

Microorganisms and products of yeast, fungi and bacteria, plant components, insect skeletal remains and feces, and waste by-products of higher animals (dander) constitute a large, diverse group of organic substances that potentially have health effects in those exposed. The best known and most feared, of course, are the infectious organisms that have a biphasic natural history (such as the Fungi Imperfecti), and those that replicate in animal tissue (*Anthrax, Coxiella burnetii, Hantavirus, Arenaviruses*) and are found in feces, urine, or decaying carcasses (Table 6-9). The life cycles of these organisms, to a large extent, have been characterized, but new agents continue to appear. More common, however, are the diverse variety of organic materials that are responsible for immunologically mediated disorders of three types: (1) conjunctival and nasal irritation (hay fever), (2) bronchial asthma and irritative bronchitis, and (3) hypersensitivity pneumonitis (allergic alveolitis).[32] Fig. 6-32 depicts the temporal prevalence pattern of a variety of common pollen allergens in the northeastern North American environment. Similarly, Fig. 6-33 shows the pattern observed for the spores of common fungi, realizing that meteorological considerations critically influence fungal growth and thus the prevalence and types of spores in the ambient air. One of the most common allergens recognized to have caused widespread disease in the industrial setting was "alcalase," a proteolytic enzyme produced from

Bacillus subtilis and used commercially as a component of detergents.[11,53,70] In general, these allergens sensitize atopic persons and are commonly responsible for the hay fever syndrome and may contribute to the development of bronchial asthma in susceptible atopic persons. Hypersensitivity pneumonitis, alternatively, is associated with unique exposures to a variety of organic materials, often in the specific work environment. The clinical and pathological features of these diseases are considered in Chapter 28.

Originally called mycotoxicosis, the term acute organic dust toxic syndrome describes a complex of acute symptoms (including chills, malaise, myalgia, dry cough, breathlessness, headache, and nausea) occurring a few hours after a heavy exposure to organic dust.[90] For example, it has been described after exposure to moldy hay and dust from grains, straw, and silage. It differs from hypersensitivity pneumonitis, in that prior sensitization is not required, and the condition is abrupt in onset with recovery usually occurring in 2 to 3 days.

Table 6-11. Average inorganic and quartz content of respirable dust from various grains processed in elevators

Grain type	Inorganic content (%) terminal	Quartz content (%)
Wheat	27.2 ± 7.0*	5.3 ± 3.3
Barley	43.4 ± 5.3	6.1 ± 3.8
All types	32.4 ± 11.4	4.8 ± 3.2

Adapted from Dosman JA, Cotton DJ: *Occupational pulmonary disease: focus on grain dust and health,* New York, 1980, Academic Press, p 501. *Standard deviation.

Table 6-13. Mean microorganism and endotoxin concentrations in mills processing dried herbs and grains

	Sage	Marjoram	Rye & Oat
Microorganisms (10^3 cfu/m^3)			
Gram-negative bacteria	5	58	26
Spore-forming bacilli	20	395	26
Other bacteria	25	10	64
Mesophilic actinomycetes	24	1	> 10
Thermophilic actinomycetes	4	55	12
Fungi	7	109	127
Total count	94	627	
Respirable fraction (%)	41	51	42
Total dust (mg/m^3)	8	946	113
Total endotoxin (μg/m^3)	4	757	55

cfu, Colony-forming units.
Adapted from Dutkiewicz J: Microbial hazards in plants. Processing grains and herbs, *Am J Ind Med* 10:300, 1986.

Table 6-12. Spores of common fungi by percent of total sample in grain and in dust around combine harvester

Spore type	Total spore content (%) Wheat	Barley	Oats	Combine harvester
Cladosporium	47	46	59	100
Alternaria	24	10	9	99
Epicoccum	1	1	1	70
Botrytis	< 1	—	< 1	67
Verticillium/Paecilomyces	6	2	7	67
Puccinia uredospores	3	4	0	70
Ustilago	2	< 1	0	55

Adapted from Dosman JA, Cotton DJ, editors: *Occupational pulmonary disease: focus on grain dust and health,* New York, 1980, Academic Press, p 426.

Table 6-14. Airborne dust and endotoxin concentrations of ambient air in selected agricultural environments

Environment	Dust (mg/m³)		Endotoxin (µg/m³)	
	Median	Range	Median	Range
Swine confinement	2.64	1.1-8	0.09	0.02-0.4
Poultry confinement	2.43	1-3.7	0.36	0.1-0.5
Compost facilities	1.48	0.7-5.5	0.0005	0.0005-0.009

Adapted from Clark S: Comparisons of organic dust exposures in agricultural occupations and waste processing industries, *Am J Ind Med* 10:286, 1986.

Agricultural workers experience exceptionally heavy exposures to a diverse variety of aerosolized particulates (Table 6-10).[13,72] It has been estimated that U.S. agricultural operations produce 1.8×10^6 tons of dust annually.[30] Grain handlers are at a particularly high risk of exposures to fragmented particles of grain, inorganic silicates and silica, fungi and bacteria (Table 6-11), insect parts, urine protein, feces from vermin, endotoxins, and pesticides. The mixture is highly variable, depending on the grain, the soil it is grown in, and the methods of harvest and storage. It is estimated that 30% to 60% of this material is respirable. It is not surprising, therefore, that the majority of grain elevator workers complain of eye and nasal symptoms.[33,73] Documented airborne dusts in grains and around combine harvesters are known to be as high as 230 mg/m³ and 2×10^8mg/m³ fungal spores of diverse genera (Table 6-12).[34] The average amounts of bacteria, fungal spore, and endotoxin in the air of processing plants for herbs and grains are illustrated in Table 6-13. The effects of organic industrial dusts and those of pollen and fungal spores are not restricted to persons living or working in immediate proximity to the source. This is exemplified by observations in a European port city where soybean dust emanating from the docks was found to be responsible for cases of asthma in the adjacent city.[3]

Modern agriculture employs intensive techniques for livestock production usually in confined quarters (swine, poultry, dairy cows, and veal calves). According to Donham and Gustafsson,[31] roughly 7×10^5 persons in the United States are occupationally exposed to the ambient air in these facilities. In addition to high concentrations of the gases, methane, hydrogen sulfide (H_2S), and ammonia, the working environment is replete with dusts from feed grains, bedding, and fecal material and derived from animal dander, urine protein, microorganisms, endotoxin, and insect parts. Table 6-14 summarizes information on the amounts of dust and endotoxin found in agricultural animal housing facilities.[31]

REFERENCES

1. Adamson IYR, Bowden DH: Pulmonary reaction to long and short asbestos fibers is independent of fibroblast growth factor production by alveolar macrophages, *Am J Pathol* 137:523, 1990.
2. Ampian SG, Virta RL: *Crystalline silica overview: occurrence and analysis,* Washington, DC, 1992, U.S. Department of the Interior, Bureau of Mines Information Circular/IC-9317.
3. Antó JM et al: Preventing asthma epidemics due to soybeans by dust-control measures, *N Engl J Med* 329:1760, 1993.
4. Artvinli M, Baris YI: Malignant mesotheliomas in a small village in the Anatollan region of Turkey: an epidemiologic study, *J Natl Cancer Inst* 63:17, 1979.
5. Ayalp A, Myroniuk D: Evaluation of occupational exposure to free silica in Alberta foundries, *Am Ind Hyg Assoc* 43:825, 1982.
6. Baris I et al: Epidemiological and environmental evidence of the health effects of exposure to erionite fibres: a four-year study in the Cappadocian region of Turkey, *Int J Cancer* 39:10, 1987.
7. Bégin R et al: Carborundum pneumoconiosis. Fibers in the mineral activate macrophages to produce fibroblast growth factors and sustain the chronic inflammatory disease, *Chest* 95:842, 1989.
8. Bennett JG et al: The relationship between coal rank and the prevalence of pneumoconiosis, *Br J Industr Med* 46:206, 1979.
9. Bignon J, editor: *Health related effects of phyllosilicates,* NATO ASI Series, Vol G21, Berlin, 1990, Springer-Verlag.
10. Blong RJ: *Volcanic hazards: a sourcebook on the effects of eruptions.* Sydney, 1984, Academic Press.
11. British Medical Association: Biological effects of proteolytic enzyme detergents, *Thorax* 31:621, 1976.
12. Casey KR et al: Zeolite exposure and associated pneumoconiosis, *Chest* 87:837, 1985.
13. Clark S: Comparisons of organic dust exposures in agricultural occupations and waste processing industries, *Am J Ind Med* 10:286, 1986.
14. Commins BT: *Asbestos fibres in drinking water.* Scientific and Technical Report—STR 1, Maidenhead, England, 1983, Commins Associates.
15. Commins BT: *The significance of asbestos and other mineral fibres in environmental ambient air.* Scientific and Technical Report—STR 2, England, 1985, Commins Associates.
16. Constantopoulos SH et al: Regional findings in metsovo lung, *Lancet* 1:452, 1987.
17. Cook PM: Semi-quantitative determination of asbestiform amphibole mineral concentrations in Western Lake Superior water samples, *Adv X-ray Anal* 18:557, 1975.
18. Cook PM, Glass GE, Tucker JH: Asbestiform amphibole minerals: detection and measurement of high concentrations in municipal water supplies, *Science* 185:853, 1974.
19. Cooper WC, Sargent EN: Study of chest radiographs and pulmonary ventilatory function in perlite workers, *J Occup Med* 28:199, 1986.
20. Craighead JE et al: The pathology of asbestos-associated diseases of the lungs and pleural cavities: diagnostic criteria and proposed grading schema. Report of the Pneumoconiosis Committee of the College of American Pathologists and the National Institute for Occupational Safety and Health, *Arch Pathol Lab Med* 106:542, 1982.
21. Craighead JE, Emerson RJ, Stanley DE: Slateworkers' pneumoconiosis. *Hum Pathol* 23:1098, 1992.
22. Craighead JE et al: Health effects of Mount St. Helens volcanic dust, *Lab Invest* 48:5, 1983.
23. Craighead JE et al: Diseases associated with exposure to silica and nonfibrous silicate minerals, *Arch Pathol Lab Med* 112:673, 1988.

24. Darwin C: An account of the fine dust which often falls on vessels in the Atlantic Ocean, *QJ Geological Society (Lond)* 2:26, 1846.
25. Davies D, Cotton R: Mica pneumoconiosis, *Br J Ind Med* 40:22, 1983.
26. de Klerk NH et al: Cancer mortality in relation to measures of occupational exposure to crocidolite at Wittenoom Gorge in Western Australia, *Br J Ind Med* 46:529, 1989.
27. De Vuyst P et al: Dental technician's pneumoconiosis. A report of two cases, *Am Rev Respir Dis* 133:316, 1986.
28. Dockery DW et al: An association between air pollution and mortality in six U.S. cities. *N Engl J Med* 329:1753, 1993.
29. Donaldson K et al: Inflammation generating potential of long and short fibre amosite asbestos samples, *Br J Ind Med* 46:271, 1989.
30. Donham KJ: Hazardous agents in agricultural dusts and methods of evaluation, *Am J Ind Med* 10:205, 1986.
31. Donham KJ, Gustafsson KE: Human occupational hazards from swine confinement, *Ann Am Conf Governmental Ind Hyg* 2:137, 1982.
32. doPico GA: Report on diseases, *Am J Ind Med* 10:261, 1986.
33. doPico GA: Health effects of occupational grain dust exposure, *Am J Ind Med* 10:298, 1986.
34. Dosman JA, Cotton DJ: *Occupational pulmonary disease focus on grain dust and health*, New York, 1980, Academic Press.
35. Driscoll RJ et al: Malignant mesothelioma. A cluster in a native American pueblo, *N Engl J Med* 318:1437, 1988.
36. Dutkiewicz J: Microbial hazards in plants processing grain and herbs, *Am J Ind Med* 10:300, 1986.
37. Eisele JW et al: Deaths during the May 18, 1980, eruption of Mount St. Helens, *N Engl J Med* 305:931, 1981.
38. Enterline PE: Letter to Editor, *Br J Ind Med* 47:145, 1990.
39. Environmental Protection Agency: (40 CFR Part 763) Asbestos-containing materials in schools; final rule and notice, *Federal Register,* Oct. 30, 1987.
40. Estes W, editor: *Man-made vitreous fibers. Nomenclature, chemistry and physical properties,* 1991, TIMA.
41. Friar JJ, Phillips AM: Exposure to ceramic man-made mineral fibres. In *Non-occupational exposure to mineral fibres.* Lyon, France, 1990, IARC.
42. Funahashi A et al: Pneumoconiosis in workers exposed to silicon carbide, *Am Rev Respir Dis* 129:635, 1984.
43. Geurin MR, Jenkins RA, Tomkins BA: *The chemistry of environmental tobacco smoke: composition and measurement,* Boca Raton, Fla, 1993, Lewis Publishers.
44. Gibbs AE et al: Talc pneumoconiosis: a pathologic and mineralogic study, *Hum Pathol* 23:1344, 1992.
45. Glover JR et al: Effects of exposure to slate dust in North Wales, *Br J Ind Med* 37:152, 1980.
46. Gloyne SR, Marshall G, Hoyle C: Pneumoconiosis due to graphite dust, *Thorax* 4:31, 1949.
47. Golden EB et al: Fly ash lung: a new pneumoconiosis? *Am Rev Respir Dis* 125:108, 1982.
48. Goodglick LA, Kane AB: Cytotoxicity of long and short crocidolite asbestos fibers in vitro and in vivo. *Cancer Res* 50:5153, 1990.
49. Hamlin LE, Weber HJ: Siderosis: a benign pneumoconiosis due to the inhalation of iron dust. Part I: a clinical, roentgenological and industrial hygiene study of foundry cleaning room employees, *Ind Med Surg* 19:151, 1950.
50. Hanoa R: Graphite pneumoconiosis. A review of etiologic and epidemiologic aspects, *Scand J Work Environ Health* 9:303, 1983.
51. HEI-Asbestos Research: *Asbestos in public and commercial buildings,* Cambridge, Mass, 1991, Health Effects Institute.
52. Hwang C-Y: Size and shape of airborne asbestos fibres in mines and mills, *Br J Ind Med* 40:273, 1983.
53. Juniper CP et al: *Bacillus subtilis* enzymes: a 7-year clinical, epidemiological and immunological study of an industrial allergen, *J Soc Occup Med* 27:3, 1977.
54. Kern DG, Hanley KT, Roggli VL: Malignant mesothelioma in the jewelry industry, *Am J Ind Med* 21:409, 1992.
55. Lapenas D et al: Kaolin pneumoconiosis. Radiologic, pathologic, and mineralogic findings, *Am Rev Respir Dis* 130:282, 1984.
56. MacFarland HN et al: Long-term inhalation studies with raw and processed shale dusts, *Ann Occup Hyg* 26:213, 1982.
57. Machta L, List JR, Hubert LF: World-wide travel of atomic debris, *Science* 124:474, 1956.
58. Martin JR et al: Pneumoconiosis in iron ore surface mining in Labrador, *J Occup Med* 30:780, 1988.
59. Massé, Bégin R, Cantin A: Pathology of silicon carbide pneumoconiosis, *Mod Pathol* 1:104, 1988.
60. McDonald JC et al: Cohort study of mortality of vermiculite miners exposed to tremolite, *Br J Ind Med* 43:436, 1986.
61. McDonald JC et al: Health of vermiculite miners exposed to trace amounts of fibrous tremolite, *Br J Ind Med* 45:630, 1988.
62. McLaughlin AIG: Pneumoconiosis in foundry workers, *Br J Tubercul Dis Chest* LI(4):297, 1957.
63. Merchant JA, editor: *Occupational respiratory diseases,* Washington DC, 1986, US Department of Health and Human Services.
64. Millette JR, Clark PJ, Pansing MF: *Exposure to asbestos from drinking water in the United States,* EPA report. Health Effects Research Laboratory, 1979.
65. Millette JR et al: Asbestos in water supplies of the United States, *Env Health Perspect* 53:45, 1983.
66. Morgan WKC: Kaolin and the lung, *Am Rev Respir Dis* 127:141, 1983.
67. Morgan WKC, Seaton A: *Occupational lung diseases,* ed 2, Philadelphia, 1984, WB Saunders.
68. Mossman BT, Adler KB, Craighead JE: Interaction of carbon particles with tracheal epithelium in organ culture, *Environ Res* 16:110, 1978.
69. Musk AW, Greville HW, Tribe AE: Pulmonary disease from occupational exposure to an artificial aluminum silicate used for cat litter, *Br J Ind Med* 37:367, 1980.
70. Newhouse ML, Tagg B, Pocock SJ: An epidemiological study of workers producing enzyme washing powders, *Lancet* 1:689, 1970.
71. Parkes WR: *Occupational lung disorders,* ed 2. London, 1982, Butterworths.
72. Popendorf W: Report on agents, *Am J Ind Med* 10:251, 1986.
73. Popendorf W et al: A synopsis of agricultural respiratory hazards, *Am Ind Hyg Assoc J* 46:154, 1985.
74. Pye K: *Aeolian dust and dust deposits,* New York, 1987, Academic Press.
75. Roggli VL, Greenberg SD, Pratt PC: *Pathology of asbestos-associated diseases,* Boston, 1992, Little, Brown.
76. Ross M: *The geological occurrences and health hazards of amphibole and serpentine asbestos.* In Veblen DR, editor: *Reviews in mineralogy, vol 9, Amphiboles.* Mineralogical Society of America, 1981.
77. Ross M, Kuntze RA, Clifton RA: *A definition for asbestos,* American Society for Testing and Materials, 1984.
78. Samimi B, Weill H, Ziskind M: Respirable silica dust exposure of sandblasters and associated workers in steel fabrication yards, *Arch Env Health* 29:61, 1974.
79. Seaton A, Louw SJ, Cowie HA: Epidemiologic studies of Scottish oil shale workers: I. prevalence of skin disease and pneumoconiosis, *Am J Ind Med* 9:409, 1986.
80. Seaton A et al: Pneumoconiosis of shale miners, *Thorax* 36:412, 1981.
81. Sherwin RP, Barman ML, Abraham JL: Silicate pneumoconiosis of farm workers, *Lab Invest* 40:576, 1979.
82. Skinner HCW, Ross M, Frondel C: *Asbestos and other fibrous materials. Mineralogy, crystal chemistry and health effects,* New York, 1988, Oxford University Press.
83. Stanton MF, Wrench C: Mechanisms of mesothelioma induction with asbestos and fibrous glass, *J Natl Cancer Inst* 48:797, 1972.
84. Stanton MF et al: Relation of particle dimension to carcinogenicity in amphibole asbestoses and other fibrous minerals, *J Natl Cancer Inst* 67:965, 1981.

85. Talcott J et al: Mesothelioma in manufacturers of asbestos-containing cigarette filters, *Lancet* 1:392, 1987.

86. Vallyathan NV, Craighead JE: Pulmonary pathology of workers exposed to nonasbestiform talc, *Hum Pathol* 12:28, 1981.

87. Vallyathan NV et al: Pulmonary fibrosis in an aluminum arc welder, *Chest* 81:372, 1982.

88. Vigliani EC, Mottura G: Diatomaceous earth silicosis, *Br J Ind Med* 5:148, 1948.

89. Vocaturo G et al: Human exposure to heavy metals. Rare earth pneumoconiosis in occupational workers, *Chest* 83:780, 1983.

90. Von Essen S et al: Organic dust toxic syndrome: an acute febrile reaction to organic dust exposure distinct from hypersensitivity pneumonitis, *Clin Toxicol* 28:389, 1990.

91. Wagner JC et al: Inhalation of china stone and china clay dusts: relationship between the mineralogy of dust retained in the lungs and pathological changes, *Thorax* 41:190, 1986.

92. Waxweiler RJ et al: A retrospective cohort mortality study of males mining and milling attapulgite clay, *Am J Ind Med* 13:305, 1988.

93. WHO/EURO Technical committee for monitoring and evaluating airborne MMMF: *Reference methods for measuring airborne man-made mineral fibers,* Copenhagen, 1985, World Health Organization.

94. Wilson CL: *Coal—bridge to the future*. Report of the World Coal Study (WOCOL), Cambridge, Mass, 1980, Ballinger Publishing Company.

95. Xu X, Wang L: Association of indoor and outdoor particulate level with chronic respiratory illness, *Am Rev Respir Dis* 148:1516, 1993.

96. Yazicioglu S et al: Pleural calcification, pleural mesotheliomas, and bronchial cancers caused by tremolite dust, *Thorax* 35:564, 1980.

Chapter 7

HIGH ALTITUDE AND HUMAN DISEASE

John T. Reeves

GENERAL CONCEPTS

Approximately 1% of the world's population lives at altitudes above 2500 m. Much of the world's mineral resources and its recreational opportunities are above this altitude. For example, although only 120,000 of Colorado's 3 million people live at high altitude, some 20 million persons come annually for recreation. Thus, many people live, work, and play at high altitude. Also, because hypoxia is important in many diseases at all altitudes, the effects of high altitude provide lessons we cannot afford to ignore. Lung and cardiovascular diseases are all associated with hypoxia in some way. Furthermore, fetal life, referred to by Barcroft as "Mount Everest in Utero," is a hypoxic state we all must experience no matter where we live. The study of humankind at high altitude provides a window to the understanding of the effects of hypoxia.

Barometric pressure

Pressure, altitude, and arterial P_{O_2}. As one leaves sea level, the atmospheric pressure falls, but because air is compressible, the fall is more rapid at first (Fig. 7-1,*A*). Because oxygen concentration is 20.94% of dry air at all altitudes, atmospheric barometric pressure (P_B) determines the oxygen pressure (P_{O_2}) in the atmosphere:

$$\text{Atmospheric } P_{O_2} \text{ (mmHg)} = 0.2094 \times P_B \text{ (mmHg)}.$$

The arterial P_{O_2} (P_{O_3}), however, is less than that in the atmosphere (Fig. 7-1, *B*) because of the alveolar partial pressures of H_2O (47 mmHg at 37° C) and CO_2 and the alveolar-to-arterial pressure gradient.

This work was partially supported by National Institutes of Health grant HL 46481.

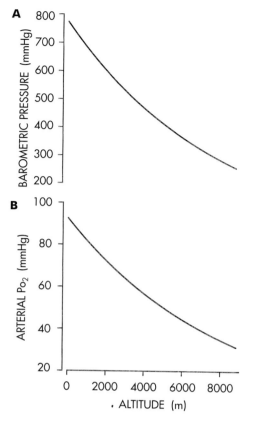

Fig. 7-1. A, Barometric pressure for increasing terrestrial elevations from sea level (0 altitude) to the summit of Mt. Everest (8848 m). **B,** Approximate oxygen pressures in arterial blood *(Pao₂)* for acclimatized subjects with increasing terrestrial elevation.

Hypoxemia. Hypoxemia accompanying exposure to reduced barometric pressure stimulates responses that begin immediately but that continue over a lifetime. Indeed, some responses develop over generations within altitude populations. For example as is shown later, Tibetans, who have the longest tenure at altitude of any population, have less polycythemia, less pulmonary hypertension, and better respiratory control, and their children have more normal birth weights than do populations more recently arrived at altitude.[43] For any one individual the normal adaptations are those arising in currently recognized oxygen sensors within the carotid body, the lungs, arteries, and kidney.

Hypoxia stimulates the carotid body to increase ventilation.[34] Concomitantly and possibly related to carotid body stimulation, there is activation of the sympathetic nervous system, which in turn initiates the cardiovascular adaptations.[3,53] Heart rate and cardiac contractility rise. The plasma volume and cardiac output fall. The peripheral resistance and arterial pressure rise. The increase in ventilation is essential and persists; the cardiovascular changes tend to be temporary and are of questionable benefit.

Pulmonary arteriolar smooth muscle senses hypoxia, causing pulmonary vasoconstriction and elevation of pul-

monary arterial pressure.[50,52] Hypoxic pulmonary vasoconstriction is necessary for the survival of the fetus and neonate but is potentially detrimental in the adult at high altitude. Although increasing pulmonary arterial pressure may have a small benefit for improving the ventilation-to-perfusion ratio (and hence arterial oxygenation) at altitude, it certainly increases the work of the right heart and the risk of lung edema.

Hypoxia stimulates release of erythropoietin from the renal juxtaglomerular apparatus. The result is an increase in red cell mass, which acts to increase the oxygen-carrying capacity of the blood to offset the reduced oxygen saturation.[66] The risk is that some persons have excessive increases in red cell production, which leads to altitude illness.[1,2,9,49]

Ventilatory acclimatization

Of the aforementioned processes, only the carotid body's stimulation of ventilation is essential for well-being of either a visitor or a resident at high altitude. Ventilation is the first and most important link in the chain transporting oxygen from atmosphere to tissue mitochondria because if oxygen is not brought to the alveolus, more distal transport is jeopardized. A key function of the increase in ventilation is the fall in carbon dioxide pressure (Pco_2). A convenient way to think of how ventilation affects alveolar oxygen is to recall that the partial pressures of the four main alveolar gases, N_2 (including other inert gases), O_2, CO_2, and H_2O, must add up to total barometric pressure. The partial pressure of water vapor (PH_2O) is a constant, and PN_2 in the body (and the alveolus) equilibrates closely to that in the ambient air, leaving only CO_2 and O_2, which can vary. Increasing ventilation blows off CO_2, in which, approximately, for each molecule of CO_2 lost, the alveolus gains a molecule of O_2. Although increasing ventilation with increasing altitude can be monitored by the fall in Pco_2, it can also be reckoned as the primary defense of arterial oxygenation. Ventilatory acclimatization requires time because of the incompatible demands of the body to defend both oxygenation and pH. On arrival at altitude, hyperventilation causes alkalosis, which limits the ventilatory response. Several days are required for the renal excretion of bicarbonate to lower pH back toward the sea level norm. With the progressive excretion of bicarbonate, the ventilation rises, reaching a stable, higher plateau after about 1 week for the visitor from sea level to 4000 m. During the acclimatization period, some persons are particularly susceptible to acute altitude syndromes.

ACUTE AND SUBACUTE ALTITUDE SYNDROMES
Acute syndromes (develop in hours to days)

Acute mountain sickness and high altitude cerebral edema. These syndromes have been defined by an international working group reporting to the Hypoxia Symposium.[17]

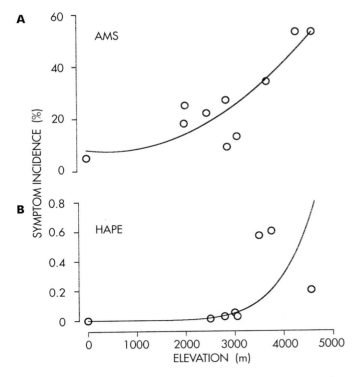

Fig. 7-2. A, Incidence of symptoms indicating acute mountain sickness *(AMS)* for increasing terrestrial elevation. (Summarized data from references 18,22,23,35,40,41,47.) **B,** Incidence of high altitude pulmonary edema *(HAPE)* for increasing terrestrial elevation. Not shown is the reported incidence of 15% in the Indian army (referred to by Hackett). (Summarized data from references 19,26,27,48.)

acute mountain sickness (AMS) in the setting of a recent gain in altitude, the presence of headache and at least one of the following symptoms: gastrointestinal (anorexia, nausea, or vomiting), fatigue or weakness, dizziness or lightheadedness, difficulty sleeping. As discussed next, the related syndrome is high altitude cerebral edema (HACE).

HACE can be considered end-stage or severe AMS. In the setting of a recent gain in altitude, the presence of a change in mental status or ataxia in a person with AMS or the presence of both mental status change and ataxia in a person without AMS.

On going from sea level to altitudes above approximately 2000 m (6500 ft), some persons experience this mysterious syndrome of symptoms, characterized principally by headache but also including (with decreasing frequency) sleeplessness, fatigue, shortness of breath, or loss of appetite.[23] The syndrome must somehow be caused by the hypoxia of altitude because incidence and severity increase with increasing altitude exposure (Fig. 7-2), the symptoms can be induced by prolonged breathing of hypoxic gas mixtures, and symptom relief occurs with relief of the hypoxia (oxygen breathing or descent from altitude.[22,49,57] Headache is by far the most frequent symptom (reported by 60% to 100% of affected subjects); severe cases are accompanied

by symptoms (vomiting, disorientation, ataxia, coma) or signs (papilledema,[59]) of increased intracranial pressure; spinal fluid pressure is sometimes increased;[21] and brain scan or autopsy findings have shown cerebral edema.

The above-mentioned findings have suggested that AMS is a syndrome, the severity of which depends on the magnitude of intracranial water accumulation. Brain scan and histology in fatal cases are most consistent with cellular swelling, suggesting intracellular rather than interstitial fluid accumulation. The mechanism remains a mystery, but time lag of several hours between hypoxic exposure and symptom development is consistent with the time required for fluid to accumulate within the brain. There are other aspects of the illness that may not increase our understanding of the mechanism but that certainly contribute to our ability to prevent or treat the syndrome. Perhaps most important is the concept that, given time, the body adapts to the hypoxic challenge. Thus, at a given altitude, as for example, in Summit County, Colorado, at 2500 to 3000 m, if the symptoms have not developed by day 2, they are unlikely to develop at all (Fig. 7-3,*B*).[18,23] If symptoms do develop but do not require evacuation of the patient, they usually subside within a day at 3000 m and within 2 to 3 days at 4300 m. Even those persons who develop symptoms but who have recovered can subsequently remain at altitude and be symptom free. Therefore the syndrome name includes the word "acute" because the symptoms occur soon after altitude exposure and usually quickly resolve.

The magnitude of a sudden altitude gain, i.e., the magnitude of the hypoxic stimulus, seems to be important.[47] For example, persons who go to Summit County (approximately 3000 m), from Denver (1600 m) have only an 8% incidence of symptoms, compared with a 28% incidence in those who come from sea level.[23] Furthermore, those who remain in Denver for 36 hours or more before going to Summit County have decreased incidence of symptoms.[23] Because of hypoventilation and periodic breathing during sleep,[13] hypoxemia is known to be greater during the night than during the waking hours. Therefore, considering the time required for altitude adaptation, the magnitude of altitude gain, and the worsening of hypoxemia during sleep, the principle has evolved that climbers should not increase their sleeping altitude more than 300 to 400 m per 24 hours.[47] Such considerations determine the rate of ascent for sportsmen and have led to the dictum that if you "climb high, sleep low."

We understand that hypoxia is a trigger for AMS, but we do not understand the variable susceptibility among persons. We are puzzled why subjects who have once had symptoms have a fourfold greater risk on reexposure than those who have not had symptoms.[23] Indeed, susceptible subjects have symptoms that occur earlier, are more severe, are more frequent, and occur at lower altitudes than resistant subjects. Other than knowing that altitude-resistant subjects tend to be older (Fig. 7-3,*A*) and in better physical condition, we know essentially nothing as to what makes

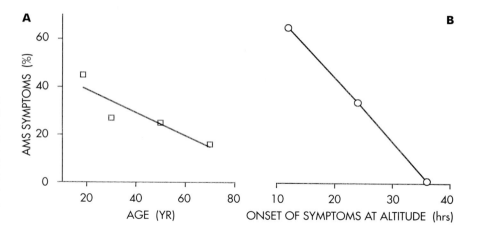

Fig. 7-3. **A,** Incidence of acute mountain sickness *(AMS)* according to age of persons going to high altitude in Summit County. **B,** The percentage of persons with AMS who develop symptoms by 12 hours (65%), between 12 and 36 hours (34%), and after 36 hours (1%). (Data replotted from Honigman B et al: Acute mountain sickness in a general tourist population at moderate altitudes, *Ann Intern Med* 118:587, 1993.)

some persons resistant to AMS and others susceptible. One could speculate that once we understand the susceptibility/resistance factor(s), we will understand mechanisms of hypoxia's adverse effect on the central nervous system.

The question is important because the cerebral cortex is the primary target organ for hypoxia. In Operation Everest II, in which over a 40-day period, healthy men were decompressed in a chamber to an altitude equivalent to that of Mt. Everest (8848 m), an important lesson was that cerebral function was maintained less well than that of other tissues.[51] Cerebral symptoms caused two of the eight men to be removed from the chamber before reaching the summit, and all six of those who reached the summit had deteriorated cognitive and coordination skills and had retinal hemorrhages. By contrast, we found no malfunction of skeletal or cardiac muscle or of peripheral nerve transmission. Although the lung was affected by these extreme altitudes, the effect was less apparent than that on the brain.

In AMS, fluid is retained. One could ask the question whether fluid retention is the cause or the result of cerebral edema. Because there is no animal model of AMS, the information about the disease has had to come from human studies, in which even the best information does not directly answer the question. Urinary output and sodium excretion increase on altitude exposure of asymptomatic persons but fall in persons destined to develop *AMS* (Fig. 7-4). Aldosterone blood levels are higher in symptomatic persons compared with asymptomatic persons at rest (Fig. 7-4), and the rise with exercise is exaggerated. Antidiuretic hormone (not shown) is normal at rest but shows an excessive increase with exercise in persons with AMS. (Exercise has been considered a precipitating factor for AMS.) Fluid retention is associated with increased levels of atrial natriuretic factor,[38] which may reflect increased right atrial stretch from higher central blood volume. Maldistribution of fluid within the body is central to the pathogenesis of all the acute altitude syndromes, but it is difficult to know which is cause and which is effect.

One could imagine that in AMS, liberation of inflammatory substances would increase vascular permeability, or activation of the sympathetics would raise vascular pressures, either or both of which would favor leak of fluid from vessels to tissues. Therefore, investigators have measured numerous eicosanoids as markers of inflammation and catecholamines as markers of sympathetic activity in blood and urine of healthy and symptomatic persons (Table 7-1). The evidence indicates that there is an increase in circulating eicosanoids such as *6-KPGF$_{1\alpha}$* (the stable metabolite of the vasodilator, prostacyclin), *TBx* (the stable metabolite of the vasoconstrictor, thromboxane), and *LTB4* (the leukotriene that is chemotactic for leukocytes). Haptoglobin and C reactive proteins, which also may be increased with inflammation, have been found increased. The increase in circulating catecholamines is not consistent among investigations. Although the data indicate that activation of these systems is likely, they do not separate cause from effect.

In addition to the aforementioned data, measurements have shown that with more severe symptoms, arterial hypoxemia is usually more severe,[6,18] and angiotensin-converting enzyme activity is better preserved (tested with hypoxic mixtures at sea level[37]). Despite the wealth of blood studies that are reported, none have demonstrated the mechanism of the disease. Inflammatory mechanisms and the sympathetics are activated at altitude, but they may be markers of altitude exposure or AMS, rather than the cause of the syndrome. Cerebral blood flow is increased in hypoxemic persons, and the increase is greater when hypoxemia is more severe in persons with AMS. An increase in flow, however, does not necessarily accompany the development of symptoms, and thus the symptoms cannot be attributed to changes in cerebral hemodynamics.[4]

Prevention and treatment of AMS have been largely nonspecific.[14,18,47] Prevention of symptoms by slow ascent allows for ventilatory acclimatization and improved oxygenation; whether there is an adaptation to hypoxia per se by the cerebral cells themselves is not clear. The carbonic an-

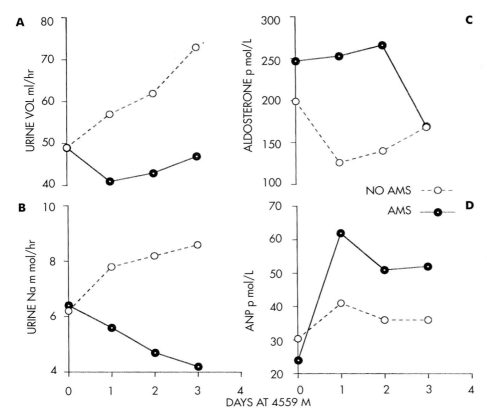

Fig. 7-4. Serial measurements at low altitude (day 0) and in subjects with and without acute mountain sickness *(AMS)* at 4559 m. **A,** Urine volume; **B,** urine sodium excretion; **C,** blood aldosterone; **D,** blood atrial natriuretic peptide *(ANP).* (Data replotted from Bèrtsch P: Aldosterone, antidiuretic hormone, and atrial natriuretic peptide in acute mountain sickness. In Sutton JR, Coates G, Houston CS, editors: *Hypoxia and mountain medicine,* Burlington, VT, 1992, Queen City Printers.)

Table 7-1. Eicosanoids as markers of inflammation and catecholamines as markers of sympathetic activity in blood of healthy and symptomatic persons

Measurement	Units	No symptoms	Acute mountain sickness	Reference no.
6-KPGF$_{1\alpha}$	pg/ml	101	236*	55
TBx	pg/ml	224	390*	55
PGE$_2$	pg/ml	37	48	55
PGF$_{2\alpha}$	pg/ml	40	47	55
LTB$_4$	pg/ml	574	2393*	55
LTC$_4$	pg/ml	1046	1067	55
Norepinephrine	ng/ml	825	446	55
Epinephrine	ng/ml	48	84	55
Haptoglobin	g/L	1.1	1.2*	6
C-reactive protein	mg/L	3.3	5.6*	6
Urinary protein	mg/hr	5.3	6.4	6
Serum protein	g/L	6.8	7.0	6
Norepinephrine	nMol/L	2.4	3.5*	6
Epinephrine	pMol/L	248	481*	6
Plasma renin	ng/L	0.4	0.8*	6

TBx, Thromboxane; *PGE$_2$*; prostaglandin E$_2$; *PGF$_2$*, prostaglandin F$_{2\alpha}$; *LTB$_4$*, leukotriene B$_4$; *LTC$_4$*; leukotriene C$_4$.
*Higher values ($P < 0.05$) in symptomatic versus nonsymptomatic persons.

hydrase inhibitor, acetazolamide (125 or 250 mg three times daily), taken orally a day or two in advance of altitude exposure, markedly reduces symptoms, probably by promoting urinary bicarbonate excretion. The resulting acidosis facilitates ventilatory response to altitude and diminishes hypoxemia on arrival. Also, by improving ventilation and arterial oxygenation, the drug can be helpful in treating established AMS.[14] Dexamethasone, which has been used extensively in other forms of cerebral edema, was found useful in persons with AMS at 2700 m but not at 2000 m in a double-blind, randomized trial.[41] Milder symptoms spontaneously resolve with rest. More severe symptoms are effectively reduced by improved oxygenation, i.e., by increasing barometric pressure by descent or portable chamber[57] or by administering oxygen-enriched air. Fatalities have occurred when severe symptoms were not treated.

High altitude pulmonary edema. High altitude pulmonary edema (HAPE) has been defined by an international working group reporting to the Hypoxia Symposium:[17]

HAPE in the setting of a recent gain in altitude, the presence of the following: symptoms (at least two of)—dyspnea at rest, cough, weakness or decreased exercise performance, chest tightness, or congestion; signs (at least two of)—rales or wheezing in at least one lung field, central cyanosis, tachypnea, or tachycardia.

Next to the cerebral cortex, the lung is the most susceptible organ to the acute adverse effects of hypoxia. HAPE may be 10-fold to 100-fold less common than AMS (Fig. 7-2), but subclinical pulmonary edema as manifested by pulmonary rales and a widened alveolar-arterial oxygen gradient in the absence of symptoms may occur in as many as 10% to 25% of climbers at 4000 m.[19] Similar to AMS and HACE, HAPE is a syndrome that is poorly understood and for which there is no animal model.

Although there were prior reports for many centuries alluding to HAPE, the succinct report by Houston in 1960[24] called modern attention to the problem. He focused on a young man without underlying disease who vigorously exercised at altitude. The usual history is an AMS syndrome for 2 to 3 days at altitudes above 2200 m before the development of chest congestion, dyspnea, cough, or fulminant edema.[19] Arterial oxygen saturation is almost invariably present and may be extreme, being most likely due to intrapulmonary mismatch of ventilation and perfusion. Fibrin formation occurs but seems to be the result of the edema formation and not the cause.[5] Because water displaces air in the lungs, the vital capacity is reduced, for example in the adult, by 200 to 300 ml at the onset of symptoms,[60] by 400 to 700 ml at the time the chest radiograph shows an infiltrate, and by 1 to 3 L when symptoms are severe and chest radiograph shows confluence of infiltrate.[46]

In 1961, Hultgren and colleagues[27] considered two main possible, but not mutually exclusive, mechanisms for HAPE: (1) increased capillary permeability and (2) in-

creased capillary pressure. Today it is not yet clear which initiates the process, which is more important, or to what extent both are operative.

With regard to lung vascular pressure, there seems to be little doubt that pulmonary hypertension is a part of the pathogenesis for several reasons previously summarized:[19,29,30]

1. Hypoxia of high altitude raises pulmonary arterial pressure immediately on ascent.
2. Most (but not all) persons who have a history of HAPE have an excessive rise in pulmonary arterial pressure (suggesting a reactive vascular bed) when exercised or given an hypoxic challenge at low altitude.[25,29,30]
3. Pulmonary arterial pressure has always been found to be above normal, and usually markedly so, during the acute episode of HAPE before treatment.
4. When there is increased lung capillary permeability, increasing the pulmonary arterial pressure worsens the leak.
5. Treatment designed to lower pulmonary arterial pressure has been effective.[19,48]

These findings indicate that pulmonary arterial hypertension precedes the development of symptoms and that it almost certainly participates in the pathogenesis.

Because the left atrial and pulmonary capillary wedge pressures in HAPE have uniformly been found to be normal or even low, however, one wonders how the elevated arterial pressure raises that in the capillary. The argument proposed is that the acute hypoxic pulmonary vasoconstriction is marked but unevenly distributed throughout the lung.[19,26,27] For example, intense vasoconstriction in some areas would redirect flow to other areas, where the increased flow would raise capillary pressure. Although the uneven distribution of intense vasoconstriction has not been shown in humans, the patchy infiltrates seen by radiographs early in the course of the syndrome are compatible with patches of overperfused lung.[64,65] Also, congenital absence of one main pulmonary artery is associated with HAPE[19,56] even at altitudes as low as 1600 m,[19] suggesting that when all blood flow must go through the one lung, the resulting overperfusion augments the risk. Work has emphasized that the thin wall structure of capillaries renders them susceptible to breakage, which would cause or contribute the leak in HAPE.[67]

There is evidence, however, that HAPE may not be entirely explained by hypoxic vasoconstriction, uneven or not. For example, two of five HAPE susceptible men, tested at sea level, did not have excessive hypoxic pulmonary pressure responses.[25] Within 24 hours of going to 3000 m, all had developed severe pulmonary hypertension, which was little affected by oxygen breathing. Thus, increased vasoreactivity to acute hypoxia was not universal at sea level, and hypoxic vasoconstriction could not account for the pulmonary hypertension at altitude. Some persons who develop severe pulmonary hypertension at altitude do not develop pulmonary edema, whereas others get HAPE with rather modest pressure elevations.[19,29,30] Furthermore, pressure elevation does not explain the high cellularity and protein content found in the edema fluid of persons with HAPE.[58]

Pulmonary vascular reactivity to hypoxia is expected to be a repeatable characteristic of an individual. Yet, persons may develop HAPE on some occasions and not on others, suggesting that there are factors in addition to hypoxia. One potentially important factor is increased lung vascular permeability, possibly caused by inflammation, a classic cause of edema. HAPE frequently coexists with upper respiratory infections,[19] and autopsy of those dying almost always reveals the presence of alveolar polymorphonuclear neutrophils. Alveolar fluid that contains high protein concentration suggests an inflammatory process, whereas a low protein content suggests hemodynamic edema as in heart failure. Alveolar fluid with high protein concentration was obtained in HAPE patients and controls by intrepid investigators using bronchoalveolar lavage of the right middle lung lobe at 4400 m on the Denali glacier near the West Buttress of Mt. McKinley.[58] Total leukocyte counts and the differential counts for monocytes, polymorphonuclear neutrophils (PMNs), and lymphocytes were normal in patients with AMS, as were the values for proteins, C5a, thromboxane, and eicosanoids.[58] In HAPE patients, however, there was a greater than fiftyfold increase in alveolar protein, PMNs, and lymphocytes. Thromboxane was increased tenfold, and leukotriene B$_4$, which was not detectable in normal persons and those with AMS, was clearly increased in persons with HAPE. The numbers of neutrophils and lymphocytes as well as the amount of protein present (Fig. 7-5) all related well to the leukotriene B$_4$ concentration. Alveolar monocytes were not increased, but rather the increase in cells was in those leukocytes (*PMNs* and lymphocytes) associated with acute inflammation. Also the high protein concentration was consistent with an inflammatory process, rather than a transudate filtered from the circulation by a high intravascular pressure. These data indicate that there is an inflammatory component to HAPE, but they do not establish that lung inflammation is the primary initiating event.

Although hypoxia, acting through some unknown mechanism, is central to the mechanism of HAPE, there are other precipitating factors in the pathogenesis.[19] Why are plasma natriuretic factor and vasopressin elevated?[8] Why, following recovery, can the subject remain at altitude or even go higher without difficulty? Does the increased pressure/permeability resolve, or does the lung adapt? In any event, the protection is quickly lost on descent to lower altitude. It is a peculiarity of children and young adults residing at altitudes of 2500 m or above that following a visit of only a few days to sea level, they risk HAPE on return home.[19] The time required for both pulmonary and cerebral adapta-

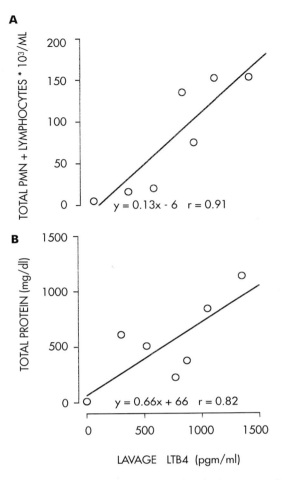

Fig. 7-5. Measurements in the bronchoalveolar lavage as related to the leukotriene B$_4$ in the lavage for persons with and without high altitude pulmonary edema on Mt. McKinley. **A,** Total counts, in thousands per milliliter, for neutrophils (polymorphonuclear neutrophils *[PMN]*) + lymphocytes in the lavage. **B,** Total protein in the lavage. (Replotted from Schoene RB et al: The lung at high altitude: bronchoalveolar lavage in acute mountain sickness and pulmonary edema, *J Appl Physiol* 64:2605, 1988.)

tion and deadaptation to hypoxia is almost exactly the same as that for ventilatory acclimatization and deacclimatization, suggesting that the ventilatory response to altitude is linked to the risk of altitude illnesses. If so, the link is not tight because some persons with a strong hypoxic ventilatory response develop HAPE, and others with poor response remain well at altitude.

Cold weather is a risk factor for HAPE. In Vail, Colorado, 90% of the HAPE cases occurred in winter months, whereas less than 10% of cases occurred in summer months, with nearly equal numbers of tourists.[61] In Summit County, Colorado, there was no seasonal or temperature-dependence for AMS, but there was a strong predilection for HAPE to occur on cold rather than warm days (Reeves, unpublished). The mechanisms by which cold had an adverse impact on the lung circulation in HAPE are not known. Other factors thought to affect HAPE adversely are exercise, sleeping medication, and excessive salt ingestion, but these have not been specifically evaluated.

High altitude retinal hemorrhage. Since 1970, it has been known that retinal hemorrhage occurs at high altitude, when it was described in newcomers to 5360 m elevation.[12] The hemorrhage was often accompanied by engorgement and tortuosity of the arteries and veins and occasionally by "cotton wool spots" or edema of the optic disk. At 5360 m elevation, hemorrhage was not seen in any of 12 persons immediately on arrival by air, but it was seen in 7 of 16 persons (44%) who arrived after 8 climbing days and in 7 of 11 persons (64%) who had resided there for at least 4 weeks, suggesting that the syndrome takes some time to develop.[36] Exercise immediately on arrival or later was associated with the development of vascular leak identified by fluorescein or of new hemorrhages in several subjects, indicating that exercise augmented the rate and incidence of the hemorrhages. The presence of fluorescein leak with the hemorrhages suggested that increased capillary permeability was an important part of the pathogenesis.

Because the hemorrhages develop following hypoxic exposure in normal subjects at altitude and resolve without apparent residual damage after the subjects return to low altitude, hypoxia is implicated in the pathogenesis. Because prior acclimatization to a lower altitude protected subjects against retinal hemorrhage when they were subsequently airlifted to higher altitude, the syndrome is somehow related to acclimatization.[59] The syndrome of retinal hemorrhage is important because the retina is the only window for an observer to see cerebral-related tissue. The cotton wool exudates probably represent ischemic neurons surrounded by edema, and the hemorrhages are probably preceded by vascular leak, implying that hypoxia may be compromising the function both of the brain cells and of the vessels.

Subacute illness (develops in weeks to months)

Right ventricular failure and pulmonary hypertension in the newborn and young child. Before birth, the placenta is the organ of oxygenation, the fluid-filled lungs are collapsed, and the pulmonary vascular resistance is higher than that in the systemic circulation. The onset of breathing at sea level expands the lungs with oxygen-rich air, thereby contributing to the rapid fall in pulmonary arterial pressure (Fig. 7-6,A) and vascular resistance and the closure of the ductus arteriosus. At high altitude, where the air is not as rich in oxygen, the fall in pulmonary vascular

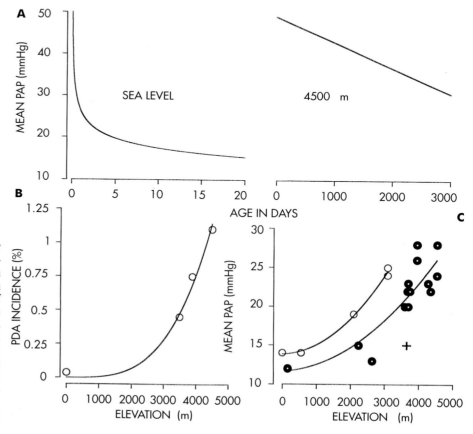

Fig. 7-6. A, The fall in mean pulmonary arterial pressure *(PAP)* after birth for children born at sea level *(left)*, and those born at 4500 m in Peru. (Summarized data from reference 51.) **B,** Increase in incidence of patent ductus arteriosus *(PDA)* in residents at increasing altitudes. (Summarized data from reference 51.) **C,** Increase in mean PAP with increasing altitude for residents of North America *(open circles)* and South America *(solid circles)*. Tibetan residents of Lhasa *(plus sign)* have the lowest pressures relative to their altitude of residence. (Summarized data from references 16,50.)

resistance and the closure of the ductus arteriosus are delayed or even may not occur. As a result, the postnatal fall in pulmonary arterial pressure is delayed (Fig. 7-6,*A*), and the sea level value in some populations is never achieved. Because the pressure remains elevated, the pulmonary arterioles remain muscularized, contributing to pulmonary vascular reactivity. High reactivity was a feature of children in Leadville, Colorado (3100 m), who have recovered from HAPE, no matter whether the edema developed following a trip to the lowlands or accompanied a viral upper respiratory illness.[11] The persistence of muscularized arterioles and pulmonary vasoconstriction at altitude probably is the cause of persisting pulmonary hypertension at altitude, which in some infants leads to right ventricular failure.[1,2]

Patent ductus arteriosus. Following expansion of the lung at birth at sea level, the ductus arteriosus closes because high oxygen in the arterial blood leads to decreased synthesis of those prostaglandins that in the fetus had maintained patency of the ductus arteriosus. Normally then, hypoxia in the fetus is associated with ductal patency, and normoxemia in the newborn is associated with ductal closure. The hypoxemia of high altitude would be expected to maintain ductal patency. The persistence of high pressure in the pulmonary artery would contribute to such patency. Indeed the hypoxemia of altitude combined with some increase in pulmonary arterial pressure is associated with an increased incidence of patent ductus arteriosus at high altitude (Fig. 7-6, *B*).

Right ventricular failure and pulmonary hypertension in young adults. A form of subacute mountain sickness has been described in soldiers who were stationed between 5800 and 6700 m for approximately 11 weeks.[2] The men developed dependent edema of the legs and thighs, and some even developed ascites. Exertional dyspnea was nearly universal, and angina of effort and cough were frequent. Right ventricular failure secondary to pulmonary hypertension was indicated by jugular venous distention, hepatomegaly, palpable pulmonary closure sound, right ventricular gallop, sternal lift, tricuspid regurgitation, and electrocardiographic right axis deviation and right ventricular hypertrophy, together with no evidence of abnormal left ventricular signs or symptoms. Also, echocardiography indicated normal left ventricular dimensions but marked dilation of the right ventricle.

That hypoxia might be the cause was suggested by the prompt diuresis that began within hours of descent to near sea level, with no other treatment being required. Electrocardiograms and echocardiograms returned toward normal over several weeks at low altitude. Similar findings and time course of illness were described for right ventricular failure secondary to pulmonary hypertension in "adolescent" cattle taken for 12 weeks to 4000 m. Until recently, however, such a syndrome had not been described in humans.

POPULATIONS AT ALTITUDE
Normal adaptations

Lung volume. Persons born and living at high altitude have increased lung vital capacity, total lung capacity, chest diameter, and probably lung diffusing capacity. Similar increases are found in dogs residing at altitude during the period of lung growth but not after growth is complete.[28] Apparently the high ventilatory effort of chronic hypoxia results in larger lungs when the hypoxia coincides with the growth of the individual but not when growth is complete. The larger lung volume and diffusing capacity contribute to the increased exercise performance observed in persons living from birth at altitude.[10,62]

Control of breathing. Although the normal response to acute hypoxia is an acute increase in ventilation, the increase becomes blunted over many years of high altitude residence.[20] The blunting is greater the higher the altitude and the longer the residence there. Although Tibetans and Sherpas develop this blunting, their resting minute ventilations are usually well maintained.[20,69]

Pulmonary circulation. The hypoxia of chronic high altitude residence raises pulmonary arterial pressure (Fig. 7-6, *B*) a response that appears to be maladaptive. In fact, populations that have lived the most generations at altitude have the least pulmonary hypertension. Populations in North America that have lived at altitude no more than two generations tend to have higher pulmonary arterial pressures than those living for many thousands of years in South and Central America and Asia (Fig. 7-6, *C*). Of particular interest are the low pulmonary arterial pressures in Tibetans,[16] who may represent the population with the longest history of altitude residence (Fig. 7-6, *C*). Animals that have evolved at high altitude (llama, high altitude deer, guinea pig) have low pulmonary arterial pressures and relatively small pulmonary pressure responses to acute hypoxia. Even the bovine species, which most of all is susceptible to pulmonary hypertension at altitude, adapts over many generations. Humans appear to participate in this general adaptation of the pulmonary circulation.

Red cell mass. Chronic hypoxia provides continuing stimulation of renal erythropoietin release, which in turn increases the bone marrow production of erythrocytes. Red cell mass therefore increases with increasing altitude residence. Work by Weil and colleagues[66] in Colorado found that arterial Po_2 values less than 65 mmHg were associated with elevated red cell mass. It follows that hematocrit increases with altitude. From published data,[68] the altitude threshold appears to be approximately 2000 m, above which hematocrit values are increased (Fig. 7-7, *A*). Examination of hematocrits shows a narrow distribution of values at sea level, but the distribution becomes broad at altitude (Fig. 7-7, *B*). The high values in the altitude population represent patients with chronic mountain sickness, as discussed subsequently.

Arterial pressure. In sea level natives who go to high

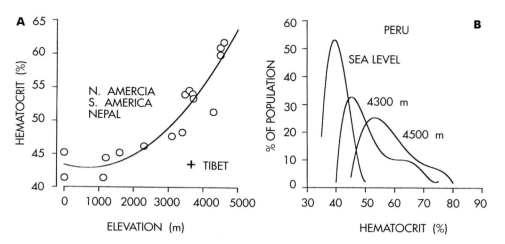

Fig. 7-7. Hematocrit at various altitudes. **A,** Hematocrit values for residents of the Americas and Nepal increase with increasing altitude *(open circles).* For their altitude of residence, values in Tibetan residents of Lhasa are less than for other peoples. **B,** Histograms of hematocrit for people at various altitudes showing skewing of the hematocrit to higher values at high altitude. (Summarized data from references 43, 66, and 68.)

altitude for 1 to 4 weeks, systemic arterial pressure is increased roughly in proportion to the increase in norepinephrine blood levels and urinary excretion, suggesting that alpha-adrenergic activity is important in blood pressure control.[53] In high altitude natives, however, neither blood pressure nor norepinephrine blood levels are increased, whether or not there is chronic mountain sickness.[3] Apparently, sympathetic stimulation is transient, lasting only a few weeks, after which blood pressure and norepinephrine excretion return to sea level values.

Pregnancy at altitude

Birth weight. At high altitude, infants are smaller at birth than at sea level (Fig. 7-8). In fact, birth weights are progressively lower with increasing altitude.[42] Duration of gestation is not decreased, but fetal growth during the last trimester is slowed. The key to fetal growth at altitude appears to be the magnitude of the oxygen transport to the pregnant uterus. Women at altitude in Colorado and Peru who have higher ventilations and higher arterial oxygen saturations tend to give birth to slightly heavier infants than women with lower saturations, suggesting that oxygen transport to the pregnant uterus is an important determinant of birth weight. Of interest, infants born to Tibetan women in Lhasa (3658 m) weigh nearly the sea level norm (Fig. 7-8), and much more than infants born to the Han Chinese, who have only recently come to Tibet. What adaptation has occurred within the Tibetan mother? Their arterial oxygen contents are not higher than those of women from Colorado or Peru at comparable altitude. Doppler studies indicate, however, that they have particularly high flow velocities in the uterine artery, suggesting that their adaptation is not maternal ventilation but is higher blood flow to the uterus. If so, the adaptation primarily involves the uterine circulation and not maternal ventilation or red cell mass.

Maternal hypertension. Pregnancy-induced systemic hypertension in Colorado[44] occurred in 12% of pregnancies at Leadville (3100 m), 4% at Aspen (2400 m), and 3% at

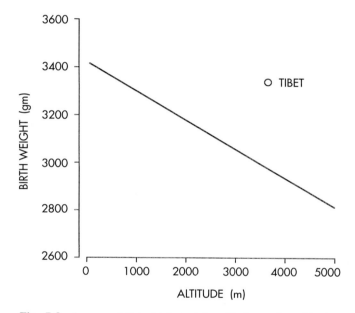

Fig. 7-8. Average fall in birth weight with increasing altitude. For the altitude of the mother's residence, Tibetan children born in Lhasa have higher weights than other populations. (Redrawn from Moore LG, et al: Are Tibetans better adapted? *Int J Sports Med* 13:586, 1992.)

Denver (1600 m). Mean arterial pressures in the third trimester were 95, 92, and 88 mmHg, respectively, compared with the normal of 80 mmHg at sea level. Frequency of proteinuria was threefold and upper extremity edema twofold higher in Leadville than in Denver. The results suggest that preeclampsia is more frequent at altitude and raise the possibility that at any altitude some hypoxic site in pregnancy may precipitate the syndrome.

Neonatal hyperbilirubinemia. Neonatal hyperbilirubinemia[33] was more frequent in Leadville (39%) than Denver (16%), and the absolute levels for all births were higher (181 versus 153 μmol/L). The concomitant elevation of erythropoietin suggested an augmented hematopoietic response, which would increase bilirubin production, and the continued elevation at day 5 suggested an impaired clearance.

Chronic mountain sickness (develops within years)

Description of the syndrome. Chronic mountain sickness (CMS) is the occurrence of symptomatic, excessive polycythemia in long-term residents of high altitude. Most high altitude clinicians have agreed on a definition of CMS: a hypoventilatory disorder affecting the high altitude native or long-term resident, which, by aggravating hypoxemia, leads to excessive polycythemia. The degree of polycythemia is defined as a hematocrit above the statistical maximum for the altitude in question.[68]

CMS is almost exclusively a syndrome affecting men. They are usually older, and they suffer with a variety of symptoms, including headache, bone pain, confusion, sleeplessness, and a subjective feeling of congestion in the head. Because they are persons who were previously well and because descent to a lower altitude is curative, this syndrome has been considered to represent the loss of the body's ability to acclimatize to high altitude.[68]

Affected men usually are over 40 years old and have lived at altitudes above 2500 m for more than 10 years. Pulmonary hypertension and right ventricular failure may be present. Of interest, the CMS syndrome is nearly identical to the pickwickian syndrome, which was described at low altitude but is due to hypoventilation accompanying obesity. Therefore it seems likely that chronic hypoventilation can result in symptomatic, excessive polycythemia at any altitude.

Hypoxia and excessive polycythemia. As noted earlier (Fig. 7-7), the distribution of hematocrits is skewed toward higher values at high altitudes.[68] Hematocrit values of 65% or more occurred in one sixth of men examined at Cerro de Pasco (4300 m) and one fourth of men examined at Morococha (4500 m). The mode (hematocrit value most frequently seen) was 48% at Cerro de Pasco and 55% at Morococha, suggesting that polycythemia was excessive in some men. Because hematocrit increases with increasing hypoxemia, an excessive hematocrit suggests excessive hypoxemia.[39] The relation of hematocrit to saturation is clear for men younger than 55 years but is not present in older men.[39] Work done in Leadville (3100 m) indicates, however, that although the daytime saturation may not explain the high hematocrit, polycythemic patients show severe, prolonged desaturation during the night, suggesting that nocturnal hypoxemia may be an important stimulus for red cell production. Therefore the broad distribution of hematocrits at a given high altitude with skewing to higher values most probably represents abnormal hypoxemia during the day or night.

Hypoventilation and hypoxemia. Hypoventilation is the cause of the hypoxemia. For the altitude of residence,

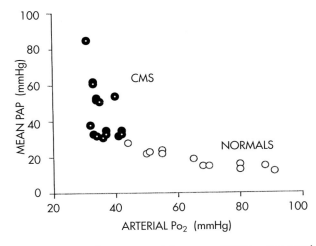

Fig. 7-9. Mean pulmonary arterial pressure *(PAP)* versus arterial oxygen pressure *(Po₂)* for residents of various altitudes. Normal values *(open circles)* and men with chronic mountain sickness *(solid circles)* appear to form a continuum. (Redrawn from Reeves JT: Pulmonary vascular reponses to high altitude, *Cardiovasc Clin* 5:81, 1973.)

most persons with CMS have Pco_2 values that average 5 mmHg more than those of healthy residents.[9,39,49,63] The Po_2 values are correspondingly reduced. Contributing to the hypoventilation are the loss of the hypoxic ventilatory response,[63] the presence of obstructive lung disease,[32] apnea or hypoventilation during sleep,[31] and small airway obstruction owing to excessive polycythemia.[9] Phlebotomy[9] and stimulation of ventilation during sleep improves oxygenation[31] in some patients, and supplemental oxygen or descent to lower altitude improves oxygenation in all CMS patients.

Pulmonary hypertension. Pulmonary hypertension is the primary cause of right ventricular failure in patients with CMS. Contributing to the hypertension is both the chronic hypoxemia and the high viscosity from the polycythemia. Chronic hypoxemia appears to be the major factor, as the patients with CMS appear as an extension of the normal curve relating pulmonary arterial pressure to Pao_2 (Fig. 7-9).

Other diseases in altitude residents

Migration of elderly. In Colorado, elderly persons do not prefer to live at high altitude. The numbers of persons above 65 years of age (as a percentage of residents) decrease with elevation.[45] Personal interviews of the residents of high and low altitude towns established an increasing migration with increasing age from high but not from low altitude towns in Colorado.[54] The "out-migration" from the high altitude towns was universally to lower altitude and overwhelmingly due to poor health, usually (81% of migrants) involving the heart or lungs. The out-migration involved the elderly because heart and lung diseases are much more common in the older age groups. (Out-migration from low altitude towns was usually to be near family members.)

Lung disease. Even though elderly with chronic lung disease leave high altitude, mortality from emphysema is always higher in Colorado than in the rest of the United States, and within the state, mortality increases with increasing altitude.[45] In addition, the illness runs a shorter course at altitude, where the cause of death is most often cor pulmonale rather than respiratory failure as at sea level. Probably the combination of lung disease plus altitude augments the hypoxemia, promoting pulmonary hypertension and right ventricular failure.

Heart disease. Altitude effects on coronary artery disease are less clear. Persons limited by angina at low altitude may find slightly greater limitation at altitude,[15] and ultrasound studies have suggested that those with ischemic heart disease may show an increase (rather than the normal decrease) in left ventricular chamber volume on ascent. Telemetry studies of 149 older men engaging in strenuous activities at high altitude, however, found "little evidence to indicate an added risk beyond what one might expect at lower altitudes." Paradoxically, lifelong high altitude residence has been reported to have a protective effect relative to arterial pressure and coronary disease.[15]

CONCLUSION

Although the arterial Po_2 and Pco_2 begin to fall as one ascends from sea level, the adverse effects of altitude on health do not appear to become significant until threshold elevations above 2000 m are reached. For the healthy young adult, the adverse effects are largely limited to the acute altitude syndromes of AMS, HACE, high altitude retinal hemorrhage, and HAPE. These are usually self-limited syndromes that improve or resolve within a few days concomitant with ventilatory acclimatization. For the high altitude resident, the adverse effects are primarily at the extremes of life, i.e., the very young or the elderly with heart or lung disease, and women in the third trimester of pregnancy. For all of these altitude syndromes in either the visitor or resident, an increase in ventilation provides the first defense of arterial oxygenation and is of crucial importance. Although physicians focus on the adverse effects of high altitude, it remains axiomatic that high altitude provides opportunities for recreation and beauties of scenery that refresh the soul. Therefore, it is no surprise that the most rapidly growing communities in Colorado are those at high altitude. Medicine must maximize benefits and minimize risks for persons who go to high altitude.

REFERENCES

1. Anand IS, Chandrashekhar Y: Subacute mountain sickness syndromes: role of pulmonary hypertension. In Sutton JR, Coates G, Houston CS, editors: *Hypoxia and mountain medicine,* Burlington, VT, 1992, Queen City Printers.
2. Anand IS et al: Adult subacute mountain sickness—a syndrome of congestive heart failure in man at very high altitude, *Lancet* 335:561, 1990.
3. Antezana AM et al: Adrenergic system in high altitude residents, *Int J Sports Med* 13:S96, 1992.
4. Baumgartner RW et al: The role of cerebral blood flow in acute mountain sickness. In Sutton JR, Coates G, Houston CS, editors: *Hypoxia and mountain medicine,* Burlington, VT, 1992, Queen City Printers.
5. Bèrtsch P: Fibrin formation: not a cause but consequence of high altitude pulmonary edema, *Fortschr Med* 110:177, 1992.
6. Bèrtsch P: Aldosterone, antidiuretic hormone, and atrial natriuretic peptide in acute mountain sickness. In Sutton JR, Coates G, Houston CS, editors: *Hypoxia and mountain medicine,* Burlington, VT, 1992, Queen City Printers.
7. Bèrtsch P et al: Enhanced exercise-induced rise of aldosterone and vasopressin preceding mountain sickness, *J Appl Physiol* 71:136, 1991.
8. Cosby RL et al: Elevated plasma atrial natriuretic factor and vasopressin in high altitude pulmonary edema, *Ann Intern Med* 109:796, 1988.
9. Cruz JC et al: Phlebotomy improves pulmonary gas exchange in chronic mountain polycythemia, *Respiration* 38:305, 1979.
10. Droma TS et al: Increased vital and total lung capacities in Tibetan compared to Han residents of Lhasa (3658 m), *Am J Phys Anthropol* 86:341, 1991.
11. Fasules JW, Wiggins JW, Wolfe RR: Increased lung vasoreactivity in children from Leadville, Colorado after recovery from high altitude pulmonary edema, *Circulation* 72:957, 1985.
12. Frayser R et al: Retinal hemorrhage at high altitude, *N Engl J Med* 282:1183, 1970.
13. Goldenberg F et al: Sleep apneas and high altitude newcomers, *Int J Sports Med* 13:S34, 1992.
14. Grissom CK et al: Acetazolamide in the treatment of acute mountain sickness: clinical efficacy and effect on gas exchange, *Ann Intern Med* 116:461, 1992.
15. Grover RF et al: The influence of environmental factors on the cardiovascular system. In Hurst JW et al, editors, *The Heart,* New York, 1990, McGraw-Hill.
16. Groves BM et al: Minimal hypoxic pulmonary hypertension in normal Tibetans at 3658 m, *J Appl Physiol* 74:312, 1993.
17. Hackett P, Oelz O: The Lake Louise concensus on the definition and quantification of altitude illness. In: Sutton JR, Coates G, Houston CS, editors: *Hypoxia and mountain medicine,* Burlington, VT, 1992, Queen City Printers.
18. Hackett PH, Rennie D: The incidence, importance, and prophylaxis of acute mountain sickness, *Lancet* 2:1149, 1976.
19. Hackett PH, Roach RC. High altitude pulmonary edema, *J Wilderness Med* 1:3, 1990.
20. Hackett PH et al: Ventilation in populations native to high altitude. In West JB, Lahiri S, editors: *High altitude and man,* Bethesda, MD, 1984, American Physiological Society.
21. Hartig GS, Hackett PH: Cerebral spinal fluid pressure and cerebral blood velocity in acute mountain sickness. In Sutton JR, Coates G, Houston CS, editors: *Hypoxia and mountain medicine,* Burlington, VT, 1992, Queen City Printers.
22. Hochstrasser J, Nanzer A, Oelz O: Altitude edema in the Swiss Alps. Observatons on the incidence and clinical course in 50 patients, *Schweiz Med Wochenschr* 28:866, 1986.
23. Honigman B et al: Acute mountain sickness in a general tourist population at moderate altitudes, *Ann Intern Med* 118:587, 1993.
24. Houston CS: Acute pulmonary edema of high altitude, *N Engl J Med* 263:478, 1960.
25. Hultgren HN, Grover RF, Hartley LH: Abnormal circulatory responses to high altitude in subjects with a history of high altitude pulmonary edema, *Circulation* 44:759, 1971.
26. Hultgren HN, Marticorena EA: High altitude pulmonary edema. Epidemiologic observations in Peru, *Chest* 74:372, 1978.
27. Hultgren HN et al: High altitude pulmonary edema, *Medicine* 40:289, 1961.
28. Johnson RL et al: Functional capacities of lungs and thorax in bea-

gles after prolonged residence at 3100 m, *J Appl Physiol* 59:1773, 1985.

29. Kawashima A et al: Hemodynamic responses to acute hypoxia, hypobaria, and exercise in subjects susceptible to high altitude pulmonary edema, *J Appl Physiol* 67:1982, 1989.

30. Kobayashi T et al: Clinical features of patients with high-altitude pulmonary edema in Japan, *Chest* 92:814, 1987.

31. Kryger M et al: Impaired oxygenation during sleep in excessive polycythemia of high altitude: improvement with respiratory stimulation, *Sleep* 1:3, 1978.

32. Kryger M et al: Excessive polycythemia of high altitude: role of ventilatory drive and lung disease, *Am Rev Respir Dis* 118:659, 1978.

33. Leibson C et al: Neonatal hyperbilirubinemia at high altitude, *Am J Dis Child* 143:983, 1989.

34. Lopez-Barneo J et al: Chemotransduction in the carotid body. K+ current modulated by PO_2 in type I chemoreceptor cells, *Science* 242:580, 1988.

35. Maggiorini M et al: Prevalence of acute mountain sickness in the Swiss Alps, *Br Med J* 301:853, 1990.

36. McFadden DM et al: High-altitude retinopathy, *JAMA* 245:581, 1981.

37. Milledge JS, Catley DM: Angiotensin converting enzyme response to hypoxia in man: its role in altitude acclimatization, *Clin Sci* 67:453, 1984.

38. Milledge JS et al: Atrial natriuretic peptide, altitude and acute mountain sickness, *Clin Sci* 77:509, 1989.

39. Monge C, Arregui A, Leon-Velarde F: Pathophysiology and epidemiology of chronic mountain sickness, *Int J Sports Med* 13:S79, 1992.

40. Montgomery AB, Mills J, Luce JM: Incidence of acute moutain sickness at intermdiate altitude, *JAMA* 261:732, 1989.

41. Montgomery AB et al: Effects of dexamethasone on the incidence of acute mountain sickness at two intermediate altitudes, *JAMA* 261:734, 1989.

42. Moore LG: Maternal O_2 transport and fetal growth in Colorado, Peru, and Tibet high-altitude residents, *Am J Hum Biol* 2:627, 1990.

43. Moore LG et al: Are Tibetans better adapted? *Int J Sports Med* 13:S86, 1992.

44. Moore LG et al: The incidence of pregnancy-induced hypertension is increased among Colorado residents at high altitude, *Am J Obstet Gynecol* 144:423, 1982.

45. Moore LG et al: Emphysema mortality is increased in Colorado residents at high altitude, *Am Rev Respir Dis* 126:225, 1982.

46. Noordeweir E: Personal communication.

47. Oelz O: Incidence, prevention, and therapy of acute mountain sickness, *Schweiz Med Wochenschr* 112:492, 1982.

48. Oelz O et al: Prevention and treatment of high altitude pulmonary edema by a calcium channel blocker, *Int J Sports Med* 13(S1):S65, 1992.

49. Penalosa D, Sime F: Chronic cor pulmonale due to loss of altitude acclimatization (chronic mountain sickness), *Am J Med* 50:728, 1971.

50. Reeves JT: Pulmonary vascular responses to high altitude, *Cardiovasc Clin* 5:81, 1973.

51. Reeves JT, Grover RF: High-altitude pulmonary hypertension and pulmonary edema. In Yu PN, Goodwin JF, editors: *Progress in cardiology,* vol 4, Philadelphia, 1974, Lea & Febiger.

52. Reeves JT, Houston CS, Sutton JR: Operation Everest II: resistance and susceptibility to chronic hypoxia in man, *J Roy Soc Med* 82:513, 1989.

53. Reeves JT et al: Increased arterial pressure after acclimatization to 4300 m: possible role of norepinephrine, *Int J Sports Med* 13:S18, 1992.

54. Regensteiner JG, Moore LG: Migration of the elderly from high altitudes in Colorado, *JAMA* 253:3124, 1985.

55. Richalet JP et al: Plasma prostaglandins, leukotrienes, and thromboxane in acute high altitude hypoxia, *Respir Physiol* 85:205, 1991.

56. Rios B, Driscoll DJ, McNamara DG: High-altitude pulmonary edema with absent right pulmonary artery, *Pediatrics* 75:314, 1985.

57. Roach R, Hackett P: Hyperbaria and high altitude illness. In Sutton JR, Coates G, Houston CS, editors: *Hypoxia and mountain medicine,* Burlington, VT, 1992, Queen City Printers.

58. Schoene RB et al: The lung at high altitude: bronchoalveolar lavage in acute mountain sickness and pulmonary edema, *J Appl Physiol* 64:2605, 1988.

59. Schumacher GA, Petajan JH: High altitude stress and retinal hemorrhages: relation to vascular headache mechanism, *Arch Environ Health* 30:217, 1975.

60. Selland MA et al: Pulmonary function and hypoxic ventilatory response in subjects susceptible to high-altitude pulmonary edema, *Chest* 103:111, 1993.

61. Sophocles AM: High-altitude pulmonary edema in Vail, Colorado, 1975-1982, *Clin Sci* 144:569, 1986.

62. Sun SF et al: Greater maximal oxygen uptakes and vital capacities in Tibetan than Han residents of Lhasa, *Respir Physiol* 79:151, 1990.

63. Sun SF et al: Decreased ventilation and hypoxic ventilatory response are not reversed by naloxone in Lhasa residents with chronic mountain sickness, *Am Rev Respir Dis* 142:1294, 1990.

64. Vock P et al: Variable radiolomorphologic data of high altitude pulmonary edema, *Chest* 100:1306, 1991.

65. Vock P et al: High-altitude pulmonary edema: findings at high altitude chest radiography and physical examination, *Radiology* 170:661, 1989.

66. Weil JV et al: The red cell mass–arterial oxygen relationship in normal man, *J Clin Invest* 47:1627, 1968.

67. West JB, Mathieu-Costello O: Stress failure in pulmonary capillaries: a mechanism for high altitude pulmonary edema. In Sutton JR, Coates G, Houston CS, editors: *Hypoxia and mountain medicine,* Burlington, VT, 1992, Queen City Printers.

68. Winslow RM, Monge C: *Hypoxia, polycythemia, and chronic mountain sickness,* Baltimore, 1987, The Johns Hopkins University Press.

69. Zhuang J et al: Hypoxic ventilatory responsiveness in Tibetan compared with Han residents of 3658 m, *J Appl Physiol* 74:303, 1993.

Chapter 8

AGRICULTURAL PESTICIDES

Vincent F. Garry
Jack Griffith

AGRICULTURE: ENVIRONMENTAL PATHOLOGY

Agriculture and agricultural development have been and remain key elements in the industrialization and improvement of living standards for the world's peoples. To increase the quantity and improve the quality of the food supply, pest and weed control by chemical or biological means is required. The development of genetically modified crop plant strains is also required. These human efforts involve manipulation and alteration of land and water to suit human needs. The work of agriculture entails risks to those working the land and to the environment, both plant and animal. To a lesser degree, the risks of agricultural food production extend to the manufacturers and processors of food and food products, the transporters, and finally to the consumer. In a certain sense, the daily life of each human depends on the safety and efficiency of agricultural work. Stewardship of this work resides mainly within the agricultural community and in industries servicing the agricultural community (Fig. 8-1).

In this chapter, a human-centered view is taken that is limited to issues pertaining to human pathology and toxicology associated with agriculture. Even within these confines, the topic is broad and cannot be treated in depth. In the United States, there are more than 3 million persons employed on farms; approximately 2.5 million are hired employees, of whom almost 58% work less than 74 days per year.[159] Migrant workers make up about 6% of the work force. Agricultural workers are exposed to an environment containing a mixture of biological and chemical agents with the potential for noxious health effects. Allergenic dusts, dander, fungi, fungal toxins, bacterial pathogens, toxicant gases generated from bacterial action, and viral pathogens are the major biologic sources of the exposure burden of

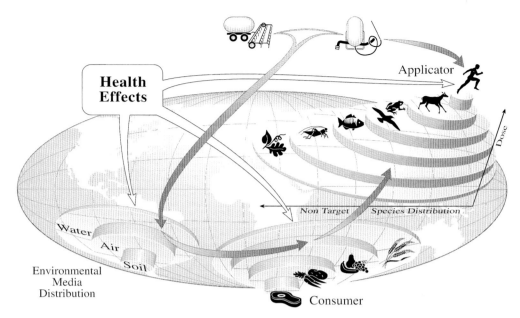

Fig. 8-1. Cycle of pesticide use and pesticide distribution among nontarget species, food products, and environmental media (soil, air, water). In the first icon *(top right),* the relative doses of pesticide to the applier, then to mammals, avian species, amphibians, fish, and finally to insects are envisioned. In this scenario, pesticides are distributed to biologically diverse nontarget species with decreasing dose. The icon in the lower center depicts the dose and dose distribution among food products. Residues are distributed more widely in the food chain but at lower levels in fruits, nuts, and grains. The distribution of pesticide residues in different environmental media is indicated in the lower left. It is expected that pesticide residue levels will follow a pattern of increasing dilution as they are more widely distributed in soil, air, and groundwater. In the upper left, health effects are generically identified as the endpoint of multiple sources of exposure. The relative contribution of each source of human exposure to pesticides and health status is thought to depend on dose, length of exposure, genetic constitution, preexisting disease, and age.

the farming community. The environmental chemical burden of farm workers is an equally diverse mixture of solvents, fuels, paints, fertilizers, and pesticides. Because almost 3 billion pounds (about 1 billion kg) of active ingredient pesticides is used in the United States each year, pesticide exposure is one of the most common chemical exposures of agricultural workers (see Laughlin and Gold.*) For this reason, our attention is focused on an examination of the major health impacts of current and past agricultural pesticide practices in relation to human health. Because the number of pesticide formulations exceeds 45,000 from over 1400 active ingredients (see Hollingworth,*) our discussion will be limited to selected groups of pesticides in common use, either currently or historically. When possible, we explore the possible biochemical mechanisms for pesticide-related health effects by chemical class. Traumatic injury, although an important element

*In Griffith J and Duncan RC: Exposure of agriculture workers to anticholinesterases. In Ballantyne B and Marrs TC, editors: Clinical and experimental toxicology of organophosphates and carbamates. Boston, 1992, Butterworth & Heinemann, pp 339-345.

in the overall health and well-being of agricultural workers, is not discussed in detail. Our discussion begins with a general description of the health of the farming community derived from epidemiological studies.

DESCRIPTIVE EPIDEMIOLOGY AND DEMOGRAPHIC HEALTH

Of all occupations in the United States, agriculture has the highest rate of injury.[107] Machinery-related mortality and enclosed space toxicant gas–related deaths are increasingly reported.[100] Specific cancers, including lip cancer; melanoma; non-Hodgkin lymphoma; leukemia; and perhaps testicular, prostate, and brain cancer, tend to be overrepresented in male members of the farming community.[14,15,171] Lung cancer, the most common neoplastic disease of men, is relatively uncommon in the agricultural setting.[15] Cancer of the ovary and myeloma appear in excess among women.[40,181] Certain birth defects, including anencephaly, limb reduction deformities, and polydactyly, may also be in excess in this population.[47,136,169] Among men in the farming community, hypertension and cardiovascular disease are less prevalent than in the community at large.[15,36,147]

Allergies, asthma, hypersensitivity diseases of the lung, and chronic lung disease are more prevalent among farmers than in the general population (see Dosman and Cockcroft[41] for a review). Certain neurological diseases, such as Parkinson's disease, peripheral neuropathy, and alterations of behavior patterns, are more prevalent in some sectors of the farming community.[68,132,135] More recently, suicide has become a significant concern in the psychosocial life of the agricultural community in some U.S. states.[62]

The health data cited point out the pattern of known health risks entailed in agricultural work. Links with some environmental agents including pesticides have been developed, at various levels of certainty, for some noxious health effects that appear in excess in this population. The laboratory chain of evidence between disease and pesticide exposure for many of these observations is restricted to animal or in vitro studies. In our further considerations, we point out where possible laboratory-based human studies have made important contributions to our understanding of the diseases affecting the agricultural community with reference to pesticide use. The relevance of laboratory biomarkers of pesticide exposure and effect is also considered.

PESTICIDES AND AGRICULTURE

Pesticides have been defined by the Environmental Protection Agency (EPA) as any substance or mixture of substances intended for preventing, destroying, repelling, or mitigating any pest and any substance or mixture of substances intended for use as a plant regulator, defoliant, or desiccant. Most pesticides are products designed to mitigate noxious weed, insect, or rodent infestation. Some are derived from plants, most are synthetic, and a few are of mineral origin (e.g., arsenates). Even fewer are of biological origin (e.g., *Bacillus thuringiensis*[59]). Similar to any other pharmacological agent, all pesticides are toxic at some dose in a given species or some sensitive subgroup. Acute and chronic toxicity can be directed to a single organ system or to effects on several organ systems with one or more pathological consequences. Each pesticide group related either by chemical structure or biological activity tends to have similar toxicological and pathobiological properties. For this reason, we explore potential health hazards of pesticides by pesticide class.

PESTICIDE CLASSES

Herbicides, insecticides, fumigants, and fungicides are the major classes of pesticides in current use. Pesticides used for weed control and eradication are termed *herbicides*. *Insecticides* are products designed to reduce insect infestation primarily by surface application (interior or exterior) or soil incorporation. *Fumigants* are used to rid enclosed spaces, including homes, barns, grain bins and silos, of insect and sometimes rodent infestation. They are typically highly volatile, are sometimes gaseous, and have high penetrability. *Fungicides* are designed primarily to protect seeds from fungal deterioration either in storage or at the time of planting. Products within each of these functional pesticide groups differ in their acute toxicity. Most herbicides are of a low order of acute toxicity. Insecticides vary from low to high levels of acute toxicity for mammalian species. As a general rule, fumigants are highly toxic. Fungicides are moderately toxic. The volatility and stability of these chemicals are determinants for the extent of environmental contamination of air, water, or soil. Chemical stability is linked to persistence and bioaccumulation in human, animal, and plant life. For example, DDT (dichlorodiphenyltrichloroethane), an organochlorine insecticide, was formerly considered to be an ideal pesticide because it is of low-order acute toxicity for mammalian species including humans. Evidence gathered in the late 1960s showed that the pesticide was harmful to certain predatory avian species.[119] Moreover, DDT was found to be persistent, bioaccumulating in fat tissue,[66] and was present in maternal milk.[124] Detectable levels of this pesticide remain today in older homes and on farms even though the chemical has not been in use in the United States for more than 20 years.[110]

Similarly, in the 1970s, the commercial grade product of the chlorophenoxy herbicide 2,4,5-T was found to be contaminated with dioxins.[77] Members of the dioxin family of chemicals are persistent, bioaccumulate in fatty tissue, and are highly toxic to sensitive mammalian species. One of the more toxic forms is TCDD (2,3,7,8-tetrachlorodibenzo-p-dioxin). 2,4,5-T and the mixture of the herbicides 2,4,5-T and 2,4-D (2,4-dichlorophenoxy acetic acid) a Vietnam-era defoliant, agent orange, produced before 1965 may have contained as much as 30 mg/kg or more TCDD.

DIOXINS AND TCDD

The highly toxic potential of dioxins (of which TCDD is one chemical family member) for immunosuppressive, teratogenic, and tumorigenic effects in animals[118] still remains controversial with respect to humans. Central to the discussion is the relatively consistent relationship between toxicity and biological receptor mediated toxic effects.[120] In 1976, Poland and colleagues[117] first described the relationship between a cytosol protein receptor with high affinity for dioxins modulated by the genetic locus controlling the enzyme aryl hydrocarbon hydroxylase, i.e., the Ah receptor. These data and subsequent studies imply a threshold for carcinogenic and teratogenic effects of these chemicals.[90] Variance in biological receptors for dioxins among species and within species adds further complexity to the issue. Studies of the interaction between dioxins and specific biological receptors may resolve these points of contention.[130]

CONSIDERATIONS IN PESTICIDE TOXICITY

The works cited previously and other published works suggest that the level of toxicity and spectrum of toxicity of commercial-grade pesticide formulations may differ at times from the pure test chemical owing to contaminants generated in the manufacturing process. Variation in storage and use conditions (temperature, length of time in storage, and reuse practices) may produce degradation or alter the composition of the commercial-grade product. Volatility, solubility, and solvent carrier or adjuvant used in conjunction with pesticides[161] influence the rate of absorption of these chemicals through skin, lungs, and gastrointestinal tract. Again the level of toxicity and spectrum of toxicity of pesticides can be altered by product formulation. Finally, these physical chemical characteristics of pesticides and pesticide formulations are determinants for possible short-term and long-term health sequelae for each pesticide. In the following discussion, we attempt to characterize pesticides according to pesticide class and biological activity.

PESTICIDE CHARACTERIZATION

See Table 8-1 at end of chapter for quick reference.

Herbicides

In 1985, herbicide production in the United States amounted to 755 million pounds, approximately equal the volume by weight of all other classes of pesticide combined.[23] The major chemical families of herbicides in current use include chloracetanilides, triazines, dinitrophenols, thiocarbamates, organic phosphorus compounds, and chlorophenoxy herbicides. Because of the sheer volume of use, concerns have been raised regarding the extent of environmental contamination of the water supply in rural and suburban areas through runoff from treated crops. More pertinent are questions regarding possible long-term health effects. An overview of the known pathobiological effects of commonly used herbicides by chemical family is given here. The herbicide product examples used in these descriptions were selected based on use, available information, and chemical structural similarity to other family members.

Chloroacetanilides: alachlor. Alachlor (2-chloro-2'-6'-diethyl-*N*-(methoxymethyl)-acetanilide), a widely used preemergent herbicide, has been shown to be tumorigenic in animals.[159] Based on these animal studies, the U.S. EPA and the National Research Council[106] calculated that concentrations of 1 mg/kg/day in humans could be carcinogenic. It is of interest that alachlor and atrazine (a triazine herbicide) are common groundwater contaminants in the upper midwest. In an in vitro (human) and in vivo (animal) cytogenetic study of this herbicide mixture in dose ranges that do occur in heavily contaminated groundwater noted by the authors, increased chromosome aberrations were found, a further suggestion of possible long-term human hazard.[98]

Triazines: atrazine. Atrazine (2-chloro-4-ethylamino-6-isopropylamine-*s*-triazine) is one of the most commonly used herbicides to control broadleaf weeds in the United States and throughout the world.[177] It is also one of the most common groundwater contaminants in the United States.[160] Based on animal and in vitro studies, atrazine is not thought to be mutagenic.[28] As with some other pesticides, atrazine is weakly estrogenic and binds estrogen receptor sites.[174] In certain strains of rats treated chronically with atrazine, females demonstrate excess breast and ovarian neoplasms.[76] One human study suggests a possible epidemiological link between use of or exposure to triazine herbicides and ovarian carcinoma.[40]

Dinitrophenols: dinoseb. Dinitrophenols are a complex group of pesticides in which minor changes in chemical structure produce significant change in the spectrum of pesticide activity. Some members of this group of pesticides are fungicides, some are insecticides, and some, such as dinoseb, are herbicides. As a general rule, dinitrophenols are uncouplers of mitochondrial oxidative phosphorylation.[114] For this reason, acute intoxication is accompanied by fever and profuse sweating.[13] Dinoseb (2-*sec*-butyl-4,6-dinitrophenol), the herbicide example of this chemical group, is spermatotoxic in animals.[87] Chemical analysis of commercial-grade dinoseb as the diethanolamine salt shows that similar to other nitrosated commercial mixtures,[51] dinoseb can contain as much as 2000 ppm N-nitrosodiethanolamine,[170] a chemical contaminant of the commercial preparation and potent animal carcinogen. These data suggest that the carcinogenic potency of commercial-grade preparations of the pesticide could differ significantly from the pure form, given the level of nitrosoamine contamination.

Organic phosphorus herbicides: glyphosate (Roundup). Glyphosate (N-[phosphonomethyl] glycine) is a postemergent herbicide with weak anticholinesterase activity[145] with no apparent biologically significant neurotoxic effects. Other work suggests that glyphosate may act as an uncoupler of oxidative phosphorylation.[111] Instances of acute intoxication have been increasingly reported in the United States,[91] Taiwan,[155] and New Zealand.[151] Most of these case reports involve ingestion with suicidal intent. Lethal intoxication is associated with cardiovascular symptoms and the development of pulmonary edema. Hemorrhages in the gastrointestinal tract are noted. Many of the features of poisoning appear to be related to the surfactant used in the formulated product[150] rather than the pesticide itself. There is little current evidence to suggest effects on long-term health.[86,107]

Chlorophenoxy herbicides. Much controversy surrounds the question of the long-term pathobiological effects of the chlorophenoxy group of herbicides, in particular with reference to the risk of non-Hodgkin lymphoma and soft tissue sarcoma among agricultural workers. Chlorophenoxy herbicides have been in use since 1944.[77] Before 1965, product mixtures containing the chlorophenoxy herbicides 2,4-D and 2,4,5-T were found to be contaminated with as much as 30 mg/kg TCDD, a potent dioxin.[77] This same product mixture was used as a defoliant (agent orange) in Vietnam. Formation of dioxins was found to be an inadvertent by-product in the synthesis of 2,4,5-T but not in 2,4-D. In the 1970s, much effort was expended to alter commercial production methods to minimize dioxin contamination.

Animal studies performed with 2,4-D in the pure form show little or no evidence of carcinogenicity.[79,103a] In vitro studies show no clear evidence of genotoxicity. Other mechanistic studies, however, indicate that 2,4-D may have properties of an epigenetic or nongenotoxic carcinogen or tumor promoter. Those studies demonstrate that 2,4-D induces dose-dependent hepatic peroxisomal proliferation.[162] Altogether, animal, in vitro, and analytic chemical studies suggest that pathobiological variability in the expression of carcinogenicity might be expected in epidemiological studies. Use of chlorophenoxy herbicides is generally confined to use on broadleaf woody weeds in agriculture and forestry in combination with other herbicides. Further variability in the expression of carcinogenicity in human populations exposed to this herbicide class can also be expected, if carcinogenic interaction with other pesticide products were possible. In Sweden, early studies by Hardell[63] and Hardell and Sandstrom[64] showed significant increase in non-Hodgkin lymphoma and soft tissue sarcoma in excess of four times the expected frequency of these tumors among workers exposed to chlorophenoxy herbicides. Similarly constructed epidemiological studies in New Zealand[116,139] failed to show a significant association between these neoplasms and chlorophenoxy herbicide exposure. In the United States, the epidemiological experience in the farming community tends to give intermediate results between these two extremes. Case-control studies in Kansas[70] and Nebraska[71] demonstrate significant increases (risk ratios 1.3 to 2.2) in non-Hodgkin lymphoma among farmers using 2,4-D, with the risk increasing in proportion to days used per year (up to sevenfold for 20 days or more per year). From this limited review and from far more extensive reviews of the epidemiological literature,[16,115] it appears that statistical variability in the risk of non-Hodgkin lymphoma is expressed in populations exposed to chlorophenoxy herbicides. Whether these statistical variations are a true reflection of pathobiologic interaction between 2,4-D and other pesticides or other environmental agents is not understood.

Insecticides

Of all genera, insects have been and remain an evolutionarily stable phylogenetic class, the impact of which on human society in terms of benefit and risk touches each individual. One part of the picture of the insect world portrays insects as plant pollinators, crop protectors, and a nutritional source. The other, more ominous side pictures an insect world of crop devastation, disease vectors, reservoirs of disease, and acute intoxication owing to envenomation. Insecticides are designed to minimize the noxious infesta-

tion of insects in the home, in the workplace, in the garden, on crop land, in forests, and in standing waters. Because the insecticide-targeted organ systems of insects bear phylogenetic relationship to other species including humans, there is some expected health risk.

The manifestations of acute, subacute, and chronic health effects of insecticides are protean. Neurological and dermatological effects have been recorded in humans. Carcinogenic and reproductive effects have been shown primarily in animal studies. The major chemical families of insecticides in current use include organophosphates, carbamates, organochlorine insecticides, and pyrethroid insecticides. Although each of these chemical families has insect control in common, each chemical family has some biologically unique properties and is considered separately.

Organophosphates. All members of this chemical group affect the primary neurotransmitter substrate acetylcholine and are irreversible inhibitors of cholinesterase. For the purpose of understanding the inhibitory effect of organophosphates on cholinesterases, three important members within this family of enzymes are identified:

1. Acetylcholinesterase, whose substrate is acetylcholine, is a major neurotransmitter in the central and peripheral nervous system. Acetylcholinesterase is present in central and peripheral nerve endings, on the surface of erythrocytes, and in the developing mammalian embryo.[137,143]
2. Pseudocholinesterase is a cholinesterase whose substrate is butrylcholine. This group of enzymes is synthesized by the liver and can be quantitated in human blood. Genetically based variance in the molecular forms of the enzyme is in part responsible for the human variation in anticholinesterase chemical sensitivity.[42,97]
3. Neurotoxic esterase is a relatively unknown group of esterases whose activity is inhibited by organophosphates that produce a delayed neuropathy. Aside from the central nervous system, neurotoxic esterases are present in detectable concentrations in human lymphocytes and platelets.[93] Interaction with cytoskeletal protein by certain organophosphates is thought to produce a myelin degenerative process and subsequent neuropathy.[1]

The acute toxicity of organophosphates is reflected by inhibition of one or more members of the cholinesterase family of enzymes. The dose at which acute toxicity is observed depends on a number of factors:

1. Organophosphate anticholinesterases phosphorylate and alkylate cholinesterase and other protein moieties. The rate at which these bonds are formed is an important determinate of the toxic dose. Similarly the rate at which the bond formed leads to irreversible binding to cholinesterase (aging) versus the rate of hydrolysis of the bond is a primary determinant of toxicity.[173] For example, the notorious ability of the

highly organophosphate chemical warfare agents (nerve agents, e.g., soman and sarin) to phosphorylate cholinesterase irreversibly is measured in minutes.[35] Recovery from organophosphate intoxication depends on the rate of new synthesis of cholinesterase enzyme, the rate of aging, and the rate of metabolic conversion of the organophosphate to an inactive form.

2. Organophosphate insecticides in common use today require biotransformation by the liver for activation and degradation. The rate of activation versus the rate of degradation is the second determinant of organophosphate acute toxicity. Nerve agents used in chemical warfare do not require biotransformation for their toxicant activity.

3. Organophosphates can be absorbed by inhalation, through the skin, and through the gastrointestinal tract. Ambient dose, carrier vehicle (solvent), duration of exposure, temperature, humidity, and degree of physical activity are collectively the third determinant of acute toxicity.

All of the factors have a common endpoint measurable by quantitative analysis of human red cell and plasma cholinesterase activity. Measurement of cholinesterase activity as a biomarker in conjunction with the clinical profile of the patient (heart rate, pupillary diameter, respiratory rate, seizures) is useful to monitor exposure-related effects and to guide therapeutic intervention with atropine and 2-PAM.[43,104]

Studies in California,[6] Nebraska,[144] and Minnesota[123] show that as many as 20% to 40% of farm workers exposed to organophosphates show significant inhibition of either red cell or plasma cholinesterase. The overall mortality rate from acute pesticide poisoning and organophosphate intoxication is not presently known. One EPA report based on vital statistics data suggests that deaths specifically related to pesticides are infrequent.[18] Another EPA report[82] of selected medical centers suggests a similar result. Both reports do indicate that organophosphates and carbamates are most frequently involved in the deaths recorded.

Case reports and collected case studies of delayed neurotoxicity, including peripheral neuropathies and neurobehavioral disturbances, are not uncommon.[132,135] Several studies point to the development of tolerance to organophosphate toxicity[30] with repeated exposure. Compensatory down-regulation of muscarinic cholinergic receptors appears to be part of this adaptive response.[73] Neurobehavioral changes (e.g., memory impairment), however, may occur independent of this adaptive mechanism.[49,89]

One of the most striking examples of mass acute intoxication involves use of commercial-grade malathion in Pakistan.[9] Studies performed on these pesticide applicators demonstrated that use of certain commercial brands of malathion were an important factor in the acute toxicant effects observed. With further study, analysis of these commercial products showed a number of contaminants. One of these contaminants was a specific inhibitor of malathion decarboxylase, one of the critical liver enzymes responsible for biological degradation of malathion. In this instance, the toxicant dose of malathion was amplified through inhibition of biodegradation.

With regard to possible carcinogenicity, few epidemiological studies suggest linkage to excess leukemia or lymphoma.[15] Because many of the organophosphates are also significant alkylating agents, in vitro studies for genotoxicity show evidence for genotoxic effects for many of these products, either in prokaryotic microbial species or in mammalian cells.

Carbamates. In contrast to organophosphates, carbamates are reversible inhibitors of cholinesterase. The acute spectrum of anticholinesterase effects is similar to that observed for organophosphates but differs generally in terms of severity and persistence. Recovery from carbamate intoxication occurs usually in a matter of hours. There is no evidence of delayed neurotoxicity for carbamate insecticides. Currently, few members of this insecticide group show evidence of genotoxicity, carcinogenicity, or teratogenic effects in animals or in vitro.[10] Along these lines, animal and in vitro studies suggest that the commonly used carbamate insecticide, carbaryl (Sevin) may have mutagenic[168] and teratogenic effects.[95] In this connection, the action of carbaryl as a mitotic spindle poison is of interest.[141] No counterpart human studies are available. Aside from these health issues, concerns are raised regarding possible immunosuppressive and hormonal alterations induced by some carbamates.

Organochlorine insecticides. Chlorinated hydrocarbon insecticides are structurally diverse but have somewhat similar biological properties. From this unique group of pesticides, we consider DDT (a biphenyl ethane), lindane (a hexachlorocyclohexane), and chlordane (a chlorinated cyclodiene) as representative members of this class of insecticide. In general, members of this pesticide class tend to be of low acute toxicity for humans, but some are much more toxic (dieldrin, endrin). They also tend to persist or bioaccumulate, predominately in tissues with high fat content, and can be excreted in milk fat. Hepatic toxicity and hepatic microsomal enzyme induction are part of the pattern of biological activities of this pesticide class. The mechanism(s) of neurotoxicity are not clearly understood. Absorption of chlorinated hydrocarbon insecticides occurs through skin, lungs, and the gastrointestinal tract.

DDT. DDT   (1,1,1-trichloro-2,2-*bis*[*p*-chlorophenyl] ethane) is a low-order, acute toxicity insecticide for humans and other mammalian species. For this reason, at the outset of its use, DDT was considered to be an ideal pesticide. As mentioned before, information gathered in the early 1960s showed that the pesticide was harmful to certain predatory avian species.[24] Moreover, DDT was found to be persistent, bioaccumulated in fat tissue, and concentrated in human and animal breast milk. Although the EPA canceled the use of DDT in 1973, residues of DDT and its metabolite, p,p'DDE, continue to be found in the serum of the general population today in the part per billion range.[60] Current work in breast cancer patients demonstrates that the serum from these patients shows significantly higher levels of DDE.[175] In this regard, similar to other members of this class, DDT has weakly estrogenic properties[108] and has other hormonal effects. This persistent, continuous source of estrogenic stimulation of breast and ovarian tissue by halogenated xenobiotics such as DDT further suggests a role for polychlorinated chemicals in the development of neoplasms of these tissues.

In ecological terms, removal of organochlorine pesticides in the 10 years following the decision on DDT has had immediate and recognizable effects (e.g., the survival of the brown pelican as a species). Subsequent increase in the use of more acutely toxic organophosphorous and carbamate pesticides has also occurred, increasing the danger to humans.[34] In some other countries, DDT remains in use for public health insect vector control.[85]

Chlordane. Chlordane (1,2,4,5,6,7,8,8,-octachloro-3a,4,7,7a-tetrahydro-4,7-methanoindan) is a representative member of the cyclodiene group of insecticides that includes heptachlor, aldrin, kepone, dieldrin, and endrin. These products are used primarily for termite control and for soil-borne insects. For chlordane as well as for other cyclodienes, signs of acute intoxication include hypothermia, hyperexcitability, tremor, and convulsions.[61] Instances of acute intoxication are relatively rare but can occur both in the residential[65] and occupational setting. More significant are reports of altered immunocompetence both in animals[17,27,31] and more recently in humans.[96] In the human study, T-lymphocyte subpopulations, mitogen response, and mixed (allogeneic) lymphocyte response of persons exposed to technical-grade chlordane in their homes or at work were found to be significantly altered compared with unexposed control subjects.

Early epidemiologic studies[78] suggest some linkage between neuroblastoma, aplastic anemia, and leukemia. More recent occupational studies in pesticide manufacturing plants suggest a relationship between cyclodiene exposure and development of liver and bile duct cancer.[19] Farm workers exposed to chlordane and other insecticides show increased risk for non-Hodgkin lymphoma.[22] Mechanistic studies suggest that chlordane may be a nongenotoxic carcinogen or a tumor promoter. Disruption of intercellular communication[133] and promotion of N-nitrosamine carcinogenesis were noted.[172]

Lindane. Chemically, lindane is the gamma isomer of benzene hexachloride (1,2,3,4,5,6-hexachlorocyclohexane). The pesticide has been used as a wood preservative, as a household fumigant, and for treatment of poultry and livestock. It is most commonly used in humans as a treatment for scabies and lice (Kwell). In terms of acute toxicity, lindane has a clinical pattern of effects similar to that of other chlorinated insecticides. Since the 1950s, documented cases of aplastic anemia in association with exposure to lindane have been consistently recorded. These occurrences do not necessarily appear to be dose related. These early case studies reviewed in current work[134] suggest that certain human leukocyte antigen phenotypes may be more sensitive to the toxicant effects of the chemical on bone marrow. Other work suggests involvement of immune dysregulation in this process.[125] Endocrine abnormalities in women leading to habitual abortions and infertility have been associated with exposure to and elevated blood and tissue levels of lindane or pentachlorophenol.[57] (Pentachlorophenol is a metabolite of lindane. It is also a pesticide and wood preservative.) Elevated levels of beta-hexachlorocyclohexane, a tissue metabolite of the gamma isomer, have been observed in breast cancer patients.[105] Altogether, these human laboratory-based studies demonstrate the same general pattern of effects seen in animal studies of chlorinated hydrocarbon insecticides.

Pyrethrums and pyrethroid insecticides. The insecticidal properties of the dried flowers from chrysanthemums have been known for more than a century. In contrast to synthetic pesticides, the dried or extracted product is a highly complex racemic mixture of chemical isomers centered on a cyclopropane ring structure. Because of the lack of stability of the natural product in sunlight, synthetic derivatives (pyrethroids) have been formulated; more than 1000 structures have been synthesized.[126] Both natural and synthetic derivatives tend to be used with a synergist such as piperonyl butoxide. Most forms of these pesticide mixtures exert their insecticidal action by stereospecifically blocking sodium channels in the cell membrane. In general, these stereospecific effects on the cell membrane favor low acute neurotoxicity for humans and specific high-level toxicity for insects. Acute occupational exposure to pyrethroids can lead to paresthesia and respiratory irritation.[25,165] More common are reports of contact dermatitis. In vitro human lymphocyte and in vivo animal studies for genotoxicity suggest that some pyrethroids are clastogenic and can induce aneuploidy.[12,148] One epidemiological study[20] suggests an association with excess leukemia among Midwestern farmers in the United States. Both natural and synthetic pyrethroids have been associated with epidemic gynecomastia in men. These health effects are thought to be related to pyrethroid binding of androgen receptors.[44]

Fumigants

Members of this class of pesticide are best characterized by high volatility and high lethality in relatively low concentrations. They are used to treat food and seed products, such as grain, coffee, and herbs, and the structures used to store and transport these agricultural products, to eliminate and prevent infestation with insects and sometimes rodent pests. Pesticides in this class are a panoply of classic toxicants that include cyanide, chloroform, carbon tetrachloride, carbon disulfide, ethylene dichloride, ethylene dibromide, ethylene oxide, methyl bromide, dibromochloropropane, chloropicrin, and phosphine. The majority of these toxicants are genotoxic and have carcinogenic effects in animals. Some are also teratogens, and a few produce delayed neurotoxic effects. Thirty years ago, a mixture of carbon tetrachloride and carbon disulfide was the most commonly used fumigant. In the 1980s, the EPA removed this product from use because of its known carcinogenic effects in animals. In the same time frame, ethylene dibromide was removed from use because of known and suspected carcinogenic effects. Most recently, methyl bromide has been removed from use because of its potential for delayed neurotoxic effects. The most commonly used fumigant currently is phosphine derived from aluminum or magnesium phosphide pellets. Phosphine accounts for approximately 80% of fumigant use. Less common is the use of chloropicrin and methyl bromide. For purposes of this discussion, the health effects of methyl bromide, chloropicrin, and phosphine are considered in some detail.

Methyl bromide. From 1953 to 1981, methyl bromide accounted for 60 fatalities and 301 cases of systemic poisoning related to its use as a fumigant.[5] Typically, symptoms related to acute intoxication are delayed, varying from a few hours to 2 days. Central nervous system symptoms predominate, varying from numbness and ataxia to seizures and personality disturbances. Recovery may be marked by persistent neurological deficits.[69] Even without acute symptomatic effects, apparent repeated low-level exposure has been associated with neurobehavioral deficits in exposed workers.[7] One of the factors accounting for the frequency of acute intoxication is the apparent lack of odor warning properties of the chemical. Selective destruction of the sensory epithelium of the olfactory nerve is an added feature of toxication.[153] Anatomical studies in animals show central neuron degeneration affecting the cerebrum and cerebellum.[46,74] Aside from these neurotoxic effects, in vitro studies in cultured human lymphocytes show that the fumigant can be genotoxic[54] in relatively high concentrations. Animal studies[129] for carcinogenicity are inconclusive.

Chloropicrin. Vapors of this volatile fumigant are extremely irritating in low concentrations. Burning skin, lacrimation, wheezing, nausea, and vomiting are initial signs and symptoms of exposure and intoxication. The primary source data on human exposure effects is derived from use of chloropicrin as a chemical warfare agent in World War I. Lethal effects of this agent include development of pulmonary edema and cardiac arrhythmias. Concentrations of 1 ppm can induce intense eye irritation without significant systemic toxicity.[127] Because of this warning property, chloropicrin is sometimes used in conjunction with methyl bromide as a fumigant mixture. The EPA [158] reported one

death in a 5-year period in 22 reported incidents involving chloropicrin intoxication. Chronic health effects in humans are poorly documented. Incidents of acute intoxication and lethality continue to be reported.[8,58] Short-term (5-day) studies in animals show that concentrations as low 8 ppm induce severe degenerative changes in the olfactory and respiratory epithelium.[21] In vitro studies for gentoxicity in human lymphocytes show some evidence for genotoxic effects at high concentrations of the chemical.[54]

Mechanistically, chloropicrin was found to bind sulfhydryl groups[127] and induce methemoglobin in vitro (Potter W, Garry VF: unpublished observations, 1992). Interestingly, chloropicrin can be formed by oxidative chlorination of the water supply.[99]

Phosphine. The fumigant phosphine is a toxicant gas derived from hydrolysis of aluminum or magnesium phosphide supplied in tablet or other like products for enclosed space applications. The toxicity of this gas is both cumulative and acute. Concentrations of the gas higher than 2.5 ppm are lethal when given to experimental animals over a course of days.[83] Higher concentrations given over shorter periods of time are also lethal. Lethal effects even at high concentrations of phosphine tend to be delayed for periods in excess of 4 hours.[83] Characteristically, intoxicated patients first become anxious, develop a significant tachycardia, may become tremulous, and develop seizures. Finally a rapidly evolving pulmonary edema occurs. Renal and hepatic damage may also occur.[26,101,102]

Morphologically, pulmonary edema and anoxic changes in the brain are frequently seen at autopsy. Persons who recover from intoxication tend to show neurobehavioral changes. Treatment for intoxication is nonspecific. Hemodialysis and exchange transfusion may be beneficial in some circumstances. Repeated relatively low-level exposures are common in the occupational setting.[52,180] Under these conditions, phosphine is thought to be genotoxic and induce chromosome rearrangements[52] in exposed workers. In vitro studies show that phosphine induces chromosome aberrations in low concentrations, and alkaline elution studies indicate that the gas induces DNA cross-links.[52] Epidemiological studies[3] demonstrate an excess risk of certain cancers in the grain industry, particularly non-Hodgkin lymphoma. Early mechanistic studies performed by Trimborn and Klimmer[156] showed that phosphine induced production of abnormal hemoglobin species other than methemoglobin. Later studies[122] demonstrate that in vitro phosphine produces a dose-dependent increase in Heinz body formation in human erythrocytes. Examination of another heme protein, myeloperoxidase, in exposed workers showed histochemically inhibition of the enzyme in neutrophils.[53]

Other work done with animals demonstrates that the gas can be an inhibitor of cholinesterase. Further work in exposed workers and in vitro demonstrates that phosphine is an inhibitor of red cell cholinesterase.[122] Altogether the data demonstrate that phosphine is a potent broad-spectrum toxicant with an affinity for heme proteins, including hemoglobin, myeloperoxidase, and cytochrome-c oxidase.[53]

Fungicides

Purchase of fungicides is responsible for more than 12% ($2.8 billion) of the $12.8 billion spent on pesticides worldwide.[176] Aside from their economic impact on crop production, fungicides form one of the most chemically diverse groups of pesticides.[142] Their major use in agriculture is to control or eradicate fungi, bacteria, viruses, and nematodes that affect plant life. In terms of spectrum function, use, and application practice, there are two major fungicide groups:

1. Nonsystemic fungicides are plant surface protectants (foliage, roots, and seeds). Early on, inorganic arsenic, copper, zinc, and sulfur were used. Organometals, including triethyl tin, were and continue to be used. More recently, chloroalkyl thio fungicides (e.g., captan, folpet) and thiocarbamates (e.g., maneb, zineb, thiram, mancozeb) have become the most commonly used nonsystemic fungicides.

2. Systemic fungicides are actively absorbed and are distributed within the plant. These relatively new products have become more widespread in their use because of their effects on a broad spectrum of fungi. Benzimidazoles (e.g., benomyl) are representative of systemic fungicides.

It is difficult in this chapter to explore the many-faceted biological and biochemical effects of fungicides because of their structural diversity. To limit the discussion, we focus on representative members of this pesticide group that are in common use today. Most health concerns for this pesticide class focus on teratogenicity and carcinogenicity. Acute toxicant effects and allergic contact dermatitis are also of concern.

Chloroalkyl thio fungicides: captan. An independent review of the anatomical pathology of two different animal studies in which animals were chronically treated with different doses of captan shows clear evidence of carcinogenicity with relatively low concentrations of the fungicide.[128] Tumors of the endocrine glands were highly prevalent. Tumors of the female reproductive system, including breast and ovary, were noted in excess. Male rodents showed severe testicular atrophy. Because of the known chemical structural relationship of chloroalkyl thio fungicides to thalidomide, (one of the few proven human teratogens), reproductive effects have been a significant concern. Thus far, animal studies have reported conflicting results. Studies in avian species[163] show teratogenic effects, whereas a study in subhuman primates does not.[166] In vitro studies show that captan is genotoxic in a broad spectrum of prokaryotic and eukaryotic cell systems, including human lymphocytes.[152,164] Mechanistic studies indicate that captan induces single-strand breaks and DNA cross-links.[140] Other work shows that captan inhibits microtubule formation.[146]

Thiocarbamate fungicides: maneb. Maneb is one of a group of widely used ethylene bis-thiocarbamates (EDBC) used in agriculture and in forestry. Ethylenethiourea (ETU), a potent teratogen in rats, is a degradation and by-product of manufacture of these pesticides. ETU can also be formed during product storage.[45] Agricultural workers exposed to EDBC aerosols metabolize these products to ETU,[84] detected in the urine. Behavioral studies in animals suggest that maneb is a central nervous system depressant with effects on the dopaminergic system.[103,127a]

Benzimidazoles: benomyl. Because systemic fungicides such as benomyl are actively taken up by treated plants, they have the potential for and do demonstrate residual levels of these pesticides in food crops.[113,167] There is no current evidence that adverse health effects in humans occur owing to ingestion of low-level residuals in foods. Animal studies, however, do show that benomyl is a significant teratogen when administered to pregnant animals early in pregnancy[32] or at later times.[72,81] Recorded anomalies include ocular and craniocerebral abnormalities. In treated male animals, degenerative changes in the genital tract and testes are noted.[69a] Investigation of the mechanism(s) of genotoxicity demonstrates that benomyl induces dose-dependent aneuploidy in treated cells, including female gametes.[4,56,92] Other mechanistic studies indicate that the fungicide is an inhibitor of liver microsomal mixed-function oxidases[33] and therefore may enhance the toxicity of other pesticides.[38]

SOME CONTINUING HEALTH CONCERNS
Reproductive effects

Earlier parts of this chapter discussed reproductive health issues raised by specific pesticide groups, including the chlorinated hydrocarbon insecticides, certain fungicides, and fumigants. Of all organ systems, the reproductive system presents an inordinately diverse set of physiological mechanisms at risk for toxicant effects. Other than induction of spontaneous abortion and the presence of placental barriers for transfer of some chemicals to the fetus, there appear to be few physiological offset mechanisms to minimize toxicant effects. Interference with the endocrine system (organochlorine insecticides), effects on sperm (dibromochloropropane), effects on the ovum (benomyl), and effects on fetal cell organization (captan) can lead to adverse reproductive outcomes.

Immunity and allergy (see Chapters 6, 25, and 28)

Exposure to potential biological and nonbiological sources of untoward immunostimulation and immunosuppression in agriculture is broad based and spans the gamut from plant, animal, viral, fungal, and bacterial sources to pesticides.[178] The intensity of these exposures is highly variable depending on season and type of agricultural work. For example, work in animal confinement buildings, grain

Table 8-1. Structure and spectrum of pathobiological activity of selected pesticides

Representative pesticide structure	Pesticide class/group	Significant acute toxicity (Ref. No.)
Alachlor	Herbicide/chloracetanilide	No
Atrazine	Herbicide/triazine	No
Dinoseb	Herbicide/dinitrophenol	Yes (114)
Glyphosate	Herbicide/organic phosphorus	Yes (91, 145, 150, 155)
2,4-D	Herbicide/chlorophenoxy	No
Malathion	Insecticide/ organophosphate	Yes (173)
Carbaryl	Insecticide/carbamate	Yes (10)

	Potential chronic health effects			
Allergy **(Ref. No.)**	**Immune** **system** **(Ref. No.)**	**Nervous** **system** **(Ref. No.)**	**Cancer and** **cancer-related** **effects (Ref. No.)**	**Birth defects** **and reproductive** **effects (Ref. No.)**
—	—	—	▲ (106, 159)	★ (98)
—	—	—	▲◇ (40 , 76)	★ (174)
★ (114)	★ (114)	★ (114)	★ (170)	★ (87)
★ (91)	—	—	—	—
★ (77)	★ (77)	No	▲◇ (15, 16, 63, 64, 70, 71, 115, 162)	★ (77, 162)
Yes (154)	Yes (154)	Yes (173)	▲◇ (15, 16, 109)	★ (137)
★ (154)	★ (154)	Yes (10)	△ (10, 168)	▲◇ (95, 141)

Closed triangle, Animal studies; *open triangle*, in vitro studies; *diamond*, human studies; *star*, unknown and questionable; *dash*, no evidence.
Numbered text references indicate suggested readings.

Continued.

Table 8-1. Structure and spectrum of pathobiological activity of selected pesticides—cont'd

Representative pesticide structure	Pesticide class/group	Significant acute toxicity (Ref. No.)
DDT	Insecticide/chloro-biphenylethane	No (138)
Chlordane	Insecticide/chlorinated cyclodiene	Yes (61, 65, 133)
Lindane	Insecticide/hexachlorocyclohexane (gamma isomer)	No
Permethrin	Insecticide/pyrethroid	No
Methyl bromide	Fumigant/bromomethane	Yes (5)
Chloropicrin	Fumigant/trichloronitromethane	Yes (8)
Phosphine	Fumigant/phosphine	Yes (83)

		Potential chronic health effects		
Allergy (Ref. No.)	**Immune system (Ref. No.)**	**Nervous system (Ref. No.)**	**Cancer and cancer-related effects (Ref. No.)**	**Birth defects and reproductive effects (Ref. No.)**
★ (154)	★ (154)	Yes (142)	▲◇ (108, 138, 175)	▲★ (108, 119)
★ (154)	Yes (96, 154)	Yes (61)	▲◇ (20, 138)	★ (133)
Yes (125, 134)	Yes (125, 132)	★ (138)	★◇ (105, 138)	★◇ (57, 138)
Yes (165)	★ (25)	★ (166)	△◇ (20, 148)	★ (44)
No	★ (53)	Yes (46, 69)	△ (54)	★ (54)
★ (21)	★ (21, 54)	Yes (8, 58)	△ (54)	★ (54)
No	Yes (54)	Yes (122)	△◇ (3, 53)	★ (53)

Closed triangle, Animal studies; *open triangle,* in vitro studies; *diamond,* human studies; *star,* unknown and questionable; *dash,* no evidence.
Numbered text references indicate suggested readings.   *Continued.*

Table 8-1. Structure and spectrum of pathobiological activity of selected pesticides—cont'd

Representative pesticide structure	Pesticide class/group	Significant acute toxicity (Ref. No.)
Captan	Fungicide/chlorothioalkyl	★ (140, 146)
Maneb	Fungicide/thiocarbamate	★ (45, 84)
Benomyl	Fungicide/benzimidazole carbamate	No

bins, and barns carries with it an enhanced opportunity for exposure to allergenic dusts, danders, and fungi.[2,11,39] Pesticide application in enclosed space work can also produce higher sustained levels of exposure to potential immunosuppressive agents.[180] In these enclosed space work activities, exposures to gaseous lung irritants and asphyxiants, such as nitrogen dioxide in silage[29] and hydrogen sulfide generated in manure holding tanks,[182] are a concern.

The known pathobiological consequences of these biological and nonbiological toxicant exposures can vary from grain dust allergy, to progressive allergic alveolitis, to rapid development of fulminant pulmonary edema owing to nitrogen dioxide exposure. In a health survey of members of the farming community, workers whose major activities involved enclosed space work demonstrated an excess of chronic lung disease, allergy, and asthma compared with other agricultural workers not involved in confined space work.[55] (See Chapter 27.)

Dermatitis. Nonallergic and allergic contact dermatitis is a common work-related disease in agriculture. The Cal-

ifornia experience[94] shows that 14% of all occupational skin disease is related to work in agriculture, particularly in workers involved in crop service. Of that number, 63% were caused by plant/animal products (inedible), and 20% were related to pesticides. A number of pesticides, including some in common use (glyphosate, benomyl, captan, and pyrethroids) have been associated with contact dermatitis.[112] More detailed work[136a] suggests that some carbamates (particularly thiocarbamates), some organophosphates, and chlorophenoxy herbicides can produce allergic contact dermatitis.

Immune dysregulation. With regard to regulation of the immune response, aflatoxin B1, a fungal toxin derived from aspergillus and not an uncommon biological contaminant in stored grain, can be a cause of immune dysregulation.[121] Animal studies show that some pesticides can alter cellular and humoral immunity.[37,50] Evidence for augmentation and suppression of different components of the cellular and humoral response have been observed, suggesting immune dysregulation.[131] Several human studies[67,179]

	Potential chronic health effects			
Allergy **(Ref. No.)**	**Immune** **system** **(Ref. No.)**	**Nervous** **system** **(Ref. No.)**	**Cancer and** **cancer-related** **effects (Ref. No.)**	**Birth defects** **and reproductive** **effects (Ref. No.)**
★ (140, 146)	★ (140, 146)	No	▲★ (128, 140, 146)	▲★ (128, 140, 146)
★ (45, 84)	★ (45, 84)	▲ (103)	▲★ (45, 84)	★ (45)
No	★ (38)	★ (32, 38)	△★ (4, 56, 92)	▲★ (32, 72)

Closed triangle, Animal studies; *open triangle,* in vitro studies; *diamond,* human studies; *star,* unknown and questionable; *dash,* no evidence.
Numbered text references indicate suggested readings.

show correlation between impairment of cholinesterase activity and impairment of neutrophil function. Most recently, Newcombe[109] speculated that inhibition of monocyte esterases and perhaps other immune cell esterases by organophosphates alters the ability of the immune system to handle retroviral pathogens important in the evolution of non-Hodgkin lymphoma. In other human studies, exposure to chlordane, an organochlorine insecticide and termitocide, has been shown to alter the proportion of certain T- and B-lymphocyte subsets in persons exposed at work or in their home.[96] Similarly, exposure to aldicarb, a carbamate, in contaminated water supplies may also affect T- and B-cell subset regulation.[48] More direct evidence for immune dysregulation in humans exposed to pesticides was put forward by Lipkowitz and colleagues.[88] In these studies, polymerase chain reaction demonstrated that a quantitative excess of specific rearrangements of DNA from the V(J) region of immunoglobulin occurred only during the pesticide use season by pesticide applicators. In parallel with pesticide applicators, patients who have a high genetic risk for non-Hodgkin lymphoma also demonstrated excess rearrangement of this DNA region associated with immunoglobulin synthesis. It appears from these data and those of others that immune dysregulation may be a factor in the evolution of non-Hodgkin lymphoma in the environment of agriculture. Immunotoxic effects exerted in one or more components of the immune system (neutrophils, monocytes, lymphocytes, or macrophages) are biomarkers for immune dysregulation.

A LOOK INTO THE FUTURE: A PERSONAL VIEW OF A LABORATORY-BASED PHYSICIAN

In preparing this final segment of the chapter, we decided to dust off an old book, *Silent Spring* by Rachel Carson,[24] to see how far we have progressed in the more than 30 years since its publication. As I turned and read the pages, yellowed with age, many all too familiar images made their appearance. Some comments made by the author are pertinent for today and for the future[24]:

It is not my contention that chemical insecticides must never be used. I do contend that we have put poisonous and biologically potent chemicals indiscriminately into the hands of persons largely or wholly ignorant of their potentials for harm. We have subjected enormous numbers of people to contact with these poisons, without their consent and often without their knowledge.

Comment: The professional pesticide applicator in the United States today is licensed through the state and is subject to a continuing education requirement conducted by state and federally supported agricultural extension services. In addition to this source, detailed information is available from pesticide manufacturers, including health-related data. The lay public is continually informed through various mass media presentations and pesticide labeling requirements. Although progress in terms of knowledge and information transfer has been made, experience speaks to some failings on the part of the nonlicensed pesticide applier (your neighbor, your employer, your housing manager) and undereducated segments of our society. A continuing problem in the urban setting is the use of pesticides on lawns and for insect infestation. Some examples from personal experience are in order: (1) A neighbor attempts to rid his home of wasps by using a bait soaked in organophosphate pesticide placed in a bowl on the turf near the wasp nest. Inadvertently a pet eats the bait and suffers many of the manifestations of organophosphate acute toxicity but recovers. (2) Several employees in a local bank building suffer a multiple sclerosis–like syndrome within 2 weeks after application of the pesticide Dursban in and about the work area. Information regarding the application was not provided to the employees or their customers. (3) An apartment manager leases an apartment to a woman with asthma. He fails to tell the woman that the apartment has recently been fumigated. Within 1 week, the woman is hospitalized with recurrent bouts of severe asthma. She recovers, and investigation reveals use of an organophosphate for fumigation.

The monthly report of the office of vital statistics for July 1959 states that malignant growths, including those of the lymphatic and blood-forming tissues, accounted for 15% of the deaths in 1958 compared with only 4% in 1900. Judging by the present incidence of this disease, the American Cancer Society estimates that 45,000,000 Americans now living will eventually develop cancer. This means that malignant disease will strike two out of three families.

Carson goes on to state[24]

Dr. Malcolm Hargraves and his associates in the Hematology Department of the Mayo Clinic report that almost without exception these patients have had a history of exposure to various toxic chemicals, including sprays which contain DDT, chlordane, benzene, lindane and petroleum distillates.

In other parts of this chapter, Carson speaks to possible relationships between pesticides and childhood cancer and to hormonal induction by pesticides and their possible relationships to cancer of the reproductive system.

Comment: In the early 1960s, these were provocative and for the most part unsubstantiated statements. They remain controversial today, but the trend in current laboratory-based and epidemiological based evidence indicates that these early statements with respect to cancer and other diseases of the hematopoietic and reproductive system may not be totally unfounded.

CONCLUSION

This chapter has explored the many health implications of pesticide use. As laboratory-based physicians, we have a unique role in the recognition and prevention of pesticide-related disease. Development and use of biomarker technologies for preclinical diagnosis and prevention of pesticide-related and other environmental disease will lead to a distinct role for pathologists in disease prevention. Large-scale studies that link laboratory and epidemiological methods of investigation offer the opportunity to resolve many of the health issues surrounding pesticide use in agriculture. The current joint National Cancer Institute, National Institute of Environmental Health and Safety (NIEHS), and EPA initiative to study farm family health is an important step on a national scale to provide answers to these continuing health questions.

REFERENCES

1. Abou-Dona M, Lapadula D: Mechanisms of organophosphorus ester-induced delayed neurotoxicity: type I and type II, *Annu Rev Pharmacol Toxicol* 30:405, 1990.
2. Abramson D: Mycotoxins in grains and dust. In Dosman J, Cockcroft D, editors: *Principles of health and safety in agriculture*, Boca Raton, 1989, CRC Press.
3. Alavanja M et al: Proportionate mortality study of workers in the grain industry, *J Natl Cancer Inst* 78:247, 1987.
4. Albertini S: Reevaluation of the 9 compounds reported conclusive positive in yeast Saccharomyces cerevisiae aneuploidy test systems by the Gene-Tox Program using strain D61.M of Saccharomyces cerevisiae, *Mutation Res* 260:165, 1991.
5. Alexceff GV, Kilgore WW: Methyl bromide, *Residue Rev* 88:101, 1983.
6. Ames R et al: Cholinesterase activity depression among California pesticide applicators, *Am J Ind Med* 15:143, 1989.
7. Anger K et al: Neurobehavioral evaluation of soil and structural fu-

migators using methyl bromide and sulfural fluoride, *Neurotoxicology* 7:137, 1986.

8. Asauliuk IK: Symptoms of acute inhalation lesions caused by trichloronitromethane, *Vrach Delo* 1:104, 1990.

9. Baker E et al: Epidemic malathion poisoning in Pakistan malaria workers, *Lancet* 1:31, 1978.

10. Baron R: Carbamate insecticides. In Hayes W, Laws E, editors: *Handbook of pesticide toxicology,* Vol 3, New York, 1991, Academic Press.

11. Barthel E, Krecklow K: Epidemiological cross-sectional study on prevalence of chronic bronchitis and lung function impairments among swine and cattle workers, *Z Erkank Atm Org* 172:143, 1989.

12. Bhunya S, Pati P: Effect of deltamethrin, a synthetic pyrethroid, on the induction of chromosome aberrations, micronuclei and sperm abnormalities in mice, *Mutagenesis* 5:229, 1990.

13. Bidstrup P, Payne D: Poisoning by dinitro-ortho-cresol, *Br Med J* 2:16, 1951.

14. Blair A, Zahm S: Cancer among farmers, *Occup Med* 6:335, 1991.

15. Blair A et al: Cancer among farmers: a review, *Scand J Work Environ Health* 11:397, 1985.

16. Blair A et al: Carcinogenic effects of pesticides. In Baker S, Wilkinson C, editors: *The effects of pesticides on human health, advances in modern environmental toxicology,* Princeton, 1990, Princeton Scientific Publishing Co.

17. Blaylock B et al: Cytotoxic T-lymphocyte and NK responses in mice treated prenatally with chlordane, *Toxicol Lett* 51:41, 1990.

18. Blondell G: Personal communication, Washington, DC, Office of Pesticide Programs USEPA, 1993.

19. Brown D: Mortality of workers employed at organochlorine pesticide manufacturing plants—an update, *Scand J Work Environ Health* 18:155, 1992.

20. Brown L et al: Pesticide exposures and other agricultural risk factors for leukemia among men in Iowa and Minnesota, *Cancer Res* 50:6585, 1990.

21. Buckley L et al: Respiratory tract lesions induced by sensory irritants at the RD50 concentration, *Toxicol Appl Pharmacol* 74:417, 1984.

22. Cantor K et al: Pesticides and other agricultural risk factors for non-Hodgkin's lymphoma among men in Iowa and Minnesota, *Cancer Res* 52:2447, 1992.

23. Cappuccilli E: *Synthetic organic chemicals,* Section XIII. US International Trade Commission Washington, DC, US Government Printing Office, 1985.

24. Carson R: *The silent spring,* Boston, 1962, Houghton Mifflin.

25. Chen S et al: An epidemiological study on occupational acute pyrethroid poisoning in cotton farmers, *Br J Ind Med* 48:77, 1991.

26. Chopra J et al: Aluminum phosphide poisoning: a prospective study of 16 cases in one year, *Postgrad Med J* 62:1113, 1986.

27. Chuang L et al: Modulation by the insecticides heptachlor and chlordane of the cell mediated immune proliferative responses of rhesus monkeys, *In Vivo* 6:29, 1992.

28. CIBA-GEIGY: *Review of mutagenicity data base for atrazine,* Greensboro, NC, 1987, Ciba-Geigy Corporation.

29. Commins B, Raveney F, Jesson M: Toxic gases in tower silos, *Ann Occup Hyg* 14:275, 1971.

30. Costa L et al: Tolerance to acetylcholinesterase compounds in mammals, *Toxicology* 25:79, 1982.

31. Cranmer J, Avery D, Barnett J: Altered immune competence of offspring exposed during development to the chlorinated hydrocarbon pesticide chlordane, *Teratology* 19:23A, 1979.

32. Cummings A et al: Developmental effects of methyl benzimidazolecarbamate following exposure during early pregnancy, *Fund Appl Toxicol* 18:288, 1992.

33. Dalvi R: Effect of the fungicide benomyl on xenobiotic metabolism in rats, *Toxicology* 71:63, 1992.

34. Davies J, Lee J: Changing profiles in human health effects of pesticides. In Greenhalgh R, Roberts T, editors: *Pesticide science and biotechnology,* Oxford, 1987, Blackwell Scientific Publications.

35. deJong L, Kossen S: Stereospecific reactivation of human brain and erythrocyte acetylcholinesterase inhibited by 1,2,2-trimethylpropyl methylphosphonofluoridate (soman), *Biochim Biophys Acta* 830:345, 1985.

36. Delzell E, Grufferman S: Mortality among white and nonwhite farmers in North Carolina, 1976-1978, *Am J Epidemiol* 121:391, 1985.

37. Desi I, Varga L, Farkas I: The effect of DDVP, an organophosphorus pesticide on the humoral and cell-mediated immunity of rabbits, *Arch Toxicol* (Suppl 4):171, 1980.

38. Dolara P et al: Sister-chromatid exchanges in human lymphocytes induced by dimethoate, omethoate, deltamethrin, benomyl and their mixture, *Mutation Res* 283:113, 1992.

39. Donham K et al: Characterization of dusts collected from swine confinement buildings, *Am Ind Hyg Assoc* 47:404, 1986.

40. Donna A et al: Triazine herbicides and ovarian epithelial neoplasms, *Scand J Work Environ Health* 15:47, 1989.

41. Dosman J, Cockcroft D, editors: *Principles of health and safety in agriculture,* Boca Raton, 1989, CRC Press, Inc.

42. Dreyfus P et al: Cross-homologies and structural differences between human cholinesterases revealed by antibodies against cDNA-Produced human butyrylcholinesterase peptides, *J Neurochem* 51:1858, 1988.

43. Duncan R, Griffith J: Screening of agricultural workers for exposure to anticholinesterases. In Ballantyne B, Marrs T, editors: *Clinical and experimental toxicology of organophosphates and carbamates,* Oxford, 1992, Butterworth & Heinemann.

44. Eil C, Nisula B: The binding properties of pyrethroids to human skin fibroblast androgen receptors and to sex hormone binding globulin, *J Steroid Biochem* 35:409, 1990.

45. Engst R, Schaak W: Residue of dithiocarbamate fungicides and metabolites on plant foods, *Residue Rev* 52:45, 1974.

46. Eustis L et al: Pathology of methyl bromide toxicity, *Toxicologist,* 6:54, 1986.

47. Field F, Kerr C: Herbicide use and incidence of neural tube defects, *Lancet* 1:1341, 1979.

48. Fiore M et al: Chronic exposure to aldicarb-contaminated groundwater and human immune function, *Environ Res* 41:633, 1986.

49. Fitzgerald B, Costa L: Modulation of muscarinic receptors and acetylcholinesterase activity in lymphocytes and in brain areas following repeated organophosphate exposure in rats, *Fund Appl Toxicol* 20:210, 1993.

50. Flipo D et al: Combined effects of selected insecticides on humoral response in mice, *Int J Immunopharmacol* 14:747, 1992.

51. Garry V et al: Integration of laboratory and epidemiologic studies to evaluate genotoxic exposure in tool and die workers. In Sorsa M. and Norppa H, editors: *Monitoring of occupational genotoxicants,* New York, 1986, Alan R. Liss, Inc.

52. Garry V et al: Human genotoxicity: pesticide applicators and phosphine, *Science* 246:251, 1989.

53. Garry V et al: Human genotoxicity in phosphine exposed fumigant applicators. In Mendelsohn M, Albertini R, editors: *Mutation and the environment, Part C,* New York, 1990, Wiley-Liss Inc.

54. Garry V et al: Preparation for human study of pesticide applicators: sister chromatid exchanges and chromosome aberrations in cultured human lymphocytes exposed to selected fumigants, *Teratogen Carcinog Mutagen* 10:21, 1990.

55. Garry V et al: Survey of health and characterization of pesticide use among agricultural pesticide appliers in Minnesota, *Arch Environ Health* (in press).

56. Georgieva V et al: Genotoxic activity of Benomyl in different test systems, *Environ Mol Mutagen* 16:32, 1990.

57. Gerhard I, Derner M, Runnebaum B: Prolonged exposure to wood preservatives induces endocrine and immunologic disorders in women, *Am J Obstet Gynecol* 165:487, 1991 (letter).

58. Gonmori K et al: A case of homicidal intoxication by chloropicrin, *Am J Forens Med Pathol* 8:135, 1987.

59. Green M et al: Public health implications of the microbial pesticide *Bacillus thuringiensis:* an epidemiologic study, Oregon, 1985-86, *Am J Pub Health* 80:848, 1990.

60. Griffith J, Duncan R: Serum organochlorine residues in Florida citrus workers compared to the national health and nutrition survey sample, *Bull Environ Contam Toxic* 35:411, 1985.

61. Grutsch J, Khasawinah A: Signs and mechanisms of chlordane intoxication, *Biomed Environ Sci* 4:317, 1991.

62. Gunderson P et al: The epidemiology of suicide among farm residents or workers in five north central states, 1980-1988, *Am J Prevent Med* 9:26, 1993.

63. Hardell L: Malignant lymphoma of histiocytic type and exposure to phenoxyacetic acids or chlorophenols, *Lancet* 1:55, 1979.

64. Hardell L, Sandstrom A: Case-control study: soft-tissue sarcomas and exposure to phenoxyacetic acids or chlorophenols, *Br J Cancer* 39:711, 1979.

65. Harrington J et al: Chlordane contamination of a municipal water system, *Environ Res* 15:155, 1978.

66. Hayes W: Pharmacology and toxicology of DDT. In Muller P, editor: *DDT: the insecticide dichlorodiphenyl-trichloroethane and its significance,* Vol 2, Basel, 1959, Birkhaeuser.

67. Hermanowicz A, Kossman S: Neutrophil function and infectious disease in workers occupationally exposed to phosphoorganic pesticides: role of mononuclear chemotactic factor for neutrophils, *Clin Immunol Immunopathol* 33:13, 1984.

68. Hertzman C et al: Parkinson's disease: a case-control study of occupational and environmental risk factors, *Am J Ind Med* 17:349, 1990.

69. Herzstein J, Cullen M: Methyl bromide intoxication in four field workers during removal of soil fumigation sheets, *Am J Ind Med* 17:321, 1990.

69a. Hess, R, et al: The fungicide benomyl (methyl 1-(butylcarbamoyl)-2-benzimidazolecarbamate) causes testicular dysfunction by inducing the sloughing of germ cells and occulusion of efferent ductiles, *Fundam Appl Toxicol* 17:733-745, 1991.

70. Hoar S et al: Agricultural herbicide use and risk of lymphoma and soft-tissue sarcoma, *JAMA* 256:1141, 1986.

71. Hoar-Zahm S et al: A case-control study of non-Hodgkin's lymphoma and the herbicide 2,4-dichlorophenoxyacetic acid (2,4-D) in eastern Nebraska, *Epidemiology* 1:349, 1990.

72. Hoogenboom E et al: Effects on rat eye of maternal benomyl exposure and protein malnutrition, *Curr Eye Res* 10:601, 1991.

73. Hoskins B, Ho I: Tolerance to organophorous cholinesterase inhibitors. In Chambers J, Levi P, editors: *Organophosphates: chemistry, fate and effects,* San Diego, 1992, Academic Press.

74. Hurtt M, Morgan K, Working P: Histopathology of acute responses in rats exposed by inhalation to methyl bromide, *Pharmacologist* 28:207, 1986.

75. Hydrogen sulfide: case report. In Zenz C, editor: *Occupational medicine,* Chicago, 1988, Year Book Medical Publishers.

76. IARC Monographs Volume 53: *Occupational exposures in insecticide application, and some pesticides.* Lyon, 1991, International Agency for Research on Cancer.

77. *IARC monograph on the evaluation of the carcinogenic risk of chemicals to man,* Vol 15, Lyon, 1977, International Agency for Research on Cancer.

78. Infante P, Epstein S, Newton W: Blood dyscrasias and childhood tumors and exposure to chlordane and heptachlor, *Scand J Work Environ Health* 4:137, 1978.

79. Innes J et al: Bioassay of pesticides and industrial chemicals for tumorigenicity in mice: a preliminary note, *J Natl Cancer Inst* 42:1101, 1969.

80. Kashi K, Chefurka W: The effect of phosphine on absorption and circular dichroic spectra of cytochrome-c oxidase, *Pestis Biochem Physiol* 6:350, 1976.

81. Kavlock R et al: Teratogenic effects of Benomyl in the Wistar rat and CD-1 mouse, with emphasis on the route of administration, *Toxicol Appl Pharmacol* 62:44, 1982.

82. Keefe T, Savage E, Wheeler H: *Third national study of hospitalized pesticide poisonings in the United States, 1977-1982,* USEPA report, Washington, DC, 1990, Office of Pesticide Programs.

83. Klimmer O: Contribution on poisoning by phosphine on the question of sub-chronic phosphine intoxication, *Arch Toxikol* 24:164, 1969.

84. Kurttio P, Vartianen T, Salvolainen K: Environmental and biological monitoring of exposure to ethylenebisdithiocarbamate fungicides and ethylenethiourea, *Br J Ind Med* 47:203, 1990.

85. Kutz F, Wood P, Bottimore D: Organochlorine pesticides and polychlorinated biphenyls in human adipose tissue, *Rev Environ Contam Toxicol* 120:1, 1991.

86. Li A, Long T: An evaluation of the genotoxic potential of glyphosate, *Fund Appl Toxicol* 10:537, 1988.

87. Linder R, Strader L, Suarez V: Endpoints of spermatotoxicity in the rat after short duration exposures to fourteen reproductive toxicants, *Reprod Toxicol* 6:491, 1992.

88. Lipkowitz S, Garry V, Kirsch I: Interlocus V-J recombination measures genomic instability in agriculture workers at risk for lymphoid malignancies, *Proc Natl Acad Sci* 89:5301, 1992.

89. Llorens J et al: Characterization of disulfoton-induced behavioral and neurochemical effects following repeated exposure, *Fund Appl Toxicol* 20:163, 1993.

90. Lucier G, Portier C, Gallo M: Receptor mechanisms and dose-response models for the effects of dioxins, *Environ Health Pers* 101:36, 1993.

91. Mack R: Roundup (glyphosphate) poisoning, *N C Med J* 54:35, 1993.

92. Mailhes J, Aardema M: Benomyl-induced aneuploidy in mouse oocytes, *Mutagenesis* 7:303, 1992.

93. Maroni M, Bleeker M: Neuropathy target esterase in human lymphocytes and platelets, *J Appl Toxicol* 6:1, 1986.

94. Mathias C: Epidemiology of occupational skin disease in agriculture. In Dosman J, Cockcroft D, editors: *Principles of health and safety in agriculture,* Boca Raton, 1989, CRC Press.

95. Mathur A, Bhatnager P: A teratogenic study of carbaryl in Swiss albino mice, *Food Chem Toxicol* 29:629, 1991.

96. McConnachie P, Zahalsky A: Immune alterations in humans exposed to the termiticide technical chlordane, *Arch Environ Health* 47:295, 1992.

97. McGuire M et al: Identification of the structural mutation responsible for the dibucaine-resistant (atypical) variant form of human serum cholinesterase, *Proc Nat Acad Sci* 86:953, 1989.

98. Meisner L, Belluck D, Roloff B: Cytogenetic effects of Alachlor and/or Atrazine in vivo and in vitro, *Environ Molec Mutagene* 19:77, 1992.

99. Merlet N, Thibaud H, Dore M: Chloropicrin formation during oxidative treatments in the preparation of drinking water, *Sci Total Environ* 47:223, 1985.

100. Milham S: *Occupational mortality in Washington state 1950-1979,* Publication 83-166, Washington, DC, 1983, US Department of Health and Human Services.

101. Misra U et al: Occupational phosphine exposure in Indian workers, *Toxicol Lett* 42:257, 1988.

102. Misra U et al: Acute poisoning following ingestion of aluminum phosphide, *Human Toxicol* 7:343, 1988.

103. Morato G, Lemos T, Takahashi R: Acute exposure to Maneb alters some behavioral functions in the mouse, *Neurotoxicol Teratol* 11:421, 1989.

103a. Mullison WR: An interim report summarizing 2,4-D toxicological research sponsored by the Industry Task Force on 2,4-D Research Data and a brief review of 2,4-D environmental effects. Washington, DC, 1986, Industry Task Force on 2,4-D Research Data.

104. Murphy S: Pesticides. In Doull J, Klaasen C, Amdur M, editors: *Casarett and Doull's Toxicology,* ed 2, New York, 1980, Macmillan.

105. Mussalo-Rauhamaa H et al: Occurrence of beta-hexachlorocyclohexane in breast cancer patients, *Cancer* 66:2124, 1990.

106. National Research Council: *Regulating pesticides in food: the Delaney paradox,* Washington, DC, 1987, National Academy Press.

107. National Safety Council: Accident Facts, Chicago, 1993, National Safety Council.

108. Nelson J: Effects of DDT analogs and polychlorinated biphenyls (PCB) mixtures on 3H-estradiol binding to rat uterine receptor, *Fed Proc Fed Am Soc Exp Biol* 32:326, 1973.

109. Newcombe D: Immune surveillance, organophosphorus exposure, and lymphomagenesis, *Lancet* 1:539, 1992.

110. Nigg H et al: Exposure to pesticides. In Mehlman M, editor: *Advances in modern environmental toxicology,* Vol 18, Princeton, 1990, Princeton Scientific Publishing.

111. Olorunsogo O, Bababunmi E: Inhibition of succinate-linking reduction of pyridine nucleotide in rat liver mitochondria in vivo by N-(phosphomethyl) glycine, *Toxicol Lett* 7:149, 1980.

112. O'Malley M, Mathias C, Coye M: Epidemiology of pesticide-related skin disease in California agriculture: 1978-1983. In Dosman J, Cockcroft D, editors: *Principles of health and safety in agriculture,* Boca Raton, 1989, CRC Press.

113. Papadopoulou-Mourkidou E: Postharvest-applied agrichemicals and their residues in fresh fruits and vegetables, *J Assoc Off Anal Chem* 74:745, 1991.

114. Parker V: Effect of nitrophenols and halogenophenols on the enzymatic activity of rat-liver mitochondria, *Biochem J* 69:306, 1958.

115. Pearce N, Reif J: Epidemiologic studies of cancer in agricultural workers, *Am J Ind Med* 18:133, 1990.

116. Pearce N et al: Non-Hodgkin's lymphoma and farming: an expanded case-control study, *Int J Cancer* 39:155, 1987.

117. Poland A, Glover E, Kende A: Stereospecific high affinity binding of 2,3,7,8-tetrachlorodibenzo-p-dioxin by hepatic cytosol. Evidence that the binding species is receptor for induction of arylhydrocarbon hydroxylase, *J Biol Chem* 251:4936, 1976.

118. Poland A, Knutson J: *Biologic mechanisms of dioxin action,* Banbury Report 18, Cold Spring Harbor, NY, 1984, Cold Spring Harbor Laboratory.

119. Porter S, Wiemeyer R: Dieldrin and DDT: effects on sparrow hawk eggshells and reproduction, *Science* 165:199, 1969.

120. Portier C et al: Ligand/receptor binding for 2,3,7,8-TCDD: implications for risk assessment, *Fund Appl Toxicol* 20:48, 1993.

121. Potchinsky M, Bloom S: Selective aflatoxin B1-induced sister chromatid exchanges and cytotoxicity in differentiating B and T lymphocytes in vivo, *Environ Molec Mutagen* 21:87, 1993.

122. Potter W et al: Phosphine-mediated Heinz body formation and hemoglobin oxidation in human erythrocytes, *Toxicol Lett* 57:37, 1991.

123. Potter W et al: Radiometric assay of red cell and plasma cholinesterase in pesticide appliers from Minnesota, *Toxicol Appl Pharmacol* 119:150, 1993.

124. Quimby G, Armstrong J, Durham W: DDT in human milk, *Nature* 207:726, 1965.

125. Rauch A et al: Lindane (Kwell)-induced aplastic anemia, *Arch Intern Med* 150:2393, 1990.

126. Ray D: Pesticides derived from plants and other organisms. In Hayes W, Laws E, editors: *Handbook of pesticide toxicology,* Vol 2, New York, 1991, Academic Press.

127. Reed DW: Chloropicrin. In Parmeggiani L, editor: *Encyclopedia of occupational health and safety,* vol 1, ed 3, Geneva, 1983, International Labor Office.

127a. Takahashi R, Rogerio R, Zanin M: Maneb enhances MPTP neurotoxicity in mice, *Res Commun Chem Pathol Pharmacol,* 66:167-170, 1989.

128. Reuber M: Carcinogenicity of Captan, *J Environ Pathol Toxicol Oncol* 9:127, 1989.

129. Reuzel P et al: Chronic inhalation toxicity and carcinogenicity of methyl bromide in Wistar rats, *Food Chem Toxicol* 29:31, 1991.

130. Reyes H, Reisz-Porszasz S, Hankinson O: Identification of the Ah receptor nuclear translocator protein (Arnt) as a component of the DNA binding form of the Ah receptor, *Science* 256:1193, 1992.

131. Rogers K, Davens B, Imamura T: Immunotoxic effects of anticholinesterases. In Ballantyne B, Marrs T, editors: *Clinical and experimental toxicology of organophosphates and carbamates,* Oxford, 1992, Butterworth & Heinemann.

132. Rosenstock L et al: Chronic central nervous system effects of acute organophosphate intoxication, *Lancet* 338:223, 1991.

133. Ruch R et al: Inhibition of hepatocyte gap junctional intercellular communication by endosulfan, chlordane and heptachlor, *Carcinogenesis* 11:1097, 1990.

134. Rugman F, Cosstick R: Aplastic anaemia associated with organochlorine pesticide: case reports and review of evidence, *J Clin Pathol* 43:98, 1990.

135. Savage E et al: Chronic neurologic sequelae of acute organophosphate pesticide poisoning, *Arch Environ Health* 43:38, 1988.

136. Schwartz D, Logerfo J: Congenital limb reduction defects in the agricultural setting, *Am J Pub Health* 12:51, 1988.

136a. Sharma V, Kaur S: Contact sensitization by pesticides in farmers, *Contact Dermatitis* 23:77-80, 1990.

137. Silver A: *The biology of cholinesterases,* Amsterdam, 1974, Elsevier-North Holland.

138. Smith A: Chlorinated hydrocarbon insecticides. In Hayes W, Laws E, editors: *Handbook of pesticide toxicology,* New York, 1991, Academic Press.

139. Smith A, Pearce N: Update on soft tissue sarcoma and phenoxyherbicides in New Zealand, *Chemosphere* 15:1795, 1986.

140. Snyder R: Effects of Captan on DNA and DNA metabolic processes in human diploid fibroblasts, *Environ Molec Mutagen* 20:127, 1992.

141. Soderpalm-Berndes C, Onfelt A: The action of carbaryl and its metabolite alpha-naphthol on mitosis in V79 Chinese hamster fibroblasts. Indications of the involvement of some cholinesterase in cell division, *Mutat Res* 201:349, 1988.

142. Somerville L: The metabolism of fungicides, *Xenobiotica* 16:1017, 1986.

143. Soreq H, Zakut H: Amplification of butyrlcholinesterase and acetylcholinesterase genes in normal and tumor tissues: putative relationship to organophosphorus poisoning, *Pharmaceut Res* 7:1, 1990.

144. Spigiel R et al: Organophosphate pesticide exposure in farmers and commercial applicators, *Clin Toxicol Consult* 3:45, 1981.

145. Stevens J, Sumner D: Herbicides. In Hayes W, Laws E, editors: *Handbook of pesticide toxicology,* New York, 1991, Academic Press.

146. Stournaras C et al: Interaction of Captan with mammalian microtubules, *Cell Biochem Function* 9:23, 1991.

147. Stubbs H, Harris J, Spear R: A proportionate mortality analysis of California agricultural workers, 1978-1979, *Am J Ind Med* 6:305, 1984.

148. Surralles J et al: Induction of mitotic micronuclei by the pyrethroid insecticide fenvalerate in cultured human lymphocytes, *Toxicol Lett* 54:151, 1990.

149. Takahashi N, Rogerio R, Zanin M: Maneb enhances MPTP neurotoxicity in mice, *Res Commun Chem Pathol Pharmacol* 66:167, 1989.

150. Talbot A et al: Acute poisoning with a glyphosate-surfactant herbicide ("Roundup"): a review of 93 cases, *Hum Exp Toxicol* 10:1, 1991.

151. Temple W, Smith N: Glyphosate herbicide poisoning experience in New Zealand, *N Z Med J* 105:173, 1992.

152. Tezuka H et al: Sister chromatid exchanges and chromosomal aberrations in cultured Chinese hamster cells treated with pesticides positive in microbial reversion assays, *Mutation Res* 78:177, 1980.

153. Thomas D, Lacy S, Morgan K: Studies on the mechanism of methyl bromide-induced olfactory toxicity, *Toxicologist* 9:37, 1989.

154. Thomas P et al: Immunologic effects of pesticides. In Baker SR, Wilkinson CF, editors: *The effects of pesticides on human health,* Princeton, 1990, Princeton Publishing Co.

155. Tominack R et al: Taiwan National Poison Center survey of glyphosate—surfactant herbicide ingestions, *J Toxicol Clin Toxicol* 29:91, 1991.

156. Trimborn H, Klimmer O: Experimental studies on chemical changes in blood pigments caused by hydrogen phosphide in vitro, *Arch Int Pharmacodyn* 137:331, 1962.

157. US Department of Commerce: *National data book and guide to sources,* Washington, DC, E. 108, 1988, Statistical Abstract of the United States.

158. US Environmental Protection Agency: *Summary of reported incidents involving chloropicrin,* Pesticide Incident Monitoring System Report No. 218, Washington, DC, 1979, US Environmental Protection Agency.

159. US Environmental Protection Agency, Office of Pesticide Programs: *Alachlor; position document 1,* Washington, DC, 1984, US Environmental Protection Agency.

160. US Environmental Protection Agency: *Methods for the determination of organic compounds in drinking water,* EPA Report No. EPA-600/4-88/039, Cincinnati, OH, 1988, Environmental Monitoring Systems Laboratory.

161. US Environmental Protection Agency: *List of pesticide products inert ingredients,* Washington, DC, 1992, Office of Pesticide Programs.

162. Vainio H et al: Hyperlipidemia and peroxisome proliferation induced by phenoxyacetic acid herbicides in rats, *Biochem Pharmacol* 32:2775, 1983.

163. Verrett M et al: Teratogenic effects of Captan and related compounds in the developing chick embryo, *Ann NY Acad Sci* 160:334, 1969.

164. Vigfusson N, Vyse E: The effect of the pesticides Dexon, Captan and Roundup on sister chromatid-exchanges in human lymphocytes in vitro, *Mutation Res* 79:53, 1980.

165. Vijverberg H, van den Bercken J: Neurotoxicological effects and the mode of action of pyrethroid insecticides, *Crit Rev Toxicol* 21:105, 1990.

166. Vondruska J, Fancher O, Calandra J: An investigation into the teratogenic potential of Captan, Folpet and Difolatan in non-human primates, *Toxicol Appl Pharmacol* 18:619, 1971.

167. Ware G: *The pesticide book,* Fresno, CA, 1989, Thomson Publications.

168. Waters M et al: *USEPA/IARC, Genetic profile database (Version 3.4),* [the database is available to the public: USEPA HERL (MD68); Research Triangle Park, NC], 1993.

169. Weisenberger D et al: *Birth defects and well water contamination by agricultural chemicals: an ecologic study,* Third International Symposium: Issues in Health, Safety and Agriculture, Saskatoon, Canada, 1992 (abstract 154).

170. Wigfield Y et al: Determination of *N*-nitrosodiethanolamine in dinoseb formulations by mass spectrometry and thermal energy analyzer detection, *J Assoc Off Anal Chem* 70:792, 1987.

171. Wiklund K et al: Risk of cancer in pesticide applicators in Swedish agriculture, *Br J Ind Med* 46:809, 1989.

172. Williams G, Numoto S: Promotion of mouse liver neoplasms by the organochlorine pesticides chlordane and heptachlor in comparison to dichlorodiphenyltrichloroethane, *Carcinogenesis* 5:1689, 1984.

173. Wilson B et al: Reactivation of organophosphorus inhibited AChE with oximes. In Chambers J, Levi P, editors: *Organophosphates: chemistry, fate and effects,* New York, 1992, Academic Press.

174. Wittliff J et al: Influence in vitro of chlorotriazines on estrogen receptors in human and rat reproductive tissues, *Toxicologist,* 12:443, 1993 (abstract).

175. Wolff M et al: Blood levels of organochlorine residues and risk of breast cancer, *J Natl Cancer Inst* 85:648, 1993.

176. Wood-McKenzie. *Agrochemical Service Edinburgh,* 1984.

177. Worthing C, Walker S, editors: *The pesticide manual: a world compendium,* ed 8, British Crop Protection Council, 1987, Thornton Heath.

178. Wright J: Lung disease in farm workers: pathologic reactions. In Dosman J, Cockcroft D, editors: *Principles of health and safety in agriculture,* Boca Raton, 1989, CRC Press.

179. Wysocki J, Kalina Z, Owczarzy I: Effect of organophosphoric pesticides on the behavior of NBT-dye reduction and E rosette formation tests in human blood. *Int Arch Occup Environ Health* 59:63, 1987.

180. Zaebst D et al: Phosphine exposures in grain elevators during fumigation with aluminum phosphide, *Appl Ind Hyg* 3:146, 1988.

181. Zahm S, Weisenberger D, Blair A: *Agriculture and multiple myeloma in men and women in Nebraska,* Third International Symposium: Issues in Health, Safety and Agriculture. Saskatoon, Canada, 1992, (Abstract 167).

182. Zeny, C: Hydrogen sulfide: case report. In Zeny C, editor: *Occupational medicine,* ed 2, Chicago, 1988, Year-Book Medical Publishers, pp 741-742.

ALIMENTARY AND NUTRITIONAL EXCESSES AND DEFICIENCIES

Imbalances in the consumption of mineral and nutritional elements have multifactorial bases, related to the complex interactions of cultural, economic, educational, and geographical influences. Widespread disease among various of the world's populations relates to these factors. The quality and characteristics of the food we consume reflect environmental influences and warrant consideration here. Classic treatises and countless texts address the common and long-recognized nutritional diseases; this information is not reconsidered here. A number of significant, contemporary nutritional public health issues, however, justify our critical evaluation, particularly in the context of evolving, new scientific insights. Elsewhere in this book, we have considered water quality as an important environmental determinant of health and disease (see Chapter 16). Some constituents of food that may serve as antioxidants are discussed in Chapter 21.

Information on minimal dietary requirements can be found in textbooks on nutrition, but dietary recommendations are ever changing. Caloric excess characterizes the diets of inhabitants of the countries of the Western world, where relatively large amounts of animal fat and simple refined carbohydrates are consumed. This diet is believed to predispose to hypertension and atherosclerosis and may trigger diabetes mellitus and certain forms of cancer. Indeed, excess body weight is a risk factor for premature death from a variety of causes. Many residents of the economically wealthy countries consume relatively small amounts of fiber and vegetable products in comparison to individuals in developing countries. These dietary characteristics serve as a focus for debate regarding their possible role in diverticulosis and colonic cancer. In the relatively affluent Eastern countries of Asia, dietary patterns and methods of food preservation and preparation appear to be factors influencing the development of certain forms of digestive tract cancer (esophagus and stomach) but seem to inhibit the occurrence of others. In certain countries of the developing world, geography, culture, and economics contribute to profound nutritional deficiencies, and diets of a substantial proportion of the populations in these regions are marginal, both nutritionally and with respect to overall energy content. The health effects of several of these nutritional problems of great public health importance are considered here.

Concepts in food toxicology

Bernard M. Wagner, Robert W. Leader

The role of food, in its broadest sense, as a factor in the evolution of acute and chronic disease has been proposed for centuries. Natural toxins; toxic additives; and adulteration owing to processing, handling, and storage all are implicated in the cause of human illness, as are a variety of microbial agents.

Even though the United States has a food supply that is as safe as any in the world, there is considerable unease on the part of the public. The Federal Food, Drug and Cosmetic Act gives the Food and Drug Administration (FDA) the authority to ensure the safety of whole foods. Under the law, those who develop and sell food have a duty to ensure the safety of the products they offer to consumers. The FDA has a broad mandate from Congress to enforce the food safety laws. Thus, the FDA can remove a food

from commerce if there is even a "reasonable possibility" that a substance added by human intervention might be unsafe for use. The FDA also has the authority to require formal premarket review and approval for food additives if there is a question of safety. Based on extensive human use and experience over the years, the safety of certain foods has been accepted. In general, foods derived from new plant varieties are not routinely subjected to scientific tests. The Congressional legislation on labeling of food (Nutrition and Education Food Label Act of 1992) requires all foods containing potential allergens to be clearly identified.

Food has been implicated as a factor in the evolution of many important chronic diseases. There is renewed interest in "natural" toxicants, believed to be produced by plants as a defense mechanism to ward off predators. Some of these naturally occurring constituents fit the criteria for potential human carcinogens. Ames[1] has said that by far the greatest source of carcinogens for humans is natural substances, many of which are foods (Table 9-1). According to Scheuplein,[11] "even a modestly effective attempt to lessen the dietary risk of natural carcinogens would probably be enormously more useful to human health than the regulatory efforts devoted to eliminating traces of pesticide residues or contaminants." The safety of the various pharmaceutical, hormonal, and chemical agents used worldwide to promote plant and animal growth and the chemicals added to food as well as the physical parameters involved in processing present complex problems for scientists and regulators. The importance of pesticide residues is considered in Chapter 8. The term "environmentally caused cancer" has been amplified and often exaggerated. As a result, there is a public perception that there are chemicals in the food chain capable of causing cancer and important chronic diseases.

Human health risk can best be defined as the probability that a given chemical exposure or series of exposures may damage the health of exposed individuals. Risk assessment is composed of four major components: hazard identification, dose-response assessment, human exposure assessment, and risk characterization. Many of these principles are generally accepted by the scientific community. Concepts, however, such as "thresholds" for carcinogens and the utility of negative epidemiological data are controversial. All human activities carry some degree of risk. Data have been collected on many known risks with a fairly high degree of accuracy, but risks associated with exposure to chemical substances in food cannot be readily assessed and quantified.

Considerable data have been gathered on the risks of some types of food exposures (including additives, flavors, colors), although such data are generally restricted to observations of acute episodes. In such situations, a single exposure results in an immediately detectable form of injury, leaving little doubt about causation. Risk assessment for food exposures that do not cause immediate clinical problems is far more complex. These types of exposures range

Table 9-1. Some natural pesticide carcinogens in food

Rodent carcinogen	Concentration (ppm)	Plant food
5-methoxypsoralen and 8-methoxypsoralen	14	Parsley
	32	Parsnip, cooked
	0.8	Celery
	6.2	Celery, new cultivar
	25	Celery, stressed
p-Hydrazinobenzoate	11	Mushrooms
Glutamyl p-hydrazinobenzoate	42	Mushrooms
Sinigrin (allyl isothiocyanate)	35-590	Cabbage
	250-788	Collard greens
	12-66	Cauliflower
	110-1560	Brussels sprouts
	16,000-72,000	Mustard (brown)
	4500	Horseradish
D-Limonene	31	Orange juice
	40	Mango
	8000	Pepper, black
Estragole	3800	Basil
	3000	Fennel
Safrole	3000	Nutmeg
	10,000	Mace
	100	Pepper, black
Ethyl acrylate	0.07	Pineapple
Sesamol	75	Sesame seeds (heated oil)
α-Methylbenzol alcohol	1.3	Cocoa
Benzyl acetate	82	Basil
	230	Jasmine tea
	15	Honey
Catechol	100	Coffee (roasted beans)
Caffeic acid	50-200	Apple, carrot, celery, cherry, eggplant, endive, grapes, lettuce, pear, plum, potato
	>1000	Absinthe, anise, basil, caraway, dill, marjoram, rosemary, sage, savory, tarragon, thyme
	1800	Coffee (roasted beans)
Chlorogenic acid (caffeic acid)	50-500	Apricot, cherry, peach, plum
	21,600	Coffee (roasted beans)
Neochlorogenic acid (caffeic acid)	50-500	Apple, apricot, broccoli, brussels sprouts, cabbage, cherry, kale, peach, pear, plum
	11,600	Coffee (roasted beans)

Modified from Ames BN, Profet M, Gold LS: Dietary pesticides (99.99% all natural), *Proc Natl Acad Sci USA* 87:7777, 1990; where a complete bibliography can be found.

from brief to extended and continuous. The safety of chemical substances in food or water has typically been defined by government as a condition of exposure under which there is a "practical certainty" that no harm will result to exposed humans.

The amount of a substance in food is the exposure concentration. The amount of the chemical received by the target organ, however, is the dose. This target organ dose may be different from the exposure amount. Ingested materials are absorbed, distributed through the body, metabolized, and excreted. These factors serve to determine the tissue dose. Animal toxicity studies are based primarily on the assumption that effects in humans can be inferred from effects in animals. This principle of generalizing animal data to humans is a basic tenet of toxicology and is accepted by the scientific and regulatory communities. The term "extrapolation" is frequently used to describe this process.

One of the most complex and important toxicity tests is the carcinogenesis bioassay. In general, the test substance is fed over most of the adult life of the animal (mouse, rat), and the animal is observed for tumors. Animals are fed the maximum tolerated dose (MTD) daily. The MTD is the maximum dose that an animal can tolerate for a major portion of its lifetime without significant impairment of growth or observable toxic effects other than carcinogenicity. The use of the MTD continues to be a matter of considerable debate. This is especially true for chemical constituents in foods.

Risk management is a complex business as are the controversies it generates. Much of risk management involves going beyond the available data, either to guess at what the facts might be or to figure how to live with uncertainty. The interpretation of risk and its management are largely political processes in the United States, resulting in sociopolitical and financial decisions. Safety assessment, however, is a largely scientific process, for the regulatory agencies concerned with food safety (U.S. Department of Agriculture and FDA) mandate animal toxicity studies. The demonstration of tissue injury owing to the ingested food must be interpreted and evaluated in terms of potential human risk. One of the more difficult decisions is to determine if cellular changes represent physiological adaptation or true injury. Knowledge of absorption, tissue distribution, metabolism, and excretion of chemicals in food is a prerequisite for determining the biological activity of a food substance.

MICROBIAL CONSIDERATIONS

Bacterial and viral contamination of natural and processed food is by far the most common cause of illness in the world today. This is often regarded as a problem of developing countries, particularly in areas subject to unusual climatic conditions and poor sanitation. Microbial contamination in the United States and other developed countries is considered to be less significant. Microbial contamination of foods even in such advanced countries as the United

States, however, is a problem of great importance.[14] In 1990, the annual rate of *Salmonella* infection in the United States was estimated to be between 7.9×10^5 to 3.7×10^6.[14] Overall, food-borne infectious disease was estimated at between 6.8×10^6 and 81×10^6 cases per annum, and the cost was calculated to be $8.4 billion. During 1993, this problem was highlighted by two disease outbreaks. One was from hamburger contaminated with *Escherichia coli* 0157:H7, which caused several deaths and more than 500 illnesses in the state of Washington. There was also a large outbreak of waterborne infection from *Cryptosporidium* in Milwaukee. Many illnesses and a considerable number of deaths occur each year from certain dairy products contaminated with *Listeria monocytogenes*. Severe enteritis from *Campylobacter* is a common sporadic disease but does not occur in large outbreaks. There has been a substantial increase in the number of cases of *Salmonella enteritidis* from contamination of eggs. From 1985 through 1990, a total of 46 outbreaks representing 10,253 cases of *S. enteritidis* were reported to the Centers for Disease Control. Thus, food-borne infections, although they have not been regarded with as much anxiety as chemical contaminations by the public, are problems of considerable dimension.

FOOD ALLERGY AND INTOLERANCE
(see Chapter 25)

According to current concepts, food allergy and hypersensitivity are synonymous when applied to a group of diseases characterized by an abnormal or exaggerated immunological response to specific food constituents, resulting in disease. Sampson and Metcalfe have reviewed this subject in detail.[10] The gastrointestinal tract is extremely efficient in preventing intact foreign antigens from entering the body, while processing ingested food. It is estimated that more than 98% of ingested antigen is blocked from entry. The 1% to 2% of intact food antigens that are absorbed, however, gain access to the entire body. In normal individuals, circulating, intact protein with immunogenic properties causes no adverse effects. Most humans develop tolerance to ingested food antigens, although the mechanisms of tolerance are incompletely understood.

Studies in mice provide interesting observations.[3] A single antigen fed to a 4-day-old mouse leads to suppression of antigen-specific systemic immunoglobulin M (IgM), immunoglobulin G (IgG), and immunoglobulin E (IgE) antibody responses and cell-mediated immune responses. Food antigens are processed by the digestive tract to a "tolerogenic" form, which is essential for the development of oral tolerance. The lymphoid population in the digestive tract appears to be required for the evolution of tolerogenic proteins. Whole-body irradiation of mice blocks this ability and infusion of normal spleen cells in irradiated mice restores it. The antigen-presenting cells of the immune system play a significant role in the development of oral tolerance.

A variety of agents that activate the immune system and stimulate antigen-presenting cell activity inhibit the generation of CD8+ lymphocytes and the development of oral tolerance. It is important to realize that low concentrations of detectable serum IgG, IgM, and immunoglobulin A (IgA) food-specific antibodies are measured in normal individuals. Patients with inflammatory digestive tract disease, however, frequently have high serum concentrations of food-specific IgG and IgM antibodies. These antibodies are responsive to individual dietary constituents and are not specific for foods that the patient cannot tolerate. A variety of in vitro T-cell responses have been reported using lymphocytes from patients with food allergy and gastrointestinal tract disease. These same responses can be elicited in normal individuals. The significance of these T-cell responses remains obscure and may only reflect a response to increased antigen penetration of the digestive tract mucosa.

Food-specific IgE antibodies can bind to high-affinity receptors on mast cells and basophils or to low-affinity receptors on macrophages, monocytes, lymphocytes, eosinophils, and platelets. The binding of the food allergen to IgE antibodies on mast cells and basophils causes the release of mediators, inducing symptoms of immediate hypersensitivity. A late-phase response also occurs and is characterized by the infiltration of eosinophils, lymphocytes, and monocytes. Again, these cells release a variety of inflammatory mediators and cytokines. Repeated exposure of the digestive tract to a food allergen causes mononuclear cells to secrete "histamine-releasing factors." In turn, these factors facilitate the release of mediators by mast cells and basophils. Clinical hyperactivity of target organs results.

What do we know about food antigens? Such antigens are usually composed of glycoproteins with molecular weights between 1×10^4 and 4×10^4. These allergens are frequently resistant to proteolysis and heat. One of the best characterized food allergens is an albumin of codfish termed Allergen M (Gad C 1).[5] This protein has been sequenced and two major epitopes defined; a three-dimensional structure is available. Foods that are closely related may contain antigens that cross-react clinically. Reports indicate that cross-reactive allergens can exist between certain foods and pollens, for example, melons and bananas with ragweed pollen; celery with mugwort pollen; and apple, carrot, and hazelnut with birch pollen. From the aforementioned, it is clear that the diverse clinical manifestations of food hypersensitivity are IgE-mediated reactions and relate to the site and extent of mast cell degranulation.

Food allergy is estimated to occur in 8% of children under 6 years of age. About 2% to 4% of these children have reproducible allergic reactions to foods. The data for adults are incomplete but suggest that 1% to 2% of the general adult population are sensitive to foods or food additives. Clinically an immediate reaction to food may be limited to the digestive tract with cramping, distention, vomiting, and diarrhea. As the antigen circulates in the body, target sites may be skin (hives, angioedema), lungs (asthma), eyes (conjunctivitis), and nose (rhinorrhea). Crucial to the clinical state is the intensity and duration of mast cell degranulation, which can result in systemic anaphylaxis. This is an acute and occasionally fatal reaction. Lethal food allergy is most often associated with the ingestion of peanuts, nuts, fish, and shellfish. Food-induced anaphylaxis can be an explosive situation, with cardiorespiratory arrest and shock occurring shortly after the onset of symptoms. The Food Label Act of 1992 enables individuals with food hypersensitivity to avoid foods associated with allergic illness.

An entity that may be more common than previously estimated is allergic eosinophilic gastroenteritis (Fig. 9-1). The ease of endoscopy and biopsy allows for confirmatory diagnosis. Biopsy reveals a marked eosinophilic infiltration of the stomach or small bowel mucosa that can extend into the muscularis and the serosa. These patients also have peripheral eosinophilia, elevated levels of IgE, and multiple food allergies.[8,9,13]

Foods most often responsible for eliciting responses in children with atopic dermatitis include eggs, milk, soy, fish, and wheat. One study showed that more than 60% of children with clinical respiratory illness and wheezing induced by food challenge had atopic dermatitis or a history of eczema. Numerous standard medical textbooks provide more details.

A key question is whether current safety assessment studies in animals can predict the presence of potential human food allergens. Immunotoxicology has undergone considerable growth since its inception in the early 1970s. It is a scientific discipline that explores the effects of physical, biological, and chemical agents on the immune system, an extremely sophisticated and self-regulated system. There is significant reciprocal interaction between the nervous, endocrine, and immune systems, complicating attempts to study responses in animals and in vitro. Intact animals are essential for accurate investigations of the immunotoxic potential of xenobiotics. At present, the ability to identify a potential food allergen is extremely limited. As a result, clinical profiles of individuals at risk and epidemiological data are used to identify children and adults in the population most likely to develop severe allergic reactions to food. Once these individuals are identified, physicians practice risk management.

FOOD ADDITIVES

Flavor modifiers are among the most ancient of food additives, especially salt and natural sugars. Spices as food additives are recorded in the Old Testament. Many of these substances were used to preserve foods or mask the process of spoilage, e.g., sugar, salt, and nitrates. Obviously, most of the additives that have been used in foods for centuries with no known adverse effects are safe for human consumption. Food additives, however, can generally be classified as follows: flavor materials (enhancers, modifiers), sweeteners (natural, artificial), colors (natural, synthetic), preservatives, stabilizers, and nutritional supplements.

In 1958, the Federal Food, Drug and Cosmetic Act was passed by the U.S. Congress to assure the American public that the food supply was safe. This legislation mandated safety assessment procedures for foods and further strengthened the role of the FDA as regulator and enforcer. Importantly the 1958 Act exempts any substance "generally recognized, among experts qualified by scientific training and experience to evaluate its safety, as having been adequately shown through scientific procedures (or, in the case of a substance used in food prior to January 1, 1958, through either scientific procedures or experience based on common use in food) to be safe under the conditions of intended use." Thus, the concept of *generally recognized as safe* (GRAS) was established. Special attention is directed to the phrase "under conditions of intended use." The "scientific procedures" in the original regulations included "not only animal, analytical and other scientific studies, but also an unprejudiced compilation of reliable information, both favorable and unfavorable, drawn from the scientific litera-

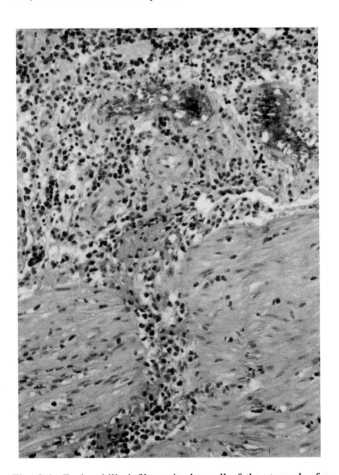

Fig. 9-1. Eosinophilic infiltrate in the wall of the stomach of a 59-year-old woman with eosinophilic gastroenteritis. The basis for sensitization is not known. (Courtesy of Caroline Compton, M.D.)

ture." In 1974, this phrase was expanded to include published or unpublished scientific studies appropriate to establish the safety of a food substance.

After its enactment in 1958, the Flavor and Extract Manufacturers Association (FEMA), with the advice and consent of the FDA, established an expert panel of scientists charged with determining the GRAS status for flavor materials and has done so since 1960. A food flavor material affirmed as GRAS by the panel is communicated to the FDA and published in the scientific literature. The criteria used by the panel for the determination of GRAS for a flavor ingredient are (1) exposure to the substance in specific foods, the total amount in the diet and the total poundage; (2) natural occurrence in food; (3) chemical identity (including purity and method of preparation) and specific chemical structure; (4) metabolic and pharmacokinetic characteristics; and (5) animal toxicity. The criteria used by the panel must be mutually supportive. The panel decision is a subjective scientific judgment based on a consideration of all relevant factors, and a designation of GRAS for each individual flavor ingredient requires a unanimous decision by the panel. The concept of GRAS for a food additive and the use of an expert panel are unique to the FDA and the United States. Only now is the European Community considering this arrangement to harmonize with the FDA approach to food safety assessment. Unless there is general agreement between nations or trading blocks as to safety assessment guidelines for food additives, there can be serious economic impacts. Of course, such decisions and recommendations can and often are overruled by political bodies.

A CONTEMPORARY ISSUE: THE DELANEY CLAUSE

The Delaney Clause of the Food, Drug and Cosmetic Act serves as a legal basis for the federal regulation of carcinogens in foods and carcinogenic color additives in cosmetics. Congressman Delaney convinced the House Commerce Committee to insert anticancer clauses into the Food Additives Amendment of 1958. These clauses represent a national commitment to minimize exposure to cancer-causing agents, regardless of the "benefits the ingredients might provide." The Delaney Clause as it pertains to food additives states

no additive shall be deemed to be safe if it is found to induce cancer when ingested by man or animal, or if it is found after tests which are appropriate for the evaluation of the safety of food additives, to induce cancer in man or animal (our emphasis)

The FDA and the Environmental Protection Agency (EPA) are the regulatory agencies charged with implement-

ing the Delaney Clause. The FDA has exclusive responsibility to implement and enforce regulations concerning nonpesticide food additives, whereas the EPA establishes regulations concerning pesticide residues in food.

Since 1958, the number of real and potential human carcinogens has increased explosively. Analytical chemists can now detect a whole new universe of substances in food at exceedingly low concentrations. Detection limits have been pushed from parts per thousand to parts per trillion. Thus, we have increased by 1×10^6 our ability to detect "chemicals" in food. Many scientists believe that almost any chemical can cause cancer in laboratory animals, if given in sufficiently high doses, by the mechanism of cytotoxicity-induced neoplasia. When the MTD is administered daily to rodents over a lifetime, about half of the chemicals tested induce cancer.

The absolute banning of every "carcinogen" that is recognized by these tests defies common sense. It has been suggested that zero-tolerance may actually be counterproductive to the policy of the FDA. Banning weak rodent carcinogens that are beneficial to the U.S. food supply could change the American diet, resulting in increased human cancer rates. To escape this paradox, the FDA asserts that, even when a substance does cause cancer in animals, the agency may find it is not a carcinogen in humans or animals within the legal meaning of the Delaney Clause.

Controversy continues regarding what is an appropriate test for determining whether a compound is "found" to induce cancer. For food additives, the test system must be appropriate to ingestion in humans. The antioxidant butylated hydroxyanisole (BHA) produces a significant increase in squamous cell tumors of the rat forestomach. Because humans do not have a forestomach, however, the FDA conceded that the ingestion study was irrelevant and inappropriate for humans. The FDA did not ban BHA from the American diet.

Probably the most famous recent case has been the safety of the artificial sweetener saccharin. Today, on every packet of sweetener containing saccharin is the warning: "Use of this product may be hazardous to your health. This product contains saccharin which has been determined to cause cancer in laboratory animals." Saccharin is an organic synthetic chemical that is very sweet to the taste. It is not metabolized following ingestion and is almost totally excreted intact. At MTD doses, however, saccharin induces tumors of the urinary bladder in male rats at statistically significant levels after 2 years of dosing.

Repeated epidemiological studies failed to demonstrate that saccharin was an independent risk factor for human cancer. Given the rat data, quantitative risk assessments were made using a variety of statistical assumptions. Predictions of increased cancer incidence in the population were made. There is no evidence that this is actually happening. At worst, saccharin is a weak carcinogen because, in rats developing tumors, dose levels of saccharin per kilogram of body weight used were up to 250 to 500 times greater than the maximum daily human consumption. Thus, under the conditions of intended use and 80 years of human consumption experience, saccharin is safe for human use. Unfortunately the Delaney Clause required the FDA to restrict public access to saccharin.

Congress was unwilling to face the issue of modifying the Delaney Clause, and the United States was moving, similar to Canada, to ban saccharin use. The public and the majority of scientists in the United States, however, refused to believe that saccharin was carcinogenic for humans. A compromise eventually was reached between Congress and the FDA, and Congress voted a waiver of the law to give the FDA time to conduct additional research. The research was performed at great expense to industry, and the mechanism of induced bladder cancer in male rats was determined. At high dosages in male rats, saccharin induces epithelial cell damage owing to precipitation of calcium salts intracellularly. Persistent injury causes hyperplasia, papilloma, and carcinoma.

The saccharin waiver has been renewed by Congress several times, and the FDA imposed a warning label on saccharin sweeteners. This impasse between Congress, the FDA, and the public is not due to lack of scientific data. A persistent demand by a variety of public groups and pseudoscientists that the Delaney Clause not be altered has intimidated elected officials. The cry is, "The Delaney Clause protects the public against cancer-causing agents." The result, unfortunately, is the public's loss of respect for the scientific establishment. Sweeteners containing saccharin carry a warning label in the United States today, whereas in Canada the ban persists.

FUTURE DIRECTION OF FOOD SAFETY RESEARCH

As long as food is internationally marketed and contact with other parts of the world increases, there will continue to be public concern about health risks related to consumption of the constantly changing foods available in the market. The importance of food safety research is underscored by a report issued by the Food Safety Research Work Group[7] that presents future directions and needs for federal food safety research. Although the report focuses on research associated primarily with domestically produced or imported foods consumed by Americans, the group acknowledged that it is increasingly difficult to separate food safety problems associated with the U.S. food supply from those occurring globally. International harmonization of food safety regulations is an important goal. What are the important questions to be asked in research programs? Where will these lead in the future? One ever-present force in decision making on the part of the public as well as regulatory authorities is the flow of stories in the news media. An excellent example of this is the incident involving Alar, a maturing factor used in ripening apples, as a potential hu-

man carcinogen. Alar is a substance that has been used for many years in the processing of apples. It is present in extremely small amounts and was never seriously considered a hazard to the health of the public until an enormous outcry occurred. Even so, its use had been scheduled to be discontinued by EPA.

We are looking at one small segment of the total panoply of toxic materials when we discuss issues in food safety. As long as public and regulatory agencies continue to be interested in food safety, there will be a need to develop more integrated programs in research and public education. The responsibility lies heavily on the government, especially the FDA and U.S. Department of Agriculture (USDA), but also on private industry and, to a significant degree, on universities. The U.S. Agriculture Department Experiment Station Committee on Organization and Policy has published a research agenda for the 1990s[6] that gives high priority to food safety.

First, one should look at the list of hazards in a roughly prioritized sequence. The federal Food Safety Research Group[7] defined "food safety research" and lists priorities as follows:

Food safety research is that work incorporating primary hypothesis testing in a systematic manner to provide information for enhancing scientific knowledge and understanding of issues involving food (including drinking water) and human health. Information obtained through the performance of food safety research is both basic and applied. Food safety research can encompass the following subject areas, to the extent that they address the safety of food:

- *Microbial hazards/parasites/disease agents*
- *Drug residues*
- *Pesticide residues*
- *Naturally occurring toxicants*
- *Environmental contaminants/industrial chemicals*
- *Heavy metals*
- *Radionuclides*
- *Decomposition and filth*
- *Biotechnologically produced/altered food*
- *Food processing and storage*
- *Food additives*
- *Food packaging and packaging materials*
- *Diet and nutrition*
- *Food production issues (preharvest to harvest)*

It is fascinating to observe that this list of priorities prepared by government experts is in sharp contrast to that of the public, who would consider pesticides and food additives to be their top priorities. It is, however, close to a similar list of priorities prepared from a survey of scientists working in food safety.

Cliver[4] summarizes priorities as follows:

1. Determine the true incidence, causes, and financial and personal impact of food-borne diseases in the United States and study how to communicate this information accurately and effectively to the public.
2. Develop more effective methods of testing foods, both for routine monitoring and in after-the-fact investigation of outbreaks.
3. Devise better methods—all the way from the food source (farm or sea) to the ultimate consumer—of controlling microbiological risks associated with foods.
4. Develop better means of hazard assessment, including degree of exposure, pathogenicity/toxicity for humans, and differential risks among special population groups—infants; the elderly; and those who are allergic, enzyme deficient, or immunoimpaired.

There should be a strong orientation toward risk evaluation and analytical methodology, which are the bases on which future decisions should be made. There must be a strong, vital program to look at the impact of newly developing production and processing methods on the ultimate safety of food. Some of these methods decrease hazards, but some may increase them. Some of the hazards that may be introduced are chemical contaminants such as pesticides and animal drugs, packaging components, microbial contaminants, and other unpredictable substances.

Outbreaks have illustrated that introduction of pathogens during the production and processing of food can be a significant factor. A controversial approach to decreasing these hazards is the irradiation of foods to eliminate pathogenic organisms.[12] The method is usually exposure to an isotope of cobalt or devices that produce x-rays. The process does not make the food radioactive and is considered by most scientists to be a valid, effective method of helping to control certain kinds of contamination. This is especially applicable to meat, poultry, shellfish, and some vegetables, although other substances, such as spices and fresh fruits, also may be effectively sterilized in this way.

Nearly 40 countries process many tons of potatoes by irradiation to prevent sprouting, and a variety of irradiated foods have been approved in the Netherlands. Food processing plants in that country have been irradiating about 20,000 tons of food per year. The United States has one large radiation facility dedicated to food protection. Food irradiation is regulated by the FDA under the terms on the 1958 Food Additive Amendment to the Food, Drug and Cosmetic Act. In the United States, radiation has been approved for (1) maturation delay of fresh foods, (2) insect disinfestation of food, (3) control of pathogens in poultry and *Trichinella spiralis* in pork, (4) control of microorganisms in dry enzymes, and (5) disinfestation of spices or other seasonings. The Food and Safety Inspection Service of the USDA has approved irradiation to control or reduce some food-borne pathogens, such as those in the genera *Salmonella, Campylobacter,* and *Listeria.* Seafood now is being considered for irradiation.

There are many factors that bear on whether irradiation will be widely used. Many environmentally active groups opposing the use of irradiation contend that it may be damaging or have unknown effects on the foods. Certain citizen groups also are taking active roles in opposing irradiation of foods, contending that there may be serious side effects. They believe that the USDA and FDA have not properly considered studies that reach these conclusions. It is clear that consumer attitudes will have a significant impact on the extent of utilization.

Many scientists contend that the antiirradiation tactics of the opposing groups constitute harassment and intimidation against the use of food irradiation. We all know, however, that the word "irradiation" is an expression that can cause fear. Not long ago, the name of "nuclear" magnetic resonance had to be changed to magnetic resonance imaging before the public accepted the technology.

Association of food and water constituents with hypertension

Harriet P. Dustan

Hypertension results from a malfunction of one or more of the many systems that control arterial pressure. There are a few types of hypertension for which the cause is known, and, to a large extent, these reflect abnormalities of the adrenal gland or of the kidney—either its parenchyma or its arteries. Most hypertension is of unknown cause and is called essential, although the elevated pressure is not essential to anything we now recognize. Currently, essential hypertension is considered to have multiple causes because normal pressure is so multifactorial in its control; the autonomic nervous system, salt active steroids, the renin angiotensin system, and sodium balance appear to be the most important of these influences.

Considering this multifaceted control, it is not surprising that many environmental factors have been implicated in the pathogenesis of hypertension (see box below). Thus, excesses—of energy, sodium chloride, alcohol, and lead—have been well established through epidemiological and

---

**Environmental factors implicated
in hypertension pathogenesis**

Excesses of	Deficiencies of
Calories → Obesity	Potassium
Sodium chloride	Calcium
Alcohol	Magnesium
Lead	Polyunsaturated fat

clinical research, whereas the deficiencies—of potassium, calcium, magnesium, and unsaturated fats—are supported by some evidence, but up to this time, attempts to implicate them have yielded variable results.

OBESITY

The maintenance of obesity is a complex clinical problem that involves much more than caloric intakes in excess of energy needs. Obesity is a major risk factor for hypertension and has an adverse effect on blood lipids, thereby adding to cardiovascular risk.[19] The data relating obesity to hypertension are not controversial; they have been gathered for longer than 50 years from millions of people worldwide. The information can be summarized to show that, in populations with age-related increases in body weight, there is an age-related increase in arterial pressure. In contrast, primitive societies show a decrease in body weight with age as well as a decrease in blood pressure.[16] There is, however, not a parallel relationship between weight gain and an increase in arterial pressure as people grow older. In a study of more than 35,000 white men and women, arterial pressure rose with advancing age, and, for the most part, the greater the body weight, the higher the blood pressure. Regression analyses, however, showed that blood pressure rose with age even among nonobese individuals, although obesity appeared to have an additive effect.[39]

There is no understanding of the mechanisms of obesity-related hypertension. The increase in body mass has cardiovascular and metabolic consequences that have the potential for being causally associated with hypertension. None occurs exclusively in hypertensive obese subjects, however, as opposed to those with normal blood pressure. Various mechanisms have been proposed.[18,21] They include (1) increased blood volume and systemic blood flow with failure of peripheral vasodilatory responses; (2) hyperinsulinemia, which causes sodium retention and increased activity of the sympathetic nervous system; (3) impairment of cell membrane pumps that regulate intracellular cation concentrations; and (4) insulin as a growth factor affecting vascular smooth muscle and cardiac myocyte growth.

SODIUM CHLORIDE

The possibility that hypertension could be related to salt intake was first suggested in the early part of the 20th century and has been the focus of much attention since (reviewed in Dustan and Kirk[23]) (Fig. 9-2). That possibility dates back even further in history if one considers the statement, "hence, if too much salt is used in food, the pulse hardens," from the Yellow Emperor's Classic on Internal Medicine, written more than 2000 years ago. The first recorded observation of the possible relationship of salt intake to high blood pressure, however, was published in 1904 by Ambard and Beaujard, who were studying chloride excretion in a variety of cardiovascular conditions.[15a] Chloride excretion was used as a measure of salt intake be-

cause, at the time, there was no method available to measure sodium. Their opening statement in a paper entitled, "Causes of Arterial Hypertension" is

among the phenomena closely related with hypertension, one of those which we have found the most constant and the most remarkable is the retention of chloride; and this to such an extent that it enables us to say that every individual capable of developing chloride retention is, because of that very fact, apt to have arterial hypertension.

In the 1920s, Allen used low-sodium diets to treat hypertension and reported his conclusion that "a general abstinence from salt" would reduce the morbidity and mortality from diseases of the blood vessels. He stated, however, that "diet does not under any ordinary conditions cause disease in an otherwise healthy renal-vascular system." The modern era of interest in the relationship of salt intake to hypertension began in the 1940s, when Kempner used a severely restricted salt and protein diet (the rice fruit diet) for the treatment of hypertension with some startlingly good results in patients otherwise destined to die. Because it was the only nonsurgical treatment available at the time, there was much interest and many studies were undertaken. Although mechanisms were not defined, about 50% of hypertensive patients responded with a reduction of blood pressure, often to normal. It is important to state that the cul-

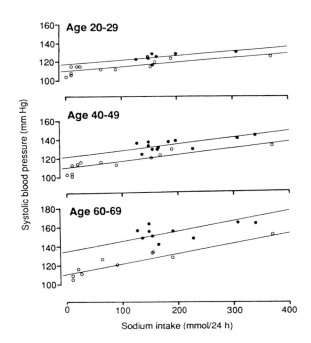

Fig. 9-2. Systolic blood pressure according to sodium intake for three age groups from developed (—) and undeveloped (○) communities. (From Law MR, Frost CD, Wald NJ: By how much does dietary salt reduction lower blood pressure: analysis of data from trials of salt reduction, *BMJ* 302:819, 1991.)

prit is sodium chloride (not any sodium salt) because the pressor effects of added sodium chloride are not duplicated by other sodium salts.

In 1954, Dahl and Love reported that the prevalence of hypertension among Alaskan Eskimos, Marshall Islanders, Americans, Southern Japanese, and Northern Japanese was directly related to the average daily salt intake. Although the paper contained little documentation, it sparked much interest. Subsequent epidemiological surveys found that, in isolated cultures with a low sodium intake, hypertension was rare or nonexistent. Further, in contrast to industrialized populations, blood pressure in these primitive cultures did not increase with age. Thus, a high dietary salt intake would appear to be a major factor in the pathogenesis of hypertension. This conclusion became a conviction despite the fact that primitive societies are different from industrialized ones in ways that could well affect the prevalence of hypertension: Their members tend not to be obese, they have a high potassium intake, they are physically active, and they are genetically homogeneous.

The chief stumbling block to the wide acceptance of dietary salt intake as a cause of hypertension in industrialized societies was the observation that data from individual populations failed, for the most part, to support that hypothesis. For example, a large epidemiological study in Wales found no relationship between arterial pressure and salt intake;[38] in the Framingham study, neither salt intake nor urinary sodium excretion correlated with blood pressure,[17] and a relationship between urinary sodium and arterial pressure was not found among blacks.[24]

There the matter lay until the late 1980s and early 1990s, when two reports strengthened the evidence relating dietary salt intake to hypertension. One was a large epidemiological study involving 10,079 subjects worldwide, and the other was a meta-analysis of epidemiological studies on approximately 47,000 individuals that reported blood pressure and salt intake relationships. The first investigation was the Intersalt study published in 1988.[26] It was an international, five-continent, cross-sectional, epidemiological study exploring the relationship of arterial pressure with sodium and potassium intake as judged by urinary excretion. Sodium intake was found to vary widely from 0.2 mmol/24 hr for the Yanomamo Indians of Brazil to 242 mmol/24 hr in Northern China. Two types of analyses were carried out, one "within populations" and the other "cross-populations." In both analyses, body mass index and alcohol consumption were positively related to arterial pressure. A significant and positive relationship between 24-hour urinary sodium excretion and systolic pressure and the urinary sodium to potassium ratio and systolic pressure was found in the within-population analyses. Diastolic pressure was not significantly related. The relationship between urinary sodium excretion and blood pressure was stronger for older than for younger adults. In cross-population analy-

ses, it was found that sodium excretion correlated with the age-related rises of both systolic and diastolic pressure.

In 1991, Law and colleagues[32] published a meta-analysis of studies involving 47,000 individuals in an effort "to obtain a coherent quantitative estimate of the effect of sodium intake on blood pressure." Data came from 24 communities separated into two equal groups by economic development criteria. The data also were analyzed by decades. It was found that the differences in mean systolic and diastolic blood pressures for 100 mmol difference in sodium intake rose with advancing age from $5 \pm 1.3/1.8 \pm 0.5$ at 15 to 19 years of age to $10.3 \pm 2.9/4.3 \pm 1.6$ at 60 to 69 years. Blood pressure was higher in developed communities than in the undeveloped, but in both groups, there was an association with sodium intake. The authors calculated the effects of reducing sodium intake by 100 mmol/day and showed that higher blood pressures fell more than lower blood pressures. In another report, the data from trials of dietary salt restriction were analyzed.[33] It was concluded that a 50-mmol reduction in salt intake per day reduces stroke incidence by 26% and ischemic heart disease by 15%.

These epidemiological reports leave the impression that everyone's blood pressure, whether normal or elevated, would be reduced by a substantially decreased dietary salt intake. Clinical investigations, however, have shown that only about 50% of people have "salt-sensitive" blood pressure.[44] This characteristic is not restricted to hypertensives, although it is more frequent in hypertensives than normotensives; it is common among blacks and appears to become more frequent with age.

The mechanism of salt sensitivity is not known. The belief is widely held that it begins with an inability to excrete sodium normally,[44] but this is not a universal characteristic of salt-sensitive hypertension.[22] Because sodium homeostasis is so vital to health, many mechanisms maintain it, and, in turn, sodium balance affects a number of systems that regulate arterial pressure: the autonomic nervous system, the renin-angiotensin system, and aldosterone. In fact, when multidimensional response modeling was used to analyze the interaction of many variables, the rise in blood pressure associated with salt loading was found to result from an interaction of variables and not from any one alone.[23]

ALCOHOL (see Chapter 14)

Although the relationship of excessive alcohol intake to hypertension was first reported in the early years of the 20th century, excessive drinking as a major factor did not become apparent until much later. Epidemiological studies now have shown that heavy alcohol intake (i.e., >6 oz/day) is associated with increased prevalence of hypertension. In fact, even a lesser amount (about 40 g of ethanol/per day) is positively associated with blood pressure. These data have been greatly strengthened by short-term trials in which alcohol consumption either was reduced or eliminated in hypertensive men who were moderate to heavy drinkers.[35,36] Without exception, these trials showed significant decreases in blood pressure. Recent alcohol intake proved to have a greater effect on blood pressure than previous alcohol consumption.[36] These findings firmly establish alcohol intake of more than 3 oz/day as a risk factor for hypertension. It has been suggested that excess alcohol consumption is the cause for 11% of essential hypertension. Mechanisms for alcohol-mediated hypertension are not known. The following possibilities have been suggested: (1) increased activity of the sympathetic nervous system, (2) sensitization of the vessel wall to circulating pressor substances, (3) increased renin release, and (4) increased cortisol production.[29]

LEAD (see Chapter 4)

Lead concentrations in many public water systems in the United States are considered unsafe by the EPA. This possibility renews concerns regarding the relationship of blood lead to hypertension. The most recent information relating lead intake to hypertension is found in the Second National Health and Nutrition Examination Survey (NHANES II). It examined a large number of the civilian, noninstitutionalized U.S. population aged 0.5 to 74 years in a pattern that allowed the results to be representative of the entire population.[25] In the analysis of the relationship of lead to blood pressure, adults were separated into three groups, depending on whether diastolic pressure was less than 90 mmHg (normotensive), 90 mmHg or more (hypertensive), and (if diastolic pressure was normal) systolic pressure 160 mmHg or more (isolated systolic hypertensive). Participants with elevated diastolic pressures had higher blood lead concentrations than normotensive or systolic hypertensive groups ($P \leq 0.05$). In addition, a positive linear relationship between blood pressure and the natural logarithm of blood lead was found for each race-gender group. These regression coefficients ranged from 0.11 to 0.22 ($P < 0.001$).

Place of residence related directly to the blood lead concentrations in both men and women, an indication that lead from automobile exhaust was a major source of human lead exposure. Dietary calcium as estimated by a 24-hour dietary recall proved to be inversely related to blood lead concentration. This analysis of data from NHANES II suggests that current lead exposure could be one of the factors responsible for the prevalence of hypertension in the United States. Because leaded gasoline is the major source of lead exposure and because this source is diminishing owing to the use of unleaded gas, future analyses should show a decline in the association.

Although this analysis of NHANES II data supports a role for lead exposure as a risk factor for hypertension in the United States, the same cannot be said for other countries. One report described results of a large-scale Belgian study in which blood pressure, blood lead, urinary lead excretion, and serum calcium were measured in 827 men and 821 women.[20] Analysis of the data showed that blood pressure was strongly dependent on age; the values positively correlated with heart rate, serum calcium concentration, and alcohol intake. In men, systolic pressure was negatively related to blood lead ($P < 0.05$) but not diastolic pressure. In women, neither systolic nor diastolic pressure correlated with blood lead. Additional data analysis included calculation of the interaction of blood lead and serum calcium with blood pressure. No correlations were found in men, but in women there was a significant interaction of blood lead with serum calcium concentration and a positive correlation with systolic pressure.

POTASSIUM

Potassium is another commonly occurring ion implicated in the pathogenesis of hypertension. In this case, however, potassium deficiency, rather than an excess, is the problem. Linas[34] has provided an excellent review concerning the role of potassium in hypertension (Table 9-2).

In 1928, Addison was the first to suggest that the prevalence of hypertension in North America is "in large part due to a Potash poor diet," along with extra use of salt for flavoring and for the preservation of meat. Modern considerations of this relationship began with studies in the southern United States. Blacks, who have a higher prevalence of hypertension than whites, were found to have lower potassium intakes than whites. These epidemiological studies

Table 9-2. Predicted change in systolic and diastolic blood pressure (mmHg) for each 100 mmol/24 hr change in sodium intake for various centiles of blood pressure distribution

Age (years)	Centile				
	5th	20th	50th	80th	95th
Systolic					
15-19	3	4	5	6	7
20-29	2	4	5	6	8
30-39	2	4	6	7	9
40-49	2	4	7	9	11
50-59	4	6	9	12	15
60-69	6	8	10	13	15
Diastolic					
15-19	1	1	2	2	3
10-29	1	2	3	3	4
30-39	1	2	3	4	5
40-49	2	3	4	4	5
50-59	2	3	5	6	7
60-69	2	3	4	6	7

From Law MR, Frost CD, Wald NJ: By how much does dietary salt reduction lower blood pressure; analysis of data from trials of salt reduction, *BMJ* 302:819, 1991.

failed to suggest that blacks differed from whites in having a higher salt intake, but they did show that the ratio of urinary sodium to potassium appeared to play a role because it positively correlated with blood pressure.

In a predominantly white community in southern California, Khaw and Barrett-Connor[29] carried out a study of the relationship of potassium to blood pressure by estimating intake by dietary recall. For men, the age-adjusted systolic and diastolic blood pressures were negatively associated with total potassium intake, whereas in women, a correlation was found for systolic pressure. In another study of the same community, these authors found not only that age-adjusted systolic and diastolic pressures were inversely related with potassium intake in both men and women, but also blood pressures positively correlated with the urinary sodium to potassium ratio.[30] Khaw and Barrett-Connor[31] additionally implicated potassium intake in stroke morbidity in this same community, the population of which was observed over a period of 12 years. Twenty-four stroke deaths occurred, and these were found to bear a relationship to potassium intake. For example, in men the relative risk of stroke was 2.6 and in women 4.8 for those consuming the lowest amounts of potassium, compared with those consuming more. Interestingly, these effects did not relate to blood pressure. This suggestion of a protective effect of an "adequate" potassium intake on stroke in this population is of interest because Tobian and colleagues[42] reported several studies indicating that a high-potassium diet reduces the incidence of cerebral hemorrhage and death without affecting blood pressure in stroke-prone hypertensive rats.

The question can be asked whether increasing potassium intake has an effect on blood pressure. The data can be summarized by saying that, in studies of short duration, little blood pressure reduction has been found, but when the period of administration was extended up to 4 or more months, a small decrease in both systolic and diastolic pressures was observed. If blood pressure is influenced by potassium intake, the question of mechanism arises. In his review of the role of potassium in the pathogenesis and treatment of hypertension, Linas[34] concluded that the most likely mechanism relates to the effect of potassium on natriuresis and its ability to prevent a positive sodium balance (Table 9-3).

CALCIUM

Among possible environmental factors involved in the pathogenesis of hypertension, calcium intake may well be the most controversial. Calcium is a major intracellular cation and is pivotal in the contraction mechanism of vascular smooth muscle. Not surprisingly, intravenous administration of calcium increases arterial pressure, as would be expected as a result of increased intracellular calcium concentration. In large epidemiological studies such as NHANES II, however, blood pressure has been found to be inversely related to calcium intake.[25,37] This, along with the obser-

Table 9-3. Effect of potassium intake on urinary sodium excretion, plasma volume, and mean arterial pressure

	High K	Normal K	Low K
Urinary sodium (mmol/day)	183.1 ± 8.1*	158.2 ± 8.9	130.7 ± 7.0
Plasma volume (%) of normotensive controls	77.8 ± 2.4*	83.5 ± 2.5	87.7 ± 2.9
Mean arterial pressure (mmHg)	103 ± 3†	114 ± 3	111 ± 3

From Linas SL: The role of potassium in the pathogenesis and treatment of hypertension, *Kidney Int* 39:771, 1991. Reprinted by permission of Blackwell Scientific Publications, Inc.
*$P < 0.002$ high potassium versus low potassium.
†$P < 0.005$ high potassium versus low potassium.

vation that some essential hypertensives have unexplained hypercalciuria, has led to the suggestion that increasing calcium intake could lower arterial pressure. A number of clinical trials have been carried out in which calcium intake was increased.[28] A few of these trials have demonstrated a small decrease in blood pressure (systolic, diastolic, or both) but the results were not sufficiently consistent to warrant recommending a population-wide increase in calcium intake.[27]

MAGNESIUM

Magnesium is predominantly an intracellular cation and appears to counteract some of the actions of calcium. In rat experiments, a low intake of magnesium can elevate blood pressure, and hypomagnesemia can potentiate vasoconstriction.[28] Further, a study by Resnick and colleagues[40] found intracellular free magnesium to be inversely related to arterial pressure (Fig. 9-3), and a more recent examination of the problem[43] showed that the platelets of hypertensives had elevated concentrations of calcium and lower levels of magnesium. A few clinical trials using magnesium supplementation as treatment for hypertension have been carried out.[28] One reported a decrease in blood pressure in hypertensives with a low serum magnesium level, but two others found no effect. What little evidence there is does not support a conclusion that magnesium deficiency is important in the pathogenesis of hypertension or that magnesium supplementation would reduce arterial pressure of hypertensives.

POLYUNSATURATED DIETARY FAT

Vegetarians have lower blood pressure than nonvegetarians. This has led to the suggestion that the ratio of polyunsaturated to saturated fat in the diet may play a role in arterial pressure regulation, presumably through production of vasodilator compounds. A review summarizes the rela-

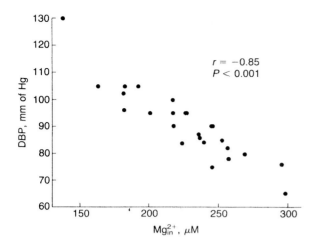

Fig. 9-3. Relationship of intracellular free magnesium (Mg^{2+}) to diastolic blood pressure *(DBP)* for all subjects. Regression analysis used the Pearson correlation coefficient and Student *t* test for level of significance. (From Resnick LM, et al: Intracellular free magnesium in erythrocytes of essential hypertension: relation to blood pressure and serum divalentcations, *Proc Natl Acad Sci USA* 81:6513, 1984; with permission.)

tionship of dietary fats to blood pressure[41] and notes "there is little convincing evidence that the amount or type of dietary fat affects blood pressure levels in persons with normal or mildly elevated blood pressure." Large amounts of omega-3 fatty acids can reduce arterial pressure.[15,27]

Iodine deficiency disorders

Laura H. McArthur

Until the 1980s, iodine deficiency generally was associated only with goiter and cretinism. It is now recognized that iodine deficiency results in a broad spectrum of physical, neurological, and intellectual deficits and is associated with increased rates of spontaneous abortions, stillbirths, neonatal and infant mortality, and learning disabilities. These features are referred to collectively as iodine deficiency disorders (IDD) and are attributable to suboptimal iodine status and inadequate synthesis of thyroxine (T_4) by the thyroid gland.[48,69,77]

When the iodine status of a community is surveyed, field workers examine the thyroid glands of a representative sample of the population to estimate the occurrence of goiters, assaying serum T_4 and thyroid-stimulating hormone (TSH) concentrations and urinary iodine excretion expressed as micrograms iodine per gram creatinine per 24 hours.[63,66,79] A community is considered at risk for hypothyroidism if mean daily urinary iodine excretion is less than 50 μg iodine/g creatinine/24 hr.[78] Neonatal screening for risk of hypothyroidism involves collection of cord blood samples at birth or capillary heel-stick samples 2 to 5 days postnatally using a filter paper blood spot method and assaying serum

for T_4 or TSH concentrations using radioimmunoassay techniques.[55,65,76,81]

Goiter is a widely recognized physical manifestation of dietary iodine deficiency (Figs. 9-4 and 9-5). A goiter is an enlargement of the thyroid resulting from its attempt to respond to TSH from the pituitary signaling the need for increased circulating T_4. Increased secretions of TSH cause a corresponding acceleration of the thyroidal iodide clearance rate. The accelerated iodide trapping rate in the presence of low iodine intake results in hyperplastic thyroid tissue with varying degrees of nodularity. When field workers examine the thyroid glands of subjects to survey the iodine status of a community or monitor the effectiveness of a prevention program, they commonly employ a classification system that assigns the thyroid glands to various grades, depending on size and potential adverse effects of this condition on health status.[75]

An area of endemic goiter is considered to be one in which more than 10% of school-aged children exhibit goiters, indicating that the problem is of public health significance.[77] In regions of severe iodine depletion, goiters first appear during childhood, a period of rapid growth, and enlarge as the child reaches adolescence and adulthood. In these communities, most of the adult population exhibit some degree of thyroid enlargement, and a high proportion present with large nodular goiters. In areas of moderate iodine depletion, goiters most often are seen in adolescents and women. In areas of mild iodine deficiency, goiters occur primarily in adolescent girls. For females living in endemic areas, goiters tend to persist and increase throughout life, whereas for males, the thyroid tends to decrease in size after puberty and the incidence of goiter declines.[51,63,74,78]

The most severe manifestation of iodine deficiency is cretinism, a syndrome featuring physical and neurological impairments. Traditionally the distinction is made between the myxedematous and neurological forms of cretinism.[71] According to this classification, neurological cretinism is characterized by euthyroidism, mental retardation, goiter, speech and hearing deficits, and abnormal gait and posture,[50] whereas myxedematous cretinism features thyroid atrophy, mental retardation, goiter, stunted growth, and sexual immaturity.[80] Chaouki and colleagues,[49] working in an endemic area in Algeria, reported stunted growth, delayed reflexes, delayed sexual development, skin myxedema, and macroglossia in myxedematous cretins and deaf-mutism, proximal spasticity, and rigidity in neurological cretins. Both groups were mentally retarded and presented with palpable thyroid glands. These authors postulate that the distinction between the neurological and myxedematous forms of cretinism is attributable to the timing of the induction of the brain lesion. Should it occur during the first trimester of gestation owing to suboptimal maternal iodine status, neurological cretinism results. Myxedematous cretinism results from the postnatal feed-

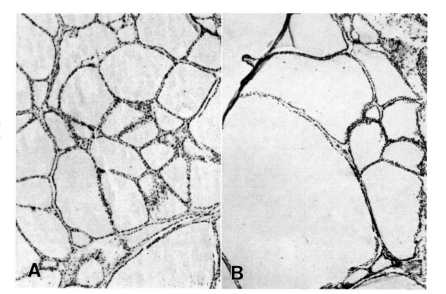

Fig. 9-4. Histology of the normal thyroid (**A**) to be compared with the thyroid of a 23-year-old woman with a goiter of 10 years' duration (**B**). (From Follis RH: *Deficiency diseases,* Springfield, IL, Charles C Thomas, 1958; with permission.)

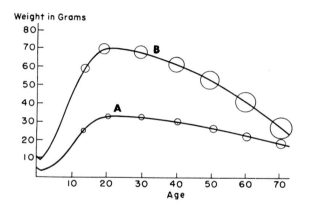

Fig. 9-5. Relationship of thyroid weight and nodularity in goitrogenic region of Europe (**A**) to normal subjects (**B**) by age. The data was originally published by Aschoff. (From Follis RH: *Deficiency diseases,* Springfield, IL, Charles C Thomas, 1958; with permission.)

ing of iodine-poor breast milk or foods high in goitrogens. Todd and colleagues[83] conducted audiometric tests on 121 primary school children living in an area of endemic goiter in Zimbabwe and found no cases of impaired hearing. They conclude that this condition is not associated with mild to moderate iodine deficiency in this population. Halpern and colleagues[61] question the accuracy and usefulness of distinguishing between the myxedematous and neurological forms of cretinism, given that neurological signs overlap and that impaired hearing is not always present. They investigated the nature and extent of the neurological deficit in 100 cretins from a predominantly myxedematous endemia in western China and in 35 cretins from a predominantly neurological endemia in central Java and found a similar pattern of neurological involvement in nearly all subjects from both endemias.

These authors hypothesize that the clinical picture of cretinism arises from an interaction of two pathophysiological events, both attributable to iodine insufficiency but acting at different stages of fetal and neonatal development. The first event reflects a deficiency of T_4 in utero, resulting in the neurological manifestations of cretinism. The second event reflects progressive postnatal thyroidal atrophy, resulting in retarded linear growth and sexual immaturity (frequently seen in myxedematous cretinism). The findings of Halpern and colleagues confirm those of DeLong,[53] who reported neurological deficits in 26 of 80 myxedematous cretins examined in Zaire.

Dietary iodine deficiency is one of the most widespread nutrient deficiency diseases in the developing world (Fig. 9-6). Data published by the World Health Organization[87] indicate that approximately 1×10^9 people living in 90 developing countries are at risk of nutritional iodine deficiency, and an estimated 2.1×10^8 people in these countries exhibit goiters. A breakdown of these estimates by geographic region indicates that in China and other Asian countries (excluding Southeast Asia), 4×10^8 people are at risk of iodine deficiency, and 3×10^7 have goiters. In Southeast Asia, 2.8×10^8 people are at risk, and 1×10^8 have goiters. In Africa, 2.3×10^8 people are at risk of iodine deficiency, and 3.9×10^7 have goiters. In Latin America, 6×10^7 people are at risk of iodine deficiency, and 3×10^7 have goiters. In the Eastern Mediterranean, 3.3×10^7 people are at risk of iodine deficiency, and 1.2×10^7 have goiters. An estimated 2×10^7 people in developing countries are thought to have some degree of mental retardation or other neurological abnormality, and approximately 6×10^6 exhibit signs of cretinism.*

*References 49, 62, 63, 64, 66, 77, 79, 85.

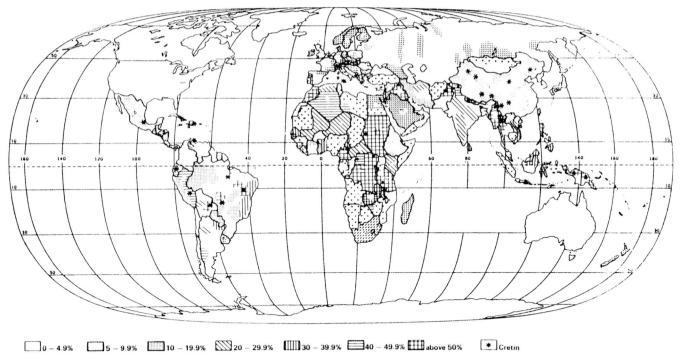

Fig. 9-6. Prevalence of goiter and occurrence of cretinism worldwide, ca. 1980. (From *Ann Rev Nutr* 3:341, 1983; with permission.)

Pandav and Kochupillai[73] reported that approximately 1.5×10^8 people in India are at risk of iodine deficiency and that an estimated 4.0×10^6 are goitrous. They noted that the incidence of neonatal hypothyroidism in endemic regions in India is more than 100-fold higher than the incidence in nonendemic regions. Eltom and colleagues[54] reported that western Sudan has a goiter prevalence of 85%. Gitau[58] observed that approximately 62% of the population of Kenya is at risk of contracting IDD. IDD are also serious public health problems in Brazil, as evidenced by goiter and cretinism prevalence data from two national surveys of schoolchildren.[68,72]

It is widely accepted that goiter is attributable to an inadequate dietary intake of iodine.[49,64,69,78] Cretinism is generally attributed to insufficient placental transfer of thyroxin during the first trimester of gestation or to iodine insufficiency postnatally.[48] The precise mechanism, however, by which iodine deficiency impairs fetal and neonatal psychomotor development has not yet been elucidated. The classic hypotheses are a direct adverse effect of iodine deficiency on fetal brain development; destruction of fetal thyroid tissue by exhaustion atrophy; and a toxic action of dietary goitrogens on thyroid gland development.[81]

Endemic goiter and cretinism are found in populations that depend on foods grown locally in iodine-poor soil (Fig. 9-7). Endemic areas typically feature mountainous terrain, heavy annual rainfall, or glaciated, eroded topsoil.[77] Jenesi and colleagues[62] observed that those at greatest risk for IDD

in Zimbabwe are subsistence farmers living on a high inland, granite-based plateau featuring eroded topsoil and erratic rainfall. Similar findings have been reported for southern Tanzania,[85] Sudan,[46] and western Kenya.[45] Jooste and colleagues[63] noted that the soil in an endemic area in eastern Namibia experiencing occasional flooding appeared sandy and of poor quality. Pang and colleagues,[74] working in a rural village in China, observed that the 176 patients diagnosed with either goiter or cretinism consumed a diet consisting largely of wheat, corn, and sweet potato. These foods, along with the local water supply, are low in iodine. Kochupillai[65] reported higher incidences of goiter and cretinism in flood-prone villages in India and lower incidences in villages that did not experience flooding.

Dietary goitrogens, such as those derived from members of the cabbage family (*Brassica species*), chelate iodine and reduce its bioavailability. They have also been studied as possible factors in the cause of IDD.[82] A few investigators[47,56,57] have found correlations between ingestion of high levels of these substances and the occurrence of goiter and cretinism. Other investigators dismiss dietary goitrogens as primary causal factors in the pathogenesis of these conditions. Mahdi and colleagues[70] analyzed water samples from four endemic areas in Sudan for the presence of naturally occurring goitrogens and found insignificant amounts of these compounds. The authors conclude that the drinking water in the Sudan plays a limited role, if any, in the cause of endemic goiter. Jooste and colleagues[63] con-

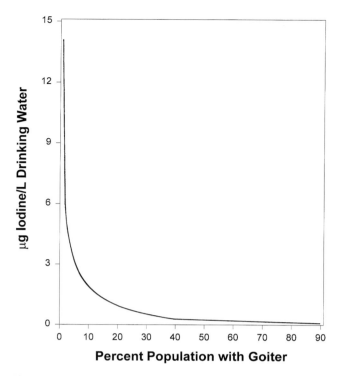

Fig. 9-7. Prevalence of goiter in relation to iodine concentrations in potable water in a goitrogenic region of the European Alps. (Adapted from von Fellenberg I: Kropf und Trinkwasser in der Schweiz, Mitt. Gebiete Lebensm, *Hyg* 24:123, 1933; with permission.)

clude that dietary goitrogens are probably not the primary cause of goiters in schoolchildren from eastern Namibia. They suggest that consumption of a nutritionally inadequate diet low in calories and micronutrients, including iodine, is most likely responsible for the occurrence of this condition in this community. Jenesi and colleagues,[62] working in an endemic area in Zimbabwe, found no significant difference in goitrogen intakes between goitrous and nongoitrous subjects overall or when subjects were subdivided by age or goiter size. The authors conclude that endemic goiter in this geographical region is attributable to iodine deficiency rather than to ingestion of dietary goitrogen. Similar findings were reported by Chaouki and colleages[49] from an endemic area in Algeria.

Factors other than insufficient iodine intake have been investigated as possible causes of IDD. Bayoumi and colleages[46] studied the occurrence of goiter among the tribes of western Sudan and found a significantly higher incidence among the offspring of affected parents than among children of nongoitrous parents. These authors propose a possible genetic predisposition to goiter. Selenium deficiency has also been studied as a factor in the cause of IDD.[52] Goyens and colleagues[59] found suboptimal serum selenium and glutathione peroxidase concentrations in subjects living in an endemic area in Zaire. They hypothesize that

subnormal cellular levels of this enzyme in the thyroid gland may result in cytotoxic concentrations of hydrogen peroxide in the gland, contributing to the pathogenesis of cretinism in this geographical area. Vanderpas and colleagues,[84] however, conclude that selenium supplementation alone is contraindicated in iodine-deficient and selenium-deficient subjects diagnosed with myxedematous cretinism because selenium would increase thyroxin metabolism, aggravating the hypothyroxinemia. They recommend concomitant selenium and iodine supplementation in these cases.

Dietary iron deficiency and excess

Robert C. Woodworth

Living organisms, with few exceptions, have an absolute metabolic requirement for iron as a trace element. During early evolution, before widespread photosynthetic activity, the atmosphere of the earth was reducing, and iron was readily available in the highly soluble ferrous form, i.e., Fe^{2+}. As the level of O_2 in the atmosphere increased, Fe^{2+} was gradually oxidized to the highly insoluble ferric hydroxide ($K_{sp} \approx 10^{-38}$ at pH7).[98,110] The oxidation-reduction potentials for iron and its complexes, however, are such that this element is ideally suited for electron transport and oxidation reduction processes in living systems. Biological evolution had to develop biochemical schema for acquiring and utilizing the inherently insoluble $Fe(OH)_3$ and variants thereof.[98,110]

In higher animals, including humans, the primary role of iron is to serve as the O_2 ligand in the hemoglobin of erythrocytes and thereby to deliver oxygen from the lungs to the peripheral tissues as the ultimate electron acceptor in the electron transport system of the mitochondria (see Chapter 23). Minor but essential roles are in the heme prosthetic groups of myoglobin in muscle, especially cardiac muscle in humans, of electron transport cytochromes in mitochondria, of cytochrome P-450s of microsomes; as the iron component of iron-sulfur proteins, as storage iron, e.g., ferritin, hemosiderin, primarily in the liver and reticuloendothelial cells; and as transport iron in the blood complexed to transferrin. Table 9-4 gives approximate distributions of iron in average males and females.[91]

Ferritin is a storage protein for iron made up of a hollow sphere of 24 subunits of two major types, H and L, the distribution depending on the organ of origin and on the degree of iron repletion of the person.[88] One 450-kDa molecule can accommodate up to approximately 4×10^3 Fe^{3+} per molecule. Found primarily in cytoplasm and secondary lysosomes of the parenchymal cells of liver and reticuloendothelial cells, ferritin serves to store in soluble form the highly insoluble ferric hydroxide. A sensitive and quite accurate measure of total body iron stores is serum ferritin, usually found in the range of 10 to 100 $\mu g/L$.[91]

Table 9-4. Approximate distribution of iron proteins in the average male and female in iron balance

Iron protein	~mg Fe/75-kg male	~mg Fe/60-kg female
Hemoglobin	2300	1800
Myoglobin	320	260
Heme enzymes (e.g., cytochromes)	80	55
Nonheme enzymes	100	80
Transferrin	4	3
Ferritin	700	220
Hemosiderin	300	80
Total	*ca.* 3800	*ca.* 2500

The origin of this glycosylated iron-poor form of ferritin is as yet unknown.

Hemosiderin appears to be a partial degradation product of ferritin with lower relative protein content. In contrast to ferritin, hemosiderin is insoluble in water. At elevated levels, it may account for some damage to membranes of secondary lysosomes and cells via Haber-Weiss chemistry (see Chapter 21). Transferrin is an 80-kDa glycoprotein of blood plasma, which can bind up to two ferric ions, one in each of two lobes, along with an accompanying synergistic anion, normally carbonate.[89,94] A major role of this protein is to transport iron in a soluble, nontoxic form among body tissues, the primary cycle being from degraded hemoglobin in the reticuloendothelial system to the red bone marrow for the synthesis of new hemoglobin.

Transferrin transports iron from absorption in the gut to the liver and other tissues for storage and heme synthesis. In addition, the normal one third saturation of transferrin with iron serves to provide a buffering system for iron such that the free concentration of free iron is vanishingly small ($K_d \simeq 10^{-20}$). The general immune function of this system is deprivation of potential pathogens of iron required for replication and growth.[92,108] Cells of the body requiring iron, i.e., rapidly dividing cells, readily obtain it from transferrin by expressing species-specific transferrin receptors on their plasma membranes. The iron-transferrin complex, but not the apoprotein, binds to these receptors and is endocytosed via clathrin-coated pits into endosomes.[107] The endosomal pH drops to approximately 5.5 via an adenosine triphosphatase (ATPase)-driven proton pump, whereupon the iron dissociates; the apoprotein binds tightly to the receptor at this pH and is recycled back to the plasma membrane and dissociates at pH 7.4. The mechanism by which the freed iron transits the endosomal membrane for synthesis of heme or ferritin is currently unknown. The entire transit cycle for the transferrin molecule takes about 3 minutes.

Iron balance in the human is almost exclusively controlled by uptake from the diet.[91] Daily losses in normal males average approximately 1 mg/day, via the bile, urine, intestinal blood loss, and sloughed cells from the skin and gut epithelium. Menstruating females lose on average approximately 1.4 mg/day, although the range is wider than in males largely owing to variable blood loss during the menses. During pregnancy, the iron requirement of women is significantly increased to provide for the needs of the fetus, placenta, and expanding maternal erythrocyte mass. These increased needs sum to about 1 g of iron per pregnancy, with the greatest requirement of 5 to 6 mg/day occurring during the last two trimesters of pregnancy. Although on the average Western diet, the normal daily iron requirement can be met from the foodstuff (6 mg Fe/1000 kcal), during pregnancy supplementation with iron compounds is required if adequate amounts of iron are to be absorbed. Iron uptake, however, is not directly proportional to iron concentration in the gut, the percent absorbed decreasing with increasing iron dose.[109]

Absorption of iron from the intestinal content is normally controlled at the gut epithelium. Although the early notion of a "mucosal block" for iron has been largely discredited by later workers, no clear mechanism has been put forth to replace it. Alternatives advanced by other investigators have included the findings that normally iron absorption is inversely related to body iron stores and that iron uptake is proportional to the plasma iron turnover rate.[99,101] It is well established that persons with latent or frank iron deficiency absorb iron more efficiently from the lumen of the small intestine into the blood stream and that persons with "iron-loading anemias," e.g., Cooley's anemia and sickle cell anemia, and with idiopathic hemochromatosis fail to control iron uptake from the gut despite inordinately high body iron stores.[90,93,103] After extensive iron loading in the liver, in the form of ferritin and hemosiderin, other organs become involved. Iron loading of the pancreas eventuates in "golden diabetes," as pigmentation of the skin increases. Loading of iron by the myocytes in cardiac tissue leads, in the end, to cardiac failure and death.

The iron content of foodstuffs can be divided into two pools, inorganic iron and heme iron.[102] The uptake of inorganic iron from the intestinal lumen appears to be biphasic, with a saturable phase that follows Michaelis-Menton kinetics and a nonsaturable phase.[105,109] The nonsaturable phase appears to be considerably more rapid in hemochromototics than in normals. Uptake of ferrous iron is much more rapid and extensive than the uptake of ferric iron.[91,102] Thus, addition of reducing substances to the diet, especially ascorbic acid, greatly enhances the bioavailability of iron to the human body. In addition, meat in the diet also greatly enhances the absorption of iron, probably by forming soluble chelates with ferric iron rather than reducing it to ferrous iron. Other proposed enhancers of iron absorption, e.g., sugars and organic acids, appear to be of little effect unless given in vast excess over iron, with the possible exception of succinic, lactic, and lactobionic acids. Certain substances in vegetable foods, such as grains, inhibit absorption of iron, e.g., phosphates, carbonates, oxalates, tannins, and phytates (although the inhibitory effects of phytates have been disputed). The absorption of heme iron is not inhibited by these substances because it is sequestered in the protoporphyrin ring of heme and is absorbed by epithelial cells of the gut as such, where it is catabolized to iron and bilirubin. Heme uptake is enhanced by meat in the diet, presumably because the heme is solubilized by peptides and thereby prevented from polymerizing at the alkaline pH of the small intestine. Therefore, even though the heme iron pool of the typical Western diet is smaller (6% to 33%) than the inorganic iron pool, the former plays a relatively greater role by supplying 30% to 74% of the absorbed iron.[91]

The picture is quite different among people of emerging nations, where the diet is largely based on cereal grains, so many of the inhibitors of iron absorption, but few of the enhancers, play a role. Inclusion in these diets of fresh fruits, high in ascorbate, is particularly important as an enhancer of iron absorption. Nevertheless, iron deficiency anemia is endemic throughout much of this population.[91,97] A study by the World Health Organization reports that in Asia iron deficiency occurs in at least 10% of men, 20% of women, 40% of pregnant women, 50% of children of all ages, and 90% of children under 2 years of age.[96] This situation is exacerbated by frequent infestation with intestinal parasites, such as hookworm, which cause increased intestinal blood loss and the resultant increased loss of iron from the body,[91] although some of this iron is recycled into the body via digestion of the lost red cells.[96] Estimates of iron deficiency among women of fertile age in Great Britain and Sweden were also in the 20% range, whereas in Georgia, it was about 10%.[100] Partly as a result of increased iron supplementation of staple foodstuffs, this frequency in Sweden has dropped to the 6% to 7% range.[91] Severe iron deficiency anemia leads not only to decreased levels of hemoglobin in the blood and thereby a decreased ability of the body to deliver O_2 to tissues, but also to demonstrable decreases in levels of cytochromes and iron-sulfur proteins.

In certain select populations, e.g., the South African Bantu, dietary iron overload leading to siderosis is caused by consumption, especially by the men, of large quantities of an acidic beer, brewed in iron drums.[91,93] The low pH solubilizes iron from the containers, most likely in the ferrous form, and the alcohol enhances iron absorption from the gut. The high iron load along with alcohol eventually leads to a high incidence of hepatic siderosis, cirrhosis and fibrosis. Associated with the hemochromatosis are also scurvy and osteroporosis. A comparison of iron contents of liver among men gives a median value of 30 mg/dl for white South Africans, 20 mg/dl for Americans, and 13 mg/dl for Swedes, but values of 500 mg/dl for at least 20% of Bantu men.[93] In contrast, the high dietary iron content, from cooking utensils, of Ethiopians does not lead to similar consequences, presumably owing to the relatively low bioavailability of this iron.

Although iron supplementation of basic foodstuffs is practiced in most Western nations, increased levels of supplementation have been opposed by those concerned about the relatively high gene frequency for hemochromatosis in the white population, i.e., from 1 in 30 to 1 in 10 of the population.[103] This gene frequency is as high as that for hemoglobin S among the black population of Africa. The hypothesis is that increased dietary iron will lead to earlier onset of iron overload in the population at risk from this genetic defect.

Although the vast majority of the world's population suffers from chronic iron deficiency, the hypothesis has been advanced that latent iron deficiency may be a better situation for general health than is "normal" iron repletion.[95,106,108] The possibility of precipitation of ischemic heart disease in Western societies by "normal" iron levels is suggested by the observations that premenopausal women are subject to a significantly lower incidence of ischemic heart disease than are men of equal age. Postmenopausal women accumulate increased iron stores, and their rate of ischemic heart disease rises to parallel that of age-matched men. A study of a group of Finnish men showed a high correlation between serum ferritin levels (an index of total bodily iron stores) and cardiovascular disease.[104] According to this hypothesis, the increased frequency of cardiovascular disease among postmenopausal women may be more directly related to increased iron stores than to decreased estrogen. Likewise, evidence exists as to low iron stores serving as a defense against neoplasia[105a,108] and microbial infections.[92,108] Clearly the final word on the benefits and hazards of iron repletion in humans has not been written, and more must be learned about the benefits and hazards of this vital trace element to human health.

Dietary selenium deficiency and excess

Orville A. Levander

Selenium is of great interest biogeochemically because both deficiency and toxicity have been observed in humans under natural conditions. The primary route of exposure to selenium in the general population is through food because air and water normally contain minor quantities.[130] Selenium enters the food chain through plants. Although some plant species (so-called accumulators) contain large amounts, the usual food and forage crops do not concentrate selenium. The level found in these plants, however, does vary with the selenium in the soil that is available for uptake. The most extreme values for the selenium content of foods have been reported from the People's Republic of China, where differences spanning three orders of magnitude have been reported for dietary staples such as corn or soybeans, depending on where they were grown. These differences in the selenium content of foods give rise to great ranges in the total dietary selenium intake in various regions of China, with corresponding differences in blood selenium concentrations also being observed (Table 9-5). Such a wide divergence in blood selenium levels is not without consequences for human health, and, indeed, frank deficiency and overt toxicity of selenium have been extensively documented in humans residing in certain parts of China.[166]

SELENIUM DEFICIENCY

The first suggestion that selenium might have beneficial nutritional properties was provided by Schwarz and Foltz,[151] who found that traces in the diet could prevent liver necrosis in vitamin E– deficient rats. Soon thereafter, selenium was shown to protect against several economically important nutritional diseases of farm animals, such as white muscle disease in sheep and cattle, hepatosis diatetica in swine, and exudative diathesis in poultry.[158] Presumptive evidence for a role in human nutrition was provided in 1973, when selenium was discovered at the active site of the peroxide-destroying enzyme, glutathione peroxidase.[148] This observation also provided a logical explanation for the long-recognized nutritional relationship between selenium and the fat-soluble antioxidant vitamin E. Both nutrients can now be regarded as part of the antioxidant defense system (see Chapter 21). An actual association, however, between selenium nutrition and human health was not demonstrated until 1979, when Chinese scientists showed the prophylactic value of selenium supplements against Keshan disease, a cardiomyopathy that affects infants, children, and women of child-bearing age in areas of China with soils of low selenium content.[134] (For a detailed description of the pathology of this condition, see Ge and colleagues[124] or Gu.[127]) The amount of dietary selenium needed to protect against Keshan disease is small, only about 19 μg/day for men and 14 μg/day for women.

Table 9-5. Dietary selenium intake and blood selenium concentration of persons living in high-selenium, adequate-selenium, and low-selenium areas of China

Area	Average selenium intake (mg/day)	Blood selenium concentration (μg/ml)
High-selenium area with chronic selenosis	4.99	3.2
High-selenium area without chronic selenosis	0.75	0.44
Selenium-adequate area (Beijing)	0.116	0.095
Low-selenium area with Keshan disease	0.011	0.021

Adapted from Yang et al: Endemic selenium intoxication of humans in China, *Am J Clin Nutr* 37:872, 1983.

Although poor selenium status has been successful in accounting for the biogeochemical features of Keshan disease, there are certain temporal characteristics of the disease that are difficult to rationalize solely based on differences in selenium status. The incidence of Keshan disease has a marked seasonal or annual fluctuation that is more typical of an infectious agent than of a nutritional deficiency. The Chinese scientists emphasized the probably multifactorial nature of Keshan disease and stressed the possible involvement of viral infection, especially infection with a cardiotoxic virus of the coxsackievirus.[123] These workers found that selenium-deficient mice were more susceptible to heart damage owing to a coxsackievirus B_4 virus isolated from a Keshan disease patient than were selenium-supplemented mice.[125] More recently, Beck and colleagues[116] showed that heart lesions caused by coxsackievirus B_3 were more severe in mice deficient in either vitamin E or selenium. Moreover, deficiency of either nutrient allowed a normally benign strain of the virus to cause significant heart lesions in mice.[115] A diet taken from a Keshan disease area produced liver necrosis in rats (Yang GQ: personal communication, 1993), a phenomenon that is seen only with diets that are deficient in both selenium and vitamin E. Additional research is needed to clarify the relative contribution of various antioxidant nutrient deficiencies and viral infection to the cause of Keshan disease.

Although the effectiveness of selenium in preventing Keshan disease could perhaps be reasonably accounted for based on its role in glutathione peroxidase, research shows that selenium has many other functions. For example, the selenium-containing phospholipid hydroperoxide glutathione peroxidase,[140] in contrast the glutathione peroxidase already discussed, specifically reduces phospholipid-bound lipid hydroperoxide. This could play a prophylactic role in Keshan disease. Furthermore, selenoprotein P, an unusual plasma protein containing several selenocysteine residues, may act to protect against free radicals in vivo.[128] The discovery that the type I iodothyronine 5′-deiodinase is a selenium-containing enzyme reveals a new function for selenium independent of its role in antioxidant defense and suggests the possibility of a bifactorial biogeochemical disease.[114] Some workers have hypothesized that selenium deficiency in an iodine-deficient area of Central Africa might favor development of myxedematous endemic cretinism over nervous endemic cretinism.[120]

Kashin-Beck disease, an osteoarthritis endemic to certain regions of the People's Republic of China and eastern Siberia,[155] has also been linked to low selenium status, but the association is less clear than the relationship of selenium with Keshan disease.[123] This permanently disabling condition develops primarily in children 5 to 13 years of age, and 2×10^6 people are affected in China alone.[164] Research on Kashin-Beck disease has been hampered by the lack of a suitable animal model, but experiments in mice fed selenium-deficient diets or given fulvic acid in the drinking water revealed histological changes in the tibial epiphysis that resemble x-ray absorption patterns seen in the finger joints of patients with this disease.[165]

Several attempts have been made to link poor selenium status with increased risk of cancer.[119,149] Some of the limitations of this hypothesis have been discussed;[136,161] one of the early proponents of this idea concluded that the question is wide open.[162] Large, prospective cohort studies have failed to demonstrate any association between selenium status as assessed by toenail selenium levels and breast cancer in the United States[129] or colorectal cancer in the Netherlands.[159] The former trial, however, was criticized because the dispersion of selenium values in the study population might not have been great enough to reveal a protective effect.[150] A Chinese study (which encompassed a wide range of cancer mortality rates and plasma selenium levels) found significant negative correlations between selenium status and esophageal and stomach cancer.[118] The potential utility of selenium as a cancer chemoprevention agent[142] is undergoing active research.[131]

Selenium supplements may be of value in the recovery of patients with kwashiorkor (reviewed in Levander[136]). Evidence from malnourished Jamaican children indicates that free radicals might play a role in the pathogenesis of kwashiorkor,[126] and South African researchers pointed out that specific selenium replacement may be required for the treatment of children with this disease.[152] It was questioned, however, whether the low selenium status of Sudanese children posed any health risk during rehabilitation from severe protein-calorie malnutrition.[112] Deficiencies of selenium or vitamin E were not consistently found in African children suffering from various clinical forms of malnutrition.[135]

The first nutritional standard for selenium, an Estimated Safe and Adequate Daily Dietary Intake (ESADDI), was established by the U.S. National Research Council in 1980.[143] This standard, 50 to 200 μg/day for adults, with progressively lower values for infants and children, was expressed as a range to reflect the lack of knowledge about human selenium requirements at that time. In fact, the ESADDI was based primarily on an extrapolation of animal data. Our understanding of human selenium requirements increased greatly in the 1980s so that, by 1989, the National Research Council was able to set a Recommended Dietary Allowance (RDA).[145]

The selenium RDA was based on data generated from a supplementation trial in China that determined the dietary intake needed to maximize plasma glutathione peroxidase activity.[137,169] Previous studies had shown that the balance technique was not suitable for estimating human selenium requirements because of the ability of people to adapt metabolically to widely diverging selenium intakes.[138] Modification of the Chinese supplementation study data with body weight and safety factors resulted in a selenium RDA of 70 μg/day for men and 55 μg/day for women.[137]

The typical diet in the United States would readily satisfy this dietary standard,[137] but not so for certain other countries. For example, New Zealand and Finland have populations whose platelet glutathione peroxidase activity responds well to selenium supplementation.[113,157] Public health authorities in Finland, a country with low-selenium soils, decided to add selenium to fertilizers in 1984 as a way of increasing the amount of selenium in the national food supply.[160] This intervention increased the mean dietary intake from 30 to 40 μg/day to more than 100 μg/day in the early 1990s. A follow-up of the situation in Finland revealed no dramatic change in the incidence or mortality from cardiovascular disease or cancer after the initiation of this program.[160]

SELENIUM TOXICITY

Interest in selenium toxicity was stimulated in the 1930s, when it was discovered that high levels of selenium in plants grown in seleniferous soils cause alkali disease, a condition of livestock raised in certain parts of the northern Great Plains of the United States.[141] Animals with chronic selenosis suffered hair loss, deformed hoofs, and eventually death. Blind staggers, once considered a form of selenium poisoning, now is thought to be due to the consumption of alkaloids.[144] Although selenium toxicity of farm animals has become rare because of effective range management, episodes of selenosis in horses in Wyoming and western Iowa demonstrate the continuing potential hazard.[147,163]

Early attempts to document human selenium poisoning were unclear in studies conducted in areas of the United States where selenosis of livestock is reported.[153,154] An investigation of possible human health effects of selenium overexposure in persons residing on seleniferous ranches of western South Dakota and eastern Wyoming revealed no deleterious effects at dietary intakes as high as 724 μg/day.[139] Examination of schoolchildren residing in a seleniferous zone of Venezuela failed to uncover health problems ascribable to high selenium intake.[133]

The most complete description available of human selenium poisoning from seleniferous foods comes from the study of an outbreak of selenosis in Hubei Province, People's Republic of China.[168] Loss of hair and nails proved to be the most characteristic feature of human selenium intoxication. Patients with more serious illness had skin lesions and possible involvement of the nervous system. A later evaluation of the situation showed that signs of selenosis occur in a sensitive individual at an intake of 910 μg/day.[167] It was concluded that a lowest observed adverse effect level (LOAEL) of 1540 μg/day could be calculated (Yang GQ: personal communication, 1993).

Ecological contamination owing to selenium assumed a sense of urgency when it was realized that subsurface irrigation wastewater draining seleniferous soils contains enough selenium to be considered hazardous.[117] Accumulation and concentration of agricultural wastewater in disposal ponds also managed as wetland habitat for waterfowl resulted in deaths, deformation, and reproductive failure in the birds. Although originally discovered at the Kesterson Reservoir in the Central Valley of California, seleniferous wastewater now has been identified at several sites in the western United States.[122] Various drainage waste management approaches have been suggested, and research is continuing in an attempt to deal with the problem.[156]

The mechanism(s) of selenium toxicity are poorly understood and there is no sensitive, specific, and reliable biochemical indicator of selenium overexposure.[130] For that reason, standard setting in selenium toxicology depends more on clinical indices of selenosis, such as changes in fingernail morphology. Based on his many years of experience in selenium toxicity research, Olson[146] suggested a maximum safe multiple oral dose of 5 μg/day per kilogram of body weight, equal to 350 μg/day for the standard 70-kg man. Yang and colleagues,[167] drawing on their extensive data about human selenium toxicosis in China, concluded that a suggested maximal daily safe dietary selenium intake should be 400 μg. Additional research is needed to clarify the upper limit of safe selenium intake.

Protein energy malnutrition

Laura H. McArthur

Protein energy malnutrition (PEM) is a term given to a range of pathological conditions resulting from deficiencies of dietary protein and calories. An international classification system used to screen high-risk cases identifies kwashiorkor, marasmus, and marasmic kwashiorkor as the most severe and less common forms of PEM.[198] Kwashiorkor, occurring most often in children aged 1 to 3 years after the termination of breast-feeding, results from the consumption of high-carbohydrate diets containing inadequate amounts of protein. These diets frequently consist of watery gruels made from staple crops such as cassava, maize, plantain, or yams. Kwashiorkor is characterized by edema in the hands, feet, or abdomen and by low body weight for height. Other clinical signs may include muscle wasting; dermatosis; hepatomegaly; discolored, sparse, and easily pluckable hair; xerophthalmia; emotional and behavioral changes; and impaired cognitive performance. Low serum protein and amino acid concentrations, reduced immunocompetence, partial villous atrophy, iron deficiency anemia, and bacterial and viral infections are found in laboratory studies. Marasmus is most often observed in infants from birth to 2 years of age who were never breast-fed or who were weaned early. The condition results from the consumption of a diet balanced in nutrient composition but deficient in calories. Clinical features include very low body weight for height, loss of subcutaneous adipose tissue, muscle wasting, infections, and an absence of edema. Other clinical findings that

also may be present are iron deficiency anemia, impaired immunocompetence, and low serum albumin and plasma retinol concentrations. Marasmic kwashiorkor exhibits the clinical features of kwashiorkor and marasmus and is attributed to the consumption of a diet inadequate in calories and protein.*

The symptoms of these three types of PEM differ markedly among geographical regions.[197] Some investigators have speculated that genetic factors play a role in the cause of PEM because not all children consuming a nutritionally inadequate diet are afflicted.[184] The majority of PEM patients present with milder symptoms featuring low weight-for-height ratios, infections, and signs of subclinical micronutrient deficiencies.

PEM is the most widespread form of malnutrition among children under the age of 5 years in developing countries. The prevalence of this heterogeneous disease is difficult to estimate because of the lack of internationally accepted diagnostic criteria, inconsistent data collection and recording practices, and the inability of health care professionals to recognize the classic features of PEM.[200] For example, Zollner and colleagues[200] found that physicians and primary health care nurses in three South African hospitals failed to recognize 25% of children with severe PEM and 50% of children with mild PEM. UNICEF data indicate that wasting affects 1% to 27% of children aged 12 to 23 months in 28 African countries, 2% to 28% of children in 12 Asian countries (not including India), and zero to 17% of children in 20 Latin American countries. For these same countries, stunting affects 13% to 61% of African children aged 24 to 59 months, 14% to 66% of Asian children, and 4% to 68% of Latin American children.[196]

Factors contributing to the onset of PEM—cultural, economic, educational, and environmental—are closely linked to poverty. In developing countries, impoverished rural families often subsist on the crops grown on small plots and have little, if any, surplus money to purchase additional food. As a result, weanlings and young children are often fed a high-carbohydrate, low-protein diet containing few animal products, predisposing them to PEM.[199] Inequitable intrahousehold food distribution practices may also contribute. In some cultures, men and older boys are favored at mealtime by serving them first and offering them the largest and choicest portions of food. Consequently, younger children consume nutritionally inadequate diets consisting of the discarded remains of the family meal. This gender and age bias has been observed by Pitt and colleagues[185] in 15 villages in Bangladesh and by Behrman[172] in India.

The use of commercial infant formulas by low-income families rather than breast milk is another widely recognized risk factor for PEM. Inadequate maternal knowledge regarding preparation of the formula often results in overdilution of the milk powder with contaminated water. This

*References 171, 174, 191, 194, 195.

practice delivers inadequate calories and nutrients to the infant and causes recurrent episodes of infection and diarrhea.[176,187]

Infectious diseases, often attributable to a contaminated home environment, lack of a potable water supply, sanitation facilities, and immunization services, frequently act synergistically with PEM to augment the course and severity of illness. These infections are rapidly transmitted in overcrowded dwellings and hospital wards and are a major cause of mortality from PEM. Tolboom and colleagues[195] reported that 55 of the 218 patients with severe PEM admitted to the Lesotho Central Hospital during 1981-1982 died within 1 week of admission and that the most frequent causes of death were acute gastroenteritis among marasmus patients and pneumonia among kwashiorkor patients. Other investigators[191] reported that 30 of 38 children aged 3 to 36 months admitted to the pediatric ward of the Obafemi Awolowo University Teaching Hospital in Nigeria for treatment of severe PEM were also diagnosed with gastroenteritis, pneumonia, or measles. Molteno and Kibel[182] reported similar findings among a group of infants in Matroosberg, South Africa.

The question of whether infectious disease precipitates an episode of PEM owing to anorexia or inappropriate feeding practices during illness or whether PEM predisposes the child to infections owing to diminished immunocompetence or damage to protective mucosal membranes remains unresolved. African investigators found that infectious diseases often occurred during the weeks preceding outbreaks of PEM.*

Inadequate maternal knowledge regarding the cause and treatment of diarrheal disease often results in the withholding of nutritious foods and the use of inappropriate management strategies, making the child more vulnerable to PEM. In a study conducted in four rural communities in the Shewa Administrative Region of Ethiopia, Ketsela and colleagues[180] found that of the 750 caretakers interviewed, fewer than 3% possessed accurate information about the causes of diarrhea, and only 6% followed appropriate management practices. Similar findings have been reported in central Thailand[175] and India.[186]

Often the child treated for PEM remains below normal in height for age, an anthropometric indicator of growth stunting. Another frequently reported consequence of PEM is partial or total blindness owing to inadequate dietary intakes of vitamin A or to a decreased hepatic synthesis of retinol binding protein.[173,181,193] Other possible consequences of PEM include impaired developmental and cognitive performance. Studies conducted in Kenya showed that children aged 30 months and 5 years who had experienced episodes of PEM earned lower scores on developmental measures and on the Bayley Mental scales than a comparison group who had never been afflicted with PEM.[183,190]

*References 170, 177, 179, 188, 189, 192.

Diet, plasma lipids, and cardiovascular disease

Russell P. Tracy

Cardiovascular disease (CVD) is a major cause of morbidity and mortality worldwide. In 1989, CVD claimed close to 1×10^6 lives in the United States, accounting for almost 44% of all deaths. Of these, approximately half were attributable to coronary heart disease (CHD), the leading single cause of death in the United States.[201] Clearly, this is a public health problem of enormous proportions, one that is directly influenced by several environmental factors, chief among which is diet.

CVD, particularly CHD, is most commonly associated with two processes: atherosclerosis and thrombosis. Three major modifiable CVD risk factors have been identified: (1) smoking, (2) hypertension, and (3) hypercholesterolemia. Hypercholesterolemia is believed to be a causal link in the chain of atherosclerotic development and may be related to thrombosis as well. In particular, elevated low-density lipoprotein levels (LDL-cholesterol) and decreased high-density lipoprotein levels (HDL-cholesterol) appear to be associated with increased risk of CVD. The National Cholesterol Education Panel has established guidelines based on plasma levels of total cholesterol, LDL-cholesterol, and HDL-cholesterol that help define three categories of relative risk: low, moderate, and high.[285] It is believed that total cholesterol levels and lipoprotein subfraction levels reflect (albeit poorly) the complex lipid metabolism of humans, which is, in turn, related to atherosclerotic development, including that in the coronary arteries. In this way, these values reflect risk for incident CVD.

Over the past decade, it has become apparent that diets high in cholesterol and saturated fats contribute to the plasma cholesterol level. Therefore, the dietary habits of Americans have come under intense scrutiny, and much public education has promoted dietary modification (principally reduction of cholesterol and saturated fat intake to reduce plasma cholesterol levels) as a means of reducing risk. The role of other plasma lipids is less well defined.

In particular, the evidence concerning plasma triglycerides, primarily transported in the large chylomicron, and very low-density lipoprotein (VLDL) particles is conflicting and unclear.[206,219,286] Partly, this may stem from the relatively large effect of eating on plasma triglyceride levels. Large epidemiology studies for the most part have used fasting samples. Another more recently identified lipid is lipoprotein (a) (Lp(a)).[301,312] This particle is similar to LDL, with the addition of apo (a), a unique protein component similar in structure to a protein associated with clot lysis.[228] Although plasma levels of Lp(a) appear to be important in defining risk,* the role of diet is probably rela-

*References 100, 204, 220, 262, 283, 291, 294, 300.

tively small because plasma levels appear to be, for the most part, genetically regulated.[263] Therefore, at this time, the key role for diet from the standpoint of plasma lipids appears to be related to the regulation of plasma LDL-cholesterol and HDL-cholesterol levels, as reviewed subsequently.

A second area of interest concerns the plasma levels of oxidants and antioxidants because an hypothesis has been developed that suggests that modified (oxidized) LDL may be scavenged by monocytes and macrophages through LDL receptor–independent pathways, allowing the formation of foam cells and the accumulation of lipid during atherosclerosis.[306,307] Some evidence, reviewed subsequently, indicates that increased oxidant levels or decreased antioxidant levels may contribute to this process.

Finally the relationship of plasma lipids to thrombosis has been a subject of interest. Evidence has identified three of the proteins important in the formation and lysis of blood clots as risk factors: fibrinogen,* factor VII,[275-277] and plasminogen activator inhibitor-1 (PAI-1).[242,243] The plasma levels of factor VII and PAI-1 and, to a much lesser extent, fibrinogen are associated with the plasma levels of triglyceride and cholesterol, although the actual mechanism(s) underlying these associations remains unclear. For factor VII, there is some evidence that changes in postprandial lipid metabolism may be related to changes in plasma levels which, in turn, are related to thrombotic risk. Therefore, as discussed subsequently, diet may be related to the thrombotic component of CVD as well as the atherosclerotic component.

EPIDEMIOLOGY

In this section, we concentrate on international studies because the dietary data are strongest in these studies. There are reviews of several large American studies with limited dietary components, such as the Framingham study,[254] and there are several ongoing longitudinal studies, the incident disease data from which will be available during the next several years[205,232] (e.g., Cardiovascular Health Study; 5000 elderly men and women). Although not strictly dietary studies, some information on the relationship of diet to CHD will be available from these studies.

Virtually the entire distribution of serum cholesterol may be higher in one culture than in another.[209] Although such a difference may well have genetic components, diet plays a major role. The position that habitual diet (and attendant hyperlipidemia) is a major preventable cause of early CVD morbidity and mortality was initially strengthened by studies of Japanese and Finnish populations.[209,256,259] Even in the face of considerable hypertension (linked at least partly to salt intake) and cigarette smoking, there was a relatively small population burden of CHD in Japan before the 1970s. At this time, the Japanese diet had the highest carbohydrate

and lowest fat content of any industrialized country.[257] This was in contrast to the population of Eastern Finland, which has the highest rate of CHD mortality of any population group yet studied in detail. Hypertension and smoking in the Finns is not substantively different from other parts of Europe with much lower CHD rates, but the diet contains a much higher percentage of calories from saturated fat and cholesterol.[209]

Although early studies suggested a link between diet and cardiovascular disease,[222,310] this notion became popularized in the 1970s and 1980s owing to several large, multipopulation epidemiological studies. In particular, the Seven Countries Study observed large differences in CHD incidence across the 15 cohorts from the seven countries involved.[257,258] In these initial analyses, the incidence of CHD was associated with plasma cholesterol and blood pressure. In more recent evaluations 46% of the variance among cohorts in all-cause mortality, 45% of the variance in stroke mortality, and 80% of the variance in CHD mortality could be explained by differences in mean age, blood pressure, serum cholesterol, and smoking habits.

The cohorts had substantially different dietary habits.[258] The percentage of total calories supplied by fats ranges from 9% in the two Japanese cohorts to approximately 38% in the cohorts from the Netherlands, East Finland, and the United States. Saturated fatty acids supplied a low of 3% of total calories to the Japanese and a high of 24% of total calories to the men from East Finland, whereas the percentages of total calories supplied from monounsaturated fatty acids ranged from 3% in the Japanese to 26% in the Greek cohort from Crete. CHD death rates were related positively to the saturated fatty acid intake, negatively to the monounsaturated fatty acid intake, and negatively to the ratio of monounsaturated to saturated fatty acids. There was little or no indication that CHD mortality was related to protein, polyunsaturated fatty acid, or alcohol intake in this study. When the ratio of dietary monounsaturated to saturated fatty acids was included with the other variables in the multiple regression analysis, 96% of the variance in CHD mortality rates could be explained.[258]

The majority of the differences in monounsaturated fatty acids between cohorts could be explained by differences in oleic acid intake, primarily in the form of olive oil (approximately 80% oleic acid), with CHD mortality lowest in the cohorts with olive oil as the main dietary source of fat. Although there are other components in olive oil, this suggested a possible protective role for oleic acid.

A different approach has been taken by Connor and Connor.[217,218] Data on national food statistics and CHD deaths have been collected from 30 different countries by the World Health Organization and the Food and Agriculture Organization of the United Nations. These data have been used to calculate correlation coefficients in men aged 55 to 59 years (Table 9-6). These correlations indicate significant positive associations between CHD mortality rates and the

*References 253, 255, 275, 277, 308, 314, 318.

Table 9-6. Correlations between the mortality rates from coronary heart disease in men aged 55 to 59 years and the intake of certain nutrients in the diet

Positive correlations (P < 0.05)

Animal protein	0.782
Cholesterol	0.762
Meat	0.697
Total fat	0.676
Eggs	0.666
Sugar	0.638
Total calories	0.633
Animal fat	0.632

No correlations (P > 0.05)

Plant sterols	0.144
Fish	0.013
Vegetable fat	0.011
Vegetables	0.009

Negative correlations (P < 0.05)

Starch	−0.464
Vegetable protein	−0.403

From Conner W, Conner S: The key role of nutritional factors in the prevention of coronary heart disease, *Prevent Med* 1:49, 1972.

intake of animal protein and fat, among other variables. The data are especially compelling for cholesterol, with a correlation coefficient between cholesterol intake (mg/day) and CHD mortality of 0.83 for 24 countries.

An analysis has examined the so-called cholesterol/saturated fat index (CSI),[217] the latest attempt to calculate a summary variable that might explain the cholesterolemic and atherogenic potential of various foods. The CSI was calculated as follows:

$$CSI = (1.01 \times g \text{ saturated fat}) + (0.05 \times mg \text{ cholesterol}).$$

Using this formula, the CSI values for a variety of foods were calculated. For comparison purposes, some examples include (per 100 g, cooked if appropriate) salmon, 5; skinless poultry, 6; ground chuck, 13; cream cheese, 26. The CSI values, expressed per 1000 kcal/day, were then calculated for 40 countries based on food disappearance data from the Food and Agriculture Organization of the United Nations. The average national CSI values ranged from 5 in Egypt to 28 in New Zealand. CHD mortality data were obtained for these same countries from the World Health Organization and ranged from a low of 45 per 100,000 male population in Nicaragua to 1030 per 100,000 in Finland. The correlation between CSI and CHD mortality rate, shown graphically in Figure 9-8, was strong, with a correlation coefficient of 0.78.

The migratory data obtained during the Ni-Hon-San Study (*Nippon-Hon*olulu-*San* Francisco) are also relevant.* Japanese were studied simultaneously in Japan, Honolulu,

*References 252, 272, 273, 316, 317.

and mainland United States for differences in lifestyle and incidence of CVD. Based on a 24-hour recall dietary assessment, the differences in intake of total fat, saturated fat and several other dietary components were striking (e.g., percentage of calories from fat: Japan, 15%; Honolulu, 33%; United States, 38%). The incidence rate of CHD mortality was progressive across the Pacific, with an approximate tripling from Japan to San Francisco (for those 60 to 64 years old at death: 2.1 Japan, CHD deaths/1000; 3.9, Honolulu; San Francisco, 4.9). This study, using comparison populations with relatively restricted genetic diversity, strongly supports the position that diet can have a significant impact on CHD risk. Follow-up studies in the Honolulu cohort (the Honolulu Heart Study) have generally supported the importance of diet and lipid levels, even in this population with a relatively low rate of CHD incidence (approximately one half that of whites on the mainland United States); however, low-fat diets in the Honolulu cohort have been associated with greater all-cause mortality, bringing into question the wisdom of attempting to lower dietary fat intake in this group.[273,274]

The data collected by Dyerberg and colleagues[227] have addressed the Greenland Eskimo population, which is characterized by a habitual diet high in cholesterol but low in saturated fats and high in so-called omega-3 polyunsaturated fatty acids (such as eicosapentanoic acid and docosahexanoic acid), to a large degree owing to the consumption of fish. This population appears to have a relatively low CHD incidence rate, which has led to the speculation that the consumption of fish and, specifically, the consumption of the omega-3 fatty acids may be protective against cardiovascular disease. The data concerning fish consumption, however, must be related to the total dietary context. As reviewed by Nordoy and Goodnight,[287] the literature concerning fish consumption and incident CHD is inconsistent and probably reflects the effects of the other components of the diet. There are studies that appear to show no relationship between fish consumption and CHD and even some that show a negative relationship. None of the populations studied, however, had a habitual diet similar to that of the Eskimos, and several had diets high in saturated fats. The story is also complicated by the fact that, when people eat fish, they are not eating beef or other meats high in animal fat. Thus, it has been difficult to distinguish the direct effect of fish consumption from the effect of less animal fat in the diet. Nonetheless, it appears that fish is an excellent substitute for animal meat in the diet and, depending on the other dietary components, may have antiatherosclerotic and antithrombotic effects as well.

One study has explored the relationship of serum cholesterol to CHD in Chinese men and women, a population with low serum cholesterol values by Western standards.[215] It is reasonable to presume that at least part of the reason for low cholesterol values in the Chinese is their traditional low-fat diet. It was discovered that there was a significant,

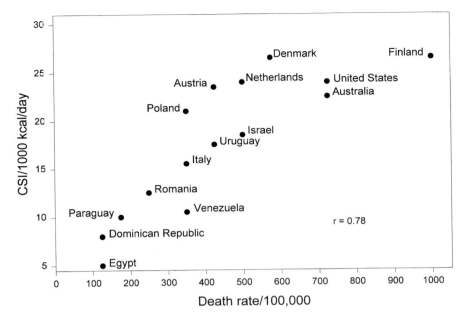

Fig. 9-8. The age-adjusted death rates from ischemic heart disease compared with the cholesterol/saturated fat index (CSI) per 1000 kcal in selected countries expressed per 100,000 population in men aged 55 to 64, 1977. The cholesterol (mg/day) and saturated fat (g/day) were computed from food balance sheets of the Food and Agricultural Organization for 1975-77. (Modified from Connor S et al: The cholesterol/saturated fat index: an indication of the hypercholesterolemic and atherogenic potential of food, *Lancet* 1:1229, 1986; with permission.)

statistically independent relationship between serum cholesterol values and CHD throughout the range of values seen. This implies that there may be benefit in lowering cholesterol, regardless of the starting cholesterol value. More work is needed in this area because several studies seem to indicate that low cholesterol values may be associated with an increased risk for non-CHD death, and lowering cholesterol levels in some populations may have unwanted side effects.[249,281]

DIETARY INTERVENTION

One of the largest intervention trials was the Multiple Risk Factor Intervention Trial (MRFIT), a study designed to test the effect of modifying three major risk factors: smoking, hypertension, and hypercholesterolemia.[282] The participants in MRFIT (middle-aged men at increased risk for CHD) were randomized into experimental and control groups, with the experimental group receiving counseling and support for risk factor modification. Although significant reductions in the three risk factors were accomplished in the experimental group, there were also unexpectedly large reductions in the controls. The overall effect of serum cholesterol reduction was not statistically significant, primarily because of the unexpected reduction in risk in the control group. In one subsequent analysis, however, the MRFIT investigators demonstrated that in both experimental and control groups, CHD mortality was associated with a lower decrease in serum cholesterol; that is, those individuals (whether control or experimental) that demonstrated the greatest reduction in cholesterol were the individuals at the lowest risk for CHD.

Although not strictly a dietary intervention study, a second study worth examining is the Lipid Research Clinics Coronary Primary Prevention Trial (LRC-CPPT), which used the drug cholestyramine in an attempt to lower cholesterol levels in hyperlipidemic men.[265] With an average of 7.4 years of follow-up, the LRC-CPPT investigators reported a 19% reduction in risk ($P \leq 0.05$) of CHD death or nonfatal myocardial infarction (the primary end point), illustrating the usefulness of cholesterol lowering. Similar to the LRC-CPPT, the Helsinki Heart Study also demonstrated a positive benefit to medical lipid lowering, using the drug gemfibrozil.[231,268] With an average of 8% lower total and LDL-cholesterol levels and 10% higher HDL-cholesterol levels, the gemfibrozil group had approximately 34% fewer CHD events than the placebo group. Both the LRC-CPPT and the Helsinki Heart Study were among the first clinical trials to suggest the added benefit of HDL elevation.

Increased dietary fiber has been examined in several studies.[223,230] As is the case with fish consumption, it has been difficult to distinguish between the direct and indirect effects of a high fiber, i.e., between any benefit caused by fiber displacing other more cholesterogenic foods in the diet versus a direct effect of fiber on cholesterol metabolism. A recent study has examined the effect of relatively large amounts of soluble versus insoluble ("lipid-neutral") fiber on biochemical risk factors in a diet already low in saturated fat and cholesterol.[248] A direct benefit of soluble fiber was seen, with blood cholesterol levels being lowered by approximately 5%. There was also a lowering of HDL-cholesterol levels, however, and the overall effect on CHD risk of the fiber component in a high-fiber, low saturated fat/cholesterol diet remains to be established.

Dietary interventions designed to increase intake of omega-3 fatty acids in patients with hypertriglyceridemia have often shown a benefit with respect to lipid profile, principally decreased VLDL and plasma triglyceride levels.[239,289,309,311] Although there are other considerations that may still warrant the use of fish oil supplementation in persons without hypertriglyceridemia,[207,240,264,287] more research is required to reach a firm conclusion on this issue. Several studies have examined the effect of lipid lowering on the progression of atherosclerosis, and have identified a benefit.[210,211] A comprehensive review by Yusuf and colleagues[320] summarized 22 randomized trials of lipid lowering by either dietary intervention or medication, looking at the effect on nonfatal myocardial infarction plus cardiac death, with a total of 40,000 subjects involved. An average 23% reduction in risk was found, with a direct relationship to the duration and extent of cholesterol lowering that was achieved. No apparent heterogeneity in the effect on CHD risk of lowering cholesterol was found, whether intervention was dietary or medical. Although there has been no consistent effect on overall mortality, a beneficial effect of lipid lowering on CHD morbidity and mortality seems likely. Benefits have been proposed for cholesterol lowering in young adults because the cholesterol level at a young age appears to predict CHD in middle age,[260] and cholesterol has been linked to CHD events in the elderly as well.[321] Finally, as has been pointed out by Rifkind and colleagues, there is also a likely benefit in lowering cholesterol levels following myocardial infarction in an effort to reduce the incidence of repeat heart attacks.[296] In all of the afore-mentioned scenarios, appropriate dietary modification seems likely to be of the greatest public health benefit because this route of lipid lowering is more universally available than medical intervention.

Not all reviews of the effectiveness of cholesterol lowering in preventing CHD have come to the same conclusions, with some offering the view that the data are not compelling, especially if mortality and not simply CHD events is used as the primary end point.[281] A general review of this question, however, has been published as a joint statement of the American Heart Association and the National Heart, Lung and Blood Institute.[241] This is not reviewed in detail here except to say that these groups believe that the data strongly support the benefits of cholesterol lowering, by diet if possible and by medical therapy if required.

PROPOSED MECHANISMS LINKING PLASMA LIPIDS TO ATHEROSCLEROSIS

The previous discussion presents the epidemiological and clinical trial data in support of the association of plasma lipid levels, as influenced by diet (among other factors), and CVD. The mechanisms that might actualize this link are less clear. The ground-breaking work of Brown, Goldstein and colleagues[212] demonstrated in biochemical terms that several lifestyle and heritable factors may lower the LDL receptor levels and raise the serum LDL-cholesterol concentration. In this way, LDL receptor regulation may be

linked to CHD risk through elevated serum lipid levels. The mechanisms by which elevated serum lipids may cause CHD, however, remain to be elucidated. There are several possible links, including obesity and hypertension. We concentrate here, however, on the evidence for a direct link to atherosclerosis.

The original "response to injury" model of Ross has remained the primary hypothesis being pursued by researchers in this field. Although the current version of this model focuses on the roles of growth and differentiation factors, such as platelet-derived growth factor (PDGF), it does list many possible "injuries," including not only physical damage, but also biochemical abnormalities.[295] In this model, plasma lipids play a role if taken up by macrophages (and possibly other cells) in a nonreceptor-mediated manner. Such lipid uptake would not participate in the regulation of LDL receptors, and because the lipid would not be metabolized in the normal manner, it might lead to the production of foam cells, key cellular "players" in atherogenesis and atherosclerotic progression. One development in this area is the recognition that there may be modified forms of plasma lipids, including oxidized LDL particles, which are taken up by macrophages and monocytes by just such a receptor-independent mechanism (Fig. 9-9).[306,307] It is clear that oxidized LDL may be taken up by the scavenger (or acetyl LDL) receptor,[238,246,307] thereby bypassing normal LDL receptor–mediated metabolism; that some LDL oxidation occurs in vivo;[288] and that oxidized LDL may be present in atherosclerotic lesions in experimental animals and in humans.[319] The primary hypothesis is that the higher the LDL concentration in plasma and the longer the LDL resides in plasma, the greater the level of modified LDL and the greater the risk of atherosclerotic development through the receptor-independent uptake pathway.[306,307]

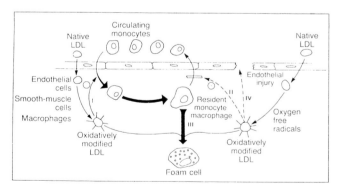

Fig. 9-9. Mechanisms by which oxidized low-density lipoprotein *(LDL)* may contribute to atherosclerosis: (1) Oxidized LDL acts as a chemoattractant to circulating monocytes; (2) inhibition of macrophage mobility, forcing increased residence in the intima; (3) scavenger-receptor-mediated uptake of LDL by resident monocyte/macrophage; (4) cytotoxicity of oxidized LDL. (From Steinberg D et al: Beyond cholesterol: modifications of low density lipoprotein that increase its atherogenicity. *N Engl J Med* 320:915, 1989; with permission.)

This hypothesis has led many to attempt to measure the oxidized LDL concentration in plasma, a difficult measurement to make for technical reasons. Nonetheless, there are many attempts underway in epidemiological studies with the goal of establishing whether or not this form of "injury" is relevant to clinical CHD.

Consistent with this model, several research groups are currently exploring the hypothesis that increased plasma oxidants or decreased plasma antioxidants are risk factors for CHD. Either condition might be expected to be associated with increased potential to form oxidized LDL and lead to atherosclerotic progression. Plasma metals have been explored as oxidants, and there are compelling data available that establish the fact that copper and iron can oxidize LDL in the presence of human cells in tissue culture.[245] Reports have indicated that high levels of both plasma iron and copper are associated with increased risk for CVD.[290,297-299] These reports, however, have not always been consistent with older literature (for example, the work of Klevay[261] indicating that low copper may be atherogenic) and need to be substantiated by further work.

Concerning plasma antioxidant levels, research has focused on vitamins E and C and β-carotene. Two large, prospective epidemiological studies are noteworthy. The first assessed vitamin E intake, both dietary and supplemental, in 87,245 female nurses aged 34 to 59.[304] Follow-up with questionnaires occurred at 2-, 4-, 6- and 8-year intervals. When CHD was assessed (nonfatal myocardial infarction or CHD death), there was a strong statistical relationship between vitamin E intake and reduced risk when intake included supplements. If only dietary intake was examined, there was no statistical significance. After age and smoking adjustments, those women in the highest quintile of total vitamin E intake had a relative risk of 0.66 (95% confidence interval = $0.50 - 0.87$; $P \leq 0.001$) compared with those in the lowest quintile. Most of the effect, however, was seen in this highest quintile. Similar results were seen in a study of 39,910 male health professionals, followed from 1986, aged 40 to 75 years at baseline.[292] In addition, this study also examined β-carotene and vitamin C intake. A significant effect was seen for β-carotene in smokers and former smokers, but no effect was observed for vitamin C, either in the total population studied or in any subgroup.

A reasonable conclusion at this point is that there are compelling epidemiological data but little or no clinical trial data to support antioxidant supplements in healthy individuals. Moreover the data that are available tend to support the use of relatively large doses of supplemental vitamins and do not seem to indicate that dietary modifications can be effective.

PROPOSED MECHANISMS LINKING PLASMA LIPIDS TO THROMBOSIS

Most CHD events have thrombosis as their proximal cause.[224] Thrombus formation is stimulated by a procoagulant surface, e.g., an ulcerated atherosclerotic plaque, which has several active components: exposed collagen and von Willebrand factor, adenosine diphosphate liberated from damaged cells and activated platelets, and tissue factor elaboration by damaged cells.

Recently, Fuster and colleagues,[233-235] Woolf and Davies,[315] and Chandler[214] have reproposed the original hypothesis of von Rokitansky,[293] Mallory,[266] Clark and colleagues[216] and Duguid[226] (see Chandler[214] for a brief review) that thrombosis may be involved with atherosclerotic development as well as with precipitating the clinical event. It appears likely that platelet and monocyte adherence to "damaged" endothelium may be an early event in atherogenesis,[236,237,295] an event similar to the adherence events that play a role in thrombosis and coagulation. Additional thrombosis comes later, at the site of ulceration of a lipid-rich atherosclerotic plaque[208,233,303]

The potential for dietary regulation of thrombosis is not well understood, but dietary lipids have been linked to thrombosis in several ways: (1) dietary saturated and monounsaturated and polyunsaturated fats may affect platelet function, (2) plasma triglyceride levels (i.e., VLDL and chylomicron particles) may affect factor VII activity, and (3) fibrinolysis appears to be inhibited in hypertriglyceridemic individuals.

The effect of saturated and polyunsaturated fatty acids on thrombosis is not yet clear.[243,264,287] Dietary and supplemental omega-3 fatty acids such as eicosapentanoic acid and docosahexanoic acid may affect thrombotic potential by one of several mechanisms. They may inhibit thromboxane A_2 production in platelets, leading to a decrease in platelet reactivity[240,313]; they may alter plasma lipoproteins, which may, in turn, have an effect on platelets directly or through thrombin generation (see later); or they may alter the lipid composition of the platelet membrane,[225,264] a structure critical for proper coagulation function.[267] The overall effect of omega-3 fatty acids is readily observed in the Greenland Eskimos, with their well-documented (and readily reversible) easy bruisability and prolonged bleeding times.[227,240,264,287] To show effects on bleeding time and other platelet parameters, dietary supplement studies have used relatively large doses of fish oil (3.6 g/day or more) for several weeks. It is not yet clear whether relatively minor diet modifications, such as substituting fish for animal meat one to two times per week, can have a significant effect on platelet function.

It has been demonstrated in several studies that factor VII activity, as assessed in a so-called one-stage clotting assay, may be affected by fat intake both in the short term (postprandially)[279] and over a longer period of time.[271,278] The composition of the fat in the diet does not seem to be of as much importance as the quantity of fat.[279] Also, it has been clearly established that in normal populations[229,275] and in populations of individuals at risk for cardiovascular disease,[221,247,280] there are associations between factor VII and plasma levels of triglyceride and cholesterol. The bivariate correlation coefficients are in the range of 0.3 to 0.4, depending on the study. Because factor VII has been reported to be an independent risk factor for CHD,[275,277] this finding may have clinical relevance. The majority of work concerning fat intake, however, has been done by one group of investigators and must be reinforced by others in the field.[244,302] In three studies reported by Marckmann and colleagues[269,270] factor VII was observed to respond to some high-fat diets but not others, which, in contrast to the results already mentioned, seems to indicate a dependence on the type of fat in the diet as well as the quantity. It seems appropriate to consider this a provocative but unresolved issue.

Finally, hypertriglyceridemia has also been associated with increased values of the antifibrinolytic protein, PAI-1, and decreased fibrinolytic potential.[202,250,251] Dietary intervention has been shown to be effective in improving fibrinolytic activity in hypertriglyceridemic individuals.[203] The exact mechanism, however, remains unknown.[243,242,284]

Vitamin A, retinoids, and carotenoids: their role in infection and cancer prevention

John E. Craighead

Xerophthalmia, the pathognomonic lesion of nutritional vitamin A deficiency, has been recognized for centuries. (see Chapter 37).[333] It continues to be a major public health problem in developing countries. According to Sommer and colleagues,[343] more than 5×10^6 Asian children develop xerophthalmia annually, and about 5% of these ultimately become blind as a complication. The association of night blindness (hemeralopia)[346] (Fig. 9-10) and xerophthalmia was recognized in 1862 by Bitot, a French physician whose name is now linked with the punctate, granular lesions of the cornea (Bitot's spots) typically found in hypovitaminosis A.[322] After the turn of the century, Mori[334] associated xerophthalmia with the fat-deficient diets of Japanese children. The recognition of vitamin A as a critical dietary component dates from 1913, when certain fats were shown to contain an essential nutrient that affected growth of rats and promoted the development of typical lesions in the external eye.[329] In 1933, Wohlbach and Howe[351] documented the development of squamous metaplasia in the mucociliary epithelium of the respiratory mucosa in vitamin A–deprived rats. This work was followed by the demonstration of similar histological changes in the genitourinary system and various accessory glands of the digestive tract of rats. These histological features uniquely simulated the finding observed in the internal organs of children with clinical hypovitaminosis A and the histological features of the conjunctiva and cornea in xerophthalmia.[324] In the discussion

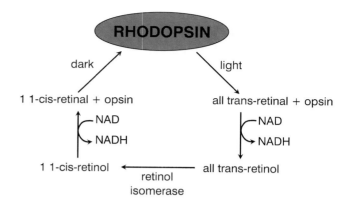

Fig. 9-10. Night vision, specifically, is dependent on vitamin A metabolism in the retinae. Circulating *trans*-retinol is isomerized and dehydrogenated enzymatically in the rod cells to 11-*cis*-retinol, which in turn reacts with the ϵ-amino moiety of lysine to form rhodopsin. Light initiates photoisomerization back to all *trans*-retinol, thus reactivating the cycle. *NAD*, Nicotinamide-adenine dinucleotide; *NADH*, nicotinamide-adenine dinucleotide (reduced form).

Major sources of preformed vitamin A and carotenoids	
Major sources of carotenoids	*Major sources of preformed vitamin A*
Carrots	Liver
Spinach	Breakfast cereal, typical
Tomatoes	Margarine
Yellow squash	Hard cheese
Broccoli	Eggs
Orange juice	Butter
Mixed peas and carrots	
Cantaloupe	
Tomato paste, sauce	

that follows, I do not address further the clinical features of hypovitaminosis A, which are adequately considered elsewhere. Rather attention focuses on the more contemporary, new information that relates vitamin A deficiency to development of certain cancers and infections in humans.

β-carotene, a provitamin, is derived from numerous dietary sources, the most common of which are yellow and leafy vegetables (see box above). It is the most biologically active member of a family of carotenoids in plant tissue, only some of which have recognized significant human health importance.[337] Carotenoids endow chicken fat and egg yolks with their characteristic color; these pigments are not believed to be otherwise biologically active. Vitamin A is derived from animal tissues and products (Table 9-7) but is formed from β-carotene as it is absorbed from the gut wall (Fig. 9-11). At this site, it is converted into two molecules of vitamin A_1, i.e., retinol, an alcohol that

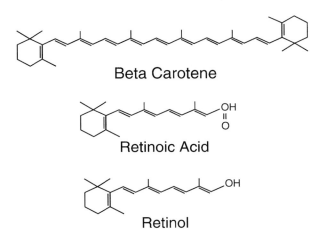

Beta Carotene

Retinoic Acid

Retinol

Fig. 9-11. β-carotene is metabolized to retinoic acid (vitamin A) in the gut and hydrolyzed to retinol in the liver.

is the active form in vivo. It is carried by retinol-binding proteins and is stored primarily in the liver and other fatty organs as retinyl ester. Serum levels of vitamin A bound to a retinol-binding protein (RBP) do not serve as a measure of vitamin A nutritional status (except in extreme deficiencies) because regulation of the serum concentration is through the liver stores of the vitamin and the synthesis of RBP in the liver.[344]

As shown by Wohlbach and Howe 60 years ago,[351] retinol dramatically influences epithelial differentiation. In the interim period, an enormous body of experimental information has accumulated that documents the essential role of retinol and its derivatives in the regulation of cell growth, differentiation and morphogenesis, and in embryogenesis. Retinol and a family of synthetic commercial compounds known as retinoids are now known to act as direct transcriptional activators controlling a myriad of regulatory target genes.[347] In doing so, retinol exhibits a mode of action similar to that of steroid and thyroid hormones. Indeed the retinol nuclear receptors belong to the steroid/thyroid superfamily.[326] In addition, these compounds have posttranscriptional effects and interact with other signal transduction pathways. In the respiratory mucosa, regulation of proliferation and differentiation by retinol appear to be separate phenomena.[328] Specifically, retinol and its derivatives act by stopping proliferation and initiating terminal differentiation, the end result of which is the development of the normal mucociliary epithelium.[341] Contrarywise, in the absence of retinol, basal cell proliferation accelerates, and the squamous phenotype is expressed. The end result of this process is squamous metaplasia (Fig. 9-12).

BRONCHOGENIC CARCINOMA

Epidemiological studies indicating a role for carotenoids and vitamin A in the natural history of cancer largely have focused on their role in the development of bronchogenic

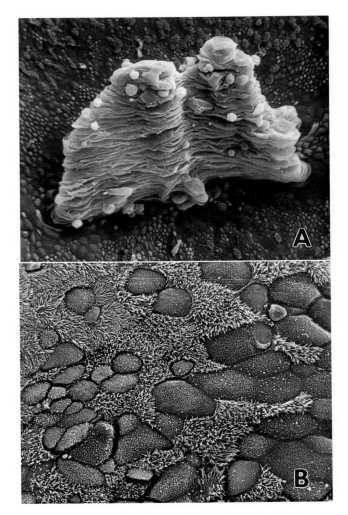

Fig. 9-12. A, Scanning electron micrograph of localized area of squamous metaplasia developing in an organ culture of a hamster trachea maintained in a highly enriched medium lacking vitamin A. Note the laminated flakes of squames, which characterize this lesion. **B,** Normal respiratory mucosa. Note the mixture of mucus-secreting and ciliated cells. (Courtesy of Craig Woodworth, Ph.D.)

carcinoma. In 1975, Bjelke[323] reported that the relative risk for developing lung cancer among male smokers (and former smokers) who consumed above-average amounts of vitamin A was only 0.4 in comparison with age-matched men whose intake was less than average (Table 9-7). This observation triggered additional studies among larger groups of men (smokers and nonsmokers) in the United States and abroad that demonstrated the ameliorating effect of dietary carotenoid consumption (but not retinol) on the occurrence of lung cancer (Fig. 9-13). Case control studies have yielded similar results as summarized in Table 9-8. In these investigations, consumption of carotenoids appeared to affect the development of both squamous carcinomas and adenocarcinomas; no information is available regarding the effects on anaplastic small cell carcinoma.

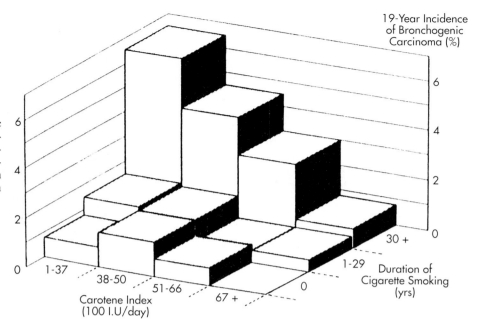

Fig. 9-13. Association of bronchogenic carcinoma with dietary intake of carotenoids in relation to cigarette consumption. (From Shekelle RB et al: Dietary vitamin A and risk of cancer in the Western Electric Study, *Lancet* 2:1186, 1981; with permission.)

Table 9-7. Rates of lung cancer among men with indices of high and low vitamin A dietary intake

Cigarette smoking status	Rate of lung cancer/*	
	≤5	≥5
Ever smoked	10.6	4.2
Current smoker, >20 cigarettes/day	21.0	7.4
Current smoker, 1 to 19 cigarettes/day	12.8	5.7
Ex-smoker	6.1	1.5
Never smoked	1.1	1.2

Adapted from Bjelke E: Dietary vitamin A and human lung cancer, Int J Cancer 15:561, 1975.
*Age adjusted 5-year cumulative index/1000 men.

Again, preformed vitamin A had no demonstrable influence, for reasons that remain unexplained.

The studies summarized here have several clearly evident shortcomings, the most important of which is the inability of the investigators to exclude effects of other possible dietary constituents or deficiencies. Similarly, subtle socioeconomic or lifestyle influences on outcomes are possible considerations. Dietary histories cannot readily be adapted to assess dosage effects, a clear requirement for establishing cause and effect relationships. To address these shortcomings, investigators next focused on attempts to correlate serum levels of retinol with cancer incidence. Although early studies provided provocative evidence, the work overall failed to establish a relationship.[349] In retro-

Table 9-8. Results of selected case control studies comparing lung cancer prevalence among persons with relatively high and low dietary consumption of carotenoids and preformed vitamin A as determined by dietary history

Sex	Reference and specifics	Relative risk	
		Vitamin A	Carotenoids
F	Pisani et al[338]	0.4	0.3
F	Wu et al[352]		
	Adenocarcinoma	0.8	0.4
	Squamous cell carcinoma	1.0	0.7
M	Ziegler et al[353]	1.3	0.8
M	Gao et al[330]	—	0.45
M/F	Byers et al[325]		
	Male	—	0.6
	Female	—	0.8
M/F	Jain et al[332]		
	Male	1.3	0.95
	Female	0.9	0.95
	Adenocarcinoma	1.2	0.85
	Squamous cell carcinoma	1.1	0.85
M/F	Samet et al[339]		
	White	1.1	0.7
	Hispanic	1.7	1.1

spect, this is not surprising because serum retinol concentrations (except in overtly vitamin A–deficient individuals) do not directly reflect dietary intake but rather regulation mediated by the liver and RBP.

One is obliged to conclude that an association exists between the dietary intake of carotenoids in orange and green leafy vegetables and the development of bronchogenic carcinoma. To date, however, the hypothesis that carotenoids play a prophylactic role remains to be tested in rigorously designed field trials in which the effect of dietary supplementation is tested.

Although chronic cigarette smoking is the major cause of metaplastic changes in the human respiratory epithelium, other exogenous inhalants such as asbestos are believed to have similar effects. Studies by the writer and his colleagues demonstrated the experimental induction of squamous metaplasia of the tracheobronchial mucosa by exposure to fiberglass (Fig. 9-14). Interestingly, the process was reversed by the synthetic retinoid, retinyl methyl ether.[335] In this model, basal cell replication was dramatically increased by the exogenous stimulus and similarly reversed by the retinoid. Susceptibility of rapidly multiplying cells (in comparison to a static cell population) to the carcinogenic effects of polycyclic aromatic hydrocarbons is known to be increased. The effect of vitamin A on this dynamic process may be at least one mechanism accounting for the prophylactic influence of vitamin A in carcinogenesis.

INFECTION

Acute respiratory infections, measles, and diarrheal disease are major causes of mortality and morbidity among infants and young children in developing countries. In the context of this section, it is noteworthy that xerophthalmia is exceedingly common in these same populations, as has been shown in numerous field surveys. Although the actual association of infection with hypovitaminosis A defies calculation, the predisposing role of vitamin A deficiency is becoming increasingly apparent. The problem is exceedingly difficult to analyze because of the confounding influences of other deficiency conditions and the effect of diarrheal disease and infections, such as measles, on retinol body stores.[348]

In studies conducted in Indonesia and India during the late 1970s and early 1980s, long-term observations were made on the survival of preschool children using the clinical marker of xerophthalmia as a nutritional indicator. Serendipitously, it was found that children with mild xerophthalmia died at an accelerated rate, in comparison to those lacking eye disease. Moreover, the severity of the ophthalmological disease correlated directly with mortality.[331] Further analysis revealed a twofold greater incidence of nonfatal lower respiratory infections in those with eye disease. Recognizing the potential role of vitamin A deficiency in this phenomenon, Sommer[342] undertook controlled, prospective trials of vitamin A therapy in large numbers of preschool Indonesian children. Death occurred at a 50% greater rate among children not receiving therapy than

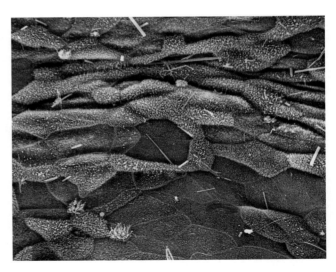

Fig. 9-14. Scanning electron micrograph demonstrating diffuse squamous metaplasia developing in an organ culture of a human trachea that was exposed to code 100 fiberglass. (Courtesy of Craig Woodworth, Ph.D.)

among treated subjects. The overall reduction in mortality attributable to vitamin A supplementation in six Asian studies was 34% (Fig. 9-15).

Common encapsulated bacterial pathogens (*Haemophilus influenzae* and *Streptococcus pneumoniae*) are the usual causes of pneumonia in the children in the study groups discussed previously. Although the causes for increased susceptibility to infection and ultimate mortality are not fully defined, the evidence clearly suggests that the epithelial changes in the respiratory mucosa of the child with hypovitaminosis A are an important factor.[324] Immune consideration also may contribute, as suggested by experimental studies that have documented depressed cell-mediated and humoral immune responsivity in vitamin A–deficient animals.[336,348] It has long been recognized that small animals with induced deficiencies exhibit an increased susceptibility to infection. Indeed, pneumonia commonly results in the death of these animals.[350]

Diarrheal disease shares with respiratory infections an ominous role as a major cause of mortality among children in developing countries throughout the world. At least in some field studies, children with diarrhea are twice as likely to exhibit the features of xerophthalmia as those without a history of diarrhea.[327] The association overall, however, is not as well established, possibly owing to the multifactorial nature of diarrheal disease. Urinary tract infections commonly have been observed in children with xerophthalmia, but an epidemiological association has yet to be established. One might envision that squamous metaplasia of the urinary tract epithelium in vitamin A–deficient children predisposes to these infections.

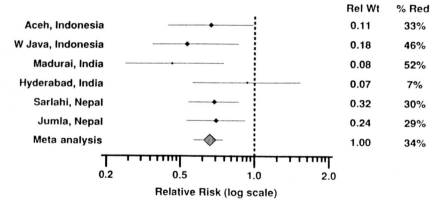

Fig. 9-15. Relative risk among children (0.5 to 6 years of age) in six different studies conducted in Asia to determine the influence of dietary supplementation with vitamin A on overall mortality. A meta-analysis of the data also is shown. Overall mortality in these children (which can largely be attributed to respiratory infections and diarrhea) was reduced 34%. (From Sommer A: Vitamin A, infectious disease, and childhood mortality: a 2¢ solution? *J Infect Dis* 167: 1003, 1993; with permission.)

Vitamin D deficiency

Laura H. McArthur

Rickets is a systemic disease of the growing skeleton characterized by defective mineralization of bone matrix and epiphyseal cartilage.[366] The features of rickets can vary between climatic zones.[356] The biochemical indicators of rickets are hypocalcemia, subnormal serum 25-hydroxycholecalciferol concentrations, secondary hyperparathyroidism, and elevated serum alkaline phosphatase activity. In moderate and severe cases, the skeleton becomes demineralized, and the child exhibits the clinical signs of rickets, including craniotabes; persistently open fontanelles; frontal or parietal bossing; bowed legs; muscular hypotonia; and beading of the ankles, knees, wrists, and rib cage.[357,366,369] Demineralization of the ribs can impede the normal functioning of the pulmonary system, making the child vulnerable to respiratory infections. In addition, severe rickets can lead to tetany and convulsions. In addition to laboratory studies referred to previously, the diagnosis of rickets is generally based on clinical evidence of skeletal deformities or radiological findings indicating wide osteoid seams at the ends of long bones (Fig. 9-16)[356,365,366,377]. Hutchison and Bell[366] maintain that the diagnosis of rickets must be based on the simultaneous occurrence of wide osteoid seams and abnormal tetracycline labeling because wide osteoid seams can occur in the absence of defective skeletal mineralization in diseases associated with hyperthyroidism, Paget's disease, and primary hyperparathyroidism (Fig. 9-17). Tetracyclines are deposited as bands in bone at the mineralization front, and the fluorescent features are detected with a fluorescence microscope in histological sections of bone biopsy samples from the iliac crest. The diagnostic criteria used by clinicians in developing countries are inconsistent and depend largely on the availability of laboratory equipment and trained personnel.

Rickets is no longer a public health problem in developed countries except among African and Asian immigrants because of vitamin supplementation and food fortification programs, reduced air pollution, health education campaigns, and construction of less crowded housing projects in low-income neighborhoods.* Rickets, however, remains one of the major nutrient deficiency diseases in developing countries. Precise, current national or regional prevalence statistics are unavailable because most studies assessing the occurrence of rickets are based on cross-sectional data from clinics or hospitals located in urban areas and because of the lack of uniform diagnostic criteria.[356] In temperate regions, neonates and infants are most susceptible to rickets because they receive fewer hours of sunlight annually,[374,375,378] whereas in the tropics, rickets is seen in neonates, infants, young children, and adolescents.[356,363]

Shawky[381] reported an incidence of rickets of 45% to 60% among a sample of Egyptian children aged 6 to 24 months. High prevalence of rickets has also been reported in Ethiopia[354] and Nigeria.[379] Klasmer[370] has reported a high occurrence of rickets in Jerusalem, and Salimpour[380] diagnosed rickets in 15% of 82 children admitted to a hospital in Tehran. Hutchison and Shah[367] examined 659 children in northern India and noted that 24% had rickets. Rickets is still a common childhood disease throughout the People's Republic of China.[384] In northern districts, most cases are moderate or severe, whereas in southern districts, most cases are mild. Jelliffe[368] observed that rickets is widespread in South America, and Miller and Chutkan[376] reported a similar finding in Jamaica.

Rickets is primarily attributable to inadequate endogenous synthesis of vitamin D owing to restricted sun exposure and to low dietary intakes of vitamin D and/or calcium. Less frequently, rickets occurs as a consequence of disorders such as vitamin D–dependent rickets types I and II, intestinal malabsorption, and hepatic or renal dysfunction.[355,357] For bone mineralization to proceed normally, the concentrations of calcium and phosphate, alkaline phosphatase activity, and pH at the site of mineralization must be optimal. The processes of bone formation and skeletal

*References 357, 361, 364, 365, 374.

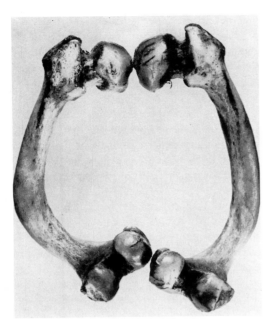

Fig. 9-16. Femoral deformities from a child dying with rickets. (From Follis RH: *Deficiency diseases*, Springfield, IL, Charles C Thomas, 1958; with permission.)

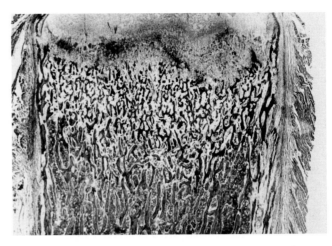

Fig. 9-17. Irregular zone of provisional calcification at the costochondral junction of a child dying with rickets. (From Follis RH: *Deficiency diseases*, Springfield, IL, Charles C Thomas, 1958; with permission.)

growth and remodeling are regulated by a complex interaction between systemic hormones, local cytokinin, prostaglandin, and vitamin D.[366] The metabolically active, hormonal form of vitamin D, 1,25-dihydroxycholecalciferol, promotes skeletal mineralization through the induction of calcium-binding proteins that facilitate intestinal absorption and renal reabsorption of calcium and excretion of excess phosphate.[355,371,383] Thus, any factors that adversely affect vitamin D status would ultimately contribute to disturbances in the plasma calcium-phosphorus ratio and to faulty skeletal development and maintenance.[359]

Cultural factors associated with the cause of rickets include the status of women in society, beliefs about the causes and prevention of illness, and infant and child feeding practices. In Moslem countries, especially in urban areas, women's activities are primarily confined to the home, offering them little sun exposure and compromising their vitamin D status. When women appear in public, they often observe the custom of the purdah or bordah, wearing the traditional veil and clothing that shields the body from view and from sunlight. Consequently, many of these women are deficient in vitamin D during pregnancy. Because fetal vitamin D and calcium status depend on placental transfer of these nutrients, their offspring, especially preterm infants, are frequently born rachitic.

Often in developing countries, when young children are taken outdoors, it is customary to wrap their bodies so no part is exposed to sunlight. Mothers in Saudi Arabia traditionally wrap their infants up to the age of 4 months before taking them outdoors in the belief that sunlight is unhealthy for infants.[360] In rural North Yemen, mothers believe they are protecting their offspring from the fatal consequences of the "evil eye" by wrapping their bodies.[382] In other cultures, lighter skin is considered more prestigious than darker skin; therefore, infants and young children are kept out of the sun. The consequence of severely restricting the amount of sunlight available to women, infants, and young children is that the initial step in the endogenous synthesis of vitamin D (the conversion of 7-dehydrocholesterol stored in the skin's melanocytes to cholecalciferol via ultraviolet (uv) irradiation) is blocked.[371] Several authors suggest that the degree of skin pigmentation is another factor linked to the cause of rickets.[355,358,373] These researchers contend that Asians and Africans typically have lower concentrations of serum 25-hydroxycholecalciferol relative to whites owing to the greater amounts of melanin in their skin, reducing the ability of uv light to irradiate the vitamin D precursor.

The dietary link to the cause of rickets is an inadequate intake of calcium and/or vitamin D by pregnant women, infants, and young children. Without the benefit of food fortification, it is difficult to obtain an adequate amount of vitamin D from the diet because food, including human and cows' milk, provides only small amounts of this nutrient. Infants living in rural communities in developing countries often are breast-fed for prolonged periods, making them vulnerable to rickets, especially if the mother's vitamin D status is inadequate. Lawson and colleagues[372] examined 54 rachitic Egyptian children and concluded that the practice of prolonged breast-feeding beyond 12 months probably exacerbated their suboptimal vitamin D status. Indian infants traditionally are breast-fed for at least 2 years; this practice contributes to the cause of rickets in India.[362] Commercial infant formulas and weaning foods generally are not fortified with vitamin D in developing countries.[355,372,374]

Henderson and colleagues[365] investigated the dietary factors associated with rickets among Asian children living in Great Britain and found that in all cases of severe rickets with deformity the child consumed a vegetarian diet high in phytate. These authors suggest that the avoidance or low intake of meat is strongly associated with Asian rickets, independent of other dietary considerations. Thus, meat may contain greater amounts of vitamin D than previously supposed, or, alternatively, it influences vitamin D metabolism in ways not yet understood. Okonofua and colleagues[377] assessed the diets of 11 Nigerian children and found that all rachitic patients had a calcium intake of less than 150 mg/day and a high phytate intake. These authors conclude that the cause of rickets in Nigeria is inadequate dietary calcium.

Environmental factors associated with the onset of rickets include crowded living conditions and air pollution. In urban residential neighborhoods where apartment buildings are close together, there is little opportunity for sunlight to penetrate into individual dwellings. The rachitic infants examined by Elidrissy[360] in Saudi Arabia lived in apartments or mud houses with high walls and small, high windows that allowed no direct access to sunlight. Underwood and Margetts[382] described similar living conditions among a group of rachitic children examined in rural North Yemen. Air pollution also reduces the amount of uv light available for endogenous vitamin D synthesis by absorbing the sun's rays before these can penetrate the skin.[356]

Even after the biochemical and radiological signs of rickets are corrected, some of the physical deformities, including frontal or parietal bossing, knock-knees, bowed legs, deformities of the thorax, and pigeon chest, may remain, along with poor linear growth.[356,369] The medical consequence of persistent defective skeletal mineralization for adults is osteomalacia, with its accompanying diffuse skeletal pain, weakness, muscle wasting, waddling gait, fractures in long bones, and loss of height. If untreated, osteomalacia may cause the individual to be confined to a wheelchair or bed.[366] The social and economic consequences for those afflicted by rickets and osteomalacia thus may include restricted physical activity and reduced productivity.

Folic acid deficiency

Richard F. Branda

Folate compounds are essential cofactors for nucleic acid and protein synthesis. Because mammalian cells are unable to synthesize the folate molecule, humans depend on dietary sources for this vitamin. Several large segments of the population have marginal intakes of folate. In addition, impaired absorption, increased metabolic requirements, and relatively small body stores contribute to the high incidence of folate deficiency worldwide. The most easily identified

clinical manifestation of folic acid deficiency is megaloblastic anemia. Because this disease is satisfactorily treated with small amounts of an inexpensive, essentially nontoxic nutrient, folic acid deficiency generally has been regarded as a diagnostic problem with little or no long-term sequelae. More recently, it has become clear that folic acid deficiency can have devastating but preventable effects on fetal development. There also is growing evidence that folate lack may play a role in carcinogenesis and tumor cell progression. These pathological effects are probably mediated by the alterations of DNA metabolism that are associated with folic acid deficiency.

Adults require approximately 1 μg per kilogram body weight of folate per day to maintain DNA metabolism.[399] The earliest indication of negative folate balance is a serum folate level below 3 ng/ml. Persistence of this negative balance for more than a few weeks usually results in reduced tissue folate stores, characterized by a red cell folate concentration below 160 ng/ml and low liver folate stores.[399] Negative folate balance for about 3 months eventuates in abnormal pyrimidine metabolism. Persistence of this process for another 2 months results in marked megaloblastic bone marrow changes and anemia.[385] Because folate compounds are needed by all dividing cells, clinical conditions characterized by increased cell growth, proliferation, or metabolism, such as pregnancy, hemolytic anemia, hyperthyroidism,[399] or cancer[385], may increase folate requirements by sixfold to eightfold.[399]

Food sources that are particularly rich in folate compounds include green leafy vegetables, liver, whole wheat products, nuts, and beans.[401] Because folate is heat labile, cooking reduces its bioavailability by 10% to 65%.[403] Evaluations of the total folacin content of composite Western diets suggest that it is difficult to attain consistently the RDA of 400 μg for adults and 800 μg for pregnant women and 600 μg for lactating women.[401]

Because body stores of folate are relatively limited and dietary intake of folacin is often marginal, folate deficiency is probably the most common vitamin deficiency in the United States and the rest of the world.[390] For example, NHANES II in the United States found that 18% of men and 15% of women, aged 20 to 44 years, had low serum folate levels (< 3.0 ng/ml), and 8% of men and 13% of women in the same age group had red cell folate levels less than 140 ng/ml.[412] Population groups with limited access to fresh fruits and vegetables, such as individuals in lower socioeconomic groups, particularly in northern climates, are at higher risk of folate depletion.[399] Nutritional surveys of pregnant women indicate that women who do not take supplemental folic acid have a high incidence of folate deficiency. Thus, in New York City, 22% of unselected pregnant patients had folate deficiency as evidenced by increased formiminoglutamic acid (FIGLU) excretion levels,[413] and in Birmingham, Alabama, 90% of pregnant adolescents had a dietary intake of folacin that was 50% of the RDA, and 52% took less than 10% of recommended folate.[391] Cancer patients are another group in which low blood folate levels are particularly common. For example, Magnus[407] described low serum folate levels in 85% of a series of patients with metastatic cancer.

Diets in many developing countries contain about 10% to 20% of the recommended allowance, and folate deficiency is predictably frequent.[410] In a rural black population in South Africa, 44% of pregnant women, 33% of nonpregnant women, and 19% of adult men were found to be folate deficient.[410] In some cultures, this propensity to folate deficiency can be traced to a change from traditional diets based on game and wild vegetation to food purchased at local stores or provided by government agencies. The latter diets often consist of maize supplemented with small, irregular quantities of meat and vegetables.[394]

Folate deficiency can occur despite an adequate dietary intake of the vitamin.[389] Intestinal disorders, such as celiac disease, tropical sprue, and short bowel syndrome, impair absorption. Various drugs interfere with the absorption or metabolism of folate compounds. Examples are anticonvulsants, oral contraceptives, and alcohol. Finally, there are rare inherited conditions that restrict metabolic utilization of folic acid.[389]

BIOCHEMICAL BASIS OF DISEASE

Dietary folate compounds are predominantly in polyglutamate form.[398] After ingestion, they are deconjugated, reduced, and methylated to 5-methyltetrahydrofolate in the small intestine.[398] This is the transport form of the vitamin, and it is incorporated into cells by a specific carrier-mediated membrane transport system. Soon after cellular uptake, 5-methyltetrahydrofolate is converted to

tetrahydrofolate, in a vitamin B_{12}–dependent step (Fig. 9-18). This interaction of folate and vitamin B_{12} metabolism accounts for the observation that deficiency of either vitamin results in identical megaloblastosis and abnormalities of DNA metabolism.[398] Simultaneously, homocysteine is methylated to methionine, some of which is incorporated into S-adenosylmethionine. Glutamic acid residues are added to tetrahydrofolate or one of its analogues intracellularly to form the active folate polyglutamate coenzymes. Various folate compounds then participate as cofactors for nucleic acid and protein synthesis (Fig. 9-19).

The principal biochemical abnormality that results in megaloblastosis is slowed DNA synthesis.[398] Measurements in folate-deficient cells showed that migration of the DNA replication fork and joining of Okazaki fragments are delayed.[416] Replication fork rate was 40% to 92% of the rate in control cells owing to impaired biosynthesis of DNA precursors.[416] Although nucleotide pool depletion has not been detected in human megaloblastic anemia,[416] there appears to be "functional compartmentation" of thymine nucleotides within the nucleus of S-phase cells.[414] Therefore, pools of nucleotides that are not available for replication may mask a deficiency of nucleotides for DNA synthesis.[414] Deoxynucleoside triphosphate pools are small, and compartmentalization can quickly restrict DNA synthesis. The reduced supply of one or more nucleotides probably impairs the cell's ability to elongate newly initiated DNA fragments by preventing gap filling.[400] In contrast to observations in humans, rats placed on folate-deficient diets have reduced cellular pools of both thymidylate monophosphate and triphosphate.[402]

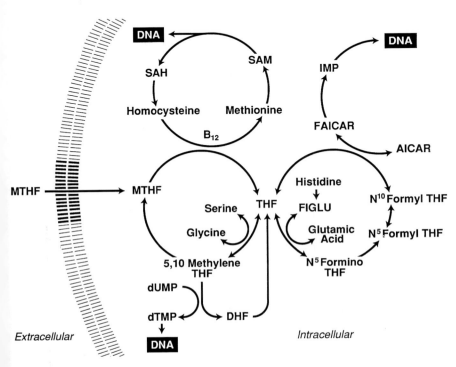

Fig. 9-18. Metabolic pathways that involve folate compounds. *MTHF,* 5-Methyltetrahydrofolate; B_{12}, vitamin B_{12}; *SAM,* S-adenosyl-L-methionine; *SAH,* S-adenosyl-L-homocysteine; *THF,* tetrahydrofolate; *dUMP,* deoxyuridylic acid; *dTMP,* thymidylic acid; *DHF,* dihydrofolate; *AICAR,* 5-amino-4-imidazolecarboxamide; *FAICAR,* formyl-AICAR; *IMP,* inosinic acid; *FIGLU,* formiminoglutamic acid.

CELL BIOLOGY

The principal clinical manifestation of folic acid deficiency is megaloblastosis. Although the cytological changes are most evident in the bone marrow, similar abnormalities occur in epithelial cells from the mouth, stomach, intestine, and uterine cervix. The megaloblastic cells are large, with a dysynchrony between nuclear and cytoplasmic maturation (Fig. 9-19). The bone marrow usually is hypercellular, but there is peripheral reticulocytopenia and varying degrees of pancytopenia. Laboratory manifestations of this ineffective myelopoiesis include

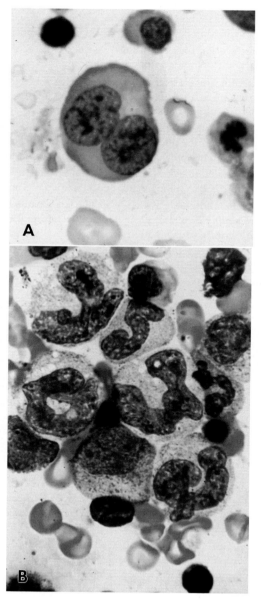

Fig. 9-19. Megaloblastic changes in human bone marrow cells. **A,** Abnormal neutrophil maturation with giant metamyelocytes. **B,** Red cell precursors showing delayed nuclear maturation with nuclear-cytoplasmic dysynchrony.

increased serum levels of unconjugated bilirubin and of lactate dehydrogenase (LDH).

Many of the studies that characterize the effects of folic acid deficiency on cell biology were performed on cultured cell lines that were often derived from tumors. Therefore, these observations should be applied cautiously to human subjects. The in vitro studies indicate that folic acid deficiency affects cellular proliferation, cell size, cell cycle traverse, and cell membrane properties and causes genetic damage (reviewed in Branda[387]).

In the absence of exogenous folate, cellular proliferation causes a progressive decrease of intracellular polyglutamyl folate levels. When folate pools are eventually depleted, cell doubling time lengthens. Initially this restriction of proliferation is reversible by the addition to the culture medium of either folic acid or the combination of thymidine and hypoxanthine (but not by either nucleotide singly). Proliferation then resumes at the same rate as before folate depletion. This observation does not support a clinical impression that folate repletion enhances tumor cell growth. If folate deficiency is prolonged, cell viability in culture eventually decreases. Nevertheless, even under the most stringent conditions of folate depletion, approximately 10% of cells survive.

Folate deficiency causes an increase in cell size both in patients and in in vitro systems. Measurements of cell volumes indicate that this increase occurs at about the time the deoxyuridine suppression test becomes abnormal and is progressive, as folate depletion becomes more severe, until growth arrest occurs. This change in cell size can be prevented by the addition of both thymidine and hypoxanthine.[387] Therefore, similar to restriction of cell proliferation, the increase in cell size appears to be mediated through an impairment of both pyrimidine and purine metabolism by folate deficiency.

Cell cycle analysis of bone marrow cells from patients with megaloblastic anemia shows prolongation of the S and G2 phases. There is evidence of DNA synthesis in later stages of cellular differentiation (myelocyte stage) than is seen in normal bone marrow. Studies in cell lines confirm that folate deficiency is accompanied by a delay in transit through S phase, resulting in an increased DNA and protein content per cell. Although the cells eventually move through the cell cycle, their viability declines unless they are rescued by supplementation with either folic acid or the combination of thymidine and hypoxanthine.

The development of folate deficiency in cell lines is accompanied by a change in membrane properties. For example, murine melanoma cells adhere more rapidly and in higher percentages to plastic or to plastic dishes coated with fibronectin or laminin. The observed increase in adherence does not appear to correlate with changes in cell cycle distribution, proliferation, or size. The addition of either thymidine or hypoxanthine modulates this effect of folate deficiency in Chinese hamster ovary (CHO) cells, suggesting that altered nucleotide pools are involved. In other experimental systems, disruption of mitochondria and endoplasmic reticulum has been described in folate-deficient rats, and abnormal erythrocyte membrane protein patterns have been reported in red cells from patients with either folic acid or vitamin B_{12} deficiency. Thus the changes in tumor cell adherence may be caused by alterations of membrane structure.

Folic acid deficiency in both humans and in cell lines is associated with several types of genetic damage. Karyotypic abnormalities are prominent. As many as one third of metaphases show chromosome breaks, gaps, acentric fragments, and dicentric forms. Centromere regions may be widely spread and cause chromatid breaks. Allocyclic chromosomes resulting from despiralization are present in 25% to 55% of lymphocyte metaphases and 40% to 70% of bone marrow metaphases in cells from patients with megaloblastic anemia. The extent of the karyotypic abnormalities is proportional to the severity of the megaloblastosis (see Chapter 20).

Incubation of human cells in folate-deficient medium can lead to expression of fragile sites. Probably the most frequent heritable cause of mental retardation in males is the fragile X syndrome. Karyotypic analysis of lymphocytes from affected individuals after culture in low folate medium shows a characteristic fragile site at the end of the long arm of the X chromosome at Xq28. Since description of the fragile X syndrome in 1979, other folate-sensitive fragile sites have been reported. Many of these fragile sites map close to breakpoints found in human cancers. It has been postulated that expression of fragile sites may predispose to malignancies, but this association remains to be proved. Fragile site breakage can lead to chromosome rearrangements. The latter observation suggests that the effects of folate deficiency may not be fully reversible with vitamin replacement and can lead to stable chromosomal abnormalities.

Bone marrow cells and peripheral blood lymphocytes from patients with megaloblastosis express a high rate of sister chromatid exchanges. These interchanges of DNA are useful to monitor mutagenesis. Oral folic acid therapy can reduce the frequency of sister chromatid exchanges, indicating that this manifestation of chromosome damage can be ameliorated by vitamin supplementation.

Studies in CHO cells, murine melanoma cells, and human fibroblasts indicate that folate deficiency is associated with DNA strand breaks, as detected by alkaline filter elution. The appearance of strand breaks coincides with the development of an abnormal deoxyuridine suppression test, and the breaks become more frequent with progressive deficiency. We have determined that folate deficiency in CHO cells caused DNA strand breaks equivalent to 26 cGy of gamma irradiation.[388]

It seems likely that the genetic damage associated with folate deficiency is caused, at least in part, by the effects of folate on nucleotide metabolism. DNA from HL60 leukemia cells grown in folate-deficient medium contained increased amounts of deoxyuridine. Misincorporation of uracil into DNA initiates excision by uracil N-glycosidase, which leaves an apyrimidinic site and strand breakage. Nucleoside supplementation of folate-deficient medium partially protects against cytogenetic abnormalities in CHO cells. Perturbation of nucleotide pools in mammalian cells leads to chromosome breaks and aberrations, chromatid gaps and breaks, and expression of fragile sites. Thus folate deficiency may represent a specialized case of the general phenomenon of chromosomal instability related to nucleotide pool imbalances.

TERATOGENESIS (see Chapter 34)

Experimentally induced folate deficiency in rodents causes fetal death or congenital malformations in 95% of newborns.[403] The latter have included abnormalities of the central nervous system, skeleton, great vessels, viscera, and eyes.[403] Studies in humans have shown that low blood folate levels correlate with low birth weight, and folate supplementation during pregnancy significantly increases birth weight.[403] Intrauterine growth retardation is associated with congenital malformations.[403] Inhibitors of folate metabolism, such as nitrous oxide (which acts by interfering with the vitamin B_{12}–dependent conversion of 5-methyltetrahydrofolate to tetrahydrofolate), methotrexate, and diphenylhydantoin, can cause fetal wastage and malformations. Mental retardation is common in patients with inborn errors of folate metabolism.[392] Epidemiological studies have shown that the incidence of neural tube defects (anencephaly, encephalocele, myelomeningocele, and spina bifida occulta) varies with socioeconomic group, season of the year, and during periods of poor maternal nutrition (war, economic depressions).[406] These studies suggest that environmental influences contribute to the risk of neural tube defects.

Most evidence now indicates that poor nutrition, particularly folate lack, is important in the cause of neural tube defects. The data supporting this conclusion come from both nutritional surveys and from vitamin intervention trials. For example, a dietary study performed in South Wales between 1969 and 1975 found that women with the poorest diets during the first trimester were most likely to have a pregnancy ending in a neural tube defect.[406] Recurrences of neural tube defects occurred only in those women who continued to have a poor diet. A case control study in the same area from 1974 through 1979 confirmed that recurrent neural tube defects were observed only in women who remained on an inadequate diet.[406] A case control study performed in Western Australia showed a protective effect of an increasing dietary intake of folate during the first 6 weeks of pregnancy.[386]

During the past 10 years, observational and interventional studies of folic acid and neural tube defects have generally supported the conclusion that folate supplementation reduces the risk of this congenital malformation.[409] Two case control studies (one in the United States and the second in Western Australia) found a 60% to 75% reduction in risk in women taking vitamin supplements before conception and during the first trimester, but a third from the United States did not find a protective effect.[409] A prospective cohort study performed in New England showed a 72% reduction in risk by use of a multivitamin and folate supplement.[409] Controlled trials of folate supplementation performed in Wales, Hungary, Cuba, and at multiple centers in the United Kingdom, have recorded effects varying from a 60% reduction in risk to complete protection.[409] The doses of folic acid used in these trials ranged from 0.36 g to 5 mg; no toxicity was reported from folate supplementation at these doses.

A case control study involving women in the United States and Canada looked at whether folate supplementation also could decrease the risk of first (as opposed to recurrent) neural tube defects.[415] Mothers of 436 infants with neural tube defects and 2615 controls were identified. Use of multivitamins containing folic acid during the period 28 days before conception to 28 days after the last menstrual period was associated with a dose-related decrease in risk according to quintile of intake. Women who took the dose of folic acid most commonly found in vitamin supplements (0.4 mg) had a relative risk of 0.3.[415] Previous studies have shown that the addition of multivitamins to folic acid does not confer additional protection.[409]

The mechanism by which folate supplementation decreases the risk of neural tube defects is unclear at present. Simple vitamin deficiency seems unlikely because measurements of serum and red cell folate and amniotic fluid folate levels have not been useful to identify women at risk or been associated with the occurrence of neural tube defects. Although it seems likely that the effect is mediated by altered DNA synthesis, other inhibitors of DNA metabolism have a less predictable influence on neural tube defects.[411] Patients with frank megaloblastic anemia do not have a higher proportion of infants with neural tube defects.[411] Consequently, it has been proposed that women at risk have an underlying abnormality of folate metabolism that predisposes them to producing a congenitally malformed infant when their dietary intake of folic acid is inadequate.[411]

DEVELOPMENT AND PROGRESSION OF MALIGNANCY (see Chapter 26)

Evidence exists that folate deficiency may be involved in the cause of some types of cancer. Clinical observations have suggested an increased risk of malignancy, particularly stomach cancer, in patients with pernicious anemia, which is caused by vitamin B_{12} deficiency but also disturbs folate metabolism. Analyses of large populations of patients with pernicious anemia in both the United Kingdom and the United States identified excesses of stomach cancer,

myeloid leukemia, head and neck cancers, melanoma, and multiple myeloma.

The possible role of folate in dysplasias of the uterine cervix, bronchus, and colon has been investigated. Folic acid supplementation of women taking oral contraceptives improved uterine cervical dysplasia scores (reviewed in Potischman[408]). Although a trial of folic acid supplementation for cervical dysplasia did not alter dysplasia status, patients with lower red cell folate levels tended to have a higher prevalence of human papillomavirus type 16 infection.[408] The authors concluded that folate deficiency may be involved as a cocarcinogen during the initiation of cervical dysplasia. Studies by other investigators have produced conflicting results. Some have described an inverse association between cervical intraepithelial neoplasia and serum and dietary folate, whereas others found no association between serum folate and risk of cervical cancer.[408] The role of folate appears to be more important in cervical dysplasia than in advanced lesions and may require interactions with other risk factors.[408]

Because cigarette smoke may inactivate folate and vitamin B_{12}, and smokers tend to have lower blood levels of these vitamins, patients with bronchial squamous metaplasia were randomly treated with either 10 mg of folate plus 500 μg of hydroxocobalamin or placebo.[397] Four months later, the supplemented group had significantly less atypia.[397] Histopathological studies of rat airways treated with methylcholanthrene showed that metaplasia, atypia of metaplastic cells, and hyperplasia with marked changes were less frequent in animals that received supplemental folate. The role of folate supplementation was investigated in a third type of dysplasia: the incidence of dysplasia and cancer in chronic ulcerative colitis. In a case control study, 35 patients with neoplasia were compared with 64 patients in whom dysplasia was never found. Folate supplementation was associated with a 62% lower incidence of neoplasia.[405] A case control study in western New York found a decreased risk of rectal cancer associated with dietary folate.[395] In addition, the risk associated with high alcohol intake and low folate ingestion was greater than the risk of either alone, suggesting an interaction.[395] In an analysis of adenomatous polyps in 15,984 women and 9490 men, Giovannucci and colleagues[396] observed that high dietary folate was inversely associated with the risk of colorectal adenoma. The combination of high alcohol ingestion and low folate was a particularly strong risk factor for small adenomas.[396] Of particular interest was the finding that the risk of adenoma formation increased at dietary levels of folate that were above those that cause megaloblastic anemia. These studies provide evidence that mild or moderate folate deficiency contributes to colorectal carcinogenesis. Investigations in rodents support this possibility. Folate-deficient rats had significantly more colonic dysplasia and carcinoma after exposure to dimethylhydrazine than folate-replete rats.[390] Rats that were folate-deficient but not exposed to carcinogen, however, did not have a higher incidence of neoplasia. The authors concluded that folate deficiency is not carcinogenic itself but increases the susceptibility to neoplastic transformation.[390] This conclusion supports the observations of Eto and Krumdieck,[393] who reviewed the role of folate and vitamin B_{12} deficiencies in carcinogenesis and noted that neither deficiency is carcinogenic by itself but that each increased susceptibility to the action of carcinogens.

Experiments in our laboratory are consistent with this interpretation. Mutant frequencies of 6-thioguanine–resistant CHO cells and of diphtheria toxin–resistant cells were not significantly increased by incubation in low folate medium.[388] Folate deficiency, however, increased the mutant frequencies of thioguanine-resistant cells about threefold and of diphtheria toxin–resistant cells 70% after exposure to alkylating agents. It appears likely, therefore, that folate deficiency alone is not mutagenic but that it acts synergistically with mutagens/carcinogens to increase genetic damage.[388]

Several mechanisms by which folate deficiency might promote carcinogenesis have been proposed (reviewed in Krumdieck[404]). They can be summarized as follows. (1) Folate coenzymes are required for de novo synthesis of methyl groups that are necessary to regenerate S-adenosylmethionine (SAM). Folate deficiency leads to decreased availability of methyl groups that are important for membrane signal transduction and DNA methylation. The latter function regulates gene expression and may cause activation of specific proto-oncogenes.[390,404] (2) Folate deficiency results in nucleotide pool perturbations, and this interferes with DNA synthesis and repair. (3) Folate deficiency prolongs the cell cycle time with accumulation of cells in S phase. These cells may be more vulnerable to initiating carcinogens. (4) Folate deficiency is associated with defective immune function and thereby may impair immune surveillance. These mechanisms are not mutually exclusive, and more than one may be operative.

There is evidence to suggest that folate deficiency also may affect the course of an established cancer. Folate-deficient murine melanoma cells produced more pulmonary and liver metastases than folate replete tumor cells (reviewed in Branda[387]). These differences were found with cell lines of both high and low metastatic potential. The increased metastatic potential of folate-deficient cells did not appear to be cell-cycle– or cell-size–dependent. Folate deficiency alters two other determinants of metastatic potential: genetic stability and membrane adhesion. A temporal relationship was found between increased DNA strand breaks and enhanced metastasis formation, suggesting that folate induced chromosome instability may contribute to potentiation of metastatic capacity.[387] Other investigators have shown that increased genetic instability promotes the generation of tumor cells with the capacity to metastasize by fostering diversity.

Diet and gastroesophageal cancers

Chung S. Yang, Wei-Cheng You

Gastroesophageal cancers are common diseases in many parts of the world. Gastric cancer is a leading type of cancer in the world.[443] About 6.7×10^5 new cases of gastric cancer are diagnosed each year around the world. Japan, Chile, Costa Rica, and the People's Republic of China currently have the highest gastric cancer mortality rates. The mortality rate among males in Japan exceeded 70 per 1×10^5 in 1985, which is eight times higher than the rate in North America. Gastric cancer mortality rates have decreased dramatically in most developed countries. Sixty years ago, gastric cancer was the leading cause of cancer among men and third among women in the United States. Presently, gastric cancer rates in the United States have dropped 80% to 90% and are among the lowest in the world.

Esophageal cancer mortality rate ranks sixth among all cancers worldwide[443] with an exceptionally high prevalence in Iran, central Asia, north China, and South Africa. In China, esophageal cancer accounts for about 22% of total cancer deaths. In China, esophageal squamous carcinoma and gastric cardia adenocarcinoma seem to occur together in many high incidence areas; whereas in the United States, these two cancers appear to have different time trends and racial distributions. In the United States, squamous esophageal cancer is considered to be a rare cancer among whites. The incidence rates of adenocarcinoma of the esophagus and gastric cardia, however, have risen sharply in the past few decades in the United States, especially among white men.[420,444]

The geographical distribution and time trend of gastroesophageal cancer incidence strongly suggest that diet is an important factor in affecting the rates of these cancers. It has repeatedly been shown that the intake of fresh fruits and vegetables is associated with reduced risk of esophageal, stomach, and other cancers.[446] This section considers the epidemiology and cause of gastroesophageal cancers with special emphasis on dietary factors.

GASTRIC CANCER

In most areas of the world, gastric cancer occurs about twice as often among males than females. It is inversely associated with socioeconomic status; the rate is approximately twice as high among lower than upper socioeconomic strata.[429] In the United States, blacks and Hispanics tend to have higher mortality rates than whites, possibly a reflection of socioeconomic differences. In the United States, immigrants from Japan and northern Europe experience a decrease in gastric cancer mortality over successive generations.[442]

Adenocarcinoma is the most common gastric neoplasia, accounting for 95% of gastric cancer. Gastric cancer is not equally distributed in the stomach. In high-risk areas, such as Japan, China, and Colombia, most tumors develop in the antrum or lower third of the stomach and in the lesser curvature of the stomach.[424,459] The intestinal histological pattern of adenocarcinoma predominates in areas where the gastric cancer mortality rate is high, especially among men and the elderly. The evidence suggests that the intestinal pattern of adenocarcinoma is a result of the transformation of gastric mucosa over many years in a multistep process; chronic atrophic gastritis and dysplasia are believed to be precancerous lesions.[424,459]

The causes of gastric cancer are not understood. The worldwide variation in mortality rates, declining rates in many countries, and the marked changes in death rates among immigrants strongly suggest that environmental factors play a major role. Dietary factors are likely to be paramount. N-nitroso compounds have received a great deal of attention.[424] Mutagenic and carcinogenic N-nitroso compounds are found in foods in some high-risk areas for gastric cancer.[424,457] The urinary excretion of N-nitroso compounds is higher in persons with advanced gastric precancerous lesions. Gastric juice pH and nitrite also increase with the increasing severity of the lesions.[418] According to Correa,[424] as the gastric pH rises, the prevalence of bacteria increases, and the bacteriocidal activity of the body results in higher concentrations of gastric juice nitrite. This in turn increases endogenous formation of N-nitroso compounds.

Excessive salt and salty food intake is considered to be a risk factor for gastric cancer.[424] High salt concentration, by irritating the gastric mucosa, may cause desquamation and atrophy, events that increase the risk of gastric cancer.[433,447] The widespread use of refrigerators in the United States since the 1930s may be partly responsible for the decline in gastric cancer rates, owing to a decrease in the consumption of salty and preserved foods and increased consumption of fresh vegetables and fruits.[442] In Japan, salt consumption has been significantly reduced in the past 20 years, and a decrease in the death rate from gastric cancer has been seen, beginning later than in the United States.

Chronic mucosal infection by *Helicobacter pylori* has been found to be associated with histological evidence of gastritis and with an increased risk of gastric cancer.[454] *H. pylori* is typically associated with what has been described as chronic superficial, chronic active, or chronic quiescent gastritis. Therefore, it is suspected that *H. pylori* may play a role in the early phases of the gastric cancer process.[419]

Cigarette smoking has been found to be a risk factor for gastric cancer in many, but not all, epidemiological studies of gastric cancer.[432,457] Smoking may also be responsible for progression to the (dysplasia) stage of gastric carcinogenesis.[432]

Both epidemiological and experimental studies consistently show that gastric cancer is strongly associated with nutritional deficiencies. Overall, gastric cancer is more common in countries where the intake of fresh vegetables

and fruits is low. More than 10 epidemiological studies in nine countries indicated that the risk of gastric cancer among those in the upper quartile of vegetable consumption was about half of those in the lowest quartile.[427] A similar association was seen for fruit intake.[427] A reduction in risk was associated with several individual vegetables, such as green vegetables and members of the *Crucifera* and *Allium* families.[458] The specific protective constituents in vegetables and fruits and their mechanisms are unclear, but micronutrients that may function as antioxidants, particularly vitamin C and β-carotene, are suspected.[440] Vitamin C can also inhibit endogenous formation of carcinogenic nitrosamines.[440] People who had low serum concentrations of vitamin C and β-carotene experienced a high risk of more advanced precancerous gastric lesions in two studies conducted in Colombia and China.[424,460]

A negative association between dietary calcium and gastric cancer was reported in a correlation study in Japan[439] and a case control study in the People's Republic of China.[457] Lower concentrations of selenium in hair were found among residents living in a high-risk area for gastric cancer than those living in a low-risk area in China.[462] Prediagnostic serum levels of selenium in gastric cancer patients was lower than in controls.[431] No association, however, between serum selenium concentrations and gastric cancer and its precancerous lesions was found in two large, population-based studies.[425,461]

ESOPHAGEAL AND GASTRIC CARDIA CANCER

Esophageal cancer is one of the most intriguing cancers from the perspective of its geographical distribution. The ratio between the incidence rate of high-risk and low-risk areas can be as great as 500:1.[423,452] Even within a general geographical area, there are distinctly high-incidence and low-incidence areas only a few hundred miles apart. A high esophageal cancer incidence belt bridges eastern Turkey, Iraq, and Iran with central Asia, and northern China.[430,452] Well-documented high esophageal cancer areas with an annual incidence of more than 50 per 100,000 are found in the Taihang mountain range areas of Henan, Hebei, and Shanxi provinces in northern China,[453] the Caspian Littoral of Iran; and the Transkei region of South Africa.[430] In Western countries, the rates of esophageal cancer are usually low. An exceptionally high incidence rate, however, is found in a few specific population groups. For example, in certain areas of Normandy and Brittany, France, annual incidence rates of up to 60 per 1×10^5 have been reported.[441] In the United States, the incidence of esophageal squamous carcinoma is fivefold higher among urban blacks (17 per 1×10^5) than whites.[417] High esophageal cancer rates are also found among heavy drinkers and smokers.[448]

In the United States, squamous cell carcinomas that occur mainly in the middle third of the esophagus have accounted for the majority of esophageal cancers. The incidence of squamous esophageal cancer is fairly stable, but adenocarcinomas of the esophagus and gastric cardia are increasing in prevalence.[421,444] The rates of adenocarcinomas in both of these locations increased fivefold to sixfold from the period of 1935 through 1971 to the period of 1974 through 1989; these results cannot be explained by improved diagnostic methods. As pathologists appreciate, adenocarcinomas of the esophagus and gastric cardia are often difficult to differentiate anatomically; indeed, they may be related disorders.[444] During the period of 1984 to 1987, adenocarcinomas accounted for 34% of all the esophageal cancer among white men, and it exceeded the rate of squamous cell cancers among white men below age 55 years.[420] Barrett's esophagus, a condition in which the normal stratified squamous epithelium is replaced by metaplastic columnar epithelium, is a frequent precursor lesion of esophageal adenocarcinoma. The reasons for the increase of Barrett's esophagus and adenocarcinomas are not known but are believed to relate to diet.

TOXIC RISK FACTORS FOR ESOPHAGEAL CANCER
Alcohol and tobacco (see Chapters 13 and 14)

In Western countries, excessive alcoholic beverage consumption and tobacco smoking are significant risk factors for esophageal cancer. A multiplicative interaction of these two risk factors has been demonstrated in several studies.[448] In Normandy, France, these two habits are believed to account for more than 95% of the esophageal cancer in men.[441] Case control studies in New York, Puerto Rico, Washington, D.C., South Carolina, Los Angeles, and Normandy all demonstrated that consumption of distilled alcoholic beverages provides a higher risk than that of comparable volumes of ethanol in the form of wine or beer.[426] The reasons are not known.[426]

Nitrosamines (see Chapter 5 and 26)

Nitrosamines have been implicated in the cause of esophageal cancer in many studies.[417,426,437,453] Either preformed nitrosamines or endogenously formed nitrosamines can be important factors. The consumption of smoked mutton, which contains N-nitrosomethylphenylamine, is believed to be a risk factor for esophageal cancer in Iceland.[426] Consumption of smoked fish and bacon, which are believed to contain high concentrations of either nitrite or nitrosamine, is a suspected risk factor for esophageal cancer in regions of Scotland and North Wales.[426] Nitrosamines and precursors of nitrosamines are believed to be major etiological factors in many high esophageal cancer incidence areas in China.[417,437,453] There is insufficient evidence, however, to demonstrate that food samples from high-risk areas have significantly higher concentrations of nitrosamines than food samples from low-risk areas. The reported presence of high concentrations of carcinogenic nitrosamines such as N-nitrosomethylbenzylamine and N-nitrosodiethylamine in cooked food in Linxian, a high incidence area of esophageal cancer in Northern China,[437] is interesting. These findings, especially the occurrence of N-nitrosomethylbenzylamine (a potent rat esophageal carcinogen) in the human diet, however, need further confirmation.

Moldy food and mycotoxins

Consumption of pickled vegetables in Linxian was believed to be a risk factor for esophageal cancer. A case control study, however, could not confirm this idea.[435] The pickled vegetables contain Roussin's red methyl ester, which is a weak mutagen and possible tumor promoter. When the concentrated juice or extracts of pickled vegetables were fed to rats and mice, esophageal carcinoma was not induced, but papilloma and carcinoma in other sites were observed.[436] The consumption of moldy corn is believed to be an important risk factor for esophageal cancer in both northern China and southern Africa. In addition to nitrogenous precursors for the formation of N-nitroso compounds, moldy corn may contain a variety of mycotoxins. *Fusarium* infection is widespread, and the strain most often associated with esophageal cancer is *Fusarium moniliform*. *F. moniliform* produces two major types of toxins, zearalenones which are estrogenic, and trichothecenes, which are associated with hemorrhagic disease and carcinogenicity. The toxicity of T-2 toxin, a trichothecene toxin, in the gastrointestinal tract and the hyperproliferative effect of trichothecene diacetoxyscirpenol on rat esophagus have been observed.[426] Esophageal carcinogenicity of these mycotoxins, however, has not been demonstrated. The wide occurrence and biological activities of fumonisin B_1 have received a great deal of attention.[428] This toxin was found in high concentrations (50 to 100 ppm) in some corn samples from Linxian.[422a] SF: Its role in esophageal carcinogenesis remains to be studied.

NUTRITIONAL DEFICIENCIES AND ESOPHAGEAL CANCER

Nutritional deficiency appears to be a common feature of many different populations at high risk for esophageal carcinoma. The high-risk populations in northern Iran, south and east Africa, northern China, and Soviet Central Asia all share the common feature of a monotonous diet.* The people consume mainly a diet of staples, which consists of corn, wheat, or millet; intake of vegetables, fruits, and animal products is usually low. The consumption of corn is high in many of these areas.[451] Low nutritional status of vitamins A, B_2, and C; molybdenum; magnesium; calcium; and selenium has been observed among these populations. In a study in China, the nutritional status of the population was correlated with the cancer mortality rates

*References 423, 439, 449, 452, 453.

in different parts of the country. Preliminary analysis showed that the esophageal cancer rate is inversely correlated with plasma levels of vitamins A, B_2, and C and selenium as well as the dietary intake of vitamin A equivalents, soybeans, and legume-related foods.[422]

In economically developed countries (although the major risk factors for esophageal cancer are the drinking of alcoholic beverages and smoking),[445,448] nutritional deficiency may still be a contributing factor to the esophageal cancer of high-risk populations, such as urban black men. A study of black men in Washington, D.C., showed that, in addition to alcohol consumption and smoking, the risk factors for esophageal cancer were low dietary intake of dairy products, fruits, and vegetables as well as general signs of undernutrition, such as relative weight.[445,463] Alcoholics may suffer from nutritional deficiencies owing to poor absorption of nutrients or liver damage[434,451] in addition to decreased intake or poor dietary habits.

To determine further the contribution of nutrient deficiencies to the high incidence of esophageal/gastric cardia cancer, a large-scale intervention study was conducted in the high incidence area of Linxian.[420] In this U.S.-China collaborative project, 3×10^4 adults in the age group of 40 to 69 years old were randomly divided into eight groups. Four groups of nutrients—(1) retinol and zinc; (2) riboflavin and niacin; (3) vitamin C and molybdenum; and (4) β-carotene, vitamin E, and selenium—were used. The dosages ranged from one to two times the U.S. RDA. Compliance was good. After 5 years of intervention, 32% of the deaths of trial participants were due to esophageal and stomach cancers. The death rate due to stomach cancer (mainly gastric cardia cancer) was significantly reduced (RR = 0.79, 95% CI = 0.64 to 0.99) (RR, relative risk; CI, confidence interval) among those receiving supplementation of β-carotene, vitamin E, and selenium. The supplementation also decreased total mortality (RR = 0.91, 95% CI = 0.84 to 0.98) and total cancer deaths (RR = 0.87, 95% CI = 0.75 to 1.00). No significant effects on the rates of mortality from esophageal/stomach cancer, all cancers, and all causes were found for supplementation with retinol and zinc, riboflavin and niacin, or vitamin C and molybdenum.

Because human carcinogenesis is a long-term, multifactorial process that may require 20 to 30 years to develop, it is remarkable that a beneficial effect was observed in 5 years. Low dietary intake and tissue concentrations of vitamin E and β-carotene have been observed in Linxian,[455,461] suggesting that marginal deficiencies may be contributing factors to the high incidence of esophageal/gastric cardia cancers in Linxian.

CONCLUDING REMARKS

Several lines of evidence illustrate the importance of diet on gastroesophageal cancer. Consumption of vegetables and fruits is a protective factor, whereas reduced intake of

vitamin C, vitamin E, and β-carotene appears to increase the risk of these cancers. The mechanism of action of these factors is not fully understood, partly because the cause of these cancers is not known. In addition to vitamin C, vitamin E, and β-carotene, other carotenoids and polyphenolic compounds are also found in vegetables and fruits. These compounds may protect against carcinogenesis by inhibiting oxidative DNA damage caused by reactive oxygen species, which are generated under a variety of irritating or inflammatory conditions. These compounds may also inhibit carcinogenesis by blocking endogenous nitrosation reactions.[454] Dietary improvement focused on increasing the consumption of fresh vegetables and fruits and by avoiding salty, moldy, and pickled foods should be effective measures for reducing the incidence of gastroesophageal cancer.

Diet and renal stones

Gary Curhan

Nephrolithiasis, or kidney stone disease, is one of the major causes of morbidity involving the urinary tract. It has been estimated that 12% of the U.S. population may form a kidney stone at some time.[476,496] Historically, bladder stones were the predominant type of urinary stone until the twentieth century when, with industrialization and dietary changes, calcium stones forming in the upper urinary tract became more common. Incidence rates of calcium stone disease continue to rise in the United States and elsewhere.[476,486,496,502]

The incidence of nephrolithiasis begins to rise in the early teens, peaks between the ages of 30 to 60 years, and then declines in later life.[474,476] Males are two to three times more likely to develop nephrolithiasis than females.[474,476] More than 85% of kidney stones in men and 70% in women contain calcium, with calcium oxalate stones the most common.[469,476] Stones due to urinary tract infection or metabolic derangements, such as hyperparathyroidism or cystinosis, constitute less than 10% of stones in men and less than 25% in women. Because dietary factors appear to play a significant role in calcium stone formation, this section focuses on calcium stone disease.

When the concentration of urinary constituents exceed their solubility, kidney stones may form. Hypercalciuria, hyperoxaluria, and hyperuricosuria are all common conditions in which crystal formation may occur. Under normal conditions, natural urinary inhibitors, such as citrate and glycoproteins, help maintain the stability of the saturated solution to prevent crystal formation.

DIETARY FACTORS

Rising incidence rates in Western countries and Japan have focused attention on changes in dietary habits. Based on physiological principles and per capita consumption

Table 9-9. Dietary factors reported to be associated with risk of kidney stone formation*

Increased risk	Decreased risk
Calcium	Calcium
Animal protein	Potassium
Sodium	Magnesium
Sucrose	Fiber
Oxalate	Fluid intake
Ascorbic acid	
Sugared cola	

*See text for details.

data, it has been suggested that several dietary factors may increase the risk of kidney stone formation, including calcium, animal protein,[490] oxalate,[479] sodium,[485] and sucrose[482] (Table 9-9). Moreover, it has been suggested that higher magnesium,[475] fiber,[472] and potassium[483] consumption may reduce risk. It has been known for quite some time that a high fluid intake decreases the risk of crystal formation, but only recently has information become available on the relative effect of individual beverages (see Beverages).

The interpretation of previous research into the association between diet and nephrolithiasis is limited by the design of the studies performed. Retrospective studies of diet and nephrolithiasis have evaluated the association between diet and recurrent stone formation. This type of study design is limited by the potential for bias of dietary recall or changes in dietary habits as a result of the disease. The majority of prospective studies have been limited to changes in the lithogenic composition of the urine and have provided no information on changes in stone formation rates. Moreover, the potential contribution of other unmeasured factors to the process of stone formation has been overlooked.

CALCIUM

For years, dietary calcium has been suspected of raising the risk of nephrolithiasis. This hypothesis derived largely from the finding of hypercalciuria in 20% to 40% of recurrent stone formers. Consequently, calcium stone formers have been advised to restrict their calcium intake to prevent stone recurrence. Although dietary calcium restriction can decrease urinary calcium excretion in stone formers with and without idiopathic hypercalciuria, there are insufficient data on the effect of these changes on the rate of stone formation. Indeed, a low calcium intake has been shown to increase oxalate absorption in the gastrointestinal tract, leading to increased urinary oxalate excretion.[503] As calcium oxalate saturation of urine increases rapidly with small increases in oxalate concentration,[466] it appears that urinary oxalate may play an even more significant role in stone formation than urinary calcium. Therefore, by increasing urinary oxalate excretion, calcium restriction actually may be harmful.

Case control studies of diet and nephrolithiasis have not demonstrated a difference in mean calcium intake in stone formers;[471,473,488,499] however, the interpretation of these studies is complicated by the lack of control for other risk factors associated with stone formation. Until recently, there were no prospective data on the relation between calcium intake and the risk of forming a kidney stone. Curhan and colleagues[470] performed the first prospective study of dietary factors and the risk of incident stone disease in a cohort of 45,619 male health professionals aged 40 to 75 years at baseline. This study found that men with a higher intake of dietary calcium had a 34% *lower* risk of incident nephrolithiasis (Table 9-10). Although the exact mechanism of this effect is unknown, it may be related to the effect of calcium on oxalate absorption.[465] Thus, there is no evidence that higher dietary calcium intake increases the risk of stone formation and in fact may reduce the risk.

ANIMAL PROTEIN

Increasing affluence is associated with an increase in the intake of animal protein.[492] Per capita consumption data from England revealed a direct relation between animal protein intake and stone disease.[490] In the prospective study

Table 9-10. Dietary factors and the multivariate relative risk of incident kidney stone formation and daily calorie-adjusted nutrient intake for the highest and lowest quintiles in a prospective study of 45,510 men

Nutrient	Multivariate relative risk	95% CI	Lowest quintile	Highest quintile
Calcium	0.66	0.49-0.90	< 605 mg	> 1049 mg
Potassium	0.49	0.35-0.68	< 2896 mg	> 4041 mg
Animal protein	1.33	1.00-1.77	< 51 g	> 76 g
Fiber	0.73	0.48-1.11	< 16.4 g	> 28.4 g
Sodium	0.89	0.66-1.20	< 2237 mg	> 3877 mg
Sucrose	0.94	0.67-1.32	< 31 g	> 61 g
Magnesium	0.86	0.57-1.28	< 304 mg	> 443 mg
Fluid intake	0.71	0.52-0.97	<1275 ml	> 2537 ml

CI, Confidence interval.

by Curhan and colleagues,[470] men with the highest animal protein intake had a 33% increased risk of stone formation (Table 9-10). Ingestion of animal protein, and thus purine, leads to increased urinary uric acid excretion,[467] a risk factor for both uric acid and calcium stone formation. In addition, an increased acid load from the metabolism of sulfur-containing amino acids leads to lower urinary citrate levels, an important inhibitor of calcium oxalate crystallization, and possibly increased urinary calcium excretion.[467]

OXALATE

Oxalate is found in many foods, but the content is typically low.[477] Excessive ingestion of foods high in oxalate, such as chocolate, nuts, tea, and spinach, can lead to hyperoxaluria and calcium oxalate stone formation.[479] Unfortunately, there are no comprehensive nutrient databases that currently include oxalate for the majority of foods; thus an analysis of oxalate as an individual nutrient and its relation to stone disease has not been performed.

SODIUM

A high sodium intake increases urinary sodium and calcium excretion,[478] apparently due to inhibition of sodium and calcium reabsorption in the proximal tubule and along the loop of Henle.[464] In a case control study of stone formers, urinary sodium excretion was highly correlated with urinary calcium excretion, and individuals with recurrent stones were more sensitive than controls to the hypercalciuric action of dietary sodium.[350] The prospective study[470] found no association between sodium intake and risk (Table 9-10); however, the lack of a significant association could be due to misclassification of sodium intake as a result of difficulty measuring sodium intake by our dietary instrument. Clearly, further investigation of the relation between sodium intake and stone formation is required.

SUCROSE

Sucrose and other refined carbohydrates may induce calciuria independent of calcium intake, thereby increasing the risk of stone formation.[482] This increase in calcium excretion appears to be the result of reduced net tubular reabsorption of calcium.[480] Retrospective and prospective studies, however, have not demonstrated a significant association between sucrose intake and the risk of stone formation (Table 9-10).

POTASSIUM

Potassium has been shown to reduce urinary calcium excretion in healthy adults,[483] presumably reducing the risk of calcium stone formation. In addition, because foods high in potassium tend to be high in alkali, consumption of these foods results in increased urinary citrate. Retrospective studies have demonstrated no differences in potassium intake between stone cases and controls.[471,473,499] In contrast, the prospective study revealed that a high potassium intake was associated with a 51% decreased risk of stone forma-

tion[470] (Table 9-10). Accordingly, although it has been suggested that the decreased risk of stone formation in vegetarians is due to the lack of consumption of animal protein, it may actually be due to a high intake of potassium-containing foods.[491]

MAGNESIUM AND FIBER

Fiber has been proposed to bind calcium in the gastrointestinal tract, consequently decreasing urinary calcium excretion.[472] Magnesium interferes with calcium oxalate lattice formation. Prospectively, no association was found between the risk of stone formation and magnesium or fiber intake[470] (Table 9-10).

ASCORBIC ACID

Ascorbic acid in large doses has been implicated in stone formation as ascorbate is metabolized to oxalate, which is then excreted in the urine. Previous measurements of urinary oxalate, however, should be viewed with caution because it is now known that the presence of ascorbic acid may falsely elevate oxalate results. In addition, there may be significant imprecision in laboratory measurements of urinary oxalate.[493] In the prospective study, men in the highest quintile of vitamin C intake (dietary and from supplements) were not at increased risk (unpublished data).

BEVERAGES

To decrease the likelihood of stone formation, patients are routinely advised to increase their urine volume by increasing their fluid intake. Although increasing fluid intake is not a proven remedy, this recommendation is supported by most authors,[468,487,497,498] although not by all.[484] An inverse association between total fluid intake and the risk of stone formation was found in the prospective cohort study.[470]

Although some information exists regarding the effect of increasing the intake of certain beverages on changes in urine composition, little information is available on changes in stone formation rates. Using a retrospective case control design to examine the relation between the intake of six beverages and a history of kidney stones, Shuster and colleagues[494] observed an inverse association for beer and coffee consumption and a direct association for carbonated beverage (soda) consumption. This study was followed by a randomized trial of decreasing soft drink (soda) use on the risk of stone recurrence.[495] A significant decrease of 6.4% in the stone recurrence rate was observed in the group advised to avoid soda consumption. Unfortunately, other risk factors for stone disease, such as other dietary variables, were not controlled for in the analysis.

To investigate whether the type of fluid ingested is important, we examined prospectively the relation between the use of 21 beverages and the risk of symptomatic kidney stones. Our data suggest that higher consumption of caffeinated and decaffeinated coffee, tea, beer, and wine decreases the risk of symptomatic kidney stones, and higher

Table 9-11. Multivariate relative risk of incident kidney stones for individual beverages per 240 ml (8 oz) serving size per day in a prospective study of 45,289 men*

Beverage	Multivariate relative risk†	95% CI
Juices		
Apple juice	1.35	1.04-1.75
Grapefruit juice	1.37	1.01-1.85
Coffee/tea		
Coffee, caffeinated	0.90	0.85-0.96
Coffee, decaffeinated	0.90	0.84-0.97
Tea	0.86	0.78-0.95
Alcoholic beverages		
Beer	0.79	0.70-0.88
Wine	0.61	0.42-0.90

CI denotes confidence interval.
*The multivariate model included age (in 5-year age categories); profession, geographic region (seven categories); use of thiazide diuretics (yes or no); dietary intake of calcium, animal protein, and potassium (quintile groups); and intake of all 21 beverages (continuous variables with each unit representing 240 ml [8 oz] per day of that beverage).
†Relative risk for a 240-ml increment in the specified beverage.

consumption of apple juice and grapefruit juice increases the risk (unpublished data, Table 9-11). The mechanism for the protective effect of caffeinated coffee and tea may be mediated through caffeine. Caffeine interferes with the action of antidiuretic hormone (ADH) on the distal nephron[489] resulting in increased urine flow and a more dilute urine, thereby reducing the risk of crystal formation. The protective effect of beer and wine may be due to the inhibitory effect of alcohol on ADH secretion,[489] also resulting in increased urine flow and decreased urinary concentration.

The inverse association for tea and coffee may seem surprising given the common belief that these beverages, particularly tea, are high in oxalate. As mentioned previously, little information on the oxalate content of foods and beverages is available. Kasidas and Rose,[477] using foods bought in England and an enzymatic method to measure oxalate content, found an 8-oz (240 ml) portion of tea contained 17 mg of oxalate, and an 8-oz serving of instant coffee contained 8 mg of oxalate. Thus, it appears that the amount of oxalate contributed to the diet by these beverages, although not trivial, is probably small.

The mechanism for the increased risk associated with apple juice and grapefruit juice consumption is not clear. Although the pH of these beverages is acidic (approximately 3.5),[500] the actual total acid load is small. These beverages also contain a substantial amount of sugar, which can increase calcium excretion.[481] Other acidic beverages, however, containing considerably more sugar, such as punch and soda, were not associated with increased risk. Further data from extended follow-up and

other populations are required to elucidate the associations with these fruit juices.

Age-adjusted data from the prospective study demonstrated an association between consumption of caffeinated sugared cola and risk of stone formation that is consistent with previous reports.[494,495] After controlling for other risk factors, however, the association was no longer significant for sugared cola or for the other types of soda. Notably the intake of caffeinated sugared cola was inversely correlated with dietary calcium and dietary potassium. Thus, it appears that the results of these previous studies on soda consumption may have been confounded by other dietary factors.

REFERENCES
Concepts in food toxicology
1. Ames BN: Dietary carcinogens and anticarcinogens, *Science* 221:1256, 1983.
2. Ames BN, Profet M, Gold LS: Dietary pesticides (99.99% all natural), *Proc Natl Acad Sci USA* 87:7777, 1990.
3. Bruce MG, Ferguson A: Oral tolerance to ovalbumin in mice: studies of chemically modified and "biologically filtered" antigen, *Immunology* 57:627, 1986.
4. Cliver DO: Research needs in food safety, *Food Technol* 47:10S, 1993.
5. Elsayet S, Apold J: Immunochemical analysis of cod fish allergen M: locations of the immunoglobulin binding sites as demonstrated by the native and synthetic peptides, *Allergy* 38:449, 1983.
6. Experiment Station Committee on Organization and Policy: *Research agenda for the 1990s*, 1992.
7. Food Safety Research Work Group: *Federal food safety research (an overview)—including the needs for the future*, Washington, DC, 1993, Food and Drug Administration.
8. Johnstone JM, Morson BC: Eosinophilic gastroenteritis, *Histopathology* 2:335, 1978.
9. Klein et al: Eosinophilic gastroenteritis, *Medicine* 49:299, 1970.
10. Sampson HA, Metcalfe DD: Food allergies, *JAMA* 268:2840, 1992.
11. Scheuplein RJ: *The FDA Redbook*. In *Toxicology Forum*, Washington, DC, 1992.
12. Steele JH, Engel RE: Radiation processing of food, *J Am Vet Med Assoc* 201:1992.
13. Steffen RM et al: The spectrum of eosinophilic gastroenteritis: report of six pediatric cases and review of the literature, *Clin Pediatr* 30:404, 1991.
14. Todd E: Epidemiology of foodborne illness. North America, *Lancet* 2:788, 1990.

Association of food and water constituents with hypertension
15a. Ambard L, Beaujard E: *Causes of arterial hypertension*. In Ruskin A, editor: *Classics in arterial hypertension*, Springfield, Ill, 1956, Charles C Thomas, pp. 297-310.
15. Appel LJ et al: Does supplementation of diet with "fish oil" reduce blood pressure? *Arch Intern Med* 153:429, 1993.
16. Chiang BN, Perlman LV, Epstein FH: Overweight and hypertension, *Circulation* 39:403, 1969.
17. Dawber TR et al: *Environmental factors in hypertension*. In Stamler J, Stamler R, Pullman T, editors: *The epidemiology of hypertension*, New York, 1967, Grune & Stratton, pp 255-288.
18. DeFronzo RA, Ferrannini E: Insulin resistance: a multifaceted syndrome responsible for NIDDM, obesity, hypertension, dislipidemia and atherosclerotic cardiovascular disease, *Diab Care* 14:173, 1991.
19. Denke MA, Sempos CT, Grundy SM: Excess body weight: an unrecognized contributor to high blood cholesterol levels in white American men, *Arch Intern Med* 153:1093, 1993.

20. Dolenc P, Staessen JA, Lauwerysrr Amery A: Short report: low-level lead exposure does not increase the blood pressure in the general population, *J Hypertens* 11:589, 1993.

21. Dustan HP: Obesity in hypertension, *Diab Care* 14:488, 1991.

22. Dustan HP, Kirk KA: Relationship of sodium balance to arterial pressure in black hypertensive patients, *Am J Med Sci* 295:378, 1988.

23. Dustan HP, Kirk KA: Corcoran Lecture: the case for or against salt in hypertension, *Hypertension* 13:696, 1989.

24. Grim CE et al: Racial differences in blood pressure in Evans County, Georgia: relationship to sodium and potassium intake and plasma renin activity, *J Chronic Dis* 33:87, 1980.

25. Harlan WR et al: Blood lead and blood pressure: relationship in the adolescent and adult U.S. population, *JAMA* 253:530, 1985.

26. Intersalt Cooperative Group: Intersalt: an international study of electrolyte excretion and blood pressure. Results for 24-hour urinary sodium and potassium excretion, *BMJ* 297:319, 1988.

27. Joint National Committee on Detection, Evaluation and Treatment of Hypertension: Vth report, *Arch Intern Med* 153:154, 1993.

28. Kaplan NM: *Clinical hypertension,* ed 4, Baltimore, 1986, Williams & Wilkins.

29. Khaw K-T, Barrett-Connor E: Dietary potassium and blood pressure in a population, *Am J Clin Nutr* 39:963, 1984.

30. Khaw K-T, Barrett-Connor E: The association between blood pressure, age and dietary sodium and potassium: a population study, *Circulation* 77:53, 1988.

31. Khaw K-T, Barrett-Connor E: Dietary potassium and stroke associated mortality. *N Engl J Med* 316:235, 1987.

32. Law MR, Frost CD, Wald NJ: By how much does dietary salt reduction lower blood pressure? I. Analysis of observational data among populations, *BMJ* 302:811, 1991.

33. Law MR, Frost CD, Wald NJ: By how much does dietary salt reduction lower blood pressure? III. Analysis of data from trials of salt reduction, *BMJ* 302:819,1991.

34. Linas SL: The role of potassium in the pathogenesis and treatment of hypertension, *Kidney Int* 39:771, 1991.

35. MacMahon S: Alcohol consumption and hypertension, *Hypertension* 9:111, 1987.

36. Maheswaran R et al: High blood pressure due to alcohol, a rapidly reversible effect, *Hypertension* 17:787, 1991.

37. McCarron DA et al: Blood pressure and nutrient intake in the United States, *Science* 224:1392, 1984.

38. Miall WE: Follow up study of arterial pressure in the population of a Welch mining valley, *BMJ* 2:1204, 1959.

39. Pan W et al: The role of weight in the positive association between age and blood pressure, *Am J Epidemiol* 24:612, 1986.

40. Resnick LM et al: Intracellular free magnesium in erythrocytes of essential hypertension: relation to blood pressure and serum divalent cations, *Proc Natl Acad Sci USA* 81:6511, 1984.

41. Sachs FM: Dietary fats and blood pressure: a critical review of the evidence. *Nutr Rev* 47:291, 1989.

42. Tobian L et al: Potassium reduces cerebral hemorrhage and death rate in rats even when blood pressure is not lowered, *Hypertension* 7(suppl I):I110, 1985.

43. Touyz RM, Schiffrn EL: The effect of angiotension 2 on platelet intracellular free magnesium and calcium ionic concentrations in essential hypertension, *J Hypertens* 11:551, 1993.

44. Weinberger MH et al: Definitions and characteristics of sodium sensitivity and blood pressure resistance, *Hypertension* 8(suppl II):II127, 1986.

Iodine deficiency disorders

45. Alnwick DJ: Prevention of iodine deficiency disorders in Kenya—a preliminary investigation of the iodine content of salt on sale in western Kenya, *East Afr Med J* 65:723, 1988.

46. Bayoumi RA, Taha TSM, Saha N: Study of possible genetic predisposition to endemic goitre among the Fur and Baggara tribes of the Sudan, *Hum Hered* 38:8, 1988.

47. Bourdoux P et al: *Antithyroid action of cassave in humans.* In Ermans AM, et al, editors: *Role of Cassave in the etiology of endemic goitre and cretinism,* Canada, 1980, International Research Centre.

48. Boyages SC et al: Iodine deficiency impairs intellectual and neuromotor development in apparently-normal persons. A study of rural inhabitants of north-central China, *Med J Aust* 150:676, 1989.

49. Chaouki ML, Maoui R, Benmiloud M: Comparative study of neurological and myxoedematous cretinism associated with severe iodine deficiency, *Clin Endocrinol* 28:399, 1988.

50. Choufoer JC, van Rhun M, Querido A: Endemic goiter in western New Guinea. II. Clinical picture, incidence anbd pathogenesis of endemic cretinism, *J Clin Endocrinol Metab* 25:385, 1965.

51. Clements FW: *Endemic goitre.* In Beaton GH, Bengoa JM, editors: *Nutrition in preventive medicine,* Geneva, 1976, World Health Organization.

52. Corvilain B et al: Selenium and the thyroid: how the relationship was established, *Am J Clin Nutr* 57 (2 suppl):244S, 1993.

53. DeLong R: *Neurological involvement in iodine deficiency disorders.* In Hetzel BS, Dunn JT, Stanbury JB, editors: *The prevention and control of iodine deficiency disorders,* Amsterdam, 1987, Elsevier.

54. Eltom M et al: Endemic goitre in the Darfur region (Sudan): epidemiology and aetiology, *Acta Med Scand* 215:467, 1984.

55. Fisher DA et al: Screening for congenital hypothyroidism: results of screening one million North American infants, *J Pediatr* 94:700, 1979.

56. Gaitan E: Water-borne goitrogens and their role in the etiology of endemic goitre, *World Rev Nutr Diet* 17:53, 1973.

57. Gaitan ER, Cooksey MD, Preson R: In vitro measurements of antithyroid compounds and environment goitrogens, *Clin Endocrinol Metab* 56:767, 1983.

58. Giau W: A review of iodine deficiency disorders in Kenya, *East Afr Med J* 65:727, 1988.

59. Goyens P et al: Selenium deficiency as a possible factor in the pathogenesis of myxoedematous endemic cretinism, *Acta Endocrinol (Copenh)* 1114:497, 1987.

60. Gyoh SK, Emergy JG: Coping with respiratory obstruction after thyroidectomy for giant gotres in Northern Nigeria, *Ann Roy Coll Surg Engl* 70:99, 1988.

61. Halpern J et al: The neurology of endemic cretinism: a study of two endemias, *Brain* 114:835, 1991.

62. Jenesi R et al: Endemic goitre in Chinamora, Zimbabwe, *Lancet* 1:1198, 1986.

63. Jooste PL et al: Endemic goitre among undernourished schoolchildren in eastern Caprivi, Namibia, *S Afr Med J* 81:571, 1992.

64. Kimiagar M, Farhud DD, Sabet-Rohani R: Thyroidal radioactive iodine uptake in Iran, *Inte J Vit Nutr Res* 58:466, 1988.

65. Kochupillai N: Neonatal hypothyroidism in India, *Mt Sinai J Med* 59:111, 1992.

66. Kochupillai N et al: Iodine deficiency and neonatal hypothyroidism, *Bull WHO* 64:547, 1986.

67. Lamberg BA: Iodine deficiency disorders and endemic goitre, *Eur J Clin Nutr* 47:1, 1993.

68. Lobo LCG et al: *Epidemiological survey of endemic goiter and cretinism in Mato Grosso, Brazil.* In Stanbury JB, editor: *Endemic goiter,* Washington DC, 1969, Pan American Health Organization.

69. Ma T, Guo J, Wang F: The epidemiology of iodine-deficiency diseases in China, *Am J Clin Nutr* 57:264S, 1993.

70. Mahdi EE et al: Water goitrogens and endemic goitre in the Sudan, *Trop Geogr Med* 38:180, 1986.

71. McCarrison R: Observations on endemic cretinism in the Chitral and Gilgit Valleys, *Lancet* 2:1275, 1908.

72. Medeiros-Filho A: *Report of the 1975 survey on endemic goiter prevalence in Brazil,* Brasilia, 1977, Ministry of Health.

73. Pandav CS, Kochupillai N: Endemic goiter in India: prevalence, etiology, attendant disability, and control measures, *Ind J Pediat* 50:1259, 1982.

74. Pang X et al: Thyroid function of subjects with goitre and cretinism in an endemic goitre area of rural China after use of iodized salt, *Acta Endocrinol (Copenh)* 118:444, 1988.

75. Perez C, Scrimshaw NS, Munoz JA: *Technique of endemic goitre surveys.* In *Endemic goiter,* WHO Monogr No 44, 1960.

76. Sava L et al: Transient impairment of thyroid function in newborn from an area of endemic goiter, *J Clin Endocrinol Metab* 59:90, 1984.

77. Scrimshaw NS: The consequences of hidden hunger: the effect on individuals and societies, *Vital Speeches of the Day* 58:138, 1991.

78. Stanbury JB et al: Endemic goitre and cretinism: public health significance and prevention, *WHO Chronicle* 28:220, 1974.

79. Swennen B et al: Epidemiology and strategy of goitre control in Malawi, *East Afr Med J* 64:759, 1987.

80. Thilly CH, Delange F, Ermans AM: Further investigations of iodine deficiency in the etiology of endemic goiter, *Am J Clin Nutr* 25:30, 1972.

81. Thilly CH et al: Fetal hypothyroidism and maternal thyroid status in severe endemic goiter, *J Clin Endocrinol Metab* 47:354, 1978.

82. Thilly CH et al: The epidemiology of iodine-deficiency disorders in relation to goitrogenic factors and thyroid-stimulating-hormone regulation, *Am J Clin Nutr* 57:267S, 1993.

83. Todd CH, Sanders D, Chimanyiwa T: Hearing in primary school children in an iodine-deficient population in Chinamhora, Zimbabwe, *Trop Geogr Med* 40:223, 1988.

84. Vanderpas JB et al: Selenium deficiency mitigates hypothyroxinemia in iodine-deficient subjects, *Am J Clin Nutr* 57:271S, 1993.

85. Wachter W et al: Prevalence of goitre and hypothyroidism in Southern Tanzania: effect of iodised oil on thyroid hormone deficiency, *J Epidemiol Commun Hlth* 40:86, 1986.

86. Wang Yan-Yon, Yang Shu-Hua: Improvement in hearing among otherwise normal school children in iodine deficient areas of Guizhou, China, following use of iodised salt, *Lancet* 2:518, 1985.

87. *World Health Organizaton draft report to the World Health Assembly,* Geneva, 1990.

Dietary iron deficiency and excess

88. Andrews SC et al: Structure, function and evolution of ferritins, *J Inorg Biochem* 47:161, 1992.

89. Baker EN, Lindley PF: New perspectives on the structure and function of transferrins, *J Inorg Biochem* 47:147, 1992.

90. Barry M: Iron overload: clinical aspects, evaluation and treatment. *Clin Haematol* 2:405, 1973.

91. Bothwell TH, Charlton RW: *Nutritional aspects of iron deficiency.* In Saltman P, Hegenauer J, editors: *The biochemistry and physiology of iron,* New York, 1982, Elsevier Biomedical.

92. Bullen JJ, Griffiths E, editors: *Iron and infection,* New York, 1987, John Wiley & Sons.

93. Charlton RW, Bothwell TH, Seftel HC: Dietary iron overload. *Clin Haematol* 2:383, 1973.

94. Chasteen ND, Woodworth RC: *Transferrin and lactoferrin.* In Ponka P, Schulman HM, Woodworth RC, editors: *Iron transport and storage.* Boca Raton, Fla, 1990, CRC Press.

95. Conrad ME: Excess iron and catastrophic illness, *Am J Hematol* 43:234, 1993.

96. Cowan B, Bharucha C: Iron deficiency in the tropics, *Clin Haematol* 2:353, 1973.

97. Dagg JH, Goldberg A: Detection and treatment of iron deficiency, *Clin Haematol* 2:365, 1973.

98. da Silva JJRF, Williams RJP: *The biological chemistry of the elements,* Oxford, 1991, Clarendon Press.

99. Flanagan PR: *Intestinal iron metabolism and absorption.* In Ponka P, Schulman HM, Woodworth RC, editors: *Iron transport and storage,* Boca Raton, Fla, 1990, CRC Press.

100. Garby L: Iron deficiency: definition and prevalence, *Clin Haematol* 2:245, 1973.

101. Jacobs A: The mechanism of iron absorption, *Clin Haematol* 2:325, 1973.

102. Layrisse M, Martinez-Torres C: *Enhancers for intestinal absorption of food iron.* In Saltman P, Hegenauer J, editors: *The biochemistry and physiology of iron,* New York, 1982, Elsevier Biomedical.

103. Powell LW, Halliday JW, Bassett ML: *The case against iron supplementation.* In Saltman P, Hegenauer J, editors: *The biochemistry and physiology of iron,* New York, 1982, Elsevier BioMedical.

104. Salonen JT et al: High stored iron levels are associated with excess risk of myocardial infarction in eastern Finnish men, *Circulation* 86:805, 1992.

105. Srai SKS, Debnam ES, Boss M, Epstein O: *The ontogeny of duodenal iron absorption in the guinea pig: clues to the aetiology of idiopathic haemochromatosis.* In Spik G, Montreuil J, Crichton RR, Mazurier J, editors: *Proteins of iron storage and transport,* Amsterdam, 1985, Elsevier Biomedical.

105a. Stevens RG et al: Moderate elevation of body iron level and increased risk of cancer occurrence and death. *Int J Cancer* 56:364, 1994.

106. Sullivan JL: The iron paradigm of ischemic heart disease, *Am Heart J* 117:1177, 1989.

107. van Renswoude J, Bridges KR, Harford JB, Klausner RD: Receptor-mediated endocytosis of transferrin and the uptake of Fe in K562 cells: identification of a nonlysosomal acidic compartment, *Proc Natl Acad Sci USA* 79:6186, 1982.

108. Weinberg ED: Iron withholding: a defense against infection and neoplasia, *Physiol Rev* 64:65, 1984.

109. Werner E, Roth EW, Kaltwasser JP: *Relationship between the dose administered and the intestinal absorption of iron from ferrous sulfate in humans.* In Saltman P, Hegenauer J, editors: *The biochemistry and physiology of iron,* New York, 1982, Elsevier Biomedical.

110. Williams RJP: *An introduction to the nature of iron transport and storage.* In Ponka P, Schulman HM, Woodworth RC, editors: *Iron transport and storage,* Boca Raton, Fla, 1990, CRC Press.

Dietary selenium deficiency and excess

111. Abernathy CO et al: *Essentiality versus toxicity: some considerations in the risk assessment of essential trace elements.* In Saxena J, editor, *Hazard assessment of chemicals,* vol 8, Washington, 1993, Taylor & Francis.

112. Ahmed HM et al: Selenium status in Sudanese children with protein-calorie malnutrition, *J Trace Elem Electrolyte Health Dis* 3:171, 1989.

113. Alfthan G et al: Selenium supplementation and platelet glutathione peroxidase activity in healthy Finnish men: effects of selenium yeast, selenite, and selenate, *Am J Clin Nutr* 53:120, 1991.

114. Arthur JR, Nicol F, Beckett GJ: Selenium deficiency, thyroid hormone metabolism, and thyroid hormone deiodinase, *Am J Clin Nutr Suppl* 57:236S, 1993.

115. Beck MA, et al: Benign human enterovirus becomes virulent in selenium-deficient mice, *J Med Virol* 43:166, 1994.

116. Beck MA, et al: Vitamin E deficiency intensifies the myocardial injury of coxsackievirus B3 infection of mice, *J Nutr* 124:345, 1994.

117. Benson SM, Delamore M, Hoffman S: Kesterson crisis, *J Irrig Drain Eng* 119:471, 1993.

118. Chen J et al: Antioxidant status and cancer mortality in China, *Int J Epidemiol* 21:625, 1992.

119. Clark LC, Combs GF Jr: Selenium compounds and the prevention of cancer: research needs and public health implications, *J Nutr* 116:170, 1986.

120. Corvilain B et al: Selenium and the thyroid: how the relationship was established, *Am J Clin Nutr* Suppl 57:244S, 1993.

121. Reference deleted in proofs.

122. Engberg RA, Sylvester MA: Concentrations, distribution, and sources of selenium from irrigated lands in western United States, *J Irrig Drain Eng* 119:522, 1993.

123. Ge K, Yang G: The epidemiology of selenium deficiency in the etiological study of endemic diseases in China, *Am J Clin Nutr Suppl* 57:259S, 1993.

124. Ge K et al: Keshan disease—an endemic cardiomyopathy in China, *Virchows Arch [Pathol Anat]* 401:1, 1983.

125. Ge K et al: *The protective effect of selenium against viral myocarditis in mice.* In Combs GF Jr et al, editors: *Selenium in biology and medicine, part B,* New York, 1987, Van Nostrand Reinhold.

126. Golden MHN, Ramdath D: Free radicals in the pathogenesis of kwashiorkor, *Proc Nutr Soc* 46:53, 1987.

127. Gu B: Pathology of Keshan disease, *Chin Med J* 96:281, 1983.

128. Hill KE et al: The cDNA for rat selenoprotein P contains 10 TGA codons in the open reading frame, *J Biol Chem* 266:10050, 1991.

129. Hunter DJ et al: A prospective study of selenium status and breast cancer risk, *JAMA* 264:1128, 1990.

130. International Programme on Chemical Safety: *Environmental Health Criteria 58. Selenium,* Geneva, 1987, World Health Organization.

131. Ip C: *Novel strategies in selenium cancer chemoprevention research.* In Burk RF, editor: *Selenium in biology and medicine,* New York, 1993, Springer-Verlag.

132. Jaffe W: Selenio, un elemento esencial y toxico. Datos de Latinoamerica, *Arch Latinoam Nutr* 42:90, 1992.

133. Jaffe WG et al: Estudio clinico y bioquimico en ninos eseolares de una zone selenifera, *Arch Latinoam Nutr* 22:595, 1972.

134. Keshan Disease Research Group: Observation on effect of sodium selenite in prevention of Keshan disease, *Chin Med J* 92:431, 1979.

135. Leichsenring M et al: *Clinical studies on polyunsaturated fatty acids and antioxidants in African children.* In Ong ASH, Packer L, editors: *Lipid-soluble antioxidants: biochemical and clinical applications,* Basel, 1992, Birkhauser.

136. Levander OA: A global view of human selenium nutrition, *Ann Rev Nutr* 7:227, 1987.

137. Levander OA: Scientific rationale for the 1989 Recommended Dietary Allowance for selenium, *J Am Dietet Assoc* 91:1572, 1991.

138. Levander OA, Morris VC: *What can balance studies tell us about human dietary selenium requirements?* In Mills CF, Bremner I, Chesters JK, editors: *Trace elements in man and animals-TEMA-5,* Slough, UK, 1985, Commonwealth Agricultural Bureaux.

139. Longnecker MP et al: Selenium in diet, blood, and toenails in relation to human health in a seleniferous area, *Am J Clin Nutr* 53:1288, 1991.

140. Maiorino M, Ursini F: *Synergistic effect of lipid hyroperoxyl radical scavenging and lipid hydroperoxide reduction in the inhibition of lipid peroxidation in biomembranes.* In Ong ASH, Packer L, editors: *Lipid-soluble antioxidants: biochemical and clinical applications,* Basel, 1992, Birkauser Verlag.

141. Moxon AL, Rhian M: Selenium poisoning, *Physiol Rev* 23:305, 1943.

142. National Cancer Institute, Division of Cancer Prevention and Control, *Workshop on Selenium Compounds in Cancer Chemoprevention Trials,* National Institute of Health, Rockville, Md, 1993.

143. National Research Council: *Recommended dietary allowances,* ed 9, Washington, 1980, National Academy of Sciences.

144. National Research Council: *Selenium in nutrition,* rev ed, Washington, 1983, National Academy Press.

145. National Research Council: *Recommended dietary allowances,* ed 10, Washington, 1989, National Academy Press.

146. Olson OE: Selenium toxicity in animals with emphasis on man, *J Am Coll Toxicol* 5:45, 1986.

147. Raisbeck MF et al: Naturally occurring selenosis in Wyoming, *J Vet Diagn Invest* 5:64, 1993.

148. Rotruck JT et al: Selenium: biochemical role as a component of glutathione peroxidase, *Science* 179:588, 1973.

149. Schrauzer GN: *Selenium in nutritonal cancer prophylaxis: an update.* In Prasad AS, editor: *Vitamins, nutrition and cancer,* Basel, 1984, Karger.

150. Schrauzer GN: Selenium and breast cancer, *JAMA* 265:28, 1991.

151. Schwarz K, Foltz CM: Selenium an integral part of Factor 3 against dietary necrotic liver degeneration. *J Am Chem Soc* 79:3293, 1957.

152. Sive AA et al: *Protein energy malnutrition: selenium, glutathione peroxidase and glutathione in children with acute Kwashiorkor and during refeeding.* In Momcilovic B, editor: *Trace elements in man and animals 7,* Zagreb, 1991, University of Zagreb.

153. Smith MI, Franke KW, Westfall BB: The selenium problem in relation to public health. A preliminary survey to determine the possibility of selenium intoxication in the rural populations living on seleniferous soil, *US Public Health Rep* 51:1496, 1936.

154. Smith MI, Westfall BB: Further field studies on the selenium problem in relation to public health, *US Public Health Rep* 52:1375, 1937.

155. Sokoloff L: Endemic forms of osteoarthritis, *Clin Rheum Dis* 11:187, 1985.

156. Tanji KK: Prognosis on managing trace elements, *J Irrig Drain Eng* 119:577, 1993.

157. Thomson CD et al: Long-term supplementation with selenate and selenomethionine: selenium and glutathione peroxidase (EC 1.11.1.9) in blood components of New Zealand women, *Brit J Nutr* 69:577, 1993.

158. Ullrey DE: Basis for regulation of selenium supplements in animal diets, *J Anim Sci* 70:3922, 1992.

159. van den Brandt PA: A prospective cohort study on toenail selenium levels and risk of gastrointestinal caner, *J Natl Cancer Inst* 85:224, 1993.

160. Varo P et al: *Nationwide selenium supplementation in Finland.* In Burk RF, editor: *Selenium in biology and medicine,* New York, 1993, Springer-Verlag.

161. Whanger PD: Selenium in the treatment of heavy metal poisoning and chemical carcinogenesis, *J Trace Elem Electrolytes Health Dis* 6:209, 1992.

162. Willett WC, Stampfer MJ: Selenium and cancer, *BMJ* 297:593, 1988.

163. Witte ST et al: Chronic selenosis in horses fed locally produced alfalfa hay, *J Am Vet Med Assoc* 202:406, 1993.

164. World Health Organization: *Kashin-Beck disease and noncommunicable diseases,* Beijing, 1990, Chinese Academy of Preventive Medicine.

165. Yang C et al: Fulvic acid supplementation and selenium deficiency disturbs the structural integrity of mouse skeletal tissues, *Biochem J* 289:829, 1993.

166. Yang G et al: Selenium-related endemic diseases and the daily selenium requirements of humans, *World Rev Nutr Diet* 55:98, 1988.

167. Yang G et al: Studies of safe maximal daily dietary Se intake in a seleniferous area in China. Part II: Relation between Se intake and the manifestation of clinical signs and certain biochemical alterations in blood and urine, *J Trace Elem Electrolytes Health Dis* 3:123, 1989.

168. Yang GQ et al: Endemic selenium intoxication of humans in China, *Am J Clin Nutr* 37:872, 1983.

169. Yang GQ et al: *Human selenium requirements in China.* In Combs

GF Jr et al, editors: *Selenium in biology and medicine,* New York, 1987, Van Nostrand Reinhold.

Protein energy malnutrition

170. Abdeljaber MH et al: The impact of vitamin A supplementation on morbidity: a randomized community intervention trial, *Am J Public Health* 81:1654, 1991.
171. Adelekan DA et al: Plasma ferritin concentration in relation to vitamin A and E status of children with severe oedematous malnutrition, *Ann Trop Paediat* 11:175, 1991.
172. Behrman J: *Intrahousehold allocation of nutrients and gender effects: a survey of structural and reduced form estimates.* In Osmani SR, editor: *Nutrition and poverty,* Oxford, 1990, Oxford University Press.
173. Bloem MW et al: A prevalence study of vitamin A deficiency and xeropthalmia in northeastern Thailand, *Am J Epidemiol* 129:1095, 1989.
174. Carlier C et al: Prevalence of malnutrition and vitamin A deficiency in the Diourbel, Fatick, and Kaolock regions of Senegal: a controlled study, *Am J Clin Nutr* 53:74, 1991.
175. Choprapawon C et al: Cultural study of diarrhoeal illnesses in central Thailand and its practical implications, *J Diarrhoeal Dis Res* 9:204, 1991.
176. Donovan P: Dangerous myths, *Hygiene* 11:7, 1992.
177. Foster A, Sommer A: Corneal ulceration, measles, and childhood blindness in Tanzania, *Br J Ophthalmol* 71:331, 1987.
178. Gordon JE, Scrimshaw NS: Nutrition and the diseases of early childhood in the tropics, *Milbank Mem Fnd Quart* 43:235, 1965.
179. Kambarami RA et al: Measles epidemic in Harare, Zimbabwe, despite high measles immunization coverage rates, *Bull WHO* 69:213, 1991.
180. Ketsela T, Asfaw M, Belachew C: Knowledge and practice of mothers/care-takers towards diarrhoea and its treatment in rural communities in Ethiopia, *Ethiop Med J* 29:213, 1991.
181. Milton RC, Reddy V, Naidu AN: Mild vitamin A deficiency and childhood morbidity—an Indian experience, *Am J Clin Nutr* 46:827, 1987.
182. Molteno CD, Kibel MA: Postneonatal mortality in the Matroosberg Divisional Council area of the Cape Western Health Region, *S Afr Med J* 75:575, 1989.
183. Neumann C et al: Relationships between morbidity and development in mildly to moderately malnourished Kenyan toddlers, *Pediatrics* 88:934, 1991.
184. Olson RE: World food production and problems in human nutrition, *Nutr Today* 24:15, 1989.
185. Pitt MM, Rosenzweig MR, Hassan MdN: Productivity, health, and inequality in the intrahousehold distribution of food in low-income countries, *Am Econ Rev* 80:1139, 1990.
186. Reddaiah VP, Kapoor SK: Epidemiology of diarrhea and its implications for providing services, *Indi J Pediatr* 58:205, 1991.
187. Rodriguez-Garcia R, Schaefer LA: Breastfeeding: an old practice or a new technique?, *Hygiene* 10:5, 1991.
188. Salomon JB et al: Malnutrition and the common communicable diseases of childhood in rural Guatemala, *Am J Pub Hlth* 58:505-516, 1968.
189. Scrimshaw NS et al: Nutrition and infection field study in Guatemalan villages, 1959-1964. V. Disease incidence among preschool children under natural village conditions, with improved diet and with medical and public health services, *Arch Environ Hlth* 16:223, 1968.
190. Sigman M et al: Prediction of cognitive competence in Kenyan children from toddler nutrition, family characteristics and abilities, *J Child Psychol Psychiat* 32:307, 1991.
191. Smith IF, Taiwo O, Golden MHN: Plant protein rehabilitation diets and iron supplementation of the protein-energy malnourished child, *Eur J Clin Nutr* 43:763, 1989.

192. Sommer A, Tarwotjo I, Katz J: Increased risk of xerophthalmia following diarrhea and respiratory disease, *Am J Clin Nutr* 45:977, 1987.
193. Stanton BF et al: Risk factors for developing mild nutritional blindness in urban Bangladesh, *Am J Dis Child* 140:584, 1986.
194. Sullivan PB et al: Chronic diarrhea and malnutrition—histology of the small intestinal lesion, *J Pediatr Gastroenterol Nutr* 12:195, 1991.
195. Tolboom JJM et al: Severe protein energy malnutrition in Lesotho, death and survival in hospital, clinical findings, *Trop Geogr Med* 38:351, 1986.
196. UNICEF: *The state of the world's children,* Oxford, 1992, Oxford University Press.
197. Victora CG: The association between wasting and stunting: an international perspective, *J Nutr* 122:1105, 1992.
198. Wellcome Trust Working Party: Classification of infantile malnutrition, *Lancet* 2:302, 1970.
199. Wharton BA: Food for the weanling: the next priority in infant nutrition, *Acta Paediat Scand Suppl* 323:96, 1986.
200. Zollner EWA et al: Protein energy malnutrition and its recognition in outpatient departments in Venda hospitals, *S Afr Med J* 81:210, 1992.

Diet, plasma lipids, and cardiovascular disease

201. American Heart Association: *1992 Heart and stroke facts,* Dallas, 1992, American Heart Association.
202. Andersen P, Arnesen H, Hjermann I: Increased fibrinolytic capacity after intervention on diet in healthy coronary high risk men, *Scand J Haematol* 30:47, 1983.
203. Andersen P et al: Increased fibrinolytic potential after diet intervention in healthy coronary high-risk individuals, *Acta Med Scand* 223:499, 1988.
204. Armstrong V et al: The association between Lp(a) concentrations and angiographically assessed coronary atherosclerosis: dependence on serum LDL levels, *Atherosclerosis* 62:249, 1986.
205. Atherosclerosis Risk in Communities (ARIC) Study: design and objectives. *Am J Epidemiol* 129:687, 1989.
206. Austin M: Epidemiologic associations between hypertriglyceridemia and coronary heart disease, *Sem Thromb Hemostas* 14:137, 1988.
207. Beynen A, West C: *Mechanisms underlying nutritional effects on serum cholesterol concentrations.* In Cliff W, G Schoefl, editors: *Coronaries and cholesterol,* London, 1989, Chapman & Hall Medical.
208. Bini A et al: Identification and distribution of fibrinogen, fibrin, and fibrin(ogen) degradation products in atherosclerosis: use of monoclonal antibodies, *Arteriosclerosis* 9:109, 1989.
209. Blackburn H: *A public health approach to nutrition, mass hyperlipidemia, and atherosclerotic diseases.* In Naito H, editor: *Nutrition and heart disease.* New York, 1982, SP Medical and Scientific Books.
210. Blankenhorn D et al: Beneficial effects of combined colestipol-niacin therapy on coronary atherosclerosis and coronary venous bypass grafts, *JAMA* 257:3233, 1987.
211. Brown G et al: Regression of coronary artery disease as a result of intensive lipid-lowering therapy in men with high levels of apolipoprotein B, *N Engl J Med* 323:1289, 1990.
212. Brown M, Kovanen P, Goldstein J: Regulation of plasma cholesterol by lipoprotein receptors, *Science* 212:628, 1981.
213. Burr M et al: Effects of changes in fat, fish and fibre intakes on death and myocardial reinfarction: Diet and Reinfarction Trial (DART), *Lancet* 2:757, 1989.
214. Chandler A: *An overview of thrombosis and platelet involvement in the development of the human atherosclerotic plaque.* In Glagov S, Newman W, Schaffer S, editors: *Pathobiology of the human atherosclerotic plaque,* New York, 1990, Springer-Verlag.

215. Chen Z et al: Serum cholesterol concentration and coronary heart disease in population with low cholesterol concentrations, *BMJ* 303:276, 1991.

216. Clark E, Graef I, Chasis H: Thrombosis of the aorta and coronary arteries with special reference to "fibrinoid" lesions, *Arch Pathol* 22:183, 1936.

217. Connor S et al: The cholesterol/saturated fat index: an indication of the hypercholesterolemic and atherogenic potential of food, *Lancet* 1:1229, 1986.

218. Connor W, Connor S: The key role of nutritional factors in the prevention of coronary heart disease, *Preventive Med* 1:49, 1972.

219. Criqui M et al: Plasma triglyceride level and mortality from coronary heart disease, *N Engl J Med* 328:1220, 1993.

220. Dahlen G et al: Association of levels of lipoprotein (a), plasma lipids, and other lipoproteins with coronary artery disease documented by angiography, *Circulation* 74:758, 1986.

221. Dalaker K, Hjermann I, Prydz H: A novel form of factor VII in plasma from men at risk for cardiovascular disease, *Br J Haematol* 61:315, 1985.

222. DeLangen C: Cholesterol exchange and pathology of race, *Presse Med* 24:332, 1916.

223. Department of Health and Human Services: *Physiological effects and health consequences of dietary fiber*, Washington, DC, 1987, Department of Health and Human Services.

224. DeWood M et al: Prevalence of total coronary occlusion during the early hours of transmural myocardial infarction, *N Engl J Med* 303:897, 1980.

225. Dratz E, Deese A: *The role of docoashexaenoic acid (22:6n3) in biological membranes: examples from photoreceptors and model membrane bilayers*. In Simopoulos A, Kifer R, Martin R, editors: *Health effects of polyunsaturated fatty acids in seafood*, Orlando, 1986, Academic Press.

226. Duguid J: Thrombosis as a factor in the pathogenesis of coronary atherosclerosis, *J Pathol Bact* 58:207, 1946.

227. Dyerberg J, et al: Eicosapentaenoic acid and prevention of thrombosis and atherosclerosis, *Lancet* 2:117, 1978.

228. Eaton D et al: Partial amino acid sequence of apolipoprotein (a) shows that it is homologous to plasminogen, *Proc Natl Acad Sci USA* 84:3224, 1987.

229. Folsom A et al: Population correlates of plasma fibrinogen and factor VII, putative cardiovascular risk factors, *Atherosclerosis* 91:191, 1991.

230. Food and Drug Administration: *Food labelling: health claims, dietary fiber and cardiovascular disease*, Washington, DC, 1991, Food and Drug Administration.

231. Frick M et al: Helsinki Heart Study: Primary prevention trial with gemfibrozil in middle-aged men with dyslipidemia, *N Engl J Med* 317:1237, 1987.

232. Fried L et al: The Cardiovascular Health Study: design and rationale, *Ann Epidemiol* 1:263, 1991.

233. Fuster V et al: Atherosclerotic plaque rupture and thrombosis: evolving concepts, *Circulation* 82:1147, 1990.

234. Fuster V et al: Pathogenesis of coronary artery disease and the acute coronary syndromes: part 1, *N Engl J Med* 326:242, 1992.

235. Fuster V et al: The pathogenesis of coronary artery disease and the acute coronary syndromes: part 2, *N Engl J Med* 326:310, 1992.

236. Gerrity R: The role of the monocyte in atherogenesis. I: transition of blood-borne monocytes into the foam cells in fatty lesions, *Am J Pathol* 103:181, 1981.

237. Gerrity R: The role of the monocyte in atherogenesis. II: migration of foam cells from atherosclerotic lesions, *Am J Pathol* 103:191, 1981.

238. Goldstein J et al: Binding site on macrophages that mediates uptake and degradation of acetylated low density lipoprotein, producing massive cholesterol deposition, *Proc Natl Acad Sci* 76:333, 1979.

239. Goodnight S et al: Polyunsaturated fatty acids, hyperlipidemia and thrombosis, *Arteriosclerosis* 2:87, 1982.

240. Gorlin R: The biological actions and potential clinical significance of dietary omega-3 fatty acids, *Arch Intern Med* 148:2043, 1988.

241. Gotto A et al: The cholesterol facts: a summary of the evidence relating dietary fats, serum cholesterol, and coronary heart disease: a joint statement by the American Heart Association and the National Heart, Lung, and Blood Institute, *Circulation* 81:1721, 1990.

242. Hamsten A et al: Increased plasma levels of a rapid inhibitor of tissue plasminogen activator in young survivors of myocardial infarction, *N Engl J Med* 313:1557, 1985.

243. Hamsten A et al: Plasminogen activator inhibitor in plasma: risk factor for recurrent myocardial infarction, *Lancet* 2:3, 1987.

244. Hayes T, Pike J, Tracy R: Factor VII assays, *Arch Pathol Lab Med* 117:52, 1993.

245. Heinecke J, Rosen H, Chait A: Iron and copper promote modification of low density lipoprotein by human arterial smooth muscle cells in culture, *J Clin Invest* 74:1890, 1984.

246. Henriksen T, Mahoney E, Steinberg D: Enhanced macrophage degradation of low density lipoprotein previously incubated with cultured endothelial cells: recognition by receptor for acetylated low density lipoproteins, *Proc Natl Acad Sci* 78:6499, 1981.

247. Hoffman C et al: Elevation of factor VII activity and mass in young adults at risk of ischaemic heart disease, *J Am Coll Cardiol* 14:941, 1989.

248. Jenkins D et al: Effect on blood lipids of very high intakes of fiber in diets low in saturated fat and cholesterol, *N Engl J Med* 329:21, 1993.

249. Johnstone J: *Controlled trials, cholesterol, coronary heart disease and health*. In Cliff W, and Schoefl G, editors: *Coronaries and cholesterol*, London, 1989, Chapman & Hall Medical.

250. Juhan-Vague I, Alessi M, Vague P: Increased plasma plasminogen activator inhibitor 1 levels: a possible link between insulin resistance and atherothrombosis, *Diabetologia* 34:457, 1991.

251. Juhan-Vague I et al: Relationships between plasma insulin, triglyceride, body mass index, and plasminogen activator inhibitor 1, *Diabetes Metab* 13:331, 1987.

252. Kagan A et al: Epidemiologic studies of coronary heart disease and stroke in Japanese living in Japan, Hawaii and California: demographic, physical, dietary and biochemical characteristics, *J Chron Dis* 27:345, 1974.

253. Kannel W, D'Agostino R, Belanger A: Update on fibrinogen as a cardiovascular risk factor, *Ann Epidemiol* 2:457, 1992.

254. Kannel W et al: Serum cholesterol, lipoproteins, and the risk of coronary heart disease: the Framingham study, *Ann Intern Med* 74:1, 1971.

255. Kannel W et al: Fibrinogen and risk of cardiovascular disease: the Framingham study, *JAMA* 258:1183, 1987.

256. Karvonen M et al: Men in rural East and West Finland, *Acta Med Scand* 460S:169, 1967.

257. Keys A et al: Epidemiological studies related to coronary heart disease: characteristics of men aged 40-59 in seven countries, *Acta Med Scand* 460S:8, 1967.

258. Keys A et al: The diet and 15-year death rate in the Seven Countries Study, *Am J Epidemiol* 124:903, 1986.

259. Kimura N: A farming and fishing village in Japan: Tanushimaru and Ushibuka, *Acta Med Scand* 460S:231, 1967.

260. Klag M et al: Serum cholesterol in young men and subsequent cardiovascular disease, *N Engl J Med* 328:313, 1993.

261. Klevay L: *Ischemic heart disease: updating the zinc/copper hypothesis*. In Naito H, editor: *Nutrition and heart disease*, New York, 1982, SP Medical & Scientific Books.

262. Kostner G et al: Lipoprotein Lp(a) and the risk for myocardial infarction, *Atherosclerosis* 38:51, 1981.

263. Kraft H et al: Apolipoprotein (a) alleles determine lipoprotein (a)

particle density and concentration in plasma, *Arterioscler Thromb* 12:302, 1992.

264. Leaf A, Weber P: Cardiovascular effects of n-3 fatty acids, *N Engl J Med* 318:549, 1988.

265. Lipid Research Clinincs Program: The Lipid Research Clinics Coronary Primary Prevention Trial. I. Reduction in incidence of coronary heart disease, *JAMA* 251:351, 1984.

266. Mallory F: *The infectious lesions of blood vessels,* Philadelphia, 1913, JB Lippincott.

267. Mann K, Lawson J: The role of the membrane in the expression of the vitamin K-dependent enzymes, *Arch Pathol Lab Med* 116:1330, 1992.

268. Manninen V et al: Lipid alterations and decline in the incidence of coronary heart disease in the Helsinki Heart Study, *JAMA* 260:641, 1988.

269. Marckmann P, Sandstrom B, Jespersen J: Effect of total fat content and fatty acid composition in diet on factor VII coagulant activity and blood lipids, *Atherosclerosis* 80:227, 1990.

270. Marckmann P, Sandstrom B, Jespersen J: Fasting blood coagulation and fibrinolysis of young adults unchanged by reduction in dietary fat content, *Arterioscler Thromb* 12:201, 1992.

271. Marckmann P, Sandstrom B, Jespersen J: Favorable long-term effect of a low-fat/high-fiber diet on human blood coagulation and fibrinolysis, *Arterioscler Thromb* 13:505, 1993.

272. Marmot M et al: Epidemiologic studies of coronary heart disease and stroke in Japanese men living in Japan, Hawaii and California. Prevalence of coronary disease and hypertensive heart disease and associated risk factors, *Am J Epidemiol* 102:514, 1975.

273. McGee D et al: Ten-year incidence of coronary heart disease in the Honolulu Heart Program: relationship to nutrient intake, *Am J Epidemiol* 119:667, 1984.

274. McGee D et al: The relationship of dietary fat and cholesterol to mortality in 10 years: the Honolulu Heart Program, *Int J Epidemiol* 14:97, 1985.

275. Meade T: *The epidemiology of haemostatic and other variables in coronary artery disease.* In Verstraete M, Vermylen J, Lijnen H, Arnout J, editors: *Thrombosis and haemostasis 1987,* Leuven, 1987, Leuven University Press.

276. Meade T et al: Haemostatic function and cardiovascular death: early results of a prospective study, *Lancet* 1:1050, 1980.

277. Meade T et al: Haemostatic function and ischaemic heart disease: principal results of the Northwick Park Heart Study, *Lancet* 2:533, 1986.

278. Miller G et al: Association between dietary fat intake and plasma factor VII coagulant activity—a predictor of cardiovascular mortality, *Atherosclerosis* 60:269, 1986.

279. Miller G et al: Plasma factor VII is activated by postproandial triglyceridemia, irrespective of dietary fat composition, *Atherosclerosis* 86:163, 1991.

280. Mitropoulos K: Hypercoagulability and factor VII in hypertriglyceridemia, *Sem Thromb Hemostas* 14:246, 1988.

281. Muldoon M, Manuck S, Mathews K: Lowering cholesterol concentrations and mortality: a quantitative review of primary prevention trials, *BMJ* 301:309, 1990.

282. Multiple Risk Factor Intervention Trial Research Group: Multiple risk factor intervention trial: risk factor changes and mortality results, *JAMA* 248:1465, 1982.

283. Murai A et al: Lp(a) lipoprotein as a risk factor for coronary heart disease and cerebral infarction, *Atherosclerosis* 59:199, 1986.

284. Mussoni L et al: Hypertriglyceridemia and regulation of fibrinolytic activity, *Arterioscler Thromb* 12:19, 1992.

285. National Cholesterol Education Panel: Report of the National Cholesterol Education Program Expert Panel on detection, evaluation and treatment of high blood cholesterol in adults, *Arch Intern Med* 148:36, 1988.

286. National Heart, Lung, and Blood Institute Consensus Development Panel: Treatment of hypertriglyceridemia, *JAMA* 251:1196, 1984.

287. Nordoy A, Goodnight S: Dietary lipids and thrombosis: relationships to atherosclerosis, *Arteriosclerosis* 10:149, 1990.

288. Palinski W et al: Low density lipoprotein undergoes oxidative modification in vivo, *Proc Natl Acad Sci* 86:1372, 1989.

289. Phillipson B et al: Reduction of plasma lipids, lipoproteins, and apoproteins by dietary fish oils in patients with hypertriglyceridemia, *N Engl J Med* 312:1210, 1985.

290. Reunanen A, Knekt P, Aaran R-K: Serum ceruloplasmin level and risk of myocardial infarction and stroke, *Am J Epidemiol* 136:1082, 1992.

291. Rhoads G et al: Lp(a) lipoprotein as a risk factor for myocardial infarction, *JAMA* 256:2540, 1986.

292. Rimm E et al: Vitamin E consumption and the risk of coronary heart disease in men, *N Engl J Med* 328:1450, 1993.

293. Rokitansky C: *A manual of pathological anatomy,* Philadelphia, 1855, Blanchard & Lee.

294. Rosengren A et al: Lipoprotein (a) and coronary heart disease: a prospective case-control study in a general population sample of middle aged men, *BMJ* 301:1248, 1990.

295. Ross R: The pathogenesis of atherosclerosis—an update, *N Engl J Med* 314:488, 1986.

296. Rossouw J, Lewis B, Rifkind B: The value of lowering cholesterol after myocardial infarction, *N Engl J Med* 323:1112, 1990.

297. Salonen J et al: Interactions of serum copper, selenium, and low density lipoprotein cholesterol in atherogenesis, *BMJ* 302:756, 1991.

298. Salonen J et al: Serum copper and the risk of acute myocardial infarction: a prospective population study in men in eastern Finland, *Am J Epidemiol* 134:268, 1991.

299. Salonen J et al: High stored iron levels are associated with excess risk of myocardial infarction in eastern Finnish men, *Circulation* 86:803, 1992.

300. Sandkamp M et al: Lipoprotein (a) is an independent risk factor for myocardial infarction at a young age, *Clin Chem* 36:20, 1990.

301. Scanu A, Fless G: Lipoprotein (a): heterogeneity and biological relevance, *J Clin Invest* 85:1709, 1990.

302. Seligsohn U et al: Evidence for the participation of both activated factor XII and activated factor IX in the cold promoted-activation of factor VII, *Thromb Res* 13:1049, 1978.

303. Smith E et al: Fate of fibrinogen in human arterial intima, *Arteriosclerosis* 10:263, 1990.

304. Stampfer M et al: Vitamin E consumption and the risk of coronary disease in women, *N Engl J Med* 328:1444, 1993.

305. Stary H: Evolution and progression of atherosclerotic lesions in coronary arteries of children and young adults, *Arteriosclerosis* 99:I19, 1989.

306. Steinberg D: Metabolism of lipoproteins and their role in the pathogenesis of atherosclerosis, *Atheroscler Rev* 18:1, 1988.

307. Steinberg D et al: Beyond cholesterol: modifications of low density lipoprotein that increase its atherogenicity, *N Engl J Med* 320:915, 1989.

308. Stone M, Thorp J: Plasma fibrinogen—a major coronary risk factor, *J R Coll Gen Pract* 35:565, 1985.

309. Sullivan D et al: Paradoxical elevation of LDL apoprotein B levels in hypertriglyceridemic patients and normal subjects ingesting fish oil, *Atherosclerosis* 61:129, 1986.

310. Thomas W, Hartroft W: Myocardial infarction in rats fed diets containing high fat, cholesterol, thiouracil and sodium cholate, *Circulation* 19:65, 1959.

311. Thompson G: Lipids, fish and coronary heart disease, *Curr Opin Cardiol* 1:827, 1986.

312. Uterman G: The mysteries of lipoprotein(a), *Science* 246:904, 1989.

313. von Schacky C, Fischer S, Weber P: Long-term effects of dietary marine omega-3 fatty acids upon plasma and cellular lipids, platelet

function, and eicosanoid formation in humans, *J Clin Invest* 76:1626, 1985.

314. Wilhelmsen L et al: Fibrinogen as a risk factor for stroke and myocardial infarction, *N Engl J Med* 311:501, 1984.

315. Woolf N, Davies M: *Interrelationship between atherosclerosis and thrombosis.* In Fuster V, Verstraete M, editors: *Thrombosis in cardiovascular disorders,* Philadelphia, 1992, WB Saunders.

316. Yano K, Reed D, Kagan A: Coronary heart disease, hypertension and stroke among Japanese-American men in Hawaii: the Honolulu Heart Program, *Hawaii Med J* 44:297, 1985.

317. Yano K, Reed D, McGee D: Ten-year incidence of coronary heart disease in the Honolulu Heart Program: Relationship to biological and lifestyle characteristics, *Am J Epidemiol* 119:653, 1984.

318. Yarnell J et al: Fibrinogen, viscosity, and white blood cell count are major risk factors for ischemic heart disease, *Circulation* 83:836, 1991.

319. Yla-Herttuala S et al: Evidence for the presence of oxidatively modified low density lipoprotein in atherosclerotic lesions of rabbit and man, *J Clin Invest* 84:1086, 1989.

320. Yusuf S, Wittes J, Friedman L: Overview of results of randomized clinical trials in heart disease: II. unstable angina, heart failure, primary prevention with aspirin and risk factor modification, *JAMA* 260:2259, 1988.

321. Zimetbaum P et al: Plasma lipids and lipoproteins and the incidence of cardiovascular disease in the very elderly: the Bronx Aging Study, *Arterioscler Thromb* 12:416, 1992.

Vitamin A, retinoids, and carotenoids

322. Bitot P: Memoire sur une lesion conjunctivale, non encore decrite, coincidant avec l'hemeralopie, *Bull Acad Med Paris* 28:619, 1862.

323. Bjelke E: Dietary vitamin A and human lung cancer, *Int J Cancer* 15:561, 1975.

324. Blackfan KD, Wolbach SB: Vitamin A deficiency in infants: a clinical and pathological study, *J Pediatr* 3:679, 1933.

325. Byers T et al: Dietary vitamin A and lung cancer risk: an analysis by histologic subtypes, *Am J Epidemiol* 120:769, 1984.

326. De Luca LM: Retinoids and their receptors in differentiation, embryogenesis, and neoplasia, *FASEB J* 5:2924, 1991.

327. Feachem RG: Vitamin A deficiency and diarrhoea: a review of the interrelationships and their implications for the control of xerophthalmia and diarrhoea, *Trop Dis Bull* 84:R1, 1987.

328. Floyd EE, Jetten AM: Retinoids, growth factors, and the tracheobronchial epithelium, *Lab Invest* 59:1, 1988 (editorial).

329. Follis RH Jr: *Deficiency disease,* Springfield, Ill, 1958, Charles C Thomas.

330. Gao C et al: Protective effects of raw vegetables and fruit against lung cancer among smokers and ex-smokers: a case-control study in the Tokai area of Japan, *Jpn J Cancer Res* 84:594, 1993.

331. Humphrey JH, West KP Jr: *Vitamin A deficiency: role in childhood infection and mortality.* In Bendich A, Butterworth CE Jr, editors: *Micronutrients in health and in disease prevention,* New York, 1991, Marcel Dekker.

332. Jain M et al: Dietary factors and risk of lung cancer: results from a case-control study, Toronto, 1981-85, *Int J Cancer* 45:287, 1990.

333. Mackenzie W: *A practical treatise on diseases of the eye,* London, 1830, Longman.

334. Mori M: Uber den sog. Hikan (xerosis conjunctivae infantum ev. Keratomalacie), *Jahrbuch f Kindheilkund* 59:175, 1904.

335. Mossman BT, Craighead JE: Asbestos-induced epithelial changes in organ cultures of hamster trachea: inhibition by the vitamin A analog, retinyl methyl ether, *Science* 207:311, 1980.

336. Nauss KM: *Influence of vitamin A status on the immune system.* In Bauernfeind JC, editor: *Vitamin A deficiency and its control,* Orlando, 1986, Academic Press.

337. Peto R: The marked differences between carotenoids and retinoids: methodological implications for biochemical epidemiology, *Cancer Surv* 2:327, 1983.

338. Pisani P et al: Carrots, green vegetables and lung cancer: a case-control study, *Int J Epidemiol* 15:463, 1986.

339. Samet JM et al: Lung cancer risk and vitamin A consumption in New Mexico, *Am Rev Respir Dis* 131:198, 1985.

340. Shekelle et al: Dietary vitamin A and risk of cancer in the Western Electric study, *Lancet* 2:1186, 1981.

341. Sherman MI: *Retinoids and cell differentiation,* Boca Raton, Fla, 1986, CRC Press.

342. Sommer A: Vitamin A, infectious disease, and childhood mortality: a 2¢ solution? *J Infect Dis* 167:1003, 1993.

343. Sommer A et al: Incidence, prevalence and scale of blinding malnutrition, *Lancet* 1:1407, 1981.

344. Sporn MB, Roberts AB, Goodman DS: *The retinoids,* vols 1,2, New York, 1984, Academic Press.

345. Wald G: *The biochemistry of vitamin A.* In *A symposium on nutrition,* Baltimore, 1953, The Johns Hopkins Press.

346. Wald G, Steven D: *Proc Natl Acad Sci USA* 25:344, 1959.

347. Warrell RP Jr et al: Acute promyelocytic leukemia, *N Engl J Med* 329:177, 1993.

348. West KP Jr, Howard GR, Sommer A: Vitamin A and infection: public health implications, *Ann Rev Nutr* 9:63, 1989.

349. Willett WC et al: *Diet, nutrition and cancer,* Washington, DC, 1982, National Academy Press.

350. Wohlbach SB, Bessey OA: Tissue changes in vitamin deficiences, *Physiol Rev* 22:233, 1942.

351. Wohlbach SB, Howe PR: Epithelial repair in recovery from vitamin A deficiency, *J Exp Med* 57:511, 1933.

352. Wu AH et al: Smoking and other risk factors for lung cancer in women, *J Natl Cancer Inst* 74:747, 1985.

353. Ziegler RG et al: Dietary carotene and vitamin A and risk of lung cancer among white men in New Jersey, *J Natl Cancer Inst* 73:1429, 1984.

Vitamin D deficiency

354. Aust-Kettis A et al: Rickets in Ethiopia, *Ethiop Med J* 3:109, 1965.

355. Belton NR: Rickets—not only the "English disease," *Acta Paediatr Scand Suppl* 323:68, 1986.

356. Bhattacharyya AK: Nutritional rickets in the tropics, *World Rev Nutr Diet* 67:140, 1992.

357. Boyle IT: Bones for the future, *Acta Paediatr Scand* Suppl 373:58, 1991.

358. Chang YT et al: Hypocalcemia in nonwhite breast-fed infants, *Clin Pediatr* 31:695, 1992.

359. Clements MR et al: The role of 1,25-dihydroxyvitamin D in the mechanisms of acquired vitamin D deficiency, *Clin Endocrinol* 37:17, 1992.

360. Elidrissy ATH: *Vitamin D-deficiency rickets in Saudi Arabia.* In Glorieux FH, editor: *Rickets,* vol 21, New York, 1991, Raven Press.

361. Garbedian M, Ben-Mekhbi H: *Is vitamin D-deficiency rickets a public health problem in France and Algeria?* In Glorieux FH, editor: *Rickets,* vol 21, New York, 1991, Raven Press.

362. Ghai OP, Koul PB: *Rickets in India.* In Glorieux FH, editor: *Rickets,* vol 21, New York, 1991, Raven Press.

363. Glorieux FH: Rickets, the continuing challenge, *N Engl J Med* 325:1875, 1991.

364. Grindulis H et al: Combined deficiency of iron and vitamin D in Asian toddlers, *Arch Dis Child* 61:843, 1986.

365. Henderson JB et al: The importance of limited exposure to ultraviolet radiation and dietary factors in the aetiology of Asian rickets: a risk-factor model, *Quart J Med* 63:413, 1987.

366. Hutchison FN, Bell NH: Osteomalacia and rickets, *Sem Nephrol* 12:127, 1992.

367. Hutchison HS, Shah JJ: The aetiology of rickets early and late, *Quart J Med* 15:167, 1922.

368. Jelliffe DB: *Infant nutrition in the tropics and subtropics*, WHO Monograph No 29, Geneva, 1955, World Health Organization.

369. Jelliffe DB: *The assessment of the nutritional status of the community*, WHO Monograph No 53, Geneva, 1966, World Health Organization.

370. Klasmer R: Serum phosphatase activity and clinical rickets in children in Jerusalem, *Am J Dis Child* 67:348, 1944.

371. Kumar R: Vitamin D and calcium transport, *Kidney Int* 40:1177, 1991.

372. Lawson DEM et al: Aetiology of rickets in Egyptian children, *Hum Nutr Clin Nutr* 41:199, 1987.

373. Lo CW, Paris PW, Holick MF: Indian and Pakistani immigrants have the same capacity as Caucasians to produce vitamin D in response to ultraviolet irradiation, *Am J Clin Nutr* 44:683, 1986.

374. Markestad T, Elzouki AY: *Vitamin D-deficiency rickets in northern Europe and Libya.* In Glorieux FH, editor: *Rickets,* vol 21, New York, 1991, Raven Press.

375. McKenna MJ: Differences in vitamin D status between countries in young adults and the elderly, *Am J Med* 93:69, 1992.

376. Miller CG, Chutkan W: Vitamin D deficiency rickets in Jamaican children, *Arch Dis Child* 51:214, 1976.

377. Okonofua F et al: Rickets in Nigerian children: a consequence of calcium malnutrition, *Metabolism* 40:209, 1991.

378. Oliveri BM et al: *Nutritional rickets in Argentina.* In Glorieux FH, editor: *Rickets,* vol 21, New York, 1991, Raven Press.

379. Oyenade GAA: Aetiological factors in genu valga, vara and varo valga in Nigerian children, *J Trop Pediatr Environ Child Health* 21:167, 1975.

380. Salimpour R: Rickets in Tehran: study of 200 cases, *Arch Dis Child* 50:63, 1975.

381. Shawky I: Prevalence and aetiology of rickets in tropical and subtropical countries, *CR Cong Int Med Trop Hyg* 2:961, 1929.

382. Underwood P, Margetts B: High levels of childhood rickets in rural North Yemen, *Soc Sci Med* 24:37, 1987.

383. Walters MR, Kollenkirchen U, Fox J: What is vitamin D deficiency? *Proc Soc Exp Biol Med* 199:385, 1992.

384. Zhou H: *Rickets in China.* In Glorieux FH, editor: *Rickets,* vol 21, New York, 1991, Raven Press.

Folic acid deficiency

385. Blakely RL: *The biochemistry of folic acid and related pteridines,* Amsterdam, 1969, North-Holland.

386. Bower C, Stanley FJ: Dietary folate as a risk factor for neural-tube defects: evidence from a case-control study in Western Australia, *Med J Aust* 150:613, 1989.

387. Branda RF: *Effects of folic acid deficiency on tumor cell biology.* In Jacobs MM, editor: *Vitamins and minerals in the prevention and treatment of cancer,* Boca Raton, Fla, 1990, CRC Press.

388. Branda RF, Blickensderfer DB: Folate deficiency amplifies genetic damage caused by alkylating agents and gamma irradiation in Chinese hamster ovary cells, *Cancer Res* 53:5401, 1993.

389. Colon-Otero G, Menke D, Hook CC: A practical approach to the differential diagnosis and evaluation of the adult patient with macrocytic anemia, *Med Clin North Am* 76:581, 1992.

390. Cravo ML et al: Folate deficiency enhances the development of colonic neoplasia in dimethylhydrazine-treated rats, *Cancer Res* 52:5002, 1992.

391. Daniel WA, Mounger JR, Perkins JC: Obstetric and fetal complications in folate-deficient adolescent girls, *Am J Obstet Gynecol* 111:233, 1971.

392. Erbe RW: Inborn errors of folate metabolism, *N Engl J Med* 293:807, 1975.

393. Eto I, Krumdieck CL: Role of vitamin B_{12} and folate deficiencies in carcinogenesis, *Adv Exp Med Biol* 206:313, 1986.

394. Fernandes-Costa FJ et al: Transition from a hunter-gatherer to a settled lifestyle in the !Kung San: effect of iron, folate, and vitamin B_{12} nutrition, *Am J Clin Nutr* 40:1295, 1984.

395. Freudenheim JL et al: Folate intake and carcinogenesis of the colon and rectum, *Int J Epidemiol* 20:368, 1991.

396. Giovannucci E et al: Folate, methionine, and alcohol intake and risk of colorectal adenoma. *J Natl Cancer Inst* 85:875, 1993.

397. Heimburger et al: Improvement in bronchial squamous metaplasia in smokers treated with folate and vitamin B_{12}, *JAMA* 259:1525, 1988.

398. Herbert V: Biology of disease: megaloblastic anemias, *Lab Invest* 52:3, 1985.

399. Herbert V: Making sense of laboratory test of folate status: folate requirements to sustain normality, *Am J Hematol* 26:199, 1987.

400. Hoffbrand AV et al: Megaloblastic anaemia: initiation of DNA synthesis in excess of DNA chain elongation as the underlying mechanism, *Clin Haematol* 5:727, 1976.

401. Hoppner K, Lampi B, Smith DC: *Data on folacin activity in foods: availability, applications, and limitations.* In *Folic acid: biochemistry and physiology in relation to human nutrition requirement,* Washington, DC, 1977, National Academy of Science.

402. James SJ, Cross DR, Miller BJ: Alterations in nucleotide pools in rats fed diets deficient in choline, methionine and/or folic acid, *Carcinogenesis* 13:2471, 1992.

403. Kristoffersen K, Rolshchau J: *Vitamin supplements and intrauterine growth.* In Briggs MG, editor: *Recent vitamin research,* Boca Raton, Fla, 1984, CRC Press.

404. Krumdieck CL: *Role of folate deficiency in carcinogenesis.* In Butterworth CE, Hutchinson ML, editors: *Nutritional factors in the induction and maintenance of malignancy,* New York, 1983, Academic Press.

405. Lashner BA et al: Effect of folate supplementation on the incidence of dysplasia and cancer in chronic ulcerative colitis, *Gastroenterology* 97:255, 1989.

406. Laurence KM: *Causes of neural tube malformation and their prevention by dietary improvement and preconceptional supplementation with folic acid and multivitamins.* In Briggs MH, editor: *Recent vitamin research,* Boca Raton, Fla, 1984, CRC Press.

407. Magnus EM: Folate activity in serum and red cells of patients with cancer, *Cancer Res* 27:490, 1967.

408. Potischman N: Nutritional epidemiology of cervical neoplasia, *J Nutr* 123:424, 1993.

409. Recommendations for use of folic acid to reduce number of spina bifida cases and other neural tube defects, *JAMA* 269:1233, 1993.

410. Sauberlich HE: *Detection of folic acid deficiency in populations.* In *Folic acid: biochemistry and physiology in relation to human nutrition requirement,* Washington DC, 1977, National Academy of Science.

411. Schorah CJ: *Importance of adequate folate nutrition in embryonic and early fetal development.* In Berger H, editor: *Vitamins and minerals in pregnancy and lactation,* New York, 1988, Vevey/Raven Press.

412. Senti FR, Pilch SM: Analysis of folate data from the Second National Health and Nutrition Examination Survey (NHANES II), *J Nutr* 115:1398, 1985.

413. Stone ML et al: Folic acid metabolism in pregnancy, *Am J Obstet Gynecol* 99:638, 1967.

414. Taheri MR, Wickremasinghe RG, Hoffbrand AV: Alternative metabolic fates of thymine nucleotides in human cells, *Biochem J* 194:451, 1981.

415. Werler MM, Shapiro S, Mitchell AA: Periconceptional folic acid exposure and risk of occurrent neural tube defects, *JAMA* 269:1257, 1993.

416. Wickremasinghe RG, Hoffbrand AV: Reduced rate of DNA replication fork movement in megaloblastic anemia, *J Clin Invest* 65:26, 1980.

Diet and gastroesophageal cancers

417. American Cancer Society: *Cancer facts and figures—1992*. 1992, American Cancer Society.
418. Bartsch H: *N-nitroso compounds and human cancer: where do we stand?* In O'Neill IK, Chen J, Bartsch H, editors: *Relevance to human cancer of N-nitroso compounds, tobacco and mycotoxins*, vol 105, Lyon, France, 1991, IARC Scientific, pp 1-10.
419. Blaser MJ: *Helicobacter pylori* and pathogenesis of gastroduodenal inflammation, *J Infect Dis* 161:626, 1990.
420. Blot WJ et al: Rising incidence of adenocarcinoma of the esophagus and gastric cardia, *JAMA* 265:1287, 1991.
421. Blot WJ et al: Linxian nutrition intervention trials: supplementation with specific vitamin/mineral combinations, cancer incidence, and disease-specific mortality in the general population, *J Natl Cancer Inst* 85:1483, 1993.
422. Chen J: *Dietary practices and cancer mortality in China*. In O'Neill IK, Chen J, Bartsch H, editors: *Relevance to human cancer of N-nitroso compounds, tobacco smoke and mycotoxins*, vol 105, Lyon, France, 1991, IARC Scientific, pp 18-21.
422a. Chu SF, personal communication, 1993.
423. Cook-Mozaffari P: The epidemiology of cancer of the esophagus, *Nutr Cancer* 1:51, 1979.
424. Correa P: A human model of gastric carcinogenesis, *Cancer Res* 48:3554, 1988.
425. Costes RJ et al: Serum levels of selenium and retinol and the subsequent risk of cancer, *Am J Epidemiol* 128:515, 1988.
426. Craddock VM: Aetiology of oesophageal cancer: some operative factors, *Eur J Cancer Prev* 1:89, 1992.
427. Forman D: *The etiology of stomach cancer*. In O'Neill IK, Chen J, Bartsch H, editors: *Relevance to human cancer of N-nitroso compounds, tobacco smoke and mycotoxins*, vol 105, Lyon, France, 1991, IARC Scientific, pp 22-32.
428. Gelderblom WCA: Fumonisins: isolation, chemical characterization and biological effects, *Mycopathologia* 117:11, 1992.
429. Howson CP, Hiyama T, Wynder EL: The decline in gastric cancer: epidemiology of an unplanned triumph, *Epidemiol Rev* 8:1, 1986.
430. Kmet J, Mahboubi E: Esophageal cancer in the Caspian Littoral of Iran: initial studies, *Science* 175:846, 1972.
431. Knekt P et al: Serum selenium and subsequent risk of cancer among Finnish men and women, *J Natl Cancer Inst* 82:864, 1990.
432. Kneller RW et al: Cigarette smoking and other risk factors for progression of precancerous stomach lesions, *J Natl Cancer Inst* 84:1261, 1992.
433. Kodama M, Kodama T, Suzuki T: Effect of rice and salty rice diets on structure of mouse stomach, *Nutr Cancer* 6:135, 1984.
434. Leevy CM et al: B complex vitamins in liver diseases of the alcoholic, *Am J Clin Nutr* 16:339, 1965.
435. Li JY et al: A case-control study of cancer of the esophagus and gastric cardia in Linxian, *Int J Cancer* 43:755, 1989.
436. Li M, Li P, Li B: Recent progress in research on esophageal cancer in China, *Adv Cancer Res* 33:173, 1980.
437. Lu SH et al: *Relevance of N-nitrosamines to oesophageal cancer in China*. In O'Neill IK, Chen J, Bartsch H, editors: *Relevance to human cancer of N-nitroso compounds, tobacco smoke and mycotoxins*, vol 105, Lyon, France, 1991, IARC Scientific, pp 11-17.
438. Mettlin C et al: Diet and cancer of the esophagus, *Nutr Cancer* 2:143, 1981.
439. Minowa S et al: Studies on the relation between cancer and calcium, *Kita Kanto Med J* 10:713, 1960.
440. Mirvish SS: The etiology of gastric cancer: intragastric nitrosamide formation and other theories, *J Natl Cancer Inst* 71:1983.

441. Muir CS, McKinney PA: Cancer of the oesophagus: a global overview, *Eur J Cancer Prev* 1:259, 1992.
442. Nomura SA: *Stomach* In Schottenfeld D, Fraumeni JFJ, editors: *Cancer epidemiology and prevention*, Philadelphia, 1982, WB Saunders, pp 624-637.
443. Parkin DM, Laara E, Muir CS: Estimates of the worldwide frequency of sixteen major cancers in 1980, *Int J Cancer* 41:184, 1988.
444. Pera M et al: Increasing incidence of adenocarcinoma of the esophagus and esophagogastric junction, *Gastroenterology* 104:510, 1993.
445. Pottern LM et al: Esophageal cancer among black men in Washington, DC. I. Alcohol, tobacco, and other risk factors, *J Natl Cancer Inst* 67:777, 1981.
446. Steinmetz KA, Potter JD: Vegetables, fruit and cancer, *Epidemiol Cancer Causes Control* 2:325, 1991.
447. Takahashi M et al: Effect of high salt diet on rat gastric carcinogenesis induced by *N*-methyl-*N*-nitro-*N*-nitrosoguanidine, *Gann* 74:28, 1983.
448. Tuyns AJ: Alcohol and cancer. An instructive association, *Br J Cancer* 64:415, 1991.
449. van Rensburg SJ: Epidemiologic and dietary evidence for a specific nutritional predisposition to esophageal cancer, *J Natl Cancer Inst* 67:243, 1981.
450. van Rensburg SJ, Hall JM, Gathercole PS: Inhibition of esophageal carcinogensis in corn-fed rats by riboflavin, nicotinic acid, selenium, molybdenum, zinc and magnesium, *Nutr Cancer* 8:163, 1986.
451. Vitale JJ, Coffey J: *Alcohol and vitamin metabolism*. In Kissin B, Begleiter H, editors: *The biology of alcoholism*, vol 1, New York, 1971, Plenum Press.
452. Warwick GP: Some aspects of the epidemiology and etiology of esophageal cancer with particular emphasis on the Transkei, South Africa, *Adv Cancer Res* 17:81, 1973.
453. Yang CS: Research on esophageal cancer in China: a review, *Cancer Res* 40:2633, 1980.
454. Yang CS, Lu S-H: *Effect of nutrition on carcinogensis: mechanisms involving nitrosamines*, In *Nutrition and cancer prevention*, Clifton, NJ, 1990, Humana Press, pp 53-70.
455. Yang CS et al: Diet and vitamin nutrition of the high esophageal cancer risk population in Linxian, China, *Nutr Cancer* 4:154, 1982.
456. Yardley JH, Pauli G: *Campylobacter pylori*. A newly recognized infectious agent in the gastrointestinal tract, *Am J Surg Pathol* 1:89, 1988.
457. You W-C et al: Diet and high risk of stomach cancer in Shandong, China, *Cancer Res* 48:3518, 1988.
458. You W-C et al: Allium vegetables and reduced risk of stomach cancer, *J Natl Cancer Inst* 81:162, 1989.
459. You WC et al: Precancerous gastric lesions in a population at high risk of stomach cancer, *Cancer Res* 53:1317, 1993.
460. Zhang L et al: Serum micronutrients in relation to precancerous gastric lesions, *Int J Cancer* 1993 56:650, 1994.
461. Zheng S et al: Nutritional status in Linxian, China: effects of season and supplementation, *Int J Vitam Nutr Res* 59:190, 1989.
462. Zhou YD et al: Hair selenium and zinc in relation to precancerous gastric lesions (in Chinese), *J Pract Oncol* 4:16, 1990.
463. Ziegler RG et al: Esophageal cancer among black men in Washington, D.C. II. Role of nutrition, *J Natl Cancer Inst* 67:1199, 1981.

Diet and renal stones

464. Agus ZS, Goldfarbb S, Wasserstein AW: Calcium transport in the nephron, *Rev Physiol Biochem Pharmacol* 90:155, 1981.
465. Bataille P et al: Effect of calcium restriction on renal excretion of oxalate and the probability of stones in the various pathophysiological groups with calcium stones, *J Urol* 130:218, 1983.
466. Borsatti A: Calcium oxalate nephrolithiasis: defective oxalate transport, *Kidney Int* 39:1283, 1991.
467. Breslau NA et al: Relationship of animal protein-rich diet to sidney

stone formation and calcium metabolism, *J Clin Endocrinol Metab* 66:140, 1988.

468. Broadus AE, Thier SO: Metabolic basis of renal-stone disease, *N Engl J Med* 300:839, 1979.

469. Coe FL, Parks JH: *Nephrolithiasis: pathogenesis and treatment.* Chicago, 1988, Year Book Medical Publishers.

470. Curhan GC et al: A prospective study of dietary calcium and other nutrients and the risk of symptomatic kidney stones, *N Engl J Med* 328:833, 1993.

471. Fellstrom B et al: Dietary habits in renal stone patients compared with healthy sujects, *Br J Urol* 63:575, 1989.

472. Gleeson MJ et al: Effect of unprocessed wheat bran on calciuria and oxaluria in patients with urolithiasis, *Urology* 35:231, 1990.

473. Griffith HM et al: A control study of dietary factors in renal stone formation, *Br J Urol* 53:416, 1981.

474. Hiatt RA et al: Frequency of urolithiasis in a prepaid medical care program, *Am J Epidemiol* 115:255, 1982.

475. Johansson G et al: iochemical and clinical effects of the prophylactic treatment of renal calcium stones with magnesium hydroxide, *J Urol* 124:770, 1980.

476. Johnson CM et al: Renal stone epidemiology: a 25-year study in Rochester, Minnesota, *Kidney Int* 16:624, 1979.

477. Kasidis GP, Rose GA: Oxalate content of some common foods: determination by an enzymatic method, *J Hum Nutr* 34:255, 1980.

478. Kleeman CR et al: Effect of variation in sodium intake on calcium excretion in normal humans, *Proc Soc Exp Biol Med* 115:29, 1964.

479. Larsson L, Tiselius H-G: Hyperoxaluria, *Miner Electrolyte Metab* 13:242, 1987.

480. Lemann J et al: Evidence that glucose ingestion inhibitsnet tubular reabsorption of calcium and magnesium in man, *J Lab Clin Med* 75:578, 1970.

481. Lemann J Jr, Adams ND, Gray RW: Urinary calcium excretion in human beings, *N Engl J Med* 301:535, 1979.

482. Lemann J Jr, Piering WF, Lennon EJ: Possible role of carbohydrate-induced calciuria in calcium oxalate kidney stone formation, *N Engl J Med* 280:232, 1969.

483. Lemann J Jr et al: Potassium administration increases and potassium deprivation reduces urinary calcium excretion in healthy adults, *Kidney Int* 39:973, 1991.

484. Ljunghall S, Fellstrom B, Johansson G: Prevention of renal stones by a high fluid intake? *Eur Urol* 14:381, 1988.

485. Muldowney FP, Freaney R, Moloney MF: Importance of dietary sodium in the hypercalciuria syndrome, *Kidney Int* 22:292, 1982.

486. Norlin A et al: Urolithiasis: a study of its frequency, *Scand J Urol Nephrol* 10:150, 1976.

487. Pak CYC et al: Evidence justifying a high fluid intake of treatment of nephrolithiasis, *Ann Intern Med* 93:36, 1980.

488. Power C et al: Diet and renal stones: a case-control study, *Br J Urol* 56:456, 1984.

489. Robertson GL: *Regulation of vasopressin secretion.* In Seldin DW, Giebisch G, editors: *The kidney, physiology and pathophysiology,* ed 2, New York, 1992, Raven Press.

490. Robertson WG et al: Dietary changes and the incidence of urinary calculi in the U.K. between 1958 and 1976, *J Chron Dis* 32:469, 1979.

491. Robertson WG et al: In Smith LH, Robertson WG, Finlayson B, editors: *Urolithiasis: clinical and basic research,* New York, 1981, Plenum Publishing.

492. Robertson WG et al: In Brockis JG, Finlayson B, editors, *Urinary calculus,* Littleton, MA, 1981, PSG.

493. Samuell CT: In Rose GA, editor: *Oxalate metabolism in relation to urinary stones,* New York, 1988, Springer-Verlag.

494. Shuster J et al: Primary liquid intake and urinary stone disease, *J Chron Dis* 38:907, 1985.

495. Shuster J et al: Soft drink consumption and urinary stone recurrence: a randomized prevention trial, *J Clin Epidemiol* 45:911, 1992.

496. Sierakowski R et al: The frequency of urolithiasis in hospital discharge diagnoses in the United States, *Invest Urol* 15:438, 1978.

497. Smith LH, van den Berg CJ, Wilson DM: Current concepts in nutrition: nutrition and urolithiasis, *N Engl J Med* 298:87, 1978.

498. Strauss AL et al: Factors that predict relapse of calcium nephrolithiasis during treatment, *Am J Med* 72:17, 1982.

499. Trinchieri A et al: The influence of diet on urinary risk factors for stones in healthy subjects and idiopathic renal calcium stone formers, *Br J Urol* 67:230, 1991.

500. van der Horst G et al: Chemical analysis of cool drinks and pure fruit juices—some clinical implications, *S Afr Med J* 66:755, 1984.

501. Wasserstein AG: Case-control study of risk factors for idiopathic calcium nephrolithiasis, *Miner Electrolyte Metab* 13:85, 1987.

502. Yoshida O, Okada Y: Epidemiology of urolithiasis in Japan: a chronological and geographical study, *Urol Int* 45:104, 1990.

503. Zarembski PM, Hodgkinson A: Some factors influencing the urinary excretion of oxalic acid in man, *Clin Chim Acta* 25:1, 1969.

Chapter 10

ULTRAVIOLET RADIATION

Cheryl F. Rosen

Ultraviolet radiation (UV) is ubiquitous because it is a component of terrestrial sunlight. UV radiation forms part of the spectrum of electromagnetic radiation, with wavelengths between x-rays and visible light (Fig. 10-1). It has been arbitrarily divided into three portions: ultraviolet A (UVA), ultraviolet B (UVB), and ultraviolet C (UVC). Only UVA (320 to 400 nm) and UVB (290 to 320 nm) reach the earth's surface. Of the total solar radiant energy that reaches the earth, approximately 3% to 5% is UV. Depending on the time of day and atmospheric conditions UVB composes 10% or less of the total. Stratospheric ozone is crucial for the protection of living organisms because it completely absorbs UVC (200 to 290 nm), absorbing UVB to a lesser extent.[47] Exposure to UVC may occur, however, from artificial sources of radiation, such as germicidal lamps.

In this chapter, the effect of UV radiation on mammalian skin is discussed. The skin functions as a barrier to UV radiation, with UVC being absorbed in the outer layer of the epidermis (stratum corneum), UVB being primarily absorbed in the epidermis, and UVA being absorbed in the dermis. UV radiation produces multiple effects in the skin, both acute and chronic in nature. For example, acute exposure to UV radiation results in the induction of erythema and pigmentation, effects known to occur within minutes to several days after exposure. In contrast, chronic exposure to sunlight may result in the development of cutaneous malignancies, including basal cell and squamous cell carcinomas and melanoma.[4]

NATURE OF EXPOSURE AND EPIDEMIOLOGY

Human skin is exposed to solar UV radiation during the course of everyday life. Clothing can provide protection, but the face, neck, and dorsal hands are routinely exposed. The degree of exposure varies greatly, with geography playing a large role in determining the extent of UV exposure. The closer the latitude to the equator, the greater the UV exposure. Altitude affects the amount of UV that reaches the earth's surface. Weather conditions, including cloud cover and humidity, also affect the amount of UV reaching the earth's surface.[105] The season of the year also plays a role. At the time of the winter solstice, the sun is at a higher zenith angle than at the summer solstice, and the UV radiation must travel through the atmosphere more obliquely, with greater scattering and absorption of the radiation by ozone. Shorter days in winter also result in less terrestrial UV.[83]

Ozone in the stratosphere above the earth absorbs UVC radiation entirely and attenuates the amount of UVB reaching the earth. The amount of ozone represents a balance between the formation of ozone through the interaction of sunlight and oxygen and the destruction of ozone by chemical reactions, which may be natural or human-made. Volcanic eruptions, and energy-derived pollutants produce an increase in sulfur in the stratosphere and are thought to play a role in determining the ozone level (Fig. 10-2). Anthro-

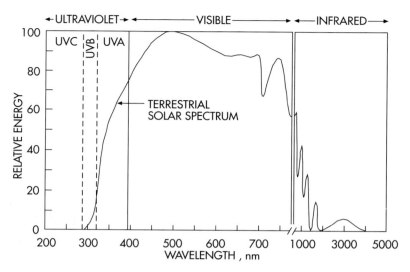

Fig. 10-1. Spectrum of solar radiation that reaches the earth's surface. Wavelengths of radiation shorter than about 290 nm are absorbed by ozone in the stratosphere. (From Kochevar I: Basic concepts in photobiology. In Parrish JA, Kripke ML, Morison WL, editors: *Photoimmunology,* New York, 1983, Plenum Medical Books.)

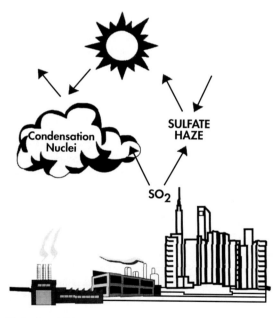

Fig. 10-2. In addition to effects on the ozone layer, anthropogenic sulfur dioxide *(SO₂),* primarily resulting from coal and fuel oil incineration, accumulates in the troposphere. The condensation nuclei and gases serve as a screen for solar ultraviolet irradiation and heat. These pollutants therefore potentially reduce ultraviolet injury to humans and reduce the tendency to earth warming.

pogenic depletion of the ozone has occurred owing to the presence of chemical compounds in the atmosphere, particularly chlorofluorocarbons (CFCs), which have a prolonged lifetime. Chlorine released from CFCs interacts with ozone, producing chlorine monoxide and diminishing the amount of ozone available to absorb UV. These chemicals

have been used for refrigeration, insulation, cleaning solvents and propellants in aerosols. It is suggested, based on mathematical models, that a 1% reduction in the quantity of atmospheric ozone results in a 1% to 2% increase in UVB reaching the earth's surface, leading to a 2% to 4% increase in the incidence of nonmelanoma skin cancers.[38,47] The increase in UVB that would result from a depletion of ozone also varies according to specific wavelength, season, and the zenith angle of the sun.[105] With a change in the zenith angle from low to high, the sunlight passes through the stratosphere at a greater angle, passing through a greater column of ozone, with a greater attenuation of UVB. In 1992, the global average total ozone was 2% to 3% lower than the previous years studied (1979 to 1991).[33] The low levels of ozone were noted in a wide range of latitudes in both the Northern and Southern hemispheres. In the Northern hemisphere, the largest decrease was found between 10° and 60° North latitude.[33] It is important to note that the current increase in incidence in skin cancer does not reflect the recent decreases in the ozone layer because skin cancer is caused by a cumulative effect of UV.[121] The great concern regarding the depletion of atmospheric ozone, however, reflects on the likely amplification of the harmful effects of UV in the future.

Window glass absorbs all UVB radiation, while transmitting UVA. Fluorescent lights emit a small amount of UV radiation, but this is mostly absorbed by fitting the tubes with diffusers or shields and is also attenuated by the distance between the fluorescent light and humans beneath.[109] Incandescent light emits no UV radiation.

Certain occupations require a great deal of outdoor work. Farmers and fishermen, for example, have a greater exposure to sunlight. Also, many people spend a large part of their leisure time outdoors. Furthermore, in certain cultures, the acquisition of a suntan is looked on with favor. Commercial tanning salons are fairly common in North American cities. Clients wishing to obtain a tan are exposed to an artificial source of UV, primarily UVA. Both the American Academy of Dermatology and the Canadian Dermatology Association have issued statements condemning the use of artificial UVA for cosmetic purposes.

SKIN CANCER EPIDEMIOLOGY

Skin cancer is an extremely common form of malignancy. Nonmelanoma skin cancers make up more than one third of all cancers in the United States. An American survey of the years 1977 to 1978 documented an annual incidence of about 500,000 basal cell carcinomas and 100,000 squamous cell carcinomas.[93] It is estimated that more than 700,000 new cases of nonmelanoma skin cancer for the United States will occur in 1994.[7] Because many of these lesions are treated without histological diagnosis, this is likely a conservative estimate.[93] In a study of people enrolled in a large prepaid health insurance program in the Northeast United States, all cases of squamous cell carcinoma and melanoma from 1960 to 1986 were reviewed.[31] In that time period, the incidence of squamous cell carcinoma increased 2.6 times in men and 3.1 times in women. The incidence of melanoma rose 3.5-fold in men and 4.6-fold in women. The American Cancer Society estimate for the number of new cases of melanoma in the United States for 1994 is 32,000.[7] In addition about 8000 cases of melanoma in situ are estimated for the same year.[7] It is estimated that 6900 people will die of melanoma in 1994, with about 2300 deaths occurring from nonmelanoma skin cancer.[7] It is of note that melanoma is the fourth most common cause of cancer-related death in men aged 15 to 34, based on data from 1990.[7]

In Canada, the National Cancer Institute of Canada estimated that 58,500 new cases of nonmelanoma skin cancer would occur in 1994, with an estimate of 3100 cases of melanoma. There were 580 deaths from melanoma predicted for 1994. In men, melanoma was the form of cancer with the greatest average annual percentage change in incidence. Australia has the highest incidence rate of melanoma in the world. In Queensland, the age-standardized incidence rate is greater than 30 per 100,000 person-years.[54]

Actinic keratoses are a common manifestation of cumulative sun exposure. These lesions appear as small, scaly patches and may become hypertrophic. Histologically, there is atypia of the epidermis, which may be limited to the basal layer or may extend throughout the thickness of the epidermis.[64] They are considered precancerous because a proportion of them go on to become squamous cell carcinomas. In a study comparing the incidence of

these lesions in white people who had lived all their lives in Australia and those who had moved to Australia after age 20, the incidence of actinic keratosis was 44.5% in the Australian-born and 15.7% in age-matched immigrants.[77] It would appear that childhood sunlight exposure is important in the development of actinic keratoses and, thus, squamous cell carcinomas.

UV exposure is strongly linked to the development of skin cancer. In white people, chronic UV exposure appears to be the major risk factor for both basal cell carcinoma and squamous cell carcinoma.[121] Both types of cancer occur primarily on sunlight-exposed areas. Risk factors for development of basal cell carcinoma and squamous cell carcinoma include older age, male sex (possibly owing to occupational differences), geographic location of residence, white skin, skin that tans poorly and burns easily, prolonged erythema after sun exposure, freckling, fair hair, and blue and light-colored eyes.[38,93,126] People who have had basal cell and squamous cell carcinomas have been found, in a series of experiments, to have a high incidence (91%) of UVB-induced inhibition of their contact hypersensitivity response to common haptens, although this trait also has been found in 40% to 45% of normal white and black people tested.[117] Maryland watermen, a group whose occupation requires extensive sun exposure, have been found to have increased risk of squamous cell carcinoma and actinic keratoses.[124] British outdoor workers have been found to have increased incidence of squamous cell carcinoma and basal cell carcinoma and an excess of melanomas of exposed skin, including head, face, and neck, whereas office workers were found to have an excess of melanomas of the trunk and limbs.[4] A higher risk of melanoma in whites is associated with painful or blistering sunburns in childhood or adolescence, a tendency to burn rather than tan, and an increased number of benign melanocytic nevi.[42,66] Exposure to UV radiation also greatly increases the development of cutaneous malignancies seen in patients with xeroderma pigmentosum, an autosomal recessive disease characterized by an inability to repair DNA damage caused by UV radiation.[95]

It is generally agreed that solar UV radiation is the major environmental cause of melanoma. The relationship between sunlight exposure and the risk of melanoma, however, is more complex than that described for basal cell carcinoma and squamous cell carcinoma. There are four types of cutaneous melanoma: superficial spreading, nodular, acral lentiginous, and lentigo maligna melanoma. Only lentigo maligna melanoma appears to be directly related to cumulative sun exposure, occurring most commonly on sun-exposed skin. In the Western Canada Melanoma Study, a significant inverse association was noted between the incidence of the other forms of melanoma and long-term occupational sun exposure in men, with the lowest risk found in men with the greatest sun exposure.[25] There is extensive epidemiological evidence, however, in support of the link between sun exposure and the non–lentigo maligna forms of melanoma. There is an inverse relationship between melanoma incidence and latitude, noted in Australia, North America, and other areas, with higher rates of melanoma noted with decreasing latitude.[38,47] Melanoma seems to be associated with acute intense exposures to UV radiation.[17,18] Studies examining the incidence of melanoma in Australian-born population, and immigrant populations in Australia have determined that the incidence of melanoma and deaths from melanoma are far higher in Australian-born individuals except for immigrants who arrived before the age of 15.[54] The risk of melanoma is greater in people with light hair and skin color and the tendency to burn easily and tan poorly.[17]

In animal models, UVB is a complete carcinogen, with numerous studies documenting the development of squamous cell carcinomas and papillomas in mice and other species.[51] There is also evidence to support a carcinogenic effect of UVA in murine models.[51,110,118] A fish model, a cross between playfish and swordfish, is susceptible to UVB-induced melanoma.[106] Melanoma has also been induced in the South American opposum *Monodelphis domestica*.[68] Transgenic mice have been produced with a construct of the tyrosinase gene promoter linked to Simian Virus 40 oncogenic sequences.[62] This transgene is expressed in melanocytes, and the mice develop both cutaneous and ocular melanomas late in life. Melanocytes from these transgenic mice are much more susceptible to UVB, becoming transformed at lower doses of UVB than are required to transform wild type cells.[62]

SKIN CANCER PATHOLOGY

In humans, basal cell carcinomas display several clinical patterns. The noduloulcerative lesion is the most common type, but the lesions may also be fibrosing or morphealike, presenting as an indurated smooth shiny plaque.[64] The lesions may also present as erythematous, scaling patches that can appear rather eczematous and are termed superficial basal cell carcinomas.[64] These lesions grow locally but have an extremely low rate of metastasis. Microscopically, there are groups of basaloid cells that are rather uniform in appearance, with a large nucleus and relatively little cytoplasm.[64] Squamous cell carcinomas are made up of irregular masses of keratinocytes, which proliferate into the underlying dermis. The keratinocytes vary in the degree of atypicality, such as nuclear atypia, mitotic figures, and pleomorphism of the size and shape of the cells.[64] Squamous cell carcinomas arising in sun-damaged skin have a low rate of metastasis, compared with squamous cell carcinomas arising in normal-appearing skin.[64] Basal cell and squamous cell carcinomas are associated with a low mortality rate. Morbidity, owing to loss of function and cosmetic alteration, from the

lesions themselves and the treatment required, however, is substantial (see Chapter 27).

ROLE OF ULTRAVIOLET RADIATION IN CUTANEOUS DISEASES

A large body of evidence attests to the important role of UV radiation in the induction of certain cutaneous diseases and in the treatment of others. Diseases such as solar urticaria, polymorphous light eruption, and actinic reticuloid all derive directly from exposure to UV radiation. In solar urticaria, hives (urticaria) develop on sun-exposed areas within minutes of exposure. The hives resolve gradually on returning to an indoor area. UVB or UVA radiation (or both) may be responsible. People with polymorphous light eruption develop erythematous papules and plaques with or without vesicles on sun-exposed areas of skin after a variable period of sun exposure. The lesions may only occur at the beginning of the spring season or after a period of intense exposure, as may occur on a vacation to an area with far greater UV flux. Again, UVB, UVA, or both may be involved. After a relatively short period of sun avoidance, the skin lesions resolve. Patients with actinic reticuloid develop a more severe UV radiation sensitivity and a more persistent cutaneous eruption, with a histological appearance that can mimic lymphoma.

The interaction of drugs or chemicals with UV radiation may also result in severe cutaneous injury, as seen in patients with photocontact dermatitis and persistent light reaction. In photocontact dermatitis, the exogenous substance may have been applied topically or ingested. The cutaneous eruption occurs only at sites that have been exposed to both the drug and UV radiation, usually UVA. Commonly implicated drugs include sulfonamides and tetracycline. The skin eruption may appear as an exaggerated sunburn or as a dermatitis. In persistent light reaction, the UV sensitivity persists even after the original contactant is removed from the environment. Exposure to UV radiation can also produce flares of the cutaneous manifestations of other diseases, including systemic lupus erythematosus and atopic dermatitis.

Despite the major role of UV radiation in the induction of certain dermatoses, the judicious use of UV radiation has proved to be of great benefit in the treatment of a number of different diseases. For example, psoriasis, a chronic disease characterized by hyperproliferation of the epidermis, can be cleared by phototherapy with UVB.[65,85] PUVA, an acronym for the combination of psoralen, a photosensitizing agent, and UVA, is also extremely effective in clearing recalcitrant psoriasis.[79] PUVA can also induce remissions in patients with the cutaneous T-cell lymphoma, mycosis fungoides.[43] In addition to the benefical effects of UV radiation in the treatment of proliferative and malignant disease, UVB has also been shown to be effective in the treatment of poorly understood but debilitating disorders, such as uremic pruritus.[29]

BIOLOGICAL EFFECTS OF ULTRAVIOLET RADIATION

UV radiation may be understood as either waves of rapidly alternating electric and magnetic fields or as discrete packets or quanta of energy. When UV radiation reaches the skin, it can be absorbed, scattered, transmitted or reflected. Scattering, in which the direction of the radiation is changed by interaction with tissue, is inversely proportional to wavelength. Most UV radiation does not pass through the skin; it is scattered back out through the stratum corneum or absorbed by a variety of chromophores in the skin. UV radiation is absorbed by individual molecules within the skin, in a precise manner that is dependent on wavelength, or energy content. This absorbed energy can excite specific molecules, enabling them to undergo various chemical reactions, including oxidation, reduction, isomerization, breakage of covalent bonds, or interactions with other molecules.

The multiple pathogenic and therapeutic effects of UV radiation have engendered much effort aimed at defining the mechanisms whereby UV radiation exerts its effects. The molecular and cellular basis for the effects of UV radiation, however, remains incompletely understood. The primary site of photon absorption may occur within DNA, cellular membranes, or organelles.

Effects on skin

The skin appears to have a set of mechanisms in place to deal with UV-induced injury. Melanin and other chromophores in the skin, such as urocanic acid, absorb chromophores absorb much of the incident UV radiation. The cutaneous response to UV radiation involves a fairly characteristic pattern of inflammation, repair, and changes in cell function and skin structure.

One of the most well-known effects of UV radiation is sunburn. The dose of radiation required to induce erythema, the qualitative nature of the erythema and the time course (onset of erythema, time to peak erythema, and time to resolution) differ for UVC, UVB, and UVA. The UVA dose to produce erythema in human skin is 1000 times greater than that required for UVB-induced erythema. UVB-induced erythema is first noted at 3 to 5 hours after exposure, peaks at 12 to 24 hours, and fades by 72 hours. With UVA, the erythema peaks at 8 hours and can persist 24 to 48 hours, depending on the dose.[30] The amount of UV radiation required to induce sunburn or erythema also varies from individual to individual, based on constitutive level of pigmentation and other factors. The erythema is accompanied by heat, edema, pain, and pruritus if the exposure is sufficiently intense. Sunburn is the clinical manifestation of histological vasodilation and edema.[97] UVB irradiation, and not UVA, results in the formation of dyskeratotic "sunburn" cells within the epidermis.[97,10] Particularly following UVA exposure, as UVA is capable of reaching further into the dermis, neutrophils and lymphocytes accumulate

in the dermis, and dermal endothelial cell damage may be noted.[37,97] UVA-induced erythema is an oxygen-dependent process.[3]

Because it is easily recognizable, erythema has long been used as an endpoint in studies of the effects of UV radiation. Visual quantitation of erythema, however, can be problematic. Of course, skin can be damaged, with detectable biochemical abnormalities, without the occurrence of erythema or sunburn. This is particularily important in the area of public education, where avoidance of sunburn cannot be equated with avoiding the harmful effects of the sun. Although sunscreen use was able to prevent the development of erythema in human volunteers exposed to UVB, other changes in the skin were not blocked, including alterations in the activity of glucose-6-phosphate dehydrogenase and succinic dehydrogenase and an increase in stratum corneum thickness.[88]

Acute epidermal changes after UVB and UVA irradiation include the depletion of Langerhans' cells and alteration of their antigen-presenting capability,[116] and thickening of the stratum corneum and stratum malpighii owing to keratinocyte proliferation, in association with an increase in pigment production by melanocytes.[102]

UV radiation is known to produce an increase in the pigmentation of skin. The immediate onset of an increase in pigmentation after exposure to UVA radiation is known as immediate pigment darkening.[45,101] This is a transient grayish brown discoloration of the skin that is due to an oxygen-dependent photochemical reaction in preexisting melanin, with no increase in melanocyte number. It is more noticeable in individuals who have constitutively darker skin. The function of immediate pigment darkening is not known. It does not appear to protect the skin against UVB-induced erythema.[5]

The delayed increase in pigmentation after UVB and UVA exposure is tanning. Melanocytes increase in number following both UVB and UVA exposure. Individual melanocytes enlarge, become more dendritic, and increase the amount of melanin that they produce and transfer to keratinocytes.[102] In both a murine model and human skin, exposure to UVB at one site led to an increase in melanocyte number at sites distant from the UVB irradiation.[98,115] In vitro studies using human melanocytes and keratinocytes have demonstrated that basic fibroblast growth factor, an important melanocyte growth factor, is produced by keratinocytes to a greater extent after UVB exposure.[35] Although a tan is part of the skin's protective mechanism against further UV exposure, a tan induced by UVA in human skin provided limited protection against solar-simulated radiation. Two to three times the minimal erythema dose was required to induce erythema in the tanned areas of skin, a skin protection factor (SPF) of 2 to 3.[48]

Long-term sun exposure produces visible changes in skin, including wrinkling, solar elastosis, solar lentigines, and pigment irregularities. Chronic exposure to UV radiation has been shown in humans and murine models to damage dermal collagen and elastin and to cause keratinocyte atypia and skin tumor formation.[46,129] In the albino hairless mouse exposed to UVA three times weekly for 32 weeks, elastic fiber hyperplasia, duplication of vascular basement membrane, and extensive endothelial cell damage was found.[129] Collagen appeared unchanged. After chronic UVB exposure, the hyperplastic elastic fibers were noted to be degraded. Vascular basement membranes were unaffected, whereas the dermal epidermal membrane was duplicated. Collagen fibers showed evidence of dissolution.[129] Thus, although chronic exposure to either UVB and UVA results in damage to the same connective tissue components, there are differences in their effects. Murine photo-aged dermis shows large increases in glycosaminoglycans and elastic tissue, degeneration of elastin into an amorphous mass, increased numbers of dermal fibroblasts and mast cells, and the appearance of inflammatory cells.[57]

Effects on skeletal system

The role of sunlight in the prevention and treatment of rickets and osteomalacia has been recognized for many years. 7-Dehydrocholesterol in the epidermis is converted by exposure to UVB to previtamin D_3. Previtamin D_3 then isomerizes by a thermally dependent process to vitamin D_3 over a period of several days. Once formed, vitamin D_3 is carried by vitamin D_3 binding protein into the circulation, ensuring efficient conversion of previtamin D_3, by shifting the equilibrium of the reaction in favor of ongoing vitamin D3 synthesis.[40] In the event of prolonged sun exposure, the synthesis of previtamin D_3 reaches a plateau at a concentration of about 10% to 15% of the original 7-dehydrocholesterol concentration, and previtamin D_3 photoisomerizes to two biologically inert compounds, tachysterol and lumisterol. These products are likely important in preventing vitamin D toxicity from prolonged UV exposure. These products are not bound to vitamin D_3 binding protein to any significant extent and are sloughed off in the usual natural exfoliation of the skin. The production of vitamin D in the skin depends on latitude and on skin pigmentation because epidermal melanin competes with 7-dehydrocholesterol in the absorption of UVB photons (see Chapter 9).

Effects on immune system

UV radiation has been shown to have multiple effects on the immune system. It is believed that the effect of UV is selective, suppressing certain cell-mediated immune responses.[81] UVB has been shown, in animal models, to inhibit the development of delayed-type hypersensitivity and contact hypersensitivity to chemicals and to induce a state of susceptibility to transplanted UV-induced tumors.[20,84] Failure to reject transplanted tumors appears to be related to a preferential induction of suppressor T-cell activity in the UVB-irradiated mice.[60] In humans, there is also evi-

dence that immunosuppression leads to an increase in skin cancer. Immunocompromised renal transplant patients have an increased rate of skin cancer in sun-exposed areas of skin.[71] As well, impaired induction of contact sensitization to dinitrochlorobenzene following UVB exposure was seen in 35% to 40% of normal white adults.[127] In humans, whole-body irradiation with one minimal erythema dose of UVB has been shown to produce an increase in serum interleukin-1 levels.[34]

Arachidonate metabolism appears to be involved in the production of UV-induced erythema. Arachidonic acid is present in membrane phospholipids. Metabolites of arachidonic acid, eicosanoids including prostaglandins (PG), are formed via two enzyme pathways, cyclooxygenase and lipoxygenase. Significant elevation of arachidonic acid and both the cyclooxygenase (PGD_2, PGE_2 and 6-oxo-PGF1$_\alpha$) and the lipoxygenase products occurs in association with the onset of erythema.[44] Inhibition of cyclooxygenase-derived prostaglandins by indomethacin resulted in a 50% decrease in UVB-induced erythema during the first 24 hours after exposure. The increase in prostaglandins between 3 and 6 hours after UVB is thought to be mediated by endogenous histamine, released from dermal mast cells.[90] Elevations of arachidonic acid, PGE_2 and PGD_2, and histamine were also found in human skin, after UVA irradiation.[37] Levels of these compounds peaked earlier after UVA than UVB exposure. In keratinocytes in vitro, UVB exposure induced the increased synthesis of a phospholipase, thus enhancing the release of arachidonate from cell membranes.[49] Eicosanoids may also be involved in other aspects of UV-induced cutaneous inflammation, apart from erythema, such as edema and the inflammatory cell infiltration to the site of injury.[44]

Effects on DNA and gene expression

There is evidence to support the role of reactive oxygen species, singlet oxygen, hydrogen peroxide, superoxide anion, and hydroxyl radical in UV-induced cutaneous damage (see Chapter 20). Because the direct absorption of UVA by DNA is far less than for UVB, alternative mechanisms for UVA-induced DNA damage have been postulated. It is proposed that the reactive oxygen species act as intermediates between various endogenous chromophores and DNA. Reactive oxygen species are known to damage normal cellular processes via lipid peroxidation, DNA damage, and altered enzyme activity. The reactive oxygen species generated damage cell membranes and organelles. UV irradiation resulted in the formation of free radicals in whole skin and skin homogenates.[108] Antioxidant enzymes, such as superoxide dismutase, catalase, and glutathione peroxidase, are found in both the dermis and the epidermis, as are α-tocopherol, ascorbic acid, glutathione, and ubiquinol.[15,108] The concentrations of these molecules are altered by UVB and UVA exposure.[82,108] Endogenous cellular glutathione is thought to be an important molecule in the protection against UVB-induced and UVA-induced damage. Levels of glutathione in mouse skin rapidly decreased after UVB exposure[108] as the level of oxidized glutathione (glutathione disulfide) increased. This was believed to support a role for glutathione as a quencher of free radical species generated during the UVB irradiation.[15] In another experimental system, glutathione depletion led to an increase in UVA-induced mutations in cultured human lymphoblastoid cells.[1]

UV radiation can cause lethal damage and induce mutations in mammalian cells, producing multiple lesions in DNA, including cyclobutane pyrimidine dimers, pyrimidine-pyrimidone(6-4) photoproducts, single-strand breaks, and DNA to protein cross-links.[9,23,87] The cyclobutane pyrimidine dimer and the (6-4) photoproduct form between adjacent pyrimidines on the same DNA strand. Lethality and mutagenesis have been attributed principally to the formation of these dimers.[8,94] Cyclobutane pyrimidine dimers have been found in human skin, after irradiation with both UVB and UVA.[24] It is interesting to note that higher levels of the dimers were found in individuals with greater sun sensitivity.[24] Enzymatic systems exist that repair these DNA lesions.[6,14,36,120] The major forms of DNA repair include excision repair, direct reversal, and postreplication repair. In excision repair, multiple enzymes are involved and result in the recognition and excision of the damaged DNA followed by synthesis of a replacement repair patch of DNA using the opposite, undamaged DNA strand as a template.

Another form of repair is known as photoreactivation. An enzyme, photoreactivating enzyme, actually requires the presence of visible light to reverse cyclobutane pyrimidine dimers.[67] This enzyme has been found in the skin of a number of different species but may not be present in human skin.[69] In several experimental systems, photoreversal of cyclobutane dimers can reverse much of the lethal and mutagenic effect of UV-induced DNA damage.[80]

The enzymatic repair processes are not foolproof, and it is the unrepaired DNA damage that results in lethality, mutagenesis, and carcinogenesis. A possible event in UV-induced carcinogenesis is the induction of mutations in oncogenes or tumor-suppressor genes.

In a murine model, chronic UVB radiation resulted in the production of squamous cell carcinomas. Twenty percent of the tumors had p53 tumor suppressor gene mutations.[59] In humans, 56% of basal cell carcinomas had mutations within the p53 gene.[128] Of the base substitutions, 100% occurred at sites of adjacent pyrimidine bases, and 80% were CC → TT double base substitutions or C → T substitutions.[59,128] These mutations appeared to be UV specific, identifying UV as the likely etiologic agent.

UV radiation has been shown to affect total DNA, RNA, and protein synthesis, causing an immediate decrease, followed by an increase that surpasses preirradiation values.[19] UV radiation has been shown to induce the expression of

multiple genes in many model systems, both in vivo and in vitro. Much of the work done aimed at understanding the molecular basis for the effects of UV radiation on cells and tissues has used wavelengths of UVC radiation. UVC, UVB, and UVA are all capable of inducing the expression of a variety of genes, but the specific genes induced are not necessarily induced by all wavebands.[96] Studies with UVC irradiation have demonstrated that there are many genes that are UVC-inducible, including keratins, plasminogen activator, interleukin 1, metallotheionein and several transcription factors.* One group of these genes is also induced by other DNA-damaging agents, and a subset is activated by the phorbol ester, 12-O-tetradecanoyl-phorbol-13-acetate (TPA).[12,28] Several of the genes that are inducible by UVC and TPA, collagenase, c-fos, and metallothionein, have been found to be regulated transcriptionally[12,32,113,114] via cis-acting UV-responsive elements that were mapped using chloramphenicol acetyltransferase reporter gene constructs. These cis-acting elements did not appear to be specific for UVC but were also targets of other signal transduction pathways. For example, c-fos transcription requires the serum response element for induction by UVC and TPA as well as serum.[12]

UVC also induced another oncogene, c-jun.[111] Expression of c-jun increased 200-fold in HeLa cells. Through the use of a nuclear run on assay, it was found that UVC regulated c-jun by an increase in transcription. UVC has been shown to regulate the expression of the promoter of the human immunodeficiency virus (HIV). In a variety of experiments linking the promoter region of the HIV-long terminal repeat gene (HIV-LTR) to reporter genes, UVC[112,114,122] was shown to increase the expression of the reporter genes, demonstrating that UVC regulates the expression of this promoter region,[13,112,114,125] possible through another transcription factor, NFkB.[112,114] The function of the gene gadd153 is not known but is induced by growth arrest and DNA damage. Its promoter is activated by UVC exposure in a dose-dependent manner.[63] The initiating event is considered to be DNA damage because the dose of UVC to induce maximally the promoter is much lower in xeroderma pigmentosa cells, which are known to be deficient in DNA repair[63] (see Chapter 19). HIV-1 LTR, collagenase, spr2, and metallothionein have also been shown to be inducible at lower doses in xeroderma pigmentosa cells.[28,114]

UVC has also been shown to increase the phosphorylation of c-jun, a transcription factor, at two serine residues, resulting in an increased ability of c-jun to activate transcription of AP-1 target genes.[16] This phosphorylation required the initial activation of Src family tyrosine kinases. Tyrosine kinase inhibitors considerably decreased the UVC induction of c-jun mRNA.[16] The UVC induction of c-fos and HIV-LTR was also obliterated by protein kinase inhib-

*References 12, 21, 41, 50, 63, 111.

itors.[113] In an attempt to demonstrate a protective effect of the so-called UV response, the addition of tyrosine kinase inhibitors to cell cultures irradiated with UVC was found to potentiate cell death by UVC.[16]

Although most of the work has focused on transcriptional regulation of genes by UVC, in human kidney cells in vitro, UVC resulted in increased mRNA stability in a dose-dependent manner.[39] The level of p53 was increased in murine 3T3 cells after UVC exposure by posttranslational stabilization, that is, a decrease in the rate of protein turnover.[76] It has been shown that induction of metallothionein after UVC exposure results from the extensive demethylation of one metallothionein allele.[72] In several studies, UV-conditioned media were found to contain a factor that led to an increase in the expression of specific genes in cells that had not been exposed to UV.[103,104] More recently, this factor was found to be a mixture of interleukin-1 α (IL-1α) and basic fibroblast growth factor.[58] Thus, one possible mechanism for the cellular effects of UV radiation may be the induction of secreted protein(s), which can communicate the UV effect to nonirradiated cells, amplifying the response to UV radiation.

The effects of UVC on gene expression are of great interest, providing useful models for the study of the molecular effects of UV radiation. Several genes appear to be regulated by both UVC and UVB, as both wavebands increased the expression of an HIV-LTR-reporter gene construct in murine skin.[13] One, however, cannot extrapolate the findings concerning UVC regulation of gene expression to UVB or UVA because substantial differences exist in the clinical and biochemical response of the skin to UVC, UVA, and UVB. For example, the dose response and time course of erythema and pigmentation induced by these wavelengths differ markedly.[86,97] Although the effects of UV radiation have been shown to be mediated to a large extent by the induction of DNA damage,[114] differences do exist in the spectra of lesions induced by UVB and UVC.[2,52] Furthermore, it has not been shown that findings derived from experimental systems that use UVC are relevant for understanding the effects of UVB. For example, the induction of c-*fos*, collagenase, and HIV-1 gene expression in fibroblasts was limited to wavelengths in the UVC range, with no induction of these genes detected in similar experiments following exposure to radiation in the UVB range.[114] The kinetics of UVC induction of gene expression may also differ markedly from that elucidated from studies using UVB. For example, UVC induces the expression of c-*fos* in Chinese hamster ovary cells, with maximum induction 2 hours after exposure. The levels of c-*fos* mRNA transcripts remained elevated for at least 16 hours after exposure to UVC.[41] Studies of the UVC induction of c-*fos* in fibroblasts, however, demonstrated that accumulation of c-*fos* mRNA transcripts peaked 10 to 15 minutes after UVC irradiation.[96] In contrast, the UVB induction of c-*fos* was similar to that obtained with serum, with an initial maximum induction being detected 60 minutes after exposure to UVB.[107] Thus, it cannot be assumed that the mechanisms by which gene expression is affected by UVC, UVB, and UVA are the same. As well, much of the work has been done in cell lines other than those derived from the skin. It is possible that there is cellular specificity in the response to UV radiation, with keratinocytes being among the cell types most commonly exposed to UV radiation.

Considerably less information is available about the effects of UVB and UVA on the regulation of gene expression. UVB radiation specifically increased IL-1 mRNA and protein in a dose-dependent fashion in cultured human keratinocytes.[61] Several cytokines, including granulocyte-macrophage colony-stimulating factor (GM-CSF), IL-1, and IL-6, have been shown to be inducible by UVB irradiation.[26,55,61] UVA has been shown to induce the synthesis of heme oxygenase in normal human fibroblasts, but the mechanism responsible remains unknown.[53] In one study, UVB irradiation and heat stress were found to induce an overlapping group of proteins in cultured mouse keratinocytes.[78] Although there were proteins that were induced by only one of the two stimuli, a group of nine proteins were induced by both stimuli that are distinct from traditional heat-shock proteins.[78]

UVB exposure is known to increase the activity of the enzyme ornithine decarboxylase (ODC).[75] ODC is the first enzyme in the mammalian polyamine biosynthetic pathway, forming putrescine by the decarboxylation of ornithine. The polyamines (spermine, spermidine, and putrescine) play an important role in cell growth[89,92] and differentiation and have been implicated in the process of carcinogenesis. Studies in mice have shown that epidermal ODC activity increases dramatically following both single and multiple UVB exposures, in a dose-dependent manner.[74] The induction of ODC activity appears to be wavelength dependent, with peak effectiveness occurring at 290 nm, with a rapid decline at wavelengths longer than 300 nm.[56] The increase in ODC activity occurs before the increase in DNA synthesis. The UVB-induced ODC activity was depressed by treatment of the mice with cycloheximide, a protein synthesis inhibitor, indicating a requirement for ongoing protein synthesis.[123] The capability of UV radiation to increase ODC activity is not specific for UVB because UVC has also been shown to induce ODC activity both in vivo and in vitro.[70,73] In contrast, UVA does not induce ODC activity, unless it is combined with phototoxic agents.[27] UVB radiation has been shown to result in an increase in ODC mRNA levels in a dose-dependent and a time-dependent manner, in keratinocytes in vitro, and in a hairless mouse model.[99,100]

After UVB exposure, c-*fos* was inducible in murine epidermal cells.[107] The response was biphasic, with an initial increase in c-*fos* mRNA that was maximal at 1 hour, with a return to control levels by 2 hours. A second maximum was found at 8 hours. Ongoing protein synthesis was not required for the initial rise but was necessary for the delayed response. Both serum and UVB resulted in an increase in c-*fos* gene transcription, with a slower rise to a lower maximum with UVB. Using chloramphenicol acetyltransferase reporter constructs, the known c-*fos* enhancer elements Dyad Symmetry Element (DSE) and AP-1 were found to enhance c-*fos* induction by UVB but to a lesser extent than with serum.[107]

The induction of genes by UV radiation appears to be specific, at least to a certain extent. It does not seem that UV induction is part of a general response to stress. Certain genes that are UV-inducible have not been induced by other causes of cellular stress or DNA damage or are regulated differently by other causes of growth arrest.[32] Several heat-shock proteins, however, are also inducible by UV.[11,22,119] One of these, Hsp27, was found to be inducible by both UVC and UVB[22] in Chinese hamster ovary cells, whereas an increase in the mRNA of another, Hsp70, was noted in murine epidermis after exposure to both UVB and solar-simulated irradiation.[11]

CONCLUDING REMARKS

Much remains to be learned concerning the mechanisms of action of UV radiation. Because UV radiation is a ubiquitous environmental carcinogen, it is difficult to avoid exposure in the context of living a normal life. UV radiation produces multiple effects in the skin, which are primarily deleterious. Some of these changes, in particular the wrinkling and altered pigmentation owing to long-term exposure, are incorrectly considered by the vast majority of the population to be inevitable, caused by chronological aging of the skin as opposed to photo-aging. The incidence of cutaneous malignancy is growing. Further work is required to fully understand the effects of UV radiation on the skin, with a view to the prevention of cutaneous malignancy and other harmful effects.

REFERENCES

1. Applegate LA et al: Endogenous glutathione levels modulate the frequency of both spontaneous and long wavelength ultraviolet induced mutations in human cells, *Carcinogenesis* 13:1557, 1992.
2. Arlett CF et al: Hypersensitivity of human lymphocytes to UV-B and solar irradiation, *Cancer Res* 53:609, 1993.
3. Auletta M et al: Effect of cutaneous hypoxia upon erythema and pigment responses to UVA, UVB, and PUVA (8-MOP + UVA) in human skin, *J Invest Dermatol* 86:649, 1986.
4. Beral V, Robinson N: The relationship of malignant melanoma, basal and squamous skin cancers to indoor and outdoor work, *Br J Cancer* 44:886, 1981.
5. Black G, Matzinger E, Gange RW: Lack of photoprotection against UVB-induced erythema by immediate pigmentation induced by 382 nm radiation, *J Invest Dermatol* 85:448, 1985.
6. Bohr VA: Gene specific DNA repair, *Carcinogenesis* 12:1983, 1991.
7. Boring CC, et al: Cancer statistics, 1994, *CA Cancer J Clin* 44:7, 1994.
8. Bourre F, Benoit A, Sarasin A: Respective roles of pyrimidine dimers and pyrimidine (6-4) pyrimidone photoproducts in UV mutagenesis of simian virus 40 DNA in mammalian cells, *J Virol* 63:4520, 1989.
9. Brash DE, Haseltine WA: UV-induced mutation hotspots occur at DNA damage hotspots, *Nature* 298:189, 1982.
10. Brenner W, Gschnait F: Decreased DNA repair activity in sunburn cell, *Arch Dermatol Res* 266:11, 1979.
11. Brunet S, Giacomoni PU: Heat shock mRNA in mouse epidermis after UV irradiation, *Mutation Res* 219:217, 1989.
12. Buscher M et al: Activation of the c-*fos* gene by UV and phorbol ester: different signal transduction pathways converge to the same enhancer element, *Oncogene* 3:301, 1988.
13. Cavard C et al: In vivo activation by ultraviolet rays of the human immunodeficiency virus type 1 long terminal repeat, *J Clin Invest* 86:1369, 1990.
14. Chao CC-K, Rosenstein BS: Use of metabolic inhibitors to investigate the excision repair of pyrimidine dimers and nondimer DNA damages induced in human and ICR 2A frog cells by ultraviolet radiation, *Photochem Photobiol* 43:165, 1986.
15. Connor MJ, Wheeler L: Depletion of cutaneous glutathione by ultraviolet radiation, *Photochem Photobiol* 46:239, 1987.
16. Devary Y et al: The mammalian ultraviolet response is triggered by activation of Src tyrosine kinases, *Cell* 71:1081, 1992.
17. Elwood JM et al: Sunburn, suntan and the risk of cutaneous malignant melanoma: the Western Canada Melanoma Study, *Br J Cancer* 51:543, 1985.
18. Elwood JM et al: Cutaneous melanoma in relation to intermittent and constant sun exposure—the Western Canada Melanoma Study, *Int J Cancer* 35:427, 1985.
19. Epstein JH, Fukuyama K, Fye K: Effects of ultraviolet radiation on the mitotic cycle and DNA, RNA and protein synthesis in mammalian epidermis in vivo, *Photochem Photobiol* 12:57, 1970.
20. Fisher MS, Kripke ML: UVB and tumour immunity, *Proc Natl Acad Sci USA* 74:1688, 1977.
21. Fornace AJ Jr, Alamo I Jr, Hollander MC: DNA damage-inducible transcripts in mammalian cells, *Proc Natl Acad Sci USA* 85:8800, 1988.
22. Fornace AJ Jr et al: Induction of heat shock protein transcripts and B2 transcripts by various stresses in Chinese hamster cells, *Exp Cell Res* 182:61, 1989.
23. Freeman SE: Variations in excision repair of UVB-induced pyrimidine dimers in DNA of human skin in situ, *J Invest Dermatol* 90:814, 1988.
24. Freeman SE, Gange RW, Sutherland JC, et al: Pyrimidine dimer formation in human skin, *Photochem Photobiol* 46:207, 1987.
25. Gallagher RP, Elwood JM, Yang CP: Is chronic sunlight exposure important in accounting for increases in melanoma incidence? *Int J Cancer* 44:813, 1989.
26. Gallo RL et al: Regulation of GM-CSF and IL-3 production from the murine keratinocyte cell line PAM 212 following exposure to ultraviolet radiation, *J Invest Dermatol* 97:203, 1991.
27. Gange RW: Epidermal ornithine decarboxylase activity and thymidine incorporation following treatment with ultraviolet A combined with topical 8-methoxypsoralen or anthracene in the hairless mouse, *Br J Dermatol* 105:247, 1981.
28. Gibbs S et al: Characterization of the human spr2 promoter: induction after UV irradiation or TPA treatment and regulation during differentiation of cultured primary keratinocytes, *Nucl Acids Res* 18:4401, 1990.
29. Gilchrest BA et al: Ultraviolet phototherapy of uremic pruritus, *Ann Intern Med* 91:17, 1979.
30. Gilchrest BA et al: Histologic changes associated with ultraviolet A-induced erythema in normal human skin, *J Am Acad Dermatol* 9:213, 1983.
31. Glass AG, Hoover RN: The emerging epidemic of melanoma and squamous cell skin cancer, *JAMA* 262:2097, 1989.

32. Glazer PM et al: UV-induced DNA-binding proteins in human cells, *Proc Natl Acad Sci USA* 86:1163, 1989.

33. Gleason JF et al: Record low global ozone in 1992, *Science* 260:523, 1993.

34. Granstein RD, Sauder DN: Whole-body exposure to ultraviolet radiation results in increased serum interleukin-1 activity in humans, *Lymphokine Res* 6:187, 1987.

35. Halaban R et al: Basic fibroblast growth factor from human keratinocytes is a natural mitogen for melanocytes, *J Cell Biol* 107:1611, 1988.

36. Haseltine WA: Ultraviolet light repair and mutagenesis revisited, *Cell* 33:13, 1983.

37. Hawk JLM et al: Increased concentration of arachidonic acid, prostaglandins E2, D2 and 6-oxo-F, and histamine in human skin following UVA irradiation, *J Invest Dermatol* 80:496, 1983.

38. Henriksen T et al: Ultraviolet-radiation and skin cancer. Effect of an ozone layer depletion, *Photochem Photobiol* 51:579, 1990.

39. Hilgers G et al: Post-transcriptional effect of ultraviolet light on gene expression in human cells, *Eur J Biochem* 201:483, 1991.

40. Holick MF et al: Photosynthesis of previtamin D_3 in human skin and the physiologic consequences, *Science* 210:203, 1980.

41. Hollander MC, Fornace AJ Jr: Induction of *fos* RNA by DNA-damaging agents, *Cancer Res* 49:1687, 1989.

42. Holly EA et al: Number of melanocytic nevi as a major risk factor for malignant melanoma, *J Am Acad Dermatol* 17:459, 1987.

43. Honigsmann H et al: Photochemotherapy for cutaneous T cell lymphoma, *J Am Acad Dermatol* 10:238, 1984.

44. Hruza LL, Pentland A: Mechanisms of UV-induced inflammation, *J Invest Dermatol* 100:35S, 1993.

45. Irwin C et al: An ultraviolet radiation action spectrum for immediate pigment darkening, *Photochem Photobiol* 57:504, 1993.

46. Johnston KJ et al: Ultraviolet radiation-induced connective tissue changes in the skin of hairless mice, *J Invest Dermatol* 82:587, 1984.

47. Jones RR: Ozone depletion and cancer risk, *Lancet* 2:443, 1987.

48. Kaidbey KH, Kligman AM: Sunburn protection by longwave ultraviolet radiation-induced pigmentation, *Arch Dermatol* 114:46, 1978.

49. Kang-Rotondo CH et al: Enhanced keratinocyte prostaglandin synthesis after UV injury is due to increased phospholipase activity, *Am J Physiol* 264(*Cell Physiol* 33):C396, 1993.

50. Kartasova T et al: Effects of UV, 4-NQO and TPA on gene expression in cultured human epidermal keratinocytes, *Nucl Acids Res* 15:5945, 1987.

51. Kelfkens G, de Gruijl FR, van der Leun JC: Tumorigenesis by shortwave ultraviolet A: papillomas versus squamous cell carcinomas, *Carcinogenesis* 12:1377, 1991.

52. Keyse SM, Amaudreuz F, Tyrrel RM: Determination of the spectrum of mutations induced by defined-wavelength solar UVB (313-nm) radiation in mammalian cells by use of a shuttle vector, *Mol Cell Biol* 8:5425, 1988.

53. Keyse SM, Tyrrell RM: Heme oxygenase is the major 32-kDa stress protein induced in human skin fibroblasts by UVA radiation, hydrogen peroxide, and sodium arsenite, *Proc Natl Acad Sci USA* 86:99, 1989.

54. Khlat M: Mortality from melanoma in migrants to Australia: variation by age at arrival and duration of stay, *Am J Epidemiol* 135:1103, 1992.

55. Kirnbauer R et al: Regulation of epidermal cell interleukin-6 production by UV light and corticosteroids, *J Invest Dermatol* 96:484, 1991.

56. Kligman LH, Kaidbey KH: Wavelength dependence for ornithine decarboxylase induction in vivo, *Photochem Photobiol* 43:649, 1986.

57. Kochevar IE et al: Effects of systemic indomethacin, meclizine, and BW755C on chronic ultraviolet B-induced effects in hairless mouse skin, *J Invest Dermatol* 100:186, 1993.

58. Kramer M et al: UV irradiation-induced interleukin-1 and basic fi-

broblast growth factor synthesis and release mediate part of the UV response, *J Biol Chem* 268:6734, 1993.

59. Kress S et al: Carcinogen-specific mutational pattern in the p53 gene in ultraviolet B radiation-induced squamous cell carcinomas in mouse skin, *Cancer Res* 52:6400, 1992.

60. Krutmann J, Elmets CA: Recent studies on mechanisms in photoimmunology, *Photochem Photobiol* 48:787, 1988.

61. Kupper TS et al: Interleukin 1 gene expression in cultured human keratinocytes is augmented by ultraviolet irradiation, *J Clin Invest* 80:430, 1987.

62. Larue L, Dougherty N, Mintz B: Genetic predisposition of transgenic mouse melanocytes to melanoma results in malignant melanoma after exposure to a low ultraviolet B intensity nontumorigenic for normal melanocytes, *Proc Natl Acad Sci USA* 89:9534, 1992.

63. Leuthy JD, Holbrook NJ: Activation of the gadd153 promoter by genotoxic agents: a rapid and specific reponse to DNA damage, *Cancer Res* 52:5, 1992.

64. Lever WF, Schaumberg-Lever G: *Histopathology of the skin,* ed 6, Philadelphia, 1993, JB Lippincott.

65. LeVine MJ, Parrish JA: Outpatient phototherapy of psoriasis, *Arch Dermatol* 116:552, 1980.

66. Lew RA et al: Sun exposure habits in patients with cutaneous melanoma: a case control study, *J Dermotol Surg Oncol* 9:981, 1983.

67. Ley RD: Photorepair of pyrimidine dimers in the epidermis of the marsupial *Monodelphis domestica, Photochem Photobiol* 40:141, 1984.

68. Ley RD et al: Ultraviolet radiation-induced malignant melanoma in *Monodelphis domestica, Photochem Photobiol* 50:1, 1989.

69. Li YF, Kim S-T, Sancar A: Evidence for lack of DNA photoactivating enzyme in humans, *Proc Natl Acad Sci USA* 90:4389, 1993.

70. Lichti U et al: Germicidal ultraviolet light induces ornithine decarboxylase in mouse epidermal cells and modifies the induction caused by phorbol ester tumor promoters, *Photochem Photobiol* 32:177, 1980.

71. Liddington M et al: Skin cancer in renal transplant patients, *Br J Surg* 76:1002, 1989.

72. Lieberman MW, Beach LR, Palmiter RD: Ultraviolet radiation-induced metallothionein-1 gene activation is associated with extensive DNA demethylation, *Cell* 35:207, 1983.

73. Lowe JN: Ultraviolet light and epidermal polyamines, *J Invest Dermatol* 77:147, 1981.

74. Lowe N, Breeding J, Russell D: Epidermal polyamine profiles after chronic ultraviolet light radiation, *J Invest Dermatol* 74:251, 1980.

75. Lowe N, Verma AK, Boutwell RK: Ultraviolet light induces epidermal ornithine decarboxylase A activity, *J Invest Dermatol* 71:417, 1978.

76. Maltzman W, Czyzyk L: UV irradiation stimulates levels of p53 cellular tumor antigen in nontransformed mouse cells, *Mol Cell Biol* 4:1689, 1984.

77. Marks R et al: The role of childhood exposure to sunlight in the development of solar keratoses and non-melanocytic skin cancer, *Med J Aust* 152:62, 1990.

78. Maytin E: Differential effects of heat shock and UVB light upon stress protein expression in epidermal keratinocytes, *J Biol Chem* 267:23189, 1992.

79. Melski J et al: Oral methoxsalen photochemotherapy for the treatment of psoriasis: a cooperative clinical trial, *J Invest Dermatol* 68:328, 1977.

80. Mitchell DM et al: Photoreactivation of cyclobutane dimers and (6-4) photoproducts in the epidermis of the marsupial, *Monodelphis domestica, Photochem Photobiol* 51:653, 1990.

81. Morison WL: Effects of ultraviolet radiation on the immune system in humans, *Photochem Photobiol* 50:515, 1989.

82. Moysan A et al: Ultraviolet A-induced lipid peroxidation and an-

tioxidant defense systems in cultured human skin fibroblasts, *J Invest Dermatol* 100:692, 1993.

83. Neer RM: Environmental light: effects on vitamin D synthesis and calcium metabolism in humans. In Wurtman RJ, Baum MJ, Potts JT Jr, editors: *The medical and biological effects of light,* New York, 1985, New York Academy of Sciences.

84. Noonan FP, De Fabo EC, Kripke ML: UVB and tumour immunity, *Photochem Photobiol* 34:683, 1981.

85. Parrish JA, Jaenicke KF: Action spectrum for phototherapy of psoriasis, *J Invest Dermatol* 176:359, 1981.

86. Parrish JA, Jaenicke KF, Anderson RR: Erythema and melanogenesis action spectra of normal human skin, *Photochem Photobiol* 36:187, 1982.

87. Peak MJ, Peak JG, Carnes BA: Induction of direct and indirect single-strand breaks in human cell DNA by far- and near-ultraviolet radiations: action spectrum and mechanisms, *Photochem Photobiol* 45:381, 1987.

88. Pearse AD, Marks R: Response of human skin to ultraviolet radiation: dissociation of erythema and metabolic changes following sunscreen protection, *J Invest Dermatol* 80:191, 1983.

89. Pegg AE, McCann PP: Polyamine metabolism and function, *Am J Physiol* 243:C212, 1982.

90. Pentland AP et al: Enhanced prostaglandin synthesis after ultraviolet injury is mediated by endogenous histamine stimulation: a mechanism for irradiation erythema, *J Clin Invest* 86:566, 1990.

91. Deleted in proofs.

92. Pohjanpelto P, Holtta E, Janne OA: Mutant strain of Chinese hamster ovary cells with no detectable ornithine decarboxylase activity, *Mol Cell Biol* 5:1385, 1985.

93. Preston DS, Stern RS: Nonmelanoma cancers of the skin, *N Eng J Med* 327:1649, 1992.

94. Protic-Sabljic M et al: UV light-induced cyclobutane pyrimidine dimers are mutagenic in mammalian cells, *Mol Cell Biol* 6:3349, 1986.

95. Robbins JH et al: Xeroderma pigmentosum: an inherited disease with sun sensitivity, multiple cutaneous neoplasms and abnormal DNA repair, *Ann Intern Med* 80:221, 1974.

96. Ronai ZA, Okin E, Weinstein IB: Ultraviolet light induces the expression of oncogenes in rat fibroblast and human keratinocyte cells, *Oncogene* 2:201, 1988.

97. Rosario R et al: Histological changes produced in skin by equally erythemogenic doses of UV-A,UV-B,UV-C and UV-A with psoralens, *Br J Dermatol* 101:299, 1979.

98. Rosdahl IK: Local and systemic effects on the epidermal melanocyte population in UV-irradiated mouse skin, *J Invest Dermatol* 73:306, 1979.

99. Rosen CF, Gajic D, Drucker DJ: Ultraviolet radiation induction of ornithine decarboxylase in rat keratinocytes, *Cancer Res* 50:2631, 1990.

100. Rosen CF et al: Ultraviolet B radiation induction of ornithine decarboxylase gene expression in mouse epidermis, *Biochem J* 270:565, 1990.

101. Rosen CF et al: Immediate pigment darkening: visual and reflectance spectrophotometric analysis of action spectrum, *Photochem Photobiol* 51:583, 1990.

102. Rosen CF et al: A comparison of the melanocyte response to narrow band UVA and UVB exposure in vivo, *J Invest Dermatol* 88:774, 1987.

103. Rotem N, Axelrod JH , Miskin R: Induction of urokinase-type plasminogen activator by UV light in human fetal fibroblasts is mediated through a UV-Induced secreted protein, *Mol Cell Biol* 7:622, 1987.

104. Schorpp M et al: UV-induced extracellular factor from human fibroblasts communicates the UV response to nonirradiated cells, *Cell* 37:861, 1984.

105. Scotto J et al: Biologically effective ultraviolet radiation: surface measurements in the United States, 1974 to 1985, *Science* 239:762, 1988.

106. Setlow RB, Woodhead AD, Grist E: Animal model for ultraviolet radiation-induced melanoma: playfish-swordfish hybrid, *Proc Natl Acad Sci USA* 86:8922, 1989.

107. Shah G et al: Mechanism of induction of c-*fos* by ultraviolet B (290-320 nm) in mouse JB6 epidermal cells, *Cancer Res* 53:38, 1993.

108. Shindo Y, Witt E, Packer L: Antioxidant defense mechanisms in murine epidermis and dermis and their responses to ultraviolet light, *J Invest Dermatol* 100:260, 1993.

109. Sontheimer RD: Fluorescent light photosensitivity in patients with systemic lupus erythematosus, *Arthritis Rheum* 36:428, 1993.

110. Staberg B et al: The carcinogenic effect of UVA irradiation, *J Invest Dermatol* 81:517, 1983.

111. Stein B et al: Ultraviolet-radiation induced c-*jun* gene transcription: two AP-1 like binding sites mediate the response, *Photochem Photobiol* 55:409, 1992.

112. Stein B et al: UV-induced transcription from the human immunodeficiency virus type 1 (HIV-1) long terminal repeat and UV-induced secretion of an extracellular factor that induces HIV-1 transcription in nonirradiated cells, *J Virol* 63:4540, 1989.

113. Stein B et al: The UV signal transduction pathway to specific genes. In Hanawalt PC, Freidberg EC, editors: *Mechanisms and consequences of DNA damage processing,* New York, 1988, Alan R. Liss, p 557.

114. Stein B et al: UV-induced DNA damage is an intermediate step in UV-induced expression of human immunodeficiency virus type1, collagenase, c-*fos* and metallothionein, *Mol Cell Biol* 9:5169, 1988.

115. Steirner U: Melanocytes, moles and melanoma, *Acta Dermatovener Suppl* 168:16, 1992.

116. Stingl G et al: Langerhans cells, *J Immunol* 127:1707, 1981.

117. Streilein JW: Sunlight and skin-associated lymphoid tissues (SALT): if UVB is the trigger and TNFα is its mediator, what is the message? *J Invest Dermatol* 100:47S, 1993.

118. Strickland P: Photocarcinogenesis by near-ultraviolet (UVA) radiation in Sencar mice, *J Invest Dermatol* 87:272, 1986.

119. Suzuki K, Watanabe M: Augmented expression of Hsp72 protein in normal human fibroblasts irradiated with ultraviolet light, *Biochem Biophys Res Commun* 186:1257, 1992.

120. Taichman LB, Setlow RB: Repair of ultraviolet light damage to the DNA of cultured human epidermal keratinocytes and fibroblasts, *J Invest Dermatol* 73:217, 1979.

121. Urbach F: Evidence and epidemiology of ultraviolet-induced cancers in man, *Natl Cancer Inst Monogr* 50:5, 1978.

122. Valerie K et al: Activation of human immunodeficiency virus type 1 by DNA damage in human cells, *Nature* 333:78, 1988.

123. Verma AK, Lowe NJ, Boutwell RK: Induction of mouse epidermal ornithine decarboxylase activity and DNA synthesis by ultraviolet light, *Cancer Res* 39:1035, 1979.

124. Vitasa BC et al: Association of nonmelanoma skin cancer and actinic keratosis with cumulative solar ultraviolet exposure in Maryland watermen, *Cancer* 65:2811, 1990.

125. Vogel J et al: UV activation of human immunodeficiency virus gene expression in transgenic mice, *J Virol* 66:1, 1992.

126. Wilson PD, Kaidbey KH, Kligman AM: Ultraviolet light sensitivity and prolonged UVR-erythema, *J Invest Dermatol* 77:434, 1981.

127. Yoshikawa T et al: Susceptibility to effects of UVB radiation on induction of contact hypersensitivity as a risk factor for skin cancer in man, *J Invest Dermatol* 95:530, 1990.

128. Zeigler A et al: Mutation hotspots due to sunlight in the p53 gene of nonmelanoma skin cancers, *Proc Natl Acad Sci USA* 90:4216, 1993.

129. Zheng P, Kligman LH: UVA-induced ultrastructural changes in hairless mouse skin: a comparison to UVB-induced damage, *J Invest Dermatol* 100:194, 1993.

Chapter 11

IONIZING RADIATION

Arthur C. Upton

This chapter reviews the pathologic effects of ionizing radiation, with particular reference to those that may result from low-level irradiation. Because of the breadth of the subject, no attempt to provide a comprehensive review is

This work was supported in part by grants ES00260 and CA13343 from the U.S. Public Health Service and grant SIG 09 from the American Cancer Society.

The author is grateful to Ms. Lynda Witte for her assistance in the preparation of the manuscript.

made herein. The chapter focuses instead on highlights and general principles, citing authoritative sources for those readers desiring further details.

HISTORICAL BACKGROUND

Within months after the x-ray was discovered by Roentgen in 1886, it was introduced widely into the diagnosis and treatment of disease. As a result, injuries from overexposure to radiation were encountered almost immediately.[9] The study of such effects has since received continuing impetus from the growing uses of radiation in medicine, science, and industry and from the military and peaceful applications of atomic energy. As a consequence, the pathological effects of ionizing radiation have come to be investigated more thoroughly than those of any other environmental agent.

The radiation injuries that were noted initially consisted predominantly of skin reactions on the hands of those working with early radiation equipment and sources, 96 cases of such injury being reported in one publication alone within barely a year after Roentgen's discovery.[29] By the dawn of the 20th century, the reactions of other tissues to irradiation also had come under intensive study. As early as 1903, for example, sterilizing effects of x-rays on male guinea pigs and rabbits were investigated,[2] leading to the important generalization by Bergonie and Tribondeau[3] that the radiosensitivity of cells varies with their rate of proliferation and inversely with their degree of differentiation. Paralleling such early studies in laboratory animals were clinical reports of oligospermia and azoospermia in radiation workers.[4]

As the thresholds for different types of pathological reactions gradually became better known, the exposure limits for radiation workers were reduced accordingly. As a result, radiation protection standards gradually evolved, which now suffice to prevent gross tissue injuries altogether, barring accidents.[12,13] Although today's exposure limits protect adequately against gross tissue injury, they cannot be assumed to protect completely against the mutagenic and carcinogenic effects of radiation, which may have no thresholds.[6,13,33]

The hypothesis that no threshold exists for the mutagenic effects of radiation dates from the 1930s, when classic experiments with the fruit fly suggested that the frequency of mutations increases in proportion to the dose of x-rays, without a threshold.[17] This concept implied that the global increases in environmental radiation resulting from the atmospheric testing of nuclear weapons in the 1950s might threaten the health of future generations, a prospect ultimately causing widespread concern among geneticists throughout the world.[1]

Further concern about the potential health impact of low-level irradiation was aroused by the observation that mortality from leukemia in atomic bomb survivors, radiologists, and patients treated with radiation for ankylosing spondylitis appeared to increase in proportion to the radiation dose. This was interpreted to imply that a significant percentage of leukemias in the general population might result from natural background irradiation.[14] The plausibility of this interpretation was reinforced by the observation of an association between the risk of leukemia in childhood and prenatal diagnostic x-irradiation.[26,27] Evidence that the dose-incidence relationship for certain other malignancies also may be of a nonthreshold nature[6,33] has since led to the conclusion that the risk of cancer from irradiation outweighs the risk of heritable abnormalities.[6,33]

RADIATION PROPERTIES AND UNITS

Ionizing radiations are of two main types: (1) electromagnetic radiations, which include x-rays and gamma rays, and (2) particulate radiations, which include electrons, protons, neutrons, alpha particles, and other atomic particles varying in mass and charge.

Quantities of ionizing radiation are measured in various units, the oldest of which, the roentgen (R), is a measure of the quantity of ionization induced in air. For expressing the dose of radiation absorbed in tissue, the principle units are the *rad* (1 rad = 100 ergs per gram of tissue) and the *gray* (1 Gy = 1 joule per kilogram of tissue = 100 rad). Particulate radiations generally cause greater injury per unit dose than do x-rays or gamma rays. Other (so-called dose-equivalent) units, the *rem* and the *sievert,* also are used; one *rem,* defined loosely, is the amount of any form of radiation that produces a biological effect equivalent to the effect produced by one *rad* of gamma rays; one *sievert* (Sv) is the amount of any radiation that causes a biological effect equivalent to that produced by 1 *gray* of gamma rays (1 Sv = 100 rem). For expressing the collective dose to a population, the units are the *person-rem* and *person-Sv,* each of which represents the product of the average dose

per person times the number of people exposed (e.g., 1 rem to each of 100 people = 100 person-rem = 1 person-Sv).

For measuring the amount of radioactivity contained in a given sample of matter, the curie (Ci) and the becquerel (Bq) are the units that are used; 1 Ci is that quantity of a radioactive nuclide in which there are 3.7×10^{10} atomic disintegrations per second, and 1 Bq is that quantity of a radioactive nuclide in which there is one atomic disintegration per second (1 Bq = 2.7×10^{-11} Ci).

POPULATIONS AT RISK

All living things are exposed to natural background radiation, the main components of which are (1) cosmic rays from outer space; (2) terrestrial radiation, emanating from the radium, thorium, uranium, and other radioactive elements in the earth's crust; and (3) internal radiation, emitted by the potassium-40, carbon-14, and other radionuclides normally contained within living cells themselves. Each of

Table 11-1. Average amounts of ionizing radiation received annually from different sources by members of the U.S. population

Source	Dose equivalent*	
	(mSv)	(mrem)
Natural		
Radon	24†	2400†
Cosmic	0.27	27
Terrestrial	0.28	28
Internal	0.39	39
Total natural	0.94	
Artificial		
Medical		
X-ray diagnosis	0.39	39
Nuclear medicine	0.14	14
Consumer products	0.10	10
Other		
Occupational	0.009	0.9
Nuclear fuel cycle	<0.01	<1.0
Fallout	<0.01	<1.0
Miscellaneous‡	<0.01	<1.0
Total artificial	0.63	0.63

From National Academy of Sciences, National Research Council, Committee on the Biological Effects of Ionizing Radiation: *Health effects of exposure to low levels of ionizing radiation (BEIR V),* Washington, DC, 1990, National Academy Press.

*Average dose equivalent to soft tissues (except for radon as noted). Doses of radiation are measured in various units, e.g., the gray (1 Gy = 1 J/kg of tissue), the rad (1 rad = 100 ergs/gm of tissue = 0.01 Gy), the sievert (Sv), and the rem (1 Sv = 100 rem). The dose equivalent of any radiation in sieverts is the dose in Gy multiplied by an appropriate quality factor *Q,* so that 1 sievert of the radiation is roughly equivalent in biological effectiveness to 1 gray of gamma rays.

†Dose equivalent from radon and its daughters to bronchial epithelium only.

‡Department of Energy facilities, smelters, phosphate fertilizer, transportation.

these three components accounts for about one third of the average total dose of natural background radiation received annually by a person residing at sea level in the United States (Table 11-1). At high elevations, however, the cosmic ray dose may be increased by a factor of two or more, and in areas where the earth is rich in radium, the terrestrial radiation dose may, likewise, be higher by a factor of two or more. It is noteworthy, moreover, that the average dose to the bronchial epithelium from inhaled radon and its daughters is larger by orders of magnitude than the dose to other soft tissues of the body (Table 11-1) (see Chapter 3).

In addition to the radiation received from natural sources, populations in the modern world receive radiation from various anthropogenic sources, the most important of which is the use of x-rays in medical diagnosis (Table 11-1). At the high altitudes of modern jet aircraft travel, persons also are exposed to cosmic rays at intensities that may exceed 0.005 mSv per hour on northerly routes and that may reach levels many times higher during solar flares.

Workers in various occupations are exposed to additional radiation, depending on their work assignments and working conditions. The average yearly dose equivalent of whole-body radiation received occupationally by monitored workers in the United States today is smaller, however, than the dose received from natural background irradiation, and fewer than 1% of such workers receive as much as the maximum permissible dose (50 mSv) in any given year.[18] Many airline crews, because of their increased exposure to cosmic rays in today's jet aircraft, accumulate doses comparable to those received by regularly monitored radiation workers.[19]

Although radiation accidents rarely have affected the public directly, they constitute another important potential source of exposure. In the two most serious recent nuclear reactor accidents—at Three Mile Island in 1978 and Chernobyl in 1986—enough radioactive material was released to deliver measurable doses to members of the public. Fortunately the maximal dose to any member of the public from the Three Mile Island accident is estimated to have been no larger than the annual dose normally received from natural background irradiation;[35] however, in the Chernobyl accident, the release of radioactivity was sufficiently great to necessitate the evacuation of tens of thousands of people from the surrounding area. It resulted in an estimated collective dose equivalent commitment of some 600,000 person-Sv for the Northern Hemisphere as a whole.[7]

CHARACTERISTICS OF RADIATION INJURY
Major types of injury

Many, if not most, clinically significant pathological reactions to radiation (such as erythema, depression of the blood count, impairment of immunity, reduction of fertility, and radiation cataract) require the killing of substantial numbers of cells in the tissues that are affected. For these types of reactions, therefore, there are threshold doses of radiation below which the injuries are not clinically detectable.[12] In contrast to these types of effects, no thresholds are presumed to exist for gene mutations, chromosome aberrations, and neoplastic transformation. Instead the latter effects are viewed as "stochastic" phenomena that may result from changes in single cells, altered individually.[6,33]

Cellular and molecular mechanisms of injury

Formation of ions and free radicals. Ionizing radiations, in contrast to other forms of radiation, can deposit enough localized energy in tissue to disrupt atoms and mol-

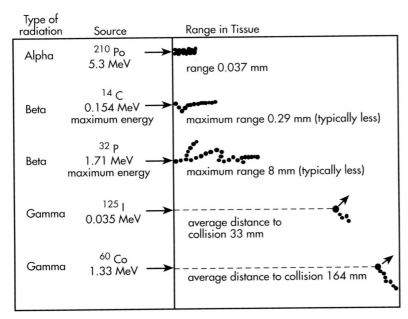

Fig. 11-1. Differences among various types of ionizing radiations in penetrating power in tissue. (From Shapiro J: *Radiation protection: a guide for scientists and physicians,* Cambridge, MA, 1972, Harvard University Press.)

ecules on which they impinge, producing ions and free radicals in the process. The distance between successive atomic collisions along the path of an impinging radiation depends on the energy, mass, and electrostatic charge of the radiation. With an alpha particle, for example, the collisions typically occur so close together that the radiation gives up all of its energy in traversing only a few cells (Fig. 11-1). Hence an alpha particle emitted externally poses little risk of injury, even to the skin. Conversely, along the track of an x-ray or gamma ray, the collisions typically occur so far apart from one another that the radiation may traverse the entire body (Figure 11-1).

DNA damage. Any molecular constituent of the cell can be altered by radiation, but DNA is the most critical biological target because of the limited redundancy of the genetic information it contains. A dose of radiation large enough to kill the average dividing cell (approximately 2 Sv) causes hundreds of lesions in its DNA molecules.[36] Such lesions include base alterations, base destruction, sugar-phosphate bond cleavage, chain breakage (single-strand, double-strand), cross-linking of DNA strands (intrastrand, interstrand), DNA-protein cross links, and DNA degradation.[36] (see Chapters 19 and 20).

The kinds of molecular changes in DNA that are produced by a given dose of radiation depend on the microscopic distribution of the delivered energy. Traversal of the DNA by a low linear energy transfer (LET) radiation is more likely to cause a simple lesion, such as a single-strand break or base damage, than a lesion of greater complexity. Because a complex and irreparable lesion is more likely to result from traversal by a high LET particle,[10] the relative

biological effectiveness (RBE) of radiation generally increases with its ion density, or LET.[20]

Mitotic inhibition. After intensive irradiation, the mitotic rate is typically depressed immediately, remains depressed for a period of minutes or hours, and then may temporarily overshoot on returning to normal (Fig. 11-2). The inhibition of mitosis is not elicited by irradiation of the cytoplasm alone, implying that it results from direct effects of radiation on the nucleus.[5]

Mutations. Unrepaired damage to DNA may be expressed in the form of mutations, the frequency of which increases in proportion with the dose, approximating 1^{-5} to 10^{-6} per locus per Sv, depending on the dose rate and other variables.[33] The linear nonthreshold form of the dose-response relationship for mutagenesis implies that the traversal of the genetic target by a single ionizing particle may, in principle, suffice to cause a mutation of the affected gene.[33]

Chromosome aberrations. Radiation, by breaking chromosomes and interfering with their normal segregation to daughter cells at mitosis, can give rise to various changes in chromosome structure and number. The combined frequency of translocations, dicentrics, and chromosome rings increases as a linear, nonthreshold function of the radiation

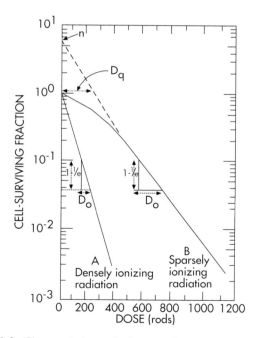

Fig. 11-3. Characteristic survival curves for clonogenic mammalian cells exposed to ionizing radiation, as scored by their ability to proliferate and form macroscopic colonies. The two parameters characterizing the curve are the slope (D_O) of the straight portion of the curve and the extrapolation number (*n*), which is a measure of the "width" of the initial shoulder; the width of the shoulder may also be expressed in terms of the quasithreshold dose (*Dq*). (From Hall EJ: *Radiobiology for the radiologist*, ed 2, New York, 1978, Harper & Row.)

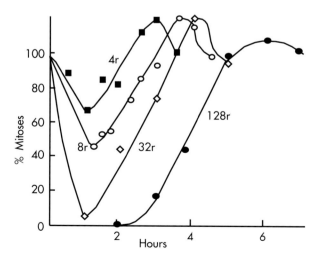

Fig. 11-2. X-ray-induced depression, "overshooting," and recovery in cells of the corneal epithelium of the rat. (From Friedenwald JS, Siglman S: The influence of ionizing radiation on mitotic activity in the rat corneal epithelium, *Exp Cell Res* 4:1, 1953.)

dose in the low-to-intermediate dose range, approximating 0.1 per cell per Sv in human lymphocytes irradiated in vitro.[15] Chromosome aberrations have also been observed to be increased in frequency in the lymphocytes of atomic bomb survivors, radiation workers, persons residing in areas of elevated natural background radiation, and radiation accident victims, the frequency of aberrations in a given individual providing a crude index of his or her radiation dose.[15]

Cell killing. Although radiation is capable of killing any cell, dividing cells are especially radiosensitive as a class. The survival of dividing cells, measured in terms of their proliferative capacity, tends to decrease exponentially with increasing dose (Fig. 11-3), 1 to 2 Gy sufficing to reduce the surviving fraction by 50% in most human tissues.[31] Noncycling cells tend to be radioresistant by comparison, but lymphocytes and oocytes represent noteworthy exceptions to this rule.[12]

Reactions of tissues

General features. The pathological changes produced by irradiation include both direct effects and indirect effects, some of which evolve slowly. Thus, although mitotic inhibition and cytological abnormalities, for example, of-

ten are detectable within minutes after intensive irradiation, atrophy and fibrosis may not become manifest until months or years later (Fig. 11-4). In general, tissues in which there is a high rate of cell turnover tend to exhibit injury more rapidly than others.[12]

Although the killing of individual cells is a stochastic process, too few cells are killed by a dose below 0.5 Gy to cause detectable histopathological changes in most tissues.[12] Furthermore, because the severity of injury is a function of the number of cells affected, the injury from a given dose generally is less severe if only a part of an organ or part of the body is exposed than if all the cells in the whole organ or the body are exposed. Also, as a result of the homeostatic effects of both intracellular repair processes and of compensatory proliferation by uninjured cells, a given dose accumulated gradually over an extended period of time tends to cause less injury than if it is absorbed in a single, brief exposure.[12]

The effects of radiation, although not strictly pathognomonic, often are sufficiently characteristic to suggest radiation in the differential diagnosis. The response to radiation can vary considerably, depending on the organ irradiated, the dose, the conditions of exposure, the time following irradiation, and other variables. Although severe

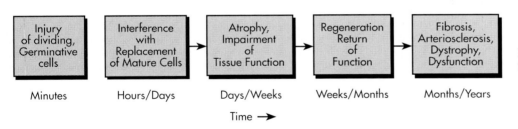

Fig. 11-4. Successive phases of tissue reaction to radiation injury.

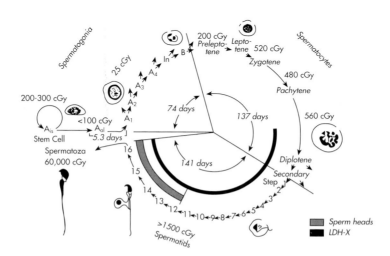

Fig. 11-5. Kinetics and radiosensitivity of mouse spermatogenic cells, as related to stage of maturation. Radiation sensitivities are given in terms of LD$_{50}$ values. (From Meistrich ML et al: Gradual regeneration of mouse testicular stem cells after exposure to ionizing radiation. *Radiat Res* 74:349, 1978.)

Table 11-2. Estimated threshold doses for various tissue reactions, based on observations in patients treated with fractionated x-irradiation or gamma-irradiation

Organ irradiated	Type of injury at 5 years	Dose causing effect in 1% to 5% of patients (Gy)	Irradiated field (area)
Skin	Ulcer, severe fibrosis	55	100 cm^2
Oral mucosa	Ulcer, severe fibrosis	60	50 cm^2
Esophagus	Ulcer, stricture	60	75 cm^2
Stomach	Ulcer, perforation	45	100 cm^2
Intestine	Ulcer, stricture	45	100 cm^2
Colon	Ulcer, stricture	45	100 cm^2
Rectum	Ulcer, stricture	55	100 cm^2
Salivary glands	Xerostomia	50	50 cm^2
Liver	Liver failure ascites	35	whole
Kidney	Nephrosclerosis	23	whole
Urinary bladder	Ulcer, contracture	60	whole
Ureters	Stricture, obstruction	75	5-10 cm
Testes	Permanent sterilization	5-15	whole
Ovary	Permanent sterilization	2-3	whole
Uterus	Necrosis perforation	>100	whole
Vagina	Ulcer, fistula	90	5 cm
Breast, child	Hypoplasia	10	5 cm^2
Breast, adult	Atrophy and necrosis	>50	whole
Lung	Pneumonitis, fibrosis	40	lobe
Capillaries	Telangiectasis, sclerosis	50-60	—
Heart	Pericarditis, pancarditis	40	whole
Bone, child	Arrested growth	20	10 cm^2
Bone, adult	Necrosis, fracture	60	10 cm^2
Cartilage, child	Arrested growth	10	whole
Cartilage, adult	Necrosis	60	whole
Central nervous system (brain)	Necrosis	50	whole
Spinal cord	Necrosis, transection	50	5 cm^2
Eye	Panophthalmitis, hemorrhage	55	whole
Cornea	Keratitis	50	whole
Lens	Cataract	5	whole
Ear (inner)	Deafness	>60	whole
Vestibulum auris	Ménière's syndrome	60	whole
Thyroid	Hypothyroidism	45	whole
Adrenal	Hypoadrenalism	>60	whole
Pituitary	Hypopituitarism	45	whole
Muscle, child	Hypoplasia	20-30	whole
Muscle, adult	Atrophy	>100	whole
Bone marrow	Hypoplasia	2	whole
Bone marrow	Hypoplasia	20	localized
Lymph nodes	Atrophy	35-45	—
Lymphatics	Sclerosis	50	—
Fetus	Death	2	whole

Data from references 12, 22, and 31.

reactions are not elicited by doses below 10 Sv in most tissues (Table 11-2), such reactions can be elicited by much smaller doses in certain organs, as described briefly in the following paragraphs.

Skin. The earliest clinically observable reaction of the skin to irradiation is erythema, resulting in histamine-like substances released by injured epidermal cells. The threshold for erythema in a 10 cm^2 field varies from 6 to 8 Sv delivered in a single, brief exposure to more than 30 Sv delivered in daily exposures over a period of weeks.[12] After rapid exposure to 6 Sv, the erythema typically appears within a day. It then lasts a few hours and is followed 2 to 4 weeks later by one or more waves of deeper, prolonged erythema, accompanied by temporary epilation. After a dose as large as 10 to 20 Sv, moist desquamation and necrosis of the skin may ensue within 2 to 4 weeks,[12,34] followed months or years later by changes in pigmentation; atrophy of the epidermis, sweat glands, sebaceous glands, and hair follicles; fibrosis of the dermis; telangiectasia; increased susceptibility to trauma; and chronic ulceration.[12]

Bone marrow and lymphoid tissue. A dose of 2 to 3 Sv delivered rapidly to the whole body causes extensive

Table 11-3. Major forms of the acute radiation syndrome

Time after irradiation	Cerebral form (>50 Gy)	Gastrointestinal form (>10 Gy)	Hemopoietic form (>2 Gy)
First day	Nausea Vomiting Diarrhea Headache Erythema Disorientation Agitation Ataxia Weakness Somnolence Coma Convulsions Shock Death	Nausea Vomiting Diarrhea	Nausea Vomiting Diarrhea
Second week		Nausea Vomiting Diarrhea Fever Erythema Emaciation Prostration Death	
Third to fourth weeks			Weakness Fatigue Anorexia Nausea Vomiting Diarrhea Fever Hemorrhage Epilation Recovery (?)

From United Nations Scientific Committee on the Effects of Atomic Radiation: *Genetic and somatic effects of ionizing radiation,* New York, 1986, United Nations.

killing of lymphocytes and their precursors, resulting within 48 hours in severe lymphopenia and immunological depression. Such a dose also causes extensive killing of hemopoietic cells, resulting in aplasia of the marrow and depression of the granulocyte and platelet counts, which fall to their lowest levels in 3 to 5 weeks.[12,33] A dose as large as 3 to 5 Sv is likely to cause death from infection or hemorrhage within 4 to 6 weeks (Table 11-3).

Gastrointestinal tract. Stem cells in the crypts of Lieberkühn are highly radiosensitive. Hence a rapidly delivered dose of 10 Sv depletes their numbers sufficiently to interfere drastically with cell renewal, resulting in denudation and ulceration of the overlying mucosa. If a large enough area of the intestinal mucosa is affected, death results within several days from a fulminating, dysentery-like syndrome (Table 11-3).

Gonads. Cells in later maturation stages of the semi-niferous epithelium are relatively radioresistant (Fig. 11-5), but acute exposure of both testes to a dose as low as 0.15 Sv suffices to deplete type A spermatogonia drastically, resulting in aplasia of the seminiferous epithelium and leading within 60 days to temporary oligospermia. A dose to both testes in excess of 2 Sv may result in permanent sterility.[12]

Mature oocytes, in contrast to spermatozoa, are highly radiosensitive. Acute exposure of both ovaries to a dose of 1.5 to 2.0 Sv may, therefore, cause temporary sterility in some women, and a dose of 2.0 to 3.0 Sv may suffice to cause permanent sterility, depending on age at the time of exposure.[12]

Lens of the eye. Radiation injury of dividing cells in the anterior epithelium of the lens can give rise to posterior polar lens opacities. The dose required to produce an opacity, or cataract, of sufficient severity to impair vision is estimated to vary, from 2 to 3 Sv absorbed in a single brief exposure to 5.5 to 14 Sv absorbed in repeated exposures over a period of months.[12]

Respiratory tract. The lung is not one of the most radiosensitive organs of the body, but intensive irradiation can cause a necrotizing reaction of alveolar cells and pulmonary vasculature.[12] Thus a dose of 8 to 10 Sv delivered to both lungs in a single, brief exposure may lead to death within 1 to 6 months from acute pneumonitis or to death years later from pulmonary fibrosis and cor pulmonale.[12,33]

Acute radiation syndrome

Intensive irradiation of a major part of the hemopoietic system, the gastrointestinal tract, or the central nervous system can give rise to the acute radiation syndrome. The syndrome takes various forms, the pathogenesis, timing, and severity of which vary, depending on the size of the dose and its anatomical distribution (Table 11-3).

Effects of prenatal irradiation on growth and development

In keeping with their undifferentiated and proliferative character, embryonal, fetal, and juvenile tissues are highly radiosensitive. Thus, doses as low as 0.25 Sv delivered to the embryo during critical stages in organogenesis have been observed to cause a wide variety of malformations in laboratory animals.[30,32] In humans, among the most noteworthy of the teratogenic effects that have been attributed to prenatal irradiation are the increased frequency of severe mental retardation and decreased intelligence quotient (IQ) test scores in atomic bomb survivors who were irradiated between the 8th and the 15th week after conception.[6,32]

Heritable (genetic) effects

Heritable radiation-induced mutations and chromosomal abnormalities are well documented in Drosophila, laboratory mice, and other organisms.[6,33] As yet, however, such changes remain to be detected in humans,[33] despite inten-

Table 11-4. Estimates of the extent to which the frequencies of different heritable disorders are attributable to natural background irradiation

Type of disorder	Natural prevalence	Contribution from natural background radiation*	
		First generation	Equilibrium
		(frequency per million live births)†	
Autosomal dominant	1000	20-100	300
X-linked	400	<1	<15
Recessive	2500	<1	Very slow increase
Chromosomal	4400	<20	Very little increase
Congenital abnormalities	20,000-30,000	30	30-300
Other disorders of complex etiology			
Heart disease	600,000	NE	NE
Cancer	300,000	NE	NE
Selected others	300,000	NE	NE

NE, Not estimated.

From National Academy of Sciences, National Research Council, Committee on the Biological Effects of Ionizing Radiation: *Health effects of exposure to low levels of ionizing radiation (BEIR V),* Washington, DC, National Academy Press, 1990.

*Equivalent to approximately 1 mSv per year (Table 11-1) or approximately 30 mSv per generation (30 years).

†Values rounded.

sive study of more than 76,000 children of the atomic bomb survivors of Hiroshima and Nagasaki, extending over four decades. These studies have failed to detect such changes as measured by (1) untoward pregnancy outcomes, (2) neonatal deaths, (3) malignancies, (4) balanced chromosomal rearrangements, (5) sex-chromosome aneuploids, (6) alterations of serum or erythrocyte protein phenotypes, (7) changes in sex ratio, and (8) disturbances of normal growth and development.[21]

The absence of detectable heritable effects in the human populations examined thus far is interpreted to signify that the dose required to double the mutation rate in human germ cells exceeds 1.0 Gy.[6] On this basis, only a small percentage of all genetic disease in the general population is thought to be attributable to natural background irradiation (Table 11-4); however, this conclusion must be qualified in the absence of quantitative dose-response data for radiation-induced mutations in human germ cells and in the face of uncertainty about the extent to which new mutations contribute to the prevalence of multifactorial diseases.

Carcinogenic effects (see Chapter 26)

It has long been known that certain types of cancer— e.g., carcinomas of the skin in x-ray workers, leukemias in radiologists, osteogenic sarcomas and carcinomas of cranial sinuses in early radium dial painters, lung cancers in pitchblende and other underground hard-rock miners— have occurred with increased frequency in radiation workers.[35] More recently, studies of atomic bomb survivors and other irradiated human populations have indicated that various other types of cancers may be increased in frequency by irradiation, depending on the conditions of exposure.

Such neoplasms, however, characteristically have required years or decades to develop. In addition, they possess no features distinguishing them individually as having resulted from radiation as opposed to other causes. With few exceptions, moreover, the induction of such cancers has been detectable only after relatively large doses of radiation (greater than 0.5 Gy) and has varied with the type of neoplasm in question as well as with the age and sex of the exposed population.[6,32] The extent to which the risk of cancer may be increased by low-level irradiation is therefore unknown and can be estimated only by extrapolation, based on assumptions about the relevant dose-incidence relationship.[6,33]

Estimates of the lifetime risks of cancer, based on analyses of the atomic bomb survivors and other irradiated human populations, depend on the extrapolation models used for the purpose (Table 11-5). Although the data for certain types of cancer are compatible with a linear, nonthreshold dose-incidence relationship, other relationships cannot be excluded. Also, quantitative human data on the comparative carcinogenicity of protracted irradiation are lacking.[18] The carcinogenicity of low LET radiation for laboratory animals is reduced by a factor of 2 to 10 if the exposure is prolonged. This implies that the estimates given in Table 11-5 may greatly exaggerate the risks attributable to dosages accumulated over extended periods of time.[6,33]

Shortening of the life span

In all species of laboratory animals investigated to date, whole-body irradiation early in life increases the age-specific mortality from cancer and other diseases. This therefore decreases longevity accordingly.[28] Similar effects

Table 11-5. Estimated lifetime risks of different cancers attributable to 0.1 Sv rapid whole-body irradiation.

Type or site of cancer	Cancer deaths per 100,000*
Lung	60-170
Stomach	90-130
Leukemia	90-100
Colon	30-80
Breast	20-40
Urinary tract	20-40
Esophagus	20-30
Ovary	20-20
Multiple myeloma	10-20
Thyroid	10-15
Remainder	90-135
Total	460-780

From United Nations Scientific Committee on the Effects of Atomic Radiation: *Sources, effects, and risks of ionizing radiation,* New York, 1988, United Nations; and National Academy of Sciences, National Research Council, Committee on the Biological Effects of Ionizing Radiation: *Health effects of exposure to low levels of ionizing radiation (BEIR V),* Washington, DC, 1990, National Academy Press.
*Values (rounded) for a population of both sexes and all ages at the time of irradiation.

have been observed in early cohorts of radiologists[23] and in atomic bomb survivors irradiated as children or young adults.[25] It is noteworthy, however, that all age-related lesions in such persons do not appear to have been affected.[25] Although the mean survival time of animals in a few experiments has appeared to be prolonged by low-level, whole-body irradiation—which has been interpreted by some observers as a hormetic effect—the survival of the controls in such experiments was usually compromised by mortality from intercurrent infection, so the significance of the findings and their implications for human health are questionable.[6]

CONCLUSION

Over the past century, studies of irradiated populations have disclosed a wide variety of pathological reactions, the details of which have varied, depending on the anatomical regions exposed, the conditions of irradiation, the age and sex of the exposed individuals, and other variables. Reactions to intensive irradiation typically evolve through a sequence of changes characterized by (1) degeneration and death of dividing, germinative cells; (2) aplasia; (3) interference with replacement of senescent cells; (4) early atrophy of the affected tissue; (5) regeneration; (6) fibrosis; (7) arteriosclerosis; (8) secondary atrophy; (9) dystrophy; and (10) dysplasia.

The reactions of tissues to large doses of radiation, such as are typically administered in the radiotherapy of cancer, have been relatively well characterized. In contrast, the reactions that may be produced by smaller doses, which include mutagenic, carcinogenic, and teratogenic effects, are less well defined. Assessment of the risks attributable to low-level environmental and occupational irradiation must therefore be based largely on assumptions and extrapolations that are fraught with uncertainty.

REFERENCES

1. Advisory Committee on the Biological Effects of Ionizing Radiation, National Academy of Sciences: *The biological effects of atomic radiation,* Washington, DC, 1956, National Academy of Sciences.
2. Albers-Schonberg HE: Ueber Line Bisher Unbekannte Wirkung der Roentgenstrahlen auf den Organismus, *Munich Med Wochschr* 50:1859, 1903.
3. Bergonie J, Tribondeau L: Interpretation de quelques resultats de la radiotherapie et assai de fixation d'une technique rationale. *C R Acad Sci* 143:983, 1906.
4. Brown FT, Osgood AT: X-rays and sterility, *Am J Surg* 18:179, 1905.
5. Cole A et al: Mechanisms of cell injury. In Meyn RE, Withers HR, editors: *Radiation biology in cancer research,* New York, 1980, Raven Press.
6. Committee on the Biological Effects of Ionizing Radiation, National Academy of Sciences: *Health effects of exposure to low levels of ionizing radiation,* Washington, DC, 1990, National Academy Press.
7. Department of Energy: *Health and environmental consequences of the Chernobyl nuclear power plant accident,* Publication No. DOE/ER-0332, Washington, DC, 1987, National Technical Information Service.
8. Friedenwald JS, Siglman S: The influence of ionizing radiation on mitotic activity in the rat corneal epithelium, *Exp Cell Res* 4:1, 1953.
9. Glasser O: *The science of radiology,* Springfield, IL, 1933, Charles C Thomas.
10. Goodhead DT: Spatial and temporal distribution of energy, *Health Phys* 55:231, 1988.
11. Hall EJ: *Radiobiology for the radiologist,* ed 2, New York, 1978, Harper & Row.
12. International Commission on Radiological Protection: *Nonstochastic effects of radiation,* ICRP Publication No. 41, Oxford, 1984, Pergamon Press.
13. International Commission on Radiological Protection: *Recommendations of the International Commission on Radiological Protection,* ICRP Publication No. 60, Ann ICRP 21:1, 1991.
14. Lewis EB: Leukemia and ionizing radiation, *Science* 125:965, 1957.
15. Lloyd DC, Purrott RJ: Chromosome aberration analysis in radiological protection dosimetry, *Radiol Protect Dosim* 1:19, 1981.
16. Meistrich ML et al: Gradual regeneration of mouse testicular stem cells after exposure to ionizing radiation. *Radiat Res* 74:349, 1978.
17. Muller HJ: The manner of production of mutations by radiation. In Hollaender A, editor: *Radiation biology,* vol 1: *High energy radiation,* New York, 1954, McGraw-Hill.
18. National Council on Radiation Protection and Measurements: *Exposures from the uranium series with emphasis on radon and its daughters,* Report No. 77, Bethesda, MD, 1984, National Council on Radiation Protection and Measurements.
19. National Council on Radiation Protection and Measurements: *Recommendations on limits for exposure to ionizing radiation,* Report No. 91, Bethesda, MD, 1987, National Council on Radiation Protection and Measurements.
20. National Council on Radiation Protection and Measurements: *The relative biological effectiveness of radiations of different quality,* Report No. 104, Bethesda, MD, 1990, National Council on Radiation Protection and Measurements.
21. Neel JV et al: The children of parents exposed to atomic bombs: estimates of the genetic doubling dose of radiation for humans, *Am J Hum Genet* 46:1053, 1990.
22. Rubin P, Casarett GW: A direction for clinical radiation pathology:

the tolerance dose. In Vaeth JM, editor: *Frontiers of radiation therapy and oncology*, Basel, 1972, Karger, and Baltimore, 1972, University Park Press.

23. Seltser R, Sartwell PE: The influence of occupational exposure to radiation on the mortality of American radiologists and other medical specialists, *Am J Epidemiol* 81:2, 1965.

24. Shapiro J: *Radiation protection: a guide for scientists and physicians*, Cambridge, MA, 1972, Harvard University Press.

25. Shimizu Y et al: *Line span study report 11, part 3. Noncancer mortality, 1950-85, based on the revised doses (DS 86)*, RERF TR 2-91, Radiation Effects Research Foundation, Hiroshima, 1991, *Radiation Res* 130:249-266, 1992.

26. Stewart A, Webb J, Hewitt D: A survey of childhood malignancies, *Br Med J* 1:1495, 1958.

27. Stewart AM et al: Preliminary communication: malignant disease in childhood and diagnostic irradiation in utero, *Lancet* 2:447, 1956.

28. Stone RS: Maximum permissible exposure standards. In Sonnenblick BP, editor: *Protection in diagnostic radiology*, New Brunswick, NJ, 1959, Rutgers University Press.

29. Stone-Scott N: X-ray injuries, *Am X-Ray J* 1:57, 1897.

30. United Nations Scientific Committee on the Effects of Atomic Radiation: *Sources and effects of ionizing radiation*, Publication No. E.77.IX.I, New York, 1977, United Nations.

31. United Nations Scientific Committee on the Effects of Atomic Radiation: *Ionizing radiation: sources and biological effects*, New York, 1982, United Nations.

32. United Nations Scientific Committee on the Effects of Atomic Radiation: *Genetic and somatic effects of ionizing radiation*, New York, 1986, United Nations.

33. United Nations Scientific Committee on the Effects of Atomic Radiation: *Sources, effects and risks of ionizing radiation*, New York, 1988, United Nations.

34. United States Nuclear Regulatory Commission: *Health effects models for nuclear power plant accident consequence analysis. Low LET radiation. Part II: Scientific bases for health effects models*, Report No. NUREG/CR-4214, SAND85-7185, Rev 1, Part 2, Albuquerque, NM, 1989, Sandia National Laboratory.

35. Upton AC et al, editors: *Radiation carcinogenesis*, New York, 1986, Elsevier Science Publishing Co.

36. Ward JF: DNA damage produced by ionizing radiation in mammalian cells: identities, mechanisms of formation and repairability, *Progr Nucleic Acid Res Mol Biol* 35:96, 1988.

Chapter 12

ELECTROMAGNETIC ENERGY

Stephen F. Cleary

Life evolved in an electromagnetic environment resulting from natural terrestrial and extraterrestrial sources. Exposure to background radiation remained essentially constant until the discovery of natural radioactivity and the generation of x-radiation at the turn of the century. Considered benign initially, it was soon recognized that ionizing-radiation or γ-electromagnetic radiation exposure induced numerous effects in living systems, including dramatic increases in the incidence of human cancer. The mechanism responsible for radiation-induced pathological change was subsequently revealed to be ionization of biomolecules resulting in, among other effects, mutational and chromosomal damage in genomic DNA (see Chapters 11, 19 and 20).

Exposure-related disease correlated with levels of environmental and occupational ionizing radiation exposure. Guidelines and standards to limit the deleterious effects of ionizing radiation were developed and promulgated based on data derived from epidemiological and experimental studies, as discussed elsewhere (see Chapters 11 and 26). Knowledge of the basic interaction mechanisms of ionizing radiation provided a basis for understanding effects on living systems that led to quantitative dosimetry and effective means of limiting exposure effects.

Fig. 12-1 indicates the electromagnetic frequency spectrum and some typical applications of man-made electromagnetic radiation, including power transmission, broadcast communication, industrial processes, and medical applications. Environmental as well as occupational exposure levels from man-made sources of nonionization electromagnetic radiation (NER) at frequencies up to 100 GHz exceed natural background radiation levels in this frequency range by factors of 10^8 or more. In industrial societies, we are thus continuously immersed in a deepening sea of variable frequency and intensity electromagnetic fields of far greater intensity than levels that existed during the evolution of life on earth. The marked departure of environmental NER exposure intensities from evolutionary levels suggests the possibility that living systems may not have developed adaptive protective mechanisms comparable to those limiting adverse effects of exposure to higher energy electromagnetic radiation such as visible light, ultraviolet light, and x-radiation and γ-radiation.

Until recently, there was limited concern about possible harmful consequences of increasing exposure to NER. The scientific basis for changing attitudes about the health effects of NER exposure is the subject of this chapter. Examples of specific sources of NER that cause concern include 60 Hz electrical and magnetic fields, hand-held cellular telephones, and police radar speed detectors.

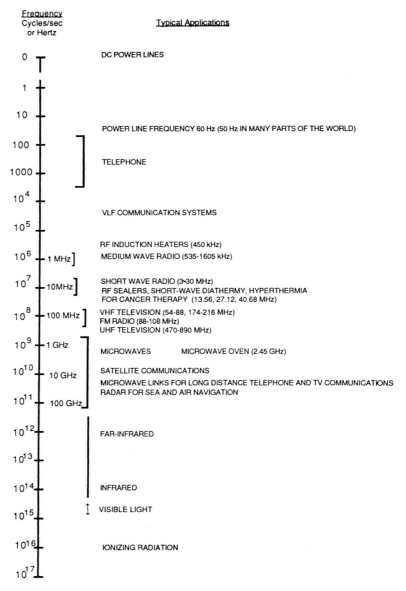

Fig. 12-1. Electromagnetic spectrum. (From Gandhi OmP: Biological effects and medical applications of electromagnetic energy, © 1990, p 4. Reprinted by permission of Prentice Hall, Englewood Cliffs, New Jersey.)

PHYSICAL AND BIOLOGICAL INTERACTION MECHANISMS

The distinction between ionizing radiation and NER is the inability of the latter to induce direct molecular disruption, such as ionization, and the associated phenomenon of bond breakage. This distinction suggests qualitatively different effects of NER and ionizing radiation on living systems. Indeed, in contrast to the well-documented induction of somatic and genetic mutations and cell killing that results from exposure to ionizing radiation, the effects of NER have until recently been ascribed to indirect heat induced by NER energy absorption. Although the underlying basic interaction mechanisms of NER leading to direct

nonthermal physiological alterations are not well understood, there is increasing evidence of their occurrence.

One reason for uncertainty regarding the mechanisms for direct NER effects relates to the highly heterogeneous and imprecisely known frequency-dependent electrical properties of living systems at the cell or tissue level. Assuming, for example, a direct NER interaction with the cell membrane surface, mechanistic understanding requires accurate information such as the magnitude of localized NER energy absorption or induced current at the interaction site. Such high-resolution dosimetric information has not been obtained experimentally. Theoretical estimates are, in turn, of uncertain accuracy owing to lack of detailed knowledge of the electrical properties of living systems at the molecular level.

Another impediment to the development of interaction mechanisms is the nonclassic nature of NER biological responses. The biological effects of other physical agents such as ionizing radiation or chemicals have generally followed classic concentration or energy-dependence and dose-response relationships over a wide dosage range. Exposure of several biological systems to NER has resulted in biphasic (1) dose responses referred to as "intensity windows"; (2) frequency or modulation responses, called "frequency windows"; and (3) complex exposure duration and postexposure time-dependence. In addition, in many instances, effects have been reported to occur under exposure conditions involving significantly lower levels of NER energy coupling than previously associated with biological activation energies associated with effects of other physical or chemical agents.

Much uncertainty surrounds the physical and biological mechanisms of NER effects on living systems. This uncertainty has generated skepticism and debate that has retarded progress in this area. Evidence of beneficial applications of NER in tissue healing and the epidemiological association of NER exposure and cancer and other adverse health effects provides the impetus for advancing the state of knowledge in this field.

BIOPHYSICAL AND BIOMEDICAL ASPECTS OF THE ASSOCIATION OF EXTREMELY LOW FREQUENCY ELECTROMAGNETIC FIELDS AND CANCER

Results of studies of residential and occupational exposure to extremely low frequency (ELF) electromagnetic fields and cancer risk add substantially to a growing body of epidemiological evidence indicating a positive association. In one such study, children exposed in their homes to time-averaged magnetic fields of 3 milliGauss (mG) or more had an almost four times greater risk of leukemia than children exposed to fields of less than 1 mG.[47] The most compelling aspect of this study with respect to an association of magnetic field exposure with cancer was the demonstration of a dose-response relationship. Magnetic field exposure at greater than 1 mG was claimed to cause a doubling of leukemia incidence, whereas exposure to magnetic field intensities of more than 2 mG was associated with a threefold increase. The childhood leukemia risk ratios in this study, after controlling for confounding influences such as socioeconomic status and air pollution, were statistically significant.[47] A 70% increase in the incidence of both acute myeloid leukemia and chronic myeloid leukemia was found in adults exposed to magnetic intensities greater than 2 mG compared with those exposed to less than 1 mG. The adult risk ratios were not statistically significant, possibly owing to sample size and uncertainty regarding the time-averaged magnetic field exposure of adults.[47]

Another significant aspect of this study was a detailed exposure assessment based on reconstruction of long-term magnetic field exposure intensities in the home for periods of up to 10 years before diagnosis. Comparison of estimated long-term exposure assessments with short-term or "spot" measurements indicated a lack of correlation. There was a tendency of "spot" measurements to overestimate past exposures, thus biasing the outcome of studies that relied on such measurements. This outcome thus supported the validity of using wire codes to estimate long-term magnetic field exposure rather than "spot" measurements. Consequently the results of this study are consistent with the results of previous studies that reported a statistically significant increase in childhood cancer incidence when residential magnetic field exposure was determined by wire code configurations.[63,90,106]

A dose-response relationship was also detected in an occupational study.[49] Based on magnetic field measurements, workers were categorized according to average magnetic field exposure. Among the most highly exposed workers, there was a fourfold increased risk of chronic lymphocytic leukemia.[49] The results of this study are of particular interest in that a leukemia dose-response relationship was detected based on measured magnetic field intensities rather than retrospective exposure estimates based on job classifications. These results, taken together with the results of previous occupational studies, including a meta-analysis that combined results of independent occupational studies,[89] indicate a consistent relationship between residential or occupational exposure to ELF magnetic fields and cancer risk.

The results of the 1992 Swedish epidemiological studies led to a formal announcement on September 30, 1993, by Sweden's National Board for Industrial and Technical Development, NUTEK, that it "will act on the assumption that there is a connection between exposure to power frequency magnetic fields and cancer, in particular, childhood cancer."[72]

In addition to an association of leukemia incidence with long-term exposure to weak residential or occupational ELF electromagnetic fields, occupational exposure has also been reported to increase the risk of brain cancer[61,93] as well as breast cancer in male workers.[39,69,94,102] Limited epidemiological evidence also indicates an association of ELF electromagnetic field exposure and adverse outcomes of reproduction,[108] altered biorhythms,[68] and neurological disorders.[36]

Trends in cancer incidence and electrical power consumption

The argument has been advanced that the reported association of exposure to weak ELF electromagnetic fields and adverse health effects is spurious because the trend during the past few decades of increased electrical power consumption has not been reflected in increased cancer morbidity or mortality. The validity of this argument rests on two premises: (1) that increased ELF electrical power consumption has resulted in parallel increases in human exposure and (2) that there has been no increase in cancer incidence during this period. Demographic changes, such as large-scale movement from urban to suburban communities, as well as changes in electrical wiring materials, installation methods, and building codes may, in fact, have acted to limit increased human exposure concomitant with increased usage as suggested by some studies.[51,107] Thus, premise (1) is unproven.

With respect to premise (2), during the past 20 years, cancer mortality in persons under age 45 has, in fact, declined in industrial nations owing to improved treatment,[41] but there has been a continuous increase in incidence.[79,103] In 16 industrial countries, the overall cancer trends indicate that the worldwide effort to combat cancer has not been successful in that there has not been a substantial reduction in overall cancer death rate. Successes in childhood cancer treatment have been offset by greater mortality in older age groups.[7] The National Cancer Institute 1989 report, *Annual Review of Cancer Statistics,* reported a 60% increase in the incidence of childhood cancers from 1950 to 1986 and a 20% decrease in mortality.[103] During the period 1969 through 1986, there was a 20% decrease in mortality in the United States for brain tumors in white males and females ages 0 to 44, but there was more than an 80% increase in brain tumor mortality in persons aged 65 to 84 over this same period.[38] Age-specific analyses of central nervous system (CNS) cancer in six major industrial countries showed significantly different trends in different age groups. There was a doubling of brain tumor rates in persons aged 75 to 84.[38] Increased multiple myeloma mortality has also persisted in people over the age of 70, whereas the rate has stabilized at younger ages in most industrial countries. These findings suggest a possible ubiquitous environmental risk factor common to all industrial countries that increased during the last quarter of the 19th century and first quarter of this century.[35] The incidence of female breast cancer and breast cancer mortality has increased at a linear rate for the past 50 years or more. Breast cancer etiological factors are generally unknown.[57]

Cancer trends during the past 20 years, especially regarding cancer incidence, contradict premise (2). Although increased cancer incidence may be attributable to multiple risk factors in industrial nations, it is not possible to exclude exposure to ELF electrical or magnetic fields as a contributory factor.

Animal studies: biorhythms/melatonin

In addition to a consistent pattern of association of ELF electromagnetic field exposure with cancer risk, as revealed by epidemiological studies, there is a body of biomedical and biophysical evidence suggesting that such fields affect numerous physiological processes in cells as well as organisms, some of which may pertain to basic mechanisms of carcinogenesis. Such laboratory studies offer the potential for accurate, precise control of experimental conditions, thus permitting unambiguous determination of cause and effect relationships and mechanisms of interaction.

The maintenance of normal biological function depends on well-controlled rhythmical variation of numerous physiological functions. Many of these controlled variations, referred to as biorhythms, occur at frequencies in the ELF range of 60 Hz or less. It is well-known that disruption of normal biorhythms can cause adverse health effects related to altered functioning of nerve and endocrine cells. Studies in humans[109] and rodents[42,87] indicate that ELF electrical fields alter biorhythms at field strengths as low as 2.5 V/m.[111]

One consequence of ELF-field altered biorhythms was the inhibition of normal nighttime rise of the pineal hormone melatonin and biosynthetic enzymes in rats exposed to 60 Hz electrical fields at 1.5 kV/m or 40 kV/m.[110-112] This effect occurred following 3 weeks of exposure.[112] In addition to reduced secretion of melatonin, phase shifts in pineal secretion of this hormone were also reported to occur as a result of exposure of young rats to 60 Hz electrical fields.[84]

The potential significance of 60-Hz electromagnetic field–induced alteration in melatonin concentrations is related to the interaction of melatonin with other hormones. A reduction in melatonin results in the elevation of circulating steroid hormones, estrogen and testosterone, and increased prolactin release by the pituitary gland.[83] Such hormonal alterations increase proliferation of breast tissue and suppress the immunological system, effects consistent with increased breast cancer risk.[94] Animal experiments have demonstrated that melatonin levels are associated with mammary tumorigenesis and decreased levels owing to pinealectomy increased breast tumor formation.[100] The effect of ELF electromagnetic field exposure on melatonin concentration in experimental animals provides a potential neuroendocrine mechanism for the observed increased breast cancer incidence in occupationally exposed workers.[40,69,94,102]

Other animal studies

Before the claim of an association of residential exposure to weak 60-Hz magnetic fields with cancer, as revealed by epidemiological studies referred to previously, primary attention focused on the potential health effects of occupational exposure to high-field-strength electrical fields. Consequently the majority of reported effects involved exposure of animals to relatively intense 60-Hz electrical fields. Little attention was focused on carcinogenic effects of long-term exposure of animals to low-intensity 60-Hz magnetic fields. One study demonstrated a tumor-promoting effect of a 60-Hz magnetic field in mouse skin carcinogenesis.[95]

Effects on neural and neuroendocrine systems, reproductive systems, cardiovascular systems, and hematopoietic systems have been investigated.[5,76] A clear response pattern has not emerged from these studies.

Effects on mammalian cells

Studies of effects of ELF electromagnetic fields on mammalian cells, referred to as in vitro studies, revealed a variety of sensitive physiological endpoints. Effects were reported on (1) DNA, RNA, and protein synthesis; (2) cell proliferation; (3) cation fluxes and binding; (4) immune responses; and (5) membrane signal transduction (i.e. hormones, enzymes, and neurotransmitters). Typically, such effects occurred as a result of short-term exposure of cells to electromagnetic fields at frequencies of 100 Hz or less and at low field intensities. The dependency on frequency or modulation as well as the apparent weak cellular interaction of ELF electromagnetic fields lacks adequate theoretic explanation. The extent to which effects are induced by either electrical or magnetic fields has not been fully determined.

Biomolecular synthesis. Low-intensity ELF electrical and magnetic fields affect cellular rates of synthesis of DNA, RNA, and proteins. Liboff and colleagues,[60] for example, noted increases in DNA synthesis in human fibroblasts exposed to low-intensity sinusoidal magnetic fields (15 to 4000 Hz). Weak ELF electrical or magnetic fields affected collagen or glycosaminoglycan synthesis in fibroblasts.[33,46,48,56] ELF electrical fields increased DNA[86] and glycosaminoglycan[58] synthesis in chondrocytes. Cell-specific biphasic stimulation of cyclic adenosine monophosphate (AMP) levels and DNA synthesis in skeletal-derived cell cultures exposed to 3-Hz electrical fields have been reported.[15]

Goodman and colleagues[53] detected increased messenger RNA synthesis in cells exposed to pulse-modulated magnetic fields at frequencies of 15 to 72-Hz. Transcriptional activity also increased after exposure to 72 Hz sinusoidal magnetic fields. The maximum magnetic and electrical field strengths were less than approximately 40 Gauss and 10 mV/m. Although the magnetic fields affected transcriptional activity, there were differences in the effects of the various magnetic field waveforms. Subsequent studies demonstrated similar effects of ELF modulated magnetic fields (including 60-Hz fields) on RNA transcription and protein synthesis in other cell types.[54]

Although ELF electrical or magnetic fields of various intensities, frequencies, and modulation altered cell biosynthetic processes, attempts to detect chromosomal alterations, such as rearrangements, single-strand breaks, point mutations, or sister chromatid exchange, have failed.[13,34,62,82] One study, however, reported significant increases in chromosomal aberrations in cells exposed to magnetic fields.[78]

Membrane calcium fluxes and binding. The most extensively investigated and well-replicated in vitro effect of ELF electromagnetic fields is altered calcium ion (Ca^{2+}) binding to chick brain tissue. Studies have revealed tissue sensitivity to extremely low intensity ELF electrical and magnetic fields characterized by multiple modulation-specific and intensity-specific responses, referred to as modulation and intensity "windows." Multiple response windows present potentially perplexing problems with respect to the development of exposure guidelines because they violate accepted dose-effect and threshold response concepts. There is also in vitro data suggesting windowed responses for other cell endpoints, such as cell proliferation[33,88] or fibroblast protein synthesis.[71]

Bawin and colleagues[11,12] reported modulation windows for Ca^{2+} efflux from chick brain exposed to 147-MHz radiofrequency (RF) electromagnetic radiation, amplitude modulated (AM) at specific frequencies between 6 and 20 Hz. Blackman and colleagues[16,17] reported intensity windows for this phenomenon and subsequently found similar responses using modulated 50-MHz RF radiation.[18] Sheppard and colleagues[91] also observed a Ca^{2+} efflux intensity window for modulated RF radiation. Dutta and colleagues[43,44] reported multiple intensity windows for Ca^{2+} efflux from neuroblastoma cells in culture exposed to 915- or 147-MHz RF radiation amplitude modulated at 16 Hz.

Sinusoidal ELF fields induced intensity-dependent and modulation-dependent windowed effects on Ca^{2+} efflux from chick brain tissue in vitro.[19] Although a 16-Hz sinusoidal field enhanced Ca^{2+} efflux at 6 and 40 V/m, 1- or 30-Hz fields were ineffective, as was a 42-Hz field at 30, 40, 50, or 60 V/m. A 45-Hz field enhanced efflux at 40 V/m, of similar magnitude to the 16-Hz field. Field strengths between 45 and 50 V/m increased efflux at 45 Hz, whereas at 60 Hz, 35 and 40 V/m were effective intensities. Holding the field strength constant at 42.5 V/m and varying the frequency resulted in Ca^{2+} efflux enhancement at 15 Hz and others in the range of 45 to 105 Hz.[19]

Blackman and colleagues[20] observed that the local DC magnetic field at the site of ELF-exposed samples determined which electrical and magnetic field frequencies were effective in inducing Ca^{2+} release from chick brain tissue in vitro. In this study, the DC magnetic field was perpendicular to the plane containing oscillating electrical and magnetic field components. In a subsequent study, Blackman and colleagues[22] observed that Ca^{2+} efflux occurred when the DC-magnetic field was perpendicular to the alternating magnetic field component of a 314-Hz, 15-V/m, 0.61-mG electromagnetic field, but not when the magnetic fields were in parallel alignment. They noted that this result is consistent with a magnetic resonance–like transduction mechanism for the conversion of electromagnetic energy into a physicochemical change, such as enhanced ion transport through helical membrane channels. It was also noted that the magnetic field alignment dependence was in direct contrast to the results of Smith and colleagues[92] who demonstrated a magnetic resonance–like effect of an alternating ELF magnetic field on the mobility of diatoms.

Diatom mobility depends on transmembrane transport of Ca^{2+}. Smith and colleagues[92] exposed diatoms to DC and alternating magnetic fields they predicted would enhance Ca^{2+} transport based on an ion cyclotron resonance theory advanced by Liboff[59] and McLeod and Liboff.[70] In agreement with theory, a mobility maximum occurred at 16 Hz when the diatoms were exposed to a DC magnetic field of 209 mG and an AC field of 209 mG, when the static and AC magnetic fields were in parallel alignment. Perpendicular magnetic field alignment had no effect on diatom mobility. The diatom experiments and chick brain experiments were conducted under different conditions. Smith and colleagues[92] exposed diatoms to a 1000-fold greater magnetic flux density than Blackman and colleagues[19,20] and with different magnetic field alignment.

The results of Blackman and colleagues[19-21] and Smith and colleagues[92] as well as observations of Thomas and colleagues[101] on the effects of ELF magnetic fields on rat behavior provide evidence of intensity-dependent and frequency-dependent responses having common features such as (1) multiple windows at frequencies less than 1000 Hz, (2) intensity windows in a range of intensities well below levels at which cellular alterations can be accounted for by well-understood physicochemical interaction mechanisms, and (3) dependence on orientation of geomagnetic and applied electromagnetic field components.

In view of these complexities and the limited number of studies that have been conducted, it is not surprising that the physiological significance of electromagnetic-induced alterations in membrane cation binding or transport has not been ascertained. The central role of Ca^{2+} fluxes in neural processes is well-known. Effects of low-intensity, low-frequency (LF) electromagnetic fields on Ca^{2+} binding to brain tissue in vitro, reported by Bawin and colleagues[11,12] and Blackman and colleagues,[16-22] suggest that such fields may affect the mammalian CNS in vivo. The results of Thomas and colleagues,[101] and behavioral changes in monkeys induced by exposure to LF electromagnetic fields reported by Gavalas-Medici and Day-Magdaleno,[52] do, in fact, implicate this phenomenon in electromagnetic-induced effects on the mammalian CNS. Further evidence derives from the observation that low-amplitude LF amplitude modulated (AM) electromagnetic radiation induced Ca^{2+} release from the brain of a live cat.[4] The potential physiological significance of ELF electromagnetic field exposure has been reviewed in detail by Adey.[1]

Cell proliferation. A significant amount of information concerning cellular effects of ELF electromagnetic radiation has been derived from studies of cell proliferation in vitro. Interest in effects on cell proliferation has been stimulated by clinical applications of such fields for the treatment of connective tissue disorders, such as bone nonunions,[9,10] fresh fractures,[104] and tendinitis,[14] as well as reported association of LF electromagnetic field exposure and cancer. Attempts to characterize and quantitate in vivo re-

sponses more fully and to establish mechanisms led to a series of in vitro studies, many of which used pulsed magnetic fields of the type reported to be clinically effective.[85]

In addition to effects of ELF pulsed magnetic fields, the results of Liboff and colleagues[60] indicated that sinusoidally varying magnetic fields at frequencies in the range 15 Hz to 4 kHz induced proliferative changes in human embryonic foreskin fibroblasts in vitro. Exposure to a 76 ± 4 Hz magnetic field, at an intensity of 160 mG, induced statistically significant time-dependent increases in DNA synthesis during exposures of up to 96 hours. Compared with sham-exposed cells, DNA synthesis in fibroblasts exposed to 10 different ELF electromagnetic frequency and amplitude combinations exhibited a time-dependent maximum after 20 hours of exposure. This exposure duration was found to correspond to the midpoint of the S phase of the fibroblast cell cycle, suggesting that electromagnetic exposure effects may be related to specific cell-cycle alterations.[60] Cell proliferation data for various combinations of magnetic field intensity and frequency provided a means of testing the hypothesis that cell proliferation was directly stimulated by eddy currents induced by sinusoidal magnetic fields. According to Faraday's law, the magnitude of the eddy currents, or induced electric fields, is proportional to the product of the magnetic field frequency and intensity. The data did not support this hypothesis, leading to the conclusion that either the magnetic field effect on fibroblast proliferation was not due to induced eddy currents or the effect was a saturable phenomenon, such as a self-limiting shift in the onset of S phase. The threshold for sinusoidal magnetic field effects on fibroblast proliferation was in the range 50 to 250 mG/s. This value was similar in magnitude to the value of approximately 100 mG/s reported to interfere with development of chick embryos.[40]

Liboff and colleagues[60] also noted that threshold magnetic field magnitudes in their study were on the order of ambient 60-Hz fields in the vicinity of devices such as fluorescent lights, fans, or electric motors. Consequently, ambient fields must be measured and controlled to ensure against artifacts in in vitro studies.

Ross[88] investigated the effect of 48-hour exposure of rabbit-ligament fibroblasts in vitro to 16-, 75-, or 100-Hz sinusoidal magnetic fields. Variation of AC magnetic field amplitude, frequency, and vertical DC magnetic field strength resulted in either stimulation or inhibition of proliferation. Proliferation was inhibited at all three frequencies when the amplitude of the AC and DC magnetic fields corresponded to cyclotron resonance conditions. The biphasic nature of the effect of sinusoidal magnetic fields on proliferation was demonstrated by varying the amplitude of a 100-Hz signal from 1 to 10 G, holding the DC magnetic field constant at 1.3 G. Proliferation was inhibited at amplitudes of 5 G or less but enhanced when the magnetic field intensity was increased to 7 G or greater, up to a maximum at 10 G, the largest amplitude reported. By varying the amplitude of the DC and AC fields while holding the frequency of the AC field at 100 Hz, Ross[88] detected a significant interaction between DC and AC magnetic fields and fibroblast proliferation. These data support the hypothesis of a cyclotron resonance–like phenomenon being associated with inhibition or stimulation of fibroblast proliferation.

Evidence that, in addition to effects of magnetic fields, electrical fields per se affect cell proliferation was reported by Noda and colleagues.[77] DNA synthesis was increased 20% in rat osteosarcoma cells exposed for 34 hours to 60-Hz electrical fields. The evidence indicated a current density "window." The results of this study are of interest because the electrical field effect depended on a number of variables. Thus the 60-Hz electrical field effect appears to depend on the mitotic status of the cell population during exposure. This finding is potentially significant because it suggests specific interaction of LF electromagnetic fields with the mammalian cell cycle.

Further evidence that electrical fields per se, of a different waveform than used by previous investigators,[60,77,88] affected cell proliferation was provided by Cleary and colleagues[33] who exposed normal chicken tendon explants in vitro to low-amplitude, unipolar, square wave pulsed electrical fields. A highly significant 32% increase in fibroblast proliferation occurred in tendon explants exposed for 96 hours to a time-averaged current density of 7 mA/m^2. Exposure to the same pulsed field at a time-averaged current density of 1.8 mA/m^2 did not affect fibroblast proliferation. Exposure to current densities of greater than 10 mA/m^2 suppressed both proliferation and collagen synthesis, without affecting noncollagen protein synthesis.

The effect of the 1-Hz pulsed electrical field on fibroblast proliferation also depended on orientation of the explant with respect to the electrical field. Fibroplasia was enhanced when the explant longitudinal axis was oriented parallel to applied E fields having current densities of 3.5 or 7 mA/m^2. For perpendicular orientation, there was no effect on proliferation. Fibroblast proliferation and collagen synthesis were inversely proportional to donor age for the 3- to 16-week-old chickens used in this study. There was no interaction, however, between donor age and the effect of ELF pulsed field exposure on these dependent variables. Subsequent studies revealed that the effect of pulsed electrical fields on proliferation of explants from chickens aged 8 to 16 weeks depended on extracellular Ca^{2+} and fetal calf serum (FCS) concentration. This was not true for explants from chickens less than 3 weeks of age.[29]

Low-intensity ELF electromagnetic fields appear to modulate proliferation of normal as well as transformed mammalian cells in vitro. Intensity (current density) windows result from exposure to magnetic as well as unipolar or bipolar (AC) electrical fields. The magnitude of the proliferative response depends on electromagnetic field intensity, exposure duration, and cellular and extracellular factors.

Cell surface effects. Phillips and colleagues[80] investigated the effect of 60-Hz electromagnetic fields on the expression of the transferrin receptor on human colon carcinoma cells in vitro. Cells were exposed for 24 hours to a 300 mA$_{rms}$/m^2 electrical field, a 1 G magnetic field, or combined E and H fields at these intensities. The rationale for this study was the association of the transferrin receptor with the receptor of natural killer cells (cytotoxic lymphocytes) and the fact that expression of this receptor is correlated with proliferation of normal and malignant cells. Phillips and colleagues[81] reported that exposure of colon cancer cells in vitro to 60-Hz electromagnetic fields significantly increased colony formation in soft agar and increased the expression of tumor-associated antigens.

Phillips and colleagues[81] reported a 24-fold increase in colony formation in colon cancer cells exposed to both E and H fields, a 14-fold increase in magnetic field exposed cells, and a 1.7-fold increase in cells exposed to the 60-Hz E field. The increased clonogenic capacity persisted for the 8-month study duration. The expression of transferrin receptors in cells exposed to the combined fields, or to the magnetic field alone, was maintained at maximal levels and was not under the normal cell density regulatory influence. The change in transferrin receptor expression was maintained in cells up to 8 months after electromagnetic exposure. Based on these data, Phillips and colleagues[81] suggested that electromagnetic exposure may affect normal cell proliferation control processes.

Luben and colleagues[64] exposed osteoblast-like mouse bone cells to either a continuous pulse train magnetic field having a pulse burst repetition rate of 72 Hz or recurrent bursts modulated at 15 Hz. These fields induced extracellular electrical field strengths of 0.1 V/m or less and current densities on the order of 10 mA/m^2 or less. Exposure to either electromagnetic signal for up to 90 hours significantly reduced the normal ability of bone cells to produce cyclic AMP in response to parathyroid hormone (PTH). There was no electromagnetic field effect on adenylate cyclase activity. Electromagnetic field exposure blocked the inhibitory effects of PTH on collagen synthesis. Inhibition of collagen synthesis by 1,25-dihydroxyvitamin D$_3$, however, was not affected. PTH acts at the site of the plasma membrane, in contrast to 1,25-dihydroxyvitamin D$_3$, which acts primarily in the cell nucleus. Luben and colleagues[64] concluded that their data supported the hypothesis that electromagnetic field effects are mediated primarily in the plasma membrane of osteoblasts, either by interfering with hormone-receptor interactions or by blocking receptor-cyclase coupling in the membrane. Support for hypothesized cell surface alterations induced by electromagnetic fields was provided by Marron and colleagues,[67] who reported that both 60-Hz electrical and magnetic fields altered the physical characteristics (surface charge, hydrophobicity) of the surface of the amoebae *Physarum*. The E and H fields acted independently and in different ways. A 60-Hz,

1 V/m electrical field exposure for 24 hours increased net negative surface charge, whereas magnetic field exposure at 1 G decreased surface hydrophobicity.

Cancer promotion (see Chapter 26). Membrane-mediated alterations, induced by 60-Hz electrical fields, have been implicated in cancer promotion. Byus and colleagues[23] reported altered activity of ornithine decarboxylase (ODC), an enzyme intimately involved in induction of proliferation of normal and tumor cells. A 1-hour exposure to a 60-Hz, 1 V/m electrical field induced a 500% increase in ODC activity in human lymphoma cells and a 200% to 300% increase in mouse myeloma cells in vitro. The magnitude and duration of ODC activation depended on cell type, E field strength, and exposure duration. For example, a 1-hour exposure of hepatoma cells to a 60-Hz field strength of 10 mV/m induced a 30% increase in ODC. Exposure for 2 hours at 1 V/m had no effect, whereas a 3-hour exposure decreased enzyme activity. Based on a comparison of the effect of electromagnetic fields and the tumor-promoting phorbol ester tetrodecanoyl phorbol acetate (TPA) on cellular ODC activity, Byus and colleagues[23] indicated that 60-Hz electromagnetic fields may function as a tumor-promoting stimulus. They noted, however, that there were significant differences in the magnitude of the effects of TPA and the electromagnetic fields used in their study on cellular ODC activity and that tumor promotion by TPA is highly dependent on the dosage time schedule. Thus direct comparisons of the tumor-promoting potential of electromagnetic fields and TPA were not possible.

Nordenson and colleagues[78] reported a significant increase in the frequency of chromosomal aberrations in human fetal cells exposed to low-intensity magnetic fields. Amniotic cells obtained by amniocentesis were exposed for 3 days to a 300-mG, 50-Hz sine wave magnetic field or to a 20-kHz, 160-mG sawtooth magnetic field. Magnetic field exposure increased the number of cells with chromosomal aberrations. In the case of 50-Hz magnetic field exposure, the increase was highly statistically significant ($P = 0.0007$), whereas the increase following sawtooth magnetic field exposure was marginally statistically significant ($P = 0.056$). It was concluded that the magnetic field effect was similar to the effect of the tumor-promoting agent TPA. As such, it may have involved an interaction of the ELF magnetic field with the cell membrane. The effect did not appear to be related to field-induced alterations in cell proliferation.[78] The results of this study thus further support the conclusion of Byus and colleagues[23] that ELF magnetic fields may act as a tumor promoter.

In addition to the possibility that ELF electromagnetic fields may act as a tumor promoter, there is in vitro evidence of an alternative but not mutually exclusive mechanism to relate electromagnetic exposure to cancer: effects on immune surveillance. Lyle and colleagues[65] detected a statistically significant 25% inhibition of allogeneic cytotoxicity of B lymphoma target cells by murine cytotoxic T

lymphocytes that were exposed for 48 hours to a 1 V/m$_{rms}$, 60-Hz sinusoidal electrical field. The magnitude of cytotoxic inhibition depended on E field strength. Exposure of T lymphocytes to 0.1 to 0.01 V/m resulted in 19% and 7% reductions in cytotoxicity. When the 4-hour cytotoxicity assay was conducted in the presence of a 1 V/m, 60-Hz E field, using previously unexposed T lymphocytes, there was a statistically nonsignificant 5% reduction in cytotoxicity. These results suggest that the electromagnetic field effect depended on exposure duration and field strength. Lyle and colleagues[65] indicated that the threshold for inhibition of cytotoxicity in clonal T lymphocytes by exposure in vitro to a 60-Hz sinusoidal electrical field is between 0.01 and 0.1 V/m.

Theoretical studies. Theories that fully explain ELF electromagnetic field effects have not been advanced. Failure to develop an adequate theoretical basis for low-intensity LF electromagnetic field effects may be due to the uniqueness of nonequilibrium living systems, which render them not directly amenable to descriptions based on classic physical or biochemical principles. The need to consider living systems from different perspectives was discussed by Fröhlich[50] and Kaiser.[55]

Weaver and Astumian[105] presented physiocochemical models to explain the coupling of weak periodic electrical fields to cells. They modeled effects of applied electrical fields on transmembrane potential under various assumptions, comparing the magnitude of induced alterations to thermally induced fluctuations. For large elongated cells with membranes having informational processing sensitivities limited to LF electromagnetic field bandwidths of 10 or 100 Hz, minimal detectable electrical fields (i.e., transmembrane-induced signals at least as great as thermal fluctuations) of 8×10^{-4} and 3×10^{-3} V/m were predicted. Phenomena such as cell membrane signal averaging and electroconformational coupling of applied electrical fields to membrane macromolecules, such as enzymes, were also considered with respect to cellular effects of ELF electromagnetic fields (see also Astumian and colleagues[6]). Weaver and Astumian[105] concluded that their estimates are consistent with experimental observations that low-intensity electromagnetic fields affect living systems via nonthermal interaction mechanisms.

Concluding remarks

In vitro studies provide direct evidence that ELF electromagnetic fields cause physiologically significant alterations in normal and transformed human and other mammalian cells. Experimental and theoretical evidence indicates that the outer surface of the cell membrane is the primary locus for electromagnetic field–induced cellular alterations.

The type and magnitude of electromagnetic field effects on cells in vitro are not inconsistent with reported effects on humans or experimental animals, principally effects on cancer incidence, behavior, and development. The limited extent of in vitro data, however, prevents the drawing of firm conclusions about the relevance to in vivo exposure effects. Although there are some uncertainties regarding electromagnetic exposure levels induced in in vitro as well as in vivo systems, it may be concluded that electromagnetic field-induced alterations in in vitro systems occur at approximately the same levels encountered in human exposures.

EFFECTS OF RADIOFREQUENCY AND MICROWAVE RADIATION ON LIVING SYSTEMS

RF and microwave radiation, although classified as NER, have physical characteristics, and hence interaction mechanisms, quite distinct from ELF electromagnetic fields, such as 60-Hz fields associated with electrical power transmission. The frequency of RF radiation extends from approximately 10 KHz (10^4 Hz) to 300 MHz (3×10^8 Hz). NER in the frequency range of 300 MHz to 300 GHz (3×10^{11} Hz) is referred to as microwave radiation. As indicated in Fig. 12-1, typical sources of RF radiation include AM, television, and FM broadcast signals, whereas the most common type of microwave radiation is generated by microwave ovens in the home that operate at a frequency of 2450 MHz. The contrast between ELF and RF/microwave NER is most apparent considering differences in wavelength. The wavelength of a 60-Hz electrical field is measured in thousands of miles compared with RF/microwave radiation having wavelengths of yards to fractions of an inch.

Based on the knowledge that the way energy is coupled from a NER source to a living system, such as the human body, relates to the NER wavelength and the size of the absorber, it would be logical to expect different biological effects of ELF versus RF/microwave radiation. Surprisingly, despite large differences in physical characteristics, there are some similarities in biological responses resulting from exposure to ELF fields and high-frequency NER. It is unlikely that there is a common mechanism for effects at such divergent frequencies, but in neither case are mechanisms well understood.

Possible association of radiofrequency and microwave exposure and cancer

In addition to the possible association of residential or occupational 60-Hz magnetic field exposure and human cancer incidence, an association has also emerged in the case of RF/microwave exposure. The use of hand-held cellular telephones that operate in the frequency range of 825 to 890 MHz has been linked with brain cancer. Exposure of police officers to microwave radiation in the frequency range of 10 to 24 GHz, used in traffic speed–detecting radar, has been associated with increases in testicular, brain, and eye cancer.

A common factor in exposure to hand-held cellular tele-

phone radiation and police radar is the localized nature of the radiation absorption. In both instances, tumors reportedly occurred at or near the apparent site of maximum microwave energy absorption. For example, parietal lobe brain tumors were reported to occur in the head region closest to the location of the hand-held cellular telephone antenna. Localized microwave exposure of testicular tissue of police officers reportedly resulted from the practice of resting the radar gun in the groin region while the unit was emitting radiation. In the case of hand-held cellular telephones or police radar, epidemiological studies have not been conducted to establish the validity of the reported effects on cancer incidence. Neither have studies been conducted of the effects of these microwave frequencies on experimental animals or mammalian cells in vitro. Therefore, in the absence of a relevant scientific database, the association of incidence and exposure to these microwave sources must be viewed in terms of effects reported from exposure to other RF or microwave frequencies. The results of epidemiological studies, studies that involved exposure of experimental animals as well as investigations of the effects of RF or microwave radiation on mammalian cells, provide evidence for a possible association of such exposure with cancer incidence.

Although the limited amount of relevant data precludes drawing conclusions, the results are consistent with the hypothesis that, under certain, presently not well-defined exposure conditions, RF or microwave radiation may act as a cancer promoter, rather than as a cancer initiator. This hypothesis is consistent with the hypothesis that exposure to another form of NER, low-intensity 60-Hz magnetic fields, may also have a tumor promotional effect.

Epidemiological studies

Until recently, there has been limited concern about the relationship of RF or microwave exposure and cancer incidence. It is thus not surprising that few epidemiological studies have been conducted to investigate this possibility. This is in contrast to the number of epidemiological studies of the relationship of residential or occupational exposure to 60-Hz magnetic fields and cancer discussed previously in this chapter.

Milham[73] analyzed death certificates of 1691 amateur radio operators from California and Washington and found 24 leukemia cases. Compared with an expected number of such cases of 12.6, this was a statistically significant excess number of leukemias among amateur radio operators. In a subsequent study, the standardized mortality ratio (SMR) for all causes of death was 71, and for combined cancers it was 89, indicating a better-than-average mortality history for amateur radio operatiors as expected from comparison of this group with professional and academic cohorts. There was a significantly elevated leukemia mortality, however, for the study group. Amateur radio operators had a SMR of 162 for cancers of lymphatic tissues, including multiple myelomas and non-Hodgkin lymphomas. The SMR of 176 for chronic myeloid leukemia was statistically significantly elevated whereas the elevated, SMR of 124 for all leukemias was not statistically significant. In addition to potential RF exposure from the operation of amateur radios, there was evidence of possible occupational RF exposure of some members of the study group from the state of Washington. Milham indicated that the elevated leukemia risk in the study group could have been related to other risk factors but that exposure to RF radiation should be considered as an etiological factor. The nature of the study was such that it was not possible to determine the extent of exposure to RF radiation.

Szmigielski and Gil[96] reviewed the association between NER exposure and cancer, including epidemiological as well as experimental studies. They observed an unexpectedly large number of cancer cases in military workers exposed to microwave radiation, including lymphomas, chronic myelocytic leukemia, acute myelocytic leukemia, and pancreatic cancer. In a retrospective epidemiological study of cancer morbidity in Polish military personnel, cancer morbidity in personnel occupationally exposed to RF/ microwave radiation was triple that of the control group.[98] Significant increases in incidence were found for lymphatic and hematopoietic malignancies and for stomach, colorectal, and skin neoplasms, including melanoma. The overall relative risk for lymphatic and hematopoietic malignancies in RF/microwave exposed workers was 6.7 ($P < 0.01$).

Evidence for an association of occupational NER exposure and brain cancer has also been reported. Lin and colleagues[61] conducted an epidemiological study of 951 cases of brain tumors among white male residents of Maryland during the period 1969 through 1982. They observed a statistically significant increase in glioma among electricians, electrical engineers, and high-voltage transmission linemen.

Epidemiological studies thus provide evidence of an association of long-term exposure to RF/microwave and lower frequency NER and cancer incidence. Although a variety of types of cancer have been reported to result from such exposure, leukemia and brain cancer appear to be the most prevalent malignancies.

Animal studies

The effects of RF and microwave radiation on psychophysiological responses in experimental animals have been reported.[26,45] Depending on species and exposure conditions, numerous physiological alterations are reported to be induced by RF or microwave exposure. The majority of these studies involved acute or relatively short-term exposure to RF field intensities that induced varying degrees of temperature elevations in the entire body, localized regions of the body, or both. Although there were indications that certain physiological alterations, such as changes in behavior, might occur in the absence of tissue heating, it was gen-

erally assumed that such effects were of little significance with respect to assessments of potential effects of RF or microwave exposure on human health. The results of more recent studies involving long-term low-intensity exposure, studies of the relationship of microwave exposure to cancer promotion, and in vitro cell studies have drawn attention to the need to reconsider health effects issues.

The potential tumor-promoting effect of microwave exposure has been investigated.[97-99] Microwave exposure of mice accelerated the growth of skin neoplasms induced by benzopyrene, suggesting a tumor-promoting effect.[97] Microwave exposure decreased the natural antineoplastic resistance of mice to implanted tumor cells. Microwave exposure also accelerated the growth of tumors induced by the carcinogens di-ethyl-nitrosoamine and methylchlorantrene.

Additional evidence of a possible association of long-term low-intensity microwave exposure and cancer in experimental animals was reported by Chou and colleagues[24] Significant alterations were reported in a number of physiological parameters. Potentially of most relevance was the finding of 18 primary malignancies in microwave-exposed rats compared with 5 such lesions in the sham-exposed animals ($P = 0.006$). There was also a statistically significant decrease in time of occurrence of tumors in exposed animals.[24]

These results support the hypothesis that long-term low-intensity microwave exposure is associated with increased incidence or growth rate of cancer in experimental animals. Although the significance of these data with respect to human cancer is uncertain, the microwave intensities used in these animal studies are in the range considered by certain regulatory and advisory bodies as safe for humans. Whole-body RF or microwave absorption rates used by Chou and colleagues[24] are assumed to be well below the level that causes tissue heating.

Cellular studies

A major impediment to assessing the effects of RF or microwave radiation on organisms is the fact that energy absorption is highly nonuniform and dependent on the wavelength of the radiation and the size and orientation of the body. Consequently, it is difficult to apply the results of studies using experimental animals directly to predict effects of RF or microwave exposure on humans. In addition to uncertain dosimetry, additional uncertainty results from interspecies physiological differences and the complex interactive nature of various organ systems. To overcome such difficulties, studies have been conducted on mammalian cells in vitro.

As with ELF NER, the effects of RF and microwave radiation on a wide variety of cellular endpoints have been investigated. Such effects include (1) membrane cation transport and binding, (2) membrane structure, (3) single ion channel kinetics, (4) neuronal activity, (5) energy metabolism, (6) proliferation and activation, and (7) transformation.[25-27,45] Because of their possible relevance to cancer, effects of RF and microwave radiation on cell proliferation and transformation are reviewed here.

To test the hypothesis that microwave radiation may interact synergistically with tumor promoters, mouse embryonic fibroblasts were exposed to low-intensity, 2450-MHz microwave radiation either in the presence or absence of the tumor promoter 12-O-tetradecanoylphorbol-13-acetate (TPA).[8] Cells were exposed to microwave radiation pulse modulated at 120 Hz for 24 hours. In the absence of TPA microwave radiation exposure had no effect on fibroblast cell survival or induction of neoplastic transformation. Neoplastic transformation was significantly enhanced, however, in cells treated with TPA. A synergistic TPA–microwave radiation dose response was detected for the frequency of neoplastic transformation in the SAR range of 0.1 to 4.4 W/kg. The neoplastic transformation frequency resulting from exposure at 4.4 W/kg, in the presence of TPA, was comparable to that induced by exposure to 1.5 Gy (1 gray (Gy) = 100 rad) of x-radiation. The authors noted that this dose of whole body x-radiation is known to result in an approximately 6% risk of tumor induction. Comparison of the effects of x-radiation exposure, with or without 4.4-W/kg, 2450-MHz microwave exposure, in the presence of TPA, indicated that the combined treatment induced two independent types of transformation damage, one due to microwave exposure and another to x-rays, both promoted by TPA.[8] This suggests separate sites of interaction for nonionizing microwave radiation versus ionizing x-radiation. Because genomic interactions of x-radiation are associated with neoplastic transformation, these data suggest the possibility of a nongenomic effect of microwave radiation leading to TPA-promoted neoplastic transformation. Biophysical considerations as well as results of studies of microwave radiation effects on other cell physiological endpoints suggests the cell plasma membrane as a likely site of interaction leading to neoplastic transformation.

In addition to evidence provided by Balcer-Kubiczek and Harrison[8] that low-intensity microwave radiation may affect neoplastic transformation of mammalian cells, in vitro studies have also revealed that such NER may alter the rate of proliferation of cells that are already transformed or malignant. Cleary and colleagues[28,30,31] exposed human or rat glioma cells for 2 hours to 27 or 2450 MHz continuous wave (CW) or pulse modulated RF radiation under isothermal (37° C ± 0.2° C) conditions. Cell proliferation was increased in a dose-rate dependent manner following exposures to either type of radiation at SARs of 0.5 to 25 W/kg. Maximum increased proliferation of 160% occurred following exposure to 25 W/kg, 27 or 2450 MHz, 5 or 3 days after exposure. The effect on glioma proliferation was biphasic in that exposures at SARs of greater than 25 W/kg decreased the rate of cell proliferation. Statistically significant time-dependent effects were detected for up to 5 days

after exposure, which suggested a kinetic cellular response to NER at these frequencies. The persistence of the RF or microwave radiation effect suggested the possibility of a cumulative effect on cell proliferation.

Evidence that NER RF or microwave radiation may have a more general effect on cell proliferation was reported by Cleary and colleagues[28,30,32] Using the same experimental procedures used to study effects on glioma, human peripheral lymphocytes were exposed isothermally (37° C ± 0.2° C) for 2 hours to 27- or 2450-MHz radiation. Exposure to CW NER at these frequencies had similar biphasic effects on the rate of proliferation of mitogen (phytohemagglutinin) stimulated lymphocytes. The maximum increase in proliferation, which occurred 3 days after exposure, was 40%, approximately one fourth the magnitude of the proliferative effect of NER RF radiation on glioma.[31] Cumulative effects were investigated by exposing lymphocyte cultures at the same SAR to two 1-hour irradiations spaced 24 hours apart. Such split-dose exposures caused similar effects but of reduced magnitude, indicating time-dependent reversal of the exposure effect on lymphocyte proliferation with a time constant of somewhat more than 24 hours.[28] Pulse modulation of 27- or 2450-MHz radiation caused generally similar effects on cell proliferation, at SARs of 5 W/kg or less, but there were differences in the dose responses. At higher SARs, pulse modulation resulted in significantly increased lymphocyte proliferation compared with CW exposures at the same SARs.[28] The effects of 27- or 2450-MHz RF radiation on glioma or lymphocyte proliferation were attributed to a nonthermal, direct RF-induced alteration of the cell cycle.[31]

In vitro studies of the effects of low-intensity RF and microwave radiation indicate dose-rate dependent increases in neoplastic transformation frequency and proliferation. In view of inherent limitations on the extrapolation of in vitro results to in vivo responses, these results cannot be related to cancer incidence in humans exposed to such radiation. These results, however, are not inconsistent with the hypothesis that human exposure to RF or microwave radiation, under presently not well defined conditions, may increase cancer incidence.

CONCLUDING REMARKS

There is increasing evidence of disease resulting from environmental exposures to NER in the home and in the workplace. Epidemiological evidence indicates possible associations of long-term NER exposure to cancer, adverse reproductive outcomes, and behavioral and neurological changes. Limitations on exposure assessment, common to epidemiological studies, provide imprecise knowledge regarding time or exposure intensity thresholds for these effects, thus making risk assessment difficult, if at all possible.

Although the results of animal experimentation and cellular studies of NER effects generally corroborate the results of epidemiological studies of the effects of NER, they provide insufficient data for meaningful risk assessment at this time.

Perhaps the most significant impediment to progress toward understanding the effects of NER on living systems has been the lack of adequate knowledge of interaction mechanisms. One consequence of this is that research in this area has been greeted with skepticism. Reviewing the diverse nature of the physical properties of the NER as well as the variety of effects induced in living systems, the large gaps in our understanding are not surprising. The potential magnitude of NER-related disease in industrial societies suggests that these gaps must be filled to provide essential perspective regarding these issues.

REFERENCES

1. Adey WR: Tissue interaction with nonionizing electromagnetic fields, *Physiol Rev* 61:435, 1981.
2. Adey WR: Physiological signalling across cell membranes and co-operative influence of extremely low frequency electromagnetic fields. In Frohlich H, editor: *Biological coherence and response to external stimuli,* Heidelberg, 1988, Springer-Verlag.
3. Adey WR: Biological effects of radio frequency electromagnetic radiation. In Lin JC, editor: *Interaction of electromagnetic waves with biological systems,* New York, 1988, Plenum Press.
4. Adey WR, Bawin SM, Lawrence AF: Effects of weak amplitude modulated microwave fields on calcium efflux from awake cat cerebral cortex, *Bioelectromagnetics* 3:295, 1982.
5. Anderson LE: Biological effects of extremely low-frequency and 60 Hz fields. In Gandhi OP, editor: *Biological effects and medical applications of electromagnetic energy,* Englewood Cliffs, NJ, 1990, Prentice Hall.
6. Astumian RD, Robertson B, Tsong TY: Charge-field interactions in cell membranes and electroconformational coupling: theory for the interactions between dynamic electric fields and membrane enzymes. In Allen MJ, Cleary SF, Hawkridge FM, editors: *Charge and field effects in biosystems,* vol 2, New York, 1989, Plenum Press.
7. Bailar JC: Death from all cancers: trends in sixteen countries. In Davis DE, Hoel D, editors: *Trends in cancer mortality in industrial countries,* vol 609, New York, 1990, New York Academy of Science.
8. Balcer-Kubiczek EK, Harrison GH: Neoplastic transformation of C3H/10T½ cells following exposure to 120-Hz modulated 2.45-GHz microwaves and phorbol ester tumor promoter, *Radiat Res* 126:65, 1991.
9. Bassett CAL, Mitchell SN, Gaston SR: Treatment of ununited tibial diaphyseal fractures with pulsed electromagnetic fields, *J Bone Joint Surg [Am]* 63A:511, 1981.
10. Bassett CAL, Mitchell SN, Gaston SR: Pulsing electromagnetic field treatment in ununited fractures and failed arthrodeses, *JAMA* 247:623, 1982.
11. Bawin SM, Adey WR: Sensitivity of calcium binding in cerebral tissues to weak environmental electric fields oscillating at low frequency, *Proc Natl Acad Sci* 73:1999, 1976.
12. Bawin SM, Kaczmarek LK, Adey WR: Effects of modulated VHF fields on the central nervous system, *Ann NY Acad Sci* 247:74, 1975.
13. Benz RD et al: Mutagenicity and toxicity of 60-Hz magnetic and electric fields. In *Final report to the New York State Power Lines Project,* Albany, NY, 1987, Wadsworth Laboratories.
14. Binder A et al: Pulsed electromagnetic field therapy of persistent rotator cuff tendinitis, *Lancet* 1:8379:695, 1984.
15. Binderman I et al: Stimulation of skeletal-derived cell cultures by different electric field intensities is cell-specific, *Biochim Biophys Acta* 844:273, 1985.
16. Blackman CF et al: Induction of calcium ion efflux from brain tissue by radiofrequency radiation: effects of modulation frequency and field strength, *Radio Sci* 14(GS):93, 1979.
17. Blackman CF et al: Induction of calcium-ion efflux from brain tissue by radiofrequency radiation: effect of sample number and modulation frequency on the power-density window, *Bioelectromagnetics* 1:35, 1980.
18. Blackman CF et al: Calcium-ion efflux from brain tissue: power-density vs internal field-intensity dependence of 50-MHz RF radiation, *Bioelectromagnetics* 1:277, 1980.
19. Blackman CF et al: Effects of ELF (1-120 Hz) and modulated (50 Hz) RF fields on the efflux of calcium ions from brain tissue in vitro, *Bioelectromagnetics* 6:1, 1985.
20. Blackman CF et al: A role for the magnetic field in the radiation-induced efflux of calcium ions from brain tissue in vitro, *Bioelectromagnetics* 6:327, 1985.
21. Blackman CF et al: Multiple power-density windows and their possible origin, *Bioelectromagnetics* 10:115, 1989.
22. Blackman CF et al: Importance of alignment between local DC magnetic field and an oscillating magnetic field in responses of brain tissue in vitro and in vivo, *Bioelectromagnetics* 11:159, 1990.
23. Byus CV, Pieper SA, Adey WR: The effects of low-energy 60-Hz environmental electromagnetic fields upon the growth-related enzyme ornithine decarboxylase, *Carcinogenesis* 8:1385, 1987.
24. Chou CK et al: Long-term, low-level microwave irradiation of rats, *Bioelectromagnetics* 13:469, 1992.
25. Cleary SF: Cellular effects of electromagnetic radiation, *IEEE Eng Med Biol* 3-06:26, 1987.
26. Cleary SF: Cellular effects of radiofrequency electromagnetic radiation. In Gandhi OP, editor, *Biological effects and medical applications of electromagnetic fields,* Englewood Cliffs, NJ, 1990, Prentice Hall.
27. Cleary SF: Biophysical mechanisms of interaction. In Stone WR, editor: *URSI Rev Radio Sci* 1990-1992, New York, 1993, Oxford University Press.
28. Cleary SF, Liu LM, Cao G: Functional alteration of mammalian cells by direct high frequency electromagnetic field interactions. In Allen MJ, Cleary SF, Hawkridge FM, editors: *Charge and field effects in biosystems,* vol 2, New York, 1989, Plenum Press.
29. Cleary SF, Liu LM, Cao G: Cellular effects of extremely low frequency electromagnetic fields. In Allen MJ et al, editors: *Charge and field effects in biosystems,* vol 3, Boston, 1992, Birkhauser.
30. Cleary SF, Liu LM, Cao G: Effects of RF power absorption in mammalian cells, *Ann NY Acad Sci* 649:166, 1992.
31. Cleary SF, Liu LM, Merchant R: Glioma proliferation modulated in vitro by isothermal radiofrequency radiation exposure, *Radiat Res* 121:38, 1990.
32. Cleary SF, Liu LM, Merchant R: In vitro lymphocyte proliferation induced by radiofrequency electromagnetic radiation under isothermal conditions, *Bioelectromagnetics* 11:47, 1990.
33. Cleary SF et al: Modulation of tendon fibroplasia by exogenous electric currents, *Bioelectromagnetics* 9:183, 1988.
34. Cohen MM et al: Effects of low-level, 60-Hz electromagnetic fields on human lymphoid cells. I. Mitotic rate and chromosomal breakage in human peripheral lymphocytes, *Bioelectromagnetics* 7:415, 1986.
35. Cuzick J: International time trends for multiple myeloma. In Davis DE, Hoel D, editors: *Trends in cancer mortality in industrial countries,* vol 609, New York, 1990, New York Academy of Science.
36. Davanipour Z: Electromagnetic field exposure and amyotrophic lateral sclerosis (ALS), *Neuroepidemiology* 10:308, 1991.
37. Davis D: Discussion comments. In Davis, DE, Hoel, D, editors:

Trends in cancer mortality in industrial countries, vol 609, New York, 1990, New York Academy of Science.

38. Davis DL et al: Is brain cancer mortality increasing in industrial countries? In Davis, DE, Hoel, D, editors: *Trends in cancer mortality in industrial countries,* vol 609, New York, 1990, New York Academy of Science.

39. Demers PA et al: Occupational exposure to electromagnetic radiation and breast cancer in males, *Am J Epidemiol* 132:775, 1990 (abstract).

40. Delgardo JMR et al: Embryological changes induced by weak, extremely low frequency electromagnetic fields, *J Anat* 134:533, 1982.

41. Doll R: Are we winning the fight against cancer? An epidemiological assessment, *Eur J Cancer* 26:500, 1990.

42. Duffy PM, Edhret CF: Effects of intermittent 60-Hz electric field exposure: circadian phase shifts, splitting, torpor, and arousal responses in mice. In *Abstracts, 4th Annual Scientific Session,* Gaithersburg, MD, 1982, Bioelectromagnetics Society.

43. Dutta SK, Ghosh B, Blackman CF: Radiofrequency radiation-induced calcium-ion-efflux enhancement from human and other neuroblastoma cells in culture, *Bioelectromagnetics* 10:197, 1989.

44. Dutta SK et al: Microwave radiation-induced calcium ion efflux from human neuroblastoma cells in culture, *Bioelectromagnetics* 5:71, 1984.

45. Elder JA, Cahill DF, editors: *Biological effects of radiofrequency radiation,* Research Triangle Park, NC, Health Effects Research Laboratory, Office of Research and Development, US Environmental Protection Agency, EPA-600/8-83-026F, 1984.

46. Farndale RW, Murray JC: Pulsed electromagnetic fields promote collagen production in bone marrow fibroblasts via athermal mechanisms, *Calcif Tissue Int* 37:178, 1985.

47. Feychting M, Ahlbom A: *Magnetic fields and cancer in people residing near Swedish high voltage power lines,* Report prepared for the Swedish National Board for Industrial and Technical Development, Stockholm, Sweden, 1992, Karolinska Institute.

48. Fitton-Jackson S, Basset CAL: The response of skeletal tissue to pulsed electromagnetic fields. In Richard RJ, Rajan KT, editors: *Tissue culture in medical research,* New York, 1980, Pergamon Press.

49. Floderus B et al: *Occupational exposure to electromagnetic fields in relation to leukemia and brain tumors. A case-control study,* Solna, Sweden, 1992, National Institute of Occupational Health.

50. Fröhlich H: General theory of coherent excitations on biological systems. In Adey WR, Lawrence AF, editors: *Nonlinear electromagnetics in biological systems,* New York, 1984, Viking Penguin.

51. Fulton JP et al: Electrical wiring configurations and childhood leukemia in Rhode Island, *Am J Epidemiol* 111:292, 1980.

52. Gavalas-Medici R, Day-Magdaleno SR: Extremely low frequency, weak electric fields affect schedule-controlled behavior of monkeys, *Nature* 261:256, 1976.

53. Goodman R, Abbott J, Henderson AS: Transcriptional patterns in the X chromosome of *Sciara coprophila* following exposure to magnetic fields, *Bioelectromagnetics* 8:1, 1987.

54. Goodman R et al: Exposure of human cells to low-frequency electromagnetic fields results in quantitative changes in transcripts, *Biochim Biophys Acta* 1009:216, 1989.

55. Kaiser F: Coherence-synchronization-chaos: cooperative processes in excited biological systems. In Chiabrera A, Nicolini C, Schwan HP, editors: *Interaction between electromagnetic fields and cells,* NATO ASI Series A97, New York, 1985, Plenum Press.

56. Kamrin BB: Induced collagenolytic activity by electrical stimulation of embryonic fibroblasts in tissue culture, *J Dent Res* 53:1475, 1974.

57. Kohlmeier L, Rehm J, Hoffmeister H: Lifestyle and trends in worldwide breast cancer rates. In Davis DE, Hoel D, editors: *Trends in cancer mortality in industrial countries,* vol 609, New York, 1990, New York Academy of Science.

58. Lee RF et al: A comparison of in vitro cellular responses to mechanical and electrical stimulation, *Am Surg* 48:567, 1982.

59. Liboff AR: Cyclotron resonance in membrane transport. In Chiabrera A, Nicolini C, Schwan HP, editors: *Interaction between electromagnetic fields and cells,* London, 1985, Plenum Press.

60. Liboff AR et al: Time-varying magnetic fields: effects on DNA synthesis, *Science* 223:818, 1984.

61. Lin RS et al: Occupational exposure to electromagnetic fields and brain tumors: an observed association, *J Occup Med* 27:413, 1985.

62. Livingston GK et al: *Reproductive integrity of mammalian cells exposed to 60-Hz electromagnetic fields.* Albany, NY, 1986, Wadsworth Laboratories.

63. London SJ et al: Exposure to residential electric and magnetic fields and risk of childhood leukemia, *Am J Epidemiol* 134:923, 1991.

64. Luben RA et al: Effects of electromagnetic stimuli in bone and bone cells in vitro: inhibition of responses to parathyroid hormone by low-energy, low-frequency fields, *Proc Natl Acad Sci* 79:4180, 1982.

65. Lyle DB et al: Suppression of T-lymphocyte cytotoxicity following exposure to 60-Hz sinusoidal electric fields, *Bioelectromagnetics* 9:303, 1988.

66. Lymangrover JR et al: Direct power frequency electric field effects on mammalian endocrine tissue, *Environ Res* 43:157-167, 1987.

67. Marron MT et al: Low frequency electric and magnetic fields have different effects on the cell surface, *FEBS Lett* 230:13, 1988.

68. Martin C et al, editors: *Electromagnetic fields and circadian rhythmicity,* Boston, MA, 1992, Birkhauser.

69. Matanowski GM, Breysse PN, Elliott EA: Electromagnetic field exposure and male breast cancer, *Lancet* 1:737, 1991 (letter).

70. McLeod BR, Liboff AR: Dynamical characteristics of membrane ions in multi-field configurations at low frequencies, *Bioelectromagnetics* 7:177, 1986.

71. McLeod KJ, Lee RC, Ehrlich HP: Frequency dependence of electric field modulation of fibroblast protein synthesis, *Science* 236:1465, 1987.

72. Slesin L: Swedish officials acknowledge EMF-cancer connection, *Microwave News* 12:1, 1992.

73. Milham S: Silent keys: leukemia mortality in amateur radio operators, *Lancet* 1:812, 1985.

74. Milham S: Increased mortality in amateur radio operators due to lymphatic and hematopoietic malignancies, *Am J Epidemiol* 127:50, 1988.

75. Murray JC, Farndale RW: Modulation of collagen production in cultured fibroblasts by a low-frequency, pulsed magnetic field, *Biochim Biophys Acta* 38:98, 1985.

76. Nair I, Morgan MG, Florig HK: *Biological effects of power frequency electric and magnetic fields—background paper,* OTA-BP-E-53, Washington, DC, 1989, US Government Printing Office.

77. Noda N et al: Effect of electric currents on DNA synthesis in rat osteosarcoma cells: dependence on conditions that influence cell growth, *J Orthop Res* 3:253, 1987.

78. Nordenson I et al: Effect of low-frequency magnetic fields on the chromosomal level in human amniotic cells. In Norden B, Ramel C, editors: *Interaction mechanisms of low-level electromagnetic fields in living systems,* Oxford, NY, 1992, Oxford University Press.

79. Office of Censuses and Population Surveys: *Cancer statistics registrations, 1985,* Series MBI, No. 18, 1990.

80. Phillips JL, Rutledge L, Winters WD: Transferrin binding to two human colon carcinoma cell lines: characterization and effect of 60-Hz electromagnetic fields, *Cancer Res* 46:239, 1986.

81. Phillips JL, Winters W, Rutledge L: In vitro exposure to electromagnetic fields: changes in tumour cell properties, *Int J Radiat Biol* 49:436, 1986.

82. Reese JA, Jostes RF, Frazier ME: Exposure of mammalian cells to 60-Hz magnetic or electric fields: analysis for DNA single-strand breaks, *Bioelectromagnetics* 9:237, 1988.

83. Reiter RJ: Effects of light on pineal function. In Wilson BW, Stevens

RG, Anderson LE, editors: *Extremely low frequency electromagnetic fields: the question of cancer,* Columbus, OH, 1990, Batelle Press.

84. Reiter RJ et al: Reduction of the nocturnal rise in pineal melatonin levels in rats exposed to 60-Hz electric fields in utero and for 23 days after birth, *Life Sci* 42:2203, 1988.

85. Robinson KR: The response of cells to electrical fields: a review, *J Cell Biol,* 101:2023, 1985.

86. Rodan GA, Bourrett LA, Norton LA: DNA-synthesis in cartilage cells is stimulated by oscillating electric fields, *Science* 199:690, 1978.

87. Rosenburg RS et al: Relationship between field strength and arousal response in mice exposed to 60-Hz electric fields, *Bioelectromagnetics* 4:181, 1983.

88. Ross SM: Combined DC and ELF magnetic fields can alter cell proliferation, *Bioelectromagnetics* 11:27, 1990.

89. Savitz DA, Calle EE: Leukemia and occupational exposure to electromagnetic fields: review of epidemiological surveys, *J Occup Med* 29:47, 1987.

90. Savitz DA et al: Case-control study of childhood cancer and exposure to 60-Hz magnetic fields, *Am J Epidemiol* 128:21, 1988.

91. Sheppard AR, Bawin SM, Adey WR: Models of long-range order in cerebral macromolecules: effects of sub-ELF and of modulated VHF and UHF fields, *Radio Sci* 14(6S):141, 1979.

92. Smith SD, McLeod BR, Liboff AR: Calcium cyclotron resonance and diatom mobility, *Bioelectromagnetics* 8:215, 1987.

93. Speers MA, Dobbins JG, Miller VS: Occupational exposures and brain cancer mortality: a preliminary study of East Texas residents, *Am J Ind Med* 13:629, 1988.

94. Stevens RG: Electric power use and breast cancer: a hypothesis, *Am J Epidemiol* 125:556, 1987.

95. Stuchly MA et al: Modification of tumor promotion in the mouse by exposure to an alternating magnetic field, *Cancer Lett* 65:1, 1992.

96. Szmigielski S, Gil J: Electromagnetic fields and neoplasms. In Franceschetti G, Gandhi OP, Grandolfo M, editors: *Electromagnetic biointeraction,* New York, 1989, Plenum Press.

97. Szmigielski S et al: Accelerated development of spontaneous and benzopyrene-induced skin cancer in mice exposed to 2450 MHz microwave radiation, *Bioelectromagnetics* 3:179, 1982.

98. Szmigielski S et al: Immunological and cancer-related aspects of exposure to low-level microwave and radiofrequency fields. In Marino A, editor: *Modern bioelectricity,* New York, 1988, Marcel Dekker.

99. Szudzinski A et al: Acceleration of the development of benzopyrene-induced skin cancer in mice by microwave radiation, *Arch Dermatol Res* 274:303, 1982.

100. Tamarkin L, et al: Melatonin inhibition and pinealectomy enhancement of 7,12-dimethylbenz (a) anthracene-induced mammary tumors in the rat, *Cancer Res* 41:4432, 1981.

101. Thomas JR, Schrot J, Liboff AR: Low-intensity magnetic fields alter operant behavior in rats, *Bioelectromagnetics* 7:349, 1986.

102. Tynes T, Andersen A: Electromagnetic fields and male breast cancer, *Lancet* 2:1596, 1990 (letter).

103. *US National Cancer Institute Cancer Statistics Review, 1973-1987,* Bethesda, MD, 1990, National Institutes of Health.

104. Wahlstrom O: Stimulation of fracture healing with electromagnetic fields of extremely low frequency (EMF of ELF), *Clin Orthop* 186:293, 1984.

105. Weaver JC, Astumian RD: The response of living cells to very weak electric fields: the thermal noise limit, *Science* 247:459, 1990.

106. Wertheimer N, Leeper E: Electrical wiring configuration and childhood cancer, *Am J Epidemiol* 109:273, 1979.

107. Wertheimer N, Leeper E: Electrical wiring configurations and childhood cancer: the authors reply, *Am J Epidemiol* 112:167, 1980.

108. Wertheimer N, Leeper E: Fetal loss associated with two seasonal sources of electromagnetic field exposure, *Am J Epidemiol* 129:220, 1989.

109. Werther R: ELF-effects on human circadian rhythms. In Persinger M, editor: *ELF and VLF electromagnetic field effects,* New York, 1974, Plenum Press.

110. Wilson BW, Chess EK, Anderson LE: 60-Hz electric field effects on pineal melatonin rhythms: time course for onset and recovery. *Bioelectromagnetics* 7:239, 1986.

111. Wilson BW et al: Chronic exposure to 60-Hz electric fields: effects on pineal function in the rat. *Bioelectromagnetics* 2:371, 1981.

112. Wilson BW et al: Chronic exposure to 60-Hz electric fields: effects on pineal function in the rat. *Bioelectromagnetics* 4:293, 1983 (erratum).

113. Winters WD: *Biological functions of immunologically reactive human and canine cells influenced by in vitro exposure to 60-Hz electric and magnetic fields.* Albany, NY, 1986, Wadsworth Laboratories.

Chapter 13

TOBACCO ABUSE

Carl G. Becker

The purpose of this chapter is to review the impact of tobacco consumption on health. As both the cost of health care and our need to have a healthy, productive, and competitive work force continue to rise, there is an increasing recognition that prevention of disease will accomplish more than advanced technological interventions. The effects of cigarette smoking are catastrophic at all stages of life. Cigarette smoking synergizes with other constitutional and environmental factors in the causation of disease, including a variety of cancers, cardiovascular and cerebrovascular disease, pulmonary disease, neonatal and perinatal disease, and accidents. It is the single most preventable cause of disease in our society. In the United States, tobacco is the most harmful product legally for sale when used as it is intended. How we deal with the use of tobacco is a measure of our commitment and resolve to address other societal ills related to addiction because the health consequences of smok-

ing are ultimately related to the potency of nicotine as an addicting substance. This chapter addresses the epidemiological association of tobacco usage with various diseases and the pathogenic mechanisms that may underlie these associations.

PUBLIC HEALTH IMPORTANCE

The use of tobacco products, principally by smoking cigarettes, is the single most avoidable cause of illness and premature death. It contributes to approximately 435,000 deaths annually in the United States (see box on next page).

It is estimated that smoking contributed to slightly more than 157,000 of the 514,000 cancer deaths occurring in the United States in 1991, accounting for 21.5% of all cancer deaths in women and 45% of all cancer deaths in men. In the same study, it was estimated that lung cancer has displaced coronary heart disease as the single leading cause of excess mortality among smokers in the United States.[184]

It is estimated that cigarette smoking contributes to 2.1 million deaths per year in developed countries. It is conservatively estimated that 21 million people will die of cigarette-related causes in developed countries in the decade 1990-1999 (United States, 5 to 6 million; European Community, 5 to 6 million; the former Soviet Union, 5 million; Eastern and other Europe, 3 million; and Australia, Canada, Japan and New Zealand, taken together, 2 million). More than half of these deaths will be between the ages of 35 and 69, or 30% of deaths in that age group. Those killed by tobacco between these ages lose on average about 23 years of life.[165] The deaths per year caused by tobacco in the United States exceed by fourfold deaths caused by alcoholic beverages and also greatly exceed combined deaths caused by automobile accidents, hard drugs, suicide, homicide, airplane crashes, and acquired immunodeficiency syndrome (AIDS).[40] It has been estimated that during the lifetime of

Deaths attributable to cigarette smoking per year for various diseases in the United States

Lung cancer	112,000
Other cancers	30,800
Cardiovascular disease	108,200
Stroke	26,300
Chronic lung disease	62,800
Other diagnoses	94,100

From U.S. Department of Health and Human Services, Public Health Service, Centers for Disease Control, Center for Chronic Disease Prevention and Health Promotion, Office of Smoking and Health: *Reducing the health consequences of smoking: 25 years of progress.* A report of the Surgeon General, DHHS Publication No. (CDC) 89-8411, 1989.

100 young adults who smoke cigarettes regularly, 1 will be murdered, 2 will be killed in traffic accidents, and 25 will die from tobacco-related diseases.[164] Because of decreasing sales of tobacco products in the United States, U.S. tobacco manufacturers have greatly increased export to underdeveloped countries. This trend has been associated with greatly increased cigarette consumption and a significant increase in tobacco-associated diseases in these countries. The incidence of these diseases may actually prove to be higher among smokers in these countries because of the prevalence of other environmental risk factors that may act synergistically with tobacco in inducing disease.[8,55,188]

Although tobacco has been used in the United States for centuries, the epidemic of cigarette smoking began to accelerate around 1918, stimulated by intense advertising campaigns of tobacco companies that still continue. Consumption peaked in 1963 when adult, per capita consumption reached 6300 cigarettes per year. Surveys in 1965 and 1966 indicated that 41% of the adult population smoked. Since the Report of the Surgeon General in 1964 focusing on the hazards of smoking to health, there has been a constant decline in overall prevalence of smoking of about 0.5%/yr to 29.1%/yr in 1987. Among women, however, smoking has only declined at the rate of 0.21%/yr compared with 0.84%/yr for men, so that by the year 2000, women will smoke more than men.[72] Rates of smoking initiation have also declined, 1.19%/yr among men and 0.28%/yr among women. The number quitting smoking has been equal between sexes. Blacks smoke more than whites, 34% versus 28.8% in 1987, but the rate of decline has been the same in both races. Of black smokers, however, 10% smoke more than 20 cigarettes/day, whereas 21% of white smokers smoke more than 20 cigarettes/day. Despite considerable progress in smoking cessation, the percentage of smokers who report smoking more than 20 cigarettes/day was 27.1% in 1985 and had not changed since 1974, indicative of the strongly addictive nature of smoking for some individuals. Overall, in 1993, 25% of American males smoked.

The largest differences in smoking rates are related to level of education. By the year 2000, it is estimated that 5% of college graduates, 16% of those with some college education, 30% of high school graduates, and 31% of high school dropouts will smoke.[194] Because those in lower educational and socioeconomic classes are likely to be exposed to greater quantities of other toxic substances in the environment either identical to those in cigarettes or capable of synergizing with them in the induction of various diseases, the impact of smoking on health in these groups will be especially severe and will greatly affect the costs of publicly financed medical care.

The costs of tobacco-related illnesses, largely due to smoking, to health care are estimated in 1985 dollars to be between 12 and 35 billion (mean 22 billion). Costs of lost productivity owing to smoking-related illnesses were estimated to be between 27 and 61 billion (mean 43 billion). Adding the mean values, the costs of health care and lost productivity were 65 billion, or 2.22 dollars per pack of cigarettes.[90]

THE TOBACCO PLANT

Tobacco belongs to the genus *Nicotiana,* which is in the family Solanaceae. This family includes the deadly nightshade as well as such commonly eaten vegetables as tomato, eggplant, and peppers, with which it shares antigenic and other chemical constituents.[12] The genus *Nicotiana* includes more than 60 different species. It is named for Jean Nicot, the French diplomat who sent tobacco seeds from Portugal to the Court of France at the end of the 16th century. *N. tabacum* and *N. rusticum* are the two species cultivated for tobacco products. *N. tabacum* is an extremely adaptive species that can be grown profitably under a wide variety of water, soil, and light conditions. A great deal of effort, much of it by the Department of Agriculture as well as industry, has been put into developing disease-resistant strains. Because the capacity of plants to resist viral, bacterial, fungal, and insect damage under varying soil and climatic conditions often depends on the ability of plants to generate defensive, often toxic chemicals, it is likely that the selection of resistant strains has also resulted in enhancement of the ability of tobacco to induce disease in the user. Tobacco is harvested as mature green leaves and cured in four ways. Virginia bright tobacco is flue or heat cured, Burley and Maryland tobaccos are air cured, and some oriental tobaccos are sun or fire cured. In the last-mentioned process, leaves are exposed to wood smoke.[206,209] With respect to the economies and ecologies of some Third World countries, it is estimated that the firewood used to cure tobacco results in the deforestation of an estimated 7 million acres/yr.[188]

CIGARETTE CONSTRUCTION

Most American and European cigarettes are made from blends of tobacco differing genetically and in the curing process. Before fine cutting, cigarette tobacco is also sprayed with a mixture of humectants, sugars, and other flavorings. The flavoring contents are held as proprietary information, and how or whether they contribute to health risk is not known. The economic advantage of using all of the tobacco purchased led to the development of using reconstituted sheet tobacco, a process resembling the manufacture of paper. How the sheet is formulated can affect the final product in terms of the amount of particulates, nicotine and so forth, produced on burning. The same is true for "puffed" or expanded tobacco, which has more filling capacity and burns more rapidly. The use of these processes has resulted in cigarettes with lower tar and nicotine content per cigarette and contributed to increased sales of cigarettes. Ventilation of the cigarette by providing more holes in the cigarette paper or filter is important to cooling the smoke and the rate of burning of the cigarette. With more ventilation, less air is drawn through the zone of pyrolysis, and the level of most mainstream components of smoke (see the next section) is reduced, and the amount of sidestream smoke produced during the smoldering period is increased. Changes in cigarette manufacture described here and the use of filters have resulted in reduction in the amount of tar and nicotine so that by 1982 the sales-weighted yields of nicotine and tar per cigarette in the United States were 1 mg and 13 mg.

CONSTITUENTS OF CIGARETTE SMOKE

The smoking cigarette is an extremely efficient drug delivery system, in which many of the products are created during the smoking process through alteration of substances originally present and distilled from the cigarette during the smoking process. Although the puff temperature of the burning tip of the cigarette may reach 900° C, smoke entering the mouth is near body temperature. This is a consequence of the porosity of the cigarette paper and moisture content owing to added humectants and storage conditions. It permits many components of tobacco to remain unburned and permits delivery of molecules of up to 100 kD in molecular mass. Mainstream smoke is generated during puffing in the burning and hot zones of the cigarette. Sidestream smoke is generated in the interval of smoldering between puffing and at temperatures of approximately 600° C. The majority of the 4865 known constituents of smoke are formed in a pyrolysis-distillation zone just behind the heat-generating combustion zone, so the tobacco granules may be thought of as exploding, the released and often altered constituents then being carried in a vapor stream where they form heterogeneous particles ($1.3 \times 10^{10}/cm^3$), which measure between 0.2 and 1.3 mm in diameter depending on the presence and type of filter.

About 30% of mainstream smoke is derived from tobacco and the remainder from air drawn through the cigarette. One cigarette yields approximately 400 to 500 mg of mainstream smoke made up of 400 to 500 gaseous components, of which nitrogen (58%), oxygen (12%), carbon dioxide (13%), and carbon monoxide (3.5%) are major components. The vapor phase also includes hydrogen, methane and other hydrocarbons, volatile aldehydes and ketones, nitrogen oxides, hydrogen cyanide, volatile nitriles, and several hundred other minor constituents.[31,94,147] The remainder consists of components of the particulate phase and other vapor phase components. In studies of cigarette smoke, the particulate phase is operationally defined as particles of greater than 0.1 μm in diameter that are trapped on a glass fiber Cambridge filter pad.[65] This material is also referred to as "tar." The majority of genotoxic and cocarcinogenic substances in cigarette smoke as demonstrated by bioassay are present in the particulate phase.[95] In this connection, the pH of cigarette smoke is important also. At about pH 5.5, the pH of mainstream cigarette smoke, the majority of nicotine is protonated and is in the particulate phase. At higher pH, pH 6.5 and higher, it follows the vapor phase.

Because nicotine is addictive and some of its derivatives are carcinogenic, it can be seen that the nature of the tobacco used and the conditions of smoking can greatly influence biological consequences.[93a] The particulate phase of cigarette smoke also contains a variety of insecticides and their derivatives as well as a variety of metals, some toxic or radioactive. These include aluminum, cadmium, lead, mercury, nickel, and polonium-210.[41,45,94] Because cigarette smoke is generated in relatively oxygen-deficient zones behind the burning tip, it has considerable reducing capacity, most prominent in sidestream smoke produced during smoldering, when there is less oxygen than during puffing. Compounds generated by reduction reactions are more common in sidestream smoke and include ammonia, aromatic amines, and volatile carcinogenic amines. Mainstream smoke also contains free radicals, one in the vapor phase, which is generated by the oxidation of nitric oxide (NO) to nitrous oxide (NO_2) and which can then react with active organic species in smoke, such as isoprene, and another, probably a quinone-hydroxyquinone complex, in the particulate phase. These may be important in direct mediation of tissue injury or indirectly through their effects on lipid peroxidation or proteins[43] and are discussed further later.

Tables 13-1 and 13-2, taken from the Report of the Surgeon General in 1989, list the major constituents of the particulate and vapor phases of cigarette smoke.[194] Table 13-3[99] lists selected compounds in nonfilter mainstream smoke and their relative distribution in sidestream smoke. Certain of these compounds are referred to when they are discussed later in relationship to the pathogens of diseases associated with the use of tobacco.

NICOTINE AND NICOTINE ADDICTION

Of the more than 4000 substances in cigarette smoke, nicotine may be viewed as the keystone to the pathogenesis of diseases associated with tobacco usage because it is

Table 13-1. Major constituents of the particulate matter of mainstream smoke of nonfilter cigarettes

Compound	µg/cigarette
Nicotine	1000-3000
Nornicotine	50-150
Anatabine	5-15
Anabasine	5-12
Other tobacco alkaloids (17)	NA
Bipyridyls (4)	10-30
n-Hentriacontane (n-$C_{31}H_{64}$)	100
Total nonvolatile hydrocarbons (45)†	300-400†
Naphthalene	2-4
Other naphthalenes (23)	3-6†
Phenanthrenes (7)	0.2-0.4†
Anthracenes (5)	0.05-0.1†
Fluorenes (7)	0.6-1.0†
Pyrenes (6)	0.3-0.5†
Fluoranthenes (5)	0.3-0.45†
Carcinogenic polynuclear aromatic hydrocarbons (11)	0.1-0.25
Phenol	80-160
Other phenols (45)†	60-180†
Catechol	200-400
Other catechols (4)	100-200†
Other dihydroxybenzenes (10)	200-400†
Scopoletin	15-30
Other polyphenols (8)†	NA
Cyclotenes (10)†	40-70†
Quinones (7)	0.5
Solanesol	600-1000
Neophytadienes (4)	200-350
Limonene	30-60
Other terpenes (200-250)†	NA
Palmitic acid	100-150
Stearic acid	50-75
Oleic acid	40-110
Linoleic acid	60-150
Linolenic acid	150-250
Lactic acid	60-80
Indole	10-15
Skatole	12-16
Other indoles (13)	NA
Quinolines (7)	2-4
Other N-heterocyclic hydrocarbons (55)	NA
Benzofurans (4)	200-300
Other O-heterocyclic hydrocarbons (42)	NA
Stigmasterol	40-70
Sitosterol	30-40
Campesterol	20-30
Cholesterol	10-20
Aniline	0.36
Toluidines	0.23
Other aromatic amines (12)	0.25
Tobacco-specific N-nitrosamines (4)‡	0.34-2.7
Glycerol	120

NA, Not available.

From Hoffmann D, Wynder EL: Chemical constituents and bioactivity of tobacco smoke, *IARC Sci Publ* 74:145, 1986; and US Department of Health and Human Services, Public Health Service, Centers for Disease Control, Center for Chronic Disease Prevention and Health Promotion, Office of Smoking and Health: *Reducing the health consequences of smoking: 25 years of progress.* A report of the Surgeon General, DHHS Publication No. (CDC) 89-8411, 1989.

*Numbers in parentheses represent individual compounds identified in a given group.

†Estimate.

Table 13-2. Major constituents of the vapor phase of the mainstream smoke of nonfilter cigarettes

Compound*	Concentration/cigarette
Nitrogen	280-320 mg (56%-64%†)
Oxygen	50-70 mg (11%-14%†)
Carbon dioxide	45-65 mg (9%-13%†)
Carbon monoxide	14-23 mg (2.8%-4.6%†)
Water	7-12 mg (1.4%-2.4%†)
Argon	5 mg (1.0%†)
Hydrogen	0.5-1.0 mg
Ammonia	10-130 µg
Nitrogen oxides (NO_x)	100-600 µg
Hydrogen cyanide	400-500 µg
Hydrogen sulfide	20-90 µg
Methane	1.0-2.0 mg
Other volatile alkanes (20)	1.0-1.6 mg‡
Volatile alkenes (16)	0.4-0.5 mg
Isoprene	0.2-0.4 mg
Butadiene	25-40 µg
Acetylene	20-35 µg
Benzene	12-50 µg
Toluene	20-60 µg
Styrene	10 µg
Other volatile aromatic hydrocarbons (29)	15-30 µg
Formic acid	200-600 µg
Acetic acid	300-1700 µg
Propionic acid	100-300 µg
Methyl formate	20-30 µg
Other volatile acids (6)	5-10 µg‡
Formaldehyde	20-100 µg
Acetaldehyde	400-1400 µg
Acrolein	60-140 µg
Other volatile aldehydes (6)	80-140 µg
Acetone	100-650 µg
Other volatile ketones (3)	50-100 µg
Methanol	80-180 µg
Other volatile alcohols (7)	10-30 µg‡
Acetonitrile	100-150 µg
Other volatile nitriles (10)	50-80 µg‡
Furan	20-40 µg
Other volatile furans (4)	45-125 µg
Pyridine	20-200 µg
Picolines (3)	15-80 µg
3-Vinylpyridine	10-30 µg
Other volatile pyridines (25)	20-50 µg‡
Pyrrole	0.1-10 µg
Pyrrolidine	10-18 µg
N-Methylpyrrolidine	2.0-3.0 µg
Volatile pyrazines (18)	3.0-8.0 µg
Methylamine	4-10 µg
Other aliphatic amines (32)	3-10 µg

From Hoffmann D, Wynder EL: Chemical constituents and bioactivity of tobacco smoke, *IARC Sci Publ* 74:145, 1986.

*Numbers in parentheses represent individual compounds identified in a given group.

†Percentage of total effluent.

‡Estimate.

Table 13-3. Concentrations of selected compounds in non-filter cigarette mainstream smoke (MS) and the ratio of their relative distribution in sidestream smoke (SS): MS$^\alpha$

Compound	Mainstream smoke	SS:MS
Vapor phase		
Carbon monoxide	10-23 mg	2.5-4.7
Carbon dioxide	20-60 mg	8-11
Carbonyl sulfide	18-42 μg	0.03-0.13
Benzene	12-48 μg	10
Toluene	160 μg	6-8
Formaldehyde	70-100 μg	0.1-50
Acrolein	60-100 μg	8-15
Acetone	100-250 μg	2-5
Pyridine	16-40 μg	7-20
3-Vinylpyridine	15-30 μg	20-40
Hydrogen cyanide	400-500 μg	0.1-0.25
Hydrazine	32 ng	3.0
Ammonia	50-150 μg	40-170
Methylamine	17.5-28.7 μg	4.2-6.4
Dimethylamine	7.8-10 μg	3.7-5.1
Nitrogen oxides	100-600 μg	4-10
N-Nitrosodimethylamine	10-40 ng	20-100
N-Nitrosopyrrolidine	6-30 ng	6-30
Formic acid	210-478 μg	1.4-1.6
Acetic acid	330-810 μg	1.9-3.9
Particulate phase		
Particulate matter	15-40 mg	1.3-1.9
Nicotine	1.7-3.3 mg	1.8-3.3
Anatabine	2.4-20.1 μg	0.1-0.5
Phenol	60-140 μg	1.6-3.0
Catechol	100-360 μg	0.6-0.9
Hydroquinone	110-300 μg	0.7-0.9
Aniline	360 ng	30
ortho-Toluidine	160 ng	19
2-Naphthylamine	1.7 ng	30
4-Aminobiphenyl	4.6 ng	31
Benz(α)anthracene	20-70 ng	2.2-4
Benzo(α)pyrene	20-40 ng	2.5-3.5
Cholesterol	14.2 μg	0.9
γ-Butyrolactone	10-22 μg	3.6-5.0
Quinoline	0.5-2 μg	8-11
Harman	1.7-3.1 μg	0.7-1.9
N-Nitrosonornicotine	200-3000 ng	0.5-3
4-(Methylnitrosamino)-1- (3-pyridyl)-1-butanone	100-1000 ng	1-4
N-Nitrosodiethanolamine	20-70 ng	1.2
Cadmium	100 ng	3.6-7.2
Nickel	20-80 ng	0.2-30
Zinc	60 ng	0.2-6.7

From International Agency for Research on Cancer: *IARC Monographs on the evaluation of the carcinogenic risk of chemicals to humans,* International Agency for Research on Cancer, Lyon, France, 1986.

so highly addicting. The Surgeon General's Report in 1988 concluded: Tobacco use is addicting; nicotine is the active pharmacological agent that causes this addictive behavior; and the pharmacological and behavioral processes that determine tobacco addiction are similar to those that determine addiction to drugs such as heroin and cocaine.[89] It is quite comparable to drugs such as heroin, cocaine, and alcohol in that it shares most of the following characteristics: psychoactive effects (pleasure, higher levels of cognitive performance, relief of anxiety, arousal), drug reinforced behavior, compulsive use (despite harmful effects), relapse after abstinence, recurrent drug cravings, tolerance, and physical dependence, as well as being an agonist useful in treating dependence.[18,89] It is estimated that one third to two thirds of starting smokers become addicted to nicotine. Relapse rates are similar between tobacco, heroin, and alcohol, in that 60% of people who quit smoking relapse in 3 months and 75% in 6 months.[96] It has been reported that 1 year after surgery for lung cancer, 48% of patients had returned to their previous smoking habit.[59] In some individuals, the likelihood of addiction to nicotine may be genetically determined,[37] although the molecular nature of this effect is unknown. It is of interest, however, that variation in the dopamine D_2 receptor gene has been associated with neuropsychiatric disorders and as a risk factor in alcohol and polysubstance abuse. These studies have not thus far included addiction to nicotine.[47,48]

Nicotine inhaled in cigarette smoke is rapidly absorbed in the lungs and enters the pulmonary circulation. It is estimated that it takes less than 19 seconds from the start of a puff to delivery of nicotine to the brain. This rapid delivery enhances rapid behavioral reinforcement and allows the smoker to control the amount of nicotine absorbed.[17]

In this connection, smokers of cigarettes of reduced nicotine content increase puff frequency and duration to adjust the level of nicotine to a level that is, for them, comfortable. Although nicotine can induce nausea, vomiting, and dizziness, tolerance begins to develop within 1 hour.[16,19]

Nicotine readily crosses the blood-brain barrier and is distributed throughout the brain. Specific binding to nicotinic receptors is greatest in the hypothalamus, hippocampus, thalamus, midbrain, brain stem, cerebral cortex, and nigrostriatal and mesolimbic dopaminergic neurons. The density of nicotinic receptors is increased in the brains of smokers as compared with nonsmokers.[20] Studies in the mouse brain indicate that nicotine binding sites increase with treatment time and treatment dosage and decrease to control levels following withdrawal, approximating changes in sensitivity to nicotine.[128] It has been demonstrated in brains of rats and mice that seven genes code for proteins with homology to the nicotinic acetylcholine receptor and five for the muscle nicotinic acetylcholine receptor. Similar sets of genes have been described in the chicken. Gamma-aminobutyric acid and glycine receptors have been cloned and are structurally related to the nicotinic receptor, raising the possibility that all ligand gated channels are members of one superfamily of related proteins (reviewed in Heinemann et al[91]). It has been reported that a specific subtype of nicotinic cholinergic receptor composed of a4 and b2 proteins is significantly increased in the cortex of rats treated with nicotine over a long-term period.[74] These observations raise the interesting possibility that the nature of nicotine addiction in different individuals may be related to variations in the structure or expression of different members of this family. Tolerance to nicotine has been shown to be genetically regulated in mice.[129]

Nicotine appears to act presynaptically, leading to the release of acetylcholine, norepinephrine, dopamine, serotonin, vasopressin, growth hormone, and adrenocorticotropic hormone (ACTH) (reviewed in Benowitz[16]). Smoking is also associated with an increase in beta-endorphin levels that increase in proportion to plasma nicotine levels[169,182] as well as increased circulating levels of growth hormone, cortisol, and prolactin. Nicotine also excites nicotinic receptors in the spinal cord, autonomic ganglia, and adrenal medulla leading to release of epinephrine and stimulates release of catecholamines and facilitates the release of neurotransmitters from sympathetic nerves in blood vessels. Release of these catecholamines contributes to the increase in heart rate and blood pressure associated with smoking, and direct and indirect effects on endothelial cells and platelets may contribute to the development of cardiovascular disease.

Another important effect of nicotine is to stimulate weight loss in humans and in experimental animals.[205] This is of historical interest in that sales campaigns of tobacco companies in the 1930s used this observation to sell cigarettes to women, and it is reflected today in current cigarette advertising (e.g., Virginia Slims). It is of current interest because the mechanisms underlying this association may also apply to the association of maternal smoking with infants of low birth weight, to be discussed later. Reduced weight of smokers appears to be related to an increase in metabolic rate owing to nicotine exposure[160,161] and to reduction in adipose tissues in smokers.[109] The precise mechanisms by which weight loss is induced are not known. It may be related to nicotine-stimulated release of epinephrine, and it may also be associated with increased lipoprotein-lipase levels in adipose tissue.[38]

Cotinine, a major metabolite of nicotine, is currently the best marker of tobacco exposure through active inhalation and passive smoke exposure.[5,84] By measuring urinary cotinine excretion, it has been demonstrated that the mean biological half-life of cotinine was 16.5 hours in smokers and 27.3 hours in never-smokers, suggesting that significant differences in nicotine binding or metabolism exist between smokers and nonsmokers.[85] It has also been shown that even when controlling for number of cigarettes, nicotine content, frequency of inhalation, weekly sidestream smoke exposure, age gender, and education, the median serum cotinine level was higher in black than white smokers, suggesting that nicotine metabolism may be different between races, perhaps accounting for the observed lower smoking cessation rates and higher rates of some smoking-related

Table 13-4. Smoking-related cancer deaths, by organ

Organ	Percent of deaths	Number of deaths
Trachea, lung, bronchus	90	123,000
Larynx	82	3,650
Lip, oral cavity, pharynx	92	5,500
Esophagus	80	7,600
Bladder and urinary tract	50	7,800
Cervix	30	1,400
Pancreas	30	8,000
Stomach	20	2,800

cancers in blacks.[196] These studies also suggest that great caution must be observed in comparing studies relating to exposure to cigarette smoke, even when as well proven a measure of nicotine exposure is available.

SMOKING AND CANCER

It has been estimated that perhaps 70% or more of cancers in the United States are a consequence of exposure to environmental carcinogens. Usage of tobacco products is an avoidable cause of approximately 30% of cancer deaths.[145,194] Combining estimates from the Surgeon General's Report of 1989[194] and Boring and colleagues,[25] smoking contributes to the percentage and number of cancer deaths listed in Table 13-4.

In addition to these cancers, epidemiological evidence indicates that 20% to 30% of leukemias are attributable to smoking, including myelogenous leukemias, lymphoma, and multiple myeloma,[79,127] and polycyclic aromatic hydrocarbon-DNA adducts have been demonstrated in significantly greater quantity in peripheral blood mononuclear cells in smokers than in nonsmokers.[178] Some studies have linked smoking to the development of hepatocellular cancer,[93] suggesting that exposure to constituents of tobacco smoke is related to the progression of cirrhosis to cancer. Malignancies in the anus, penis, and vulva are also more common in smokers than nonsmokers (reviewed in Newcomb and Carbone[145]).

The relationship between smoking and cancer has been established primarily through epidemiological methods that took into account dose-response relationships among groups of smokers and nonsmokers, including cumulative exposure. There are no consistently reproducible experimental animal models of cancer induced by exposure to cigarette smoke. The tumorigenic activity of some of the more than 4000 known constituents of tobacco smoke has been identified for the most part by such techniques as direct application to the skin of mice or other rodents. In addition, the metabolic effects of these substances have been studied with respect to their capacity to induce cytochrome P-450 monooxygenases in tissues of exposed animals, and their potentially mutagenic effects have been studied in a variety of in vitro systems, including the Ames assay, sister chromatid exchange assays (in vivo and in vitro), and cell transformation assays[99] (see Chapters 5, 17, and 26).

Based on these studies a number of classes of tumorigenic substances have been identified in cigarette smoke. These include the following classes of compounds: polyaromatic hydrocarbons; aza-azarenes; N-nitrosamines; aromatic amines, including 4-aminobiphenyl; aldehydes; other organic compounds, including benzene; and inorganic compounds, including hydrazine and polonium-210.[95,194] The basis of the tumorigenicity of many of these compounds is that they are or can become highly reactive electrophiles as a consequence of oxidation and form adducts with DNA, causing errors in transcription, replication, or repair[4] resulting in activation of oncogenes or inactivation of tumor suppressor genes.[22] It follows that in most instances these chemicals are also mutagens and are considered tumor initiators. In addition, cigarette smoke contains a large number of substances, e.g., phenolics, that function as tumor promoters, resulting in expansion of cell populations that contain altered DNA. Tumor promoters are not in themselves carcinogenic or genotoxic but serve to stimulate cell replication directly or indirectly, in some instances by stimulating release of growth-promoting cytokines from other cells, such as activated macrophages. Nicotine has been reported to inhibit apoptosis and may in that way both serve as a tumor promoter and decrease the efficiency of anticancer therapies.[208] In addition, inflammatory responses to constituents of tobacco smoke result in the generation of toxic oxygen species from pulmonary macrophages that can also result in damage to DNA. The synergy that exists between tobacco exposure and exposure to certain forms of asbestos in the pathogenesis of pulmonary cancers and malignant mesothelioma may be related, in part, to this shared mechanism.[52,100]

The long period between initiation of smoking and the appearance of cancer as well as the slow and incomplete[88] decline in cancer risk with cessation of smoking (it begins to become evident within 5 years and never reaches the same risk as nonsmokers) are the result of the accumulation of tobacco product–DNA adducts and the effects of promoters.[133,155] This model can be modified in the direction of tumorigenesis by exposure to other environmental risk factors, such as genotoxic chemicals or radiation, e.g., polyaromatic hydrocarbons from automobile exhaust or industrial exposure[156,158] and radon, and exposure to other promoters, including some drugs, e.g., barbiturates. Progression to tumor formation can be retarded or inhibited by certain dietary constituents, especially beta-carotene, vitamin A, retinoids, and antioxidants.[198]

Bioactivation of carcinogens, such as polycyclic aromatic hydrocarbons and polychlorinated biphenyls, depends on monooxygenases of the P-450 family of isoenzymes (reviewed in Kikkawa[108]). Among individuals with presumably equal exposures, however, the number of adducts demonstrable can vary widely.[159] It has been suggested that

this variation may be due to host polymorphism in the P-450 system.[97] Further, it has been shown that exposure of rats neonatally to phenobarbital can alter the metabolic profile of liver P-450 activity into adulthood,[6] a phenomenon called imprinting, raising the possibility that neonatal exposure to P-450-inducing substances can raise the risk of environmentally induced cancers later in life.

These observations, taken together, may provide a partial explanation of why some smokers seem to be at especial risk for the development of smoking-associated cancers. They may also provide an explanation of why no reproducible experimental models of smoking-induced carcinogenesis have been developed. Simply, experimental animals are relatively inbred and short-lived and do not share the same environmental experience as humans, so that for genetic and epigenetic reasons, it is perhaps unreasonable to think that they would respond in a similar manner to smoke exposure. These may be the same reasons that contribute to the difficulty in evaluating studies of exposure to environmental tobacco smoke and its relationship to lung or other cancers, in which many studies report an association and many others do not (reviewed in Byrd[36] and in Smith and colleagues[185]). It has been estimated that in the United States, 3700 deaths from lung cancer may be attributable to passive smoking.[200] In 1986, the Committee on Passive Smoking of the National Research Council (NRC) reviewed the available literature concerning environmental tobacco smoke and lung cancer and concluded that 13 studies provided adequate information for comparative analysis. The results of this analysis revealed that the overall risk of lung cancer in association with environmental tobacco smoke exposure was 1.34 (95% confidence interval, 1.18 to 1.53); the relative risk for women was 1.32 (95% confidence interval, 1.16 to 1.51); and for men, the relative risk was 1.62 (95% confidence level, 0.99 to 2.64). The NRC estimated that confounding factors associated with both lung cancer and living with a smoking spouse may lower the relative risk for nonsmokers exposed to environmental tobacco smoke to 1.25.[49]

As in all pooled studies, comparability of populations is critical. As pointed out by Angell,[2] "although there are statistical methods for neutralizing confounding variables, they are not perfect, and they are no use whatsoever unless the confounding variables are known and measured." One approach has been to compare individuals with and without smoking spouses as an attempt at neutralizing confounding variables. In 31 such studies discussed in a review by Carr and colleagues,[39] relative risk of developing lung cancer if a spouse smoked ranged between 0.7 and 2.55. Twenty-five studies showed no increase in risk. Among the six that did, relative risk was generally less than 2.0, or approximately the same magnitude as confounding lifestyle factors. The major question that arises then is what factors must be considered in ensuring comparability of populations? These should include such factors as histological definition of the tumor; a "best estimate" of lifetime environmental tobacco smoke, exposure taking into account home, workplace, parental smoking habits, and other exposure; the nature of the environment in which exposure occurred, which can affect the properties of smoke; lifestyle, including diet; social class; where one lives or works, e.g., near a freeway; occupation, especially exposure to other potential carcinogens; demographic information concerning age, gender, ethnic or racial origin, and body mass index; and medical history and family medical history, i.e., is there a genetic predisposition to cancer. To this must be added biological measures of exposure. An approach to the latter has been suggested by Perera et al[157] that proposes the use of nested case-control studies to evaluate the relationship of biological markers and cancer risk. It involves storing biological samples that remain stable among the study cohort and when cancer develops measuring chemically specific dosimeters (DNA and protein adducts) and nonspecific biological markers, e.g., oncogene activation and sister chromatid exchange, to give an integrated estimate of the genotoxic/procarcinogenic effect of exposure.[157]

Whether a study that takes into account all of the abovementioned factors can actually be accomplished is open to question. It might be prudent to accept the proposition that some individuals, for a variety of reasons, are especially susceptible to the development of cancer and that environmental tobacco smoke acting alone or in synergy with other environmental exposures increases their risk of cancer and that public policy should continue to be directed toward cessation of smoking. For these individuals, the relative risk of exposure may be much higher than in any of the published studies. The question is how can they be identified and does the possibility of such identification exceed current knowledge and epidemiological analytical capabilities? It is important to determine if environmental tobacco smoke increases the risk of cancer, either directly or indirectly. At this time, however, there is no unassailable study that demonstrates this.

SMOKING AND CARDIOVASCULAR DISEASE

Cardiovascular disease is the leading cause of death and disability in the United States. Its increase in this century parallels the trends observed in smoking prevalence. Approximately 1 million people died of various cardiovascular diseases in 1987, and it is estimated that 200,000 of these were directly related to cigarette smoking.[131,194]

In the last 25 years, there has been a decrease in deaths from cardiovascular disease amounting to a 50% decline over this period.[92,210] It is estimated that 50% to 60% of this decrease is related to changes in lifestyle and that 24% of the overall decline in deaths was related to reduction in cigarette smoking.[83,190] Smoking is associated with disease in all segments of the systemic arterial tree. The percentage of various types of cardiovascular diseases attributable to cigarette smoking is shown in Table 13-5.

Table 13-5. Cardiovascular diseases attributable to cigarette smoking

Cardiovascular disease	Percent smoking attributable*	Number of deaths†
Ischemic heart disease		108,179
<65 years	27	
>65 years	13	
Other heart diseases		42,141
Cardiac arrest	37	13,695
Cerebrovascular disease	12	26,313
Arteriosclerosis	29	8,256
Aortic aneurysm	59	7,233
Hypertension	15	

*Data from Ref. 210.
†Data from Ref. 88.

It is of interest that younger smokers appear to be at more risk of ischemic heart disease than older smokers. This may be because with advancing age, other diseases have more of an effect on mortality. It may also be that certain individuals are at especial risk of developing smoking-associated cardiovascular diseases and, if they smoke, die at younger ages.

With respect to the development of cardiovascular disease, there appears to be no level of safe exposure to cigarette smoke.[130] For each 10 cigarettes smoked per day, there is an incremental increase in cardiovascular mortality in men (18%) and in women (31%).[103] In the Nurses' Health Study, smoking as few as one to four cigarettes/day was associated with a doubling of risk for coronary heart disease.[204]

The strength of the association between cigarette smoking and the development of coronary heart disease is because smoking is by itself a major independent risk factor for coronary heart disease, equivalent to either hypercholesterolemia or hypertension, and it synergizes with these other major risk factors in induction and progression of vascular disease.[60,69] In fact, smoking in humans appears also to exert an effect on these other risk factors in that it results in an elevation in plasma cholesterol and low-density lipoprotein levels and a reduction in high-density lipoprotein levels.[29] In this connection, it has also been reported that chronic cigarette smokers are insulin resistant, hyperinsulinemic, and dyslipidemic (elevated plasma very-low-density lipoprotein triglycerides and cholesterol and lower high-density lipoprotein cholesterol) compared with a matched group of nonsmokers.[69] Changes in hormonal status, i.e., menopause or use of birth control pills, also increase the likelihood of smoking-associated cardiovascular disease in a synergistic manner,[166] probably by elevating levels of various clotting factors and decreasing functional activity of the regulatory protein, antithrombin III[80,81,202] (see Chapter 9). A number of autopsy studies have established a positive relationship between smoking and severity of atherosclerosis in coronary arteries, the aorta, and cerebral arteries.[189] A large number of both in vivo and in vitro studies have demonstrated the effects of various smoke constituents on vascular endothelial cells and platelets and interactions between these components that would favor thrombus formation as well as effects on vascular smooth muscle cells. Other reports have described the effect of tobacco smoke or constituents thereof on the immune system and major mediator pathways that might contribute to either atherogenesis or thrombogenesis. These are reviewed here in an attempt to explain how these various mechanisms might (1) interact in the pathogenesis of atherosclerosis and superimposed thrombotic events and (2) account for the apparent increased susceptibility of some individuals to cardiovascular disease associated with smoking.

The pathogenesis of atherosclerosis is currently viewed by many as a process that begins with endothelial perturbation or injury and involves platelets and their products; mononuclear cells from blood including monocytes/macrophages and their products, especially various cytokines and lymphocytes; and vascular smooth muscle cells. These cellular elements and their products stimulate alteration of the vessel wall, leading to lipid accumulation, proliferation of smooth muscle cells, increased production of connective tissue, and growth of the arteriosclerotic plaque. Necrosis and hemorrhage in the plaque may contribute to further plaque growth. Endothelial function in the now narrowed vessel may be altered by changes in flow and shear stress and in response to cytokines and growth factors elaborated by the cellular constituents of the plaque. Some of the changes in endothelial function may promote thrombus formation.[50,174,197]

Endothelial injury associated with exposure to tobacco smoke has been reported by a number of investigators, reviewed in Pittilo.[167] The nature of the injurious stimulus is unknown and has been attributed variously to nicotine and carbon monoxide, although the other constituents of smoke may be as, or more, important. More recently, it has been demonstrated that treatment of human umbilical vein endothelial cells with plasma from human volunteer smokers or with plasma exposed to cigarette smoke resulted in activation of the pentose monophosphate pathway, increased extrusion of glutathione, a decrease in intracellular adenosine triphosphate (ATP), and release of angiotensin-converting enzyme. The authors interpreted these data as indicating that endothelial injury was mediated by the oxidative burden imposed by free radicals in cigarette smoke.[148] Perhaps via a related mechanism, it has also been reported that exposure of hamsters to cigarette smoke elicited rolling and subsequent adhesion of leukocytes to endothelium of arterioles and postcapillary venules in skin fold chambers. This was preceded by increased plasma xanthine oxidase activity and evidence of intravascular hemolysis. All of these effects were significantly attenuated by treatment with

CuZn-superoxide dismutase.[116] The presence of free radicals in cigarette smoke has been cited previously.[43]

The role of oxidants in cigarette smoke in the pathogenesis of vascular injury and the development of atherosclerosis may also be related to their effect on plasma low-density lipoproteins. The biological properties of oxidized low-density lipoproteins[151a] include the ability to be taken up via the "scavenger receptor" of macrophages, a receptor expressed in macrophages in atherosclerotic plaques in which oxidized low-density lipoprotein can also be demonstrated. Oxidized low-density lipoprotein can also inhibit release of endothelially derived relaxing factor (EDRF) by endothelial cells or response to EDRF,[113] presumably leading to changes in regulation of vessel tone that would tend to augment the responses to catecholamines released as a consequence of exposure to nicotine. Oxidized low-density lipoprotein is also autoantigenic, and it has been reported that the titer of autoantibodies to malondialdehyde–low-density lipoprotein was an independent predictor of the progression of carotid atherosclerosis in Finnish men.[177] Oxidized low-density lipoprotein has also been reported to induce endothelial expression of granulocyte and macrophage colony-stimulating factors.[56] It has also been demonstrated that administration of oxidized low-density lipoprotein stimulated leukocyte/endothelial adherence in hairless mice. This adherence was inhibited by prior administration of an inhibitor of leukotriene synthesis or of monoclonal antibodies to the CD11b/CD18 adhesion receptor complex of leukocytes. Adhesion of leukocytes to endothelium of precapillary venules and arterioles was observed in these experiments.[117]

The aforementioned observations may, in part, be related to the described effects of tobacco smoke on activation of the complement system. Exposure of serum to cigarette smoke was observed to alter the third component of complement (C3) specifically by cleaving the internal thioester bond resulting in activation of this molecule.[104,105] In vivo rats exposed to cigarette smoke had significantly elevated levels of chemotactic activity for neutrophils and monocytes in their lung fluids. Prior treatment of rats with cobra venom factor, which depleted complement, blocked this smoke-induced chemotactic activity.[106] The nature of the complement-activating material in cigarette smoke is unknown. It has also been observed that nicotine is chemotactic for neutrophils and enhances neutrophil responsiveness to chemotactic peptides.[193] These data taken together suggest that components of cigarette smoke may, by activating the complement system and generating C5a, indirectly up-regulate expression of integrin molecules on the surface of leukocytes, including polymorphonuclear neutrophiles, monocytes, lymphocytes, and natural killer cells (reviewed in Springer[187] and Carlos and Harlan[36a]).

One of the consequences of increased expression of integrin molecules by leukocytes would be enhanced adherence of these cells to vascular endothelial cells that have been induced to express members of the immunoglobulin superfamily such as ICAM-1 (intercellular adhesion molecule-1), ICAM-2, and VCAM (vascular cell adhesion molecule) (reviewed in Butcher[34] and Bevilacqua[21]). Leukocytes, via surface carbohydrate ligands, can also bind to activated endothelium expressing members of the selectin family of protein (P and E selectins). It is known that histamine, bradykinin, and thrombin can stimulate release of P-selectin from Weibel-Palade bodies of endothelial cells. P-selectin can bind to carbohydrate ligands on neutrophils, monocytes, and some T cells, mediating adhesion and rolling under conditions of shear. In this connection, activation of complement by smoke constituents could generate anaphylotoxic fragments (C3a and C5a), causing release of histamine from mast cells and basophils. Further, polyphenol-containing glycoprotein constituents of cigarette smoke have been shown to be highly allergenic in humans[12] and, via their polyphenol-like or tanninlike epitopes, to activate coagulation factor XII–dependent pathways of coagulation, fibrinolysis, and bradykinin generation, which could also lead to surface expression of P-selectin.[11] It has been demonstrated that bradykinin increases the expression of kininogen binding sites on endothelial cells, possibly amplifying locally the effects of kinin generation on endothelial cells.[211]

It has also been shown that the cytokines interleukin-1-beta (IL-1β) and tumor necrosis factor-alpha (TNFα) can stimulate increased synthesis and expression of E-selectin and ICAM-1 by endothelial cells (these are normally constitutively expressed) and that TNFα can stimulate expression of VCAM-1 by endothelial cells. The transcription factor family nuclear factor-κB (NF-κB) regulates this expression, and, as hypothesized by Collins,[46] the participation of this family of regulatory proteins may be critical to the pathogenesis of atherosclerosis and thrombotic complications thereof.

Tobacco glycoprotein, described earlier,[11,12] has been shown to be at least as potent as bacterial lipopolysaccharide in stimulating production of IL-1α and IL-1β by macrophages.[77] Thus a number of constituents of tobacco smoke, acting in concert, may be able to activate major inflammatory mediator pathways and trigger synthesis and release of cytokines that initiate adhesion and emigration of inflammatory cells into the walls of blood vessels and stimulate the conversion of the endothelial cell surface from an antithrombotic to a prothrombotic surface (reviewed in Pober and Cotran[168]). These changes in endothelial function include increased production of tissue factor, downregulation of expression of thrombomodulin and the anticoagulant and profibrinolytic effects of protein C and protein S, decreased expression of tissue plasminogen activator, and increased expression of the inhibitor of tissue plasminogen activator, reviewed in Nachman.[141]

The expression of tissue factor in response to TNF stimulation has been shown in experiments using cultured endothelial cells to occur in subendothelial matrix vessels but not on the apical surface. This observation suggests a scenario in which components of smoke capable of initiating endothelial injury coming in contact with cytokine-activated endothelium might produce focal injury exposing a source of tissue factor and resulting in activation of the extrinsic pathway of coagulation. Because other components of smoke cited earlier are capable of activating the intrinsic pathway, the combined result, reviewed in Davie and colleagues[58] would favor thrombogenesis on an endothelial surface that had diminished capacity to lyse developing thrombi. This hypothesis might explain the elevated levels of coagulation factor VII found in the plasma of smokers.[134] The elevated levels of fibrinogen in smokers described in the same study might be a consequence of the effect of IL-1 generated by pulmonary macrophages in response to smoke constituents on the synthesis of coagulation factors by hepatocytes, reviewed in Dinarello.[63]

Allergic reactions to tobacco were first described in 1932, and it was hypothesized that such reactions might be involved in the pathogenesis of vascular disease.[86] Immediate cutaneous hypersensitivity responses were elicited in approximately one third of smokers and nonsmokers challenged with a polyphenol-containing, glycoprotein antigen (TGP) isolated from flue-cured tobacco leaves and from cigarette smoke condensate.[12] The same incidence of hypersensitivity to this antigen was demonstrated among Canadian subjects.[62] The high incidence of immediate cutaneous hypersensitivity to this antigen may be due to exposure to environmental tobacco smoke, but it may also be due to exposure to similar polyphenol-containing, immunologically cross-reacting antigens in commonly eaten vegetables,[14] including those in the family Solanaceae to which tobacco belongs.[12] Other investigators have also demonstrated immunogenicity of smoke-derived antigens in experimental animals.[118] Polyphenols, which structurally resemble tannins and flavonoids, are important defensive compounds in plants and have a wide range of biological activities, reviewed in Havsteen.[87] They also have a number of effects on the immune system, many of which are immunosuppressive.[137] The proinflammatory actions of cotton bract tannins are thought to contribute to the pathogenesis of byssinosis[172] and can, similar to TGP, stimulate IL-1 production by human peripheral blood monocytes.[176]

Tobacco leaves contain large amounts of polyphenol, and the high content and large variety of phenolic compounds in tobacco smoke, 200 or more, represent breakdown products of plant polyphenols. In addition, a number of intact polyphenols, including chlorogenic acid and scopoletin, are also present in smoke.[95] The polyphenols and many of their products, especially when oxidized, bind readily to proteins and can function as haptens. It has been shown that TGP, or models of it prepared by coupling the polyphenol rutin to bovine serum albumin, can selectively induce expression of immunoglobulin E (IgE) in mice, guinea pigs, and rabbits.[13,75] The mechanism underlying selective stimulation of IgE production appears to be related to the ability of polyphenol epitopes to stimulate TH2, a subset of T helper cells, reviewed in Fitch and colleagues,[73] to proliferate and to express IL-4, thereby influencing switching of B lymphocytes to production of antibodies of the IgE class.[10] IL-4 has also been shown to induce adherence of human eosinophils and basophils but not neutrophils to endothelium by inducing expression of VCAM-1.[179] It is of interest that expression of VCAM-1 is also induced in aortic endothelium of rabbits fed an atherogenic diet,[124] raising the possibility of synergy between tobacco-stimulated IL-4 release and dietary lipid in altering arterial endothelium.

Epidemiological observations indicate that smokers have higher levels of serum IgE. In men, a history of smoking correlated better with elevated IgE level than did a personal history of allergy.[54] Further the IgE concentration did not fall with increasing age as it did in nonsmokers. In a previous study, it was reported that the level of IgE was positively associated with cardiovascular diseases, including myocardial infarction, stroke, and large-vessel peripheral arterial disease in men.[53] This observation may be pertinent to an understanding of the relationship of smoking to the pathogenesis of cardiovascular disease in two ways. First, allergens in smoke might trigger vasospasm, dysrhythmia, and sudden death via cardiac anaphylaxis in the sensitized smoker in whom arteriosclerotic vessels might be more sensitive to inflammatory mediators such as histamine. The pathophysiology of cardiac anaphylaxis is reviewed in Levi.[122] Experimentally, cardiac and pulmonary anaphylaxis were induced in rabbits and guinea pigs by tobacco glycoprotein isolated from tobacco leaves and cigarette smoke condensate. These effects were IgE mediated.[123] Second, it has been reported that mast cells, in addition to releasing mediators of acute inflammatory responses such as histamine and leukotrienes, can, on antigenic challenge, release cytokines such as TNFα and IL-1 from preformed pools and synthesize them, reviewed in Galli.[78] These observations define a new role for basophils and mast cells in late phase of allergic reactions such as asthma.

It has been demonstrated that endothelial-leukocyte adhesion molecule-1 (E-selectin) is expressed on endothelium in vivo during late phase allergic reactions and that this expression in organ cultures could be blocked by antibodies to TNFα and IL-1.[121] These studies, taken together with those described in the paragraph earlier, may also define a role for IgE, mast cells, and basophils in the pathogenesis of arteriosclerosis. In this scenario, antigenic constituents of tobacco smoke could sensitize certain smokers. Inhalation of these same constituents would trigger enhanced release of cytokines from mast cells in the lung that in addition to mediating local effects might immediately downstream affect the endothelium of coronary and systemic arteries. The same endothelium would presumably also be affected by cytokines released from pulmonary macrophages as well. In this connection, it has been demonstrated that treatment of human alveolar macrophages with tobacco glycoprotein antigen stimulates release of IL-1 and IL-6 and elevation of the steady-state levels of IL-1α and IL-1β, IL-6, platelet-derived growth factor-A (PDGF-A) and PDGF-B mRNA.[76] This hypothesis would imply that those smokers with elevated levels of tobacco antigen specific IgE would be at especial risk of cardiovascular disease. It would also suggest that the population of smokers at especial risk for cardiovascular disease would be the same population at especial risk for inflammatory lung disease associated with smoking. Studies of this kind have not been described.

Although this discussion has focused primarily on the vascular endothelium, it is important to point out that platelet function is also altered in the blood of smokers, in part because of altered function of the vessel wall. Excessive thromboxane A$_2$ generation and increased excretion of prostacyclin metabolites have been described in smokers.[149] Platelet sensitivity to prostacyclin has also been described in blood of active smokers and individuals passively exposed to cigarette smoke.[32] These altered functions might contribute to the process of atherogenesis by helping to provide a source of PDGF or to thrombus formation over the altered endothelium of atherosclerotic plaques.

The hypothesis that proposes that atherosclerotic plaques arise as monoclonal proliferations of smooth muscle cells following a mutational event[15] must also be considered in relation to the association between cigarette smoking and the pathogenesis of atherosclerosis because of the large number of mutagens in cigarette smoke. It has been demonstrated in transfection experiments that DNA from human atherosclerotic plaques is capable of completing the transformation of NIH 3T3 cells[154] and that cultured human atherosclerotic plaque smooth muscle cells retain transforming potential and display enhanced expression of the *myc* proto-oncogene.[151] It was also shown that cockerels injected with 7,12-dimethylbenz(α)anthracene, a polynuclear aromatic hydrocarbon, in nontumorigenic doses developed atherosclerotic plaques. DNA from these plaques also induced transformation of NIH 3T3 cells.[152] Again using cockerels, it has been shown that inhalation of sidestream cigarette smoke accelerates development of arteriosclerotic plaques.[153] In this construction, mutagenic constituents of tobacco smoke might alter DNA of vascular smooth muscle cells, and the same or other constituents that stimulate accumulation of inflammatory cells and release of cytokine growth factors might cooperate in plaque growth.

The issue of the contribution of environmental tobacco smoke to risk of death from coronary heart disease or myocardial infarct disease, similar to that of its relationship to cancer, is still controversial. Combining a number of studies, a relative risk of approximately 1.3 was obtained with 95% confidence intervals of approximately 1.1 to 1.6 in two meta-analyses.[82,200] Of the 13 studies used in the analyses, all but one showed a relative risk greater than one. Three of the studies in men and five in women showed a relative risk that included one. Further, similar parameters were not controlled in all of the pooled studies, and in only five there was evidence of a dose-response relationship. Because other data seem to indicate that certain smokers are at greater risk than other smokers to the development of cardiovascular disease, it would seem prudent to assume that environmental tobacco smoke is of significant risk to some subsets of smokers. The lack of conclusiveness of the studies described earlier is simply because we do not currently have any understanding of the mechanisms that might underlie enhanced individual risk, and, as the reference cited reviews in detail, a wide range of biological effects are mediated by smoke constituents. It is also true that our understanding, even in a descriptive mode, of the total number of different biological effects of the constituents of smoke is extremely limited, and the most important ones may be unknown. This may be one reason for the lack of reproducible experimental models.

SMOKING AND PULMONARY DISEASE

Chronic obstructive pulmonary disease (COPD) accounts for approximately 62,000 deaths per year, of which 90% are related to cigarette smoking. It is part of a spectrum of change in the lung involving bronchitis and bronchiolitis at one extreme and emphysema at the other, both brought about as a consequence of inflammatory responses triggered by inhalation of cigarette smoke and, at some point, recurrent or chronic infection. Asthma may also contribute to both the initiation and the progression of the disease process. In addition, changes in pulmonary vessels may also occur, most probably through the same mechanisms, adding a component of pulmonary hypertension to the constellation of anatomical and functional changes that occur in the lungs of smokers.[207] The changes of COPD, emphysema, and asthma are described in Cotran et al.[51] The mechanisms initiating the release or generation of mediators of inflammation, the inflammatory process itself, tissue destruction, and fibrosis[1] have been discussed earlier in the section on cardiovascular disease and can be applied to the pathogenesis of smoking-associated pulmonary disease (see Chapters 24 and 28).

Because the lung is the portal of entry for tobacco smoke and because some pulmonary functions are relatively easily measured, i.e., forced expiratory volume and flow measurements, the effects of both active and passive smoking can be most easily quantitated,[114,183] and the most convincing evidence for pathogenic effects of environmental tobacco smoke concern its effect on inflammatory airway disease.[150,199,203]

Although COPD is relatively rare outside of smokers, it is also true that the majority of smokers do not develop COPD, suggesting that there is an idiosyncratic component

predisposing to the development of these inflammatory changes. Exposure to environmental tobacco smoke, quantified by measuring urinary cotinine levels, has been shown to be positively correlated with the development of asthma and decreases in pulmonary function.[42] These observations are in keeping with other observations that children of smoking parents have an increased frequency of respiratory symptoms, bronchitis, and pneumonia early in life associated with small abnormalities of pulmonary function tests.[150] Because of the involvement of IgE in the pathogenesis of some forms of asthma, and the fact that smokers have elevated IgE levels,[54] it is tempting to attribute the increased incidence of asthma to tobacco-specific IgE responses, especially given the familial inheritance pattern of allergy[24] and epidemiological studies that suggest the role of genetic factors in addition to deficiency of alpha-1-antitrypsin in the pathogenesis of COPD.[107]

There are no published data, however, that support or refute a hypothesis based purely on specific IgE responses to tobacco-specific antigens. Several studies, however, suggest a more complex effect of smoking on the immune system that may be pertinent to the pathogenesis of COPD. Smoking, although associated with increased levels of IgE, may result in decreased levels of other classes of immunoglobulins.[33] This immunosuppressive effect might contribute to the component of chronic infection in the pathogenesis of asthma and COPD. In this connection, elevated levels of IgE against *Streptococcus pneumoniae* have been reported in smokers,[23] as has increased skin test reactivity against other environmental allergens,[195] suggesting that smoking may influence the immune response in a way that results in enhanced allergic responses to a wide variety of environmental allergens but decreased protective immunity to local, mucosal infection. Research in immunity to infection has focused on the role of differential expression of cytokines by TH1 cells, producing IL-2 and interferon-gamma (IFN-γ), and TH2 cells, producing IL-4, IL-5, and IL-10, in determining the outcome of infection.[73,139] The cytokines produced by TH2 cells (type 2 cytokines) favor production of IgE but down-regulate cell-mediated immunity to infection. Although clinical studies exploring this area have focused on mycobacterial, protozoal, and helminth infections, it is possible that immunity to common bacteria of the respiratory tract is also altered as a consequence of expression of these cytokines. The fact that polyphenol constituents of tobacco can selectively stimulate TH2 cells to proliferate and express IL-4[10] may be highly relevant in this respect. Although the mechanism is unknown, cigarette smoking has also been reported as stimulating the development of AIDS in human immunodeficiency virus-1 (HIV-1)–seropositive individuals.[146]

Cigarette smoke, through a variety of mechanisms cited in the preceding section, and perhaps undiscovered ones as well, can produce mucosal injury. These changes, by altering the cellular milieu, may affect how antigen is recognized and presented. A hypothesis has been constructed concerning the first report of hay fever by Bostock in 1819,[26] suggesting that it emerged as a clinical entity in England as a consequence of mucosal injury produced by the smoky environment of the Industrial Revolution, which enhanced the likelihood of developing allergic responses to pollens.[71] The use of tobacco, principally pipe smoking, was also increasing at this time, and it is intriguing to think that the appearance of respiratory allergy to pollens as a clinical entity represented synergy between coal smoke and tobacco smoke.

Bronchiolar fibrosis and emphysema appear to be separable, although overlapping phenomena.[1] The degree of overlap may be modified by the immune system, i.e., whether asthma becomes a component, or genetic factors such as abnormalities of alpha-1-antitrypsin, an inhibitor of elastase produced by polymorphonuclear neutrophils. It has been demonstrated that toxic oxygen radicals present in smoke or generated by leukocytes can inhibit normal alpha-antitrypsin, making pulmonary elastic tissue susceptible to destruction by leukocyte elastase.[101] It has been hypothesized that this leads to the development of emphysema. Although this is an important contributory mechanism, several mechanisms are probably involved. The elastolytic activity produced by macrophages is not inhibited by alpha-1-antitrypsin. Further, it has been demonstrated that plasminogen activator enhances the destruction of pulmonary elastin by activating latent proteinases in tissue and that expression of alveolar macrophage plasminogen activator activity is associated with functional changes in the lungs of young smokers.[171] Macrophage urokinase expression has been shown to be protein kinase C dependent and stimulated by polyanions.[70] It is of interest that the polyphenol-containing constituents of smoke that can activate macrophages to produce various cytokines are also polyanionic and capable of activating plasminogen through factor XII–dependent pathways.[11,12,76,77] The structural similarity between polyphenols and tannins is also of interest because it has been shown that tannins can make some proteins more susceptible to digestion by trypsin by altering the structure of the former.[140] Thus the destruction of pulmonary elastic tissue may be the result of a number of different processes affecting the protease-antiprotease balance and greatly amplified by the effects of tobacco constituents on pulmonary macrophages.

SMOKING AND DISEASES OF THE FETUS AND NEONATE

Although smoking has declined in frequency, the greatest proportional increase in smokers has been in young women in child-bearing years. Approximately 31% of women smoke before pregnancy, and 25% smoke during pregnancy. Smoking is the most harmful known environmental exposure affecting pregnancy.[170,201] A study of late fetal death and early neonatal mortality in Sweden reported

the same risk of late fetal death (1.4) with smoking as with high maternal age or nulliparity. The risk doubled if mothers were more than 35 years old and smoked.[44] For an excellent and encyclopedic treatment of the relationship of smoking to disorders of the placenta, fetus, and neonate, the reader is also referred to Naeye's text on this subject[144] (see also Chapters 33 and 34).

The influence of smoking may begin at the time of conception. Data in the Collective Perinatal Study (CPS) suggest that the decreased fertility observed in smokers may be due to the fact that the women were older and had "blue collar"–type jobs and perhaps less frequent coitus.[144] A more direct relationship, however, is suggested by observations that smoking decreased fertilization rates in vitro and that those ova with high cotinine levels in the ovarian follicular fluid were less fertile than those with low levels of cotinine.[173]

A strong association has been reported between maternal cigarette smoking and spontaneous abortion. In contrast to early spontaneous abortions, these did not have an increased incidence of chromosomal abnormalities or congenital anomalies. Eleven percent of the abortions in the CPS could be attributable to smoking.[144] The mechanism underlying this association is unknown; however, it may be associated with direct or indirect effects of tobacco constituents on blood vessels because smoking is associated with an increased incidence of premature separation of the placenta and placenta previa. The former may be associated with the increased incidence of microinfarcts of the placenta and necrosis of the decidua at the edge of the placenta, which is associated with current smoking.[142] The latter is associated with previous smoking habits and may be the result of chronic scarring of endometrial vessels.[142] Uteroplacental blood flow is reduced during smoking, possibly through the effect of nicotine on secretion of catecholamines, and this may also contribute to placental injury.[119] Other possible effects, direct and indirect, of constituents of tobacco smoke on blood vessels have been discussed earlier. In this connection, ultrastructural lesions of the endothelium have been described in umbilical arteries from newborns of smoking mothers.[3]

It has long been recognized that smoking is associated with an increased incidence of low birth weight (reviewed in Werler et al[201] and Naeye[144]). The mechanisms underlying this association are unknown but may be related to the effects of nicotine on energy consumption discussed previously.

Cigarette smoking also appears to be associated with the development of the sudden infant death syndrome (SIDS). In the CPS, smoking during pregnancy accounted for 16% of the SIDS deaths. The association is attributed to abnormalities of brain stem and autonomic nervous system function.[143] Both intrauterine exposure to smoke constituents and passive exposure after birth have been found to increase the risk of SIDS by as much as threefold.[138,180] The mechanisms underlying this association are unknown.

SMOKING AND GASTROINTESTINAL DISEASE
Peptic ulcer disease

A number of epidemiological studies have shown that smoking contributes to the development of, delayed healing of, and recurrence of peptic ulcers even with treatment with histamine H_2 receptor antagonists such as cimetidine.[64,111,115,186] The pathogenetic mechanisms underlying the association of smoking with peptic ulcer disease are presently unknown. Studies of the effect of smoking on gastric acid secretion have been inconclusive. Smoking can reduce pancreatic secretion of bicarbonate, which could contribute to the development of duodenal ulcers.[30,35] Smoking may also contribute to incompetence of the pyloric sphincter leading to reflux, which might contribute to the pathogenesis of gastric ulcers.[175] More recently, it has been shown in the rat that intravenously administered nicotine exacerbated injury of the gastric mucosa induced by hypertonic saline administration by a mechanism that involved inhibition of injury-induced hyperemia by a mechanism independent of effects on cylooxygenase activity.[66] This observation is interesting because it suggests that smoking may not produce initial mucosal injury in the stomach but can aggravate injury. This might explain the association between smoking and failure to heal ulcers and recurrence of ulcers. It might also explain how the development of an ulcer is enhanced in smokers no matter what the inciting injury to the mucosa. In this connection, it has been shown that many gastric ulcers are associated with infection of the mucosa with *Helicobacter pylori*.[163] Again, it is not known whether *H. pylori* incites injury or colonizes and invades the already injured gastric mucosa, potentiating development and persistence of ulcers. It can be hypothesized, however, that the immunosuppressive effects of tobacco constituents on the immune system, discussed earlier, might contribute to persistence of infection with *H. pylori*.

Crohn's disease

From epidemiological studies, it appears that cigarette smoking is a risk factor for the development[192] and progression of Crohn's disease. The progression of the disease is related to the amount smoked.[125] It is of particular interest that an increased risk of Crohn's disease was found in those exposed to environmental tobacco smoke as children.[162] The mechanism underlying this association is unknown, but it is again tempting to think that effects of tobacco constituents on the immune system, particularly cellular mucosal immunity, are involved. If an infectious agent is involved in the granuloma formation associated with Crohn's disease, as *Mycobacterium paratuberculosis* is involved in the pathogenesis of Johne's disease, a form of granulomatous colitis in ruminants,[61] constituents of tobacco smoke that stimulate TH2 helper

cells to express type 2 cytokines, cited previously, might be involved as discussed previously.[10,139]

Ulcerative colitis

The relationship of smoking to ulcerative colitis is paradoxical. Some reports indicate that smoking ameliorates ulcerative colitis,[102] but others have not observed this effect.[28] Epidemiological studies indicate that current smokers have a decreased risk of developing ulcerative colitis as compared with nonsmokers but that former smokers have an increased risk of developing ulcerative colitis compared with nonsmokers. In this study, the relative risk of ulcerative colitis among former smokers increased in proportion to the cumulative number of cigarettes smoked before the onset of disease, suggesting a causal relationship.[27] Others have made similar observations concerning the increased risk of ulcerative colitis in former smokers and have commented on a rebound effect.[126] These data suggest that the effect of smoking on the immune system may be involved, but as in so many smoking-associated diseases, one is left with interesting, but insufficiently tested, hypotheses.

SMOKING AND OSTEOPOROSIS

Smoking has been associated epidemiologically with the earlier appearance of menopause and with osteoporosis.[7,132] Furthermore, smoking has been reported as reducing the risk of endometrial cancer in female smokers.[120] These data taken together suggest that smoking induces a relative estrogen deficiency. Irreversible, increased 2-hydroxylation of estradiol has been demonstrated in female and male smokers, leading to an increase of estrogen metabolites that have minimal peripheral estrogenic activity and are rapidly cleared from the circulation.[135,136] It should be noted that this change in pattern of estrogen metabolism in smokers might also be related to increased risk of cardiovascular disease. Further indirect support for the antiestrogenic effects of smoking in the pathogenesis of osteoporosis comes from the observations that thin individuals are more at risk for the development of osteoporosis than are obese individuals. Although this may be explained by the effect of weight bearing on enhancing bone strength, it can be argued that estrogen levels are higher in obese people because of conversion of androgens to estrogens in adipose tissue. This may be of significance in understanding the mechanisms of smoking-associated osteoporosis because smokers tend to weigh less than nonsmokers. In addition, smoking and increased alcohol consumption have been reported as increasing osteoporosis and the incidence of vertebral fractures in men. The effect of the two habits are additive in their contribution to risk of osteoporosis.[181] It was also reported that bone mineral density of the radius was inversely related to number of packs per years of smoking in postmenopausal women and that this was statistically significant. Bone density of the femoral neck, os calcis, and spine were also decreased, but in this sample of patients, these changes did not achieve statistical significance. It was also shown in this study that intestinal absorption of calcium was decreased among the smokers.[112] The mechanism of the decreased calcium absorption was unknown. It has been demonstrated that addition of IL-1 to bone cultures in vitro induces resorption and shrinking of bone matrix,[68] and systemic administration of IL-1 in mice pretreated with tritiated tetracycline induces bone resorption as measured by release of the labeled tetracycline.[110] Because constituents of cigarette smoke can stimulate IL-1 release from macrophages, it is possible that this mechanism may also contribute to the pathogenesis of smoking-associated osteoporosis.

SMOKING AND THYROID DISEASE

Smoking has been associated with toxic goiter in a number of studies over the last decade. In one study, it was observed that the incidence of smoking among women diagnosed as having nontoxic goiter, toxic nodular or adenomatous goiter, or Hashimoto's disease was the same as the normal population, about 30%. Among individuals with Graves's disease, however, it was 48% and among those with Graves's ophthalmopathy, it was 64%.[9] It has also been reported that the association between smoking and Graves's disease was more common among Europeans as opposed to Asians and that smokers were more likely to develop Graves's ophthalmopathy and that the latter was related to the amount smoked.[191] Others have reported an increased incidence of both nontoxic and toxic goiter among smokers.[67] The mechanisms underlying the association of smoking with thyroid disease are not known, but a number of possibilities have been suggested. These include the presence of goitrogens in smoke such as thiocyanate ions, indirect effects of catecholamines released in response to nicotine, and effects of smoking on the immune system that might lead to Graves's disease. The fact that tobacco smoke constituents can trigger pathways that lead to polyclonal activation of B lymphocytes, discussed earlier, is supportive of the last hypothesis. The effects of smoking on the thyroid are also of interest because the hyperthyroid state is associated with osteoporosis in postmenopausal women, raising the question of whether subtle but long-term changes in thyroid function in smokers may also contribute to the pathogenesis of smoking-associated osteoporosis.[57]

CONCLUDING REMARKS

Consumption of tobacco products is the single largest cause of premature death. The association of tobacco products, especially cigarette smoking, has been appreciated for many decades. Continuing epidemiological studies have demonstrated that all stages of life are affected by tobacco smoke either through direct inhalation or through exposure to environmental tobacco smoke. To prevent morbidity and premature mortality, especially when controlling the rate of

increase in health care costs is a major concern of government, it would seem reasonable to begin to implement the planned demise of the tobacco industry. Those already addicted to nicotine could receive treatment for their addiction under any new health plan, but the number of new nicotine addicts would be progressively decreased. In some ways, it might be easier to reduce nicotine addiction than it would be to cure the addiction of government for money associated with taxes on tobacco. The fact that the federal government plans to support health care spending in part on taxes on tobacco products without plans for an alternative source of funding is disturbing because it implies economic dependence on the industry and continuing inability of government to deal with a difficult political and major public health problem.

From a scientific standpoint, the various epidemiological approaches identifying the use of tobacco products with disease have provided important information that has led to the development of smoking cessation programs and has given direction to a large number of initiatives in basic science. A good example of this has been the progress made in the understanding at the molecular level of the complexity of the nicotine receptor protein family. These observations have also demonstrated the need for epidemiological studies that are tied to biological, biochemical, or functional measures of exposure that have stimulated the growth of the rapidly expanding field of molecular toxicology and have provided paradigms for epidemiological studies of the cause of environmental diseases other than those associated with tobacco, but which might act synergistically with those in tobacco. Although smoke is an extremely complex mixture of substances, the patient chemical analysis and definition of these substances have provided important insights into the structure and function of other hazardous environmental carcinogens in addition to carcinogens in tobacco. Finally, epidemiological studies have demonstrated synergy between risk factors in the pathogenesis of tobacco-associated diseases and the fact that some individuals are at increased risk of developing these diseases. The contributions of tobacco chemistry in identifying the constituents of tobacco, an increasing understanding of the biological activities of these substances, characterization of the mechanisms underlying these synergies, and information that will emerge from the human genome project will likely provide means of identifying those at increased risk of developing diseases associated with exposure to different substances in the environment, including those from tobacco or those that resemble substances in tobacco. An understanding of the increased risk of certain individuals could lead to the development of more specific preventive strategies.

REFERENCES

1. Adekunle AM et al: Bronchiolar inflammation and fibrosis associated with smoking. A morphologic cross-sectional population analysis, *Am Rev Respir Dis* 143:144, 1991.

2. Angell M: The interpretation of epidemiologic studies, *N Engl J Med* 23:823, 1990.

3. Asmussen I, Kjledsen K: Intimal ultrastructure of human umbilical arteries, *Circ Res* 36:579, 1975.

4. Au WW et al: Factors contributing to chromosome damage in lymphocytes of cigarette smokers, *Mutat Res* 260:137, 1991.

5. Axelrad CM et al: *Biochemical validation of cigarette smoke exposure and tobacco use,* New York, 1987, Plenum.

6. Bagley DM, Hayes JR: Xenobiotic imprinting of the hepatic monoxygenase system. Effects of neonatal phenobarbital administration, *Biochem Pharmacol* 34:1007, 1985.

7. Baron JA: Smoking and estrogen related diseases, *Am J Epidemiol* 119:9, 1984.

8. Barry M: The influence of the U.S. tobacco industry on the health, economy, and environment of developing countries, *N Engl J Med* 324:917, 1991.

9. Bartalena L et al: More on smoking habits and Graves' ophthalmopathy, *J Endocrinol Invest* 12:733, 1989.

10. Baum CG et al: Cellular control of IgE induction by a polyphenol-rich compound, *J Immunol* 145:779, 1990.

11. Becker CG, Dubin T: Activation of factor XII by tobacco glycoprotein, *J Exp Med* 146:457, 1977.

12. Becker CG, Dubin T, Wiedemann HP: Hypersensitivity to tobacco antigen, *Proc Natl Acad Sci USA* 73:1712, 1976.

13. Becker CG, Levi R, Zavecz JH: Induction of IgE antibodies to antigen isolated from tobacco leaves and from cigarette smoke condensate, *Am J Pathol* 96:249, 1979.

14. Becker CG, Van Hamont N, Wagner M: Tobacco, cocoa, coffee, and ragweed: cross reacting allergens that activate factor XII dependent pathways, *Blood* 58:861, 1981.

15. Benditt EP, Benditt JM: Evidence for a monoclonal origin of human atherosclerotic plaques, *Proc Nat Acad Sci USA* 70:1753, 1973.

16. Benowitz NL: Pharmacologic aspects of cigarette smoking and nicotine addiction, *N Engl J Med* 319:1318, 1988.

17. Benowitz NL: *Clinical pharmacology of inhaled drugs of abuse: implications in understanding nicotine dependency,* In Chiang CN, Hawks RL, editors: *Research findings on smoking of abused substances,* Nida Research Monograph 99, Washington, DC, 1990.

18. Benowitz NL: Cigarette smoking and nicotine addiction, *Med Clin North Am* 76:415, 1992.

19. Benowitz NL, Porchet H, Jacob P III: *Nicotine dependence and tolerance in man: pharmacokinetic and pharmacodynamic investigations,* 1989, New York, Elsevier Science Publishers.

20. Benwell MEM, Balfour DJK, Anderson JM: Evidence that tobacco smoking increases the density of (-)-(3H)nicotine binding sites in human brains, *J Neurochem* 50:1243, 1989.

21. Bevilacqua MP: Endothelial-leukocyte adhesion molecules, *Ann Rev Immunol* 11:767, 1993.

22. Bishop JM: The molecular genetics of cancer, *Science* 235:305, 1987.

23. Bloom JW et al: Pneumococcus-specific immunoglobulin E in cigarette smokers, *Clin Allergy* 16:25, 1986.

24. Borecki IB et al: Demonstration of a common major gene with pleiotropic effects on immunoglobulin E levels and allergy, *Gen Epidemiol* 2:327, 1985.

25. Boring CC, Squires TS, Tong T: Cancer statistics, *Cancer* 41:9, 1991.

26. Bostock J: Case of a periodical affection of the eyes and chest, *Medico-Chirurg Trans* 19:161, 1819.

27. Boyko EJ et al: Risk of ulcerative colitis among former and current cigarette smokers, *N Engl J Med* 316:707, 1987.

28. Boyko EJ et al: Effects of cigarette smoking on the clinical course of ulcerative colitis, *Scand J Gastroenterol* 23:1147, 1988.

29. Brischetto CS et al: Plasma lipid and lipoprotein profiles of cigarette smokers from randomly selected families: enhancement of hy-perlipidemia and depression of high density lipoprotein, *Am J Cardiol* 62:675, 1983.

30. Brown P: The influence of smoking on pancreatic function in man, *Med J Austral* 2:290, 1976.

31. Brunnemann KD, Hoffmann D: Pyrolytic origins of major gas phase constituents of cigarette smoke, *Recent Adv Tobacco Sci* 8:103, 1982.

32. Burghuber OC et al: Platelet sensitivity to prostacyclin in smokers and non-smokers, *Chest* 90:34, 1986.

33. Burrows B, Lebowitz MD, Barbee RA: Interactions of smoking and immunologic factors in relation to airways obstruction, *Chest* 84:657, 1983.

34. Butcher EC: Leukocyte-endothelial cell recognition: three (or more) steps to specificity and diversity, *Cell* 67:1033, 1991.

35. Bynum TE et al: Inhibition of pancreatic secretion in man by cigarette smoking, *Gut* 13:361, 1972.

36. Byrd JD: Environmental tobacco smoke: medical and legal issues, *Med Clin North Am* 76:377, 1992.

36a. Carlos TM, Harlan JM: Membrane proteins involved in phagocyte adherence to endothelium, *Immunol Rev* 114:5, 1990.

37. Carmelli D et al: Genetic influence on smoking–a study of male twins, *N Engl J Med* 327:829, 1992.

38. Carney RM, Goldberg AP: Weight gain after cessation of cigarette smoking, *N Engl J Med* 310:614, 1984.

39. Carr JS et al: Environmental tobacco smoke: current assessment and future directions, *Toxicol Pathol* 20:289, 1992.

40. Chandler WU: Banishing tobacco, *Worldwatch Paper* World Watch Institute, 1986, p 13.

41. Chiba M, Masironi R: Toxic and trace elements in tobacco and tobacco smoke, *Bull World Health Organ* 70:269, 1992.

42. Chilmonczyk BA, Salmun LM, Megathlin KN: Association between exposure to environmental tobacco smoke and exacerbations of asthma in children, *N Engl J Med* 328:1665, 1993.

43. Church DF, Pryor WA: Free-radical chemistry of cigarette smoke and its toxicological implications, *Environ Health Perspect* 64:111, 1985.

44. Cnattingius S, Haglund B, Meirik O: Cigarette smoking as a risk factor for late fetal and early neonatal death, *Br Med J* 297:258, 1988.

45. Cohen BS, Eisenbud M, Harley NH: Alpha radioactivity in cigarette smoke, *Radiat Res* 83:190, 1979.

46. Collins T: Biology of disease. Endothelial nuclear factor-κB and the initiation of the atherosclerotic lesion, *Lab Invest* 68:499, 1993.

47. Comings DE et al: The dopamine D2 receptor locus as a modifying gene in neuropsychiatric disorders, *JAMA* 266:1793, 1991.

48. Comings DE et al: The dopamine D2 receptor gene: a genetic risk factor in substance abuse, *Drug Alcohol Depend* 34:175, 1994.

49. Committee on Passive Smoking of the National Research Council: *Environmental tobacco smoke. Measuring exposures and assessing health effects,* Washington, DC, 1986, National Research Council.

50. Cotran RS, Kumar V, Robbins SL: *Arteriosclerosis.* In Cotran RS, Kumar V, Robbins SL, editors: *pathologic basis of disease,* ed 4, Philadelphia, 1989, WB Saunders.

51. Cotran RS, Kumar V, Robbins SL: *Pathologic basis of disease,* ed 4, Philadelphia, 1989, WB Saunders.

52. Craighead JE: The epidemiology and pathogenesis of malignant mesothelioma, *Chest* 96:92S, 1989.

53. Criqui MH et al: IgE and cardiovascular disease, *Am J Med* 82:964, 1987.

54. Criqui MH et al: Epidemiology of immunoglobulin E levels in a defined population, *Ann Allergy* 64:308, 1990.

55. Crofton J: Tobacco and the third world, *Thorax* 45:164, 1990.

56. Cushing SD et al: Minimally modified low density lipoprotein induces monocyte chemotactic protein I in human endothelial cells and smooth muscle cells, *Proc Natl Acad Sci USA* 87:5134, 1990.

57. Daniell HW: Replacement treatment of hypothyroidism, *N Engl J Med* 291:202, 1982.
58. Davie EW, Fujikawa K, Kisiel W: The coagulation cascade: initiation, maintenance and regulation, *Biochemistry* 30:10363, 1991.
59. Davison G, Duffy M: Smoking habits of long term survivors of surgery for lung cancer, *Thorax* 37:331, 1982.
60. Dawber TR: *The Framingham Study. The epidemiology of atherosclerotic disease,* Cambridge, Mass, 1980, Harvard University Press.
61. DeKesel M et al: Cloning and expression of portion of the 34-kilodalton protein gene of mycobacterium paratuberculosis: its application to serological analysis of John's disease, *J Clin Microbiol* 31:947, 1993.
62. Denburg J et al: Hypersensitivity to tobacco glycoprotein in human peripheral vascular disease, *Ann Allergy* 47:8, 1981.
63. Dinarello CA: Interleukin-1 and interleukin-1 antagonism, *Blood* 77:1627, 1991.
64. Doll R, Avery Jones F, Pygott F: Effect of smoking on the production and maintenance of gastric and duodenal ulcers, *Lancet* 1:657, 1958.
65. Dube MF, Green CR: Methods of collection of smoke for analytical purposes, *Recent Adv Tobacco Sci* 8:42, 1982.
66. Endoh K, Kauffman GL Jr, Leung FW: Mechanisms of aggravation of mucosal injury by intravenous nicotine in rat stomach, *Am J Physiol* 261 *(Gastrointest Liver Physiol* 24):G1037, 1991.
67. Ericsson U-B, Lindgarde F: Effects of cigarette smoking on thyroid function and the prevalence of goitre, thyrotoxicosis, and autoimmune thyroiditis, *J Int Med* 229:67, 1991.
68. Evans DB, Bunning RA, Russell RG: The effects of recombinant IL-1 beta on cellular proliferation, and the production of PGE, plasminogen activator, osteocalcin and alkaline phosphatase by osteoblast-like cells derived from human bone, *Biochem Biophys Res Commun* 166:208, 1990.
69. Facchini FS et al: Insulin resistance and cigarette smoking, *Lancet* 339:1128, 1992.
70. Falcone DJ, McCaffrey TA, Vergillio J: Stimulation of macrophage urokinase expression by polyanions is protein kinase C–dependent and requires protein and RNA synthesis, *J Biochem* 33:22726, 1991.
71. Finn, R: John Bostock, hay fever, and the mechanisms of allergy, *Lancet* 340(8833):1453, 1992.
72. Fiore MC: Trends in cigarette smoking in the United States, *Med Clin North Am* 76:289, 1992.
73. Fitch FW et al: Differential regulation of murine T lymphocyte subsets, *Annu Rev Immunol* 11:29, 1993.
74. Flores C et al: A subtype of nicotinic cholinergic receptor in rat brain is composed of α4 and β2 subunits and is up-regulated by chronic nicotine treatment, *Mol Pharmacol* 41:31, 1992.
75. Francus T, Siskind GW, Becker CG: The role of antigen structure in the regulation of IgE isotype expression, *Proc Natl Acad Sci* 80:3430, 1983.
76. Francus T et al: IL-1, IL-6 and PDGF mRNA expression in alveolar cells following stimulation with a tobacco-derived antigen, *Cell Immunol* 145:156, 1992.
77. Francus T et al: Two peaks of IL-1 expression in human leukocytes cultured with tobacco glycoprotein, *J Exp Med* 170:327, 1989.
78. Galli SJ: New concepts about the mast cell, *N Engl J Med* 328:257, 1993.
79. Garfinkel L, Boffetta P: Association between smoking and leukemia in two American Cancer Society prospective studies, *Cancer* 65:2356, 1990.
80. Gitel SN, Stephenson RC, Wessler S: The activated Factor X-Antithrombin III reaction rate: a measure of the increased thrombotic tendency induced by estrogen-containing oral contraceptives in rabbits, *Haemostasis* 7:10, 1978.
81. Gitel SN, Wessler S: Do natural estrogens pose an increased risk of thrombosis in postmenopausal women, *Thromb Res* 13:279, 1978.
82. Glantz SA, Parmley WW: Passive smoking and heart disease, *Circulation* 83:1, 1991.
83. Goldman L, Cook F: The decline in ischemic heart disease mortality rates. An analysis of the comparative effects of medical interventions and changes in lifestyle, *Ann Intern Med* 101:825, 1984.
84. Haley NJ, Axelrad CM, Tilton KA: Validation of self-reported smoking behavior: biochemical analyses of cotinine and thiocyanate, *Am J Public Health* 93:1204, 1983.
85. Haley NJ, Sepkovic DW, Hoffmann D: Elimination of cotinine from body fluids: disposition in smokers and nonsmokers, *Am J Public Health* 79:1046, 1989.
86. Harkavy J, Hebald S, Silbert S: Tobacco sensitiveness in thrombangiitis obliterans, *Proc Soc Exp Biol Med* 30:104, 1932.
87. Havsteen B: Flavonoids, a class of natural products of high pharmacological potency, *Biochem Pharmacol* 32:1141, 1985.
88. *The health benefits of smoking cessation.* US Department of Health and Human Services, Centers for Chronic Disease Prevention and Health Promotion, Office on Smoking and Health, 1990.
89. *The health consequences of smoking: nicotine addiction. A report of the Surgeon General,* DHHS (CDC), Washington, DC, 1988.
90. Health Program Office of Technology Assessment: *Smoking related deaths and financial costs.* Washington, DC, 1989, US Government Printing Office.
91. Heinemann S et al: The nicotinic receptor genes, *Clin Neuropharmacol* 14:s45, 1991.
92. Higgins M, Thom T: Trends in CHD in the United States, *Int J Epidemiol* 18:S58, 1989.
93. Hirayama T: A large-scale cohort study on risk factors for primary liver cancer with special reference to the role of cigarette smoking, *Cancer Chemother Pharmacol* 23:114, 1989.
93a. Hoffmann D, Hecht SS: Perspectives in cancer research. Nicotine-derived *N*-nitrosamines and tobacco-related cancer: current status and future directions, *Cancer Res* 45:935, 1985.
94. Hoffmann D, Wynder EL: Chemical constituents and bioactivity of tobacco smoke, *IARC Sci Publ* 74:145, 1986.
95. Hoffmann D et al: Model studies in tobacco carcinogenesis with the Syrian golden hamster, *Prog Exp Tumor Res* 24:370, 1979.
96. Hunt WA, Barnett LW: Relapse rates in addiction programs, *J Clin Psychol* 27:455, 1971.
97. Idle JR: Is environmental carcinogenesis modulated by host polymorphism, *Mutat Res* 247:259, 1991.
98. International Agency for Research on Cancer: *IARC monographs on the evaluation of the carcinogenic risk of chemicals to humans,* International Agency for Research on Cancer, Lyon, France, 1986.
99. International Agency for Research on Cancer: *IARC monographs on the evaluation of the carcinogenic risk of chemicals to humans. Tobacco smoking. Biological data relevant to the evaluation of carcinogenic risk to humans,* Lyon, France, 1986, IARC.
100. Jackson JH et al: Role of oxidants in DNA damage: hydroxyl radial mediates the synergistic DNA damaging effects of asbestos and cigarette smoke, *J Clin Invest* 80, 1987.
101. Janoff A: Emphysema: proteinase-antiproteinase imbalance. In Gallin J, et al, editors: *Inflammation: basic principles and clinical correlations,* New York, 1987, Raven Press.
102. Jick H, Walker AM: Letter, *N Engl J Med* 308:1476, 1983.
103. Kannel WB, Higgins M: Smoking and hypertension as predictors of cardiovascular risk in population studies, *J Hyperten* 8:S3, 1990.
104. Kew RR, Ghebrehiwet B, Janoff A: Cigarette smoke can activate the alternative pathway of complement in vitro by modifying the third component of complement, *J Clin Invest* 75:1000, 1985.
105. Kew RR, Ghebrehiwet B, Janoff A: Characterization of the third component of complement after activation by cigarette smoke, *Clin Immunol Immunopathol* 44:248, 1987.

106. Kew RR, Janoff A, Ghebrehiwet B: Cleavage of the third component of complement (C3) in lung fluids after acute cigarette smoke inhalation, *Am Rev Respir Dis* 127:154, 1983 (abstract).

107. Khoury MJ et al: Familial aggregation in chronic obstructive pulmonary disease: use of log linear model to analyze intermediate environmental and genetic risk factors, *Gen Epidemiol* 2:155, 1985.

108. Kikkawa Y: Diverse role of pulmonary cytochrome P-450 monooxygenase, *Lab Invest* 67:535, 1992.

109. Klesges RC et al: Smoking status: effects on the dietary intake, physical activity, and body fat of adult men, *Am J Clin Nutr* 51:784, 1990.

110. Konig A, Muhlbauer RC, Fleisch H: Tumor necrosis factor and interleukin-1 stimulate bone resorption in vivo as measured by 3-H tetracycline excretion from prelabeled mice, *J Bone Min Res* 3:621, 1988.

111. Korman MG et al: Influence of cigarette smoking on healing and relapse in duodenal ulcer disease, *Gastroenterology* 85:871, 1983.

112. Krall EA, Dawson-Hughes B: Smoking and bone loss among postmenopausal women, *J Bone Min Res* 6:331, 1991.

113. Kugiyama K et al: Impairment of endothelium-dependent arterial relaxation by lysolecithin in modified low density lipoprotein, *Nature* 344:160, 1990.

114. Kuller LH et al: The epidemiology of pulmonary function and COPD mortality in multiple risk factor intervention trial, *Am Rev Respir Dis* 140:S76, 1989.

115. Lane MR, Lee SP: Recurrence of duodenal ulcer after medical treatment, *Lancet* 1:1147, 1988.

116. Lehr H-A et al: Cigarette smoke elicits leukocyte adhesion to endothelium in hamsters: inhibition by CuZn-SOD, *Free Rad Biol Med* 14:573, 1993.

117. Lehr H-A et al: Stimulation of leukocyte/endothelium interaction by oxidized low-density lipoprotein in hairless mice. Involvement of CD11b/CD18 adhesion receptor complex, *Lab Invest* 68:388, 1993.

118. Lehrer SB, Wilson MR, Selvaggio JE: Immunologic properties of tobacco smoke, *J Allergy Clin Immunol* 62:368, 1978.

119. Lehtovirta P, Forss M: The acute effect of smoking on intervillous blood flow of the placenta, *Br J Obstet Gynaecol* 85:729, 1978.

120. Lesko SM et al: Cigarette smoking and the risk of endometrial cancer, *N Engl J Med* 313:593, 1985.

121. Leung DYM, Pober JS, Cotran RS: Expression of endothelial-leukocyte adhesion molecule-1 in elicited late phase allergic reactions, *J Clin Invest* 87:1805, 1991.

122. Levi R: Cardiac anaphylaxis: models, mediators, mechanisms and clinical considerations. In Marone G et al, editors: *Human inflammatory disease,* Toronto, 1988, BC Decker.

123. Levi R et al: Cardiac and pulmonary anaphylaxis in guinea pigs and rabbits induced by glycoprotein isolated from tobacco leaves and cigarette smoke condensate, *Am J Pathol* 106:318, 1982.

124. Li H et al: An atherogenic diet rapidly induces VCAM-1, a cytokine-regulatable mononuclear leukocyte adhesion molecule, in rabbit aortic endothelium, *Arterioscler Thromb* 13:197, 1993.

125. Lindberg E, Jarnerot G, Huitfeldt B: Smoking in Crohn's disease: effect on localization and clinical course, *Gut* 33:179, 1992.

126. Lindberg F et al: Smoking and inflammatory bowel disease. A case control study, *Gut* 29:352, 1988.

127. Linet MS, et al: Is cigarette smoking a risk factor for non-Hodgkin's lymphoma or multiple myeloma? Results from the Lutheran Brotherhood Cohort Study, *Leuk Res* 16:621, 1992.

128. Marks MJ, Stitzel JA, Collins AC: Time course study of the effects of chronic nicotine infusion on drug response and brain receptors, *J Pharmacol Exp Ther* 235:619, 1985.

129. Marks MJ et al: Nicotine-induced tolerance and receptor changes in four mouse strains, *J Pharmacol Exp Ther* 237:809, 1986.

130. Maron DJ, Fortmann SP: Nicotine yield and measures of cigarette smoke exposure in a larger population: are lower yield cigarettes safer? *Am J Public Health* 77:546, 1987.

131. McBride PE: The health consequences of smoking: cardiovascular diseases, *Med Clin North Am* 76:333, 1992.

132. McKinlay SM, Bifano NL, McKinlay JB: Smoking and age at menopause in women, *Ann Intern Med* 103:350, 1985.

133. McLemore TL: Expression of CYP1A1 gene in patients with cancer: evidence for cigarette smoke-induced gene expression in normal lung tissue and for altered gene regulation in primary pulmonary carcinomas, *J Natl Cancer Inst* 82:1333, 1990.

134. Meade TW, Imeson J, Stirling Y: Effects of changes in smoking and other characteristics on clotting factors and the risk of ischaemic heart disease, *Lancet* 2:986, 1987.

135. Michnovicz JJ et al: Increased 2-hydroxylation of estradiol as a possible mechanism for the anti-estrogenic effect of smoking, *N Engl J Med* 315:1305, 1986.

136. Michnovicz JJ et al: Cigarette smoking alters hepatic estrogen metabolism in men: implication for atherosclerosis, *Metabolism* 38:537, 1989.

137. Middleton E Jr, Kandaswami C: Effects of flavonoids on immune and inflammatory cell functions, *Biochem Pharmacol* 43:1167, 1992.

138. Mitchell EA, et al: Smoking and the sudden infant death syndrome, *Pediatrics* 91:893, 1993.

139. Modline RL, Nutman TB: Type 2 cytokines and negative immune regulation in human infections, *Curr Opin Immunol* 5:511, 1993.

140. Mole S, Waterman P: Stimulatory effects of tannins and cholic acid on trypic hydrolysis of proteins: ecological implications, *J Chem Ecol* 11:1323, 1985.

141. Nachman RL: Thrombosis and atherogenesis: molecular connections, *Blood* 79:1897, 1992.

142. Naeye RL: Abruptio placentae and placenta previa: frequency, perinatal mortality, and cigarette smoking, *Obstet Gynecol* 55:701, 1981.

143. Naeye RL: Sudden infant death syndrome, is the confusion ending, *Mod Pathol* 1:169, 1988.

144. Naeye RL: *Disorders of the placenta, fetus, and neonate,* St. Louis, 1992, Mosby-Year Book.

145. Newcomb PA, Carbone PP: The health consequences of smoking, *Med Clin North Am* 76:305, 1992.

146. Nieman RB et al: The effect of cigarette smoking on the development of AIDS in HIV-1-seropositive individuals, *AIDS* 7:705, 1993.

147. Norman V: An overview of the vapor phase, semivolatile and nonvolatile components of cigarette smoke. *Recent Adv Tobacco Sci* 3:28, 1977.

148. Noronha-Dutra AA, Epperlein MM, Woolf N: Effect of cigarette smoking on cultured human endothelial cells, *Cardiovasc Res* 27:774, 1993.

149. Nowak J et al: Biochemical evidence of a chronic abnormality in platelet and vascular function in healthy individuals who smoke cigarettes, *Circulation* 76:6, 1987.

150. O'Connor GT, Sparrow D, Weiss ST: The role of allergy and nonspecific airway hyperresponsiveness in the pathogenesis of chronic obstructive pulmonary disease, *Am Rev Respir Dis* 140:225, 1989.

151. Parkes JL et al: Cultured human atherosclerotic plaque smooth muscle cells retain transforming potential and display enhanced expression of the myc protooncogene, *Am J Pathol* 138:765, 1991.

151a. Parthasarathy S, Steinberg D, Witztum JL: The role of oxidized low-density lipoproteins in the pathogenesis of atherosclerosis, *Ann Rev Med* 43:219, 1992.

152. Penn A, Hubbard FC Jr, Parkes JL: Transforming potential is detectable in arteriosclerotic plaques of young animals, *Arterioscler Thromb* 11:1053, 1991.

153. Penn A, Snyder CA: Inhalation of sidestream cigarette smoke ac-

celerates development of arteriosclerotic plaques, *Circulation* 1993 (in press).

154. Penn A et al: Transforming gene in human atherosclerotic plaque DNA, *Proc Natl Acad Sci USA* 83:7951, 1986.

155. Perera F: Perspectives on the risk assessment for nongenotoxic carcinogens and tumor promoters, *Environ Health Perspect* 94:231, 1991.

156. Perera FP, Boffetta P, Nisbet ICT: *What are the major carcinogens in the etiology of human cancer?, Important Adv Oncol* 249-265, 1991.

157. Perera F et al: *Macromolecular adducts and related biomarkers in biomonitoring and epidemiology of complex exposures,* Lyon, France, 1990, International Agency for Research on Cancer.

158. Perera F et al: Molecular epidemiology and cancer prevention, *Cancer Detect Prev* 14:639, 1990.

159. Perera FP et al: Detection of polycyclic aromatic hydrocarbon-DNA adducts in white blood cells of foundry workers, *Cancer Res* 48:2288, 1988.

160. Perkins KA et al: The effect of nicotine on energy expenditure using light physical activity, *N Engl J Med* 320:898, 1989.

161. Perkins KA et al: Acute effects of nicotine on resting metabolic rate in cigarette smokers, *Am J Clin Nutr* 50:545, 1989.

162. Persson P-G, Ahlbom A, Hellers G: Inflammatory bowel disease and tobacco smoke–a case-control study, *Gut* 31:1377, 1990.

163. Peterson WL: Helicobacter pylori and peptic ulcer disease, *N Engl J Med* 324:1043, 1991.

164. Peto R, Doll R: The control of lung cancer, *New Scientist* 105:26, 1985.

165. Peto R et al: Mortality from tobacco in developed countries: indirect estimation from national vital statistics, *Lancet* 339(8804):1268, 1992.

166. Petti DB et al: Risk of cardiovascular disease in women. Smoking, oral contraceptives, noncontraceptive estrogen, and other factors, *JAMA* 242:1150, 1979.

167. Pittilo RM: *Cigarette smoking and endothelial injury: a review.* In Diane JN, editor: *Tobacco smoking and atherosclerosis in advances in experimental medicine and biology,* New York, 1989, Plenum, pp 61-78.

168. Pober JS, Cotran RS: Cytokines and endothelial biology, *Physiol Rev* 70:427, 1990.

169. Pomerleau OF et al: Neuroendocrine reactivity to nicotine in smokers, *Psychopharmacology* 81:61, 1983.

170. Prager KH et al: Smoking and drinking behavior before and during pregnancy of married mothers of liveborn infants and stillborn infants, *Pub Health Rep* 99:117, 1984.

171. Reilly JJ, Chapman HA Jr: Association between alveolar macrophage plasminogen activator activity and indices of lung function in young cigarette smokers, *Am Rev Respir Dis* 138:1422, 1988.

172. Rohrbach MS et al: *Plant polyphenols,* New York, 1992, Plenum Press.

173. Rosevear SK et al: Smoking and decreased fertilization rates in vitro, *Lancet* 340(8829):1195, 1992.

174. Ross R: The pathogenesis of atherosclerosis: a perspective for the 1990's, *Nature* 362:801, 1993.

175. Rovelstad RA: The incompetent pyloric sphincter, *Am J Dig Dis* 21:165, 1976.

176. Sakagami H et al: Stimulation of monocyte iodination and IL-1 production by tannins and related compounds, *Anticancer Res* 12:377, 1992.

177. Salonen J et al: Autoantibody against oxidized LDL and progression of carotid atherosclerosis, *Lancet* 339(8798):883, 1992.

178. Santella RM: Cigarette smoking related polycyclic aromatic hydrocarbon-DNA adducts in peripheral mononuclear cells, *Carcinogenesis* 13:2041, 1992.

179. Schleimer RP et al: IL-4 induces adherence of human eosinophils and basophils but not neutrophils to endothelium, *J Immunol* 148:1086, 1992.

180. Schoendorf KC, Kiely JL: Relationship of sudden infant death syndrome to maternal smoking during and after pregnancy, *Pediatrics* 90:905, 1992.

181. Seeman E et al: Risk factors for spinal osteoporosis in men, *Am J Med* 75:977, 1983.

182. Seyler LE et al: Pituitary hormone response to cigarette smoking, *Pharmacol Biochem Behav* 24:159, 1986.

183. Sherman CB: Health effects of cigarette smoking, *Clin Chest Med* 12:643, 1991.

184. Shopland DR, Eyre HJ, Pechacek TF: Smoking-attributable cancer mortality in 1991: is lung cancer now the leading cause of death among smokers in the United States?, *J Natl Cancer Inst* 83:1142, 1991.

185. Smith CJ et al: Environmental tobacco smoke: current assessment and future directions, *Toxicol Pathol* 20:289, 1992.

186. Sontag S et al: Cimetidine, cigarette smoking, and recurrence of duodenal ulcer, *N Engl J Med* 311:689, 1984.

187. Springer TA: Adhesion receptors of the immune system, *Nature* 346:425, 1990.

188. Stebbins KR: Transnational tobacco companies and health in underdeveloped countries: recommendations for avoiding a smoking epidemic, *Soc Sci Med* 30:227, 1990.

189. Strong JP, Oatman MC: *Effects of smoking on the cardiovascular system, Cardiovascular Clinics* 20 (3):205, 1990

190. Sytkowski PA, Kannel WB, D'Agostino RB: Changes in risk factors and the decline in mortality from cardiovascular disease. The Framingham Heart Study, *N Engl J Med* 322:1635, 1990.

191. Tellez M, Cooper J, Edmonds C: Graves' ophthalmopathy in relation to cigarette smoking and ethnic origin, *Clin Endocrinol* 36:291, 1992.

192. Tobin MF et al: Cigarette smoking and inflammatory bowel disease, *Gastroenterology* 93:316, 1987.

193. Totti N et al: Nicotine is chemotactic for neutrophiles and enhances neutrophil responses to chemotactic peptides, *Science* 223:169, 1984.

194. U.S. Department of Health and Human Services, Public Health Service, Centers for Disease Control, Center for Chronic Disease Prevention and Health Promotion, Office of Smoking and Health: *Reducing the health consequences of smoking: 25 years of progress.* A report of the Surgeon General, DHHS Publication No. (CDC) 89-8411, 1989.

195. Vollmer WM et al: Relationship between serum IgE and cross-sectional and longitudinal FEV in two cohort studies, *Chest* 90:416, 1986.

196. Wagenknecht LE et al: Racial differences in serum cotinine levels among smokers in the coronary artery risk development in (young) adults study, *Am J Public Health* 80:1053, 1990.

197. Ware JA, Heistad DD: Seminars in medicine of the Beth Isreal Hospital, Boston. Platelet-endothelium interactions, *N Engl J Med* 328:628, 1993.

198. Weisburger JH: Nutritional approach to cancer prevention with emphasis on vitamins, antioxidants, and carotenoids, *Am J Clin Nutr* 53:226S, 1991.

199. Weiss ST et al: The health effects of involuntary smoking, *Am Rev Respir Dis* 128:933, 1982.

200. Wells A: An estimate of adult mortality in the United States from passive smoking, *Environ Int* 14:249, 1988.

201. Werler MM, Pober B, Holmes LB: Smoking and pregnancy, *Teratology* 32:473, 1985.

202. Wessler S et al: Estrogen-containing oral contraceptive agents. A basis for their thrombogenicity, *JAMA* 236:2179, 1976.

203. White JR, Froeb HF: Small-airways dysfunction in nonsmokers chronically exposed to tobacco smoke, *N Engl J Med* 302:720, 1980.

204. Willett WC et al: Relative and absolute excess risks of coronary heart disease among women who smoke cigarettes, *N Engl J Med* 317:1303, 1987.

205. Winders SE, Grunberg NE: Nicotine, tobacco smoke, and body weight: a review of the animal literature, *Ann Behav Med* 11:125, 1989.

206. Worldwide use of smoking tobacco. *IARC Monographs on the Evaluation of Carcinogenic Risk of Chemicals to Humans* 38:47, 1986.

207. Wright JL, Churg A: Effect of long-term cigarette smoke exposure on pulmonary vascular structure and function in the guinea pig, *Exp Lung Res* 17:997, 1991.

208. Wright SC et al: Nicotine inhibition of apoptosis suggests a role in tumor promotion, *FASEB J* 7:1045, 1993.

209. Wynder EL, Hoffman D: *Tobacco and tobacco smoke: studies in experimental carcinogenesis,* New York, 1967, Academic Press.

210. Anonymous, Years of life lost from cardiovascular disease, *MMWR* 35:653, 1986.

211. Zini JM, Schmaier AH, Cines DB: Bradykinin regulates the expression of kininogen binding sites on endothelial cells, *Blood* 81:2936, 1993.

Chapter 14

ALCOHOL ABUSE

Emanuel Rubin

If an environmental disease is defined as a disorder resulting from an exposure to a physical or chemical hazard present predominantly in food, water, or air, then alcoholism in the Western world may well be the most widespread environmental disease. It is estimated that 12 to 14 million persons in the United States abuse alcohol, or about 10% of the population are at risk. Roughly one quarter of all hospital admissions in the United States record some alcohol-related problem, and the addiction is estimated to cost American society about $130 billion a year. Diseases associated with excess alcohol consumption are entirely avoidable because the amounts of naturally occurring ethanol in foods other than alcoholic beverages are trivial. Attempts to prohibit the consumption of alcoholic beverages, however, have been uniformly unsuccessful except for societies in which reli-

gious strictures against alcohol consumption are taken seriously, for example, certain fundamentalist Moslem countries. It is, therefore, likely that attempts to control other forms of environmental pollution, such as chemical carcinogens, radioactive materials, and air pollutants, will succeed more quickly than exhortations for temperance in the use of alcoholic beverages or outright prohibition.

Most environmental hazards are associated with specific disorders. For example, ionizing radiation and chemical carcinogens cause cancer, occupational dusts are associated with pneumoconioses, and excess salt aggravates hypertension in susceptible persons. Tobacco, which causes a variety of cancers, lung disease, and ischemic heart disease, is a special case because it is composed of a myriad of compounds and pyrolysis products. By contrast, excess exposure to ethanol, a simple two-carbon alcohol, leads to a bewildering variety of diseases that involve many systems and organs (see box on next page).

Although the criteria for the diagnosis of alcoholism are inexact, there are few subtleties when the physician is confronted with a person who consumes large amounts of alcoholic beverages every day, is often inebriated, and suffers withdrawal symptoms when deprived of alcohol. As in the case of many environmental toxins, individual susceptibility to the deleterious effects of ethanol vary widely. As a rule of thumb, however, the consumption of more than 1 g/kg body weight per day of ethanol probably places at least some persons at risk for organ damage. For a 70-kg man, this amount of alcohol corresponds to 7 ounces of 86-proof whiskey, about seven 3-ounce glasses of red wine, or six 12-ounce bottles of beer. Popular folklore to the contrary notwithstanding, there is no evidence that the type of alcoholic beverage is important, and only its content of ethanol needs to be considered.

The underlying mechanisms for ethanol-induced tissue

This work was supported in part by National Institute of Alcohol Abuse and Alcoholism (NIAAA) grants AA7186 and AA7215.

injury remain obscure, despite a wealth of experimental studies and a plethora of theories. We briefly review the most important and widespread medical consequences of alcoholism and describe some of the contemporary theories.

CENTRAL NERVOUS SYSTEM EFFECTS

Most environmental toxins affect people who are passively exposed, but alcohol is avidly consumed by many for its effects on the central nervous system. The acute effects vary directly with the blood alcohol concentration. In persons who are abstainers or occasional drinkers, blood levels up to 100 mg/dl lead to euphoria and signs of mild incoordination.[66] Between 100 and 200 mg/dl, incoordination becomes more pronounced and the inebriated person becomes ataxic. With higher blood alcohol concentrations, confusion and stupor supervene, and above 300 mg/dl many persons become comatose. At concentrations above 400 mg/dl, deep anesthesia is the rule, and death from respiratory failure is common.

The situation is somewhat different in habitual drinkers because such persons exhibit central nervous system (CNS) tolerance to the effects of alcohol. In other words, at any given blood alcohol concentration, the alcoholic displays a lesser effect than the casual drinker. In persons addicted to alcohol, blood alcohol concentrations up to 700 mg/dl are encountered by medical examiners in cases of drunken driving, and concentrations as high as 1200 mg/dl have been reported.

Although a single bout of alcohol intoxication does not cause permanent injury to the brain, chronic alcohol abuse is associated with a number of degenerative conditions. These disorders, however, are mostly associated with nutritional deficiencies; a direct toxic effect of alcohol that leads to permanent damage of the central nervous system has yet to be proved. Whether these nutritional deficits are caused by inadequate intake of nutrients, by ethanol-induced malabsorption, or both, is probably variable from person to person.[26,27,41]

Diseases associated with chronic alcoholism

Nervous system
NUTRITIONAL DISEASES
  Wernicke-Korsakoff disease
  Alcoholic cerebellar degeneration
  Optic neuropathy
  Peripheral neuropathy
UNKNOWN PATHOGENESIS
  Alcoholic dementia
  Cerebral atrophy
  Central pontine myelinolysis
  Marchiafava-Bignami syndrome

Liver
  Steatosis (fatty liver)
  Alcoholic hepatitis
  Cirrhosis
  Secondary iron overload

Gastrointestinal tract
ESOPHAGUS
  Peptic esophagitis
  Esophageal varices (portal hypertension)
  Mallory-Weiss syndrome
STOMACH
  Erosive gastritis
  Chronic nonerosive gastritis
  Peptic ulcer (especially with cirrhosis)
SMALL INTESTINE
  Malabsorption
RECTUM
  Anorectal varices (portal hypertension)
PANCREAS
  Acute pancreatitis
  Chronic calcifying pancreatitis

Cardiovascular system
  Alcoholic cardiomyopathy
  Hypertension

Muscle
  Alcoholic myopathy

Blood
  Megaloblastic anemia (nutritional)
  Thrombocytopenia
  Splenomegaly (portal hypertension)
  Pancytopenia (hypersplenism)

Bone
  Osteoporosis
  Aseptic necrosis of the femur

Endocrine system
MEN
  Hypogonadism
  Feminization
  Pseudo-Cushing syndrome
WOMEN
  Amenorrhea
  Anovulation
  Luteal phase dysfunction

Fetal Alcohol Syndrome

The Wernicke-Korsakoff syndrome, which is attributed to thiamine deficiency, is probably the most well-known of the CNS disorders associated with chronic alcoholism.[28,109] Wernicke's encephalopathy refers to the triad of ophthalmoplegia, ataxia, and disturbances of consciousness and cognition. Korsakoff's psychosis describes a particularly severe loss of memory in a person who is otherwise alert.[110] These conditions are usually found together and both respond dramatically to the administration of thiamine, although recovery may not be complete.

The most dramatic pathological lesions in Wernicke-Korsakoff syndrome are found in the mamillary bodies, periaqueductal gray matter, inferior and superior colliculi, fornices, and the floor of the fourth ventricle. The most severe lesions exhibit necrosis of most elements, whereas milder lesions show only destruction of neuronal cell bodies and axon cylinders, together with reactive gliosis. Advanced lesions are often hemorrhagic.

Degeneration of the cerebellar cortex is common in alcoholics and is reflected in ataxia of gait and incoordination of the arms. Alcoholic cerebellar degeneration is also associated with thiamine deficiency and is often found in conjunction with Wernicke-Korsakoff syndrome. The cerebellar cortex displays a loss of Purkinje cells, with concomitant reactive gliosis. In advanced disease, nerve cells are lost in the granular layer of the cerebellum, and the molecular layer is thinned. Gross examination of the brain reveals atrophy of the anterior and superior portions of the vermis and anterior lobes.

Central pontine myelinolysis refers to potentially fatal spastic bulbar paralysis and quadriplegia in severely ill alcoholics. The disease is characterized pathologically by a large focus of demyelination in the pons. The condition is thought to be caused by an excessively rapid correction of hyponatremia and can be demonstrated experimentally.

Cerebral atrophy, characterized by enlargement of the ventricles and sulci, is not uncommon among alcoholics.[8,29,108] Cerebral atrophy in alcoholics, however, has not been sufficiently differentiated from Wernicke-Korsakoff syndrome, concurrent Alzheimer's disease, and a number of complex medical conditions associated with alcoholism. It is clear that the subject requires further study.

Other rare diseases associated with alcoholism include nutritional optic neuropathy (alcoholic amblyopia) and a primary degeneration of the corpus callosum (Marchiafava-Bignami disease), which is of unknown origin.

ALCOHOLIC LIVER DISEASE

Liver disease is the most common fatal complication of chronic alcoholism, and cirrhosis of the liver remains one of the major causes of death in regions where alcohol is freely consumed. The spectrum of alcoholic liver disease has traditionally been categorized as fatty liver, alcoholic hepatitis, and cirrhosis, although the three conditions often overlap.

Excess ethanol consumption almost invariably results in the accumulation of hepatic triglycerides,[83] with resulting hepatomegaly. Microscopic examination reveals that the cytoplasm of the hepatocytes is distended by fat and that the nucleus is displaced to one pole of the cell. Little inflammation is present. Hepatic steatosis (fatty liver) is entirely reversible on the discontinuation of alcohol intake, and there is no evidence that fat per se is injurious to the hepatocyte. Factors that promote the accumulation of fat within the hepatocyte include an increased reducing power within the cytoplasm (increased NADH/NAD ratio [nicotinamide-adenine dinucleotide (reduced form)-to-nicotinamide-adenine dinucleotide]), depressed mitochondrial oxidation of fatty acids and decreased synthesis and excretion of lipoproteins.[82]

Some patients with fatty liver develop a far more dangerous and potentially lethal complication termed alcoholic hepatitis. This disorder features fever, malaise, right upper quadrant pain, jaundice, and leukocytosis. On microscopic examination, the liver displays steatosis, necrosis of hepatocytes particularly in the centrilobular zones, Mallory's alcoholic hyalin, numerous polymorphonuclear leukocytes, and expanded portal tracts, which contain mononuclear and polymorphonuclear leukocytes. On discontinuation of alcohol intake, the disease regresses in most cases, although some patients progress to cirrhosis and 10% to 20% die during the acute phase. In those who survive and continue to drink, many eventually develop extensive fibrosis and cirrhosis.

The final stage of alcoholic liver disease is cirrhosis, characterized by the formation of well-developed collagenous septa and regenerative nodules. With continued ethanol consumption, alcoholic cirrhosis leads to the complications of portal hypertension (ruptured esophageal varices, ascites) or hepatic failure, or both. Interestingly, patients with alcoholic cirrhosis who have not experienced the extrahepatic complications of that disease may look forward to a near-normal life expectancy if they abstain from the consumption of alcohol.

As is the case for many diseases associated with alcoholism, the pathogenesis of alcoholic cirrhosis is obscure. At one time it was fashionable to ascribe the development of cirrhosis to nutritional deficiencies, based on experiments with choline deficiency in the rat. A fatty liver and characteristic ultrastructural changes, however, have been produced by alcohol in well-nourished human volunteers fed adequate diets,[59] and cirrhosis has similarly been produced experimentally by feeding alcohol to baboons.[84] In human alcoholics, evidence has been presented that the incidence of cirrhosis varies directly with the total lifetime dose of ethanol.[55]

ALCOHOLIC PANCREATITIS

Acute and chronic pancreatitis are common occurrences among chronic alcoholics. In fact, alcoholism is considered to be the major cause of pancreatitis in men and second only to gallbladder disease in women. Typically the affected person experiences the sudden onset of unremitting, severe abdominal pain, which radiates to the back. In severe cases, shock ensues. The mortality rate is as high as 30%. The attack lasts anywhere from 2 days to a month, and recurrences are not infrequent. In many patients, destruction of pancreatic tissue leads to chronic pancreatitis, in which destruction of acinar and islet tissue causes malabsorption and diabetes. Some patients suffer from the insidious onset of chronic pancreatitis and do not report any acute episodes.

The pathogenesis of both acute and chronic pancreatitis in general has been controversial for the better part of a century. The major theories have related pancreatitis to obstruction of the pancreatic duct by gallstones, to spasm of the sphincter of Oddi with reflux of bile into the pancreatic duct, to secretion of pancreatic juice against an obstruction (gallstone or a spasm of the sphincter of Oddi), or to an obstruction of small ducts and ductules in the pancreas by proteinaceous plugs.[87] There is evidence for and against all of these theories, and none has been definitively proved. Regardless, all forms of pancreatitis seem to be characterized by the inappropriate activation of proenzymes within the pancreas, where they digest the protein and lipid constituents of the cells.

ALCOHOLIC CARDIOMYOPATHY

Cardiomyopathy is defined as an intrinsic degenerative disease of the myocardium in persons without occlusive coronary disease. In many instances, cardiomyopathy occurs without known cause, and in some cases antecedent viral infections or exposure to drugs or toxins can be identified. Based on epidemiological studies, however, chronic alcoholism is thought to cause more cardiomyopathy in Western industrialized countries than all other causes combined. At one time, congestive heart failure (CHF) in alcoholics was attributed to thiamine deficiency (beriberi), but this theory was abandoned after it was demonstrated that the condition did not respond to thiamine administration.[80] As many as one third of chronic alcoholics have lower-than-normal ejection fractions, and the extent of myocardial damage is directly related to the total lifetime dose of ethanol.[107] Alcohol actually appears to be toxic to all striated muscle, reflected clinically in acute and chronic alcoholic myopathy.[72,106]

The symptoms associated with alcoholic cardiomyopathy are not specific and are similar to those associated with other forms of dilated or congestive cardiomyopathy. Typically the malady remains asymptomatic for years, even in the presence of hypertrophy and dilatation of the left ventricle. The onset of CHF is often sudden. When the patient undergoes cardiac catheterization, an increased left ventricular end-diastolic pressure and a decreased ejection fraction are usually observed. There is no specific treatment for alcoholic cardiomyopathy, and the prognosis depends princi-

pally on the duration of symptoms, the severity of heart disease when it is discovered, and the readiness of the patient to abstain from alcohol.

On gross examination, the heart of the male alcoholic who dies from cardiomyopathy is enlarged, weighing between 400 and 900 g. All chambers of the heart are dilated, and grossly visible scars may be present in both ventricles. Microscopic examination reveals, subendocardial scarring and, often, occasional interstitial inflammatory cell infiltrates. Scattered foci of necrotic myocytes may be present. Variable degrees of hypertrophy and atrophy of myocytes are invariable features of alcoholic cardiomyopathy.

The pathogenesis of alcoholic cardiomyopathy is not understood, and research has been hampered by the lack of a suitable experimental model. Acutely, ethanol depresses cardiac contractility, although enhanced catecholamine release in the intact animal may mask this effect.[39,65,77,79] Using the isolated, perfused rat heart[23,61,88] and isolated muscle preparations in vitro,[23,25,31,50] ethanol in concentrations frequently encountered in the circulation of alcoholics and occasional drinkers interferes with the contractile activity of cardiac muscle. Potential loci of ethanol action on excitation-contraction coupling that have been suggested include (1) the ion channels that generate the action potential,[23,25,47,114] (2) calcium flux between the sarcoplasmic reticulum and the cytosol,[70,78,98,102] and (3) the calcium-dependent activation of contractile proteins.[74]

Fisher rats fed ethanol chronically for 8 months exhibited profound remodeling of the myocardium and an increase in left ventricular diastolic volume.[9] Chronic ethanol feeding has been reported to result in a number of metabolic alterations of the heart, but whether any of these are related to cardiomyopathy is unknown. A consistent finding with perfused hearts from rats chronically fed ethanol is that the positive inotropic responses to beta-adrenergic stimulation are reduced.[9,11] In the absence of an adequate experimental model, the relationship of the acute reversible effects of ethanol to eventual necrosis of cardiac myocytes, if any, remains obscure.

FETAL ALCOHOL SYNDROME

The effects of maternal alcohol abuse on the developing fetus have been recognized for only several decades.[56,92] The full-blown syndrome encompasses (1) growth retardation; (2) neurological abnormalities, including microcephaly, brain malformations, and mental retardation; and (3) facial dysmorphology. These features represent the severe end of the spectrum, and there is reason to believe that more subtle changes exist in the offspring of alcoholic mothers, such as cognitive and emotional defects.[96,97] In fact, it has been proposed that maternal alcohol abuse is the most common form of preventable mental retardation in Western societies.[13] Half of children born with fetal alcohol syndrome have IQ (intelligence quotient) scores below 70, and the

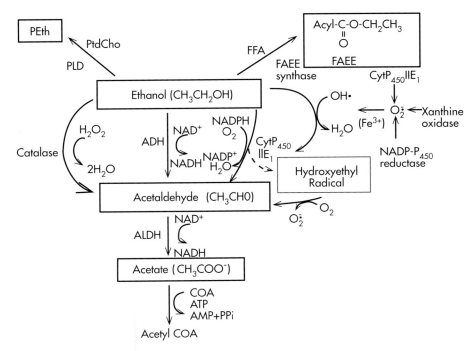

Fig.14-1. The metabolism of ethanol and the production of potentially harmful metabolites. *PEth,* Phosphatidylethanol; *PLD,* phospholipase D; *Ptd Cho,* phosphatidylcholine; *FFA,* free fatty acids; *FAEE,* fatty acid ethyl esters; *Cyt* cytochrome; *ADH,* alcohol dehydrogenase; *NAD$^+$,* nicotinamide-adenine dinucleotide (oxidized form); *NADH,* nicotinamide-adenine dinucleotide (reduced form) *NADPH* nicotinamide-adenine dinucleotide phosphate (reduced form); *NADP$^+$,* nicotinamide-adenine dinucleotide phosphate (oxidized form); *ALDH,* aldehyde dehydrogenase; *CoA,* coenzyme A; *ATP,* adenosine triphosphate; *AMP,* adenosine monophosphate; *PPi,* inorganic pyrophosphate.

mean IQ is 70.[1] Cardiac anomalies,[1] skeletal defects, and urogenital anomalies[1,76,93] are also occasionally encountered (see Chapters 30 and 34).

PATHOGENETIC MECHANISMS OF ETHANOL-INDUCED TISSUE INJURY

Despite at least a half century of serious attempts to unravel the basis of organ and tissue injury found in alcoholics, the underlying mechanisms have not been elucidated. A wide range of biochemical effects at the cellular level have been demonstrated in experimental models of acute and chronic alcohol intoxication, but an adequate experimental model for ethanol-induced irreversible tissue injury remains elusive. To date, the structural and functional changes observed experimentally after acute and chronic ethanol exposure are reversible on discontinuation of ethanol, and it has yet to be proved that any of them are directly related to cell necrosis. It is intuitively reasonable, however, to assume that chronic injury follows repeated acute injuries and that the former eventually leads to necrosis and irreversible damage.

Given the fact that chronic alcoholics suffer injury to many organs, it may be assumed that the basic molecular mechanisms responsible for injury are unique to each organ, depending on its differentiation and the presence or absence of ethanol metabolism. A more parsimonious theory holds that ethanol likely produces the same alterations in all cells, but that each organ responds differently according to its structure and function. The merits of these approaches are still controversial. A few of the major theories, a number of which involve the metabolism of ethanol (Fig. 14-1), are summarized in subsequent paragraphs.

Altered redox state

The oxidation of ethanol by alcohol dehydrogenase, and of its primary metabolite acetaldehyde by aldehyde dehydrogenase, is accomplished by the transfer of H$^+$ to NAD. As a result, the NADH to NAD ratio in the cytosol, a measure of reducing capacity, is increased. Reducing equivalents are then delivered to the mitochondria via biochemical shuttles, after which they are oxidized by the respiratory chain. The increased NADH in the mitochondria, derived from the cytosol and from the oxidation of acetaldehyde by mitochondrial aldehyde dehydrogenase, leads to inhibition of beta-oxidation of fatty acids and of the Krebs cycle.[10] The increased NADH also produces an increase in glycerol-3-phosphate, which presumably results in the accumulation of triacylglycerol.

Hypoxia

It has been proposed that chronic ethanol ingestion causes a relative hypoxia of the centrilobular zones of the liver,[42] owing to narrowing of the sinusoids by hepatocytes enlarged with water and fat. Hypoxia is thought to aggravate the shift in the redox state of the liver cells, particularly in the centrilobular zones.[72] The shift in the redox state, however, is conspicuously attenuated after chronic ethanol consumption, and its importance in the pathogenesis of irreversible liver injury remains to be determined.

Ethanol and free radical formation

More than 25 years ago, the acute administration of ethanol was reported to induce lipid peroxidation in the liver;[14,17] however, these observations became mired in controversy. More recently, attention has again been focused on lipid peroxidation caused by the generation of free radicals during the metabolism of ethanol.[16,19,69] Free radicals have been produced in vitro by microsomal oxidation of ethanol via the inducible P-450 isoform CYP2E1. Activated oxygen species can also be theoretically generated during ethanol metabolism by the activities of aldehyde oxidase and xanthine oxidase[67,89,90,95] and the mitochondrial respiratory chain.[69] The formation of superoxide anions,[7,18] hydroxyl radicals,[16,49] and hydrogen peroxide[58,103] has been reported to be increased after chronic ethanol intoxication.

Lipid peroxidation induced by ethanol would presumably be enhanced by a lack of antioxidant defenses in the liver cell. Chronic ethanol feeding has been reported to decrease hepatic GSH (reduced glutathione) levels in rats,[91] pigs,[121] and baboons.[60] When alcohol is fed to rats together with a diet deficient in vitamin E, hepatic levels of this antioxidant vitamin fell,[48] and chronic alcoholics are reported to have reduced plasma levels of vitamin E.[3,63,99,112] The theories that invoke hypoxia and lipid peroxidation in the pathogenesis of alcoholic liver injury intersect because experimental hypoxia augments lipid peroxidation,* presumably via the conversion of xanthine dehydrogenase to xanthine oxidase, the latter producing free radicals through the oxidation of acetaldehyde[57,117] (see Chapters 17 and 21).

Acetaldehyde-protein adducts

The primary metabolite of ethanol oxidation is acetaldehyde, a highly reactive compound that is rapidly converted to acetate by aldehyde dehydrogenase. Although circulating levels of acetaldehyde are negligible (<1 μM), this metabolite is present in higher quantities in hepatocytes, the principle site of ethanol oxidation. It has been proposed that the covalent binding of acetaldehyde to proteins may underly the pathogenesis of alcoholic liver injury.[45,94] Acetaldehyde has been shown to bind to proteins via unstable and stable adducts.[104] Lysine residues are particularly sus-

ceptible to forming adducts with acetaldehyde, and proteins that are rich in reactive lysine residues, e.g., alpha-tubulin, may be particularly affected. In vitro the covalent binding of acetaldehyde has been demonstrated to inhibit the catalytic activity of lysine-dependent enzymes.[64] Acetaldehyde has also been shown to cross-link membrane proteins[21] and to inhibit the activity of calmodulin.[46] In addition acetaldehyde-protein adducts have been reported to elicit antibody production,[43] and antibodies directed against acetaldehyde-protein adducts have been detected in human alcoholics.* Such studies have suggested that the covalent binding of acetaldehyde proteins may stimulate an immune response. Indeed, it has been shown that lymphocytes from patients with alcoholic liver disease are cytotoxic for hepatocytes in vitro.[44,73] Thus the hypothesis that alcoholic liver injury is, in a way, an autoimmune disease has a basis in experimental studies.[105]

Phosphatidylethanol

The plasma membranes of many cell types contain phospholipase D (*PLD*), an enzyme that is coupled to a G protein and is activated by the occupation of certain receptors by appropriate ligands.[4,5] The control of receptor-PLD coupling is not entirely understood, but there are several potential sites of interaction between ethanol and this signal transduction system.[35] A number of short-chain alcohols can act as alternate substrates to water during PLD-mediated hydrolysis of the phospholipid head group, thereby leading to the formation of the corresponding phosphatidyl alcohol. When ethanol is the substrate, the product is the unusual phospholipid, phosphatidylethanol (*PEth*). Compared with its rate of synthesis, the degradation of PEth is slow, and 1% to 2% of the total phospholipid pool in cellular membranes can be composed of this abnormal phospholipid after prolonged ethanol exposure.

The effects of PEth accumulation on cellular function are still obscure. This compound is a negatively charged phospholipid, generated principally from positively charged phosphatidylcholine. Its accumulation may therefore affect the membrane surface charge. PEth also promotes the local formation of nonbilayer structures.[71] Its introduction into artificial lipid bilayers induces resistance to fluidization by ethanol.[71] If PEth accumulates preferentially in specific membranes or microdomains, its functional effects may be magnified.

Fatty acid ethyl esters

The fact that alcoholics suffer considerable disease in organs that do not metabolize ethanol, e.g., heart and pancreas, led to a search for nonoxidative ethanol metabolites.[53] Free fatty acids condense with ethanol to form fatty acid ethyl esters in a reaction mediated by several fatty acid ethyl ester syntheses, which exhibit properties of glutathi-

*References 20,90,91,117-119.

*References 37,43,68,115,116.

one S-transferases.[6] The fatty acid ethyl esters have been reported to decrease the respiratory rate of hepatic and cardiac mitochondria and to uncouple oxidative phosphorylation.[54] The following scenario has been suggested:[52] (1) Free fatty acids within the cell are released from their binding sites by esterification and become associated with mitochondrial membranes; (2) mitochondrial lipase then hydrolyzes the esters to free fatty acid; and (3) in turn the fatty acids, which are known to be injurious to mitochondria, damage the mitochondria. Fatty acid ethyl esters also have been demonstrated to exert a disordering effect on membranes, possibly influencing lipid-protein interactions. In vitro these esters inhibit protein synthesis in hepatoma cell cultures. Although conclusive evidence for a toxic role for fatty acid ethyl esters remains to be established, the possibility is intriguing.

ETHANOL AND SIGNAL TRANSDUCTION

Biological membranes in all tissues are targets for the action of ethanol, owing to its interaction with lipid membranes. Ethanol tends to decrease the molecular order of the phospholipid acyl chains,[100] a process that has been termed *fluidization*. The intercalation of ethanol in the membrane bilayer may change lipid-protein interactions, thereby affecting the activity of membrane-bound proteins. Such proteins include those involved in receptor-linked signal transduction, a mechanism for the transfer of messages that arrive at the cell membrane in the form of hormones or growth factors. There is substantial evidence that ethanol affects signal transduction processes at the level of the membrane in a manner unrelated to its oxidation.[35] The most intensively studied signal transduction systems that have been studied with respect to ethanol are the adenylyl cyclase cyclic adenosine monophosphate (cAMP) system and the phosphoinositide system.

Adenylyl cyclase (AdCyc)

AdCyc is a membrane-bound enzyme that generates cAMP in response to hormone receptor occupancy. In turn, cAMP activates protein kinase A, with the subsequent phosphorylation of intracellular proteins. Receptor-AdCyc coupling is mediated through the trimeric guanine nucleotide-binding protein G_s.

In a number of isolated cells and membrane preparations in vitro, ethanol has been demonstrated to activate AdCyc.[34,38] The locus of ethanol action involves a G protein because this stimulation is absent in Cyc⁻ mutant cells, which lack G_s.[75] The concentrations of ethanol required for AdCyc activation, however, are quite high compared with the levels found in human alcoholics, which is less than 100 mM. Studies of the effects of ethanol on hepatic cAMP levels in vivo have resulted in reports of both stimulatory[113] and inhibitory[51,111] actions. In view of the potential indirect effects of ethanol (e.g., on catecholamine levels), these studies are difficult to interpret. In contrast to neuronal

cells, ethanol does not increase cAMP levels in isolated hepatocytes at concentrations of up to 200 mM.[36,51,120] In most systems, ethanol enhances the maximal stimulation of G_s without a shift in the sensitivity to guanine nucleotides.[12,62,75] It has been suggested that ethanol enhances the efficiency of $alpha_s$ in stimulating AdCyc.[62,75] Because data derived from studies in different tissues are not consistent, it is possible that ethanol has multiple sites of action in stimulating AdCyc. Other membrane-fluidizing agents, e.g., benzyl alcohol, short-chain alcohols, and general anesthetics, also activate AdCyc,[34,40] and it is therefore possible that the membrane-fluidizing effects of ethanol may play a role. The correlations between the molecular order of membranes and AdCyc activity, however, are not simple; it is probable that effects other than those that involve changes in bulk fluidity are involved.

Phosphoinositide signaling system

In addition to the AdCyc/cAMP system, there is a major signal transduction system that couples hormone-receptor interaction to the activation of a specific phospholipase C (PLC). This enzyme cleaves phosphatidylinositol 4,5-bisphosphate (PIP_2) in the membrane to yield inositol 1,4,5-trisphosphate (INS-1,4,5-P_3) and diacylglycerol (DAG).[2] Calcium ion (Ca^{2+}) is released from intracellular storage sites by INS-1,4,5-P_3, thereby increasing the free Ca^{2+} concentration in the cytosol. In the other arm of the system, DAG activates protein kinase C.[2] The receptors that are specific to this system are coupled to a PIP_2-specific PLC through a G protein that is distinct from G_s.[101] This PLC-dependent system, in which phosphoinositides play a key role, is considerably more sensitive to ethanol than the AdCyc/cAMP system.

Studies of the phosphoinositide system in excitable cells have been contradictory, whereas those involving hepatocytes and other nonexcitable cells have been more consistent.[35] The addition of ethanol to hepatocytes in vitro activates PLC, as evidenced by a decrease in PIP_2 and a transient accumulation of INS-1,4,5-P_3 and other inositol phosphates.[30,36,86] The same is true for human platelets, pancreatic acini, alveolar macrophages, and turkey erythrocytes.[32,34] In isolated hepatocytes and other cells, ethanol, in the absence of other agonists, initiates the complete spectrum of responses associated with receptor-mediated stimulation of the phosphoinositide-linked signaling system. The activation of PLC by ethanol involves activation of the appropriate G protein.[81,85] There is evidence that ethanol stimulates the exchange of guanosine triphosphate for guanosine diphosphate bound to the alpha subunit, although the mechanism for this effect remains to be identified.[81] The effects of ethanol on the inositol phospholipid-dependent signaling system could be brought about by direct interactions of ethanol with individual protein components but might also result from more general modifications of the physical properties of the membrane bilayer. A linear correlation between PLC activation and the calculated membrane partition coefficients for a number of alcohols[85] suggests that an altered lipid environment may mediate the effects of ethanol. There are significant differences, however, between the actions of short-chain alcohols and the effects of a general anesthetic, such as halothane, on PLC, and other factors clearly must play a role. It appears that ethanol interacts with PLC-mediated signal transduction at various sites and that cells or membrane preparations may vary in the predominant locus of ethanol action and in their sensitivity to this compound. Owing to feedback inhibition by protein kinase C, and perhaps other mediators, both homologous and heterologous desensitization to ethanol have been described.[15,24,30,33]

SUMMARY

Chronic alcoholism is associated with a wide variety of diseases, including cirrhosis of the liver, CNS disorders, pancreatitis, and cardiomyopathy. It is not clear whether these effects reflect different pathogenetic mechanisms or whether ethanol affects all organs in the same way but that specific tissues respond according to their differentiation. Much current research is directed toward the role of ethanol metabolites and to the direct effects of ethanol on biological membranes. Both acute and chronic ethanol intoxication have significant effects on signal transduction. However, the importance of these perturbations in the pathogenesis of alcohol-related disease remains to be determined.

REFERENCES

1. Abel EL: *Fetal alcohol syndrome,* Oradell, NJ, 1990, Medical Economics Company.
2. Berridge MJ: Inositol trisphosphate and diacylglycerol: two interacting second messengers, *Annu Rev Biochem* 56:159,193, 1987.
3. Bjornehoe G-E et al: Some aspects of antioxidant status in blood from alcoholics, *Alcoholism Clin Exp Res* 12:806, 1988.
4. Bocckino SB, Wilson PB, Exton JH: Ca^{2+}-mobilizing hormones elicit phosphatidylethanol accumulation via phospholipase D activation, *FEBS Lett* 225:201, 1987.
5. Bocckino SB et al: Phosphatidate accumulation in hormone-treated hepatocytes via a phospholipase D mechanism, *J Biol Chem* 262:15309, 1987.
6. Bora PS, Spilburg CA, Lange LG: Identification of a satellite fatty acid ethyl ester synthase from human myocardium as a glutathione *S*-transferase, *J Clin Invest* 84:1942, 1989.
7. Boveris A et al: Increased chemiluminescence and superoxide production in the liver of chronically ethanol-treated rats, *Arch Biochem Biophys* 227:534, 1983.
8. Brewer C, Perrett L: Brain damage due to alcohol consumption: an air-encephalographic, psychometric and electroencephalographic study, *Br J Addict* 66:170, 1971.
9. Capasso JM et al: Left ventricular dysfunction induced by chronic alcohol ingestion in rats, *Am J Physiol* 261:H212, 1991.
10. Cederbaum AI et al: Effect of chronic ethanol ingestion on fatty acid oxidation by hepatic mitochondria, *J Biol Chem* 250:5122, 1974.
11. Chan TCK, Sutter MC: The effects of chronic ethanol consumption on cardiac functions in rats, *Can J Physiol Pharmacol* 60:777, 1982.
12. Chatelain P et al: Modulation by n-alkanols of rat cardiac adenylate cyclase activity, *J Membr Biol* 93:23, 1986.
13. Clarren SK, Smith DW: The fetal alcohol syndrome, *N Engl J Med* 298:1063, 1978.
14. Comporti M, Hartman A, Di Luzio NR: Effect of in vivo and in vitro ethanol administration on liver lipid peroxidation, *Lab Invest* 16:616, 1967.
15. Diamond I et al: Basal and adenosine receptor-stimulated levels of cAMP are reduced in lymphocytes in alcoholic patients, *Proc Natl Acad Sci USA* 84:1413, 1987.
16. Dicker E, Cederbaum AI: Hydroxyl radical generation by microsomes after chronic ethanol consumption, *Alcoholism Clin Exp Res* 11:309, 1987.
17. DiLuzio NR, Kalish GH: Enhanced peroxidation of lipid in the pathogenesis of acute ethanol-induced liver injury, *Gastroenterology* 50:392, 1966.
18. Ekstrom G, Ingelman-Sundberg M: Rat liver microsomal NADPH-supported oxidase activity and lipid peroxidation dependent on ethanol-inducible cytochrome P-450 (P-450IIE1), *Biochem Pharmacol* 38:1313, 1989.
19. French SW: *Nutritional factors in the pathogenesis of alcoholic liver disease.* In Watson RR, Watzl B, editors: *Nutrition and alcohol,* Ann Arbor, 1992, CRC Press, pp. 337-362.
20. French SW: Biochemistry of alcoholic liver disease, *Crit Rev Clin Lab Sci* 29:83, 1992.
21. Gaines KC et al: Reaction of acetaldehyde with human erythrocyte membrane proteins, *FEBS Lett* 75:115, 1977.
22. Gaja G et al: Phosphorylation and redox states in ischemic liver, *Exp Mol Pathol* 19:248, 1973.
23. Gimeno AL, Gimeno MD, Webb JL: Effects of ethanol on cellular membrane potentials and contractility of isolated rat atrium, *Am J Physiol* 203:194, 1962.
24. Gordon AS, Collier K, Diamond I: Ethanol regulation of adenosine receptor-stimulated cAMP levels in a cloned cell line: an in vitro model of cellular tolerance to ethanol, *Proc Natl Acad Sci USA* 83:2105, 1986.
25. Guarnieri T, Lakatta EG: Mechanism of myocardial contractile depression by clinical concentrations of ethanol, *J Clin Invest* 85:1462, 1990.
26. Halsted CH, Robles EA, Mezey E: Decreased jejunal uptake of labeled folic acid (^{3}H-PGA) in alcoholic patients: roles of alcohol and nutrition, *N Engl J Med* 285:701, 1971.
27. Halsted CH, Robles EA, Mezey E: Intestinal malabsorption in folate-deficient alcoholics, *Gastroenterology* 64:526, 1973.
28. Harper CG: The incidence of Wernicke's encephalopathy in Australia: a neuropathological study of 131 cases, *J Neurol Neurosurg Psychiatry* 46:593, 1983.
29. Haug JO: Pneumoencephalographic evidence of brain damage in chronic alcoholics: a preliminary report. In Retterrstol N, Magnussen F, editors: Report on the Fifteenth Congress of Scandinavian Psychiatrists in Geilo, Norway, 1967, *Acta Psychiatr Scand Suppl* 203:135, 1968.
30. Higashi K, Hoek JB: Ethanol causes desensitization of receptor-mediated phospholipase C activation in isolated hepatocytes, *J Biol Chem* 266:2178, 1991.
31. Hirota Y, Bing OHL, Abelmann WH: Effect of ethanol on contraction and relaxation of ioslated rat ventricular muscle, *J Mol Cell Cardiol* 8:727, 1976.
32. Hoek JB, Rubin E: Alcohol and membrane-associated signal transduction, *Alcohol Alcohol* 25:143, 1990.
33. Hoek JB, Rubin R, Thomas AP: Ethanol-induced phospholipase C activation is inhibited by phorbol esters in isolated hepatocytes, *Biochem J* 251:865, 1988.
34. Hoek JB, Taraschi TF, Rubin E: Functional implications of the interaction of ethanol with biologic membranes: actions of ethanol on hormonal signal transduction systems, *Semin Liver Dis* 8:36, 1988.

35. Hoek JB et al: Ethanol and signal transduction in the liver, *FASEB J* 6:2386, 1992.

36. Hoek JB et al: Ethanol-induced mobilization of calcium by activation of phosphoinositide-specific phospholipase C in intact hepatocytes, *J Biol Chem* 262:682, 1987.

37. Hoerner M et al: The role of alcoholism and liver disease in the appearance of serum antibodies against acetaldehyde adducts, *Hepatology* 8:569, 1988.

38. Hoffman PL, Tabakoff B: Ethanol and guanine nucleotide binding proteins: a selective interaction, *FASEB J* 4:2612, 1990.

39. Horwitz LD, Atkins JM: Acute effects of ethanol on left ventricular performance, *Circulation* 49:124, 1974.

40. Houslay MD, Gordon LM: The activity of adenylate cyclase is regulated by the nature of its lipid environment, *Curr Top Membr Transp* 18:179, 1983.

41. Hoyumpa AM: Mechanisms of vitamin deficiencies in alcoholism, *Alcoholism Clin Exp Res* 10:573, 1986.

42. Israel Y et al: Experimental alcohol-induced hepatic necrosis: suppression by propylthiouracil, *Proc Natl Acad Sci USA* 72:1137, 1975.

43. Israel Y et al: Monoclonal and polyclonal antibodies against acetaldehyde-containing epitopes in acetaldehyde-protein adducts, *Proc Natl Acad Sci USA* 83:7923, 1986.

44. Izumi N, Hasumura Y, Takeuchi J: Lymphocyte cytotoxicity for autologous human hepatocytes in alcoholic liver diseases, *Clin Exp Immunol* 53:219, 1983.

45. Jennett RB, Tuma DJ, Sorrell MF: *Effect of acetaldehyde on hepatic proteins.* In Popper H, Schafner F, editors: *Current progress in liver disease,* Philadelphia, 1990, WB Saunders, pp. 325-333.

46. Jennett RB et al: Increased covalent binding of acetaldehyde to calmodulin in the presence of calcium, *Life Sci* 45:1461, 1989.

47. Katz AM: Effects of ethanol on ion transport in muscle membranes, *FASEB J* 41:2456, 1982.

48. Kawase T, Kato S, Lieber CS: Lipid peroxidation and antioxidant defense systems in rat liver after chronic ethanol feeding, *Hepatology* 10:815, 1989.

49. Klein SM et al: Increased microsomal oxidation of hydroxyl radical scavenging agents and ethanol after chronic consumption of ethanol, *Arch Biochem Biophys* 223:425, 1983.

50. Kobayashi M, Furukawa Y, Chiba S: Effects of ethanol and acetyldehyde on the isolated blood-perfused canine atrium, *Arch Int Pharmacodyn Ther* 239:109, 1979.

51. Kuriyama K: Ethanol-induced changes in activities of adenylate cyclase, guanylate cyclase and cyclic adenosine 3′,5′-monophosphate dependent protein kinase in the brain and liver, *Drug Alcohol Depend* 2:335, 1977.

52. Lange LG: Mechanism of fatty acid ethyl ester formation and biological significance, *Ann NY Acad Sci* 625:802, 1991.

53. Lange LG, Bergmann SR, Sobel BE: Identification of fatty acid ethyl esters as products of rabbit myocardial ethanol metabolism, *J Biol Chem* 256:12968, 1981.

54. Lange LG, Sobel BE: Mitochondrial dysfunction induced by fatty acid ethyl esters, myocardial metabolites of ethanol, *J Clin Invest* 72:724, 1983.

55. Lelbach WK: Cirrhosis in the alcoholic and its relation to the volume of alcohol abuse, *Ann NY Acad Sci* 252:85, 1975.

56. Lemoine P et al: Les enfants de parents alcooliques: anomalies observees a propos de 127 cas (The children of alcoholic parents: anomalies observed in 127 cases) *Quest Medicale* 21:476, 1968.

57. Lewis KO, Paton A: Could superoxide cause cirrhosis? *Lancet* July 24:188, 1982.

58. Lieber CS, DeCarli LM: Hepatic microsomal ethanol-oxidizing stem: in vitro characteristics and adaptive properties in vivo, *J Biol Chem* 245:2505, 1970.

59. Lieber CS, Rubin E: Alcoholic fatty liver in man on a high protein and low fat diet, *N Engl J Med* 200:705, 1969.

60. Lieber CS, et al.: *S*-adenosyl-L-methionine attenuates alcohol-induced liver injury in the baboon, *Hepatology* 11:165, 1990.

61. Lochner A, Cowley R, Brink A: Effect of ethanol on metabolism and function of perfused rat heart, *Am Heart J* 78:770, 1969.

62. Luthin GR, Tabakoff B: Activation of adenylate cyclase by alcohol requires the nucleotide-binding protein, *J Pharmacol Exp Ther* 228:579, 1984.

63. Majumdar SK, Shaw GK, Thompson AD: Plasma vitamin E status in chronic alcoholic patients, *Drug Alcohol Depend* 12:269, 1983.

64. Mauch TJ et al: Covalent binding of acetaldehyde selectively inhibits the catalytic activity of lysine-dependent enzymes, *Hepatology* 6:263, 1986.

65. Mendoza L et al: The effect of intravenous ethyl alcohol on the coronary circulation and myocardial contractility of the human and canine heart, *J Clin Pharmacol* 11:165, 1971.

66. Miles WR: *Psychological effects of alcohol on man.* In Emerson H et al, editors: *Alcohol and man,* New York, 1932, Macmillan, p.224.

67. Muller A, Sies H: Role of alcohol dehydrogenase activity and of acetaldehyde in ethanol-induced ethane and pentane production by isolated perfused rat liver, *Biochem J* 206:153, 1982.

68. Niemala O et al: Antibodies against acetaldehyde-modified protein epitopes in human alcoholics, *Hepatology* 7:1210, 1987.

69. Nordmann R, Ribiere C, Rouach H: Implication of free radical mechanisms in ethanol-induced cellular injury, *Free Rad Biol Med* 12:219, 1992.

70. Ohnishi ST, Flick JL, Rubin E: Ethanol increases calcium permeability of heavy sarcoplasmic reticulum of skeletal muscle, *Arch Biochem Biophys* 233:588, 1984.

71. Omodeo-Sale F et al: Role of phosphatidylethanol in membranes. Effects on membrane fluidity, tolerance to ethanol, and activity of membrane-bound enzymes, *Biochemistry* 30:2477, 1991.

72. Perkoff GT et al: A spectrum of myopathy associated with alcoholism. I. Clinical and laboratory features, *Ann Intern Med* 67:481, 1967.

73. Poralla T et al: Cellular cytotoxicity against autologous hepatocytes in alcoholic liver diseases, *Liver* 4:117, 1984.

74. Puszkin S, Rubin E: Adenosine diphosphate effect on contractility of human muscle acytomyosin: inhibition by ethanol and acetaldehyde, *Science* 188:1319, 1975.

75. Rabin RA, Molinoff PB: Multiple sites of action of ethanol on adenylate cyclase, *J Pharmacol Exp Ther* 227:551, 1983.

76. Randall CL, Taylor WJ: Prenatal ethanol exposure in mice: teratogenic effects, *Teratology* 19:305, 1979.

77. Regan TJ et al: The acute metabolic and hemodynamic responses of the left ventricle to ethanol, *J Clin Invest* 45:270, 1966.

78. Retig JN et al: Effects of ethanol on calcium transport by microsomes phosphorylated by cyclic amp-dependent protein kinase, *Biochem Pharmacol* 26:393, 1977.

79. Riff D, Jain A, Doyle J: Acute hemodynamic effects of ethanol on normal human volunteers, *Am Heart J* 78:592, 1969.

80. Robin E, Goldschlager N: Persistence of low cardiac output after relief of high output by thiamine in a case of alcoholic beriberi and cardiac myopathy, *Am Heart J* 80:103, 1970.

81. Rooney TA et al: Short chain alcohols activate guanine nucleotide-dependent phosphoinositidase C in turkey erythrocyte membranes, *J Biol Chem* 264:6817, 1989.

82. Rubin E, Farber JL: *Pathology,* ed 1, Philadelphia, 1988, JB Lippincott, p. 757.

83. Rubin E, Lieber CS: Alcohol-induced hepatic injury in non-alcoholic volunteers, *N Engl J Med* 278:869, 1968.

84. Rubin E, Lieber CS: Fatty liver, alcoholic hepatitis and cirrhosis produced by alcohol in primates, *N Engl J Med* 290:128, 1974.

85. Rubin R, Hoek JB: Alcohol-induced stimulation of phospholipase C

in human platelets requires G-protein activation, *Biochem J* 254:147, 1988.

86. Rubin R, Hoek JB: Ethanol-induced stimulation of phosphoinositide turnover and calcium influx in isolated hepatocytes, *Biochem Pharmacol* 37:2461, 1989.

87. Sarles H et al: Observations of 205 confirmed cases of acute pancreatitis, recurring pancreatitis, and chronic pancreatitis, *Gut* 6:545, 1965.

88. Schulman SP et al: Contractile metabolic and electrophysiologic effects of ethanol in the isolated rat heart, *J Mol Cell Cardiol* 23:417, 1991.

89. Shaw S: Lipid peroxidation, iron mobilization and radical generation induced by alcohol, *Free Rad Biol Med* 7:541, 1989.

90. Shaw S, Jayatilleke E: Acetaldehyde-mediated hepatic lipid peroxidation: role of superoxide and ferritin, *Biochem Biophys Res Commun* 143:984, 1987.

91. Shaw S et al: Ethanol-induced lipid peroxidation: potentiation by long-term alcohol feeding and attenuation by methionine, *J Lab Clin Med* 98:417, 1981.

92. Sokol RJ, Clarren SK: Guidelines for use of terminology describing the impact of prenatal alcohol on the offspring, *Alcoholism Clin Exp Res* 13:597, 1989.

93. Sokol RJ, Miller SI, Reed G: Alcohol abuse during pregnancy: an epidemiologic study, *Alcoholism Clin Exp Res* 4:135, 1980.

94. Sorrell MF, Tuma DJ: Hypothesis: alcoholic liver injury and the covalent binding of acetaldehyde, *Alcoholism Clin Exp Res* 9:306, 1985.

95. Stege TE: Acetaldehyde-induced lipid peroxidation in isolated hepatocytes, *Res Commun Chem Pathol Pharmacol* 36:287, 1982.

96. Streissguth AP: *The behavioral teratology of alcohol: performance, behavioral and intellectual deficits in prenatally exposed children.* In West JR, editor: *Alcohol and brain development,* New York, 1986, Oxford University Press, pp. 3-44.

97. Streissguth AP et al: IQ at age four in relation to maternal alcohol use and smoking during pregnancy, *Devel Psychol* 25:3, 1989.

98. Swartz MH et al: Effects of ethanol on calcium binding and calcium uptake in cardiac microsomes, *Biochem Pharmacol* 23:2369, 1974.

99. Tanner AR et al: Depressed selenium and vitamin E levels in an alcoholic population: possible relationship to hepatic injury through increased lipid peroxidation, *Dig Dis Sci* 31:1307, 1986.

100. Taraschi TF, Rubin E: Effects of ethanol on the chemical and structural properties of biologic membranes, *Lab Invest* 52:120, 1985.

101. Taylor SJ et al: Activation of the β1 isozyme of phospholipase C by α subunits of the Gq class of G proteins, *Nature (London),* 350:516, 1991.

102. Thomas AP et al: Effects of ethanol and cocaine on electrically-triggered calcium transients in cardiac muscle cells, *Ann NY Acad Sci* 625:395, 1991.

103. Thurman RG: Induction of hepatic microsomal reduced nicotinamide adenine dinucleotide phosphate-dependent production of hydrogen peroxide by chronic prior treatment with ethanol, *Mol Pharmacol* 9:670, 1973.

104. Tuma DJ, Hoffmann T, Sorrell MF: The chemistry of acetaldehyde-protein adducts, *Alcohol Alcohol* 1(suppl):271, 1991.

105. Tuma DJ, Klassen LW: Immune responses to acetaldehyde-protein adducts: role in alcoholic liver disease, *Gastroenterology* 103:1969, 1992.

106. Urbano-Marquez A et al: On alcoholic myopathy, *Ann Neurol* 17:418, 1985.

107. Urbano-Marquez A et al: The effects of alcoholism on skeletal and cardiac muscle, *N Engl J Med* 320:409, 1989.

108. Victor M, Adams RD: *The alcoholic dementias.* In Vinken PJ, Bruyn GW, Klawans HL, editors: *Neurobehavioral disorders,* vol 2, Handbook of clinical neurology, Amsterdam, 1985, Elsevier Science Publishers, pp. 335-352.

109. Victor M, Laureno R: *The neurologic complications of alcohol abuse: epidemiologic aspects.* In Schoenberg BS, editor: *Neurological epidemiology: principles and clinical applications,* vol 19, Advances in neurology, New York, 1978, Raven Press, pp. 603-617.

110. Victor M, Yakovlev PI: S.S. Korsakoff's psychic disorder in conjunction with peripheral neuritis: a translation of Korsakoff's original article with brief comments on the author and his contribution to clinical medicine, *Neurology* 5:394, 1955.

111. Volicer L, Gold BI: Interactions of ethanol with cyclic AMP, *Adv Exp Med Biol,* 56:221, 1975.

112. Ward RJ et al: Nutritional selenium and alpha-tocopherol status of alcohol abusers with and without chronic skeletal muscle myopathy, *Adv Biosci* 71:93, 1988.

113. Whetton AD et al: Forskolin and ethanol both perturb the structure of liver plasma membranes and activate adenylate cyclase activity, *Biochem Pharmacol* 32:1601, 1983.

114. Williams ES, Mirro MJ, Bailey JC: Electrophysiological effects of ethanol, acetyldehyde, and acetate on cardiac tissues from dog and guinea pig, *Circ Res* 47:473, 1980.

115. Worrall S et al: Antibodies against acetaldehyde-modified epitopes: an elevated IgA response in alcoholics, *Eur J Clin Invest* 21:90, 1991.

116. Worrall S et al: Antibodies against acetaldehyde-modified epitopes: presence in alcoholic, non-alcoholic liver disease and control subjects, *Alcohol Alcohol* 25:509,1990.

117. Younes M, Strubelt O: Enhancement of ethanol-induced hepatotoxicity by hypoxia, *Adv Biosci* 71:165, 1988.

118. Younes M, Strubelt O: Enhancement of hypoxic liver damage by ethanol: involvement of xanthine oxidase and the role of glycolysis, *Biochem Pharmacol* 36:2973, 1987.

119. Younes M, Wagner H, Strubelt O: Enhancement of acute ethanol hepatotoxicity under conditions of low oxygen supply and ischemia/reperfusion. The role of oxygen radicals, *Biochem Pharmacol* 38:3573, 1989.

120. Zederman R, Low H, Hall K: Effect of ethanol and lactate on the basal and glucagon-activated cyclic AMP formation in isolated hepatocytes, *FEBS Lett* 75:291, 1977.

121. Zidenberg-Cherr S et al: The effect of chronic alcohol ingestion on free radical defense in the miniature pig, *J Nutr* 120:213, 1990.

Chapter 15

ILLICIT DRUG ABUSE

Charles V. Wetli

Any psychoactive drug or substance can, has been, or will be abused or, at the very least, misused. The distinction between abuse and misuse is not always clear. In general, however, misuse may be defined as the use of a licit or legal drug in an inappropriate fashion. Usually, this is manifest as an inappropriate indication for a drug or an inappropriate dose or dosage schedule. Drug abuse may occur with either licit or illicit drugs and refers to drug ingestion for the purpose of achieving an altered mental state that is either a secondary effect of the drug (e.g., ingestion of several capsules of propoxyphene) or in which significant mental or motor impairment results (e.g., with alcohol, a legal drug whose sole purpose is to provide an altered mental and physiological state).

An illicit drug may be defined as any substance prohibited or unauthorized by law or custom. Some drugs, such as heroin and marijuana, have been clearly banned by laws in the United States. Others, such as fentanyl and cocaine, have legitimate medical uses and are restricted in their use. What makes these drugs illegal is (by law and custom) their unauthorized manufacture and use. Hence, by law and custom, cocaine is a local anesthetic manufactured by licensed pharmaceutical firms with appropriate quality controls. When cocaine is manufactured in a South American jungle laboratory, smuggled into Europe or the United States, and primarily used for its euphoric effects, the drug becomes defined as illicit.

This chapter therefore addresses the pathological states resulting from the abuse of legally and customarily unsanctioned drugs. The resultant pathological changes depend on several factors: the acute toxic effects of the specific drug or drugs abused, the frequency and chronicity of use, the altered mental state produced in conjunction with environmental interaction, the route of administration, and the addictive propensity of the drug.

The modern criteria for addiction are (1) evidence of compulsive use (craving), (2) loss of control over consumption (to what extent will one go to obtain the substance), and (3) continued use despite any potential or realized consequences (social, economic, or medical).[10,44,60] The addictive propensity of a drug therefore contributes to the ultimate pathological changes in two ways. First, the constant craving drives a frequent consumption of the drug for prolonged periods. Second, efforts to obtain the drug itself, or funds to obtain the drug, often result in antisocial behavior (e.g., burglary, robbery, murder, prostitution), all of which may lead to a variety of injuries and diseases that become superimposed on the basic pathological changes of illicit drug abuse. Notable among these is the spread of penicillin-resistant gonorrhea and other venereal diseases. The medical and pathological consequences of drug abuse are therefore but a morphological expression of the disease of addiction.[60]

DEMOGRAPHICS

The types of illicit drugs that are abused vary widely from one region of the United States to another[15] and often depend on what is simply popular at a particular time.[19,21] By 1975, it was clear that heroin use had reached epidemic proportions throughout the United States. In the late 1960s, marijuana use was steadily increasing, and the trends for

259

cocaine abuse were unclear.[19] By the early 1990s, cocaine abuse had reached epidemic proportions. In the 1980s, marijuana use was beginning to decline,[21] and a resurgence in heroin use became evident.[17,28,53] In addition to drug availability and notions as to what is popular, social and racial factors become determinant factors. In 1989, the Drug Abuse Warning Network (DAWN) indicated that medical examiners nationwide reported 7162 drug abuse deaths.[21] One third of these decedents were black. Because blacks compose only 12% of the population of the United States, however, they are obviously disproportionately represented in these deaths. In the same report, it was noted that white high school seniors were more than twice as likely as black high school seniors to have ever tried cocaine. Yet blacks accounted for 46% of cocaine deaths in 1989.[21]

The 1991 National Household Survey on Drug Abuse has reported a steady decline in the past-month use of any illicit drug.[43] In 1979, the prevalence rate for past-month use of an illicit drug was approximately 14%, and this had dropped to 6.9% for major metropolitan areas by 1991. This, however, has not necessarily been the trend for emergency room mentions or drug-induced deaths.[20] DAWN reported in their 1989 series that emergency rooms recorded 153,650 drug abuse episodes.[41] The most frequently mentioned drugs were cocaine (61,665 mentions), alcohol-in-combination (46,735 mentions), heroin/morphine (20,566 mentions), and marijuana/hashish (9867 mentions). Nearly three fourths of the patients were between 20 and 40 years of age, and whites accounted for 40% of the emergency room episodes, blacks for 39%, and Hispanics for 11%. Cocaine, heroin, and phencyclidine (PCP) were reported more among black patients than either whites or Hispanics. DAWN reported there were 6601 drug abuse deaths in 1991.[42] Whites constituted 55% of these deaths, blacks 31%, and Hispanics 12%. Cocaine was mentioned in 46% of the drug-related deaths and heroin/morphine in 35%.

PATHOLOGICAL CHANGES BY ROUTE OF ADMINISTRATION

As summarized in Table 15-1, pathological changes arise because of the route of administration and the toxic or pharmacological actions of the drug itself. Thus the osteocartilaginous necrosis of the sinonasal region from snorting cocaine is thought to be the result of localized ischemia induced by the vasoconstrictive property of cocaine. Similarly, necrotizing sialometaplasia is thought to be due to cocaine-induced ischemia.[54]

Smoking of various drugs may, by their irritant effects, easily result in chronic bronchitis and hemoptysis. It must be remembered, however, that many abusers of illicit drugs also smoke cigarettes, which contributes to the clinical signs and symptoms. Intense Valsalva maneuvers while smoking marijuana or cocaine may lead to a pneumothorax or pneumomediastinum.[5,7]

Intravenous drug abusers generally dissolve the drug in

Table 15-1. Pathological changes resulting from drug abuse

Route of administration	Medical consequences
Nasal insufflation ("snorting")	Cocaine: erosions and perforation of nasal septum
Smoking	Marijuana: bronchitis, possible cancer
	Cocaine: hemoptysis, pneumothorax
Oral	Cocaine: necrotizing sialometaplasia, gastrointestinal bleeding
Intravenous	Systemic infections (viral hepatitis, malaria, AIDS), localized infections, (cellulitis, abscess) venous and perivenous scarring, necrotizing fasciitis, bacterial endocarditis, fungal cerebritis, pulmonary granulomas, hemopneumothorax (subclavian injection), vasospasm
Subcutaneous injection (skin popping)	Localized abscesses, necrotizing fasciitis

AIDS, Acquired immunodeficiency syndrome.

a small amount of water (usually ordinary tap water, but toilet water has also been used) in a "cooker" (bottle cap or spoon). The concoction is then heated with a match or lighter until dissolution of the powder takes place. If some particles do not dissolve, the addict may draw the mixture into a syringe through cotton or a cigarette filter attached to the end of the needle. The unhygienic nature of the intravenous drug abuser is compounded by the fact that the abuser often uses the same needle and syringe repeatedly. Between uses "the works" (syringe, cooker, tourniquet, needle) are stored in any convenient place (e.g., pockets, socks, purse). The most dangerous practice among intravenous drug abusers is the sharing of needles and syringes, thereby spreading diseases such as acquired immunodeficiency syndrome (AIDS), hepatitis, and malaria.

The subcutaneous injection of illicit drugs is a practice known as "skin popping." This is done by individuals who either do not want to bother with an intravenous injection or who would prefer to avoid the scars and needle marks on their arms and hands that are so obvious and typical for intravenous drug abuse. Initially, these individuals inject directly into the thigh or buttocks. The intensity of the euphoria in "skin popping" is not as great as with intravenous injection. Granulomas, abscesses, and scarring are typical among "skin poppers." Because the abscess is in an anaerobic environment, these individuals are predisposed to clostridial infections, which could lead to tetanus or gas gangrene.

PATHOLOGICAL CHANGES RELATED TO THE ABUSE OF INDIVIDUAL ILLICIT DRUGS
Heroin

Heroin was introduced into the United States in the early 1900s as a cough suppressant and, interestingly, as a cure for morphine addiction (which, of course, it is). When heroin was introduced into the United States, there were two major population groups addicted to opiates. One group was addicted to opiates iatrogenically, and the other group was the Chinese, who brought the practice of opium smoking to the United States. At that time, the Chinese were at the bottom of the socioeconomic scale, and they introduced opium smoking to those who would associate with them (e.g., prostitutes, thieves). Eventually the opium laws were passed and physicians began administering morphine more judiciously. Those addicted to morphine by their physicians began to die off, leaving the remaining opiate addicts to search for an opiate substitute. Heroin quickly became that substitute, and, by 1920, intravenous injection was the preferred route of administration of heroin. The early history of opiate addiction in the United States has been extensively reviewed by Courtwright[12] and the more recent history and contemporary usage patterns by Inciardi.[24]

Today, heroin (diacetylmorphine) is illegal in the United States except by special research license. Street heroin is actually a mixture of heroin, quinine, and a variety of sugars. The quinine imparts a bitter taste and thereby masks the quality (purity) of the product being sold. Allegedly, quinine was chosen as a diluent after World War II in an attempt to stop the spread of needle-transmitted malaria among the heroin addicts of New York City.

In 1972, a $5 packet of heroin contained an average of 3.4% anhydrous heroin (5.1 mg per bag).[13] Today, however, the heroin content varies widely, and samples for street sale have been as high as 80% pure and sell for $90 to $200 per gram.[57] Opium is grown and converted into heroin in a number of different countries, particularly Mexico, Southeast Asia (the famed "Golden Triangle" of heroin production), and now Colombia. The profit margins for the smugglers are tremendous. In 1981, the price for heroin outside the United States was $20,000/kg; this kilogram, once processed (diluted, or "cut") and sold on the streets, would gross $2 million.[51] Traditionally, Colombia has been known for its exports of cocaine. Heroin production however, has an even higher profit margin. In recent years, the Colombian National Police have seized several heroin laboratories and destroyed more than 2500 acres of poppy fields.[2] Also the morphine content of opium grown in Colombia is nearly 45% as compared with 18% to 33% in other heroin-producing countries.[2]

An acute heroin overdose may result from simply injecting a large amount of the drug or by injecting the usual amount of heroin after having gone through heroin withdrawal. Heroin addicts typically develop a high tolerance for the drug. Should they be forced to undergo withdrawal (e.g., when incarcerated), they lose that drug tolerance. An injection of the previously customary amount of heroin could then result in an overdose.

Generally an acute pharmacological overdose of heroin (or any narcotic) induces a massive acute pulmonary edema. Typically the victim has a prominent accumulation of a white, sometimes blood-tinged froth of pulmonary edema fluid over the nose and mouth. This is sometimes referred to as a "foam cone." At autopsy, the combined lung weights average more than 1000 g,[61] and the cut surfaces of the lungs are usually congested and spontaneously exude copious amounts of pulmonary edema fluid. Because the process forms so acutely, the edema fluid has little or no protein, and therefore the microscopic appearance is that of pulmonary congestion only. Sometimes, however, a neutrophilic exudate may be seen, and this may closely resemble bronchopneumonia.[61] Presumably, this finding occurs in those addicts whose death has been somewhat prolonged. When death occurs acutely, it is common to find the syringe resting on the forearm and the needle still in the antecubital vein (Fig. 15-1).

In the 1960s and early 1970s, at the height of the latest heroin epidemic in the United States, a number of excellent review articles appeared that described the medical complications and pathological changes from chronic intravenous narcotism.* Most of these medical complications are

*References 9, 22, 31, 32, 50, 61.

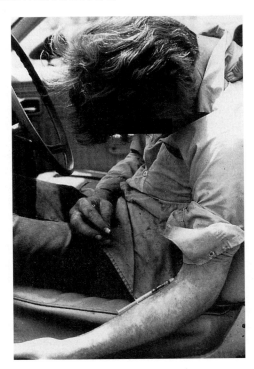

Fig. 15-1. In narcotic overdose, consciousness may be lost rapidly. In this case, the partially injected syringe and needle remains in place.

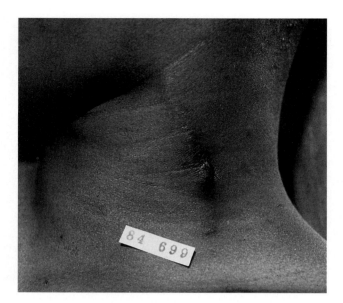

Fig. 15-2. The jugular vein may be used by heroin addicts when peripheral venous access is no longer possible. Perivenous scarring develops at this site as well. Injection into the jugular vein also poses the additional hazard of an inadvertent injection into the carotid artery, which may result in a temporary or permanent neurological deficit.

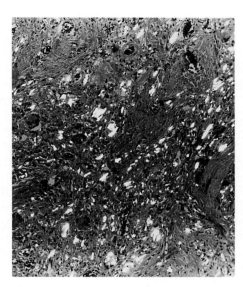

Fig. 15-3. Subcutaneous tissues in the heroin addict often contain optically active excipients and a foreign body granulomatous reaction. The white particles are excipients as seen with partially polarized light. (Hematoxylin and eosin, medium power.)

seen among intravenous heroin users today. Some, such as tetanus and malaria, would be quite unusual in the 1990s. Half of all hospitalized intravenous drug abusers who die of infections, however, actually have succumbed to the complications of AIDS.[26] This same study also revealed that chronic alcoholism contributed significantly to the deaths of these patients, and only 11% (of the 274 patients studied) died from drug overdose or drug-related organ abnormalities. Thus the pathology of heroin addiction is always modified by a variety of other systemic diseases, including chronic alcoholism in many cases.

Aside from the superimposed systemic diseases, the gross autopsy findings of intravenous heroin abusers are quite characteristic.[61] Externally, typical "track marks" of hypopigmented scars are usually seen over and around veins of the upper extremities. These look and feel like subcutaneous "ropes" of the backs of the hands, forearms, and antecubital fossae. Sometimes, similar changes may be seen involving the jugular vein (Fig. 15-2). Incising the areas of prior injection sites often discloses extensive perivenous scarring in the subcutaneous tissues. Freshly extravasated perivenous and subcutaneous blood marks the site of a fresh injection site. It is noteworthy that fresh injection sites may not be obvious externally, and "blind" incisions may be required for their detection. Internally, mild hepatosplenomegaly (which is usually not clinically apparent) is common. The cut surface of the liver, however, appears normal, whereas the cut surface of the spleen frequently re-

veals lymphoid hyperplasia.[61] On histological examination, the liver almost invariably has a portal infiltrate of lymphocytes and histiocytes ("triaditis"). The infiltrate may be quite dense, even to the point of germinal center formations.[61] One of the most characteristic, but not diagnostic, findings is a hyperplastic enlargement of lymph nodes in the porta hepatis and around the celiac axis. This nodal enlargement as well as the lymphoid hyperplasia of the spleen may be related to the immunological abnormalities frequently seen in heroin addicts.[64]

The perivenous scars so typical of the heroin addict are the result of excipients that have leaked into the subcutaneous tissue during an injection of street heroin.[30,61] Excipients are additives used in the manufacture of drugs (licit or illicit) intended for oral consumption. They may function as binders, lubricants, disintegrators, or fillers.[47] The two excipients that present the most trouble for the heroin addict are talc and starch.[47,61] The talc and starch may be added to dilute ("cut") the heroin as it is being prepared for street sales, or it may be added by the user who wishes to combine crushed oral medications to the heroin to achieve some euphoriant effect. Once the talc and starch are introduced into the subcutaneous tissues, they incite an inflammatory, often granulomatous response. The excipients cannot be destroyed, and the inflammatory process becomes chronic. Eventually scar tissue is formed, sometimes with deposits of hemosiderin. As this process is repeated over the next few years, the typical track marks of heroin

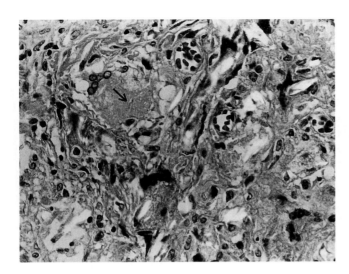

Fig. 15-4. The polarizable excipient may be intracellular *(arrow)* or extracellular *(white particles)*. (Skin, hematoxylin and eosin, high power, partial polarization.)

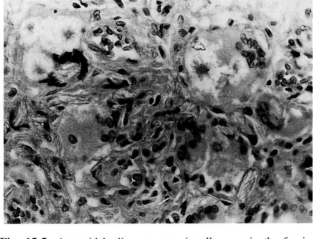

Fig. 15-5. Asteroid bodies are occasionally seen in the foreign body granulomas in the skin (or lung) of heroin addicts. (Skin, hematoxylin and eosin, high power.)

addiction appear. Microscopically, excipients are best visualized under polarized light as optically active extracellular and intracellular crystals in a foreign body granuloma (Figs. 15-3 and 15-4).[23,61] These foreign body granulomas also may contain rather striking asteroid bodies similar to those seen in the granulomas of sarcoidosis (Fig. 15-5).

In an attempt to strain out undissolved particles from the treated opiate mixture, the addict may draw the solution through cotton or a cigarette filter. These fibers, too, incite a foreign body granulomatous reaction.

The intravenously injected particles embolize to the lung, where they are trapped in the pulmonary capillary network. The trapped foreign particles then incite a granulomatous reaction just as in the skin. The identification of polarizable foreign particles in the lung and the presence of pulmonary foreign body granulomas are typical of the heroin addict. Other pulmonary complications related to these foreign particles include angiothrombosis and vascular changes suggestive of pulmonary hypertension.[29,55] Not all particles, however are trapped in the pulmonary capillaries, and therefore the polarizable material may be disseminated to other organs and even cause a systemic granulomatosis.[33,46]

A much less frequent cutaneous complication of the intravenous or subcutaneous infection of street heroin is the formation of prominent ulcers.[4,23,37] These develop at an injection site when not all of the syringe contents enter the vein. The area becomes edematous, a blister forms, and within 24 hours a necrotic nonsuppurative ulcer develops. Although these ulcers appear mostly on the extremities,[23,31,37] they can develop at any injection site, including the penis (from injecting in the dorsal vein of the penis).[4] The exact cause of the ulcers is not clear. Because

they sometimes appear a short distance away from the injection site, some have speculated on the presence of a caustic additive to the street heroin.[23,37]

Intravenous drug abusers clearly have a higher incidence of bacterial endocarditis than the population at large, and there is a distinct tendency for involvement of the tricuspid valve.[25] It is thought that valvular endothelial trauma results in the formation of small thrombi and therefore predisposes the addict to a subsequent infection of the valve. Although the source of the trauma has not been identified, one might conjecture that the insoluble particulate matter (e.g., excipients, cotton) injected along with the opiate concoction may be the offending agent. The source of the bacteria isolated from heroin addicts with bacterial endocarditis has also been the subject of speculation and research. One possible source for the bacteria is the heroin itself. At least two separate studies, however, have addressed this issue.[39,64] In short, about half the samples of street heroin yielded no microbial growth, and the remainder grew common, usually nonpathogenic organisms, especially *Bacillus* sp. and *Aspergillus* sp. Furthermore, none of the organisms cultured correlated with the usually polymicrobial infections seen in addicts in two different cities.[39] Also, heroin addicts are extremely unhygienic and therefore likely to get localized infections,[17,43] which, in turn, could infect a damaged heart valve. The most frequent organism associated with bacterial endocarditis in the heroin addict is *Staphylococcus aureus.* It has been shown that about one third of intravenous drug abusers are carriers of *S. aureus,* and the phage types matched those of organisms isolated from blood cultures of addicts with bacterial endocarditis.[56] Therefore the most likely sequence for the development of bacterial endocarditis in the heroin addict is bacterial seed-ing from the addict's own body (carrier or localized infection) of a thrombotic vegetation covering a damaged portion of heart valve. The vegetations tend to occur at the line of closure of the valve, again suggesting that foreign insoluble particles may be the cause of the initial endocardial damage.

Renal complications associated with heroin abuse are frequently secondary to other medical problems, such as bacterial endocarditis, rhabdomyolysis, or chronic skin infections (leading to renal amyloidosis). The development of a relentlessly progressive nephrotic syndrome in heroin addicts, however, has come to be called heroin-associated nephropathy (HAN).[25,45] The morphological features most often linked with HAN are focal segmental glomerulosclerosis and focal global sclerosis. The cause of HAN is uncertain but may well be immunological.[25,45]

Cocaine

Cocaine is an alkaloid derived from the leaves of *Erythroxylon coca,* a shrub grown primarily in South America. Chewing the leaves, a centuries-old practice of South American Indians, provides a mild stimulant effect and a feeling of increased energy along with a suppression of appetite. Coca tea, often served to tourists visiting a coca-growing area, has a similar effect.

When cocaine was first isolated from the coca leaves in the late 1800s, its pharmacological properties created much interest among medical professionals as well as the lay public. Considering the times, the discovery that cocaine was a true local anesthetic was sensational news. The drug could be used to soothe a teething baby and allow surgery on the eye and nasopharynx. It was even applied to the genitalia of young girls in an attempt to control the urge to masturbate.[12] Another property of cocaine, localized vasoconstriction, enhanced the surgical benefit of the anesthetic property because intraoperative bleeding was easily controlled. The stimulant effect of cocaine on the central nervous system, along with its mood-altering effects, attracted Sigmund Freud, who espoused its use in the treatment of mental disorders and morphine addiction. The stimulant property of cocaine also spawned the creation of extremely popular tonics sold to the general public, the most popular of which were Vin Mariani and Coca-Cola. Cocaine, used both medicinally and in commercial beverages, was also noted to produce a stimulant effect on the cardiovascular system, resulting in a usually mild elevation of heart rate and blood pressure. The interesting early history of cocaine has been the subject of several excellent reviews.[1,25,34]

Unfortunately, two other properties of cocaine were not appreciated at the turn of the century. One was that cocaine is a highly addictive drug (albeit without the physical withdrawal properties characteristic of opiates). The other was that the stimulant effects on the central nervous system and the cardiovascular system could result in severe, sudden, and unpredictable grand mal seizures; psychotic and behavioral abnormalities; and cardiovascular crises, all of which could be lethal. These dangers were finally realized in the early twentieth century, and the nonmedical use of cocaine was forbidden with the Harrison Narcotics Act of 1914.

Interest in the nonmedical use of cocaine was rekindled in the early 1970s as a result of an interest in recreational drug use by Americans in the 1960s. The existing scientific and medical data of 20 years ago provided nothing but anecdotal evidence from the turn of the century that cocaine might be a dangerous drug. Because there was no scientific evidence to the contrary, it was easy to regard cocaine as a safe, nonaddicting, short-lived stimulant. Also the drug did not have to be injected, was relatively scarce, and expensive (about $125 per gram). The drug quickly became popular with those who desired a safe recreational drug that was a stimulant and who could afford it. Therefore, in contrast to heroin, which initially became popular among those at the lower socioeconomic groups, cocaine was initially popular among the wealthier elite. As the drug became more available and prices dropped, however, the illicit use of cocaine spread to all socioeconomic groups in America and eventually Europe as well. This widespread, almost unrestricted, use of cocaine by an unsuspecting lay public quickly led to the recognition of the myriad of medical dangers from acute toxicity as well as the effects of chronic use. Unfortunately the realization of the medical dangers of cocaine did not occur until a great many individuals had already become addicted.

Results of administration. Cocaine hydrochloride is a water-soluble salt and is therefore readily absorbed from any mucosal surface. The vasoconstrictive effect of the drug, however, often inhibits complete absorption unless it is applied to a large surface area. Nasal ingestion (snorting) is perhaps the most common method of using cocaine hydrochloride. Lines of cocaine powder are made on a smooth surface and inhaled through a straw or through rolled paper currency with one end placed in the nose. The drug may also be snorted from various spoons or other implements created solely for that purpose. Cocaine hydrochloride is also quite readily absorbed from the gastrointestinal tract, although this route is generally used by those who swallow the drug to avoid police detection rather than for recreational purposes. Intravaginal application of cocaine, presumably for its local anesthetic and purported aphrodisiac effects, results in a rapid absorption into the blood. Naturally, water solubility also means the drug may be injected intravenously for a nearly instantaneous and intense reaction.

Cocaine hydrochloride is destroyed at its vaporization point of 200° C. By eliminating the hydrochloride part of the molecule, however, cocaine base is created, and this vaporizes at 98° C and can therefore be smoked. One method of doing this is to dissolve the cocaine hydrochloride in alkalinized water and extract the cocaine base with ether. The material obtained after evaporating the ether is usually referred to as freebase cocaine. This method of preparing cocaine is cumbersome and dangerous because of the volatility of the ether. The highly popular method used today simply requires an aqueous solution of cocaine hydrochloride and baking soda, which is heated. The water-insoluble base precipitates out and is referred to as rock or crack cocaine. Various base pipes have been created to inhale the fumes of the heated cocaine base. The simplest are fashioned from beverage cans (beer or soda) or from plastic vials and aluminum foil.

Cocaine and sudden death. In contrast to most drugs, cocaine does not have a fairly well-defined therapeutic and toxic range, and there is no approximate lethal dose or lethal blood level of cocaine.[52] Dose, route of administration, rapidity of absorption, and tolerance and reverse tolerance ("kindling") are factors determining the lethality of cocaine.[25] Kindling, or reverse tolerance, is a hyperaccentuated response to a low or usual dose of a drug. For example, repeated administration of a subconvulsant dose of a drug may eventually lead to convulsions. The phenomenon has been demonstrated in animals given repeated subconvulsant doses of cocaine. Kindling is also thought to play a role in fatal reactions to cocaine in humans, but this has not been proved.[25]

Sudden death from snorting or swallowing cocaine (usually to avoid police detection) is often preceded by the sudden onset of grand-mal seizures.[65] The seizures often occur about 20 to 30 minutes after the last line of cocaine has been snorted. The time lag may be the result of delayed absorption owing to the vasoconstriction caused by cocaine. The seizures may be of sudden onset or preceded by other signs of cocaine toxicity. These include hyperthermia, visual or tactile hallucinations, agitation, and photophobia (owing to mydriasis). Autopsy findings are generally those nonspecific signs seen in asphyxial deaths: petechiae of the epicardium and visceral pleura, pulmonary edema and congestion, and generalized visceral congestion. In addition, the preterminal seizures may result in bite marks (contusions or lacerations) of the tongue, lower lip, or inside of the cheek. Postmortem blood concentrations of cocaine are often high, about 5 mg/L.

Cocaine may also result in sudden death owing to intracranial hemorrhage.[25,36] This is presumably the result of cocaine-induced hypertension. Subarachnoid hemorrhage is usually due to the rupture of a saccular aneurysm, and intracerebral hemorrhage is often due to the rupture of an arteriovenous malformation. Basal ganglionic hemorrhage, typical for a hypertensive crisis, has also occurred. It is noteworthy that there are a number of instances of cocaine-induced intracranial hemorrhage in which no vascular abnormality is found. A cocaine-induced cerebral vasculitis, similar to that induced by amphetamines, has been proffered as a possible explanation for at least some of these cases.[25,36]

Ischemic strokes have also been associated with cocaine abuse.[36] The cerebral infarcts are often lacunar and may be located in the thalamus or rostral midbrain. Some are associated with small vessel occlusions. Possible mechanisms include vasculitis, altered perfusion, and vasospasm.[43]

Sudden cocaine-induced cardiac death may result from rhythm disturbances or myocardial ischemia.[18,25] The anesthetic effect of cocaine blocks sodium influx and potassium efflux, which in turn impair the cardiac conduction of electrical impulses. Furthermore, cocaine is associated with catecholamine release and also prevents the reuptake of catecholamines. Consequently, virtually any cardiac rhythm disturbance may result from the combined anesthetic and catecholamine effects of cocaine, particularly in high doses.[18] Because of the excess catecholamines, the fatal cocaine-induced cardiac dysrhythmia may be associated with contraction band necrosis or a mononuclear infiltrate (thought to be the result of prior microvascular damage).[18,25] The sudden death caused by myocardial ischemia and infarction has been linked to cocaine-induced coronary artery vasospasm even in the absence of coronary arteriosclerosis.[18]

Aortic dissections resulting in sudden death have also been associated with cocaine use.[18] Presumably this too is the result of a cocaine-induced hypertensive crisis.

Cocaine-induced excited delirium has been associated with sudden death, probably owing to a sudden cardiac rhythm disturbance.[62] The cocaine toxicity is manifested by bizarre, frequently violent and destructive behavior often accompanied by complete disrobing and hyperthermia (temperatures of 106° F or more have been recorded). Usually, several police officers are required to restrain the individual because of an unexpected increase in strength. Shortly after being restrained, the victim suddenly collapses and dies. Occasionally, paramedic rescue units may record residual electrical cardiac activity but no pulse. The only abnormalities seen at autopsy are injuries incurred during the melee. The injuries are usually not serious and most often are from struggling against handcuffs or ankle restraints. Postmortem concentrations of cocaine in the blood are generally less than 1 mg/L, and benzoylecgonine concentrations are often more than 1 mg/L. Should initial resuscitative attempts be successful, with death occurring 24 hours or more later, myoglobinuric nephrosis owing to rhabdomyolysis may be evident at autopsy.[48]

The paranoia that may accompany cocaine toxicity can lead to violent death, such as drowning or a fall from a building. In one instance, a small stove fire caused a paranoid cocaine user to cower in a closet, where he died from carbon monoxide poisoning.

Body packers or "mules" are individuals who ingest packets of cocaine to smuggle them into the United States.[63] The packets are made from condoms, fingers of latex gloves, thin hermetically sealed plastic, or a combination of these. Although the packets are usually swallowed (along with a constipating agent), they may be inserted into the vagina or rectum. The packets are usually evident radiographically, especially when gas seeps between the latex wrappings.[3] Death from cocaine toxicity occurs when a packet breaks open or when cocaine seeps out through the wrapping (i.e., by dialysis, especially when the packets are made from condoms or balloons). At autopsy, it is not unusual to remove a half kilogram of high-grade (about 90% purity) cocaine from throughout the gastrointestinal tract. An intense hyperemia may be seen where the cocaine has come into contact with the gastric or rectal mucosa. Body packers from Colombia have been encountered with heroin instead of cocaine.

Effects of chronic cocaine abuse. Perforations of the nasal septum are not uncommon among individuals who habitually snort cocaine. Proposed mechanisms include prolonged vasoconstriction and acidity produced by the hydrochloride part of the molecule.[38] Also, animal experiments have shown that cocaine is directly toxic to capillary endothelial cells and can induce coagulative necrosis.[6] The perforations may range from a few millimeters to complete dissolution of the entire nasal septum. Histologically the margins of the perforation have a typical coagulation necrosis. Similar mechanisms would also account for necrotizing gingivitis and sialometaplasia when cocaine is applied orally.[38]

Fresh intravenous injection sites are characterized by a puncture mark surrounded by a halo of normal-appearing skin, which in turn is surrounded by an ecchymotic zone.[38] Eventually the ecchymosis becomes diffuse and attains variegated colors before it disappears. Also, ecchymoses from several injection sites may coalesce. The chronic intravenous cocaine abuser eventually may develop flat atrophic scars along venous tracts. Because they are not usually injecting insoluble excipients, they do not develop the rope-like scars more typical of heroin addicts. Cutaneous ulcers, which eventually heal into round or atrophic scars, may also be seen among intravenous cocaine users. The mechanism is probably the same as that which produces nasal septal perforations in those who snort cocaine. These same scars, however, are sometimes seen in cocaine users where an injection is unlikely or virtually impossible (e.g., the back). The mechanism by which these form is obscure. One possibility is peripheral cutaneous vasoconstriction that inhibits blood flow and the healing process to foci of cutaneous infection.

Chronic necrotizing fasciitis, often accompanied by lymphedema, is occasionally observed among intravenous cocaine users. These frequently involve large areas and may eventuate in autoamputation.[38] Necrotizing fasciitis has also been reported in heroin addicts. A review of the literature, however, revealed that these addicts were also injecting cocaine (when the actual drugs used were specified).[59] Whether the necrotizing fasciitis is an exaggerated coagulation necrosis owing to the cocaine or is the result of a superimposed infection is not known.

The cardiovascular pathology of chronic cocaine abuse

has been extensively reviewed by Karch.[25] Intimal hyperplasia of the coronary arteries leading to cardiac ischemia and left ventricular hypertrophy has been most commonly linked to the chronic use of cocaine. Animal experiments as well as autopsy observations now strongly suggest that cocaine can induce and accelerate the development of atherosclerosis. Cocaine users also appear to have an increased number of mast cells in the adventitia of the coronary arteries. More tenuous are reports linking cocaine use to dilated cardiomyopathy and eosinophilic myocarditis. Bacterial endocarditis is known to occur among intravenous cocaine users, but, to date, no systematic studies have been undertaken to compare the disease seen in cocaine users to that seen in heroin addicts and nondrug abusers who contract endocarditis.

Primary fungal cerebritis has been reported with chronic intravenous cocaine users.[66] This appears to be a rare complication that has a fulminant, usually fatal course. The cases reported occurred before human immunodeficiency virus (HIV) testing was possible, but since then at least one unreported case is said to have been free of HIV.[38] In all cases, the organisms have been opportunistic fungi (e.g., *Acremonium* sp., *Rhizopus* sp.).

Maternal use of cocaine has been associated with placental abruption and spontaneous abortion[18,38] because of placental vasoconstriction. Although a variety of congenital anomalies have been reported in the fetus exposed to cocaine in utero, urogenital anomalies seem to predominate.[8]

Miscellaneous drugs

The gross and histopathological alterations resulting from the abuse of marijuana have not been adequately studied. In a review of the pathology of drug abuse, Karch[25] notes ". . . that there isn't enough good anatomic pathology to write about [marijuana]." Pneumothorax and pneumopericardium have been reported[5] from the Valsalva maneuver used with marijuana smoking. Clinically, smoked cannabinoids are a respiratory irritant and pose similar effects and potential hazards as tobacco. Of perhaps greater concern is the effect of acute marijuana intoxication on driving ability.[14,27] Altered perception of time, distance, and speed (particularly if the marijuana is smoked while alcohol is simultaneously consumed) creates at least a serious potential for motor vehicle crashes.

Most other illicit drugs that are popularly abused do not result in direct anatomical alterations that can be appreciated at autopsy or with the light microscope. Actually, their main effect is to alter perceptions and motor functions that diminish the ability to interact adequately with the environment. This was particularly true with the abuse of methaqualone in the late 1970s and early 1980s when the drug was frequently linked etiologically to a rising number of motor vehicle fatalities.[58]

Hallucinogenic drugs such as psilocybin, mescaline,

PCP ("angel dust"), and lysergic acid diethylamide (LSD, "acid") also alter environmental perceptions. Because the hallucinations produced may be quite bizarre, death may occur in the user or nearby individuals because of the resultant bizarre behavior. For example, hallucinations caused by PCP have resulted in deaths by drowning, falls from a building (the victim believing he could fly), and mutilating homicides. Deaths from this drug in particular are often violent and bizarre.[16,40]

Finally, it should be noted that amphetamines are basically pharmacological stimulants and have an effect on the body much like cocaine. This is particularly true of the cardiovascular effects. Also, amphetamines have been linked to brain damage by effects on the cerebral microvasculature,[49] and there may be a propensity for primary fungal cerebritis[35] and vasculitis.[11]

REFERENCES

1. Aldrich MR, Barner RW: *Historical aspects of cocaine use and abuse.* In Mule SJ, editor: *Cocaine: chemical, biological, clinical, social and treatment aspects,* Cleveland, 1976, CRC Press, pp 3-11.
2. Attarosio A: Heroin: Colombia's newest export, *The Narc Officer* May 1992, p. 21.
3. Beirmam R, Nunez D, Wetli CV: Radiographic evaluation of the cocaine smuggler, *Gastrointest Radiol* 11:351, 1986.
4. Bennett RG, Decherd JW: The heroin ulcer—new addition to the differential diagnosis of ulcers of the penis, *Arch Dermatol* 107:121, 1973.
5. Birrer RB, Calderon J: Pneumothorax, pneumomediastinum, and pneumopericardium following Valsalva's manuever, *NY State J Med* 84:619, 1984.
6. Bruckner JV et al: Histopathological evaluation of cocaine-induced skin lesions in rat, *J Cutan Pathol* 9:83, 1982.
7. Bush MN et al: Spontaneous pneumomediastinum as a consequence of cocaine use, *NY State J Med* 84:618, 1984.
8. Chavez GF, Mulinare J, Cordero JF: Maternal cocaine use during pregnancy as a risk factor for congenital urogenital anomalies, *JAMA* 262:795, 1989.
9. Cherubin C: The medical sequelae of narcotic addiction, *Ann Intern Med* 67:23, 1967.
10. Ciancutti CJ: Defining addiction: more than an academic issue, *Street Pharmacol* 8:1, 1985.
11. Citron BP et al: Necrotizing angiitis associated with drug abuse, *N Engl J Med* 283:1001, 1970.
12. Courtwright DT: *Dark paradise,* Cambridge, Mass, Harvard University Press, 1982.
13. Cushman P: Street heroin in Washington, DC, *N Engl J Med* 289:1151, 1973.
14. Davis JH: Marijuana and automobile driving, *JAMA* 221:714, 1972.
15. DeSeve P: Drugs on the street where you live, *Emerg Med* 18:128, 1986.
16. Garey RE: PCP abuse in New Orleans: a six year study, *Am J Drug Alcohol Abuse* 13:135, 1987.
17. Gehrke D: Heroin use continues rise in Dade; drug now rivals cocaine in deaths, *The Miami Herald* January 28, 1993.
18. Goldfrank LR, Hoffman RS: *The cardiovascular effects of cocaine—update 1992. In Acute cocaine intoxication: current methods of treatment,* NIDA Research Monograph No. 123, Rockville, Md, 1993, National Institute of Drug Abuse.
19. Greene MH, Nightingale SL, DuPont RL: Evolving patterns of drug abuse, *Ann Intern Med* 83:402, 1975.
20. Hall J: *Drug use in Miami (Dade County), Florida,* Up Front Drug Information Center, December 1991.
21. Hall JN: Drug trends: good news, bad news, *Street Pharmacol* 14:2, 1991.
22. Helpern M: Fatalities from narcotic addiction in New York City—incidence, circumstances and pathologic findings, *Hum Pathol* 3:13, 1972.
23. Hirsch CS: Dermatopathology of narcotic addiction, *Hum Pathol* 3:37, 1972.
24. Inciardi JA: *The war on drugs—heroin, cocaine, crime and public policy,* Palo Alto, Calif, 1986, Mayfield Publishing Co.
25. Karch SB: *The pathology of drug abuse,* Boca Raton, Fla, 1993, CRC Press.
26. Klatt EC, Mills NZ, Noguchi TT: Causes of death in hospitalized intravenous drug abusers, *J Forensic Sci* 35:1143, 1990.
27. Klein AW, Davis JH: Marijuana and automobile crashes, *J Drug Issues* 1:18, 1971.
28. Kouri J: Organized crime: resurgence of the heroin trade in America, *The Narc Officer,* Vol 7, No 9, September 1991, pp 16-17.
29. Kringsholm B, Christoffersen P: Lung and heart pathology in fatal drug addiction. A consecutive autopsy study, *Forensic Sci Int* 34:39, 1987.
30. Kringsholm B, Christoffersen P: The nature and the occurrence of birefringement material in different organs in fatal drug addiction, *Forensic Sci Int* 34:53, 1987.
31. Lerner AM, Oerther FJ: Characteristics and sequelae of paregoric abuse, *Ann Intern Med* 65:1019, 1966.
32. Louria DB, Hensle T, Rose J: The major medical complications of heroin addiction, *Ann Intern Med* 67:1, 1967.
33. Mariani-Costantini R, Jannotta FS, Johnson FB: Systemic visceral talc granulomatosis associated with miliary tuberculosis in a drug addict, *Am J Clin Pathol* 70:785, 1982.
34. McLaughlin GT: Cocaine: the history and regulation of a dangerous drug, *Cornell Law Rev* 58:537, 1973.
35. Micozzi MS, Wetli CV: Intravenous amphetamine abuse, primary mucormycosis and acquired immunodeficiency, *J Forensic Sci* 30:504, 1985.
36. Miller BL et al: *Cerebrovascular complications from cocaine: possible long-term sequelae. In Acute cocaine intoxication: current methods of treatment,* NIDA Research Monograph No. 123, Rockville, Md, 1993, National Institute of Drug Abuse.
37. Minkin W, Cohen HJ: Dermatologic complications of heroin addiction—report of a new complication, *N Engl J Med* 277:473, 1967.
38. Mittleman RE, Wetli CV: The pathology of cocaine abuse, *Adv Pathol Lab Med* 4:37, 1991.
39. Moustauras NR et al: Contaminated street heroin—relationship to clinical infections, *Arch Surg* 118:746, 1983.
40. Nakamura GR, Noguchi TT: PCP: a drug of violence and death, *J Police Sci Admin* 7:459, 1979.
41. National Institute of Drug Abuse: *Annual data 1989,* Drug Abuse Warning Network (DAWN), Statistical Series 1, No. 9, Rockville, Md, 1990, National Institute of Drug Abuse.
42. National Institute of Drug Abuse: *Annual medical examiner data 1991,* Statistical Series 1, Nos. 11-13, Rockville, Md, 1991, National Institute of Drug Abuse.
43. National Institute of Drug Abuse: *Overview of the 1991 national household survey on drug abuse,* Rockville, Md, National Institute of Drug Abuse.
44. Newman RG: The need to redefine "addiction," *N Engl J Med* 308:1096, 1983.
45. Pardo V et al: The renal complications of drug abuse and human immunodeficiency virus. In Tisher CL, Brenner BM, editors: *Renal pathology,* ed 2, Vol 1, Chapt 12, Philadelphia, 1994, JB Lippincott, pp 390-418.
46. Racela LS et al: Systemic talc granulomatosis associated with disseminated histoplasmosis in a drug abuser, *Arch Pathol Lab Med* 112:557, 1988.

47. Rhodes EF, Thornton JI: Occurrence of excipient materials in illicit tablet manufacture, *Microgram* 12:98, 1979.

48. Roth D et al: Acute rhabdomyolysis associated with cocaine intoxication, *N Engl J Med* 319:673, 1988.

49. Rumbaugh CL et al: Cerebral microvascular injury in experimental drug abuse, *Invest Radiol* 11:282, 1976.

50. Sapira JD: The narcotic addict as a medical patient, *Am J Med* 45:555, 1968.

51. Sen S: Heroin trafficking in the Golden Triangle, *Crim Just Int* 8:11, 1992.

52. Smart R, Anglia R: Do we know the lethal dose of cocaine? *J Forensic Sci* 32:303, 1986.

53. Swarns RL: Another drug scourge for South Florida—diversification of cocaine cartels brings influx of heroin, *The Miami Herald* March 27, 1992.

54. Taskin M, Tchertkoff V, Ramaswamy G: Necrotizing sialometaplasia. *ASCP Check Sample* 17:APII 93-3, Chicago, 1993, American Society of Clinical Pathologists.

55. Tomashefski JF, Hirsch CS: The pulmonary vascular lesions of intravenous drug abuse, *Hum Pathol* 11:133, 1980.

56. Tuazon CU, Sheagren JN: Staphylococcal endocarditis in parenteral drug abusers: source of the organism, *Ann Intern Med* 82:788, 1975.

57. US Department of Justice/Drug Enforcement Administration: From the source to the street—current prices for cannabis, cocaine and heroin, *The Narc Officer* Vol 6, No 3, March 1990, pp 55-67.

58. Wetli CV: Methaqualone-related deaths—a survey of 246 fatalities, *JAMA* 249:621, 1982.

59. Wetli CV: *Fatal reactions to cocaine.* In Washton AM, Gold MS, editors: *Cocaine, a clinician's handbook,* New York, 1987, Guilford Publications, pp. 33-54.

60. Wetli CV: The medical risks of cocaine, *West J Med* 148:456, 1988.

61. Wetli CV, Davis JH, Blackbourne BD: Narcotic addiction in Dade County, Florida—an analysis of 100 consecutive autopsies, *Arch Pathol* 93:330, 1972.

62. Wetli CV, Fishbain DA: Cocaine-induced psychosis and sudden death in recreational cocaine users, *J Forensic Sci* 30:873, 1985.

63. Wetli CV, Mittleman RE: The body packer syndrome—toxicity following ingestion of illicit drugs packaged for transportation, *J Forensic Sci* 26:492, 1981

64. Wetli CV, Noto TA, Fernandez-Carol A: Immunologic abnormalities in heroin addiction, *South Med J* 67:193, 1974.

65. Wetli CV, Wright RK: Death caused by recreational cocaine use, *JAMA* 241:2519, 1979.

66. Wetli CV et al: Fungal cerebritis from intravenous drug abuse, *J Forensic Sci* 29:260, 1984.

Chapter 16

WATER QUALITY AND POLLUTION

Kenneth P. Cantor
Gunther F. Craun

This chapter is composed of two major sections. In the first section, infectious diseases known to be related to microorganisms conveyed by drinking water are described. Following this, the evidence pointing to associations between several types of drinking water contaminants and occurrences of malignant neoplasms are discussed. There are important differences in our knowledge of causal factors of infectious and chronic diseases, in particular, the degree of available information that bears on water-related exposures. These differences are discussed in greater detail in the the second section of this chapter, on Water Contaminants and Cancer.

Students of epidemiology are aware that the first well-designed epidemiological investigations had as their focus infectious disease of waterborne origin. These were the seminal studies of Dr. John Snow on cholera in midnineteenth century London. In 1855, Snow[150] published the second edition of *On the Mode of Communication of Cholera*. This work culminated an intensive investigation of 7 years in which he personally evaluated conditions surrounding thousands of cholera deaths. Snow's conclusions regarding the cause and spread of this disease are recognized today as being essentially correct. Snow's hypothesis that cholera was caused by a "poison" conveyed by particular drinking waters arose from observations of disease progression and numerous anecdotal accounts of the occurrence and local spread of the disease. It took a carefully designed and executed epidemiological study, however, to convince the medical and public health community that contaminated water was implicated in the spread of the disease. In examining cholera mortality rates, Snow observed that areas served by the Lambeth Company, with a new water intake in the Thames, upriver of London, fared much better in an 1854 epidemic than in an earlier 1849 episode, before the intake was moved upstream. He therefore carried out a care-

Portions of this chapter are adapted from Craun GF: *The epidemiology of waterborne disease: the importance of drinking water disinfection*. In Talbott E, Craun GF, editors: *Introduction to Environmental Epidemiology*, Chelsea, Mich, 1994, in press; Lewis Publishers; and from Cantor KP, Shy C, Chilvers C: *Water contaminants. In Schottenfeld D, Fraumeni JF Jr, editors: Cancer epidemiology and prevention*, Philadelphia, 1994, WB Saunders, in press.

ful house-to-house survey of cholera deaths in the 1854 epidemic in districts served by both the Lambeth Company and the Southwark and Vauxhall Company, which had not moved its Thames River intakes from central London. In Snow's words, he was able to conduct this study because[150]

the intermixing of the water supply . . . admitted of the subject being sifted in such a way as to yield the most incontrovertible proof on one side or the other. . . . The pipes of each company go down all the streets, and into nearly all the courts and alleys. . . . In many cases a single house has a supply different from that on either side. Each Company supplies both rich and poor, both large houses and small; there is no difference either in the condition or occupation of the persons receiving the water of the different companies.

These were ideal conditions for making unbiased observations of disease rates in the human population unlikely to be influenced by differences in extraneous factors, such as income, occupation, or diet. Control of such potential "confounding factors" continues to be a major issue in the design and conduct of epidemiological studies. A confounding factor, one of several possible systematic biases in epidemiological studies, is often cited as a reason for cautious interpretation of small relative risks (less than 2.0). Snow's meticulous investigation showed that the mortality rate among households with water from the Southwark and Vauxhall Company was 7.1 times that of households using Lambeth Company water. In modern parlance, the relative risk was 7.1.

WATER-RELATED INFECTIOUS DISEASE

Waterborne diseases that are transmitted through ingestion of contaminated water are spread by the fecal-oral route of transmission, and contaminated water is only one of several possible vehicles of infection. Epidemiology studies are required to establish the vehicle. The epidemic* and endemic† occurrences of waterborne diseases have been documented.

Contaminated surface or groundwater sources used for public or individual water supplies, water in recreational areas not intended for drinking, or water accidentally consumed while swimming or bathing can cause illness. The importance of the waterborne route of transmission in any location depends on the general level of sanitation and the protection and treatment of water supplies. In the United States, waterborne diseases have largely been controlled through use of multiple barriers of protection: wastewater treatment, protection of source water quality, and treatment of drinking water by disinfection and filtration[40] Occasion-

ally, waterborne outbreaks occur when these systems fail. In developing countries, however, in which the multiple barrier concept is often overlooked, waterborne disease transmission occurs relatively frequently, and improvements in water supplies and waste disposal can significantly reduce morbidity and mortality from infectious diseases.

Waterborne disease symptoms can range from slight discomfort to severe reactions depending on the etiological agent and host response. Asymptomatic infections are also common. The general mobility of world populations has provided opportunities for the waterborne transmission of many pathogens, which may be carried by refugees, immigrants, and returning travelers from throughout the world. For waterborne diseases, water acts as the passive carrier of the pathogen. Possible exposures include ingestion of contaminated water; dermal contact through bathing, swimming, or wading;[53] and inhalation of organisms in aerosols from contaminated water.[37,81,109] Schistosomiasis, dracontiasis, and primary amebic meningoencephalitis are considered water-based diseases because the pathogen spends an essential part of its life in water or is dependent on aquatic organisms for completion of its life cycle.[10]

The availability of water is more important than its quality for diseases that are closely related to poor sanitation. The lack of water for bathing and handwashing contributes to diseases such as trachoma, conjunctivitis, scabies, and diarrhea.[38] Water-vectored diseases, such as yellow fever, dengue, filariasis, malaria, onchocerciasis, and sleeping sickness, are transmitted by insects that breed in water or bite near water.[38]

Water-based disease

Schistosomiasis, a blood fluke infection with adult worms living in the host for many years, is not indigenous to North America, but immigrants to the continental United States have been found infected.[10] Eggs of the female worm produce granulomata and scars in organs where they are deposited. Millions of people in Asia, Africa, the Middle East, South America, and the Caribbean are infected. The three major species causing disease are *Schistosoma haematobium, S. mansoni,* and *S. japonicum.* Hepatic and intestinal symptoms, including diarrhea and abdominal pain, are common with *S. mansoni* and *S. japonicum,* whereas *S. haematobium* causes urinary complications, including hematuria. The important pathological effects from chronic infection include liver fibrosis, obstructive uropathy, and possibly bladder cancer.[10] Humans are the principal reservoir of infection for these species; domestic animals and wild rodents are potential hosts of *S. japonicum.* Infection is acquired from free swimming cercariae, which have developed in snails, a required intermediate host. Eggs are deposited in water sources through urine or feces of infected individuals, and after hatching, the liberated larvae infect freshwater snail hosts. After several weeks, the cercariae emerge from the snail and can penetrate human skin while

*References 37, 39, 41, 74, 80, 81, 110, 153.
†References 14, 32, 64, 67, 76, 108, 137, 165, 169.

the person is working, swimming, or wading in water. Entering the blood stream, they are carried to the lungs and migrate to the liver, where they develop to maturity.

Primary amebic meningoencephalitis is caused by species of free living amebae, *Naegleria* and *Acanthamoeba*, ordinarily found in water, soil, and vegetation.[10] *Naegleria* trophozoites invade the brain and meninges via the nasal mucosa and olfactory nerve.[10] Infection is acquired by exposure of the nasal passages to contaminated water while bathing, diving, or swimming in public pools, ponds, and lakes in areas of warm climates, thermal springs, or waters warmed by effluents of power plants. More than 100 cases have been reported in the United States and almost all have been fatal.[10] *Acanthamoeba* reach the brain without involvement of the nasal passages, probably through entry from a skin lesion, and infect primarily chronically ill or immunosuppressed individuals who have not been swimming.[10]

The only disease transmitted exclusively through contaminated drinking water is dracontiasis or guinea worm infection of the subcutaneous and deeper tissues with a large nematode, *Dracunculus medinensis*.[10] The disease occurs in India, Pakistan, and Africa, where people obtain water from step wells and ponds. Humans are the only reservoir of infection, and an intermediate host, crustacean copepods, is required for transmission. A blister appears, usually on the foot, when the adult female worm is ready to discharge larvae as individuals wade into step wells and ponds to obtain water. Larvae discharged into the water are ingested by the copepods and develop into the infective stage in about 2 weeks. Infected copepods are swallowed by humans, and larvae are liberated in the stomach or duodenum, migrate through the viscera, and become adults. The female develops to maturity in the tissue of the lower extremities.

Waterborne disease

Pseudomonas folliculitis, pharyngitis, external otitis, and schistosome dermatitis have been associated with recreational activities and water contact. Folliculitis from hot tubs and whirlpools is preventable if water is maintained at pH 7.2 to 7.8 with adequate levels of free chlorine.[80] Nontuberculosis *Mycobacterium*, ubiquitous in nature and found in water, may cause disease in humans; however, their epidemiology and the importance of contaminated water have not been clearly defined.[10] A pulmonary disease resembling tuberculosis and a systemic disease in individuals with severe immunodeficiency such as acquired immunodeficiency syndrome (AIDS) have been associated with the *M. avium* complex. The reservoir for *Legionella* is primarily aqueous. Conditions in many drinking water systems are favorable for survival and growth. The organism can survive for months in tap water and may be aerosolized into the air environment.[10,109] Hot water systems, air conditioning cooling towers, and evaporative condensers have been implicated in the transmission of legionellosis. Fourteen

serogroups of *Legionella pneumophila* are currently recognized, but serogroup 1 is most commonly associated with disease.[10] Pontiac fever and Legionnaires' disease are the two recognized, distinct epidemiological syndromes.[10] The overall case fatality rate can be 15% in hospitalized cases of Legionnaires' disease. Pontiac fever does not result in pneumonia or death, and patients usually recover without treatment. Pontiac fever caused by *Legionella* has been associated with use of whirlpools.[80,81]

Cholera, the classic waterborne disease, is caused by the 01 strains that produce an enterotoxin.[10,45] Infected persons can be asymptomatic; have mild-to-moderate diarrhea; or experience severe watery diarrhea, vomiting, and dehydration, which may lead to death. Contaminated drinking water is an important source of infection in developing countries. The seventh cholera pandemic, which began in 1961 in Asia, has now spread to the Americas. In 1991, cholera was introduced to Peru. It has since spread to other South American countries and Mexico and has been imported into the United States by infected tourists. A limited waterborne outbreak of 17 cases of cholera was reported on an oil rig off the Texas coast in 1981.[45] Typhoid fever (*Salmonella typhi*), another historically important waterborne disease, usually causes fever, headache, and abdominal pain.[10] Paratyphoid fever (*Salmonella paratyphi* serotypes A, B, and C) presents a similar clinical picture but tends to be milder.[10] Cholera and typhoid are transmitted exclusively among humans by the fecal-oral route of exposure. Domestic animals, such as dairy cattle, may also be a reservoir of infection for paratyphoid fever. Few cases of waterborne typhoid fever are now reported in the United States, but outbreaks occasionally occur. In 1973, 210 cases of typhoid fever occurred in Florida after contamination of an untreated well serving a migrant labor camp,[146] and in 1985, 60 cases were reported from contamination of water mains in a housing development in the Virgin Islands.[153]

Two enteric diseases commonly transmitted by drinking water, *Shigella* and *Salmonella* gastroenteritis, have similar symptoms: diarrhea, abdominal cramps, fever, and vomiting. *Shigella* frequently causes bloody stools and rectal pain.[10] For *Salmonella*, both humans and domestic and wild animals are important sources of infection; however, humans are the only significant source for *Shigella*. The protozoan *Giardia lamblia*, a frequent cause of waterborne disease outbreaks in the United States, produces a diarrhea of several weeks' duration, accompanied by fatigue, weight loss, epigastric pain, bloating, and flatulence.[10,112] Many infections are asymptomatic. Reservoirs of infection include both humans and animals. Beavers have frequently been implicated as a source of infection, but other wild and domestic animals may also be important.[42,44] Amebiasis (*Entamoeba histolytica*) and balantidiasis (*Balantidium coli*) are also protozoan infections that can be transmitted by contaminated drinking water. Similar to *Giardia*, these protozoa exist in a cyst form that is resistant to the usual drinking water disinfection practices. The waterborne transmission of these two pathogens, however, has not been important in the United States.[37] Humans are the source of infection for *E. histolytica,* and pigs are the principal reservoir of *B. coli.*[10]

Several viral agents cause hepatitis infections.[10] Hepatitis A has long been recognized to be transmitted by drinking water, and the virus has been identified in water samples collected during outbreaks.[152] Symptoms include fever, nausea, vomiting, muscle aches, and jaundice. The disease varies in severity from a mild illness to a severely disabling disease; many infections are asymptomatic. Hepatitis A outbreaks are often not recognized because the long incubation period may obscure the relationship between illness and consumption of water. Waterborne outbreaks of viral hepatitis E (non-A non-B hepatitis) have been reported outside the United States.[10]

Often an etiological agent is not identified for waterborne outbreaks of gastroenteritis. During the past decade in the United States, a cause was not determined in almost half of the outbreaks.[80,81] In many outbreaks, the search for an etiological agent was limited, or clinical specimens could not be collected in a timely manner; in others, extensive clinical analyses failed to identify an agent. Although the symptoms and incubation period suggest viral illness in some outbreaks, it is believed that outbreaks of acute gastroenteritis of undetermined cause include illnesses of viral, bacterial, and parasitic etiologies.

Acute infectious nonbacterial gastroenteritis occurs primarily in two epidemiologically distinct forms. In infants and young children, the 70-nm rotaviruses typically cause severe diarrhea for 5 to 8 days accompanied by fever and vomiting.[10] Infants may become severely dehydrated. In developing countries, rotavirus is responsible for an estimated 870,000 deaths each year.[10] Other viruses associated with acute nonbacterial gastroenteritis include at least three serologically distinct 27-nm viruslike particles, such as the Norwalk and Norwalk-like agent(s), which generally cause epidemics among older children and adults in families and communities.[38] Gastroenteritis caused by these viruses is explosive but self-limiting, usually lasting 24 to 48 hours, and symptoms include vomiting, diarrhea, nausea, abdominal cramps, headache, low-grade fever, anorexia, and malaise.[10] One third of the epidemics of viral gastroenteritis that occur in the United States are thought to be caused by Norwalk agents.[10]

Several bacterial agents may be responsible for gastroenteritis of undetermined cause. Strains of *Escherichia coli* that cause diarrhea are of four major categories: enterotoxigenic, enteroinvasive, enteropathogenic, and enterohemorrhagic.[10] Humans are reservoirs of infection for all four types, but cattle are believed to also be a reservoir for enterohemorrhagic *E. coli.* Although its waterborne transmission had been suspected and it had been isolated from water, enterohemorrhagic *E. coli* 0157:H7 had not been doc-

umented as a cause of waterborne disease until 1989, when an outbreak of 243 cases occurred in Cabool, Missouri; one third of the patients had bloody diarrhea, 32 were hospitalized, and 4 died.[81] Contamination of the water distribution system was identified as the likely source. A smaller waterborne outbreak of 0157:H7 was reported in Tarves, England, in 1990 after use of a supplemental water supply that may have been contaminated by cattle wastes.[52]

The most common symptoms of *Yersinia enterocolitica* infection in humans are fever, abdominal pain, headache, and watery diarrhea. This pathogen is frequently found in surface and well waters, and wild and domestic animals are principal reservoirs of infection.[39] Individual cases of suspected waterborne transmission have been reported (similar serotypes are isolated from the patient and water), but few outbreaks are recognized, investigated, and reported.[25,54]

Campylobacter jejuni is thought to be an important cause of bacterial gastroenteritis and travelers' diarrhea.[10,39] In developed countries, most infections are seen in young adults, but in developing countries, children are most often affected.[10] Symptoms of mild infections may resemble those seen in viral gastroenteritis, but *C. jejuni* may also cause a typhoidlike illness. Illness is frequently self-limiting, but a prolonged illness or relapse can occur. *Campylobacter* species are widespread in animals, and organisms found in water are likely due to contamination by wild or domestic animals. The first well-documented waterborne outbreak of *C. jejuni* gastroenteritis affected more than 3000 people in Bennington, Vermont, in 1978.[162]

Even after extensive laboratory analyses, a causative agent has not been identified for a distinctive chronic diarrheal illness characterized by dramatic, urgent watery diarrhea persisting for many months. The first reported outbreak of this illness occurred in Brainerd, Minnesota, in 1984 after consumption of unpasteurized milk.[134] In 1987, the first waterborne outbreak of a similar gastroenteritis occurred; untreated well water in an Illinois restaurant was implicated as the vehicle of transmission.[136] Nonbloody diarrhea with a median frequency of 12 stools per day persisted in 87% of patients after 6 months. No bacterial, mycobacterial, viral, or parasitic agents known to be enteropathogenic were detected in stools or well water. A second outbreak also associated with untreated well water occurred in a small Oklahoma community in 1988, but again no agent could be isolated.[81] The increased availability of specialized laboratory procedures and additional research are needed to recognize and identify newly suspected agents such as this.

The potential importance of the waterborne route of transmission of *Cryptosporidium,* an intestinal protozoan parasite, has only recently been recognized.* Both animals and humans serve as sources of environmental contamination and human infection, with calves being an important

---

*References 6, 10, 15, 48, 51, 60, 77, 109, 110.

reservoir. Individuals with normal immune function generally have a self-limiting diarrhea, but patients with immunological abnormalities can develop severe, irreversible diarrhea, which may lead to death.[151] There is no known drug treatment therapy, so prevention is important.[151] The first documented waterborne outbreak of cryptosporidiosis in July 1984 was traced to the contamination of a well used by a Texas community.[51] Dye introduced into the community's sewage system was detected in the well water. *Cryptosporidium* was also responsible for one of the largest waterborne outbreaks reported in the United States, causing an estimated 13,000 cases of diarrheal illness in 1987 in Carrollton, Georgia.[77] This community used surface water treated by filtration and chlorination. Water quality limits were not exceeded for turbidity or coliform, and disinfection was not interrupted, but *Cryptosporidium* oocysts were identified in the water system. Certain operational practices associated with filtration were believed responsible for passage of oocysts into the treated water. Waterborne outbreaks of cryptosporidiosis have been reported in Oregon[106] and England, Wales, and Scotland[6] in filtered and unfiltered water systems. More than 350,000 cases of illness occurred in April 1993 during a waterborne outbreak of cryptosporidiosis in Milwaukee, Wisconsin; this water supply was filtered and met all current drinking water quality regulations (Fox K, Environmental Protection Agency [EPA], Cincinnati, personal communication, 1993). Limited studies indicate this protozoan is highly resistant to chlorination, much more than *Giardia*.[6,15] Water filtration is effective in removing oocysts when properly designed and operated, and the treated water must be protected from contamination in distribution mains and during storage.[6,15]

Other newly recognized etiological agents may cause waterborne disease.[81] Cyanobacteria-like bodies (CLB), also referred to as *Cyclospora*, have been identified in stool specimens from patients around the world. The role of CLB in causing diarrheal illness is currently being investigated. An outbreak in 1990 in a Chicago hospital was associated with drinking water in a building in which open-air, roof-top storage tanks were used to maintain water pressure. Ill persons had remissions and relapses of explosive watery diarrhea. CLB were found in stool specimens, and algae were found in a storage tank.[81]

Diseases only occasionally transmitted by contaminated drinking water include echinococcosis, tularemia, acute poliomyelitis, and leptospirosis.[10] Other vehicles of infection are more important for these diseases, and when drinking water is implicated, it is generally the ingestion of water not intended for drinking or contaminated water consumed in recreational areas. Leptospirosis can, however, be an important water-related disease for aquatic farmers, rice and sugarcane field workers, and sewer workers, where there is frequent contact with water contaminated by urine of domestic and wild animals.[10] Recreational exposures for swimmers and sportsmen in the United States have also caused leptospirosis. Limited evidence for the transmission of polio is provided by an outbreak that occurred in Lincoln, Nebraska, in 1952, when the community water system was contaminated with sewage through a cross-connection.[7]

Endemic waterborne disease. Epidemiology studies have shown endemic cases of giardiasis, cryptosporidiosis, and gastroenteritis to be associated with drinking water.

Untreated drinking water, from surface water sources appears to be an important cause of endemic giardiasis in the United States; in New Mexico, cryptosporidiosis was associated with use of untreated surface water.* In New Hampshire, increased risk of endemic giardiasis was also associated with the use of shallow well water. In Vermont, municipalities using unfiltered surface water or wells and individuals with a private water system had a higher incidence of endemic giardiasis than municipalities with filtered surface waters. In Dunedin, New Zealand, the importance of filtration as a barrier for protection against waterborne giardiasis was shown.[65] The incidence of laboratory-confirmed endemic giardiasis was found to be lower in areas where surface water was treated by coagulation, flocculation, and dual media filtration in addition to chlorination.[65] The potential importance of endemic waterborne illness is illustrated by epidemiological studies in Montreal, Canada, where it was estimated that 35% of unreported diarrhea was likely associated with use of municipal water that met all water quality standards. A randomized intervention trial found a higher incidence of self-reported gastrointestinal illness over a 15-month period among members of 307 eligible households consuming municipal tap water compared with 299 eligible households supplied with reverse osmosis water filters at their tap to remove microbial and chemical contaminants.[137,138] The households were served by a municipal water system that uses a sewage-contaminated river, conventionally treated with predisinfection, alum, coagulation, flocculation, rapid sand filtration, ozone, and chlorine.

Waterborne disease outbreaks in the United States

Statistics. During 1981-1990 in the United States, 291 waterborne outbreaks were reported in community (43%) and noncommunity (33%) systems and from the ingestion of contaminated water from recreational (14%) and individual (10%) water sources causing 65,442 cases of disease.[43] Contaminated, untreated groundwater or inadequately disinfected groundwater was responsible for 43% of all reported waterborne outbreaks; contaminated, untreated surface water or inadequately treated surface water was responsible for 24% of all reported outbreaks (Table 16-1). In surface water systems, outbreaks were found to occur primarily because of inadequate or interrupted disinfection in systems that did not provide filtration. Outbreaks were also

---

*References 14, 32, 67, 76, 108, 165, 169.

Table 16-1. Causes of waterborne outbreaks in the United States, 1981-1990

Cause of outbreak	Number of outbreaks
Untreated groundwater	77
Inadequate disinfection of groundwater	48
Ingestion of contaminated water while swimming	41
Inadequate disinfection of surface water	44
Contamination of distribution system	36
Filtration deficiencies	17
Unknown; miscellaneous	18
Untreated surface water	10
Total	291

Table 16-2. Waterborne disease outbreaks in the United States, 1981-1990

Disease	Number of outbreaks
Gastroenteritis (undefined etiology)	128
Giardiasis	71
Shigellosis	22
Chemical poisoning	18
Gastroenteritis (viral)	15
Hepatitis A	11
Campylobacteriosis	10
Salmonellosis	4
Cryptosporidiosis	2
Yersiniosis	2
Gastroenteritis (chronic)	2
Gastroenteritis (*E. coli* 0157:H7)	1
Typhoid fever	1
Dermatitis (chlorine)	1
Gastroenteritis (CLB)	1
Cholera	1
Amebiasis	1
Total	291

reported in filtered water systems because of improper design and operation of filtration facilities.

Inadequate or interrupted disinfection of groundwater caused 17% of all outbreaks. Outbreaks in disinfected groundwater systems may be due to the increased use of disinfection with little or no effort to reduce or eliminate sources of contamination and the lack of attention to providing effective, continuous disinfection.

Etiologies. The causes of outbreaks differed in community and noncommunity systems. In community systems, most outbreaks were caused by inadequate disinfection of surface water (28%) and contamination of water in the distribution systems (24%), primarily through cross-connections and repairs of mains. In noncommunity systems, almost all outbreaks (77%) were caused by contaminated, untreated, and inadequately disinfected groundwater.

Giardia is the most frequently identified organism causing waterborne outbreaks (Table 16-2). During the past decade, some 65% of waterborne giardiasis outbreaks were caused by contaminated surface water, especially inadequate disinfection of unfiltered water and ineffective filtration or pretreatment. *Giardia* can be inactivated by disinfection but only if stringent conditions are met and consistently maintained.[41] Effective disinfection also requires large concentrations and longer contact times. The occurrence of *Cryptosporidium* is widespread in water supplies in the United States, and additional research is required to determine why fewer waterborne outbreaks have been reported for cryptosporidiosis than giardiasis.[143] Most acute waterborne chemical poisonings resulted in mild, self-limited illness.[74] Fluoride and heavy metals cause vomiting, usually within 1 hour after consumption of the contaminated water. The symptoms of other chemical poisonings vary with the substance ingested. Infantile methemoglobinemia associated with high nitrate levels occasionally results in death.[110] Although no single type of acute chemical poisoning is common, chemical poisonings are among the most commonly recognized cause of waterborne outbreaks in the United States. Chemical poisonings usually occur because of cross-connections in the water distribution system and locally contaminated groundwater sources, but outbreaks of acute illness have also been caused by mechanical failures in adding fluoride to drinking water for prevention of dental caries.

WATER CONTAMINANTS AND CANCER

Establishing the microbiological causes of infectious disease has been guided for more than 100 years by the Henle-Koch postulates of causation[79,100] and evolving modifications.[57,58] Important elements of these guidelines are the specificity of the effect and the necessary presence of the microorganism among diseased individuals. Establishing causality is usually aided by the relatively short induction or incubation period between the time of initial exposure to the infectious organism and disease occurrence, typically measured in hours, days, or at most weeks. In consequence, for most waterborne infections, the causal link between microorganisms and disease is unambiguous.

Establishing an etiological role for environmental carcinogens poses an entirely different set of issues. The fundamental cellular event underlying a malignant growth is considered to be a somatic mutation resulting in loss of genetic control over cell replication. This can be caused, however, by many different environmental exposures, and once underway, uncontrolled cellular growth is influenced by a variety of host characteristics, including immunological, dietary, hormonal, and genetic factors. The multifactorial nature of cancer etiology implies that investigators must consider many other factors that can cause the disease or influence its progression, so as not to attribute causation wrongly to an exposure statistically linked to an etiological agent but not itself in the causal pathway. Understanding and controlling for the influence of such confounding factors is a major objective of epidemiological study design. In infectious diseases, the presence of a specific organism at the time of diagnosis is usually required to establish causality. For cancer, it is unusual that a specific factor is found. In further contrast with most infectious diseases, the time period for tumorigenesis is measured in years or decades, and establishing the etiological factors of importance among newly diagnosed cases usually requires evaluation of exposure events that occurred many years in the past. A strong association between disease and a putative risk factor, reflected in a high relative risk (at least above 2.0), is helpful in supporting a causal interpretation and in reducing the possibility of confounding by other factors. The relative risks for water contaminants that have been linked with human cancer are generally below 2.0, leading to cautious interpretation of most study findings. For all of these reasons, the descriptions of water-related carcinogenesis that follow are set in more tentative language than our discussion of infectious disease. This has important implications for disease control, especially with regard to quantifying the benefits of various alternatives for action. Until our understanding is further advanced, the most effective control methods will often remain elusive or lack adequate quantification.

We summarize the epidemiological evidence for a variety of drinking water contaminants and include relevant information on the types, amounts, and their environmental distribution. In this discussion, potential carcinogens in drinking water are grouped in five general categories: (1) microbiological agents, (2) radionuclides, (3) asbestiform particles, (4) inorganic solutes, and (5) organic chemicals.

Microbiological agents

Microbial pathogens found in water are not considered to be important as carcinogens, and they are usually discussed as infectious agents.[130] Mounting evidence suggests that several viruses (principally hepatitis B, papillomavirus, Epstein-Barr virus, and human immunosuppressive virus-1 [HIV-1]) are associated with human cancer, but there has been no evidence of waterborne transmission. At least one waterborne microorganism, *Schistosoma haematobium,* however, has been associated with elevated bladder cancer in many tropical and subtropical countries where schistosomiasis is endemic,[26] such as Egypt[128] and Zimbabwe.[156] Schistosomiasis-related bladder cancer is usually of squamous cell origin, whereas the histology of most other bladder carcinomas is transitional cell. In endemic areas, infections with *S. haematobium* start at an early age and persist for many years. Schistosomiasis-associated bladder cancer occurs at a relatively early age. In a series of Egyptian blad-

der cancer patients, the average age of those found with schistosome eggs at cystoscopy was 46.7 years.[56] In places where schistosomal infection is not endemic, the median age of bladder cancer patients is 69 years.[21] It is not yet known whether the carcinogenic effects of *S. haematobium* infections are due to chronic inflammation of the bladder epithelium or the release of chemical carcinogens from the eggs, such as N-nitroso compounds.[5,26,157] Infections with *S. mansoni* and *S. japonicum,* which primarily effect the liver, are thought to possibly increase hepatocellular carcinoma risk, but the evidence is weak (see Chapter 26).

Radionuclides

Traces of natural and man-made radioactivity from radionuclides are found in drinking water supplies throughout the world. The principal naturally occurring species are Radium-226, Radium-228, Uranium, Radon-222, Lead-210, Polonium-210, Thorium-230, and Thorium-232.[35] Levels vary geographically with local soil and rock conditions and may be increased by industrial and other point discharges.

Waterborne radon is responsible for most of the population dose of alpha radiation from drinking water, with the primary exposure being to the lungs via airborne releases from dishwashers and clothes washers, showers, baths, and toilets and cooking, drinking, and cleaning.[133] Ingested radon or other radionuclides are not thought to be important as environmental determinants of cancer.[130] The predominant source of indoor Rn-222 in U.S. houses is the soil underlying and adjacent to the foundation, with water contributing less than 2% on the average. In some circumstances, however, groundwater can constitute the predominant source of indoor airborne radon.[82] Although several studies have examined the association of airborne radon in homes with lung cancer risk (see Chapter 3), the contribution of radon in household drinking water to total exposure has not been considered separately. The direct contribution of ingested waterborne radon to the total body burden of radiation from all sources is small.

The few investigations of cancer and radioactivity in drinking water have ecological designs. In ecological studies, the geographical or temporal distribution of disease or mortality rates is examined with respect to the distribution of a putative risk factor and the degree of correlation measured. A Florida study of county leukemia incidence rates found a relative risk of 1.5 for total leukemia and 2.0 for acute myeloid leukemia in counties with high versus low levels of groundwater radium.[114] Associations with average county radon concentrations in water were found for county lung cancer rates among females in Maine.[82] In Iowa, the lung and bladder cancer incidence rates among males and lung and breast cancer incidence among females were elevated in towns with a water supply Ra-226 level exceeding 5.0 pCi/L.[8] The Iowa associations could not be explained by regional smoking patterns, water treatment factors, or sociodemographic factors. A subsequent study in 59 Iowa towns revealed a small, increasing trend of leukemia incidence with radium content in drinking water, but the strength of the association was small and consistent with no effect or a small effect.[66]

Asbestiform particles

Considerable epidemiological evidence, primarily from occupational settings, shows that airborne asbestos is a human carcinogen of the respiratory tract. It has been assumed that asbestos plays a role in cancer of the gastrointestinal tract, but the evidence is inconclusive. Asbestos fibers are also found in drinking water. Sources include weathering of natural deposits, such as serpentine rock formations, release from asbestos-cement pipes, and from processes associated with mining and production of iron ore.[106,123] Concentrations vary enormously, ranging from a barely detectable background level of 10^4 fibers/L to over 10^{11} fibers/L.[123] For human carcinogenesis, the size, shape, and crystalline structure of the fibers are as important as their concentration, and these characteristics are modified by physicochemical processes resulting from exposure to water or gastric fluid (see Chapter 6).[147]

Epidemiological studies of populations served by water containing high concentrations of asbestos have failed to yield results as conclusive as occupational studies of the airborne contaminant. All but one study involving waterborne asbestos are ecological, comparing the geographical distribution of asbestos levels in drinking water with cancer incidence or mortality rates. Two related studies in census tracts of the San Francisco Bay area, by Kanarek[98] and Conforti[34] and colleagues, found associations between measured levels of (naturally occurring) asbestos in drinking water and incidence of cancer of the esophagus, stomach, pancreas in both sexes,[34] lung (males), and female gallbladder and peritoneum.[98] However, factors such as diet, smoking, and occupation that might confound these associations could not be adequately controlled. Mortality in Quebec communities was associated with asbestos in drinking water for cancers of the stomach (males), pancreas (females), and lung (males).[166] An ecological study[140] and a case-control study[139] in the Puget Sound region, based on incident cancer, evaluated the risk of imbibing drinking water from a river with high levels of naturally occurring asbestos. Neither found overall patterns of association consistent with an asbestos effect. Positive associations for male stomach cancer and pharyngeal cancer that were based on small numbers, however, were observed in the case-control study. These studies included relatively few subjects, and their statistical power was small.

Duluth, Minnesota, had high levels of asbestos in its drinking water from 1955 to 1973, owing to contamination of Lake Superior with iron ore tailings from a processing facility 60 miles away. Cancer mortality[117] and incidence[111,148] in Duluth or its county were compared with rates of other Minnesota cities (or their respective counties). Some excesses of gastrointestinal mortality and morbidity were observed, but patterns were inconsistent. The variability of these results may be related to the relatively brief time period between first exposure and the observation of cancer mortality and incidence.

Cancer incidence as related to drinking water distributed by asbestos-cement water mains has been evaluated in Connecticut,[72,121] Utah,[144] and Woodstock, New York,[86] and mortality evaluated in Escambria County, Florida,[124] with inconsistent findings. In Utah, an association was found for male kidney cancer and female leukemia, and in Woodstock, for cancer of the oral cavity. Experimental toxicological studies of asbestos exposure cannot provide conclusive evidence, principally because of methodological problems, including the absence of suitable animal models.[130] Epidemiologic and experimental research on this topic should nevertheless continue because none of the available data can rule out adverse health effects of asbestos fibers present in water. Asbestos is considered a lung carcinogen, but the carcinogenic risk to the gastrointestinal tract of asbestos fibers at waterborne levels remains undetermined. Furthermore, these substances are widespread in the aqueous environment, and 20 to 40 years may be required before effects in humans are seen.

Inorganic solutes

A wide variety of inorganic solutes are found in drinking waters, and several are suspected to increase cancer risk in exposed populations. Among the inorganics associated with cancer risk are several metals and transition elements, including arsenic, and nitrate. A section on fluoride is included because of broad population exposure and equivocal evidence from animal studies suggesting a carcinogenic risk.

Metals and transition elements. Metals are present in a wide range of concentrations in drinking waters in the United States (usually under 100 µg/L). The sources include leaching from soil, industrial activities or mining activities. In some instances, metal salts such as alum are added during water treatment for chemical coagulation to remove particulates during settling and filtration. This may result in an increased concentration of aluminum in finished water. When drinking waters are corrosive (low pH, low concentration of divalent cations), metals such as lead and copper may be leached into water from distribution piping. Several metals and transition elements are considered to be carcinogenic in humans (arsenic, chromium, and nickel). Others are carcinogenic in animals.[12]

With the exception of arsenic, there has been relatively little study of cancer risk and trace metals in water. An early correlational study.[12] found some significant links between site-specific cancer mortality in U.S. sites and drinking water concentrations of eight trace metals in 16 major water basins. The most frequent associations were with beryllium, cadmium, and lead. An Iowa study observed geographical correlations between town-level cancer incidence of lung and bladder cancers and levels of nickel in drinking water.[92] The authors suggested that nickel was not directly implicated but an indicator of other contamination. A Norwegian study in 97 municipalities evaluated the correlation of 17 inorganic ions in drinking water with 16 groups of cancer morbidity.[62] Not unexpectedly, many statistically significant associations were found, however, the biological significance of these associations is uncertain.

The strongest epidemiological evidence regarding metals in water comes from studies of arsenic. Initial investigations reported elevated prevalence of skin cancer in areas of chronic arsenicism from contaminated water supplies in Mexico,[24] Argentina,[13] Taiwan,[158,159] and Chile.[15] A study by Tseng and co-workers[159] used a cross-sectional design and detected a dose-response association between arsenic concentrations (approximately 0.5 ppm) in wells and the prevalence of skin cancer (sampled data on water pollutants is also exceptional in these studies). These results were substantiated by additional studies in the same area of Taiwan,[158] but the role of arsenic has been questioned because physiologically active humic acids have also been found in arsenic-contaminated waters.[113] Interestingly, skin cancer prevalence or incidence has not been found elevated in all places where populations are exposed to elevated arsenic levels in drinking water,[73,127] suggesting that sunlight, diet, or other cofactors may play a role in mediating the effects.

Further study in Taiwan revealed geographical associations of arsenic in drinking water with risk of mortality from several other cancers, most notably cancers of the bladder, kidney, lung, nasal cavity, and liver in both sexes and prostate.[27,28,170] The most extensive study[27] extended the correlations to the whole of Taiwan (excepting Taipei City and 30 townships that had surface water or small populations), using data from 83,000 wells in 314 precincts and townships. Bladder and kidney cancers showed the strongest correlations, with the multivariate-adjusted regression coefficients indicating an increase in age-adjusted mortality per 100,000 person years of 3.9 and 4.2 (bladder) for every 0.1 ppm increase in arsenic level of well water and 1.1 and 1.7 (kidney) among males and females. In a case-control study, Chen and co-workers[29] found positive dose-response associations for bladder cancer, lung cancer, and liver cancer among those who had used contaminated water for 40 years or longer, as compared with never users. The bladder cancer findings are supported by excess bladder cancer mortality among a cohort of patients treated with Fowler's solution (potassium arsenite).[50]

The Taiwanese studies strengthened the evidence that arsenic causes human cancer of several sites by ingestion of ambient trace amounts. Additional studies of internal cancers in other populations exposed to waterborne arsenic are needed to confirm these observations, especially in view of the broad distribution of arsenic and other metals in drinking water.

Nitrate. Nitrate ion occurs in surface waters and groundwaters in concentrations ranging from less than 1.0 mg/L to over 100 mg/L. The U.S. EPA has established a maximum contaminant level (MCL) for nitrate–nitrogen (NO_3–N) in drinking water of 10 mg/L (equivalent to 45 mg/L of nitrate), primarily to protect against methemoglobinemia in infants. Nitrate in drinking water comes from numerous natural and man-made sources, including some wastewaters and agricultural and urban runoff. It is seldom removed during treatment. Nitrogen fertilizers have been implicated as an increasingly important source of drinking water nitrate, and more than 20% of rural wells may have nitrate levels above the EPA limit,[71,96,118] especially if their depth is less than 30 m. When drinking water nitrate-nitrogen is well below 10 mg/L, most ingested nitrate comes from dietary sources and averages about 100 mg/day. When water levels are near or exceed the MCL, however, water may increase total nitrate intake to 200 mg/day or more. At levels near the MCL, about 30% of ingested nitrate comes from water, and at levels between 12 and 25 mg/L NO_3–N, this rises to almost 70%.[31]

Nitrate can interact with secondary amines and amides to form a variety of N-nitroso compounds, after reduction in the saliva of nitrate to nitrite.* Many N-nitroso compounds are powerful carcinogens in several species of laboratory animals.[89] The urinary concentration of N-nitrosoproline (NPRO), a noncarcinogenic N-nitroso amine, was significantly associated with drinking water and urine nitrate levels among Nebraskan men dosed orally with 500 mg L-proline, showing the potential for in vivo N-nitroso formation.[125] In a high-risk area for gastric cancer in China, premalignant histological changes in the gastric mucosa were related to nitrate in drinking water, which ranged above 100 mg/L[171] (see Chapter 26).

This suggests the carcinogenic potential of nitrate in drinking water. Direct epidemiological evidence for its role in human cancer, however, is equivocal. Epidemiological studies, most of them of ecological design, have shown associations between nitrate concentrations in drinking water and gastric cancer. Brain cancer is also of concern, although there is less evidence. Positive geographical associations of nitrate with gastric cancer have been found in studies from Chile, Hungary, Columbia, Italy, and Denmark.† Several others, however, have not demonstrated a positive association for gastric cancer.[11,63,141] Geographical associations of this type may be subject to "publication bias," whereby positive associations may be more likely to find their way into print than null findings. Retrospective cohort studies of fertilizer workers who are presumably exposed to nitrate dusts do not show excess cancer risk.[2,65,142] Among the few

---

*References 55, 75, 126, 163, 164.
†References 3, 47, 68, 95, 97.

studies that use health outcome and exposure data from individuals is a case-control study of gastric cancer deaths from Wisconsin. This study did not show a link with nitrate level of the water source at the last residence of decedents.[141] Until more information is available from drinking water studies of nitrate conducted on the individual level, in which diet and other factors can be taken into account, the epidemiological evidence for this association must be considered weak. In view of the widespread and increasing contamination of water supplies with nitrate, however, especially in agricultural regions, and the potential for forming N-nitroso compounds, this area of epidemiological research is receiving continuing attention.

Fluoride. Fluoride is present in most natural waters, usually at concentrations well below 1.0 mg/L. In the United States, the principal source in an increasing number of communities over the past four decades has been its successful addition to drinking water to prevent dental caries. The usual dosage is in the range of 0.7 to 1.2 mg/L.

In an early study, the overall and some site-specific cancer mortality rates of the 10 largest U.S. cities that practiced water fluoridation were significantly higher than those of the 10 largest that did not.[19] Subsequent analyses of the same data[30,84] showed that these associations disappeared when relevant sociodemographic variables were controlled. Many additional investigations, almost all of ecological design, provided no supporting evidence. Given the public health implications, epidemiological findings on fluoridation and cancer risk were independently reviewed by an international panel[90] and by three separate expert committees convened in the United States[131,161] and Great Britain.[99] These reviews concluded that the available evidence does not support a link between fluoride in drinking water supplies and cancer risk. Concern was later raised by a finding of "equivocal evidence" of carcinogenicity from a lifetime sodium fluoride rodent feeding study. Three of 50 male rats in the highest dose category (79 ppm) and 1 of 50 in the next-to-highest group (45 ppm) had a rare bone tumor (osteosarcoma)[17] with no osteosarcomas found in the lower dose groups, nor in female rats or male or female mice. In the brief period since, epidemiological assessments have found no time trend nor geographical pattern of bone cancer or osteosarcoma consistent with a causal role for fluoride in drinking water.[85,87,116,120] This continues to be an area of active research interest (see Chapter 31).

Organic chemicals

Synthetic organic chemicals in drinking water can be divided into two major groupings: man-made chemicals from industrial, agricultural, commercial, or domestic sources; and chemicals produced during water disinfection from the interaction of chlorine or other chemical disinfectants with organic chemical precursors in the untreated water. These precursors are primarily naturally occurring substances in surface waters, but they are also found at lower levels in most groundwaters. Both types of organic substances have received epidemiological evaluation. Epidemiological studies of chlorination by-products have been facilitated by the widespread use of chlorine to disinfect drinking water and our ability to estimate past exposures, using available historical records of water source and treatment. The more sporadic contamination of drinking water with anthropogenic chemicals, however, has rendered these other organic chemical exposures less amenable to systematic evaluation.

Advances in analytic chemistry methods have resulted in the detection of hundreds of man-made organic chemicals in U.S. drinking waters, most occurring infrequently and at low concentration (below 1 ppb). Among these, at least 40 have been characterized as known or suspected carcinogens in experimental animals, and three are associated with human cancer: vinyl chloride, benzene, and chloromethyl ether.[91]

Organic chemicals of industrial, agricultural, commercial, and domestic origin. Contamination of underground and surface water with organic chemicals from industrial, agricultural, commercial, and domestic sources, as well as from hazardous waste disposal sites, is increasingly found. Usually the contamination is geographically restricted, but some chemicals may affect extensive aquifers.[160] There are relatively few epidemiological assessments of the health impact of such contaminants in drinking water owing to the difficulty in estimating the levels, timing, and specific chemicals involved in past exposures; the relatively small populations usually exposed to high contaminant levels; and the problem of deciding which health endpoints, or intermediate biological markers, to examine. When effects are observed, it is often impossible to sort out the specific exposures involved.

Geographical correlational studies have been conducted to evaluate county and local cancer mortality and incidence rates in places with hazardous waste sites, where the major routes of exposure have not been elucidated, or with municipal water supplies with documented contamination. In a nationwide study, age-adjusted cancer mortality rates from 339 U.S. counties with 593 hazardous waste sites listed by EPA were compared with rates from 2726 other counties.[70] Significant associations were found for lung, bladder, stomach, large intestine, and rectal cancers in white males and females, esophagus in white males, and breast in white females. In New Jersey, significant positive associations between chemical toxic waste disposal sites and eight cancer sites, especially stomach and lung, were found in one or more subpopulations living in 194 municipalities with over 10,000 population, after adjustment for sociodemographic characteristics.[129] In another New Jersey study that examined geographical correlations, female (but not male) leukemia incidence rates in 27 towns were associated with an index of volatile organic chemicals in municipal drinking water.[59]

Cancer incidence and mortality and other health-related

impacts have also been evaluated among populations near specific toxic waste sites, where there may be routes of exposure other than drinking water. Lung cancer incidence near the infamous Love Canal site in New York State for the period 1955-1977 was elevated but inconsistent across age groups.[94] Other cancers were not elevated,[94] but the statistical power to detect elevated rates of less common sites was limited. Rates of chromosomal aberrations and sister chromatid exchange frequencies were as expected.[78] In Clinton County, Pennsylvania, the location of the Drake superfund site, bladder cancer mortality among white males was significantly elevated.[18]

A Finnish community in which drinking water was contaminated with chlorophenols, probably from sawmills, had elevated incidence of soft-tissue sarcoma and non-Hodgkin lymphoma.[104] These tumors have been linked in other studies with exposure to the closely related chlorinated phenoxy-acetic acids or their dioxin contaminants.[112] Exposure to tetrachloroethylene leachate from improperly cured vinyl lined distribution pipes was studied in a population-based, case-control study in Massachusetts.[4] Nonsignificant risk elevations for bladder cancer and leukemia were found.

A cluster of childhood leukemia cases associated with contaminated community drinking water in Woburn, Massachusetts, has been the subject of scientific, legal, and political controversy.[20,49,103,115] Two of eight drinking water wells were discovered in 1979 to be contaminated with trichloroethylene (267 ppb), tetrachloroethylene (21 ppb), trichlorotrifluoroethane (23 ppb), and dichloroethylene (28 ppb). Forty-eight EPA priority pollutants and elevated levels of 22 metals were found in 61 additional test wells drilled to sample the groundwater.[103] Elevated childhood leukemia was found and statistically linked in space and time to the contamination. In addition, lymphocyte abnormalities were noted among family members of cases.[20]

A health survey in Hardeman County, Tennessee, where leachate from a pesticide waste dump contaminated the drinking water, found significant differences in hepatic profiles of exposed and unexposed members of the population that included alkaline phosphatase, albumin, total bilirubin, and serum glutamic-oxaloacetic transaminase (SGOT).[33] This may be of relevance to cancer induction because detoxification of potentially carcinogenic compounds or conversion of procarcinogens to direct-acting carcinogens may be linked to these enzyme profiles. In view of the many methodological issues involved, including the potential for bias and confounding, results from the epidemiological studies on cancer and man-made organic chemical contaminants of drinking water (other than chlorination by-products) can only be considered suggestive at this time. There is a great need for investigations to address the challenging task of more clearly defining past exposures to these chemicals and for biomarker and other studies that will as-

sist in understanding the biochemical toxicology of this large, diverse group of compounds.

Chlorination by-products. Chlorination by-products are found in almost every chlorinated drinking water in the United States. The concentration of chloroform and other trihalomethanes, accounting for 20% to 80% of the halogen covalently bound to organics, ranges from less than 1 ppb (in treated water from deep wells low in organics) to several hundred parts per billion (certain chlorinated surface waters). The remaining halogenated organics include a large number (typically greater than 200) of higher molecular weight, nonvolatile compounds, such as a variety of carboxylic acids, aldehydes, ketones, and ethers, each occurring at extremely low concentration.[149,154]

The observation of elevated chlorination by-products in treated surface water, as contrasted to well water, has served as the basis for epidemiological evaluation of these exposures. Three types of studies have been conducted.

The first were geographical correlation (ecological) studies in which both the exposure and the outcome measures (cancer mortality or incidence) were estimated for populations, not individuals. In most, the county was the geographical unit of observation. Age-adjusted, site-specific, sex-specific, and race-specific county cancer mortality rates were used as outcomes, and characteristics (chlorinated versus nonchlorinated, surface versus ground, trihalomethane [THM] of the predominant county drinking water source as the exposure variable.* Incidence rates were used in studies of water quality and cancer in Iowa towns,[9,92] Norwegian municipalities,[61] and Finnish cities.[101] In these ecological studies, the cancer sites most commonly associated with surface water, chlorination, or THM level were bladder, colon, and rectum.[132,168]

Later studies were of case-control design and used mortality records as the source of case and control subjects. In the earliest,† the exposure variable was a characteristic of the water supply (surface/ground, chlorinated/nonchlorinated, Mississippi River/other source) that served the decedent's most recent residence, abstracted from death certificate records. Results were largely supportive of the findings from the earlier ecological studies, showing associations with bladder, colon, and rectal cancers. In later studies, attempts were made to also gather information about previous residences and their sources of drinking water.[107,174] In one of these that focused on colorectal cancer,[107] no association was found between type of water source or imputed past THM level.

The third group of investigations were based on information from individuals. In these, past exposures were estimated through linking historical community water supply records with residential history information gathered in personal interviews. One community cohort follow-up study

---

*References 23, 83, 102, 135, 145.
†References 1, 16, 46, 69, 172.

and five case-control studies used this approach.* Three of the five case-control studies also gathered information about the tap water consumption of individuals.[22,129,173] In a population of 31,000 in Washington County, Maryland, Wilkins and Comstock[167] found elevated (but not statistically significant) bladder cancer incidence among men and cancer of the liver among women in the drinking water subcohort supplied with chlorinated surface water at home, as compared with users of untreated groundwater. A later nested case-control study of cancer of the pancreas from the same cohort[88] found a significantly elevated odds ratio of 2.2 (confidence interval of 1.2 to 4.1).

Colon cancer was the subject of case-control interview studies in North Carolina[36] and Wisconsin.[173] In the former, an association was observed with use of chlorinated surface water but only among cases more than 60 years old. In Wisconsin, where the authors estimated trihalomethane ingestion at various times in the past, no associations with colon cancer were noted.

Bladder cancer risk as related to water source and tap water consumption was evaluated in a large case-control interview study of 3000 cases and 6000 controls in 10 areas of the United States.[22] A lifetime profile of home drinking water source and treatment was developed for each respondent by merging individual residential histories with water utility information. Bladder cancer risk increased with the amount of tap water consumed. This increase was strongly influenced by the duration of living at residences served by chlorinated surface water. Among respondents who resided for 60 or more years at places served by surface water, a risk of 2.0 was found for persons in the highest tap water consumption quintile relative to those in the lowest quintile, after adjustment for smoking, occupation, and other factors. There was no association of bladder cancer risk with water consumption among respondents who used little or no drinking water from surface sources. Similar findings were reported from a smaller case-control study of bladder cancer and disinfection methods in Colorado.[119]

These studies support a link between bladder cancer risk and long-term consumption of water from chlorinated surface waters, which have much higher levels of chlorination by-products than chlorinated or nonchlorinated groundwater. Other contaminants in surface water sources may also be important exposures. The findings for cancer of the rectum are weaker, in that most studies are death-certificate based, with little detailed exposure information. Results for colon cancer are inconclusive.

Concluding remarks

Drinking water contains a complex mixture of many chemicals, some of which may be carcinogenic. When present, these known or suspected carcinogens are usually found in trace concentrations (<10 ppb). Human exposure

---

*References 22, 36, 88, 119, 167, 173.

to these substances has been difficult to determine, and epidemiological studies to date have relied primarily on surrogate measures to estimate exposure differences, for example, residential histories to estimate duration of exposure to a particular water supply and use of the information that chlorinated surface water contains higher levels of by-products than chlorinated groundwater. When interpreting results of the epidemiology studies, it must be remembered that surrogate measures may not adequately represent actual exposure to the water contaminant of interest. For example, the quality of ground water and surface water may differ for many other contaminants in addition to chlorination by-products. In addition, it can be difficult to assess historical exposures to many contaminants of interest over the appropriate time period 20 to 40 years, or more, before diagnosis of the cancer. With these important limitations for many of the studies, it has been difficult to establish a causal relationship for the epidemiological associations observed. Nevertheless, we believe that the following associations between water quality and cancer are suggested and should be further explored by additional epidemiological and toxicological research:

1. Arsenic with nonmelanoma skin cancers and possibly with cancer of several internal sites, including bladder, kidney, and lung.
2. Synthetic organic chemicals, especially those found in chlorinated surface waters, with cancer of the bladder and rectum.
3. Nitrate with cancer of the gastrointestinal tract, especially stomach, and possibly brain cancer.
4. Asbestiform fibers with cancer of the stomach and kidney.
5. Radon in water that contributes to airborne levels in homes, linked to increased lung cancer risk.

REFERENCES

1. Alavanja M, Goldstein I, Susser M: *A case control study of gastrointestinal and urinary tract cancer mortality and drinking water chlorination.* In, Jolley RL, Gorchev H, Hamilton DH JR, editors: *Water chlorination: environmental impact and health effects,* vol 2, Ann Arbor, Mich, 1978, Ann Arbor Science.
2. Al-Dabbagh S, Forman D, Bryson D, et al: Mortality of nitrate fertiliser workers, *Br J Ind Med* 43:507, 1986.
3. Armijo R, Coulson AH: Epidemiology of stomach cancer in Chile—the role of nitrogen fertilizers, *Int J Epidemiol* 4:301, 1975.
4. Aschengrau A, et al: Cancer risk and tetrachloroethylene (PCE) contaminated drinking water in Massachusetts, *Arch Environ Health* 48:284, 1993.
5. Badawi AF, Mostafa MH, O'Connor PJ: Involvement of alkylating agents in schistosome-associated bladder cancer: the possible basic mechanisms of induction, *Cancer Lett* 63:171, 1992.
6. Badenoch J: *Cryptosporidium in water supplies: report of an expert group,* London; 1990, Her Majesty's Stationery Office.
7. Bancroft PM: Poliomyelitis in Huskerville (Lincoln) Nebraska, *JAMA* 164:836, 1957.
8. Bean JA et al: Drinking water and cancer incidence in Iowa: II. Radioactivity in drinking water, *Am J Epidemiol* 116:924, 1982.
9. Bean JA et al: Drinking water and cancer incidence in Iowa: I.

Trends and incidence by source of drinking water and size of municipality, *Am J Epidemiol* 116:912, 1982.

10. Benenson AS, editor: *Control of communicable diseases in man,* 15th ed, Washington, DC: 1990, American Public Health Association.

11. Beresford SAA: Is nitrate in the drinking water associated with the risk of cancer in the urban UK? *Int J Epidemiol* 14:57, 1985.

12. Berg JW, Burbank F: Correlations between carcinogenic trace metals in water supplies and cancer mortality, *Ann NY Acad Sci* 199:249, 1972.

13. Bergoglio RM: Mortalidad por cancer en zonas de aguas arsenicales de la Provincia de Cordoba, Republica Argentina, *Pren Med Argent* 51:994, 1964.

14. Birkhead G, Vogt RL: Epidemiologic surveillance for endemic Giardia lamblia infection in Vermont, *Am J Epidemiol* 129:762, 1989.

15. Borgono JM, Grieber R: Estudio epidemiologicalo del arsenicismo en la ciudad de Antofagasta, *Rev Med Chil* 99:702, 1971.

16. Brenniman GR et al: *Case-control study of cancer deaths in Illinois communities served by chlorinated or nonchlorinated water.* In Jolley RL, Brungs WA, Cumming RB, editors: *Water chlorination: environmental impact and health effects,* vol 3, Ann Arbor, Mich, 1980, Ann Arbor Science.

17. Bucher JR et al: Results and conclusions of the National Toxicology Program's rodent carcinogenicity studies with sodium fluoride, *Int J Cancer* 48:733, 1991.

18. Budnick LD et al: Cancer and birth defects near the Drake Superfund Site, Pennsylvania, *Arch Environ Health* 39:409, 1984.

19. Burk D, Yiamouyiannis J: Fluoridation and cancer, *Congressional Record* July 21:1975.

20. Byers VS et al: Association between clinical symptoms and lymphocyte abnormalities in a population with chronic domestic exposure to industrial solvent-contaminated domestic water supply and a high incidence of leukaemia, *Cancer Immunol Immunother* 27:77, 1988.

21. *Cancer statistics review: 1973-1989,* NIH Pub. No.92-2789, Bethesda, Md: 1992, National Cancer Institute.

22. Cantor KP et al: Bladder cancer, drinking water source, and tap water consumption: a case-control study, *J Natl Cancer Inst* 79:1269, 1987.

23. Cantor KP et al: Associations of cancer mortality with halomethanes in drinking water, *J Natl Cancer Inst* 61:979, 1978.

24. Cebrian ME et al: Chronic arsenic poisoning in the north of Mexico, *Human Toxicol* 2:121, 1983.

25. Centers for Disease Control: Outbreak of Yersinia enterocolitica—Washington state, *MMWR* 31:562, 1982.

26. Cheever AW: Schistosomiasis and neoplasia, *J Natl Cancer Inst* 61:13, 1978 (guest editorial).

27. Chen C-J, Wang C-J: Ecological correlation between arsenic level in well water and age-adjusted mortality from malignant neoplasms, *Cancer Res* 50:5470, 1990.

28. Chen C-J et al: Malignant neoplasms among residents of a blackfoot disease-endemic area in Taiwan: high-arsenic artesian well water and cancers, *Cancer Res* 45:5895, 1985.

29. Chen C-J et al: A retrospective study on malignant neoplasms of bladder, lung and liver in blackfoot disease endemic area, *Br J Cancer* 53:399, 1986.

30. Chilvers C: Cancer mortality and fluoridation of water supplies in 35 US cities, *Int J Epidemiol* 12:397, 1983.

31. Chilvers C et al: A survey of dietary nitrate in well-water users, *Int J Epidemiol* 13:324, 1984.

32. Chute CG, Smith RP, Baron JA: Risk factors for endemic giardiasis, *Am J Public Health* 77:585, 1987.

33. Clark CS et al: An environmental health survey of drinking water contamination by leachate from a pesticide waste dump in Hardeman County, Tennessee, *Arch Environ Health* 37:9, 1982.

34. Conforti PM et al: Asbestos in drinking water and cancer in the San Francisco Bay area: 1969-1974 incidence, *J Chron Dis* 34:211, 1981.

35. Cothern CR, Lappenbusch WL, Michel J: Drinking-water contribution to natural background radiation, *Health Phys* 50:33, 1986.

36. Cragle DL et al: *A case-control study of colon cancer and water chlorination in North Carolina.* In Jolley RL et al, editors: *Water chlorination: chemistry, environmental impact and health effects,* vol 5, Chelsea, Mich, 1985, Lewis Publishers.

37. Craun GF: *Health aspects of ground water pollution.* In Bitton G, Gerba CP, editors: *Groundwater pollution microbiology,* New York, 1984, John Wiley & Sons.

38. Craun GF: *Waterborne diseases in the United States,* Boca Raton, Fla, 1986, CRC Press.

39. Craun GF: *Statistics of waterborne outbreaks in the U.S. (1920-1980).* In Craun GF, editor: *Waterborne diseases in the United States,* Boca Raton, Fla, 1986, CRC Press.

40. Craun GF: Surface water supplies and health, *J Am Water Works Assoc* 80:240, 1988.

41. Craun GF, editor: *Methods for the investigation and prevention of waterborne disease outbreaks,* Cincinnati, 1991, Environmental Protection Agency.

42. Craun GF: *Waterborne giardiasis.* In Meyer EA, editor: *Giardiasis,* Amsterdam, 1990, Elsevier.

43. Craun GF: Waterborne disease outbreaks in the United States of America: causes and prevention, *World Health Stat Q* 45:192, 1992.

44. Craun GF, Jakubowski W: *Status of waterborne giardiasis outbreaks and monitoring methods.* In Tate J Jr, editor: *Proc. International Symposium on Water Related Health Issues,* Bethesda, Md, 1993, American Water Resources Association.

45. Craun GF et al: Prevention of cholera in the United States, *J Am Water Works Assoc* 83:40, 1991.

46. Crump KS, Guess HA: Drinking water and cancer: review of recent epidemiological findings and assessment of risks, *Annu Rev Public Health* 3:339, 1982.

47. Cuello C et al: Gastric cancer in Colombia. I. Cancer risk and suspect environmental agents, *J Natl Cancer Inst* 57:1015, 1976.

48. Current WL: Cryptosporidium: its biology and potential for environmental protection, *CRC Critical Reviews in Environmental Control* 17:21, 1986.

49. Cutler JJ et al: Childhood leukemia in Woburn, Massachusetts, *Publ Health Rep* 101:201, 1986.

50. Cuzick J, Sasieni P, Evans S: Ingested arsenic, keratoses, and bladder cancer, *Am J Epidemiol* 136:417, 1992.

51. D'Antonio RG et al: A waterborne outbreak of Cryptosporidiosis in normal hosts, *Ann Intern Med* 103:886, 1985.

52. Dev VJ, Main M, Gould I: Waterborne outbreak of *Escherichia coli* 0157, *Lancet* 337:1412, 1991.

53. Dufour AP: *Diseases caused by water contact.* In Craun GF, editor: *Waterborne diseases in the United States,* Boca Raton, Fla, CRC Press.

54. Eden KV et al: Waterborne gastroenteritis at a ski resort—isolation of Yersinia enterocolitica from drinking water, *Publ Health Rep* 92:245, 1977.

55. Eisenbrand G, Speigelhalder B, Preussmann R: Nitrate and nitrite in saliva, *Oncology* 37:227, 1980.

56. El-Bolkainy MN et al: The impact of Schistosomiasis on the pathology of bladder carcinoma, *Cancer* 48:2643, 1981.

57. Evans AS: Causation and disease: the Henle-Koch postulates revisited, *Yale J Biol Med* 49:175, 1976.

58. Evans AS: Causation and disease: effect of technology on postulates of causation, *Yale J Biol Med* 64:513, 1991.

59. Fagliano J et al: Drinking water contamination and the incidence of leukemia: an ecological study, *Am J Public Health* 80:1209, 1990.

60. Fayer R, Ungar LP: Cryptosporidium spp. and cryptosporidiosis, *Microbiol Rev* 50:458, 1986.

61. Flaten TP: Chlorination of drinking water and cancer incidence in Norway, *Int J Epidemiol* 21:6, 1992.

62. Flaten TP, Bolviken B: Geographical associations between drinking water chemistry and the mortality and morbidity of cancer and some other diseases in Norway, *Sci Total Environ* 102:75, 1991.

63. Fraser P, Chilvers C: Health aspects of nitrate in drinking water, *Sci Total Environ* 18:103, 1981.

64. Fraser GG, Cooke KR: Endemic giardiasis and municipal water supply, *Am J Public Health* 81:760, 1991.

65. Fraser P et al: Further results from a census based mortality study of fertiliser manufacturers, *Br J Ind Med* 46:38, 1989.

66. Fuortes L, McNutt LA, Lynch C: Leukemia incidence and radioactivity in drinking water in 59 Iowa towns, *Am J Public Health* 80:1261, 1990.

67. Gallaher MM et al: Cryptosporidiosis and surface water, *Am J Public Health* 79:39, 1989.

68. Gilli G, Corrao G, Favilli S: Concentrations of nitrates in drinking water and incidence of gastric carcinomas: first descriptive study of the Piemonte region, Italy, *Sci Total Environ* 34:35, 1984.

69. Gottlieb MS, Carr JK: Case-control cancer mortality study and chlorination of drinking water in Louisiana, *Environ Health Perspect* 46:169, 1982.

70. Griffith J et al: Cancer mortality in U.S. counties with hazardous waste sites and ground water pollution, *Arch Environ Health* 44:69, 1989.

71. Hallberg GR: *Agricultural chemicals and groundwater quality in Iowa: status report 1985*, Cooperative Extension Service, Iowa State University, 1985.

72. Harrington JM et al: An investigation of the use of asbestos cement pipe for public water supply and the incidence of gastrointestinal cancer in Connecticut, 1935-1973, *Am J Epidemiol* 107:96, 1978.

73. Harrington JM et al: A survey of a population exposed to high concentrations of arsenic in well water in Fairbanks, Alaska, *Am J Epidemiol* 108:377, 1978.

74. Harris JR: *Clinical and epidemiological characteristics of common infectious diseases and chemical poisonings caused by ingestion of contaminated drinking water*. In Craun GF, editor: *Waterborne diseases in the United States,* Boca Raton, Fla, 1986, CRC Press.

75. Hart RJ, Walters CL: The formation of nitrite and *N*-nitroso compounds in salivas in vitro and in vivo, *Food Cosmet Toxicol* 21:749, 1983.

76. Harter L, Frost F, Jakubowski W: Giardia prevalence among 1 to 3 year old children in two Washington state counties, *Am J Public Health* 72:386, 1982.

77. Hayes EB et al: Large community outbreak of Cryptosporidiosis due to contamination of a filtered public water supply, *N Engl J Med* 320:1372, 1989.

78. Heath CW et al: Cytogenetic findings in persons living near the Love Canal, *JAMA* 251:1437, 1984.

79. Henle J: *On Miasmata and Contagie* (translation, with introduction by George Rosen), Baltimore, 1938, Johns Hopkins Press.

80. Herwaldt BL et al: Waterborne-disease outbreaks, 1989-1990, *MMWR* 40:1, 1991.

81. Herwaldt BL et al: Outbreaks of waterborne disease in the United States: 1989-1990, *J Am Water Works Assoc* 84:129, 1992.

82. Hess CT, Weiffenbach CV, Norton SA: Environmental radon and cancer correlations in Maine, *Health Phys* 45:339, 1983.

83. Hogan MD, Chi P-Y, Hoel DG: Association between chloroform levels in finished drinking water supplies and various site-specific cancer mortality rates, *J Environ Pathol Toxicol* 2:873, 1979.

84. Hoover RN, McKay FW, Fraumeni JF: Fluoridated drinking water and the occurrence of cancer, *J Natl Cancer Inst* 57:757, 1976.

85. Hoover RN et al: *Appendix F. Time trends for bone and joint cancers and osteosarcomas in the surveillance, epidemiology and end results (SEER) Program, National Cancer Institute*. In *Review of fluoride: benefits and risks. Report of the Ad Hoc Subcommittee on Fluoride of the Committee to Coordinate Environmental Health and Related Programs,* Washington, DC, 1991, Public Health Service, DHHS.

86. Howe HL et al: Cancer incidence following exposure to drinking water with asbestos leachate, *Publ Health Rep* 104:251, 1989.

87. Hrudey SE et al: Drinking water fluoridation and osteosarcoma, *Can J Public Health* 81:415, 1990.

88. IJsselmuiden CB et al: Cancer of the pancreas and drinking water: a population-based case-control study in Washington County, Maryland, *Am J Epidemiol* 136:836, 1992.

89. International Agency for Research on Cancer: *IARC monographs on the evaluation of the carcinogenic risk of chemicals to humans, vol 17: some N-nitroso compounds,* Lyon, France, 1978, International Agency for Research on Cancer.

90. International Agency for Research on Cancer: inorganic fluorides. In *IARC monographs on the evaluation of carcinogenic risk of chemicals to humans, vol 27: some aromatic amines, anthraquinones and nitroso compounds, and inorganic fluorides,* Lyon, France, 1982, International Agency for Research on Cancer.

91. International Agency for Research on Cancer: *Overall evaluations of carcinogenicity: an updating of IARC monographs,* vol 1 to 42, Lyon, France, 1987, International Agency for Research on Cancer.

92. Isacson P, et al: Drinking water and cancer incidence in Iowa: III. association of cancer with indices of contamination, *Am J Epidemiol* 121:856, 1985.

93. Isacson P, Bean JA, Lynch C: *Relationship of cancer incidence rates in Iowa municipalities to chlorination status of drinking water.* In Jolley RL et al, editors: *Water chlorination: environmental impact and health effects vol 4,* Ann Arbor, Mich, 1983, Ann Arbor Science.

94. Janerich DT et al: Cancer incidence in the Love Canal area, *Science* 212:1404, 1981.

95. Jensen OM: Nitrate in drinking water and cancer in northern Jutland, Denmark, with special reference to stomach cancer, *Ecotoxicol Environ Safety* 6:258, 1982.

96. Johnson CJ, Kross BC: Continuing importance of nitrate contamination of groundwater and wells in rural areas, *Am J Ind Med* 18:449, 1990.

97. Juhasz L, Hill MJ, Nagy G: Possible relationship between nitrate in drinking water and incidence of stomach cancer, *IARC Sci Publ* 31:619, 1980.

98. Kanarek MS et al: Asbestos in drinking water and cancer incidence in the San Francisco Bay area, *Am J Epidemiol* 112:54, 1980.

99. Knox EG: *Fluoridation of water and cancer: a review of the epidemiological evidence,* London, 1985, Report of a Working Party, Her Majesty's Stationery Office.

100. Koch R: Die aetiologie der tuberculose, *Mitt Kaiser Gesundh* 2:1, 1884.

101. Koivusalo M et al: Drinking water mutagenicity and gastrointestinal and urinary tract cancers: an ecological study in Finland, *Am J Health* 84:1994.

102. Kuzma RJ, Kuzma CM, Buncher CR: Ohio drinking water source and cancer rates, *Am J Public Health* 67:725, 1977.

103. Lagakos SW, Wessen BJ, Zelen M: An analysis of contaminated well water and health effects in Woburn, Massachusetts, *J Am Stat Assoc* 81:583, 1986.

104. Lampi P et al: Cancer incidence following chlorophenol exposure in a community in southern Finland, *Arch Environ Health* 47:167, 1992.

105. *Large outbreak of cryptosporidiosis in Jackson County, Communicable Disease Summary,* Oregon Health Division, 1992.

106. Langer AM : The contamination of Lake Superior with amphibole gangue minerals, *Ann NY Acad Sci* 330:549, 1979.

107. Lawrence CE et al: Trihalomethanes in drinking water and human colorectal cancer, *J Natl Cancer Inst* 72:563, 1984.

108. Laxter MA: Potential exposure of Utah Army National Gaurd personnel to giardiasis during field training exercises: a preliminary survey, *Mili Med* 150:23, 1985.

109. *Legionella,* Washington, DC, 1984, American Society for Microbiology.

110. Levine WC, Craun GF: Waterborne-disease outbreaks, 1986-1988, *MMWR* 39:1, 1990.

111. Levy BS et al: Investigating possible effects of asbestos in city water: surveillance of gastrointestinal cancer incidence in Duluth, Minnesota, *Am J Epidemiol* 103:362, 1976.

112. Lilienfeld DE, Gallo MA: *2,4-D, 2,4,5-T, and 2,3,7,8-TCDD: an overview.* In Armenlan HK et al, editors: *Epidemiologic reviews,* vol 11, Baltimore, 1989, American Journal of Epidemiology.

113. Lu FJ: Blackfoot disease: arsenic or humic acid? *Lancet* 336:115, 1990 (letter).

114. Lyman GH, Lyman CG, Johnson W: Association of leukemia with radium groundwater contamination, *JAMA* 254:621, 1985.

115. MacMahon B et al: Comments and rejoinder on Lagakos, Wessen, and Zelen article on contaminated well water and health effects in Woburn, Massachusetts, *J Am Stat Assoc* 81:597, 1986.

116. Mahoney MC et al: Bone cancer incidence rates in New York State: time trends and fluoridated drinking water, *Am J Public Health* 81:475, 1991.

117. Mason TJ, McKay FW, Miller RW: Asbestos-like fibers in Duluth water supply, *JAMA* 228:1019, 1974.

118. McDonald DB, Splinter RC: Long-term trends in nitrate concentration in Iowa water supplies, *J Am Water Works Assoc* 74:437, 1982.

119. McGeehin MA et al: A case-control study of bladder cancer and water disinfection methods in Colorado, *Am J Epidemiol* 138:492, 1993.

120. McGuire SM et al: Is there a link between fluoridated water and osteosarcoma? *J Am Dent Assoc* 122:38, 1991.

121. Meigs JW et al: Asbestos cement pipe and cancer in Connecticut 1955-1974, *J Environ Health* 42:187, 1980.

122. Meyer EA, editor: *Giardiasis,* Amsterdam, 1990, Elsevier.

123. Millette JR et al: Asbestos in water supplies of the United States, *Environ Health Perspect* 53:45, 1983.

124. Millette JR et al: Epidemiology study of the use of asbestos-cement pipe for the distribution of drinking water in Escambia County, Florida, *Environ Health Perspect* 53:91, 1983.

125. Mirvish SS et al: *N*-Nitrosoproline excretion by rural Nebraskans drinking water of varied nitrate content, *Cancer Epidemiol Biomark Prev* 1:455, 1992.

126. Moller H et al: Endogenous nitrosation in relation to nitrate exposure from drinking water and diet in a Danish rural population, *Cancer Res* 49:3117, 1989.

127. Morton W et al: Skin cancer and water arsenic in Lane County, Oregon, *Cancer* 37:2523, 1976.

128. Mustacchi P, Shimkin MB: Cancer of the bladder and infestation with *Schistosoma hematobium, J Natl Cancer Inst* 20:825, 1958.

129. Najem GR et al: Clusters of cancer mortality in New Jersey municipalities; with special reference to chemical toxic waste disposal sites and per capita income, *Int J Epidemiol* 14:528, 1985.

130. National Research Council: *Drinking water and health,* vol 1. Washington, DC, 1977, National Academy of Sciences.

131. National Research Council: *Inorganic solutes.* In *Drinking water and health,* vol 1, Washington, DC, 1977, National Academy of Sciences.

132. National Research Council: *Epidemiological studies.* In *Drinking water and health,* vol 3, Safe Drinking Water Committee, Washington, DC, 1980, National Academy Press.

133. Nazaroff WW et al: Potable water as a source of airborne 222Rn in U.S. dwellings: a review and assessment, *Health Phys* 52:281, 1987.

134. Osterholm MT et al: An outbreak of newly recognized chronic diarrhea syndrome associated with raw milk consumption, *JAMA* 256:484, 1986.

135. Page T, Harris RH, Epstein SS: Drinking water and cancer mortality in Louisiana, *Science* 193:55, 1976.

136. Parsonnet J et al: Chronic diarrhea associated with drinking untreated water, *Ann Intern Med* 110:985, 1989.

137. Payment P et al: Gastrointestinal health effects associated with the consumption of drinking water produced by point of use domestic reverse osmosis filteration units, *Appl Environ Microbiol* 57:945, 1991.

138. Payment P et al: A randomized trial to evaluate the risk of gastrointestinal disease due to consumption of drinking water meeting current microbiological standards, *Am J Public Health* 81:703, 1991.

139. Polissar L, Severson RK, Boatman ES: A case-control study of asbestos in drinking water and cancer risk, *Am J Epidemiol* 119:456, 1984.

140. Polissar L et al: Cancer incidence in relation to asbestos in drinking water in the Puget Sound region, *Am J Epidemiol* 116:314, 1982.

141. Rademacher JJ, Young TB, Kanarek MS: Gastric cancer mortality and nitrate levels in Wisconsin drinking water, *Arch Environ Health* 47:292, 1992.

142. Rafnsson V, Gunnarsdottir H: Mortality study of fertiliser manufacturers in Iceland, *Br J Ind Med* 47:721, 1990.

143. Rose JB, Gerba CP, Jakubowski W: Survey of potable water supplies for Cryptosporidium and Giardia, *Environ Sci Technol* 25:1393, 1991.

144. Sadler TD et al: The use of asbestos-cement pipe for public water supply and the incidence of cancer in selected communities in Utah, *J Commun Health* 9:285, 1984.

145. Salg J: *Cancer mortality rates and drinking water in 346 counties of the Ohio River Valley Basin,* Chapel Hill, NC, 1977, University of North Carolina, Ph.D. Thesis.

146. Saslow MS et al: Typhoid fever, public health aspects, *Am J Public Health* 65:1184, 1975.

147. Seshan K: How are the physical and chemical properties of chrysotile asbestos altered by a 10-year residence in water and up to 5 days in simulated stomach acid? *Environ Health Perspect* 53:143, 1983.

148. Sigurdson EE et al: Cancer morbidity investigations: lessons from the Duluth study of possible effects of asbestos in drinking water, *Environ Res* 25:50, 1981.

149. Singer PC, Chang SD: Correlations between trihalomethanes and total organic halides formed during water treatment, *J Am Water Works Assoc* 81:61, 1989.

150. Snow J: *On the mode of communication of cholera,* 2nd ed, London, 1855, Churchill.

151. Soave R: Treatment strategies for cryptosporidiosis, *Ann NY Acad Sci* 616:442, 1990.

152. Sobsey MD, Fuji T, Hall RM: Inactivation of cell-associated and dispersed hepititis A virus in water, *J Am Water Works Assoc* 83:64, 1991.

153. St. Louis ME: Water-related disease outbreaks, 1985, *MMWR* 37:15, 1988.

154. Stevens AA, Moore LA, Miltner RJ: Formation and control of non-trihalomethane disinfection by-products, *J Am Water Works Assoc* 81:54, 1989.

155. Sykora JL, Craun GF, editors: *The taxonomy, detection, epidemiology and waterborne control of Cryptosporidium,* Pittsburgh, 1989, University of Pittsburgh.

156. Thomas JE et al: Relationship between bladder cancer incidence, Schistosoma haematobium infection, and geographical region in Zimbabwe, *Trans R Soc Trop Med Hyg* 84:551, 1990.

157. Tricker AR et al: Urinary nitrate, nitrite and *N*-nitroso compounds

in bladder cancer patients with schistosomiasis (bilharzia), *IARC Sci Publ* 105:178, 1991.

158. Tseng W-P: Effects and dose-response relationships of skin cancer and blackfoot disease with arsenic, *Environ Health Perspect* 19:109, 1977.

159. Tseng WP, Chu HM, How SW: Prevalence of skin cancer in an endemic area of chronic arsenicism in Taiwan, *J Natl Cancer Inst* 40:453, 1968.

160. US Environmental Protection Agency, Office of Pesticide Programs: *Pesticides in ground water data base: 1988 interim report,* Washington, DC, 1988.

161. U.S. Public Health Service, Committee to Coordinate Environmental Health and Related Programs, Subcommittee on Fluoride: *Review of fluoride: benefits and risks,* Washington, DC, 1991, Department of Health and Human Services.

162. Vogt RL et al: Campylobacter enteritis associated with contaminated water, *Ann Intern Med* 96:292, 1982.

163. Walters CL: The exposure of humans to nitrite, *Oncology* 37:289, 1980.

164. Walters CL, Smith PLR: The effect of water-borne nitrate on salivary nitrite, *Food Cosmet Toxicol* 19:297, 1981.

165. Weiss HB et al: Giardiasis in Minnesota, 1971-1975, *Minn Med* 60:815, 1977.

166. Wigle DT: Cancer mortality in relation to asbestos in municipal water supplies, *Arch Environ Health* 32:185, 1977.

167. Wilkins JRIII, Comstock GW: Source of drinking water at home and site-specific cancer incidence in Washington County, Maryland, *Am J Epidemiol* 114:178, 1981.

168. Wilkins JRIII, Reiches NA, Kruse CW: Organic chemical contaminants in drinking water and cancer, *Am J Epidemiol* 110:420, 1979.

169. Wright HB et al: Giardiasis in Colorado: an epidemiological study, *Am J Epidemiol* 105:330, 1977.

170. Wu M-M et al: Dose-response relation between arsenic concentration in well water and mortality from cancers and vascular diseases, *Am J Epidemiol* 130:1123, 1989.

171. Xu G, Song P, Reed PI: The relationship between gastric mucosal changes and nitrate intake via drinking water in a high-risk population for gastric cancer in Moping county, China, *Eur J Cancer Prev* 1:437, 1992.

172. Young TB, Kanarek MS, Tsiatis AA: Epidemiologic study of drinking water chlorination and Wisconsin female cancer mortality, *J Natl Cancer Inst* 67:1191, 1981.

173. Young TB, Wolf DA, Kanarek MS: Case-control study of colon cancer and drinking water trihalomethanes in Wisconsin, *Int J Epidemiol* 16:190, 1987.

174. Zierler S et al: Bladder cancer in Massachusetts related to chlorinated and chloraminated drinking water: a case-control study, *Arch Environ Health* 43:195, 1988.

Part II

PATHOGENIC MECHANISMS OF ENVIRONMENTAL AND OCCUPATIONAL DISEASE

MECHANISMS OF CELL INJURY

John L. Farber

The mechanisms whereby toxic chemicals injure cells have long been a subject of interest to toxicologists and other biologists. The last two decades have witnessed a remarkable proliferation of publications dealing with the events in toxic cell injury. These studies have detailed many biochemical and morphological changes that occur when a variety of cell types are exposed to a large number of toxic agents. It has been a more difficult task, however, to elucidate which, if any, of these perturbations are casually related to the biological endpoints at issue.

This chapter reviews the literature and presents the current concepts regarding the mechanisms that may underlie toxic cell injury. It is generally assumed that the destruction of the integrity of the plasma membrane with the loss of its permeability barrier function is the critical event leading to a loss of cellular viability. Thus, this discussion focuses on the mechanisms whereby toxic chemicals produce membrane damage. Xenobiotic compounds, either directly or as a result of the generation of electrophilic metabolites, bind covalently to macromolecular components of cellular membranes, peroxidize the phospholipids of these membranes, or deplete membrane-bound protein thiol groups. These reactions are the best-known mechanisms proposed to account for the pathogenesis of membrane injury and cell death following exposure to a toxic chemical. The support for these concepts is discussed, and the still controversial role of alterations in calcium homeostasis in cell injury is reviewed. A discussion of the relationship between damage to DNA or to mitochondria and the loss of cellular viability concludes the chapter.

REACTION OF CELLS TO CHEMICALS AND OTHER STRESSES

Cells encounter many stresses as a result of changes in their internal and external environments. Potentially hazardous changes in environmental conditions include the exposure of cells to foreign chemicals, radiation, changes in the oxygen content of the blood, or extreme fluctuations in temperature. The pattern of response to these stresses constitutes the cellular basis of disease. Fortunately, all cells have efficient mechanisms to deal with such stresses. Thus foreign chemicals are metabolized, and various control mechanisms are elicited to maintain normal intracellular conditions. Injury or damage to a cell, however, occurs when environmental changes exceed the ability of the cell to adapt to those changes. If the stress is not pronounced or is removed in sufficient time, the injury is reversible, and the cell recovers functional and morphological integrity. If the stress is severe, acute irreversible injury results, followed by death of the cell. The precise moment when injury progresses to irreversible damage cannot be identified at present, but reversible injury is easily distinguished from necrosis. Necrosis is the result of irreversible injury seen on gross and microscopic examination. In other words, necrosis is the morphological expression of cell death.

Reversible cell injury

The most characteristic change seen in reversible injury is cell swelling due to an increased intracellular water content. Known as hydropic swelling, or degeneration, this condition is identified by a large pale cytoplasm and a normally located nucleus. Cells demonstrating hydropic degeneration show distinctive ultrastructural morphology, including dilation of the cisternae of the endoplasmic reticulum, which results from a shift in ions and water from the cytosol into the cisternae. The increased volume presumably results from an impairment of cellular volume regulation most likely at the level of the plasma membrane. The number of organelles does not change, but they appear more scattered in the larger cell volume.

The plasma membrane is the primary organelle that maintains cytoplasmic ionic homeostasis. In turn, ionic concentrations, particularly those of sodium and potassium, regulate the intracellular water content. The plasma membrane acts as a regulator at two levels. First, the plasma membrane provides a semipermeable barrier against the influx of sodium (Na^+) and the efflux of potassium (K^+) against their concentration gradients; however, because the membrane is semipermeable, some ions can leak passively across the membrane. The second regulatory level compensates for this leakiness. The plasma membrane sodium pump (i.e., Na^+, K^+-ATPase), fueled by adenosine triphosphate (ATP), actively exchanges sodium for potassium.

Injurious agents can interfere with this plasma membrane–associated regulatory mechanism by (1) increasing the permeability of the membrane itself, (2) damaging the sodium-potassium pump, or (3) interfering with the generation of the ATP necessary to drive the pump. As a result of one or more of these actions, sodium accumulates in an injured cell. Water then follows to maintain isosmotic conditions, and the cell subsequently swells (see Chapter 18).

Another indicator of reversible injury, known as fatty change or "fatty degeneration," is defined as any abnormal accumulation of fat in a parenchymal cell. It is less universal, primarily encountered in those cells involved in or dependent on fat metabolism, such as the hepatocyte and myocyte. Morphologically, fatty change is manifested by the appearance of non–membrane-bound fat droplets in the cytoplasm, which may eventually fuse to produce larger "cleared spaces." This increase in cellular fat reflects an imbalance in the metabolic utilization of fat in the injured cell.

In addition to hydropic swelling and fatty change, a number of characteristic alterations in the structure of cellular organelles can accompany reversible injury. As noted previously, one of the earliest ultrastructural changes seen in acutely injured cells is dilation of the endoplasmic reticulum. The dilation of the cisternae is most likely due to the redistribution of water and ions. In addition, membrane-bound polysomes may detach from the surface of the rough endoplasmic reticulum. Mitochondria also display typical changes during reversible injury: they appear swollen, with expansion of the matrix compartments. In contrast, a marked condensation of the cristae has also been described. These types of changes probably reflect loss of volume control at the mitochondrial level. Despite these morphological alterations, the mitochondria still retain their ability to respire.

A phenomenon known as cell surface blebbing is often seen during the reversible phase of cell injury. These blebs are evaginations of the plasma membrane containing cytoplasmic material, which can be pinched off and released from the cell without a loss of viability. Such blebbing appears to result directly from alterations of the cytoskeletal apparatus (microtubules and microfilaments) located beneath the plasma membrane, the function of which is to maintain normal cell shape. In turn, alterations in the cytoskeleton may relate to changes in cytosolic calcium ion concentration.

In addition to cell surface blebbing, rapid clumping of the nuclear chromatin and enlargement of the acidic vacuolar apparatus are other characteristic changes that constitute reversible injury processes. It is important to emphasize that, by definition, all of these ultrastructural changes can be reversed once the initiating stress is removed.

The morphological changes that constitute acute reversible cell injury should not be confused with those seen under conditions of persistent sublethal injury. Such "chronic cell injury" is still reversible because the cells involved are not dead, and removal of the stress generally results in restoration of normal integrity. In contrast to acute reversible injury, however, persistent sublethal injury reflects adaptation of the cell to a hostile environment. Such adaptations include atrophy, hypertrophy, hyperplasia, metaplasia, and dysplasia. Although these changes are generally not lethal, they can lead to dysfunction of the exposed cells or tissue, a consequence that eventually may or may not be lethal for the whole organism.

Irreversible cell injury

If the acute stress to which a cell must react is too great, the resulting changes in structure and function lead to death of the cell. Among the more common causes of cell death are exposure to xenobiotics (chemical and biological compounds that are foreign to the organism), ischemia, radiation, physical injury (trauma, extremes of temperature), and infectious agents. Importantly, cell death is almost always accompanied by a series of characteristic changes recognizable by gross and microscopic inspection. These changes, collectively labeled coagulative necrosis, are the most widely used criterion by which cell death is identified. In other words, when a tissue is examined for morphological evidence of irreversible injury, coagulative necrosis is the criterion by which cell death is identified. This is not to deny that there is a definable point before the appearance of coagulative necrosis when the cell injury is irreversible. If such a point exists, however, it cannot be appreciated in any morphological alteration of the injured cell.

Morphology of necrosis. A cell that has undergone coagulative necrosis exhibits increased cytoplasmic eosinophilia when stained with hematoxylin and eosin. This change is due to a loss of normal cytoplasmic basophilia, usually associated with cytoplasmic RNA, and an increased binding of eosin to the denatured proteins. In addition, the cell often displays an opaque homogeneous appearance with the loss of glycogen particles, which normally impart a granular appearance to the cytoplasm. Large eosinophilic globules represent severely swollen mitochondria. Eventually the cell becomes vacuolated, as organelles are digested by lysosomal enzymes. Calcification may also occur.

Characteristic alterations of the nucleus also accompany coagulative necrosis. The nucleus of a dead cell becomes shrunken and deeply basophilic. This change, called pyknosis, reflects pronounced clumping of chromatin. The pyknotic nucleus may eventually break up into smaller fragments and become scattered within the cytoplasm (karyorrhexis) or undergo progressive dissolution and disappear (karyolysis).

A hallmark of coagulative necrosis is the preservation of the basic shape and architecture of the dead cell, at least long enough to allow identification. The necrotic tissue is then usually removed by inflammatory processes, unless too large a volume of necrotic material is present. Large ischemic areas may be walled off to form a sequestrum of dead tissue because the inflammatory cells are unable to enter the necrotic area and remove the debris because of the low oxygen tension. When necrotic cells are removed, the void left is replaced either by a scar or by functional parenchyma depending on the regenerative capacity of the surrounding cells.

Coagulative necrosis is distinguished by some from apoptosis, or programmed cell death, a pattern of cell killing that characteristically affects scattered single cells similar to a process occurring during embryonic development and metamorphosis. The morphological features that define apoptosis include progressive contraction of cellular volume, chromatin condensation, and preservation of the integrity of the organelles. The affected cells usually disintegrate into membrane-bound fragments (apoptotic bodies), which are rapidly consumed by adjacent cells. Inflammatory cells such as neutrophils and macrophages are not involved in the removal of these apoptotic bodies.

It has been argued that apoptotic cell death occurs by a mechanism distinct from coagulative necrosis. Programmed cell death seems to depend on the triggering of an endogenous suicide program that requires gene transcription and messenger RNA translation. According to one hypothesis, the newly synthesized proteins act by inserting into the plasma membrane to create a hydrophilic channel, a situation similar to the action of complement and perforin, the mediator of cell killing by cytotoxic lymphocytes. In turn, an influx of calcium ions (see the section on Biochemical Mechanisms of Cell Injury) has been specifically related to the subsequent loss of viability of the cells.

Whether toxic chemicals can trigger the endogenous suicide program and subsequent apoptosis is largely unexplored. There is evidence that dioxins can bind to the glucocorticoid receptors of postthymic lymphocytes in vitro and thus trigger the death of these cells. However, whether such a phenomenon occurs in intact animals and whether other agents can similarly act on different cells is not known.

Pathogenesis of coagulative necrosis. As with the development of reversible injury, loss of the integrity of the plasma membrane is also closely related to the genesis of coagulative necrosis. Living cells exist in marked disequilibrium with their external environment. The plasma membrane governs the numerous passive and active mechanisms that maintain this disequilibrium. With cell death, the various ionic gradients existing between the inside and outside of the cell are dissipated. Therefore, cell death can be thought of as an equilibration of the intracellular and extracellular ionic concentrations because the plasma membrane is unable to maintain the ionic concentration gradients necessary for life.

The largest gradient in all cells is calcium. The intracellular concentration of calcium is on the order of 10^{-7} M compared with the extracellular concentration of 10^{-3} M, some 10,000-fold greater. This large gradient is maintained primarily by the plasma membrane. Its inherent impermeability to calcium coupled with the active extrusion of calcium by membrane-bound pumps provides an effective defense against the leakage of calcium into the cell. In turn, an accumulation of large amounts of intracellular calcium accompanies cell death. The influx of calcium activates numerous calcium-dependent enzymes, such as proteases, ribonucleases, and lipases, which degrade cellular constituents. Thus, the influx and accumulation of calcium can account for some of the common morphological changes recognized in coagulative necrosis.

Any further role of changes in intracellular calcium content in the development of necrosis remains controversial. One can envision at least two scenarios describing the genesis of necrosis. The first involves (1) severe biological stress, (2) irreversible injury, (3) cell death and the loss of plasma membrane integrity, (4) accumulation of calcium into the cell, and (5) the appearance of coagulative necrosis. With such a scheme, calcium accumulation and necrosis occur after irreversible injury and the death of the cell.

The second scenario gives calcium a more active role in cell death. In particular, potentially reversible injury to the plasma membrane leads to dysfunction and the subsequent leakage of extracellular calcium into the cell. The accumulated calcium then initiates processes that kill the cell. Here cell death is not distinct from necrosis and an accumulation of calcium is proposed as the critical transition converting reversible to irreversible injury.

A correlation between accumulation of calcium ions and the extent of coagulation necrosis exists in experimental liver injury. It remains to be established definitively, however, whether such calcium accumulations do indeed convert reversible injury to irreversible cell injury. There are few studies in the intact animal that have addressed this point. Existing data suggest that an influx and accumulation of calcium converts a potentially reversibly injured liver cell into an irreversibly injured necrotic hepatocyte in vitro. Such a role for calcium ions clearly needs more study in vivo.

It is clear that disruption of the permeability function of the plasma membrane seems to be a critical event in cell death and the development of necrosis. Loss of this barrier function results in equilibration of the cell's internal and external environments and transforms the cell into necrotic debris. Calcium may play a passive role in the pathogenesis of necrosis, in which case it is responsible for some of the common morphological changes. Alternatively, calcium may assume a more causal role in the genesis of toxic cell death. Regardless of the role of calcium, loss of plasma membrane integrity mediates necrosis of the cell.

ROLE OF METABOLISM IN TOXIC CELL INJURY

Many toxic chemicals are biologically inert and must be activated by cellular metabolism for injury to occur. Indeed, relatively few xenobiotics are sufficiently reactive to initiate direct cell injury on their own. Those that do are usually mitochondrial poisons, corrosive compounds (strong acids and bases), and reactive electrophiles.

The cytochrome P-450–linked monooxygenase system, a heterogeneous collection of enzymes, is responsible for the biotransformation of the majority of xenobiotics (see Chapters 5 and 26). Also known as the mixed-function oxidase system, the cytochrome P-450 system carries out the oxidative metabolism of diverse endogenous and exogenous substrates, such as fatty acids, steroids, drugs, and other foreign chemicals. Cytochrome P-450 is also responsible for the reductive metabolism of a few compounds, as occurs with the bioactivation of halothane. The term *cytochrome P-450* actually refers to a series of related hemo-

proteins containing iron-protoporphyrin IX as their prosthetic group. The various forms of cytochrome P-450 differ with respect to the primary structure of the apoprotein and, as a consequence, with respect to their substrate specificity.

In conjunction with cytochrome P-450, monooxygenase activity depends on another enzyme, nicotinamide-adenine dinucleotide phosphate (reduced form) (NADPH)–cytochrome P-450 reductase. This flavoprotein transfers electrons to cytochrome P-450 and uses NADPH as its source of reducing equivalents. Also associated with the mixed-function oxidase system is another hemoprotein called cytochrome b_5. The role that cytochrome b_5 and its respective reductase, however, play in the activity of P-450–linked oxidations has not been clearly established.

Cellular and tissue distribution of cytochrome P-450

The monooxygenase activity most commonly associated with the metabolism and toxicity of foreign compounds is localized in the membranes of the smooth endoplasmic reticulum. It should be noted that mitochondrial and nuclear monooxygenase activities have also been described. The activities of these systems, however, are low compared with that of the system in the endoplasmic reticulum. The activities of cytochrome P-450 in association with its NADPH-cytochrome P-450 reductase depend on an intact phospholipid matrix. Thus alterations in the membrane structure of the endoplasmic reticulum result in a change or loss of activity.

Among the various organs of the body, the endoplasmic reticulum of the liver hepatocytes contains the highest content of cytochrome P-450. The concentration of cytochrome P-450 in the liver of a rat or a rabbit is 30 to 40 nmol heme/g wet weight tissue. To date, at least 10 distinct isozymes of P-450 have been identified in rat liver, each with differing substrate specificities. Clearly the liver is the most active site of xenobiotic metabolism. This organ contains the widest variety and highest content of cytochrome P-450s and receives a generous flow of blood.

A significant amount of cytochrome P-450 is also present in the kidney, nasal epithelium, lung, and intestinal mucosa. Thus these organs also contribute to the metabolism of foreign compounds. Although most other tissues possess demonstrable mixed-function oxidase activity, they seem to play a minor role in xenobiotic metabolism. The biotransformation carried out by most other tissues is limited in terms of the number of substrates metabolized and the relative rate at which these reactions occur.

Enzymatic cycle of cytochrome P-450

The P-450 catalytic cycle is an electron transport system that mediates, in the presence of molecular oxygen, the oxidation of a variety of organic substrates. Our present knowledge of the reactions involved in the catalytic cycle of cytochrome P-450 can be briefly summarized. A molecule of substrate reversibly combines with oxidized (ferric) cytochrome P-450 with its iron in the low-spin state; that is, all the outer valence electrons are paired. The binding energy derived from the formation of an enzyme-substrate complex is used to convert the ferric iron to ferrous iron, and molecular oxygen readily binds to the reduced enzyme-substrate complex to form oxycytochrome P-450, a triad of enzyme, substrate, and oxygen. This complex can apparently exist in a number of electronic configurations depending on the distribution of electrons among the three components. The addition of another electron follows to yield a two electron–reduced complex termed peroxycytochrome P-450. This second electron is donated by either nicotinamide-adenine dinucleotide (reduced form) (NADH)–cytochrome P-450 reductase or cytochrome b_5 (from NADH via NADH-cytochrome b_5 reductase). The reductive activation of oxygen is followed by cleavage of the oxygen-oxygen bond. Finally, one atom of molecular oxygen is transferred to the substrate, while the other atom is incorporated into water. The newly oxidized substrate is then released, with the regeneration of oxidized (ferric) cytochrome P-450.

Two further features of this cycle are worthy of note. It is well-known that carbon monoxide interacts strongly with the ferrous iron of hemoglobin. Similarly, carbon monoxide can also bind to the one electron–reduced substrate-enzyme complex of cytochrome P-450. In the presence of substrate and carbon monoxide, reduced cytochrome P-450 displays characteristic absorption maximum at 450 nm. Denaturation of cytochrome P-450 produces a shift in the absorption maximum from 450 to 420 nm.

Cytochrome P-450 can also act as an oxidase in the presence of certain substrates, a reaction that generates partially reduced forms of oxygen, such as superoxide radical (O_2-) and hydrogen peroxide (H_2O_2). Importantly, when P-450 functions as an oxidase, the cycle is uncoupled, and bound oxygen is released without being incorporated into the substrate. Uncoupling can occur either at the level of oxycytochrome P-450 or peroxycytochrome P-450. The released oxygen retains the electron(s) donated by NADPH and is partially reduced and thus activated. Uncoupling at peroxycytochrome P-450 generates peroxide directly; uncoupling at oxycytochrome P-450 generates superoxide radicals, two of which dismutate to form peroxide and oxygen. With the release of activated oxygen, ferric cytochrome P-450 is regenerated; the substrate may or may not remain bound to the enzyme.

A wide variety of oxidative reactions are catalyzed by P-450–linked monooxygenases. These reactions are referred to as phase I of biotransformation. The primary outcome of cytochrome P-450 activity is the addition of an atom of oxygen to the substrate. The rates at which cytochrome P-450–linked metabolism in the whole animal can be increased to a varying extent by the administration of agents known to induce cytochrome P-450. These compounds, most notably phenobarbital and 3-methyl-

cholanthrene, can markedly increase the content of cytochrome P-450 in tissues by stimulating its de novo synthesis. By contrast, a number of cytochrome P-450 inhibitory agents have also been described. These inhibitors reduce the rates of mixed-function oxidation either by displacing oxygen at the heme moiety (carbon monoxide, ethylisocyanide) or by competing with substrate at the active site (SKF 525A, metyrapone, piperonyl butoxide).

The cytochrome P-450 oxidase system may be viewed as the body's toxicological immune system. Induction of a specific cytochrome P-450 enzyme may be analogous to monoclonal antibody production, whereas the general induction of the whole system, similar to what follows phenobarbital treatment, may be analogous to immunostimulation by Freund's adjuvant. It is intriguing to think that the mammalian body can respond to toxic stimuli in a manner similar to the one with which it responds to infectious agents. The liver could, therefore, be viewed as the toxicological defense system.

The metabolites that result from mixed-function oxidation are generally more hydrophilic than the parent compound. The hydrophilicity promotes the excretion of xenobiotics from the body. Furthermore, the insertion of an oxygen atom into the parent molecule allows the resulting metabolites to undergo other metabolic transformations more readily, known as phase II or conjugation reactions. Phase II reactions are enzymatic reactions that covalently link the products derived from the cytochrome P-450 oxidation of the parent xenobiotic to an endogenous compound. Such conjugates are quite water soluble and are readily excreted in either the bile or the urine. The endogenous compounds commonly used for conjugation reactions with xenobiotic metabolites include glucuronic acid, sulfate, amino acids, acetyl groups, and the tripeptide glutathione. The enzymes that catalyze these conjugation reactions are primarily found in the cytosol.

Of particular importance is the reaction between xenobiotics and glutathione. The free sulfhydryl group contained in the cysteinyl moiety of glutathione (gamma-glutamylcysteinyl-glycine) is nucleophilic and readily reacts with xenobiotics containing an electrophilic carbon center. Although the reaction between glutathione and electrophiles can occur nonenzymatically, conjugation is greatly facilitated by a group of enzymes known as the glutathione *S*-transferases, found primarily in the cytosol.

The glutathione conjugates formed by the action of glutathione *S*-transferase are further metabolized to produce mercapturic acid derivatives that are, in turn, excreted into the blood and urine. The formation of mercapturic acids involves removal of both the glutamate and the glycine residues followed by *N*-acetylation of cysteine. Importantly the formation of an adduct between glutathione and electrophilic metabolites prevents their interaction with cellular components.

By limiting the reactivity of electrophilic metabolites of

foreign chemicals, glutathione *S*-conjugate formation is an important cellular detoxification mechanism. Under certain conditions, however, glutathione *S*-conjugates may be toxic. For example, glutathione *S*-conjugate formation is now recognized as the first step in metabolic activation of nephrotoxic halogenated alkenes. Cysteine *S*-conjugates formed in the liver from glutathione conjugates are excreted in the blood and bile. On glomerular filtration, the cysteine *S*-conjugates are actively reabsorbed by the proximal tubule cells and converted by a B-lyase into toxic products that, in turn, mediate the renal injury.

Formation of reactive metabolites by cytochrome P-450

The combination of phase I and phase II metabolism converts lipophilic xenobiotics into forms that can readily be excreted from the body; hence this metabolism promotes the elimination of compounds that would ultimately prove toxic if allowed to accumulate in the body. For this reason, mixed-function oxidation is widely perceived as a detoxification mechanism. There is little doubt, however, that cytochrome P-450–dependent mixed-function oxidation can convert foreign compounds into more reactive metabolites. This biotransformation produces species that are clearly more toxic than the original substrate. In these cases, mixed-function oxidation is acting as a toxification rather than a detoxification system.

Isolation and characterization of reactive metabolites produced by cytochrome P-450 activation are difficult. Nevertheless, their transient presence in biological systems can be inferred from the appearance of the more stable conjugates that these reactive intermediates form with glutathione or other phase II substrates. Examination of phase II conjugates is a useful tool in evaluating the production of these metabolites and has been particularly useful in the study of some carcinogens or unknown carcinogenic mixtures.

Three chemicals whose toxicities depend on their cytochrome P-450–dependent biotransformation to reactive metabolites have been extensively studied as models of the mechanism by which xenobiotics produce lethal cell injury. Carbon tetrachloride, acetaminophen, and bromobenzene produce necrosis of the centrilobular zone of the liver and, to a lesser extent, of the proximal tubule cells of the kidney. The damage initiated by each of these chemicals is related to their cytochrome P-450–dependent metabolism in the target tissue. Interestingly, these compounds differ with respect to the reactive intermediates generated by their metabolism and thereby in the way they cycle through the cytochrome P-450 pathway.

Cytochrome P-450 catalyzes the reductive dehalogenation of carbon tetrachloride to produce a reactive intermediate, the trichloromethyl radical. Carbon tetrachloride binds readily to cytochrome P-450. This binding promotes the conversion of low-spin to high-spin ferric iron and its

reduction to ferrous iron by the addition of one electron. Before the entry of oxygen into the cycle, the added electron is transferred to one of the carbon-chlorine bonds, a reaction that produces the heterolytic cleavage of the bond to yield the trichloromethyl radical product and a chloride anion. Therefore the metabolism of carbon tetrachloride uses only the initial sequence of the P-450 enzymatic cycle.

The analgesic acetaminophen is another hepatotoxin whose metabolism is not typical of mixed-function oxidation. Acetaminophen is metabolized primarily by a specific isozyme of cytochrome P-450 induced by 3-methylcholanthrene, ethanol, isoniazid, and acetone. In the new nomenclature based on gene families, this enzyme has been named cytochrome P-450IIE. The specific details of the metabolism of acetaminophen to the reactive electrophile *N*-acetyl-*p*-quinone imine (NAPQI) are still being debated. There are several possible mechanisms by which this could occur. Acetaminophen may bind to cytochrome P-450 and proceed through the cycle up to the formation of oxycytochrome P-450, the one electron–reduced complex of enzyme, acetaminophen, and oxygen. Then, and for reasons presumably associated with the chemical structure of acetaminophen, acetaminophen may be oxidized by P-450 to give an acetaminophen radical (the semiquinone) and the two electron–reduced state of oxygen, hydrogen peroxide. Ferric cytochrome P-450 would be regenerated. The acetaminophen radical would rapidly lose the unpaired electron in a reaction with molecular oxygen to yield NAPQI and a superoxide anion.

Alternatively, NAPQI may be formed directly via a reaction that extracts two electrons from acetaminophen. With the two electrons added to the reaction from NADPH, two molecules of water (the four electron–reduced state of oxygen) in addition to NAPQI would be produced. By either mechanism, the mixed-function oxidation of acetaminophen is associated with the formation of a reactive intermediate (NAPQI), which presumably mediates the liver cell injury.

Bromobenzene is a typical cytochrome P-450 substrate, the metabolism of which yields a reactive electrophile. Cytochrome P-450 adds an atom of oxygen to the skeleton of bromobenzene to form either the 2,3-epoxide or 3,4-epoxide. The new electrophilic 2,3-epoxide is highly unstable and nonenzymatically rearranges to form either 2-bromophenol or 3-bromophenol, each of which is readily excreted. The 3,4-epoxide is electrophilic but more stable. Although epoxide hydrolase can convert the 3,4-epoxide to the nontoxic bromophenyldihydrodiol, any epoxide that is not converted binds either glutathione or tissue macromolecules.

For each of the three toxins discussed previously, conversion to reactive intermediates by cytochrome P-450 is the initial event in the development of liver necrosis. In other words, the trichloromethyl radical NAPQI, and bromobenzene-3,4-epoxide are the ultimate toxins produced during the metabolism of carbon tetrachloride, acetaminophen, and bromobenzene.

Non–cytochrome P-450 metabolism of toxic xenobiotics

Although cytochrome P-450 appears to mediate the formation of reactive intermediates for most toxins requiring bioactivation, other enzyme systems are also important in toxification reactions. By way of example, allyl alcohol is a hepatotoxin for which the development of liver cell injury is related to its metabolism by alcohol dehydrogenase. This enzyme converts allyl alcohol to the reactive electrophile, acrolein. Alcohol dehydrogenase is concentrated in the periportal zones of the liver. Thus, allyl alcohol produces periportal necrosis in contrast to the centrilobular liver necrosis produced by cytochrome P-450–dependent hepatotoxins.

The neurotoxin MPTP (1-methyl-4-phenyl-1,2,3,6-tetrahydropyridine) represents another example of an agent whose cytotoxicity depends on metabolism by an enzyme other than cytochrome P-450. In this case, the toxic pathway involves oxidation of MPTP to 1-methyl-4-phenylpyridinium (MPP^+) by monoamine oxidase type B, mostly in the central nervous system (see Chapter 30).

COVALENT BINDING HYPOTHESIS OF CELL INJURY

The quest for the mechanisms by which reactive intermediates mediate the loss of cellular viability remains an active and controversial area of research. One hypothesis to explain the link between metabolic activation and cell injury that has particularly dominated biochemical toxicology for almost two decades is the covalent binding hypothesis of cell injury. This hypothesis was derived from earlier studies of the metabolism of chemicals that cause cancer.

The experimental production of cancer by chemicals dates to 1915, when Japanese investigators produced skin cancers in rabbits with coal tar. Since that time, the list of organic and inorganic carcinogens has grown exponentially. Yet a curious paradox existed for many years. Many compounds known to be potent carcinogens are relatively inert in terms of chemical reactivity. The solution to this riddle became apparent in the early 1960s, when it was shown that most chemical carcinogens require metabolic activation before they can react with cell constituents. Today, it is widely believed that the biotransformation of procarcinogens to products that irreversibly bind to DNA is a critical step in the mechanism of chemically induced cancer. Alkylated or arylated DNA causes misreplication, which, if not repaired, leads to permanent alterations of the genome, for example, point mutations, frame-shift mutations, and codon rearrangement.

During the early 1970s, a similar mechanism was postulated to account for the acute organ-specific toxicities of a wide range of chemical compounds. The covalent binding hypothesis states that the injurious effects of numerous xenobiotic agents are related to their ability to bind irreversibly to nucleophilic sites in cellular macromolecules, such as the sulfhydryl groups of proteins. Furthermore, such alkylation or arylation events render the protein in question nonfunctional. In essence, the covalent binding of reactive metabolites to those proteins that have a critical role in the maintenance of cellular viability results in the loss of viability. Therefore the covalent binding hypothesis explains how chemically divergent compounds produce similar kinds of organ-specific lesions. The only important chemical characteristic demanded by this hypothesis is that the substance be sufficiently reactive to form covalent bonds or that it be converted by cellular metabolism to a product that can mediate the binding.

The covalent binding hypothesis was developed primarily from studies in rodents of the hepatotoxicity of acetaminophen and bromobenzene. The administration of a toxic dose of radiolabeled acetaminophen or bromobenzene is accompanied by an accumulation of irreversibly bound radiolabel in liver protein. NAPQI from acetaminophen and bromobenzene-3,4-epoxide from bromobenzene, reactive metabolites formed by cytochrome P-450–dependent processes, can covalently bond to molecules in the manner just described.

The extent of both the liver necrosis and the covalent binding can be manipulated by pretreating the animals with inducers or inhibitors of cytochrome P-450. Under such conditions, P-450 induction accelerates metabolism, increases the amount of covalently bound radiolabel, and exacerbates the resulting liver necrosis. By contrast, inhibition of metabolism has the reverse effect. Little covalent binding is seen, and the injury is markedly reduced. In this way, the necrosis produced by acetaminophen and bromobenzene correlates with the covalent binding of their metabolites to protein.

An important feature of the covalent binding hypothesis is the protective effect of glutathione. The reaction of electrophilic metabolites with glutathione serves as a sink for these toxic intermediates, thereby preventing their interaction with cellular proteins. As long as sufficient glutathione is present to scavenge the reactive xenobiotics or their metabolites, toxicity does not develop. Thus doses of acetaminophen or bromobenzene that do not exhaust the cellular stores of glutathione do not produce liver necrosis. Under these conditions, the covalent binding of the metabolites is also limited. Toxic doses of acetaminophen and bromobenzene, however, deplete glutathione to an extent that allows significant covalent binding to occur.

The protective role of glutathione is also demonstrated by the observations that administration of the glutathione precursor cysteine reduces the extent of both covalent binding and the necrosis seen with acetaminophen and bromobenzene. By stimulating glutathione synthesis, cysteine also reduces the extent of glutathione depletion. Prior depletion of glutathione with diethylmaleate sensitizes the liver to both toxins and increases the levels of covalent binding.

The observation that covalent binding of the reactive metabolites of acetaminophen and bromobenzene parallels the extent of liver cell injury led to the demonstration of similar correlations with a large number of other organ-specific toxins. Although the covalent binding hypothesis can be used to explain the toxicity of most xenobiotics, an essential feature of this hypothesis remains to be defined: the nature of the critical targets to which reactive metabolites bind.

In the attempt to identify proteins whose alkylation results in lethal cell injury, changes have been sought in the activities of proteins associated with the regulation of intracellular calcium homeostasis. Some compounds that generate an oxidative stress in hepatocytes have been shown to inhibit calcium translocases that are involved in the maintenance of intracellular calcium homeostasis. A sustained elevation of the cytosolic calcium ion concentration results, activating various Ca^{2+}-dependent degradative enzymes, including phospholipases, proteases, and nucleases. It has been argued that these activities may combine to cause irreversible damage. Accordingly the covalent binding hypothesis has been revised to implicate specifically those membrane proteins that are involved in the maintenance of intracellular calcium homeostasis as the relevant targets of reactive electrophiles. As a corollary, it follows that the covalent binding of reactive metabolites to other cellular macromolecules may be simply an epiphenomenon and thus unrelated to the toxicity of the parent xenobiotic.

The validity of the covalent binding hypothesis as an explanation of the metabolism-dependent toxicity of xenobiotics is as difficult to establish as it is to deny. Ultimately, confirmation must rest on confirmation of the mechanisms hypothesized to couple covalent binding to its relevant toxic consequence, for example, alteration in calcium homeostasis. It has been possible to dismiss some experimental data, seemingly inconsistent with the covalent binding hypothesis, as simply the binding of substances to proteins other than the critical targets. More difficult to dismiss, however, is the fact that toxic cell injury can occur even when the toxic agent cannot covalently bind. For example, the quinone imine metabolite of the 3,5-dimethyl derivative of acetaminophen cannot covalently bind because the electrophilic site of the molecule is masked by a methyl group. Nevertheless, 3,5-dimethyl acetaminophen is hepatotoxic.

Similarly the cytochrome P-450–dependent deethylation of ethoxycoumarin does not yield an electrophilic intermediate, but metabolism-dependent killing of cultured hepatocytes occurs. Such dissociations between covalent binding and cell injury have prompted investigators to search for other mechanisms by which xenobiotic metabolism may

be coupled to cell death. One hypothesis that has gained increasing support is the idea that the toxicity of many xenobiotics is related to oxidative stress.

OXYGEN RADICALS AS MEDIATORS OF TOXIC CELL INJURY (See also Chapter 21)

Molecular oxygen, necessary for the survival of aerobic organisms, is a diradical in its ground state. Despite oxygen's radical nature, its reactivity is surprisingly low. The two unpaired electrons of molecular oxygen possess the same spin. Thus the reaction of oxygen with electron donors to form covalent bonds is kinetically unfavored and slow; however, oxygen can readily participate in one-electron reductions.

The stepwise reduction of oxygen to water produces a variety of potentially toxic intermediates. The addition of a single electron produces the superoxide anion. In turn, a second electron reduces superoxide to the peroxide ion. At physiological pH, the peroxide ion exists primarily as hydrogen peroxide. Addition of the third electron splits the oxygen-oxygen bond to form the hydroxyl radical (and a hydroxide anion that is essentially water). Addition of the final electron to the hydroxyl radical yields another molecule of water.

These partially reduced, and thereby activated, forms of oxygen are continuously generated in all aerobic cells as a result of oxidative processes, both autocatalytic and enzymatic. Superoxide anion and hydrogen peroxide are produced by various oxidases (e.g., xanthine oxidase and cytochrome P-450) as well as by the nonenzymatic redox cycling of electron transport carriers, thiols, and catecholamines. Activated phagocytes also generate superoxide anions and hydrogen peroxide. The formation of these activated oxygen species is, in turn, related to the bacteriocidal activity of these cells and can contribute to the development of cell injury in tissues in which these inflammatory cells accumulate. By contrast, cytochrome oxidase mediates the complete reduction of oxygen to water. It is a well-coupled system and does not represent a source of activated oxygen species under normal conditions.

Aerobic organisms have developed numerous mechanisms that protect the cell from the physiological generation of activated oxygen. When the generation of such species overwhelms the cell's ability to detoxify them, however, cell injury can result. The superoxide dismutases dispose of superoxide anions. As illustrated in Equation 1, these metal-containing enzymes catalyze the dismutation of two molecules of the superoxide anion to give hydrogen peroxide and dioxygen:

$$O_2^- + O_2^- + 2H^+ \rightarrow H_2O_2 + O_2 \qquad (1)$$

In eukaryotic cells, there are two distinct superoxide dismutase enzymes, a copper-zinc–containing enzyme found in the cytosol and a manganese-containing enzyme found in the mitochondria. The superoxide dismutases present in prokaryotic cells contain either iron or manganese at the active site. Obligatory anaerobes have no superoxide dismutase activity. Superoxide dismutase activity can be induced under conditions of excess oxygen radical formation. For example, pulmonary superoxide dismutase can be induced by hyperbaric oxygen administration. This induction has been related to a protection of the organism from the deleterious effects of oxidative stress. In turn, inhibition of superoxide dismutase with, for example, disulfiram, is known to sensitize a cell to oxidative stress.

The hydrogen peroxide produced by the action of superoxide dismutases or other oxidative processes can be detoxified by two different systems. The enzyme catalase converts hydrogen peroxide to water:

$$2H_2O_2 \rightarrow 2H_2O + O_2 \qquad (2)$$

Importantly, this reduction of hydrogen peroxide by catalase occurs without the intermediate formation of the hydroxyl radical. Catalase is a hemoprotein, which is found almost exclusively within peroxisomes. Similar to the inhibition of superoxide dismutase, inhibition of catalase with aminotriazole potentiates oxidative cell injury.

The enzyme glutathione peroxidase also catalyzes the reduction of hydrogen peroxide to water. Reduced glutathione is the source of reducing equivalents necessary to drive this reaction. In the process, two molecules of glutathione are oxidized to yield one molecule of glutathione disulfide. Glutathione disulfide is efficiently reduced to glutathione by glutathione reductase. In this reaction, NADPH serves as the source of the reducing equivalents. The glutathione peroxidase–reductase system seems to be the first line of defense against hydrogen peroxide, and catalase is a secondary system. Catalase is also a specific defense against hydrogen peroxide formed within the peroxisomes.

Glutathione peroxidase is found in the cytosol of most cells as well as within mitochondria. Glutathione peroxidase also shows considerable activity toward organic hydroperoxides, converting them to their corresponding alcohols. By contrast, catalase catabolizes only hydrogen peroxide. The cytosolic and mitochondrial forms of glutathione peroxidase depend on the metal selenium for activity. Thus, it is not surprising that selenium deficiency has been demonstrated to exacerbate oxidant-stress injury.

The importance of glutathione reductase is emphasized by the observation that inhibition of this enzyme also potentiates the cytotoxicity of an oxidative stress. With the inhibition of glutathione reductase, oxidized glutathione is not converted to reduced glutathione, a result that limits the effectiveness of the peroxidase by limiting the supply of glutathione. The chemotherapeutic alkylating agent BCNU (N,N-bis(2-chloroethyl)-N-nitrosourea) inhibits glutathione reductase without effect on glutathione peroxidase and catalase. This compound sensitizes a number of cell types to the toxicity of hydrogen peroxide and other organic hydroperoxides. It should also be noted that during severe oxidative stress, NADPH levels are markedly depleted, an effect related to the consumption of NADPH by glutathione reductase. Such a depletion may exert a substrate-level inhibition of the reductase. Thus the NADPH depletion that results from oxidative stress may actually sensitize the cell to the further oxidative injury.

Hydroxyl radical in oxidant-stress injury

Oxidative stress can be defined as any situation in which there is an accumulation of partially reduced oxygen species or their equivalent, such as organic hydroperoxides. Neither hydrogen peroxide nor superoxide anions however, are reactive in aqueous solution; hence, they are unlikely to mediate directly the cell injury accompanying oxidative stress.

Ferrous iron can react with hydrogen peroxide to yield the extremely reactive hydroxyl radical. The hydroxyl radical is a potent oxidizing species, which rapidly interacts with cellular constituents such as DNA, protein, and lipids. For this reason, it has been proposed that the hydroxyl radical is the ultimate toxin generated during oxidative stress. Although the role of the hydroxyl radical in oxidative-stress cell injury remains somewhat controversial, substantial experimental evidence indicates that it, or an equivalently reactive species such as a perferryl radical, is indeed the final mediator of such toxic processes. The reduction of hydrogen peroxide by ferrous iron (Equation 3), called the Fenton reaction:

$$H_2O_2 + Fe^{2+} \rightarrow OH + OH^- + Fe^{3+} \qquad (3)$$

Other transition metals (e.g., copper) can participate in this reaction. It appears, however, that in most cases only iron plays a significant role in generation of hydroxyl radicals within a cell. The hydroxyl radical can also be produced without the participation of iron during the radiolysis of water. Hydroxyl radical formation is thought to be the mechanism that initiates the events whereby ionizing radiation kills cells (Chapter 11). It should also be noted that organic hydroperoxides can replace hydrogen peroxide in Equation 3 and react with ferrous iron to produce a radical product. For example, the cytotoxicity of tert-butyl hydroperoxide appears to be related to the formation of tert-butyl alkoxyl radicals from the reaction of this organic peroxide with ferrous iron.

The Fenton reaction requires ferrous iron, and there is little free (nonprotein bound) ferrous iron with cells. Most of the iron within cells is found in hemoproteins or as ferric iron bound to ferritin. Thus, if hydroxyl radicals participate in the toxicity of oxidative stress, one must account for the iron needed for their formation. Studies have shown that chelation of dynamic pools of ferric iron protects a variety of cell types from the toxicity of oxygen radicals.

Cells receive iron from the blood as ferric iron bound in the transport protein transferrin. Transferrin attaches to specific cell surface receptors and is subsequently internalized by endocytosis, and the acidic environment of the endocytic vacuolar compartment releases ferric iron from transferrin. This "free" (non–protein-associated) ferric iron can then be used for the synthesis of iron-containing proteins or stored within the cell as ferritin. The transferrin-receptor complex devoid of ferric iron is recycled to the cell surface. When there is a need for the iron stores of the body, iron can be mobilized from ferritin by the autophagocytosis of the protein. This process involves sequestration of cytosolic ferritin with a phagosome, followed by fusion of the phagosome with a lysosome to form a phagolysosome. The dual action of low pH and proteolytic activity releases the iron from the ferritin molecule, which then enters the free ferric iron pool. The ferric iron released from transferrin or mobilized from ferritin transiently exists in a non–protein-bound pool. This iron pool is required for cell injury by oxygen radicals and removed by ferric iron chelators.

As has just been seen, in its ferric state, iron enters and is stored in cells. A search for the mechanisms of generation of ferrous iron required for hydroxyl radical formation has implicated a role for the superoxide ion. A requirement for superoxide anions in oxidative injury is evidenced by the protective effect of superoxide dismutase. This protection is explained by the proposal that superoxide anions serve as the intracellular reductant for the formation of ferrous iron from ferric iron. In the presence of increased levels of superoxide anions, ferrous iron is formed and participates with hydrogen peroxide in the generation of hydroxyl radicals by the Fenton reaction. Equations 4 through 6 summarize the chemical reactions involving all three cellular reactants—O_2^-, H_2O_2, and ferric iron—that are believed to mediate the formation of hydroxyl radicals within cells:

$$Fe^{3+} + O_2^- \rightarrow Fe^{2+} + O_2 \tag{4}$$
$$Fe^{2+} + H_2O_2 \rightarrow Fe^{3+} \; OH + OH^- \tag{5}$$
$$\text{Net: } O_2^- + H_2O_2 \rightarrow OH + OH^- + O_2 \tag{6}$$

The sum of these reactions (Equation 6) is referred to as the iron-catalyzed Haber-Weiss reaction. It can be seen from these equations that removal of any one of the three reactants (i.e., superoxide anion, ferric or ferrous iron, or hydrogen peroxide) would prevent hydroxyl radical formation.

Sources of oxidative stress

Toxic agents oxidatively injure cells in two general ways. On the one hand, they may impose an oxidative stress on a cell, that is, cause the formation of excess superoxide anions or hydrogen peroxide. Alternatively, they may impair the protective mechanisms of the cells such that the normal flux of activated oxygen species becomes toxic. Examples of agents whose cytotoxicity is related to the first mechanism are the pulmonary toxin paraquat and the diabetogenic agent alloxan. On the other hand, the toxic effects of alkylating agents, and very likely of bromobenzene,

may be a consequence of their ability to deplete cellular stores of glutathione. Abrupt glutathione depletion sensitizes a cell to its constitutive flux of partially reduced oxygen species.

The toxicity of quinonoid compounds, such as menadione, adriamycin, or paraquat, is a good example of an imposed or exogenous oxidative stress. Quinones undergo an enzymatic, one-electron reduction to yield the corresponding semiquinone radical. Auto-oxidation of the semiquinone radical by molecular oxygen produces superoxide anions with regeneration of the parent quinone. The enzymatic or spontaneous dismutation of superoxide anions yields hydrogen peroxide. Thus, quinones repeatedly cycle through oxidation-reduction reactions that generate toxic concentrations of reduced oxygen species. Alloxan, a toxin that destroys the islets of Langerhans in the pancreas, can also generate activated oxygen species. Alloxan is reduced within a cell by a variety of NADH-linked enzymes to the corresponding hydroquinone, dialuric acid. In turn, dialuric acid spontaneously auto-oxidizes, a reaction that generates superoxide anions and hydrogen peroxide.

As discussed earlier, the liver and kidney necrosis produced by acetaminophen depends on its cytochrome P-450–mediated metabolism in the target cells. Acetaminophen is oxidized to a quinone imine, NAPQI. The metabolism of acetaminophen is associated with covalent binding, loss of glutathione, and the formation of partially reduced oxygen species. Although the relative role of each of these effects in the toxicity of acetaminophen is the basis of a decade-long controversy, oxidative stress increasingly appears to be an important factor. The covalent binding of the electrophilic metabolite of acetaminophen, NAPQI, was dissociated from the appearance of liver necrosis by the use of liposome-encapsulated superoxide dismutase. Such data document that the toxicity of acetaminophen in the intact animal is related to an oxidative stress that is imposed by some consequence of the metabolism of this chemical.

The xenobiotics just discussed are capable of imposing oxidative stress by generating activated oxygen species as a consequence of their cellular metabolism. There are other chemicals that irreversibly injure cells by mechanisms related to oxidative injury. They do not seem to increase, however, the exposure of cells to partially reduced oxygen species. As noted, aerobic cells continuously generate partially reduced oxygen species as a result of the spontaneous auto-oxidation of electron transport carriers in the mitochondria or as a result of the action of cytoplasmic oxidases. A variety of toxic chemicals may act by depleting their target cells of glutathione, thereby allowing this constitutive flux of partially reduced oxygen species to initiate mechanisms that result in the loss of viability. Primary electrophiles, such as the alkylating agents, or chemicals that are metabolized to an electrophilic derivative may cause toxicity by such a mechanism. Allyl alcohol and bromobenzene are examples of chemicals that may act in this manner.

Bromobenzene is metabolized to an epoxide, apparently without an accompanying formation of activated oxygen species. Similarly, allyl alcohol is converted to acrolein by a process that does not generate activated oxygen. Nevertheless, these compounds most likely produce liver cell necrosis by mechanisms that are related to oxidative cell injury. In both cases, the liver cell necrosis is iron dependent and prevented by antioxidants. The metabolic products of both these compounds are extremely electrophilic and readily react with and deplete cellular stores of glutathione. For both bromobenzene and allyl alcohol, evidence specifically links the depletion of glutathione to the ensuing oxidative cell injury.

Criteria for oxidative cell injury

Several criteria are commonly used to establish a causal link between an oxidative stress and the accompanying cell injury: (1) a requirement for ferric iron, (2) potentiation of the injury by inhibition of glutathione reductase, and (3) protection by either superoxide dismutase or catalase.

Depletion of the nonprotein-bound ferric iron pool with chelators such as deferoxamine protects against the toxicity of an oxidative stress. Deferoxamine binds specifically to ferric iron to form a complex that will not catalyze the Haber-Weiss reaction (Equation 6). Thus the elimination of a critical iron pool prevents the formation of hydroxyl radicals from hydrogen peroxide. Interestingly, deferoxamine does not interfere with the mixed-function oxidation of either acetaminophen or bromobenzene. Deferoxamine decreases the toxicity of these compounds without decreasing the formation of their reactive electrophilic metabolites, a result that emphasizes a role for oxidative stress in their toxicities.

Inhibition of glutathione reductase with BCNU is known to sensitize cells to the toxicity of hydrogen peroxide by inhibiting the redox cycling of glutathione. Hydrogen peroxide is detoxified by the enzyme glutathione peroxidase, accompanied by the oxidation of glutathione to glutathione disulfide. The reduction of glutathione disulfide by glutathione reductase restores the glutathione necessary for continued peroxidase activity. With the inhibition of the reductase by BCNU, the efficient redox cycling of glutathione no longer occurs. In the absence of sufficient glutathione for peroxidase activity, hydrogen peroxide accumulates to an extent that it can now imitate cell injury. The central role of hydrogen peroxide in the toxicity of acetaminophen, bromobenzene, allyl alcohol, paraquat, and alloxan is suggested by the ability of BCNU to exacerbate the toxicity of each compound. Importantly, BCNU effects a biochemical event that occurs secondary to the metabolism of the toxin—catabolism of hydrogen peroxide; the increased toxicity is not accompanied by increased covalent biding.

BIOCHEMICAL MECHANISMS OF CELL INJURY

The biochemical events coupling an initial toxic event (be it oxidative stress, tissue alkylation, or an alternative mechanism) to the genesis of lethal cell injury are of continuing interest. Several biochemical alterations have been described and, in turn, proposed as bases for irreversible cell injury. These include alterations in intracellular calcium homeostasis, altered protein thiol content, DNA damage and repair, changes in mitochondrial function, and the peroxidation of cellular lipids.

Peroxidation of membrane lipids

The peroxidative decomposition of lipids is a complex series of events whereby the fatty acyl chains of membrane phospholipids are converted to a variety of fragmented products. Lipid peroxidation is one of the best-known manifestations of oxidative cell injury. Nevertheless the role that lipid peroxidation plays in the pathogenesis of irreversible cell injury with an acute oxidative stress is a matter of continued debate.

The chemistry of lipid peroxidation can be divided into three distinct steps: initiation, propagation, and termination. Initiation begins with abstraction of a hydrogen atom from an unsaturated fatty acid of membrane phospholipids. Allylic hydrogens are most readily removed because that carbon-hydrogen bond is made relatively acidic by the adjacent carbon-carbon double bond. Such hydrogen abstraction leaves an unpaired electron, forming a lipid radical species.

Carbon-centered, sulfur-centered, nitrogen-centered, and oxygen-centered radicals are capable of extracting hydrogen atoms from the fatty acids of membrane, phospholipids, and thus of initiating lipid peroxidation. Among the activated forms of oxygen, the hydroxyl radical is the most widely implicated initiator of lipid peroxidation. This species is extremely reactive and readily abstracts hydrogens from fatty acids forming lipid radicals and water. In contrast to the hydroxyl radical, the superoxide anion radical is not sufficiently reactive to carry out hydrogen abstraction. Superoxide ions, however, can participate in the formation of the hydroxyl radical via Haber-Weiss chemistry (Equation 6). Superoxide-generating systems have been demonstrated to cause lipid peroxidation.

The propagation of lipid peroxidation starts with the reaction of a lipid radical with molecular oxygen to yield a lipid peroxide radical. These lipid peroxides are extremely reactive and abstract a second hydrogen from a neighboring intact lipid to generate a lipid hydroperoxide and a new lipid radical, thus propagating the peroxidation. Decomposition of the unstable lipid hydroperoxide generally follows. Low-molecular-weight fatty acid fragments, such as alkenals, ketones, and alkanes, arise from the breakdown of the lipid hydroperoxides. Some of these products are sufficiently stable to allow their use as quantitative markers of lipid peroxidation. For example, the accumulation of malondialdehyde in tissue and biological fluids is commonly used to assay the extent of peroxidation.

Termination of lipid peroxidation, the final step, occurs when two radical substrates react to give nonradical products. It is clear from this simplified scheme that the peroxidation of cellular lipids is an autocatalytic cascade that will continue until the substrate is exhausted, sufficient terminating has occurred, or the process is stopped with antioxidant.

Lipid peroxidation causes loss of the structural and functional integrity of the membrane. The unsaturated fatty acids of the membrane lipids are converted to lower molecular weight products, and lipid-lipid and lipid-protein cross-links are formed. Thus the biophysical properties of the membrane change. Membrane fluidity and permeability are generally increased, and lysis of the membrane can eventually occur.

In addition to the deleterious effects on lipids, the peroxidation of membranes also has pronounced effects on their proteins. Membrane-associated enzymatic activities can be decreased or lost. Most membrane-bound activities can be decreased or lost. Most membrane-bound enzymes require an intact bilayer for optimum activity. Thus, alterations in the physical properties of the membrane as a consequence of peroxidation of the lipids can result in alterations in enzyme activity. Lipid hydroperoxides decompose to low molecular weight compounds, many of which are electrolytic. Alkylation of proteins by these products of lipid peroxidation can alter enzyme function. Lipid decomposition products of particular note are the 4-hydroxyalkenals. These unsaturated compounds are generated in large amounts during lipid peroxidation and readily alkylate cellular nucleophiles, such as the thiol groups of proteins. Thiols play an important role in regulating enzymatic activity, and their depletion can result in the loss of enzyme function. In fact, many of the biochemical effects observed in cells intoxicated with xenobiotics that induce lipid peroxidation can be reproduced by the alkenal products alone. For example, liver cells exposed to carbon tetrachloride manifest decreased protein synthesis and a loss of glucose-6-phosphatase activity. These same effects can also be produced, at least in vitro, by exposing liver cells to 4-hydroxynonenal, the major product identified when membrane peroxidation is initiated with carbon tetrachloride.

Cells are continuously exposed to a variety of oxidative processes that could potentially lead to lipid peroxidation. As a result, aerobic organisms possess effective defense mechanisms against the peroxidation of membrane lipids and thereby circumvent toxic cell injury. These protective mechanisms fall into two broad categories: (1) those that prevent the initiation of lipid peroxidation and (2) those that prevent its propagation.

Superoxide dismutase and catalases provide antioxidant protection by inhibiting the formation of the hydroxyl radical. Chelation of the ferric iron necessary for the forma-

tion of the hydroxyl radical and direct removal of this species by radical scavengers (e.g., mannitol) are also protective. The generation of species capable of initiating lipid peroxidation may exceed the capacity to remove them effectively. Thus, there are other defenses to prevent the uncontrolled propagation of lipid peroxidation. These include water-soluble antioxidants, such as ascorbic acid (vitamin C) and reduced glutathione, and fat-soluble antioxidants, most notably α-tocopherol (vitamin E). It appears that vitamins E and C and glutathione combine in some as yet poorly defined cycle to donate hydrogen atom to lipid or peroxy radicals, thereby preventing further propagation of the lipid peroxidation.

Reduced glutathione also has an important antioxidant role as a substrate for glutathione peroxidase. As previously discussed, glutathione peroxidase catalyzes the reduction of hydrogen peroxide to water. This enzyme can also reduce lipid hydroperoxides to more stable lipid alcohols. Lipid hydroperoxides rapidly decompose and their reduction by the glutathione peroxidase system prevents disruption of membrane fatty acids.

Although these cellular defense mechanisms provide a highly effective defense against a low level of lipid peroxidation, severe oxidative stress can result in exhaustion of the key elements required for optimal function of these systems. Therefore, if the rate of the oxidation of endogenous antioxidants exceeds the rate of their reduction, the cell becomes more susceptible to peroxidation. The importance to the cell of an intact antioxidant system is demonstrated by the fact that rodents made deficient in selenium (to inactivate glutathione peroxidase), vitamin E, or ascorbic acid are more susceptible to the development of lipid peroxidation and cell injury under a variety of toxic conditions.

Experimental evidence suggests that a number of xenobiotics exert their toxic effects, at least in part, through lipid peroxidation. For example, the liver necrosis seen with carbon tetrachloride, acetaminophen, and bromobenzene as well as the pulmonary toxicities of ozone and nitrogen dioxide appear to be related to the peroxidation of cellular membranes (see Chapter 18). For the liver toxins, lipid peroxidation and necrosis depend on metabolism. The reductive cleavage of carbon tetrachloride by cytochrome P-450 produces the trichloromethyl radical, a potent initiator of lipid peroxidation in vitro and in vivo. The metabolism of acetaminophen is associated with superoxide and hydrogen peroxide production, which, in turn, can react to form the hydroxyl radical. The appearance of lipid peroxidation following bromobenzene intoxication has been linked to the abrupt depletion of glutathione that follows its reaction with the epoxide intermediate. Ozone and nitrogen dioxide appear to interact directly with membranes to initiate radical formation.

Because lipids can peroxidize after cell death, the mere presence of lipid peroxidation does not necessarily indicate a casual role for this process. In the four examples noted, however, lipid peroxidation occurs before evidence of cell death. Exogenous antioxidants prevent the peroxidation of lipids in parallel with prevention of cell injury. In addition, the peroxidation of lipids and the severity of liver and lung necrosis are exacerbated in rodents fed selenium-deficient (to inactive glutathione peroxidase) or α-tocopherol–deficient diets.

Protein thiol depletion

There are other circumstances under which lipid peroxidation is clearly unrelated to the course of oxidative cell injury. The nature of such peroxidation-independent mechanisms of oxidative cell injury is not well understood. A popular hypothesis is the depletion of protein-bound thiol groups.

Support of this hypothesis has been derived from studies of the toxicity of quinonoid compounds, particularly menadione and adriamycin, in isolated cell and organ systems. Menadione (2-methyl-1,4-naphthoquinone) can undergo an enzyme-catalyzed single-electron reduction to generate the corresponding menadione radical. Reduced menadione rapidly gives up its unpaired electron to molecular oxygen, a reaction that regenerates the parent compound. In turn, the reduction of molecular oxygen produces superoxide anion and hydrogen peroxide by dismutation. Thus the redox cycling of menadione generates oxidative stress, and the ensuing toxicity fits the criteria of oxidative cell injury. Because menadione itself is an antioxidant, however, the toxicity seen with this compound occurs without evidence of the peroxidation of lipids. It has been suggested that the cytotoxicity of menadione is due, at least in part, to a depletion of protein thiol groups.

What mechanisms mediate the loss of protein thiol groups? The redox cycling of quinones yields hydrogen peroxide. On the reduction of hydrogen peroxide to water by glutathione peroxidase, glutathione is depleted as a result of its oxidation to glutathione disulfide. Glutathione disulfide can undergo disulfide exchange reactions with the free thiol moiety of proteins, a process that produces a glutathione mixed disulfide. In addition, protein thiols may be depleted as a result of their direct oxidation to disulfites, presumably by partially reduced oxygen species, such as the hydroxyl radical, or by arylation by the quinine itself. A loss of protein thiols has also been proposed as the ultimate insult in covalent binding of alkylating agents to proteins.

That a loss of protein thiol groups may represent a cause of oxidative cell injury is based on two experimental observations. First, depletion of protein thiols generally precedes the loss of viability. In turn, conditions that accelerate the loss of protein thiols aggravate the toxicity of these quinones. Second, sulfhydryl reagents prevent the loss of protein thiols and prevent the loss of viability. Sulfhydryl reagents can reduce protein disulfides. In addition, exogenous thiol reagents can serve as a trap for the electrolytic

quinones to prevent their reaction with cellular thiols. The protective action of sulfhydryl reagents has been interpreted as a consequence of this sequestration of electroplates. It still must be established, however, whether the protective effect of exogenous thiols is specifically related to the prevention of protein thiol depletion. In particular, if exogenous thiols scavenge hydroxyl or lipid radicals, their ability to protect against oxidative cell injury may not relate to an effect on the loss of protein thiols.

In this regard, it is noteworthy that changes in protein thiols could be dissociated from the killing of cultured hepatocytes by an oxidative stress. Three mechanisms were identified by which protein thiols were lost with the oxidative killing of cultured hepatocytes. Two of these mechanisms, the formation of mixed disulfides and the arylation of protein thiols, were observed to deplete protein thiols on exposure to menadione. The reduction of protein thiols by these two mechanisms, however, did not correlate with the extent of cell killing.

Similarly the metabolism of acetaminophen by cultured hepatocytes depleted protein thiols as a result of the formation of glutathione mixed disulfides and by arylation. In the presence of deferoxamine, however, there was little or no cell killing for up to 8 hours despite a loss of 60% of the total protein thiols. Thus, current evidence suggests that the loss of protein thiols that accompanies exposure of cells to an oxidative stress is likely an epiphenomenon to the mechanism of lethal injury.

Alterations in calcium homeostasis

Inhibition of the activity of the major calcium regulating proteins has been suggested as the primary link between protein thiol oxidation and cell death. This notion is similar to the role of calcium regulating proteins as toxicological targets in the covalent binding theory. An alteration in intracellular calcium hemostasis has been proposed as a common toxic consequence of the action of agents that generate activated oxygen species as well as reactive electrophiles.

The plasma membrane is a primary regulator of the intracellular calcium concentration. Additionally, calcium can be sequestered within intracellular compartments, most notably the mitochondria and the endoplasmic reticulum. Thus the ability of the mitochondria and the endoplasmic reticulum to sequester calcium actively contributes to the maintenance of the low cytosolic calcium concentration. It has been shown that oxidative stress is accompanied by an elevated cytosolic calcium concentration as a result of both the mobilization of intracellular stores of calcium and an influx from extracellular sources. The activities of the various calcium-associated translocases are decreased with oxidative stress. The loss of protein thiols contained in these proteins can be specifically related to the changes in calcium homeostasis. Restoration of protein thiols restores the activity of these proteins and prevents the accumulation of calcium. Similarly the covalent binding of reactive intermediates has been directly related to alterations in calcium transport functions of isolated membrane fractions.

The hypothesis that protein thiol loss has a causal relationship with oxidative cell injury as well as with cell injury produced by covalent binding relates to the postulated role of calcium. That is, it depends on the demonstration that the intracellular accumulation of calcium is a cause of cell death, but still the role of altered intracellular calcium homeostasis in lethal cell injury owing to oxidative stress remains a matter of continued debate.

As noted previously, the mechanisms that result in depletion of both soluble and protein-bound thiols during oxidative stress and thus perturb intracellular calcium homeostasis do not depend on a cellular source of ferric iron. Chelation of iron does not prevent the changes in either thiol or calcium metabolism that accompany oxidative stress. Thus, when chelation of iron prevents irreversible cell injury, changes in viability can be readily dissociated from changes in intracellular calcium homeostasis. Thus, changes in calcium homeostasis occur without accompanying irreversible injury. Conversely, irreversible injury can occur without changes in calcium homeostasis.

When oxidative cell killing is an iron-dependent process, the accompanying changes in intracellular calcium homeostasis are again most likely an epiphenomenon. The increasing evidence for a central role of intracellular iron metabolism in oxidative cell injury simply emphasizes the significance of this conclusion.

Are there iron-independent mechanisms of oxidative cell killing? Iron dependence has not been examined in many studies of oxidative cell injury. Clearly, there are nonoxidative mechanisms of toxic cell injury that are not iron dependent. An excellent example of non–iron/copper-dependent toxicity is the toxicity of metals. Interestingly, evidence implicates glutathione as an endogenous defense against the toxicity of such metals, and glutathione depletion potentiates their toxicity. This raises the possibility that protein thiols may be a biochemical target of these metals. Further examination of this question is needed.

Mitochondria as target organelles: iron-dependent nonperoxidative cell injury

The peroxidation of membrane phospholipids is not the only way that the iron-dependent generation of potent oxidizing species can lethally injure cells. Nonperoxidative mechanisms of lethal cell injury can be readily demonstrated by exposing cells to activated oxygen species in the presence of antioxidants that prevent the peroxidation of cellular lipids. Under such a circumstance, irreversible cell injury develops in the absence of detectable lipid peroxidation.

The circumstances that determine whether a given cell is injured by lipid peroxidation or by a nonperoxidative mechanism are important to note. Acetaminophen kills cul-

tured hepatocytes by peroxidizing membrane lipids. Acetaminophen itself, however, is an antioxidant. Thus, as its concentration is raised, lipid peroxidation is inhibited. The cells, however, are still lethally injured by larger doses of acetaminophen, and the cell killing is still mediated by activated oxygen species. Clearly the antioxidant activity of any given dose of acetaminophen determines which mechanism will predominate. A similar explanation accounts for the absence of lipid peroxidation with the killing of cultured hepatocytes by menadione.

Evidence suggests that mitochondrial damage is the biochemical basis of the nonperoxidative mechanism of oxidative cell injury. That the loss of mitochondrial function can lead to the development of irreversible cell injury is, of course, attested to by the effects of ischemia on cells. In this situation, cell killing is correlated with a loss of mitochondrial energization rather than with the depletion of ATP alone. A similar loss of mitochondrial energization occurs in cultured hepatocytes intoxicated with hydrogen peroxide, t-butyl hydroperoxide, or menadione. Importantly, in each case, the collapse of the mitochondrial membrane potential and the cell killing were iron dependent. This iron-dependent loss of mitochondrial energization occurred in the absence of lipid peroxidation.

Thus, it is likely that the nonperoxidative mechanism whereby cells are irreversibly injured by activated oxygen species is similar to the mechanism whereby they are injured in the absence of oxygen, that is, by anoxia. Such a conclusion is supported by the observation that manipulations that modify the toxicity of mitochondrial poisons similarly modified the killing of cultured hepatocytes by t-butyl hydroperoxide in the presence of an antioxidant.

DNA AS THE TARGET MOLECULE

A number of different lesions in DNA can be produced by such potent oxidizing species as the hydroxyl radical. Reaction with deoxyribose results in fragmentation with loss of the base and the appearance of a strand break. Alternatively, reaction with thymine produces a variety of lesions removed by repair enzymes that similarly produce single-strand breaks in DNA. Thus the appearance of single-strand breaks in DNA is a common consequence of the interaction of oxygen radicals with DNA. Single-strand breaks have been reported to accumulate in bacteria and in a variety of mammalian cells on exposure to oxygen radicals generated by a number of different mechanisms.

In turn, oxidative DNA damage has been implicated in the killing of both bacterial and mammalian cells by oxygen radicals. Mammalian cell lines exposed to H_2O_2 showed a dose-dependent relationship between the accumulation of DNA single-strand breaks and the extent of cell killing. Superoxide dismutase decreased the number of thymine glycols produced by benzo(a)pyrene in epithelial cells while it increased cell survival. The EM9 mutant of the Chinese hamster ovary (CHO) cell line was more sensitive to the toxicity of H_2O_2, a situation that correlated with a decreased ability of the cells to repair lesions in DNA. Finally, inhibition of poly(ADP-ribose) polymerase, an enzyme that is activated by DNA strand breaks, protected $P388D_1$ cells from the toxicity of hydrogen peroxide. This result was interpreted as indicating that the metabolic responses to DNA damage may initiate a sequence of events that result in cell killing.

Several concerns are raised by these studies of the relationship between oxidative DNA damage and cell killing. First, manipulations that alter the formation or reactivity of oxygen radicals, such as the use of iron chelators or hydroxyl radial scavengers, did not distinguish between radical-mediated DNA damage and other lesions in the cell that may relate more directly to the loss of viability. Thus the protective effect of iron chelations against the lethal cell injury occurring with an oxidative stress cannot necessarily be attributed to the protective effect against the accumulation of single-strand breaks in DNA. Clearly the other chemical effects of the hydroxyl radical (or alkoxyl radical in the case of t-butyl hydroperoxide) are also prevented by iron chelation as well as by radical scavengers. Thus, to assess specifically the role of DNA damage in the cell killing by an oxidative stress, it is necessary to manipulate the sensitivity of the cell to activated oxygen species by means that act on events that occur after the formation of the hydroxyl radical.

When such a concern is observed, it can be shown that damage to DNA can be dissociated from the mechanisms of the oxidative killing of cultured hepatocytes. Stated differently, the killing of cultured hepatocytes by an acute oxidative stress does not necessarily result from the evident damage to the DNA. This was shown by manipulating the toxicity of t-butyl hydroperoxide at a point after the iron-dependent formation of the t-butyl alkoxyl radical, the species that is believed to be responsible for initiating the damage to DNA.

The appearance of single-strand breaks in the DNA of hepatocytes intoxicated with t-butyl hydroperoxide required a cellular source of ferric iron. The pretreatment of the cells with deferoxamine protected the hepatocytes from the accumulation of single-strand breaks. In a number of other models of oxidative stress, DNA damage has similarly been shown to depend on a source of ferric iron.

The antioxidant N,N-diphenyl-1-4-phenylene-diamine (DPPD) acts at a point distal to the formation of the t-butyl alkoxyl radical to inhibit lipid peroxidation. Thus the hepatocytes are protected from lethal injury at a step subsequent to the formation of the radical that damages DNA. DNA damage still occurred in hepatocytes exposed to t-butyl hydroperoxide in the presence of DPPD, despite the fact that the cells did not die. Similarly, acidification of the culture medium prevented the cell killing by t-butyl hydroperoxide without any effect on the extent of the DNA damage.

Another interpretation of the effects of both DPPD and extracellular acidosis would argue that both manipulations act to prevent some mechanism that couples DNA damage to lethal cell injury. Such a conclusion, however, would have to postulate that the presumed coupling mechanism acts to initiate lipid peroxidation. Evidence for such a mechanism is lacking in hepatocytes.

A mechanism coupling single-strand breaks in DNA to lethal cell injury has been proposed to operate in the killing of $P388D_1$ cells, a murine macrophagelike tumor cell line, exposed to hydrogen peroxide. Inhibitors of poly(ADP-ribose) polymerase, a nuclear enzyme activated under various conditions of DNA damage and repair, prevented the killing of $P388D_1$ cells by H_2O_2. Single-strand breaks in DNA activated poly(ADP-ribose) polymerase in the attempt to repair this damage. The consequent binding of ADP-ribose to proteins was responsible for a depletion of cellular stores of NAD and ATP. In turn, the latter is argued to lead to an accumulation of intracellular Ca^{2+} ions, actin polymerization, and finally cell death.

There is no evidence for a role of activation of poly(ADP-ribose) polymerase in the killing of cultured hepatocytes by an oxidative stress. By contrast, the killing of L929 mouse fibroblasts by hydrogen peroxide was prevented by inhibitors of poly(ADP-ribose) polymerase. Thus the role of DNA damage and an activation of poly(ADP-ribose) polymerase plays in oxidative cell killing depends on the cell type. The differing consequences of oxidative damage to DNA in fibroblasts and hepatocytes can be related to another important feature distinguishing these cells. L929 fibroblasts are proliferating cells, whereas hepatocytes are resting cells, which do not normally divide. Single-strand breaks inhibit DNA replication and thereby cellular proliferation. Thus, it might be expected that a proliferating cell, such as the L929 fibroblast, would rapidly repair any damage to its DNA, an activity that requires poly(ADP-ribose) polymerase. By contrast, hepatocytes would be expected to be less attentive to single-strand breaks because they are not usually replicating their DNA.

CONCLUDING REMARKS

The metabolism of toxic chemicals by mixed-function oxidation or other mechanisms leads to irreversible cell injury through mechanisms that have been related to the covalent binding of reactive metabolites, to changes in protein thiols, to alterations in intracellular calcium homeostasis, or to the formation of partially reduced oxygen species. The relative roles that each of these mechanisms plays in any particular example of toxic cell injury remains controversial and a subject of continuing investigation. In the case of two of the most widely studied hepatotoxins, bromobenzene and acetaminophen, a common theme of membrane damage resulting primarily from the peroxidation of the constituent phospholipids is emerging. Lipid peroxidation is initiated by iron-dependent mechanisms involving activated oxygen species that are formed constitutively or as a consequence of metabolism of the toxin itself.

SUGGESTED READING

Bellomo G, Orrenius S: Altered thiol and calcium homeostasis oxidative hepatocellular injury, *Hepatology* 5:876, 1985.

Casini AF, Pompella A, Comporti M: Liver glutathione depletion induced by bromobenzene, iodobenzene, and diethylmaleate poisoning and its relation to lipid peroxidation and necrosis, *Am J Pathol* 118:225, 1985.

Comporti M: Lipid peroxidation and cellular damage in toxic liver injury, *Lab Invest* 53:599, 1985.

Comporti M: Glutathione depleting agents and lipid peroxidation, *Chem Phys Lipids* 45:143, 1987.

DiGiuseppi J, Fridovich I: The toxicology of molecular oxygen, *CRC Crit Rev Toxicol* 12:315, 1984.

Estabrook RW: *Cytochrome P-450, and oxygenation reactions: a status report*. In Mitchell JR, Horning MO, editors: *Drug metabolism and drug toxicity*, New York, 1982, Raven Press.

Farber JL: Membrane injury and calcium homeostasis in the pathogenesis of coagulative necrosis, *Lab Invest* 47:114, 1982.

Hinson JA, Roberts DW: Role of covalent and noncovalent interactions in cell toxicity: effects on proteins, *Ann Rev Pharmacol Toxicol* 32:471, 1992.

Machlin LJ, Bendich A: Free radical tissue damage: protective role of antioxidant nutrients, *FASEB J* 1:441, 1987.

Nakae D, et al: Liposome-encapsulated superoxide dismutase prevents liver necrosis induced by acetaminophen, *Am J Pathol* 136:787, 1990.

Nelson SD, Pearson PG: Covalent and noncovalent interactions in acute lethal cell injury caused by chemicals, *Ann Rev Pharmacol Toxicol* 30:169, 1990.

Nicotera P, Bellomo G, Orrenius S: Calcium-mediated mechanisms in chemically induced cell death, *Ann Rev Pharmacol Toxicol* 32:449, 1992.

Packer L: *Methods of enzymology*, Orlando, Fla, 1984, Academic Press.

Reed DJ: Glutathione: toxicological implications, *Ann Rev Pharmacol Toxicol* 30:603, 1990.

Rubin E, Farber JL: *Cell injury*. In Rubin E, Farber JL, editors: *Pathology*, Philadelphia, 1994, JB Lippincott.

Sipes IG, Gandolfi AJ: *Biotransformation of toxicants*. In Klassen CD, Amdur MO, Doull J, editors: *Casarett and Doull's toxicology*, ed 4, Elmsford, NY, 1991, Pergamon Press.

Wylie AH, Kerr JFR, Currie AR: Cell death: the significance of apoptosis, *Int Rev Cytol* 68:251, 1980.

Chapter 18

CELL MEMBRANES

Elizabeth D. Dolci
Thomas R. Tritton

Cellular membranes compose a selectively permeable barrier between the cell and its environment. Only nonpolar molecules can readily diffuse through the matrix of lipids, proteins, and carbohydrates. As a consequence of this physical barrier, the membrane must also regulate the flow of information from the cell's exterior to its interior. To facilitate this process, membranes contain specific receptors to receive signals from the environment; additionally some cells may generate signals to regulate intercellular and intracellular communication. Any perturbation in the fluidity or stability of this matrix compromises cellular integrity and could ultimately culminate in cell injury or death. The plasma membrane can therefore be viewed as the cell's first line of defense against assault by toxic biological and chemical agents. Likewise the membrane is also the initial cellular target of many cytotoxic compounds.

This discussion begins with an overview of membrane structure and function to obtain a more comprehensive understanding of the mechanisms and consequences of membrane damage. Then a series of mechanisms of membrane-induced cell injury is described. The chapter is not intended to be an exhaustive analysis of all agents that induce membrane damage because the bibliography of such a treatment would contain many thousands of references. Alternatively the goal is to survey the current knowledge and understanding of this rapidly expanding field.

The text has relatively few direct references to environmental toxins. Rather the membrane-perturbing actions of pharmacological and medicinal substances are featured. By analogy, it is probable that many environmental pollutants act through similar mechanisms of action. An exhaustive computer search of the scientific literature, however, reveals that the cellular mechanisms of action of most environmental toxins remain relatively unelucidated compared with their cousin pharmacological agents. Thus, although it is known what agents are toxic, a detailed description of how they kill cells through membrane action is not readily available.

MEMBRANE STRUCTURE AND FUNCTION

Any discussion of cellular membranes begins with a model of a fluid phospholipid bilayer (Figs. 18-1).[45] The common general structure of a cell membrane is a bilayer of lipids and proteins held together by noncovalent, cooperative interactions.[1,47] The lipid component of membranes usually includes phospholipids, cholesterol, glycolipids, and a variety of minor species. The protein composition is diversified among membrane types, and this variety is responsible for the differential functions of membranes and cells.

The physical properties of the lipid molecules promote a spontaneous assembly into a fluid bilayer structure. Phospholipids are amphipathic molecules composed of a hydrophilic polar head group and two hydrophobic long-chain fatty acyl tails, which vary in both length and saturation. In a physiological environment, phospholipids aggregate so the hydrophobic tails are segregated from the polar water molecules, while the phosphate-containing head groups are

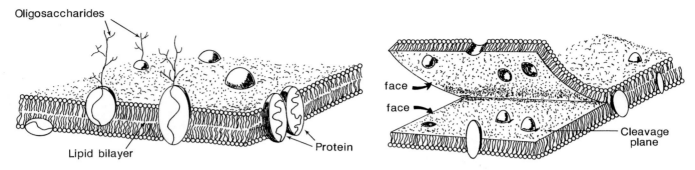

Fig. 18-1. The typical cell membrane in the fluid mosaic model is made up of a phospholipid bilayer with surface polar head groups (0) and associated hydrophilic tails. Specific glycoprotein receptors inserted into the bilayer account for the diversity among cells and their character. The lipid bilayer is fluid, and these proteins can move within it.

exposed to the aqueous medium. To minimize exposure to an aqueous environment further, the hydrocarbon tails of phospholipids close on themselves forming a sealed compartment. This inherent property of self-assembly into either spherical micelles or thin sheetlike structures with the tails segregated on the inside of the sheet and the polar head groups exposed to water is the basic foundation of the cellular membrane. Disruption of such an assembly could clearly have untoward consequences for a cell.

Fluidity is also regulated by phospholipid composition. The bilayer exhibits viscoelastic properties capable of fluctuation between fluid and solid states.[13] Phospholipids with short unsaturated hydrocarbon side chains undergo a phase transition from the gel-like solid state to a more liquidlike fluid state at lower temperatures than longer, saturated fatty acyl chains.[13] The double bonds in an unsaturated fatty acid produce kinks in the molecule, and consequently the weak attractive van der Waals interactions, which normally maintain the lipid monolayer, are disrupted. Additionally a shorter fatty acyl side chain has fewer hydrocarbon bonds capable of bonding to neighboring fatty acid tails. The phospholipid content therefore dictates the viscoelastic properties of a membrane and is capable of change in response to fluctuation in the environment; for example, a cell might resist the action of a toxic agent by changing its lipid composition.

To contribute further to the complexity of membrane organization, current evidence suggests the two leaflets of the bilayer are distinct cellular compartments. Although the two leaflets combine to form a single functional membrane, they are distinct, each capable of its own interaction with the immediate environment. Contributing to this difference is an asymmetrical distribution of lipids between the two faces of the bilayer.[32] This transverse distribution of lipids has been most extensively studied in the erythrocyte membrane, in which phosphatidylethanolamine, phosphatidylserine, and phosphatidylinositol are found in higher concentrations in the inner leaflet, and phosphatidylcholine and sphingomyelin are preferentially distributed on the outer face (re-

viewed in Bishop and Bell[6]). With the exception of cholesterol, little transverse migration of lipids occurs spontaneously.[53] Specific transport proteins, however, capable of catalyzing flip-flop of phospholipids from one layer to the other have been identified.[6]

As might be deduced, asymmetry in lipid composition between the two bilayer halves leads to changes in other physical properties of membranes. In model membranes, phosphatidylcholine and sphingomyelin, preferentially localized on the outer leaflet, are more fluid than the phosphatidylserine, phosphatidylinositol, and phosphatidylethanolamine, which are present in higher concentrations on the inner face of the bilayer.[49] Similarly a differential in fluidity has been reported in biological membranes.[42]

Although the phospholipids are the framework of the fluid bilayer, cholesterol serves several other functions. When cholesterol intercalates into a fluid lipid bilayer, its rigid steroid ring structure increases the order of other membrane components and decreases the flexibility of the hydrocarbon tails of neighboring phospholipid molecules.[53] The result is a decrease in membrane fluidity and an increase in stabilization of the bilayer. Conversely, insertion of cholesterol into a solid bilayer disrupts the ordered packing of phospholipids and increases the fluidity. Cholesterol is distributed in both leaflets of the bilayer and is capable of flip-flopping from one leaflet to the other, thereby readily controlling the overall stability of the intact membrane. Furthermore, studies suggest that cholesterol influences more than the stability of lipid bilayers. This sterol also modulates the activities of at least two ion pumps, the sodium, potassium−adenosine triphosphatase (Na^+, K^+-ATPase) and calcium (Ca^{2+})-ATPase (reviewed in Chin and Goldstein[11]). Consequently, some of the fundamental concepts concerning the role of lipids in the function of biological membranes are still in flux.

The third class of lipids present in membranes, the glycolipids, function in yet another capacity. Glycolipids are localized only on the outer leaflet of the bilayer, exposing the carbohydrate moieties to the extracellular surface. Thus,

Table 18-1. Mechanisms of membrane-induced injury

Holes	Burns	Poisons
Toxic agents		
Pore-forming bacterial toxins	Free radicals	Drugs, i.e., doxorubin hydrochloride (adriamycin)
Complement	Superoxide	Pesticides
Drugs, i.e., gramicidin	Peroxide	Neurotoxins
Cytolytic T lymphocytes	Hydroxyl	Dioxins
		Alcohol and anesthetics
Cellular consequence		
Increased permeability across bilayer	Protein oxidation	Activation of cellular lipases
	Protein cross-linking	Membrane fluidity changes
Collapse of transmembrane potential	Lipid peroxidation	Altered membrane protein function
		Increase in intracellular calcium concentration
		Compromise of signal transduction pathways

their primary role is to facilitate intercellular communication. These glycoconjugates are targets for cellular entry by some bacterial toxins, and this mechanism of cellular injury is discussed subsequently.

The molecular organization of these lipids is so efficient that few molecules can readily diffuse through this self-sealing barrier. The cell's solution to this problem is the integration into the lipid bilayer of specific membrane proteins, which transport essential nutrients, molecular signals, and other factors from the external milieu to intracellular targets. All biological membranes contain proteins, although the concentration and types vary according to membrane location. Most integral membrane proteins can tolerate a lipid bilayer because of the high concentration of nonpolar amino acids present in the membrane-spanning region.[21] Furthermore, studies of membrane protein function have produced evidence of extensive protein-lipid interactions in cellular membranes. Several proteins require annular or boundary lipid to effect optimal functional activity; cholesterol regulation of several ion pumps illustrates this dependence.

Because of the natural thermal (brownian) motion of molecules, lipids and proteins diffuse laterally within the bilayer leaflet. The rapid rate of diffusion of protein molecules is illustrated in the classic study of Frye and Edidin,[16] in which immunofluorescence was used to monitor the rapid intermixing of membrane proteins in a heterokaryon formed by fusion of human and mouse cells.

Not all molecular movement within a bilayer is unrestricted, however. Many cells contain both lipid-based and protein-based regions in their plasma membranes, where movement is confined to specific domains. The size of these regions can vary from local aggregation of membrane receptors to the larger differentiated domains of epithelial cells. Lateral movement can be restricted through self-aggregation of membrane proteins, by anchoring to the cytoskeleton or extracellular matrix, and by barriers, i.e., in-

tercellular junctions and protein fences.[23] These kinds of organizational domains in a membrane could also be sensitive to disruption by toxic agents that disorganize membrane structure.

Cellular membranes contain many potential targets by which toxic agents could exert their effects. Because of the diversity in the chemical properties of membrane constituents, a broad range of chemically unrelated agents can induce membrane damage. These disruptive agents induce damage by a variety of mechanisms. We classify the mechanisms of membrane-induced cell injury into three categories: (1) those that produce holes in membranes, (2) those that essentially burn the membrane via reactive oxygen radicals, and (3) those that lead to cellular poisoning. A summary of these mechanisms is presented in Table 18-1.

PORES

A number of cytotoxic agents directly affect cell membranes by the formation of discrete and stable pores in the lipid bilayer. This group of cytotoxic agents includes the (1) pore-forming bacterial exotoxins, such as *Staphylococcus aureus* α toxin, *Clostridium perfringens* θ toxin, and *Escherichia coli* hemolysin;[26] (2) cytolysin, the lytic component of cytotoxic T lymphocytes;[3] (3) the ninth component of complement;[55] and (4) some drugs, i.e., gramicidin.[51] The apparent consequences of toxic action are an increase in nonselective permeability across the bilayer and a collapse of transmembrane potential.[4] The degree of membrane permeabilization is proportional to the concentration of toxin; pore size is often small enough to prevent leakage of large cytosolic molecules, i.e., lactate dehydrogenase (monomer MW of 30,000 Da), but not of smaller metabolites, i.e., ions, ATP.[3,26,28] More extensive membrane damage can induce cell lysis. Secondary cellular reactions consequent to the initial membrane insult produce critical pathophysiological conditions ranging from stimulation of eicosanoid production to release of cytokines and activation of endonucleases.[5] Cellular pathology also depends on extracellular Ca^{2+} because this and other divalent ions effectively block cytoplasmic leakage apparently by closing preformed pores.[3,4,26]

Which of the cellular modifications directly triggers cell death probably depends on the extracellular environment and cell type. What is quite clear here is that disruption of the semipermeable lipid bilayer initiates a cascade of secondary pathophysiological events, which, if unchecked, culminate in cell death.

BURNS

Oxidation of membrane components is another route of membrane-induced cellular damage. Because this topic is extensively covered in Chapter 21, only a brief summary is provided here.

Most of us view oxygen as a requirement for life, but it is actually a toxic gas. Organisms that exist in aerobic environments have developed cellular detoxication mechanisms to inactivate reactive oxygen molecules

Oxygen exists in several toxic forms, including (1) singlet oxygen, (2) superoxide free radicals (O^{-2}.), (3) hydrogen peroxide (H_2O_2), and (4) hydroxyl free radicals (OH·). Aerobic organisms use the enzymes superoxide dismutase, catalase, and peroxidase to neutralize the reactive species. Toxicity results from the ability of these oxygen molecules to steal electrons from neighboring molecules in the bilayer membrane. Both lipids and proteins are susceptible to attack; the consequences of this oxidative stress include cross-linking and oxidation of proteins and peroxidation of lipids.

The antitumor agent doxorubicin hydrochloride (Adriamycin) can induce both lipoperoxidative damage and membrane-initiated modulation of second messenger signaling pathways. The latter mechanism is discussed under cellular poisons. Reaction of Adriamycin with iron catalyzes the production of hydrogen peroxide and superoxide radicals. In a biological membrane system, Adriamycin-iron complexes bind to erythrocyte membranes, and local concentrations of peroxide and free radicals ultimately induce cell lysis.[27]

POISONS

A third major route of inducing cellular injury is through the action of membrane poisons. Included in this category are a broad range of chemically unrelated agents each with its own mode of action. The ultimate consequence is membrane-mediated cellular injury. Some biological toxins, pesticides, alcohol and other anesthetics, and certain classes of drugs fall into this category.

One mode of action elicited by cellular poisons is activation of cellular phospholipases. Phospholipases are a group of enzymes that hydrolyze phospholipids; each class of lipase targets a specific cleavage site on phospholipid molecules. The degradative end products of this chemical

reaction, particularly free fatty acids and lysolipids, are unstable molecules that compromise membrane integrity. A group of biological neurotoxins induces membrane disruption through their endogenous phospholipase activity and ultimately blocks neurotransmission.[20,31,44,46] Included in this category are the classic neurotoxins, β-bungarotoxin, and notexin. A strong correlation has been established between the destructive effect of the lipase-generated degradative products and loss of plasma membrane integrity.[52] The precise relationship between the permeabilization of the cell membrane and the specificity of the neuropathology that ensues remains to be defined, however.

A number of reports have suggested that the human immunodeficiency virus type 1 (HIV-1) virus may mimic neurotoxins in its ability to interact with transmembrane ion channels.[15] Ultrastructural studies have revealed the formation of cell membrane pores following viral attachment,[15] and biochemical analyses indicate a flux in plasma membrane ion concentrations before induction of viral protein synthesis.[12,17] These modifications could promote a cytotoxic reaction, and some evidence suggests HIV-infected cells are induced to undergo apoptosis or programmed cell death.[19]

Another target of cellular poisons is membrane fluidity or ordering of the lipids in the bilayer and is regulated by phospholipid composition and cholesterol content. Four different parameters contributing to membrane mobility have been discussed and include (1) the flexibility of the fatty acyl side chains, (2) the lateral diffusion of molecules, (3) transverse diffusion, and (4) phase transition. Compromise of any of these parameters effectively disrupts membrane structure and function.

One group of drugs that effectively "fluidizes" the membrane is the anesthetics. Their potency highly correlates with solubility in biological membranes.[43] Anesthetics may have either an ordering or disordering action on biological membranes dependent on anesthetic type and concentration and membrane composition (reviewed in Goldstein[18]). For example, the gaseous anesthetic, halothane, disorders phosphatidylcholine cholesterol–containing lipid vesicles at surgical concentrations.[24] In synaptic vesicles, the anesthetic exhibits a concentration-dependent disordering effect. At low concentrations of halothane, an increase in phospholipid ordering is observed with the process reversing to an increase in disorder as the concentration is raised.[36,37]

Alcohols also possess anesthetic qualities and likewise modulate membrane fluidity. Studies on both phospholipid bilayers in vitro and biological membranes reveal a correlation between membrane disorder and intoxication suggesting a causal relationship.[43] In some investigations, however, high concentrations of ethanol elicit only small changes in membrane disorder.[14]

Furthermore, it is uncertain whether the disordering of membrane lipids by ethanol and anesthetics is responsible for the toxic or medicinal actions of these substances. More recent hypotheses propose that membrane proteins, particularly annular lipids, are the primary physiological sites of ethanol and anesthetic action.[14]

Chronic exposure to ethanol produces tolerance of and physical dependence on the drug. Chronic administration also alters the chemical and physical properties of biological membranes, and the membranes become resistant to the disordering effect of the alcohol.[9] Cellular accommodation to this disordering effect could be affected by an increase in cholesterol content. As discussed earlier, this sterol is responsible for decreasing membrane fluidity and maintaining rigidity in the lipid bilayer. As predicted, addition of cholesterol to lipid bilayers reduces the disordering effect of ethanol.[11] Furthermore, changes in the steady-state distribution of cholesterol across the two lipid faces and an increase in cholesterol content both have been reported in membranes of ethanol-tolerant animals.[10] More recently, Rottenberg and colleagues[40] have observed changes in the composition of all phospholipid classes in ethanol resistance.

A number of drugs also possess the ability to modulate cellular membranes. Because a comprehensive review would not be practical here, a single drug type is summarized. The cytotoxic and antitumor anthracyclines are a class of amphipathic drugs capable of interacting with both DNA and cellular membranes.[38,48] Both structural and functional alterations of the cell membrane are reported at therapeutic concentrations of Adriamycin.[48] A current hypothesis predicts that interaction of Adriamycin with the cell surface initiates a cascade of cytotoxic events, which ultimately compromise nuclear function.[48] Cytotoxicity results from the aberrant stimulation of the normal signal transduction events that control cell growth. The sequence is stimulated by the initial physical interaction of Adriamycin with the cell membrane. The model proposes that the anthracycline disrupts membrane structure by forcing the phospholipids into a suboptimal and strained orientation. A number of investigations have reported that Adriamycin increases membrane fluidity,[29,33] and indeed the physical perturbation of the membrane probably produces the fluidity changes. This flux triggers an increase in the turnover of phosphatidyl inositol and an accumulation of diacylglycerol.[35] The cascade continues with diacylglycerol activation of protein kinase C and the consequent phosphorylation of several cellular substrates.[35] One potentially critical intracellular target appears to be topoisomerase II, a nuclear enzyme responsible for the production and repair of double-stranded breaks in DNA during replication.[41] Modulation of this enzyme disrupts DNA replication and results in cell death.

This scheme effectively links two mechanisms of cellular damage and illustrates the importance of maintaining membrane integrity in biological systems. The initial physical interaction of Adriamycin with the cellular membrane triggers a series of signal transduction events with the consequent cytotoxic action on nuclear targets.

Perturbation of membrane protein function is another target of some cellular disruptive agents. One particular mode of action we address here is the calcium-mediated mechanisms in chemically induced cell death. Calcium is an intracellular messenger crucial to the normal physiology and regulation of many cellular processes. Disruption of Ca^{2+} homeostasis is often an initial cellular modification associated with cellular kill. Calcium levels are routinely regulated by the joint, cooperative interaction of cellular membrane Ca^{2+} transporters (Ca^{2+} channel, ATP-dependent Ca^{2+} pump, and the Na^+/Ca^{2+} exchanger) and intracellular compartments (i.e., mitochondria, endoplasmic reticulum) that store the divalent cation.[8] Intracellular Ca^{2+} concentration is normally maintained at 0.05 to 0.2 μM, many times lower than the extracellular concentration. The second messenger signaling pathways regulated by Ca^{2+} are sensitive to small, transient changes in the divalent ion concentration. Modulation of this Ca^{2+} balance consequently results in an increase in the influx of the ion across the plasma membrane and the obliteration of the normal, physiological fluctuations in intracellular Ca^{2+} concentration; the result is a disruption of a broad range of cellular processes. These alterations are reviewed by Orrenius and colleagues[30] and include (1) masking of the normal transient responses initiated by growth factors and hormones, (2) activation of Ca^{2+}-activated proteases and phospholipases, (3) mitochondrial damage, and (4) cytoskeletal alterations.

Intracellular Ca^{2+} accumulation is induced by a variety of cytotoxic agents, some of which have been discussed in this chapter (i.e., Adriamycin, neurotoxins). Another potent environmental contaminant that elicits a similar response is 2,3,7,8-tetrachlorodibenzo-p-dioxin (TCDD).[7,25] The increase in the cytosolic Ca^{2+} levels induced by this halogenated aromatic hydrocarbon initiates a cascade of intracellular events leading to DNA fragmentation and apoptosis.[25] The heart, with its high concentration of mitochondria, appears to be a target organ of TCDD action.[7] (Similar pathophysiologies are also observed with other agents that increase intracellular Ca^{2+}, i.e., Adriamycin.)

In many cases, the specific mechanism of Ca^{2+} influx has not been precisely defined. These toxic agents may directly perturb the membrane proteins responsible for Ca^{2+} transport or exert their disruptive effect on the boundary lipids, which are essential for optimal protein activity.

One group of environmental toxins that disrupts both the lipid organization and protein conformation of plasma membranes (as well as intracellular Ca^{2+} levels) is the hexachlorocyclohexane (HCCH) pesticides.[50] These organochlorine pesticides physically distort the tertiary structure and annular lipids of membrane proteins, thereby compromising function. As with many of the other membrane-perturbing agents, HCCH pesticides are highly lipophilic compounds and can influence multiple properties of the lipid bilayer. These include a potential generation of free radicals,[2] increase in membrane fluidity,[34] and mobilization of cellular Ca^{2+}.[22]

CONCLUSION

Cellular membranes are a mixture of chemically and physically diverse molecular species interacting to produce a functional lipid bilayer and a semipermeable barrier protecting the cell from its exterior environment. In addition, the plasma membrane provides a highly organized milieu in which biological reactions can take place. These molecular properties, however, are also the potential targets of a variety of cytotoxic agents and on disruption produce a wide range of pathophysiologies. As illustrated in this chapter, many membrane-perturbing agents share a common set of destructive cellular actions, which includes changes in bilayer fluidity, influx of Ca^{2+}, lipoperoxidation, and altered membrane protein function. The ultimate cause of cellular damage or death, however, may differ depending on membrane composition and toxic agent.

Comprehensive analysis of the structure and function relationships among membrane constituents facilitates a more thorough understanding of the mechanisms of action of membrane-induced cellular injury.

REFERENCES

1. Alberts B et al, editors: *Molecular biology of the cell,* New York, 1989, Garland.
2. Baker MT, Nelson RM, Van Dyke RA: The formation of chlorobenzene and benzene by the reductive metabolism of lindane in rat liver microsomes, *Arch Biochem Biophys* 236:506, 1985.
3. Bashford CL et al: Cell damage by cytolysin: spontaneous recovery and reversible inhibition by divalent cations, *J Immunol* 141:3965, 1988.
4. Bashford CL et al: Membrane damage by hemolytic viruses, toxins, complement and other toxic agents, *J Biol Chem* 261:9300, 1986.
5. Bhakdi S, Tranum-Jensen J: Alpha-toxin of *Staphylococcus aureus, Microbiol Rev* 55:733, 1991.
6. Bishop WR, Bell RM: Assembly of the endoplasmic reticulum phospholipid bilayer: the phosphatidylcholine transporter, *Cell* 42:50, 1985.
7. Canga L, Levi R, Rifkind AB: Heart as a target organ in 2,3,7,8-tetrachlorodibenzo-*p*-dioxin toxicity: decreased beta-adrenergic responsiveness and evidence of increased intracellular calcium, *Proc Nat Acad Sci USA* 85:905, 1988.
8. Carafoli E: Intracellular calcium homeostasis, *Ann Rev Biochem* 56:395, 1987.
9. Chin JH, Goldstein DB: Drug tolerance in biomembranes: a spin label study of the effects of ethanol, *Science* 196:684, 1977.
10. Chin JH, Goldstein DB: Increased cholesterol content of erythrocyte and brain membrane in ethanol tolerant mice, *Biochim Biophys Acta* 513:358, 1978.
11. Chin JH, Goldstein DB: Membrane disordering action of ethanol: variation with membrane cholesterol content and depths of the spin label probe, *Molec Pharmacol* 19:425, 1981.
12. Cloyd MW, Lynn W: Perturbation of host-cell membrane is a primary mechanism of HIV cytopathology, *Virology* 181:500, 1991.
13. Darnell J, Lodish HF, Baltimore D: *Molecular cell biology,* New York, 1990, Scientific American Books.
14. Dietrich RA et al: Mechanism of action of ethanol: initial central nervous system actions, *Pharmacol Rev* 41:489, 1989.
15. Fermin CD, Garry RF: Membrane alterations linked to early interactions of HIV with the cell surface, *Virology* 191:941, 1992.
16. Frye LD, Edidin M: The rapid intermixing cell surface antigens after formation of mouse-human heterokaryons, *J Cell Sci* 7:319, 1970.
17. Garry RF: Potential mechanisms for the cytopathic properties of HIV, *AIDS* 3:683, 1989.
18. Goldstein DB: The effects of drugs on membrane fluidity, *Annu Rev Pharmacol Toxicol* 24:43, 1984.
19. Gougeon M-L, Montagnier L: Apoptosis in AIDS, *Science* 260:1269, 1993.
20. Halliwell JV, Dolly JO: Preferential action of beta-bungarotoxin at nerve terminal regions in the hippocampus, *Neurosci Lett* 30:321, 1982.
21. Jennings ML: Topography of membrane proteins, *Ann Rev Biochem* 58:999, 1989.
22. Kaplan SS et al: Inhibition of cell movement and associated changes by hexachlorocyclohexanes due to unregulated intracellular calcium increases, *Blood* 71:677, 1988.
23. Kuo SC, Sheetz MP, Edidin M: Lateral movements of membrane glycoproteins restricted by dynamic cytoplasmic barriers, *Science* 254:1379, 1991.
24. Mastrangelo CJ et al: Effect of clinical concentrations of haloethane on phospholipid-cholesterol membrane fluidity, *Molec Pharmacol* 14:463, 1978.
25. McConkey et al: 2,3,7,8-tetrachlorodibenzo-*p*-dioxin kills immature thymocytes by calcium mediated endonuclease activation, *Science* 242:256, 1988.
26. Menestrina G, Bashford CL, Pasternak CA: Pore forming toxins: experiments with *S. aureus* alpha-toxin, *C. perfringens* theta-toxin and *E. coli* haemolysin in lipid bilayers, liposomes and intact cells, *Toxicon* 28:477, 1990.
27. Meyers CE et al: Oxidative destruction of erythrocyte ghost membranes catalyzed by the doxorubicin-iron complex, *Biochemistry* 21:1707, 1982.
28. Micklem KJ et al: Protection against complement mediated cell damage by calcium and zinc, *Complement* 5:141, 1988.
29. Murphree SA et al: Adriamycin-induced changes in the surface membrane of sarcoma 180 ascites cells, *Biochim Biophys Acta* 649:317, 1981.
30. Nicotera P, Bellomo G, Orrenius S: Calcium mediated mechanisms in chemically induced cell death, *Annu Rev Pharmacol Toxicol* 32:449, 1992.
31. Oberg SG, Kelly RB: The mechanism of beta-bungarotoxin action. I. Modification of transmitter release at the neuromuscular junction, *J Neurobiol* 7:129, 1976.
32. Op denKamp JAF: Lipid asymmetry in membranes, *Annu Rev Biochem* 48:47, 1979.
33. Oth D et al: Induction, by adriamycin and mitomycin C, of modifications in lipid composition, size distribution, membrane fluidity and permeability of cultured RDM4 lymphoma cells, *Biochim Biophys Acta* 900:198, 1987.
34. Perez-Albarsanz MA et al: Effects of lindane on fluidity and lipid composition in rat renal cortex membranes, *Biochim Biophys Acta* 1066:124, 1991.
35. Posada J, Vichi P, Tritton TR: Protein kinase C in adriamycin action and resistance in mouse sarcoma 180 cells, *Cancer Res* 49:6634, 1989.
36. Rosenberg PH, Eibl H, Stier A: Biphasic effects of haloethane on phospholipid and synaptic membranes: a spin label study, *Molec Pharmacol* 11:879, 1975.
37. Rosenberg PH, Jansson J-E, Gripenberg J: The effects of haloethane, thiopental, and lidocaine on fluidity of synaptic plasma membranes and artificial phospholipid membranes, *Anesthesiology* 46:322, 1977.
38. Ross WE: DNA topoisomerases as targets for cancer chemotherapy, *Biochem Pharmacol* 34:4191, 1985.

39. Rothman JE, Lenard J: Membrane asymmetry: the nature of membrane asymmetry provides clues to the puzzle of how membranes are assembled, *Science* 195:743, 1977.
40. Rottenberg H, Bittman R, Li H-L: Resistance to ethanol disordering of membranes from ethanol fed rats is conferred by all phospholipid classes, *Biochim Biophys Acta* 1123:282, 1992.
41. Sayhoun N et al: Protein kinase C phosphorylates topoisomerase II: topoisomerase action and its possible role in phorbol ester induced differentiation of HL60 cells, *Proc Nat Acad Sci USA* 83:1603, 1986.
42. Schroeder F: Differences in fluidity between bilayer halves of tumor cell plasma membranes, *Nature* 276:528, 1978.
43. Seeman P: The membrane actions of anesthetics and tranquilizers, *Pharmacol Rev* 24:583, 1972.
44. Sen I et al: Mechanism of action of notexin and notechis-5 on synaptosomes, *J Neurochem* 31:969, 1978.
45. Singer SJ, Nicholson GL: The fluid mosaic model of the structure of dell membranes, *Science* 175:720, 1972.
46. Strong PN et al: Beta-bungarotoxin, a presynaptic toxin with enzymatic activity, *Proc Nat Acad Sci USA* 73:178, 1976.
47. Stryer L: *Biochemistry,* New York, 1988, WH Freeman & Co.
48. Tritton TR: Cell surface actions of adriamycin, *Pharmacol Ther* 49:293, 1991.
49. Vaughan DJ, Keough KM: Changes in phase transitions of phosphatidylethanolamine- and phosphatidylcholine-water dispersions induced by small modifications in the headgroup and backbone regions, *FEBS Lett* 47:158, 1974.
50. Verma SP, Rastogi A, Lin P-S: Hexachlorocyclohexane pesticides reduce survival and alter plasma membrane structure of Chinese hamster V79 cells, *Arch Biochem Biophys* 298:587, 1992.
51. Weinstein S et al: Conformation of the gramicidin A channel in phospholipid vesicles: a fluorine-19 NMR study, *Biochemistry* 24:4374, 1985.
52. Yates SL et al: Phospholipid hydrolysis and loss of membrane integrity following treatment of rat brain synaptosomes with beta-bungarotoxin, notexin, and *Naja Naja atra* and *Naja nigricollis* PLA$_2$, *Toxicon* 28:939, 1990.
53. Yeagle PL: Cholesterol and the cell membrane, *Biochim Biophys Acta* 822:267, 1985.
54. Yeagle PL: Lipid regulation of membrane structure and function, *FASEB J* 3:1833, 1989.
55. Zalman LS et al: Mechanism of cytotoxicity of human large granular lymphocytes: relationship of the cytotoxic lymphocyte protein to the ninth (C9) of human complement, *Proc Nat Acad Sci USA* 83:5262, 1986.

Chapter 19

DNA DAMAGE AND REPAIR

Bennett Van Houten
Richard Albertini

The faithful duplication and transmission of genetic information is essential for life. Humans are being constantly bombarded by endogenous and exogenous genotoxic agents that damage our genetic material. This DNA damage, if left unrepaired, can lead to cell death, somatic mutations, or cellular transformation, which, at the organismal level, can result in cancer, aging, and decreased immunocompetency.*

* References 4, 20, 49, 50, 63, 72, 130.

Genotoxic injury is an important source of chronic human disease. Its study in relation to disease, however, is relatively recent. Until the 1960s, the science of toxicology was largely directed toward acute disease and cellular injury. Assays for environmental toxins were based on acute changes such as organ malfunction in animals or on cytotoxicity in cells. Although recognized much earlier,[11] it became apparent by the 1960s that certain classes of environmental agents were capable of interacting with DNA, altering its structure and function at dosages that were cytotoxic. Cells survived the acute toxic effects of these agents and lived to show later genetic and phenotypic changes. It was also during this era that the relationship between environmental mutagens and environmental carcinogens was becoming apparent.[2]

The 1960s saw the development of genetic toxicology. Scientific concern was mobilized and directed to assessing the health consequences of environmental mutagens, not only at the somatic level as manifest by cancer, but also at the germinal level, with particular concern directed at possible deleterious effects on the human gene pool. In more recent years, genotoxic injury has been implicated in several diseases and in the aging process.[4,99,130] Although most studies have involved nuclear genes, there is also concern about mitochondrial DNA mutations.[74]

In this chapter, we will consider several important environmental genotoxic agents and the DNA damage these agents inflict. We also examine how these DNA lesions are repaired and some of the associated mutagenic consequences of these genotoxicants. "Pathology" is viewed from the levels of the DNA, the cell, and the intact organism, i.e., the human. Chapters 20 and 26 also consider genetic injury to the intact organism.

GENOTOXIC INJURY AT THE LEVEL OF DNA

DNA is made up of basic building blocks called nucleotides, the linear order of which gives genetic material its robust coding potential in the form of genes.[30] Nucleotides consist of a sugar phosphate backbone and one of four bases: guanine, adenine (purines), cytosine, and thymine (pyrimidines). Nucleotides are linked together by the sugar phosphate backbone to form one strand with a specific polarity. The DNA double helix is formed by two self-complementary strands of nucleotides, with bases on one strand forming hydrogen bonds with bases on the other strand, such that adenine pairs with thymine, and guanine pairs with cytosine. DNA replication is a semiconservative process by which each strand of the parent molecule is used as a template for the production of a new strand. DNA damage arises by altering the chemical structure of the nucleobase. This damage, if not repaired by an intricate correcting mechanism, can lead to mutations or alterations in the coding potential of the DNA. The distinction between DNA damage and mutations is an important one. Various physical and chemical agents interact with DNA and produce alterations in the coding potential of the nucleobase. The DNA replication machinery, on encountering the damaged nucleotide, stalls and, after a time, bypasses the lesion. During the translesion synthesis, the polymerase may lower its proofreading activity and insert a wrong base across from the DNA damage, leading to a mutation. Thus, mutations are a consequence of DNA damage. This chapter outlines some of the important endogenous and exogenous agents of DNA injury.

Cells possess two major pathways for removing genotoxic injury: base excision repair (BER) and nucleotide excision repair (NER).* The route by which a specific type of DNA damage is removed ultimately depends on the nature of the DNA lesion itself. As is considered in detail later, damage to DNA resulting from either endogenous or exogenous agents may be repaired. If repair is complete, there are no lasting consequences. DNA repair, however, is a host function under genetic control and may therefore exhibit interindividual differences in efficiency.[3,9,40,130] This host susceptibility factor strongly influences the outcome of interactions between DNA and, potentially, mutagenic agents. The host-cell pathways for removing DNA damage are discussed after briefly reviewing various agents of DNA injury.

Agents of injury

Endogenous agents

Oxidative damage. DNA is under continuous chemical assault from normal cellular processes. For example, oxygen consumption, which is essential for life, can be activated to highly reactive active oxygen species (AOS), such as superoxide (O_2^-), hydroxyl-free radicals (OH·), and hydrogen peroxide (H_2O_2), all of which react with DNA. Estimates of the frequencies of endogenous oxidative injury range from 100 per cell per day to severalfold this value.[5,75] In addition to metabolic respiration, several biological processes have been shown to produce AOS: ischemia-reperfusion injury, cellular growth stimulation with phorbol esters, neutrophil and macrophage activation, and peroxisomal enzymes.[55] The types of DNA lesions produced by AOS are described later (also see Chapter 21).

Deamination and methylation. In addition to oxidative damage, DNA is susceptible to hydrolytic deaminations, especially of cytosines and 5-methylcytosines.[41,75] The resulting products, i.e., uracils and thymines, are both capable of causing mutations, although with quite different efficiencies owing to repair. Daily frequencies of premutagenic lesions resulting from hydrolytic deaminations approximate those resulting from oxidative damage. 5-Methylcytosine may also arise enzymatically through the action of DNA methyltransferase, an action that itself may contribute to mutations. Endogenous chemical agents also may produce other DNA alkylations, i.e., the methyl group donor S-adenosylmethionine (SAM), which can yield 7-methylguanine, 3-methyladenine, or O6-methylguanine lesions in DNA. The last type of damage can lead to specific mutations, which can give rise to G → A transitions. Thus, the endogenous chemical environment of the genetic material produces a host of agents of genotoxic injury.

Defects in DNA processing. In addition to chemical milieu, the several enzymatic processes operating on DNA can also be endogenous agents of genotoxic injury. A clear endogenous source of mutations is the process of DNA replication itself.[112] Mistakes here can result from the function of the DNA polymerase, i.e. in altered base selection, in strand-slippage, in altered proofreading, or in some change in mismatch repair.[45,67,79,97] In addition to the enzymology of DNA replication, a propensity to misreplication can result from the structure of the DNA, i.e., its overall architecture or primary sequence.[94] Enzymes that normally nick or otherwise modify DNA may go awry, i.e., topoisomerases, recombinases, or methylases. For example, it has been shown that the V(D)J recombinase responsible for rearranging immunoglobulin and T cell receptor genes in B lymphocytes and T lymphocytes is responsible for mutational events that underlie many carcinogenic and noncarcinogenic somatic mutations in lymphocytes.*

Considerations of genotoxic injury usually bring to mind exogenous genotoxic agents. Certainly, environmental mutagenesis deals with external agents that damage the DNA. Mutagenesis owing to exogenous agents, however, is on a continuum with those "spontaneous" mutations resulting from endogenous agents. Therefore, environmental genotoxic effects should be viewed as additional stresses to the continuous endogenous assault on the DNA.

*References 41, 47, 101, 121, 122, 125.

*References 7, 13, 19, 44, 76, 119.

Exogenous agents. Exogenous agents of genotoxic injury can be considered under the headings of physical, chemical, and biological. Each can, in turn, be divided into several subclasses. Consideration of these agents here is not exhaustive but rather concentrates on essential aspects. Several in-depth reviews are available.*

Physical agents of DNA injury. Radiation exists over a wide range of wavelengths and can interact either directly or indirectly with biological systems. For example, visible light represents only a small portion of the spectrum. Energy travels at longer wavelengths, such as infrared (a source of heat), and still longer wavelengths, such as microwaves and radiowaves. UV light exists at wavelengths shorter than visible light and can be directly absorbed by DNA. Energy traveling at wavelengths shorter than UV are ionizing radiations. Cosmic radiation contains the highest energy radiation of extremely short wavelengths. Below are listed two important types of physical agents that can interact directly with DNA and cause specific types of DNA damage; also listed are three other physical agents that might be human mutagens.

1. *Ionizing radiation.* The first exogenous agent shown to be a mutagen was ionizing radiation. Muller[89] showed that x-rays were mutagenic to *Drosophila melanogaster* in 1927, and since then, an enormous database has developed.[84,102-105] It is generally accepted that ionizing radiations produce no "new" types of mutations over those occurring "naturally." Moreover, there is no apparent threshold dose for mutations, and the induced mutational events occur stochastically (see Chapter 11).

There has been widespread concern over radiation effects on human health, especially the fear of large-scale human exposures. In former times, the concern

*References 14, 31, 51, 84, 102-105, 126.

energy was nuclear warfare; more recently, fears center on sources. The largest reported concentrated mass human exposures to ionizing radiation have been the atomic bomb explosions at Hiroshima and Nagasaki and the nuclear energy catastrophe at Chernobyl.

Despite the alarm over potential disasters, most human exposures to ionizing radiations come from *natural* sources.[84] These include internal radiations from radioactive isotopes in the body and from external sources on earth, such as radioactive rocks and from cosmic radiation. One external source on earth is radon, which accounts for twice as much radiation exposure to humans than do all other *natural* sources combined. The average background radiation level in the United States is estimated as approximately 3 mSv per year (see Chapters 3 and 11).

In contrast to natural sources of ionizing radiations, *man-made* sources probably account for less than 20% of total human exposure.[84] Of these, most, by far, result from medical applications, with a small amount from products such as tobacco. The disasters noted previously plus other occupational exposures amount to approximately 1% of total human exposure doses.

Ionizing radiation, such as X-rays, gamma-rays, and beta-emissions, appears to mediate its damage to DNA in large part through the generation of AOS, primarily the hydroxyl radical.[84,104] AOS can lead to various types of DNA damage, including frank DNA strand breaks, the production of abasic sites by the loss of bases, DNA-protein cross-links, and a spectrum of base damages. More than 40 different base products have been identified following irradiation of DNA with X-rays.[125] Some of the most common forms of oxidation damage are the purine products, 8-oxoguanine *(8-oxoG)* and 2,6-diamino-4-hydroxy-5-formamidopyrimidine *(FAPYG)* (Fig. 19-1). Ring saturation of pyrimidines includes thymine glycol *(TG)*, dihydrothymine

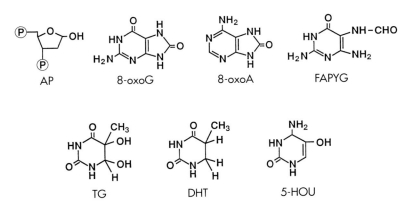

Fig. 19-1. Common base damages resulting from active oxygen species and ionizing radiation. Loss of base, apurinic/apyridimic sites, 8-oxoguanine *(8-oxoG)*, 8-oxoadenosine *(8-oxoA)*, 2,6-diamino-4-hydroxy-5-formamidopyrimidine *(FAPYG)*, thymine glycol *(TG)*, dihydrothymine *(DHT)*, and 5-hydroxyuracil *(5-HOU)*.

*(DHT),*5-hydroxycytosine *(5-HOC),* and 5-hydroxy-uracil, *(5-HOU)* (Fig. 19-1). 8-oxoG is an important lesion that is produced by endogenous and exogenous sources of AOS and has been found to be highly mutagenic, leading to G → T transversions.

Another source of radiation are neutrons and alpha emitters such as radon (see also Chapter 3). These high-energy particles produce a large amount of damage per collision and can lead to both single and double strand breaks and can even generate secondary ionizing events. Neutrons have a sevenfold to eightfold greater relative biological effectiveness in terms of cell lethality as compared with an equal dose of x-irradiation.

2. *Ultraviolet light.* The other physical genotoxic agent with a wealth of information concerning mutagenicity is UV light.[84] UV light is an unequivocal mutagen and carcinogen. This radiation can be subdivided into three different ranges, all of which are mutagenic: UVA, which is long wave UV light (320 to 400 nm); UVB, which is midrange or sunburn UV light (290 to 310 nm); and UVC (200 to 290 nm), which is short-wave or germicidal UV light. The most important source of UV exposure for humans is the sun, and from this source, little UVC traverses the atmosphere because it is absorbed by the ozone layer. There is wide concern over the seasonal and regional decreases in the ozone layer. Sunlight is clearly linked to the cause of skin cancer,[57,115] and it has been suggested that for every 1% decrease in the ozone layer, there will be a concomitant 2.5% increase in skin cancer.[65] There are, of course, man-made sources of UV light, including "tanning-parlor" lights. These are currently of concern as human mutagens (see Chapter 10).

The sun is probably one of the most important contributors to DNA damage in humans. UV light produces two major photoproducts in DNA; these include the cyclobutane dimer and the 6-4 pyrimidine pyrimidone at adjacent pyrimidines. The ratio of these two lesions is 3:1 for cyclobutane dimers and 6-4 photoproducts (Fig. 19-2, *A*). It is estimated that a 1-hour exposure to noonday sun in the midlatitudes produces approximately 250,000 of these photoproducts in the epithelium of the skin. Humans contain a collection of repair proteins that vigilantly monitor DNA for bulky lesions such as pyrimidine dimers. Once these lesions are identified by these repair proteins, they are actively removed in a process called nucleotide excision repair (described later in this chapter).

3. *Other physical agents.* There have been fears that three other physical agents might be human mutagens. These are: microwave radiation, electromagnetic radiation,[1] and ultrasound. Despite intriguing epidemiological reports of the carcinogenicity of microwave and electromagnetic radiation, however, there is little to no convincing evidence that either of these physical agents can function as mutagens or carcinogens (see Chapter 12).

Chemical agents of DNA injury. Concerns about environmental mutagens have shifted somewhat over the past several years from physical to chemical agents. The recognition that chemicals can mutate DNA occurred after the demonstration that X-rays were mutagenic; i.e., chemical mutagenesis was first described in the 1940s[10] (see Chapters 17 and 26).

It is estimated that humans live in a universe of chemicals, i.e., in the tens to hundreds of thousands, and that many of these can interact with DNA to alter its structure and function. Although all organisms have had to evolve mechanisms to cope with endogenous DNA damage, the fear is that "new" exogenous chemicals are being produced and released in such abundance that homeostatic mechanisms will be overwhelmed. Also, there is concern that

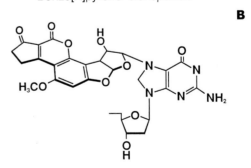

Pyrimidine dimer   6-4 Pyrimidine - Pyrimidone   **A**

Benzo[A]pyrene diol epoxide

B

Aflatoxin - B1

Fig. 19-2. Common "bulky-type" DNA lesions. **A,** Common DNA damage resulting from ultraviolet light: pyrimidine dimer, 6-4-pyrimidine-pyrimidone photoproducts. The most common sites for these two DNA lesions are adjacent thymines and pyrimidine-cytosine for PD and 6-4 photoproducts. **B,** Two common types of DNA damage resulting from environmental chemicals: and benzo[a]pyrene diol epoxide-N2-G and aflatoxin B1-N7-G.

novel exogenous chemicals may damage the DNA in ways that defy successful repair.

There are several classifications of chemical mutagens.[51] Most of these agents alter DNA by reacting chemically with it. The DNA is an electron-rich or nucleophilic substance, whereas chemicals (endogenous or exogenous) that form covalent adducts with it are electron-poor or electrophilic. Some exogenous chemicals are directly reactive with DNA, forming covalent adducts. Many or most, however, do not directly react with DNA but must be metabolized in vivo to electrophilic intermediates. These intermediates then react with DNA. For these chemicals, it is the host metabolism that converts the exogenous chemical to a mutagen (and often a carcinogen) (see Chapter 26).

In vivo metabolism operates to convert exogenous chemicals, which are often quite hydrophobic to hydrophilic compounds and which can be eliminated from the body. In vivo metabolism eliminates and detoxifies but, in the process, also converts many chemicals to DNA-damaging agents. For exogenous mutagens requiring in vivo metabolism, host factors, which are themselves under genetic control, are important determinants of susceptibility.

Some chemicals react with DNA, either directly or after in vivo metabolism, to form covalent adducts. Among these, simple alkylating agents decompose spontaneously in aqueous solutions to form direct-acting methylating or ethylating agents. These are subclassified according to whether the DNA alkylation occurs by a unimolecular (S_N1) or a bimolecular (S_N2) mechanism of nucleophilic substitution.[70] This subclassification has relevance because agents that react by the latter mechanism produce the most selective in DNA nucleophilic substitutions, methylating or ethylating the most nucleophilic atoms, i.e., N7 guanine or N3 adenine. Neither are hydrogen bonding atoms. Chemicals that react by the S_N1 mechanism, however, react with both highly and less highly nucleophilic atoms, including O6 guanine and the phosphodiesters. The O6 position of guanine normally hydrogen bonds with cytosine. O6-alkylguanine is the lesion most likely to produce mutations if unrepaired.[80]

A common classification of chemicals that form covalent adducts with and modify DNA bases orders these agents according to whether they act directly without host metabolism or whether they require metabolic activation to form electrophilic intermediates.[51] Direct-acting agents include the simple direct-acting methylating and ethylating agents considered previously, i.e., multifunctional alkylating agents. Several cancer chemotherapeutic agents, such as the chloroethylnitrosoureas, the platinum derivatives, and the nitrogen mustards and their derivatives, several epoxides, aldehydes, and a diverse group of agents can lead to DNA damage. Many mutagens of environmental importance, however, do not react directly with DNA but require in vivo metabolism to become active. Several of the DNA adducts formed by agents in this group are large and bulky.

Among these agents are the *N*-nitrosamines, some of the substituted hydrazines and triazenes, the carbamates, the halogenated hydrocarbons, the arylamines and arylamides, the azodyes and heterocyclic amines, the polycyclic aromatic hydrocarbons, the methylated and nitropolycyclic aromatic hydrocarbons, the nitroheterocyclic compounds, and mycotoxins (see Chapters 5 and 26).

Two environmentally important classes of agents in the group requiring metabolic activation are the polycyclic aromatic hydrocarbons (PAHs) and the mycotoxins. Benzo[a]pyrene (BaP), which is produced during combustion of fossil fuels, wood, and tobacco, is an example of the PAHs. Benzo[a]pyrene diol epoxide is the metabolically activated form, produced from BaP through the P-450 system. Once BaP is activated to the diol epoxide, it can react with the N2 position of guanine (Fig. 19-2, *B*). The PAHs, after metabolic activation, form bulky adducts on the DNA. The sites of adduction have been worked out for many of these agents.

Many of the DNA-damaging chemicals that require metabolic activation are man-made; many are natural products in the environment. An important example are the aflatoxins (AFB), which are mycotoxins produced by several species of the fungus, *Aspergillus,* which grows on grains and nuts. AFB is one of the most potent carcinogens known and is implicated in much of the world's hepatic cancer. AFB is activated in the liver, where it can bind to the N7 position of guanine (Fig. 19-2, *B*) (see Chapters 26 and 29).

In general, chemicals modify DNA bases so that they miss-pair (i.e., G pairs with T), or they are altered so that they do not pair well with any of the four bases. In the latter instance, the DNA polymerase must somehow bypass the site of adduction during replication, or a lethal event occurs. Bypass, however, can result in mutation. Also, chemical adducts on the DNA backbone can result in damage and breaks at this level.

Some exogenous mutagens do not react with DNA to form covalent adducts.[51] Among these are the base analogues, i.e., 5-bromouracil, which is an analogue of thymine. These agents are so like normal bases that they are incorporated during DNA replication. They have alternative base pairing preferences, however, and so may cause base substitutions in the DNA; i.e., 5-bromouracil may pair with guanine.

Another class of exogenous chemical mutagens causes its damage by intercalating into the DNA. These agents are usually flat, polycyclic compounds that bind to the purine and pyrimidine bases in DNA and alter "stacking" in the double helix. The result is often the addition or deletion of one or more base pairs in the double helix, resulting in a frameshift mutation.[95]

Exogenous chemicals can alter the DNA in a variety of additional ways. Some modify endogenous deoxynucleotide precursor pools, either directly or indirectly, thereby "tipping" a balance toward base mis-incorporations. Oth-

Table 19-1. Some common environmental genotoxicants and associated cancers

Agent	Source	Lesions	Repair	Cancer
Active oxygen species	Mitochondrial respiration, ischemia-reperfusion injury, UV light, phagocytosis, neutrophil activation, H_2O_2	Broad spectrum	BER	Lung, colorectal, stomach, skin
Aflatoxin-B1	Fungus	Purine adducts	NER	Liver
Ionizing radiation	Radon, uranium, cosmic rays	Broad spectrum	BER	Lymphoreticular, lung
Polycyclic hydrocarbons	Fossil fuels, cigarette smoke	Purine adducts	NER	Lung, skin
Ultraviolet light	Sun, tanning booths	Pyrimidine dimers	NER	Skin

H_2O_2, hydrogen peroxide: *BER*, base excision repair; *NER*, nucleotide excision repair.

ers may modify DNA indirectly, i.e., by the generation of reactive oxygen species (see endogenous agents previously). Other agents alter normal cellular processes or enzymatic functions and thereby change the DNA. Virtually any chemical that can modify the in vivo processes of DNA replication or repair can produce genotoxic injury.

Biological agents of DNA injury. Viruses and transposable genetic elements are another class of mutagens. These poorly understood agents exhibit characteristics of both endogenous and exogenous mutagenic influences. Retroviruses may be exogenous or endogenous; transposable elements are endogenous. To complicate precise classification of these further, the various genetic elements responsible for the mutations may themselves be influenced by other exogenous agents, such as chemicals. Biological agents of genotoxic injury are mentioned here for completeness but are reviewed elsewhere.[14]

There are a multiplicity of endogenous and exogenous agents responsible for DNA injury. These are produced by normal cellular metabolism or arise from external sources. Among the latter are physical, chemical, and biological agents of injury. Some of the chemical agents themselves require in vivo metabolic activation before they become mutagenic. Table 19-1 lists some sample agents, their sources, the lesions that they produce in the DNA, their mechanism of repair, and the associated genotoxic concerns.

Repair of DNA lesions

Humans, similar to all organisms, contain a complex system of DNA repair proteins that act like molecular sentries to seek out damaged nucleotides within the DNA helix. DNA damage, once identified, is removed by cellular repair machinery which faithfully restores the DNA to its normal coding potential. Two major repair pathways, BER and NER, are discussed subsequently. Several excellent reviews have been written, and the reader is directed to these articles for more information.*

*References 41, 47, 101, 121, 122, 125.

Base excision repair pathway. Repair of base damages is mediated by specific enzymes that recognize particular damaged bases.[41,101,125] These enzymes act first to remove the damaged base by breaking the glycosidic bond attaching the base to the sugar, generating an abasic site (Fig. 19-3). This abasic site is further processed by an apyrimidinic/apurinic (AP) endonuclease, which breaks the phosphodiester bond either 5′ (type I AP endonuclease) or 3′ (type II AP endonucleases). This AP endonuclease II, which is more appropriately called an AP lyase activity, is sometimes associated with the glycosylase activity. Thus, one common intermediate in the processing of all base damages is the AP site. Concomitant action of 3′ and 5′ endonucleases facilitates the removal of the baseless sugar, leaving behind a one base gap. This gap can be filled by a DNA polymerase and ligated to the parental DNA, leading to a short repair patch.[33] Some of the most important substrates for BER are oxidative damages, which arise "spontaneously" within a respiring cell.[117,125]

Nucleotide excision repair pathway. All cells in the human body remove bulky lesions through the NER pathway.* NER proceeds in five basic steps: damage recognition, incision, excision, repair synthesis, and ligation (Fig. 19-4). Damage recognition is achieved by a multiprotein complex in a specificity cascade in which the repair machinery actively discriminates normal DNA bases from damaged bases. Once a damaged site has been found and marked, an endonuclease is recruited to this site, and the phosphate backbone is cleaved. Studies on bacteria have revealed that the incision mechanism occurs on both sides and some distance away from the damaged nucleotide. Studies in human cell extracts have revealed a similar activity that incises the DNA approximately 22 bases 5′ and 5 nucleotides 3′ to the damaged site.[54] These dual incisions thus facilitate the excision of the damaged site and surrounding nucleotide during the excision step. Concomitant with excision, a DNA polymerase fills the excised region using the other strand as a template. This repair synthesis step generates a small patch approximately 25 to 30 nucleotides in

*References 41, 42, 47, 101, 121, 122.

A

B

C

D

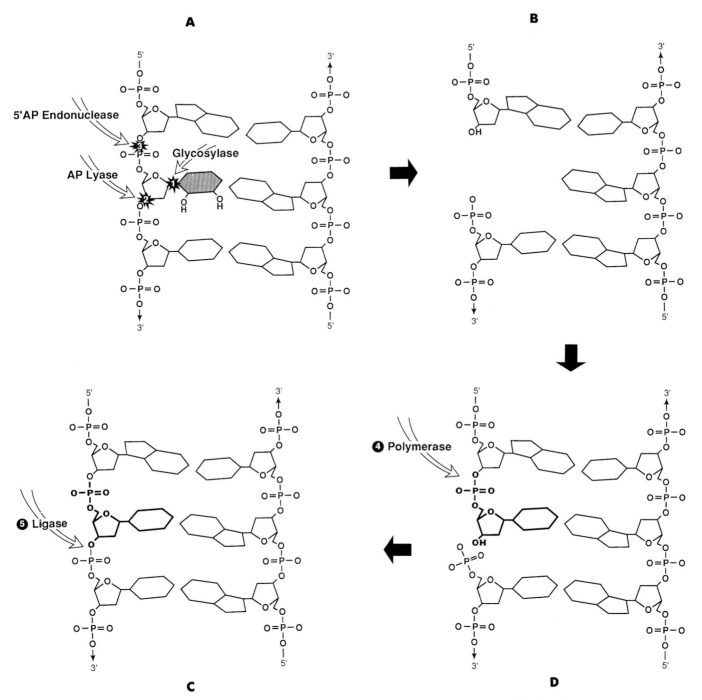

Fig. 19-3. Base excision repair (BER) pathway. **A-D,** Repair of base damage is initiated by a damage-specific glycosylase, which breaks the glycosidic bond between the damaged base and the deoxyribose sugar. In this example, a thymine glycol is illustrated as the damaged base. In the second step (2) in what is sometimes a concerted reaction with the glycosylase step (as is the case for the *Escherichia coli* DNA repair enzyme, endonuclease III), an apurinic/apyrimidinic lyase causes cleavage of the bond between the sugar and the oxygen of the phosphate. The action of a 5′ AP endonuclease (3) liberates the sugar moiety leading to a one base gap with a 3′OH. DNA polymerase (4) can fill in this gap, creating a one base repair patch, which is closed by the action of DNA ligase (5).

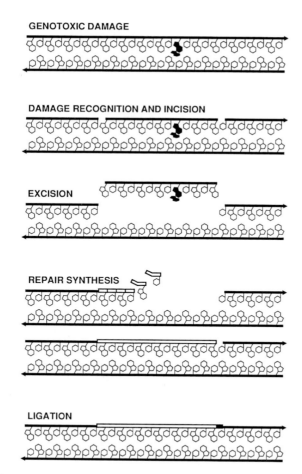

GENOTOXIC DAMAGE

DAMAGE RECOGNITION AND INCISION

EXCISION

REPAIR SYNTHESIS

LIGATION

Fig. 19-4. Nucleotide excision repair (NER) pathway. NER is a generalized repair system capable of removing a large number of different DNA lesions induced by genotoxic agents. Repair proteins survey the DNA for "bulky" damage and recognize the local distortion. Recruitment of other proteins at the damaged site result in two incisions of the phosphodiester backbone in the vicinity of the damaged nucleotide. During the excision step, an oligonucleotide containing the damaged site is removed, and a DNA polymerase fills in the resulting gap using the other DNA strand as a template. DNA ligase closes the newly generated repair patch in the last step.

length. Finally the newly created repair patch is ligated into the parental DNA.

One of the most intriguing aspects of the NER repair system is its ability to act on a wide variety of DNA lesions, which differ dramatically in chemical structure and conformation.[121] It has been suggested that the NER repair complex examines the DNA helix for damage-induced conformational changes rather than the specific damaged nucleotide.

It has been estimated that as many as 50 different gene products are necessary for NER in human cells.[43] Through the efforts of many laboratory groups, several human genes encoding these DNA repair proteins have been cloned and sequenced (Table 19-2). Based on homology with yeast re-

pair proteins, some of these gene products appear to function as enzymes that unwind the DNA, DNA helicases. Furthermore, some of these proteins may serve multiple roles in the cell's protein machinery, which mediate macromolecular processes such as DNA repair and transcription.[15] For example, it has been shown that genes that are actively transcribed are repaired faster than genomic regions that are inactive.[111] It is believed that the inhibition of the transcription machinery at the site of a bulky DNA lesion leads to the recruitment of DNA repair enzymes at this site.[108-110] Coupling of repair to transcription thus helps the cell to fix the genes it needs to maintain its normal cellular functions.[35] The human proteins encoded by the *ERCC-2* and *ERCC-3* (Excision Repair Cross-Complementing) genes are good candidates for this coupling factor (Table 19-2).[106]

One prediction of transcription-mediated repair[111] that has been borne out by specific experiments is that the repair occurs primarily in the DNA strand that is transcribed.[83] One implication of this model is that the nontranscribed strand is repaired more slowly and, as a consequence, is more prone to the formation of mutations. Experiments designed to test this hypothesis have yielded positive results.[66,93,124]

Consequences of genotoxic injury: mutations

DNA replication is characterized by remarkable fidelity. This is because the genetic information encoded in DNA must be transmitted precisely from generation to generation. Despite high fidelity, however, mistakes are made and mutations occur. Mutations are "events" that alter the primary information content of DNA by changing its primary structure. Once changed, the new DNA structure is permanent and, unless again changed by mutation, is inherited by all progeny of the cell in which the mutation arose.

Strictly speaking, mutations include all heritable changes in DNA. By convention, however, the term usually is restricted to submicroscopic changes. Microscopically visible alterations of chromosome structure or number are considered separately. This convention is followed here (see Chapter 20).

Classification according to type. The submicroscopic mutations are classified according to type. "Large" mutations may involve hundreds to thousands of base pairs of DNA and may involve more than a single gene.[27] The kinds of changes that produce these large-scale events are deletions, insertions, gene amplifications, and translocations or inversions. Obviously, DNA changes of this magnitude merge into chromosome-level alterations. For example, it has been demonstrated that mutations arising in human T lymphocytes may encompass two megabases. If looked for, these should be microscopically visible.[77] Large deletions at the somatic level characterize many tumors that have lost function of tumor suppressor genes and at the germinal level, many heritable genetic disorders.[29,32,92,98]

At the other end of the scale are small mutations, which

Table 19-2. Cloning and characterization of human repair genes involved in NER

Gene	Mutant	Chromosome	Size (Kb)	Protein	Yeast†	XP	Potential function
XPAC*	XP-A	9q34.1	25	273aa	RAD14	A	Recognize DNA damage
ERCC-1[120]	CHO-1	19q13.2	15-17	297aa	RAD10	—	Endonuclease (?)
ERCC-2[127] (XPDC*)	CHO-2	19q13.2	20	760aa	RAD3	D	Helicase
ERCC-3[88,128,129] (XPBC)	CHO-3	2q21	45	782aa	RAD25	B	Helicase (?)
ERCC-5[34,106] (XPGC)	CHO-5	13q	32	1196aa	RAD2	G	Endonuclease (?)
ERCC-6[118]	UV-61	10q.11 CS del	100	1473aa	?	—	Helicase (?)

Molecular cloning techniques have led to the identification of several genes whose protein products work together to remove "bulky-type" DNA adducts via the nucleotide excision repair system. Further characterization of these genes and protein products hold great promise for the development of a biochemical understanding of how these specific proteins work as a large multiprotein machine to identify and remove DNA damage.

*This gene encodes a protein that can complement the defect in xeroderma pigmentosum group A cells and hence are designated XPAC for XPA complementing (XPAC). Similarly, other cloned repair genes can complement other XP cells.

†RAD (radiation sensitive) mutants of yeast have been used to identify specific DNA repair genes. The gene products show striking homology to human DNA repair proteins. Biochemical characterization of the yeast proteins currently underway in several laboratories may help elucidate the specific details of eukaryotic nucleotide excision repair.

are often referred to as *point mutations*.[95] These include simple single base substitutions in coding or noncoding sequences of the DNA. An example of the latter would be a base substitution occurring in a donor-acceptor splice site. Other "point mutations" include deletions or additions of one or a few base pairs to the DNA, which, if they occur in anything except multiples of three, produce frame-shift mutations. Clearly, just as the distinction between chromosome alterations and large mutations is not precise but depends on the method of detection, neither is the distinction between point mutations and large changes. Operationally, differentiation between these two is usually made by Southern blot analysis, in which the latter give detectable changes and the former do not.

Classification of mutations by type has utility for inferring mechanisms and assigning causes.[1,25] For example, if it can be determined that a certain kind of DNA damage produced by a given exogenous agent produces a characteristic type of mutation, detections of mutations of this type indicate exposure to the agent.

For these reasons, point mutations are subclassified more precisely.[95] For example, base substitutions in which one base is exchanged for another are classified into transitions and transversions. Transitions are simple base change mutational events in which one purine is substituted for another (i.e., G for A or vice versa) or one pyrimidine is substituted for another (i.e., C for T or vice versa). Obviously, transitions result in A:T ↔ G:C interchanges but preserve the purine:pyrimidine orientation of the DNA strands. By contrast, transversions are simple base change mutational events in which a purine is substituted for a pyrimidine or vice versa (i.e., A for C or T or vice versa, or G for C or T or vice versa). There are six possible transversions, all of which reverse the orientation of purines and pyrimidines on the DNA strand.

Additions or subtractions of bases in the DNA probably arise by mechanisms other than base pair substitutions. As noted previously, these usually give rise to frame-shift mutations, but the term is usually restricted to those in the point-mutation class. Small additions or subtractions are most likely to occur in those DNA sequences in which there is a "run" of the same bases; i.e., the same base is present in a linear array. It is easily visualized that one endogenous mechanism of these frame-shift mutations could be a strand slippage of the DNA polymerase as it catalyzes replication. Exogenous chemicals that function as intercalating agents are also likely to produce frame-shift mutations.

Several mechanisms have been implicated in large mutations such as deletions or rearrangements.[24,100] In some cases, recombinations between homologous DNA sequences are implicated. An extensive literature is developing also on gene amplifications in which studies are aimed at understanding mechanisms by which these unusual mutations are generated.

Classification according to cell lineage: somatic versus germinal. An entirely different method of classifying mutations orders them according to cell type in which they arise, i.e., germinal or somatic. The relevance of making such distinctions has to do with the consequences of the mutation. For humans, the dictum is that somatic mutations affect only the individual in whom they occur, whereas germinal mutations affect the gene pool and hence subsequent generations. At the level of DNA, germinal and somatic mutations are usually considered together, and mechanisms that produce DNA changes in one cell type are likely to be operative also in others. Meiotic reduction cell divisions in germ cells may produce kinds of heritable alterations not seen in somatic cells, but they are usually at the chromosomal level. It must be remembered that mutations in early embryonic and fetal life can enter the heritable gene pool.[48]

"Spontaneous" versus "induced." From the point of view of genetic toxicology, a distinction is made between "spontaneous" and "induced" mutations. Unfortunately, this is often a dichotomy based on ignorance. Causes of mutations, certainly in humans, usually are not known. This loose terminology is frequently compounded by equating "spontaneous" mutations with endogenous mutations and "induced" mutations with exogenous mutations. As discussed earlier, however, there are many endogenous agents of genotoxicity that induce mutations. Probably the term "background" mutations, used to distinguish those preset before known exposures to genotoxic agents, is the best that can be suggested.

Most of the endogenous premutagenic DNA lesions in cells result from the hydrolytic deaminations of cytosine or 5-methylcytosine, or from oxidations of guanine, as discussed earlier.[75,95] The former produce uracils or thymines from cytosine or 5-methylcytosine, whereas the latter produces 8-oxoguanine. These lesions determine the kinds of "spontaneous" mutations that arise.

Uracils are rapidly repaired via uracil DNA glycosylase and should produce no mutation. Thymines, however, are "normal" bases and are not repaired but pair with adenines. This produces a C $\rightarrow$ T transition mutation. Furthermore, because CpG dinucleotide sites in DNA frequently contain 5-methylcytosine residues, such sites are particularly vulnerable to this hydrolytic deamination and the resultant C $\rightarrow$ T transversion. The DNA methyltransferase that catalyzes the methylation of cytosine may itself contribute to mutations at this site. The 8-oxoguanine in DNA, if unrepaired, may pair with adenine and create a G $\rightarrow$ T transversion mutation.[117] It is in this way that mutational spectra are helpful in inferring mutational mechanisms, including possible causes of the mutations.

The utility of molecular mutational spectra for determining exposures to exogenous agents of genotoxic injury is being actively investigated.[2,21,25] Certain exogenous agents do seem to provide a mutational "signature." For example, exposures to ionizing radiations produce large numbers of large-scale mutations, i.e., deletions and translocations.[2,103,104] It has been known for decades that ionizing radiations are "clastogenic," i.e., produce chromosome aberrations. The submicroscopic large mutations are probably on a continuum with the larger events. Ionizing radiations also induce point mutations, probably as a result of oxidative damage from the radiation.

The other known exogenous physical agent of genotoxicity, i.e., UV light, may be the most studied of all mutagens. This agent produces pyrimidine dimers and 6-4 photoproducts at dipyrimidinic sites in the DNA. Because of the nature of the repair of these lesions, the characteristic mutation produced by UV light is the C $\rightarrow$ T transition (giving G:C $\rightarrow$ A:T base pair substitutions) at dipyrimidinic sites.* The "signature" mutation for UV light is the double C,C $\rightarrow$ T,T transition. These characteristic mutations are

*References 8, 16, 36, 82, 85.

observed in suppressor gene mutations in human skin cancers, presumably induced by sunlight.[17] It is interesting to note that a large proportion of UV-induced pyrimidine dimers can be found in newly replicated DNA in mammalian cells.[113] This translesion synthesis is expected to be mutagenic in the case of TC dipyrimidine sites.

Mutations induced by exogenous chemical agents of genotoxic injury produce largely "targeted" mutations; i.e., the mutations involve the bases altered by the agent.[51] For example, the direct-acting alkylating agent ethyl methanesulfonate (EMS) produces G $\rightarrow$ A transitions because of the O6-ethyl guanine produced by this S_N1 agent. Chemicals that produce bulky adducts at guanine residues, such as benzo[a]pyrene diol epoxide (BPDE), produce base substitutions involving guanines. Flat planar compounds produce frame-shift mutations.[95] Given the thousands of chemicals in the environment, however, and the almost infinite number of possible combinations to which humans are exposed, the ability to determine chemical mutagen exposures from mutational spectra is not yet a reality except in the simplest of situations.

Mutations then are heritable alterations in the primary structure of the DNA that change its information content. These alterations form the final common pathway for the translation of genotoxic injury to pathological effects.

GENOTOXIC INJURY AT THE LEVEL OF THE CELL
Physical responses

Treatment of cells with genotoxic agents results in complex changes to the cell's physiology. These highly regulated physiological changes can be grouped into two major endpoints: cytotoxic and adaptive responses.

Cytotoxicity and apoptosis. If a cell incurs sufficient damage, it initiates and undergoes a series of events culminating in its own destruction. This programmed cell death or apoptosis pathway, although lethal to the cell, represents a cellular triage that is beneficial to the organ or host organism because it destroys cells that are severely damaged.[20,123] Apoptosis is characterized by the activation of cellular endonucleases that produce double strand breaks in the cellular DNA and cause the chromosomes to shatter such that the DNA takes on a discrete ladder appearance.[12,37] As would be expected following DNA degradation, all major physiological aspects of the cell, such as active transport, ion flux, energy production, and eventually membrane integrity, cease to function, and the cell literally digests itself from the inside out. How does a cell sense that it has received irreparable damage and decide to undergo apoptosis? This question cannot be answered unequivocally at this time; however, it is clear that during the life of the cell, there are specific checkpoints that monitor the health of the cell. If the cell's DNA becomes injured, these cell cycle checkpoints cause a delay in cell growth and division until the damage is fixed. Cells destined for destruction appear to exit from one of the checkpoint control points. Thus, genotoxic agents cause damage that is monitored by sentries, (checkpoint control points), which arrest the cell in a specific phase of the cell cycle until the damage is repaired.[90] Several candidate proteins that act as "guardians of the genome"[68] have been isolated, one of the most important being the p53 protein (which is discussed in more detail subsequently).

Adaptive responses: gene activation and cell cycle checkpoint control. DNA damage causes the induction of a large number of genes. The prokaryote *Escherichia coli* has been used extensively to map and characterize the genetic circuitry (regulons) involved in different responses to DNA-damaging agents. Thus, oxidative stress can induce a complex circuit of genes, *SoxR*[116] and *OxyR*[46] response, whereas UV light induces a different series of genes in the SOS response.[78] Similar types of genetic circuits have been looked for in mammalian cells and several specific genes (growth-arrest and DNA damage-inducible [GADD]), which are induced after exposure to DNA-damaging agents has been found, some of which are transcription factors and, in one case, a DNA metabolizing enzyme.*

Besides the GADD genes just mentioned, several other important genes that have been implicated in the cause of specific tumors have also been shown to be induced by a wide variety of DNA-damaging agents; these include c-*fos* and p53. The human c-*fos* oncogene encodes a transcription factor that has been shown to be induced in proliferating cells before DNA synthesis and after DNA damage. It is interesting to note that the mineral dust, asbestos, which is associated with specific types of lung cancer, causes a persistent induction of the c-*fos* and c-*jun* oncogenes.[52] Thus, asbestos may mediate its carcinogenesis effect by stimulating quiescent cells to undergo cell division. Furthermore, asbestos has been shown to cause AOS, which may cause direct DNA damage.[86,87]

This paradoxical proliferation response of c-*fos* induction, following cellular exposure to DNA-damaging agents, is not fully understood. It is known that the cell undergoes discrete changes as it goes through specific phases of the cell cycle. For example, during the G1 stage, the cell increases in size and synthesizes necessary components for cell growth. During the next phase, S-phase (DNA synthesis phase), the cell replicates its genome. The cell prepares to divide in the G2 phase, in which the 4×10^9 bp of the human genome condenses into discrete chromosomes (46 + 46). Finally, in the last phase, M-phase (mitosis), the nuclear membrane dissolves, and the cell divides into two daughter cells, each with a complement of 46 chromosomes in the case of human cells.

Treatment of cells with genotoxic agents leads to discrete alterations in this cell cycle. For example, DNA damage results in a transient decrease in DNA synthesis. Inter-

estingly, cells from patients with the disease ataxia telangiectasia do not show this characteristic delay in DNA synthesis, and it is thought that cells from these patients are deficient in this checkpoint control.[59,64]

Following the DNA synthesis phase, there is a cell-cycle checkpoint at the G2/M phase before the time in mitosis when the duplicated chromosomes separate into the two daughter cells. There is also a G1 checkpoint that causes cells to arrest before commitment to DNA synthesis. The tumor suppressor gene encoding the p53 protein is intimately involved in this G1 arrest.[58] It is interesting to note that about 50% of all human cancers are associated with mutations in the p53 gene. Even more intriguing is the fact that certain mutations in the p53 gene are associated with specific environmental genotoxic agents.[53] For example, Brash and coworkers[17] have found specific mutations in the p53 gene isolated from skin cancer biopsy specimens that are characteristic of UV-induced DNA damage.

Mutant phenotypes

The final common pathway of genotoxic injury in cells that is responsible for chronic disease is mutation. As noted earlier, mutation alters the structure of the DNA and heritably changes the genetic information. Cells with altered information are mutants. The mutational event therefore changes the genotype; the result of the altered genotype is an altered phenotype.

It is important to state that cells may alter their phenotype by epigenetic means. An epigenetic change in phenotype is usually the acquisition of expression of a trait or the loss of expression of a trait. Gene functions are "turned-on" or are "turned-off." This, of course, occurs in the normal processes of differentiation of multicellular organisms. Epigenetic changes in phenotype may also underlie some diseases. One well-studied mechanism is DNA methylation and the production of 5-methylcytosines. As discussed earlier, however, this can also have mutagenic consequences, but the mutations are rare events. Epigenetic changes in cells are frequent, involve large numbers of cells, and do not involve alterations of the DNA structure.

The phenotype alterations resulting from mutation can involve virtually any structural or functional alteration that is heritable over the somatic or germinal line. These include changes in protein structure that confer antigenic changes or changes in enzymatic capabilities, alterations in growth characteristics, differentiation status, adherence characteristics, and so forth. Inherited phenotype alterations owing to mutation involve all cells in the body and frequently result in genetic diseases. Somatic phenotypic alterations owing to mutations involve only the cell lineage in which the mutation occurred. Usually, these are harmless. Humans have many mutant clones of cells in genes that do not lead to disease, with usually mutant frequencies for reporter genes (nondisease) being of the order of 10^{-5} to 10^{-6}.[2] If the cellular mutant phenotype is one that can produce dis-

*References 6, 39, 60, 64, 115.

Table 19-3. Xeroderma pigmentosum

Group	Skin cancer	Frequency	Comments
XP-A	++	Common	Most severe
XP-B	+/−	3 patients	CS
XP-C	+	High	Limited domain
XP-D	+	Intermediate	TTD, XP-H
XP-E	−	Rare	
XP-F	−	Rare	
XP-G	+	Rare	CS, vital gene

Genetic complementation studies have revealed that xeroderma pigmentosum can be caused by mutations in one of seven different genetic loci. *CS*, Cockayne's syndrome; *TTD*, trichiothiodystrophy.
From Van Houten B, Kow YW: DNA damage, mutations, cancer and age. American Association Cancer Research Special Conference: Cellular Responses to Environmental DNA Damage. December 1-6, 1991, *New Scientist* 4:306, 1992.

ease, however, even when present in a single cell lineage, disease results. Cancer is, of course, the most feared somatic "mutational phenotype," although many different phenotypes are involved.

There are variations and combinations on this theme. It is now well recognized that inherited and somatic mutations arising separately can conspire to cause cancer.[23,61] Also, multiple mutations arising in a single cell lineage can progressively change the cellular phenotype, as in the evolution of a normal cell to a cancer cell.[38]

GENOTOXIC INJURY AT THE LEVEL OF THE INTACT ORGANISM

Genotoxic injury at the level of the intact organism is relevant to this chapter when it results in human disease. There are literally thousands of inherited genetic diseases. At the somatic level, cancer is the least understood genetic disease, but others are becoming so, such as neurological disorders and aging. The genotoxic components of the many environmental diseases are considered in several chapters. There is increasing awareness that mitochondrial as well as nuclear gene mutations can lead to human disease.[74]

Two examples of genetic injury at the level of the intact organism are discussed here because they illustrate the relationships among DNA lesions, DNA repair or its lack, and DNA damage in the form of mutations and human disease. One group of diseases is uncommon but is the best current example of this relationship. The other is quite common and illustrates in addition the importance of endogenous agents of DNA injury.

Xeroderma pigmentosum and skin cancer

It is clear that many human diseases arise by alterations in the genetic material. Genetic alterations can arise either spontaneously in somatic cells or be inherited in the germ line. There are several human disorders that have been as-

sociated with altered or reduced capacity for DNA repair.* These tragic syndromes help to illustrate the adverse consequences of genotoxic injury, in that some of these individuals, as a consequence of aberrant DNA repair, are predisposed to certain types of diseases, most notably cancer. These syndromes include: xeroderma pigmentosum (XP), Cockayne's syndrome (CS), trichothiodystrophy (TTD), and ataxia telangiectasia (AT). The first three of these diseases, XP, CS, and TTD, show a marked sensitivity to sunlight and exhibit many skin abnormalities, including hyperpigmented maculas and hypopigmented (achromic) spots as well as a premalignant condition known as actinic keratoses (Table 19-3). In addition to increased erythema and freckling, XP patients exhibit a 3000-fold increased incidence of basal cell and squamous cell carcinomas on sun-exposed areas of their body.[62] The median onset of skin cancer in XP patients is 8 years old. About 20% of XP patients show progressive neurological problems, including impaired fine motor control, abnormal gait, progressive mental deterioration, progressive deafness, diminished tendon reflexes, and mental retardation.[96] CS patients also show progressive neurological disorders and dwarfed stature.[43] TTD patients exhibit brittle sulfur-deficient hair, short status, mental retardation, and ichthyosis.[18] XP is a genetically complex disease in which mutations in one of seven different genes (A through G) can give rise to this syndrome (Table 19-3). The biochemical basis of XP is the inability to perform the recognition and incision steps of NER efficiently (Fig. 19-4). Thus, patients with this disorder accumulate DNA damage and have a high in vivo mutant frequency,[26] which correlates with the severity of the disease. For example, patients from complementation group XP-A have less than 10% repair capacity of a normal individual and have an exceedingly high incidence of cancer and neurological defects.[96]

As stated earlier, DNA damage and repair occur heterogeneously throughout the genome, and patients with CS lack the ability to perform gene-specific repair but can remove DNA damage from other regions of the genome at the same rate as normal individuals. There is some evidence that the protein factor that couples DNA repair to transcription may be part of the transcription machinery itself, and thus alterations in this protein could give rise to many pleotrophic effects seen in this disease. It has been suggested that patients with CS can remove 6-4 photoproducts but not pyrimidine dimers. Thus the lack of repair of 6-4 photoproducts in XP cells may more strongly correlate with somatic mutations and the development of skin cancer.

Careful complementation studies have shown that XP-D and TTD appear to share a common gene mutation. Identification of patients with both XP (groups B, D, or G) and CS appear to suggest a similar genetic defect in both diseases. An enigma that grows out of these studies is why do

---

*References 34, 41, 56, 62, 71-73, 96, 114.

only XP patients show an increased incidence in skin cancer? It has been suggested that the immune system, possibly natural killer cells, may be defective in XP patients, which accounts for the increased susceptibility to skin cancer.[91] This model would suggest that a defect in either the immune system or DNA repair may not result in cancer, but that alterations in both predispose a person to cancer. Thus, the lack of DNA repair may be necessary but not sufficient to cause cancer. Other factors might be important.

Work in several laboratories has led to the isolation and characterization of several repair genes that function in nucleotide excision repair (Table 19-2). Many of these repair genes functionally complement the genetic defects associated with XP.

Neurodegeneration, aging, and oxidative DNA damage

As organisms age, it might be expected that DNA damage may accumulate, either owing to a decrease efficiency in DNA repair pathways or increased environmental exposure.[49,81] A large body of literature supports the hypothesis that accumulation of DNA damage in older patients can lead to neuronal degeneration. As mentioned earlier, 20% of patients with the DNA repair disorder XP develop progressive neural degeneration. One hypothesis is that XP patients accumulate DNA damage in neuronal tissue, which cannot be repaired and leads to nerve loss. Ames and colleagues[5] reviewed the evidence for the role of oxidative DNA damage in the aging process. For example, 8-oxoguanine, a common DNA lesion resulting from oxidative damage, has been found to accumulate in older rats. A series of mutations has been found in the copper/zinc superoxide dismutase of the nervous system in some cases of Parkinson's disease and familial amyotrophic lateral sclerosis (Lou Gehrig's disease), two degenerative disorders of motor neurons.[99] Superoxide dismutase is an important enzyme that converts superoxide to H_2O_2, which, in turn, is broken down into water by catalase. Probably the most compelling case for a direct role of oxidative DNA damage in aging are experiments with the nematode, *Caenorhabditis elegans*. It has been found that nematodes carrying the recessive mutation, *age-1,* increase the mean life span by 65% and increase their maximum life expectancy by 110%.[69] Examination of cells from these nematodes indicates that *age-1* mutants have an elevated amount of superoxide dismutase as compared with wild-type nematodes. Thus, increased superoxide dismutase clearly lengthens the age of nematodes and supports the hypothesis that accumulation of oxidative DNA damage can lead to aging.

BIOMARKERS FOR DETECTING GENOTOXIC INJURY IN HUMANS

Many endpoints serve as biomarkers for detecting DNA damage in humans. These endpoints can be ordered according to a stage in the process of genotoxicity described in this chapter and related to cancer.[28] According to the model, genotoxic chemicals (carcinogens) in the environment enter the body to be metabolized, if necessary, to a genotoxic intermediate. This intermediate then reacts with macromolecules, i.e., proteins and the target DNA. Reactions in the DNA result in lesions that may not be perfectly repaired. To this point we are considering environmental chemicals, but once lesions are induced in DNA, the genotoxic pathway for physical and chemical agents is the same. Nonrepaired or imperfectly repaired lesions induce DNA-damaging events such as chromosome changes or mutations, which can be measured in surrogate tissues, using surrogate endpoints, i.e., nonspecific chromosome aberrations or somatic mutations in reporter genes that have no pathological role but do report mutagenic events.

Cancer-specific, DNA-damaging events may also be measured directly at the molecular level in oncogenes or tumor suppressor genes. These endpoints then merge into markers of early frank pathology, such as altered cell structure or function, metaplasia or dysplasia, early carcinoma in situ, and finally cancer. This scheme of using biomarkers to assess the stages in genotoxicity from exposure to disease (cancer) is shown in Fig. 19-5.

This ordering of biomarkers according to progressive induction of disease has several useful features. It orientates human biomonitoring to the stage in the process being assessed. Importantly, it separates the biomarkers themselves from disease endpoints. It also allows a choice of biomarkers for a particular study according to the question(s) being asked.

The overall goal of human biomonitoring is prevention of genotoxic diseases such as cancer. There are intermediate goals, however. One is detection of individuals who have been exposed to environmental genotoxins. Another is to identify individuals in whom exposures have had a deleterious effect and to do so before there is evidence of disease. Finally, it may be important to find individuals with an unusual sensitivity to genotoxic agents. Exposure plus effect in a susceptible individual are the requirements for disease.

With this in mind, it is useful to classify biomarkers according to type. Those to the left in the pathway depicted in Fig. 19-5 can be considered to be exposure/dose biomarkers. Relevant endpoints include detection of chemicals or their metabolites in body fluids or protein (e.g., hemoglobin) or DNA adducts. Although DNA adducts reflect primarily exposure/dose, repair can modify this end point. This group of biomarkers should be the most sensitive for detecting environmental exposures. It requires biomarkers of effect, however, to measure the consequences of exposure directly. Effect biomarkers include nonspecific chromosome aberrations, micronuclei, and mutations in reporter genes. Sister chromatid exchanges (SCE), which are cytogenetic endpoints, are primarily indicators of exposure/dose.

It is also important to identify individuals who might be

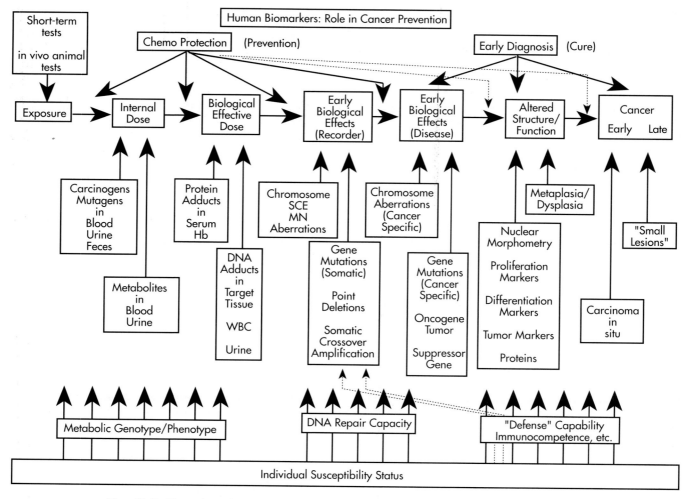

Fig. 19-5. Biomarkers for detecting genotoxic injury in humans. Pathway of production of genotoxic disease (cancer) in humans. Indicated are the many endpoints that may serve as biomarkers to assess this pathway at various points. (From NRC Committee on Biological markers in environmental health research, *Environ Health Perspec* 74:3-9, 1987; with permission.)

at increased risk of developing disease owing to exposures to genotoxic agents, and for this, there are susceptibility biomarkers as indicated at the bottom of Fig. 19-5. Some individuals have a heightened or decreased ability to metabolize xenobiotics and as a consequence have heightened or diminished genotoxic responses to certain agents. Also, as discussed in this chapter, DNA repair is critical for the maintenance of genetic integrity. Therefore, individuals with a limited capacity to repair DNA damage suffer increased genotoxic effects from exposures that may be harmless to others. Finally, even after genotoxic damage has occurred to convert a normal cell to a cancer cell, there are a variety of protective host responses. For example, some individuals may be more susceptible to cancer than others because of a defect in tumor immunity.

There is therefore no "best" biomarker for human monitoring. Exposure/dose endpoints would seem to be the most sensitive for first-line assays when the goal is exposure assessment or dose reconstruction. By contrast, effect biomarkers are the assays of choice for deciding if an exposure actually has a detectable in vivo genotoxic effect. There are caveats, of course, because one kind of biomarker is often used because there are no others for the purpose. Certainly, chromosome aberrations are the standard "internal dosimeters" for acute ionizing irradiations. It would be better, however, if there were more sensitive indicators of exposure, especially for chronic low-dose irradiations. Finally, susceptibility biomarkers are required to interpret interindividual differences in response to environmental agents and, in some cases, to protect specific persons from environmental harm.

Therefore, many of the mechanisms of DNA damage

and injury discussed in this chapter are amenable to study in humans, and the pathway from exposure to disease can be assessed at several points. This may allow targeted interventions. It should soon be possible to realize the goal of human biomonitoring, which is the prevention of environmental disease. A better understanding of the mechanisms considered in this chapter is directed at this goal.

CONCLUDING REMARKS

We have seen that physical and chemical agents in the environment can damage genetic material. This DNA damage can be repaired by a complex array of specific proteins that act as sentinels to guard the genome from the harmful effects of these lesions. Acute genotoxicity can lead to "programmed cell death," whereas low levels of DNA damage can be misread by the DNA replication machinery to produce mutations. An accumulation of mutations, such as in critical cell cycle control genes, can lead to neoplastic transformation and tumors. DNA repair in human cells is orchestrated by a large number of gene products (more than 50). Defects in any one of these genes can lead to inefficient repair and an accumulation of genetic damage. Several rare human disorders are associated with defects in DNA repair capacity. Patients with these defects experience a higher rate of neoplasms as a result of exposure to environmental genotoxic agents. Aging is another important process that may be accelerated by DNA damage. It has been suggested that endogenous production of AOS is one of the most important genotoxicants involved in the aging process. The implications for the general human population is that certain individuals in our society may have inefficient repair systems and may be particularly prone to the harmful effects of genotoxicants in our environment. Screening approaches to identify high-risk groups would permit appropriate educational and medical interventions.

REFERENCES

1. Ager DD, Radul JA: Effect of 60-Hz magnetic fields on ultraviolet light-induced mutation and mitotic recombination in Saccharomyces cerevisiae, *Mut Res* 283:279, 1992.
2. Albertini RJ, et al: In vivo somatic mutations in humans: Measurement and analysis, *Ann Rev Genet* 24:305, 1990.
3. Alcalay J, et al: Excison repair of pyrimidine dimers induced by simulated solar radiation in the skin of patients with basal cell carcinoma, *J Invest Dermatol* 95:506, 1990.
4. Ames BN, Gold LS: Endogenous mutagens and the causes of aging and cancer, *Mut Res* 250:3, 1991.
5. Ames BN, Shigenaga MK, Hagen TM: Oxidants, antioxidants, and the degeneration diseases of aging, *Proc Natl Acad Sci USA* 90:7915, 1993.
6. Amstad PA, Krupitza G, Cerutti PA: Mechanism of c-*fos* induction by active oxygen, *Cancer Res* 52:3952, 1992.
7. Aplan PD, et al: Disruption of the human SCL locus by "illegitimate" V(D)J recombinase activity. Science 250:1426, 1990.
8. Armstrong JD, Kunz BA: Site and strand specificity of UVB mutagenesis in the *SUP4-o* gene of yeast, *Proc Natl Acad Sci* 87:9005, 1990.
9. Athas WF, et al: Development and field-test validation of an assay for DNA repair in circulating human lymphocytes, *Cancer Res* 51:5786, 1991.
10. Auerbach C: The chemical production of mutations, *Science* 158:1141, 1967.
11. Auerbach C, Robson JM: Chemical production of mutations, *Nature* 157:302, 1946.
12. Barry MA, Behnke C, Eastman A: Activation of programmed cell death (apoptosis) by cisplatin, and other anticancer drugs, toxins, and hyperthermia, *Biochem Pharmacol* 40:2355, 1990.
13. Boehm T, Rabbitts TH: A chromosomal basis of lymphoid malignancy in man, *Eur J Biochem* 185:1, 1989.
14. Boone LR: *Biological mutagens.* In Li AP, Heflich RH, editors: *Genetic toxicology,* Boca Raton, Fla, 1991, CRC Press.
15. Bootsma D, Hoeijmakers JH: DNA repair. Engagement with transcription, *Nature* 363:114, 1993.
16. Brash DE, et al: Photoproduct frequency is not the major determinant of UV base substitution hotspots or coldspots in human cells, *Proc Natl Acad Sci (USA)* 84:3782, 1987.
17. Brash DE, et al: A role for sunlight in skin cancer: UV-induced *p53* mutations in squamous cell carcinoma, *Proc Natl Acad Sci USA* 88:10124, 1991.
18. Broughton BC, et al: Relationship between pyrimidine dimers, 6-4 photoproducts, repair synthesis and cell survival: studies using cells from patients with trichothiodystrophy, *Mut Res* 235:33, 1990.
19. Brown L, et al: Site-specific recombination of the tal-1 gene is a common occurrence in human T-cell leukemia, *EMBO J* 9:3343, 1990.
20. Bursch W, Oberhammer F, Schulte-Herman R: Cell death by apoptosis an its protective role against disease, *Trends Physiol Sci* 13:245, 1992.
21. Cariello NF, Skopek TR: Analysis of mutation occurring at the human *hprt* locus, *J Molec Biol* 231:41, 1993.
22. Casciano DA: *Introduction: historical perspectives of genetic toxicology,* In Li AP, Heflich RH, editors: *Genetic toxicology,* Boca Raton, Fla, 1991, CRC Press.
23. Cavenee WK, et al: Genetic origin of mutations predisposing to retinoblastoma, *Science* 228:501, 1987.
24. Clark AJ: rec genes and homologous recombination proteins in *Escherichia coli, Biochimie* 73:523, 1991.
25. Cole J, Skopek TR: ICPEMC Committee on Spontaneous Mutation: Working Paper 3: somatic mutant frequency, mutation rates and mutational spectra in the human population in vivo, *Mut Res* 304:33, 1993.
26. Cole J et al: Elevated *hprt* mutant frequency in circulating T-lymphocytes of xeroderma pigmentosum patients, *Mut Res* 273:171, 1992.
27. Collins FS, Weissman SM: The molecular genetics of human hemoglobin, *Prog Nucl Acids Res Molec Biol* 31:315, 1984.
28. Committee on Biological Markers of the National Research Council: Biological Markers in Environmental Health Research, *Environ Health Perspect,* 74:3, 1987.
29. Dao DD, et al: Genetic mechanisms of tumor-specific loss of 11 pDNA sequences in Wilms tumor, *Am J Hum Genet* 41:202, 1987.
30. Darnell J, Lodish H, Baltimore D. *Molecular cell biology,* New York, 1986, Scientific American Books, Freeman & Company.
31. DeMarini DM: *Environmental mutagens/complex mixtures.* In Li AP, Heflich RH, editors: *Genetic toxicology,* Boca Raton, Fla, 1991, CRC Press.
32. Den Dunnen JT, et al: Topography of the Duchenne muscular dystrophy (DMD) gene: FIGE and cDNA analysis of 194 cases reveals 115 deletions and 13 duplications, *Am J Hum Genet* 45:835, 1989.
33. Dianov G, Price A, Lindahl T: Generation of single-nucleotide repair patches following excision of uracil residues from DNA, *Molec Cell Biol* 12:1605, 1992.
34. Donovan A, Wood RD: Identical defects in DNA repair in xero-

derma pigmentosum group G and rodent ERCC group 5, *Nature* 363:185, 1993.

35. Downes CS, Ryan AJ, Johnson RT: Fine tuning of DNA repair in transcribed genes: mechanisms, prevalence and consequences, *Bioassays* 15:209, 1993.

36. Drobetsky EA, Grosovsky AJ, Glickman BJ: The specificity of UV-induced mutations at an endogenous locus in mammalian cells, *Proc Natl Acad Sci (USA)* 84:9103, 1987.

37. Eastman A, Barry MA: The origins of DNA breaks: a consequence of DNA damage, DNA repair, or apoptosis? *Cancer Invest* 10:229, 1992.

38. Fearon ER, Vogelstein B: A genetic model for colorectal tumorigenesis, *Cell* 61:759, 1990.

39. Fornance AJ, et al: Genotoxic-stress-repsonse genes and growth-arrest genes, *Ann NY Acad Sci* 139, 1992.

40. Freeman SE: Variations in excision repair of UVB-induced pyrimidine dimers in DNA of human skin in situ, *J Invest Dermatol* 90:814, 1988.

41. Friedberg E: *DNA repair,* New York, 1985, WH Freeman & Company,

42. Friedberg EC: Eukaryotic DNA repair: glimpses through the yeast Saccharomyces cerevisiae, *Bioassays* 13:295, 1991.

43. Friedberg EC: Xeroderma pigmentosum, Cockayne's syndrome, helicases, and DNA repair: what's the relationship? *Cell* 71:887, 1992.

44. Fuscoe JC, et al. V(D)J recombinase-like activity mediates *hprt* gene deletion in human fetal T-lymphocytes, *Cancer Res* 51:6001, 1991.

45. Goodman MF: DNA replication fidelity: kinetics and thermodynamics, *Mut Res* 200:11, 1988.

46. Greenberg JT, et al: Positive control of a global antioxidant defense regulon activated by superoxide generating agents in *Escherichia coli, Proc Natl Acad Sci USA* 87:6181, 1990.

47. Grossman L, Thiagalingam S: Nucleotide excision repair, a tracking mechanism in search of damage, *J Biol Chem* 268:16871, 1993.

48. Hall JG: Somatic mosaicism: Observations related to clinical genetics. *Am J Hum Genet* 43:355, 1983.

49. Hanawalt PC, et al: Genomic heterogeneity of DNA repair. Role in aging? *Ann NY Acad Sci* 663:17, 1992.

50. Harris CC: Interindividual variation among humans in carcinogen metabolism, DNA adduct formation and DNA repair, *Carcinogenesis* 10:1563, 1989.

51. Heflich RH: *Chemical mutagens.* In Li AP, Heflich RH, editors: *Genetic toxicology,* Boca Raton, Fla, 1991, CRC Press.

52. Heintz NH, Janssen YMW, and Mossman BT: Persistent induction of c-*fos* and c-*jun* protooncogene expression by asbestos, *Proc Natl Acad Sci USA* 90:3299, 1993.

53. Holstein M, et al: p53 mutations in human cancers, *Science* 253:49, 1992.

54. Huang J-C, et al: Human nucleotide excision nuclease removes thymine dimers from DNA by incising the 22nd phosphodiester bond 5′ and the 6th phosphodiester bond 3′ to the photodimer, *Proc Natl Acad Sci* 89:3664, 1992.

55. Janssen YMW, et al: Cell and tissue responses to oxidative damage, *Lab Invest* 69:261, 1993.

56. Johnson RT, Squires S: The XPD complementation group: insights into xeroderma pigmentosum, Cockayne's syndrome and trichothiodystrophy, *Mut Res* 273:97, 1992.

57. Karagas MR, et al: Risk of subsequent basal cell carcinoma and squamous cell carcinoma of the skin among patients with prior skin cancer, *JAMA* 267:3305, 1992.

58. Kastan MB, et al: Participation of p53 protein in the cellular response to DNA damage, *Cancer Res* 51:6304, 1991.

59. Kastan MB, et al: A mammalian cell cycle checkpoint pathway utilizing p53 and GADD45 is defective in ataxia-telangiectasia, *Cell* 71:587, 1992.

60. Kedar PS, et al: The ATF/CREB transcription factor-binding site in the polymerase beta promoter mediates the positive effect of *N*-methyl-*N′*-nitro-*N*-nitrosoguanidine on transcription, *Proc Natl Acad Sci* 88:3729, 1991.

61. Knudson AG: Mutation and cancer: Statistical study of retinoblastoma, *Proc Natl Acad Sci (USA)* 68:820, 1971.

62. Kraemer KH, Lee MM, Scotto J: Xeroderma pigmentosum. Cutaneous, ocular, and neurological abnormalities in 830 published cases, *Arch Dermatol* 123:241, 1987.

63. Kraemer KH, Lee MM, Scotto J: DNA repair protects against cutaneous and internal neoplasia: evidence from xeroderma pigmentosum, *Carcinogenesis* 5:511, 1984.

64. Kramer M, et al: Radiation-induced activation of transcription factors in mammalian cells, *Radiat Environ Biophys* 29:303, 1990.

65. Kripke M: *Effects on human health.* In *UV-B monitoring workshop: a review of the science and status of measuring and monitoring programs,* Washington, DC, 1992, Science and Policy Associates.

66. Kunala S, Brash DE: Excision repair at individual bases of the *Escherichia coli* lacI gene: relation to mutation hot spots and transcription coupling activity, *Proc Natl Acad Sci* 89:11031, 1992.

67. Kunkel TA: Misalignment-mediated DNA synthesis errors, *Biochemistry* 29:8003, 1990.

68. Lane DP: p53 guardian of the genome, *Nature* 358:15, 1992.

69. Larsen PL: Aging and resistance to oxidative damage in *Caenorhabditis elegans, Proc Natl Acad Sci* 90:8905, 1993.

70. Lawley PD: *Carcinogenesis by alkylating agents.* In Searle CE, editor: Chemical carcinogens, Vol I, Washington, DC, 1984, American Chemical Society.

71. Lehmann AR: Cockayne's syndrome and trichothiodystrophy: defective repair without cancer, *Cancer Rev* 7:82, 1987.

72. Lehmann AR, Norris PG: DNA repair and cancer: speculations based on studies with xeroderma pigmentosum, Cockayne's syndrome and trichothiodystrophy, *Carcinogenesis* 10:1353, 1989.

73. Lehmann AR, et al: Trichothiodystrophy, a human DNA repair disorder with heterogeneity in the cellular response to ultraviolet light, *Cancer Res* 48:6090, 1988.

74. Lestienne P: Mitochondrial DNA mutations in human diseases: a review, *Biochimie* 74:123, 1992.

75. Lindahl T: Instability and decay of the priary structure of DNA, *Nature* 362:709, 1993.

76. Linger LR, et al: A common mechanism of chromosomal translocation in T- and B-cell neoplasia, *Science* 234:982, 1986.

77. Lippert ML, Albertini RJ, Nicklas JA: Megabase scale mapping of the *hprt* region of the human X-chromosome (Xq26) by pulsed field gel electrophoresis, *Environ Molec Mutag* 19:S20, 1992.

78. Little JW, Mount DW: The SOS regulatory system of *Esherichia coli, Cell* 29:11, 1982.

79. Loeb LA, Cheng KC: Errors in DNA synthesis: a source of spontaneous mutations, *Mut Res* 238:297, 1990.

80. Loveless A: Possible relevance of 0-6 alkylation of deoxyguanosine to the mutagenicity and carcinogenicity of nitrosamines and nitrosamides, *Nature* 223:206, 1969.

81. Mazzarello P, et al: DNA repair mechanisms in neurological diseases: facts and hypotheses, *J Neurol Sci* 112:4, 1992.

82. McGregor WG, et al: Cell cycle-dependent strand bias for UV-induced mutations in the transcribed strand of excision repair-proficient human fibroblasts but not in repair-deficient cells, *Molec Cell Biol* 11:1927, 1991.

83. Mellon I, Hanawalt PC: Induction of the *Escherichia coli* lactose operon selectively increases repair of its transcribed DNA strand, *Nature* 342:95, 1989.

84. Meltz ML: *Physical mutagens.* In Li AP, Heflich RH, editors: *Genetic toxicology* Boca Raton, Fla, 1991, CRC Press.

85. Miller JH: Mutagenic specificity of ultraviolet light, *J Mol Biol* 182:45, 1985.

86. Mossman BT, Marsh JP: Evidence supporting a role for active ox-

ygen species in asbestos-induced toxicity and lung disease, *Environ Health Perspect* 81:91, 1989.

87. Mossman BT, et al: Asbestos: scientific developments and implications for public policy, *Science* 247:294, 1990.

88. Mounkes LC, et al: A drosophilia model of xeroderma pigmentosum and Cockayne's syndrome: haywire encoded the fly homolog of ERCC3, a human excision repair gene, *Cell* 71:925, 1992.

89. Muller HJ: Artificial transmutation of the gene, *Science* 66:84, 1927.

90. Murray AW: Creative blocks: cell-cycle checkpoints and feedback controls, *Nature* 359:599, 1992.

91. Norris PG, et al: Immune function, mutant frequency, and cancer risk in the DNA repair defective genodermatoses xeroderma pigmentosum, Cockayne's syndrome, and trichothiodystrophy, *J Invest Dermatol* 94:94, 1990.

92. Ohzeki T, et al: Long QT syndrome with insulin-dependent diabetes mellitus: contiguous gene syndrome on chromosome 11p, *J Int Med* 234:227, 1993.

93. Oller AR, et al: Transcription-repair coupling determines the strandedness of ultraviolet mutagenesis in *Escherichia coli*, *Proc Natl Acad Sci* 89:11036, 1992.

94. Ripley LS: Frameshift mutation: determinants of specificity, *Ann Rev Genet* 24:189, 1990.

95. Ripley LS: *Mechanisms of gene mutations*. In Li AP, Heflich RH, editor: *Genetic toxicology*, Boca Raton, Fla, 1991, CRC Press.

96. Robbins JH: Xeroderma pigmentosum, *JAMA* 260:384, 1988.

97. Roberts JD, Kunkel TA: Mutational specificity of animal cell DNA polymerases, *Environ Mutagen* 8:769, 1986.

98. Rose EA, et al: Complete physical map of the WAGR region of 11p13 localizes a candidate Wilms' tumor gene, *Cell* 60:495, 1990.

99. Rosen DR, Siddique T, Paterson D: Mutations in Cu/Zn superoxide dismutase genes are associated with familial amyotropic lateral sclerosis, *Nature* 362:59, 1993.

100. Roth D, Wilson J: *Illegitimate recombination in mammalian cells*. In Kucherlapti R, Smith GR, editors: *Genetic recombination*, Washington, DC, 1988, American Society for Microbiology.

101. Sancar A, Sancar G: DNA repair enzymes, *Ann Rev Biochem* 57:29, 1988.

102. Sankaranarayanan K: Ionizing radiation and genetic risk. I. Epidemiological, population genetic, biochemical and molecular aspects of Mendelian diseases, *Mut Res* 258:3, 1991.

103. Sankaranarayanan K: Ionizing radiation and genetic risk. II. Nature of radiation-induced mutations in experimental mammalian in vivo systems, *Mut Res* 258:51, 1991.

104. Sankaranarayanan K: Ionizing radiation and genetic risk. III. Nature of spontaneous and radiation-induced mutations in mammalian in vitro systems and mechanisms of induction of mutations by radiation, *Mut Res* 258:75, 1991.

105. Sankaranarayanan K: Ionizing radiation and genetic risk. IV. Current methods, estimates of risk of Mendelian disease, human data and lessons from biochemical and molecular studies, *Mut Res* 258:99, 1991.

106. Schaeffer L, et al: DNA repair helicase: a component of BTF2 (TFIIH) basic transcription, *Science* 260:58, 1993.

107. Scherly D, et al: Complementation of the DNA repair defect in xeroderma pigmentosum group G cells by a human cDNA related to yeast RAD2, *Nature* 363:182, 1993.

108. Selby CP, Sancar A: Transcription preferentially inhibits nucleotide excision repair of the template DNA strand in vitro, *J Biol Chem* 265:21330, 1990.

109. Selby CP, Sancar A: Transcription-repair coupling and mutation frequency decline, *J Bacteriol* 175:7509, 1993.

110. Selby CP, Sancar A: Molecular mechanism of transcription-repair coupling, *Science* 260:53, 1993.

111. Smith CA, Mellon I: Clues to the organization of DNA repair system gained from studies of intragenomic repair heterogeneity, *Adv Mutagen* 1:153, 1989.

112. Smith KC: Spontaneous mutagenesis: experimental genetic and other factors, *Mut Res* 277:139, 1992.

113. Spivak G, Hanawalt PC: Translesion DNA synthesis in the dihydrofolate reductase domain of UV-irradiated CHO cells, *Biochemistry* 31:6794, 1992.

114. Stefanini M, et al: Xeroderma pigmentosum (complementation group D) mutation is present in patients affected by trichothiodystrophy with photosensitivity, *Hum Genet* 74:107, 1986.

115. Strickland PT, et al: Quantitative carcinogenesis in man: solar ultraviolet B dose dependence of skin cancer in Maryland Watermen, *J Natl Cancer Inst* 81:1910, 1989.

116. Stortz G, Tartaglia LA, Ames BN: Transcriptional regulaor of oxidtive stress-inducible genes: direct activation by oxidation, *Science* 248:189, 1990.

117. Tchou J, Grollman AP: Repair of DNA containing the oxidatively-damaged base, 8-oxoguanine, *Mut Res* 299:277, 1993.

118. Troelstra C, et al: ERCC6, a member of a subfamily of putative helicases, is involved in Cockayne's syndrome and preferential repair of active genes, *Cell* 71:939, 1992.

119. Tycko B, Sklar J: Chromosome translocations in lymphoid neoplasia. A reappraisal of the recombinase model, *Cancer Cell* 2:1, 1990.

120. Van Duin M, de Wit J, Odijk H: Molecular characterization of one human excision region gene ERCC-1, *Cell* 44:913, 1986.

121. Van Houten B: Nucleotide excision repair in *Escherichia coli*, *Microbiol Rev* 44:18, 1990.

122. Van Houten B, Kow YW: DNA damage, mutations, cancer and aging. American Association Cancer Research Special Conference: Cellular Responses to Environmental DNA Damage. December 1-6, 1991, *New Scientist* 4:306, 1992.

123. Vaux DL: Toward an understanding of the molecular mechanism of physiological cell death, *Proc Natl Acad Sci*, 90:786, 1993.

124. Vrieling H, et al: DNA strand specificity for UV-induced mutations in mammalian cells, *Molec Cell Biol* 9:1277, 1989.

125. Wallace SS: AP endonucleases and DNA glycosylases that recognize oxidative DNA damage, *Environ Molec Mutagen* 12:431, 1989.

126. Wakabayashi K, Sugimura T, Nagao M: *Mutagens in foods*. In Li AP, Heflich RH, editors: *Genetic toxicology*, Boca Raton, Fla, 1991, CRC Press.

127. Weber CA, et al: ERCC2: cDNA cloning and molecular characterization of a human nucleotide excision repair gene with high homology to yeast RAD3, *Embo* 9:1437, 1990.

128. Weeda G, et al: A presumed DNA helicase encoded by *ERCC-3* is involved in the human repair disorders xeroderma pigmentosum and Cockayne's syndrome, *Cell* 62:777, 1990.

129. Weeda G, et al: Structure and expression of the human XPBC/ERCC-3 gene involved in DNA repair disorders xeroderma pigmentosum and Cockayne's syndrome, *Nucl Acids Res* 19:6301, 1991.

130. Wei Q, et al: DNA repair and aging in basal cell carcinoma: a molecular epidemiology study, *Proc Natl Acad Sci* 90:1614, 1993.

Chapter 20

GENETIC INJURY

R. Julian Preston

Genetic toxicology, the study of genetic outcomes (mutations and chromosomal alterations) following exposure to
environmental agents, in particular ionizing radiations, has
been a field of research for almost a century. Many of these
research efforts have been devoted to defining response, and
it is only more recently that determination of the mechanism underlying the response has been a major component
of the field. This latter approach has, of course, been considerably aided by the developments in molecular biology
that have allowed the research scientist to describe the genetic outcome of exposure at the DNA sequence level. This
holds true for point mutations and chromosomal alterations.
Having defined the nature of genetic toxicology, what then
is the utility of the data that can be accumulated? The over-
riding use is for estimating potential genetic or carcinogenic
risk to humans from environmental and occupational exposures to radiations and chemicals, i.e., risk assessment.

This generally takes the form of extrapolation from responses in rodents to predicted outcomes in humans using
either the appropriate response directly, cancer or birth defects, or surrogates for the specific response, such as chromosomal alterations or specific locus mutations. Where data
for humans are available, this is sensibly incorporated.
Thus, the approach for estimating human risk is broadly described as a parallelogram (Fig. 20-1).

Whether the direct approach (step 1 in Fig. 20-1) is the
only one or whether mechanistic data (steps 2 to 6) must
be incorporated where available is frequently debated. Suffice it to say that a combination of both approaches would
seem to be readily defendable, especially as more data (genetic, molecular, carcinogenic, and epidemiological) become available.

Having described the long-range use of data obtained
from studies in genetic toxicology, what are the short-range
goals? A wide range of prokaryotic and eukaryotic assays
have been developed for assessing the mutagenicity of
chemicals, either for product development guidance or for
potential risk identification. Such information has also been
used to develop predictive information for chemicals of unknown genetic activity by using structure-activity relationships for chemical groups and classes. There are clearly attendant uncertainties associated with this type of approach,
but they are not the subject of this discussion. Additionally, and perhaps unfortunately, mutagenicity data have
been used frequently as a predictor of carcinogenicity, together with the corollary, no mutagenicity, no carcinogenicity (see Chapter 26). Again, there are many confound-
ers that make such an approach quite equivocal, not least
of which is that there is a large set of chemicals that are
labeled as "nongenotoxic" carcinogens. A nongenotoxic
carcinogen is basically one that shows no mutagenicity in
one or more of the many short-term assays. It is apparent,

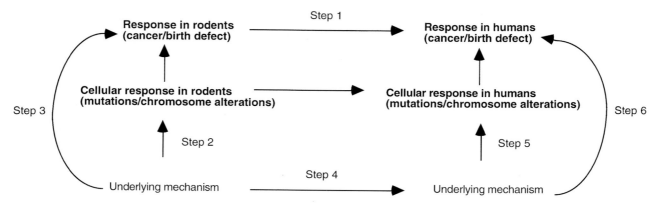

Fig. 20-1. The parallelogram approach for estimating human risk from whole animal and cellular studies.

however that such agents can cause secondary mutagenic responses, and so they might be better defined as "non-DNA reactive." A later section in this chapter further considers the role of non-DNA reactive carcinogens.

Perhaps the greatest utility of genotoxicity (mutagenicity) assay systems is for identifying the mechanisms of induction of the particular end points (e.g., mutations/chromosomal aberrations) either as a unique observation or in a comparative mode among cell types or among species to provide a basis for extrapolation of response, ultimately to humans. This chapter concentrates on the latter aspect of genotoxicity assay systems, a discussion of the possible mechanisms of induction of mutations and chromosomal alterations by radiation and chemical agents, how genotoxicity assays aid in this process, and what additional information is needed to further the development of reliable, complete genetic/carcinogenic risk assessment models. In particular, emphasis is placed on the importance of collecting data that can be directly related to specific end points of relevance in cells of the target tissue for adverse health outcomes in humans.

There may be overlap of information with other chapters, but it is hoped that the reader sees this as complementary and not repetitive. In addition, no discussion of this type can be exhaustive and inevitably contains some personal biases. It is hoped that this does not detract from the utility of the discussions. Finally, reviews often are used to indicate sources of additional information, although it is appreciated that these are only the compilation of a large number of original research publications.

DNA DAMAGE AND REPAIR, AND GENETIC ALTERATIONS

This section only briefly describes the major types of DNA damage and their repair because this subject is discussed in detail in Chapter 19. It is necessary, however to provide an overall framework for discussion of the mechanism of formation of mutations and chromosomal alterations following exposure to radiation or chemicals.

Ionizing radiation

Ionizing radiation (see Chapter 11) induces single-strand breaks (ssb) and double-strand breaks (dsb) and a broad range of DNA base damage. The relative proportion of these different types of alterations depends on the radiation quality, as described by the linear energy transfer (LET), with the proportion of dsb being highest with high LET radiation such as α particles and neutrons.[73,78,80] It is generally presumed that ssb are repaired by a triple enzyme process (phosphodiesterase, polymerase, ligase) that is both rapid and error-free[58]; therefore, this class of damage does not contribute significantly to the production of point mutations or chromosomal alterations. The induced dsb are repaired either by a ligational process or a recombinational process that involves the undamaged sister chromatid DNA double helix or that of the homologous chromosome[58]; either of these repair modes has the potential to be error-prone and thus result in the production of genetic alterations; therefore dsb are considered to be a major DNA lesion involved in mutation and chromosomal aberration induction. In the broadest terms, there are three outcomes for an induced dsb: it can be repaired correctly to restore the original, undamaged DNA molecule; it can be "misrepaired" (either as misligation or misrecombination) to produce mutated DNA molecules; or it can remain unrepaired at the time of cellular DNA replication or chromosomal condensation at mitosis/meiosis, for which the consequences are mutations and/or chromosomal aberrations (as discussed in more detail in a subsequent section).

The category of DNA base damage contains a broad range of different types of alterations, of which only a relatively small number have been identified.[22,78] It is proposed that the majority are removed by an excision repair process,[38] which also has the potential to be error-prone either during the resynthesis step ("misrepair") or as a result of remaining unrepaired at the time of replication, possibly leading to a replication error on a damaged template. It has also been shown that a glycosylase can convert a base damage into an apurinic or apyrimidinic site that can be repaired by an excision process.[79] The outcomes are the same as those described for excision repair of base damage itself.

Nonionizing radiation

The consequences of DNA damage induced by nonionizing radiation (see Chapter 10) are similar to those from ionizing radiation, although the specific damage is different. Ultraviolet (UV) light serves as the model nonionizing radiation, and the most significant DNA lesions induced are the pyrimidine dimer, whereby adjacent pyrimidines can be linked together, or the 6-4 pyrimidine, pyrimidine photoproduct. These can be repaired by several different processes, most frequently by photoreactivation or excision repair. Here, as for ionizing radiations, the excision repair process has the potential to be error-prone. In addition, as with ionizing radiation–induced dsb damage and base damage, replication errors can arise if repair is incomplete at the time of cellular DNA replication. Thus, in a general sense, the understanding of how genetic alterations arise relates more to the efficiency and accuracy of DNA repair and replication processes rather than to the particular types of damage produced.

Chemical agents

Although the types of DNA damage induced by radiation fall into relatively few, fairly distinct categories, those formed by chemical agents are many and varied and are frequently chemical-specific or chemical class–specific (see Chapter 5). The biological outcomes, to be discussed, can frequently be influenced by the particular type of DNA damage produced.

In the broadest terms, chemicals can be classified as radiomimetic or nonradiomimetic. This classification is largely based on the similarity of the pattern of chromosomal alterations and mutations induced and the cell cycle response: a mutational response can be produced in cells in any cell cycle stage at the time of treatment for radiomimetic compounds, whereas for nonradiomimetic chemicals there is an enormously higher probability of this response requiring DNA replication on a damaged template. In part, such a distinction is indirectly based on the particular types of DNA damage produced: radiomimetic compounds induce direct DNA strand breaks, together with altered bases,[13] whereas nonradiomimetic compounds produce DNA adducts and cross-links. Thus, mechanisms of formation of chromosomal aberrations and mutations for radiomimetic chemical exposures are similar to those proposed for ionizing radiation, whereas those for nonradiomimetic chemicals are similar to those for nonionizing radiation. Examples of radiomimetic chemicals are antitumor antibiotics, such as bleomycin, streptonigrin, and neocarzinostatin, and 8-ethoxycaffeine, and 8-methoxycaffeine.

For this chapter, what happens to chemically-induced DNA lesions that are not repaired before DNA replication is of greater significance. Clearly, this is influenced by the efficiency and fidelity of DNA repair processes in particular cell types or for a particular species. The reader is referred to Chapter 19 for details of the various repair processes.

GENERAL MECHANISM OF CHROMOSOMAL ABERRATIONS AND POINT MUTATION FORMATIONS: RELEVANCE TO SENSITIVITY
Ionizing radiation

The majority of the information and hypotheses related to the mechanism of formation of chromosomal aberrations are provided by ionizing radiation studies. In part, this is due to the long history of radiation research, but also to the fact that the dosimetry for ionizing radiation is quantitative, and the nature of distribution of energy in cells is well established. This background of information for radiation has been used to provide approaches for studying the induction of genetic alterations by chemicals. This has at times been beneficial, but also quite misleading because of some marked differences in mechanism that can be involved. The critical components of any model for the formation of chromosomal alterations and mutations are errors made during the repair of DNA damage or during replication on a damaged template and the relationship between DNA repair and replication, i.e., efficiency and time of repair versus entry into replication. The role of a number of genes in all these processes is currently being investigated and will have an impact on the various models for mutagenesis and relative sensitivity to genetic alterations. As a starting point for any discussion of the mechanism of production of chromosomal alterations and mutations, it is appropriate to present a review of information from ionizing radiation exposures.

The study of the production of chromosomal aberrations following exposure to ionizing radiation has been ongoing for more than 50 years, and that for mutations even longer, but still leaves a great deal to speculation and stirs up vigorous discussion. A major factor in this uncertainty of action is that it has not been established which of the DNA damages are explicitly involved in chromosomal aberration and mutation formation. Furthermore, the nature of the repair of DNA damage induced by ionizing radiation has received somewhat limited attention, especially at the molecular level.

The original mechanism for the production of chromosomal aberrations proposed by Karl Sax was known as "breakage first," which implied that DNA was "broken" by radiation and that the breaks either failed to rejoin or rejoined in a variety of ways to produce the range of chromosomal aberrations—in general terms, deletions and exchanges.[64,65] The two broad categories of aberration types—chromosome type and chromatid type—would thus be the consequence of breakage in an unreplicated or replicated chromosome, respectively. This model certainly

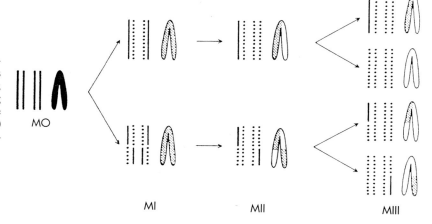

Fig. 20-2. Illustration of the mechanism underlying observation of sister chromatid exchanges (SCE). Solid line is thyrmidine-containing DNA; broken line is bromodeoxyuridine containing DNA. Switches of light and dark chromatids are SCE depicted in the second *(MII)* and third *(MIII)* metaphases after the initiation of BrdU incorporation.

has simplicity on its side and was, in fact, quite remarkable because it was developed in the absence of knowledge about the structure of DNA, specific types of radiation-induced DNA damage, and the concept of repair.

An alternate model was developed some 20 years later by Revell[59,60] to explain the nonlinear dose response curves for chromatid-type deletions and the production of so-called isochromatid deletions, in which both chromatids were deleted at apparently identical points but as the result of a process taking place in a replicated chromosome. He proposed that chromatid-type deletions were produced as the incomplete product of an intrachromosomal exchange (the so-called exchange hypothesis). If it was further assumed that all such exchanges occurred at the base of a loop, it was readily possible to produce all types of chromatid deletion, including isochromatid ones. This model was further extended by Brewen and Brock[6] to explain the formation of chromosome-type deletions, again proposed to be the product of an incomplete exchange. No specific DNA lesion was presumed to be involved, but it can readily be seen that this does not matter for the presentation of the exchange hypothesis.

The fervent debate that has surrounded the issue of which hypothesis is the "right" one has not resolved the issue. The principles of the hypotheses have frequently been lost in the dust of battle. The elegant experiments of Duncan and Evans,[15] which measured the switches of light and dark differentially stained BrdU-substituted chromatids (sister chromatid exchange [SCE], Fig. 20-2) at the site of chromatid deletions following bleomycin treatment, concluded that both hypotheses could be viable. Based on the exchange hypothesis, 40% of all deletions would be associated with a SCE (Fig. 20-3), whereas with the breakage first mechanism none would be. In fact, the observations indicate a value of about 20%, suggesting some deletions could be produced by direct breakage and a failure to rejoin and others as a result of an incomplete exchange, possibly involving DNA damage other than that *directly* induced.

Is a distinction between these mechanisms of any significance? The answer is yes, for two reasons. (1) Although they are not mutually exclusive, the exchange hypothesis is more inclusive of the types of DNA damage that it involves in aberration formation, DNA strand breaks and base damages, (2) furthermore the exchange hypothesis allows for a mechanistic link between chromosomal aberration formation from exposure to chemicals as well as to radiation, with DNA replication (normal semiconservative or repair replication) being the link.[54] Although this discussion has been restricted to chromosomal aberration formation, it needs to be appreciated that included within this is the deletion mutation category. The fact that a proportion of these can be quite small in chromosomal terms influences the shape of the dose response curve rather than the mechanism of formation.

It becomes important to consider which radiation-induced DNA lesions are involved in the process of the production of chromosomal aberrations. In support of the "breakage first" hypothesis, it has largely been presumed, with purported support from a variety of experimental approaches, that directly induced dsb are the singular lesion involved in the conversion from DNA damage to aberration (misrepair leading to exchanges, failure to repair leading to deletions).[29,47] Although this also has the attractiveness of simplicity, it does not allow for a consideration of the total spectrum of induced DNA damage. A number of studies have used restriction endonucleases to induce specific types (blunt-end or overlapping-end) of dsb in specific target sequences.[9,45,84] Following such treatments, chromosome-type or chromatid-type aberrations are formed depending on the stage of the cell cycle at the time of treatment. Many of these studies have been used as an argument for the unique role of dsb in the formation of chromosome aberrations. A more correct interpretation would

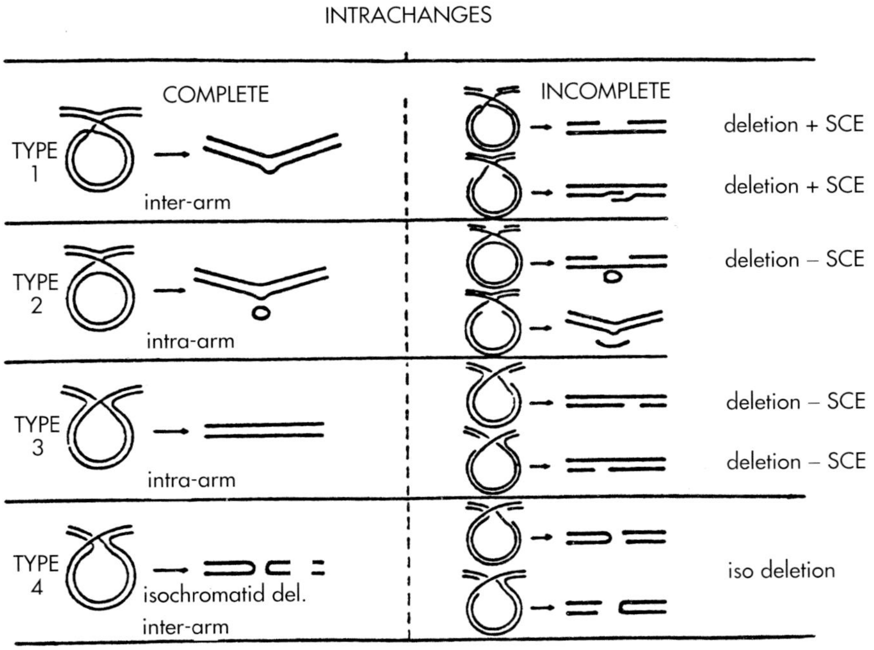

INTRACHANGES

Fig. 20-3. Formation of chromatid and isochromatid deletions by the exchange hypothesis and the proportion of deletions associated with a SCE (40%).

be that dsb are involved in aberration formation, but that other lesions cannot be excluded because they were not induced.

An interesting addition to this hypothesis is provided by studies of Winegar and Preston (unpublished) with combinations of restriction endonucleases. They showed that when cells were treated with pairs of enzymes that produced either blunt-end cuts or two-base overlap cuts, the resulting dsb could interact to produce chromosome aberrations because their frequency following the combined treatment was significantly above additivity. In contrast, the dsb produced by enzymes that made four-base overlap cuts could not interact to produce aberrations with any other cut end structure. This observation could be extended to suggest that low LET radiation that generally produce dsb with several base overlapping ends can only interact (misrepair) in aberration formation with a homologous cut end; i.e., exchanges would be predicted to involve homologous DNA sequences on homologous or nonhomologous chromosomes, such as repetitive sequences.

In a series of studies, Preston has developed the hypothesis that for low LET radiation misrepair during the coincident excision repair of induced base damage can result in exchange aberrations, and that failure to repair at the site of an exchange or otherwise can lead to a deletion (reviewed in Preston[53]). Thus, radiation-induced chromosomal aberrations can arise from this process as well as from misrepair or failure to repair dsb. This hypothesis has been further extended to show that at low exposures and/or low exposure rates of low LET radiation, the aberrations are

formed exclusively from dsb, based on probability considerations, whereas at higher acute exposures, an increasing contribution from base damage repair would be expected. This can be restated: aberrations produced by a one-track process (the linear component of the observed quadratic dose response) are a consequence of directly induced dsb, whereas that proportion produced from base damage represents the two-track component of the dose response curve.[54]

Repair of the dsb, as evidenced from studies with restriction endonucleases, can lead to point mutations at the site of the dsb.[83] To a much lesser extent, point mutations can be produced during the excision repair of base damage as a result of a replication resynthesis error.

These considerations largely reflect what is taking place in G_1 and G_2 cell populations, in which errors in DNA repair are the major mode of formation of chromosomal aberrations. Although similar errors are a component of aberrations produced during the S-phase, especially for dsb whose repair is relatively rapid, there is the additional and significant involvement of errors being produced by replication on a damaged DNA template, especially as a consequence of induced base damage. Again, failure to rejoin fully all DNA breaks produced as a consequence of replication error can lead to deletions, whereas incorrect rejoining at the sites of two or more coincident (temporally and spatially) replication error sites can lead to exchanges, involving one, two, or more chromosomes. An additional predictable outcome is that point mutations can arise from replication errors on a template containing damaged bases where incorrect base pairing can occur.[33] It is feasible that point mutations can also occur at the sites of unrepaired dsb, but these are more likely to represent a block to replication.

For high LET radiation, such as neutrons and α particles (e.g., radon), because the chromosomal alterations and mutations (deletions and point) are produced by a one-track process, independent of dose, it is reasonable to assume that dsb are almost exclusively the induced lesion involved in their formation. For this reason, sensitivity is largely a feature of DNA content because frequency of dsb is proportional to DNA content, with the kinetics of repair being less influential than is the case for low LET radiation. Furthermore, there is predicted to be, and, of course, is, little difference in sensitivity between acute and chronic exposures.

Thus, one can arrive at the simple concept that errors of repair for radiation-induced DNA damage can lead to chromosomal alterations, deletions and exchanges, and that either directly induced dsb or base damage can be involved; the relative involvement being partially dependent on the dose and dose rate. Point mutations can be produced as errors of repair, most frequently at sites of dsb. At the same time, DNA replication errors during the S-phase caused by a damaged DNA template can lead to chromosomal alterations and point mutations, with damaged bases being a more significant substrate for this process.

How does this information impact on the interpretation of genotoxicity assays and the extrapolation of clastogenicity/mutagenicity from animal or cellular model systems to humans? It is reasonable to presume that the mechanism of formation of the various genetic alterations is similar across species and from one cell type to another. For low LET radiation, such as x-rays and γ rays, it is necessary to consider relative DNA contents for comparisons among species of sensitivity to DNA damage induction, for the same or different cell types, as part of an extrapolative risk approach. This is a readily measurable value and is generally available. It is also necessary to have a knowledge of the kinetics of repair, particularly for base damage, because variation in rates of incision (and resynthesis) greatly influences the frequency of chromosomal alterations and probably the ratio of exchanges to deletions.[26] Such information is generally lacking, and for extrapolative purposes one is left with the pragmatic approach, based on a knowledge for one particular cell type, for one species pair. This information is also needed for estimating, for asynchronous populations or for noncycling populations that are stimulated to cycle by a mitogenic or cytotoxic process, the extent of repair that takes place between exposure and replication. This is a part of the determination of sensitivity and aberration type (and hence biological consequence). Thus, it is important not only to understand mechanism, but also to have quantitative information on the various components of the process to extrapolate from species to species or cell type to cell type or to begin to develop factors for estimating genetic or somatic risk in humans.

For high LET radiation, relative sensitivity depends largely on DNA content and to a much lesser extent on the kinetics of repair of the various induced DNA damages. It could be argued that estimation of risk would be simplest for high LET radiation, exempt the measurement of internal dose.

These mechanistic considerations have been greatly enhanced in the past few years by the enormously increased understanding of the control of the cell cycle and the relationship of this to DNA repair. Rather than give an in-depth review here, the reader is directed to excellent reviews by Weinert and Lydall[82] and Lane.[35] A consideration of a concept, however is appropriate at this point. An important component of sensitivity to genetic alterations, as discussed earlier, is the relative extent of repair before replication: the greater the extent of repair, the fewer the replication errors. Teliologically speaking, the cell has appreciated this fact and has developed a series of processes to help ensure fidelity of replication, the so-called checkpoints and cell arrest genes. The cell has accepted the fact that such a process of genome checking is not infallible, especially for heavily damaged DNA, and that repair itself can be an error-prone process by developing ways by which damaged cells can be removed and not contribute to an increased cellular mutation rate. One such process is the so-called apoptotic pathway (programmed cell death)—although selective cell killing might be more accurate in such cases.

The tumor suppressor gene, p53, serves as the sentinel example of a cell checkpoint gene, although it is only one component of what appears to be a rather complex, or at least multi-step, pathway (see Chapter 26). The expression of p53 is induced by DNA damage, reported to be DNA single-strand and double-strand breaks, and results in a "checking" of the cell cycle, at least preventing the cell from entering the S-phase.[1] This provides sufficient, or more, time for repair before replication. It is plausible that the function of p53 as a transcription factor could in part be related to a repair function involving GADD45, which could be enhanced in the presence of increased p53.[85] Cells containing mutant p53 genes do not show this radiation-induced cell cycle checking, but the effect of this on cell killing by ionizing radiation is rather equivocal, with resistance being reported. This puzzling observation is an important area for future study. In the absence of induced DNA damage, however, genomic instability is enhanced when p53 is mutant. It is also possible, although not yet demonstrated, that p53 is involved in the overall control of entry of undamaged cells into mitosis (Preston, unpublished).

Once a cell has repaired its induced DNA damage to an "acceptable" level, the p53 checkpoint is abrogated, and the cell can proceed into the S-phase. If a cell is too heavily damaged to be sufficiently repaired, it appears to pass into the apoptotic pathway (reviewed by Kastan[31]).

Clearly, p53 (and other genes involved in cell checkpoints or cell cycle controls) can modulate the degree of mutational alterations in irradiated cells but certainly cannot prevent them altogether. The fidelity of repair is an influential factor in this regard. This can be evidenced by the fact that in transgenic mice containing an homologous knockout of the DNA repair gene ERCC-1, a greatly increased p53 expression could not prevent a high degree of genomic instability.[41] An understanding of the function and efficiency of damage modulating genes such as p53 in different species and different cell types would greatly enhance the ability to predict or explain radiation sensitivity — a necessary component of human risk assessment. An extension of this general concept to considerations of chemically induced DNA and cellular damage is certainly appropriate.

Nonionizing radiation and chemical agents (nonradiomimetic)

The DNA damaging agents to be discussed here are combined into one section because they share a common mode of response. When cells are exposed to nonionizing radiation (such as UV light) or a nonradiomimetic chemical agent, chromatid-type aberrations are observed at mitosis regardless of the stage of the cell cycle in which the cell resides at the time of exposure. Furthermore, there is an apparent *requirement* for DNA synthesis between exposure and mitosis, and cells exposed in the S-phase are by far the most sensitive compared with those in G_1 or G_2.[17] This strongly suggests that the primary mechanism of formation of chromosomal aberrations and mutations following exposure to chemical agents is via errors of DNA replication on a damaged DNA template.

Preston and Gooch[56] demonstrated that there was not an absolute requirement for DNA replication in S-phase for aberration formation. They showed that unequivocal chromosome-type aberrations could be produced in G_1 by 4NQO or MMS provided that DNA repair was inhibited by cytosine arabinoside (araC). Preston and Gooch concluded that there was a much higher probability of a DNA replication error being involved in aberration formation under normal circumstances, but that if the probability of a DNA repair error was increased, aberrations could also be produced by this process. Suffice it to say that the major difference between the mechanism of aberration formation following chemical or radiation treatments is related to repair kinetics. All DNA lesions have the potential to be converted into aberrations in G_1, S, or G_2, but the probabilities are different for different DNA lesions. In addition, Preston[51] showed that there was a synergistic effect on aberration induction when cells were treated with X-rays and 4NQO together with the DNA repair inhibitor, araC, indicating that DNA lesions induced by radiation could interact through misrepair (or misreplication) with those induced by an alkylating agent. These studies suggest that the DNA lesions, per se, are of less significance in terms of aberration formation than how they are processed during their repair.

This particular consideration will have considerable impact on the estimation of potential risk to humans because it provides a mechanistic basis for not considering exposures singly but rather as a complex set of interactions.

To provide additional parallels between outcome from exposures to ionizing radiation and chemicals (plus UV light), it is necessary to consider the response for chronic exposures. It should be immediately clear from the previous discussion of mechanisms that the consequences are different for noncycling cells. Because chromosomal aberrations can be induced directly in nondividing (G_0) cells following exposure to ionizing radiation as a result of errors of repair, they accumulate over time following long-term exposure, with, as noted earlier, dsb being the most likely DNA damage being involved and, as observed frequently, a linear dose response curve, regardless of aberration type. With chemicals, there is little or no accumulation of aberrations or mutations over the duration of a chronic exposure, provided that the cells remain in G_0, because there is no S-phase available for conversion of DNA damage into a genetic alteration. In cycling cells, there is a probability of both ionizing radiation and chemicals being able to produce genetic alterations, by any or all of the processes described previously. Various predictions, however would allow that the dose reduction factor for chronic versus acute exposures would be considerably greater for chemical agents than radiation because there is a clear one-track component (independent of dose rate) to the dose response curve for ionizing radiations but none predicted for exchanges for chemicals. A dose-squared response or some higher power of dose is generally observed and predicted for exchange aberrations following exposure to a nonradiomimetic chemical. When the S-phase is a small fraction of the total cell cycle, however it can be argued that chronic exposures of chemicals would be more effective than acute ones for the production of recovered (i.e., observed) nonlethal chromosomal aberrations (e.g., reciprocal translocations and inversions). This would be a consequence of a much lower probability with chronic exposures of producing a lethal and nonlethal chromosomal aberration in the same cell in the small sensitive, S-phase population. This proposition still requires experimental confirmation. The outcome will certainly have an impact on the estimation of genetic risk. An expanded version of this discussion can be found in Preston.[53,54]

As mentioned at the beginning of this section, UV light was considered together with nonradiomimetic chemicals based on several similarities of aberration production. It should be noted, however that for UV the DNA lesions induced have been well characterized (thymine dimers and 6-4 photoproducts in particular); the repair of these has been equally well described; and several of the enzymes involved in the excision repair process and the photoreactivation have been cloned, been sequenced, and had a function ascribed (see short reviews by Bootsma and Hoeijmakers[4] and Hoeijmakers[28]). Despite these detailed, elegant studies, it is still not possible to describe the mechanism by which UV-induced chromosomal aberrations are formed at the molecular level. The potential role of transcription in the process should not be disregarded.[66,67]

The majority of mutations induced by nonradiomimetic chemical agents and UV-light are point mutations because they appear to be produced by errors of replication on a damaged template. This is a clear oversimplification, however because there certainly are exceptions, for example, chemical agents that induce a significant proportion of deletions along with point mutations. Whether a proportion of the deletion mutations are produced by a misrepair process rather than during S-phase replication is not clear. The proportion of total mutations that are deletions varies with the chemical (i.e., type of DNA lesion) and the cell cycle stage treated. Current studies on establishing mutational spectra for different loci (preferably autosomal, for deletion detection) for a range of chemicals should clarify the picture and aid in a further understanding of mutation induction. It is important to establish mutational spectra for risk assessment practices because the consequences of point mutations and deletions can be different, with the probability of a particular deletion causing an adverse phenotype in vivo being greater than that for a point mutation based on the concept of expressed versus silent mutations. Again, it is appreciated that this is a rather generic discussion, but within the space limitations here, it is hoped that it does at least provide a framework on which to hang the idea of importance of mechanisms and outcome at the molecular level following exposure.

MECHANISM OF FORMATION OF SPECIFIC ALTERATIONS

The concentration in the previous section was on the components of a general model for the formation of chromosomal aberrations and point mutations following exposure to ionizing radiation, chemicals, and nonionizing radiation. It can be argued, however, that what is of particular importance in considerations of predicting adverse health outcomes is the presence of specific chromosomal alterations. It has become increasingly apparent that a high proportion of birth defects and tumors have a specific chromosomal alteration as a component of their genotype or in some cases the sole genetic alteration involved in their phenotype.[5,43] Particularly in the case of tumors, it has been debated as to whether chromosomal alterations arise at random and cells containing specific ones are selected based on an advantageous phenotype such as more rapid growth or whether specific aberrations are much more frequently produced than predicted from randomness.[52] What one is considering then is, are there "hot spots" for aberration formation? There are many examples in the literature of hot spots for mutation induction/selection, for example, background mutations at CpG sites and chemically induced ones

such as frame shifts in nucleotide repeat sequences.[77] The information for chromosomal alterations is much less plentiful, and what is available can argue for either point of view. One of the difficulties for in vivo situations is to separate induction from selection when the end point for observation is a tumor. The types of experimental data that would improve an understanding would be to assess breakpoints for "spontaneous" and induced chromosomal aberrations in vitro, but at this time this presents some insurmountable problems.

If one is attempting to assess specificity of induction of chromosomal alterations as opposed to random induction with subsequent selection, it would be most advantageous to demonstrate repeatability of exactly the same mechanism for the same phenotype; i.e., are the identical DNA sequences involved in translocation breakpoints for many tumors of a particular tumor type, in which any number of different breakpoints could produce the same end result of altered gene expression for example.

Two examples might serve to demonstrate that, in fact, both processes might well be operating for different phenotypes depending perhaps on the absolute specificity of the genetic alteration involved in the tumor phenotype.

The first of these examples is for chronic myelogenous leukemia in humans for which greater than 85% of cases are associated with the presence of a chromosome 9/22 translocation (reviewed in Heisterkamp and colleagues[27]). This translocation involves chromosomal regions of the *bcr* (breakpoint cluster region) on chromosome 22 and the *abl* oncogene on chromosome 9 (Fig. 20-4). The translocation produces a chimeric *bcr/abl* gene that is expressed as the chimeric *bcr/abl* message that is further translated into a chimeric protein that attains kinase activity.[69] The breakpoints that have been located in the *bcr* region are also close together in molecular terms (within a 2 kb region), whereas those in the *abl* region cover a much larger domain. Groffen and colleagues,[23] however, localized the breakpoint itself to an Alu sequence for both the *bcr* and *abl* regions. (A description of Alu sequences can be found in Lewin[37]). Although the mechanism of involvement of this particular sequence could not be ascertained, it could be argued that the homology at the breakpoints could bring about a close association between regions on nonhomologous chromosome that in the additional presence of a chromosomal breakage (either endogenously or exogenously induced) could result in the translocation observed. The specificity of the breakpoint would be a reflection of homologous pairing over a short region.

In a recent report, Riggins and colleagues[61] designed a study to determine if a particular repeating DNA sequence in the *bcr* region (a CGG repeat) when present in variable copy number altered the potential site for nonrandom breakage. The authors concluded that this was not the case, and that random "breakage" and selection was the more likely mechanism for the involvement of the 9/22 translocation in

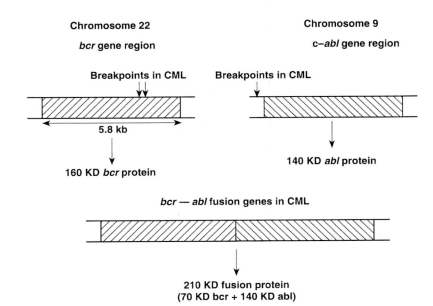

Fig. 20-4. Diagrammatic representation of translocation between chromosomes 9 and 22 in *bcr* and *abl* gene regions associated with development of chronic myeloid leukemia *(CML).*

chronic myelogenous leukemia. It can also be argued, however, that homologous or specific DNA sequences need not be the site of translocation breakpoints but rather the means by which nonhomologous chromosomes can be proximately associated in the interphase nucleus and that the breakpoint could be close by this associated region. The phenotype would be expected to be the result of the translocation not necessarily the specificity of the breakpoint. In addition, this was a rather small study that could not rule out a low-frequency association between repeat length and Ph′ translocation.

The second example is of particular interest because not only does it describe the mechanism for production of a specific translocation breakpoint, but also it might well provide the underlying mechanism for how chromosome alterations, in general, are produced. Croce and colleagues[68,74] conducted an elegant study of the breakpoints in translocations associated with B cell lymphomas and identified two regions that were frequently involved, given the designations of *bcl*-1 and *bcl*-2. Although these regions (genes) have been the subject of considerable study, especially as related to their identified functions in important cellular processes, for example, normal *bcl*-2 expression as an inhibitor of apoptosis and *bcl*-1 as cyclin D1, it is the nature of the breakpoints that is of particular interest here. The breakpoint on chromosome 14, in the 18/14 translocation involved in human follicular B cell lymphomas, is within the J_H region of the IgH locus and is part of the V(D)J recombination process of active Ig genes (Fig. 20-5). The other breakpoint on chromosome 18 is proximate to or within the *bcl*-2 gene that results in a translocation of this gene juxtaposition of the powerful enhancer elements of the IgH locus. The breakpoints on chromosome 18 were almost exclusively within a short stretch of DNA, approximately 2.1

kb in length. The significant aspect is that the translocation involves an error of the V(D)J recombinase system, and DNA sequence motifs at the sites of the two translocation breakpoints support this hypothesis.[74]

The role of a recombination process involving the V(D)J system for immunoglobulin joining reactions is further exemplified by studies of Tsujimoto and colleagues,[75] in which the breakpoints in B cell chronic lymphocytic leukemia (B-CLL) associated translocation were analyzed. The t (11; 14) (q13; q32) translocation is frequently observed in B-CLL and in several lymphomas. Because band 14q32 was involved in one form of Burkitt's lymphoma, which had been characterized at the molecular level, it was presumed that interruption of the Ig heavy-chain locus at band 14q32 was involved in B-CLL also. The breakpoint in chromosome 14 did indeed involve the J segment of the immunoglobulin heavy-chain locus. What was of particular interest was that the breakpoints on chromosome 11 from two tumors were within eight nucleotides of each other at the so-called *bcl*-1 locus and involved a 7-mer, 9-mer DNA sequence that was homologous to the sequence involved in V(D)J rejoining except with a 12-base space between the chromosome 11 7-mer, 9-mer sequences as opposed to 23 between the normal V(D)J recognition 7-mer, 9-mer (chromosome 14) (Fig. 20-6). The translocation would thus be proposed to arise from an error of V(D)J recombination involving the homologous sequences on chromosome 11 and 14.

Not only do these studies show how a specific translocation might be formed in a lymphocyte, in which V(D)J recombination is a normal cellular process, and is error prone, but also it might represent a general model for formation of chromosomal alterations. Such a mechanism could involve a recombination repair or replication process

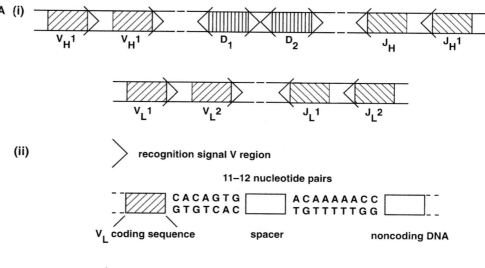

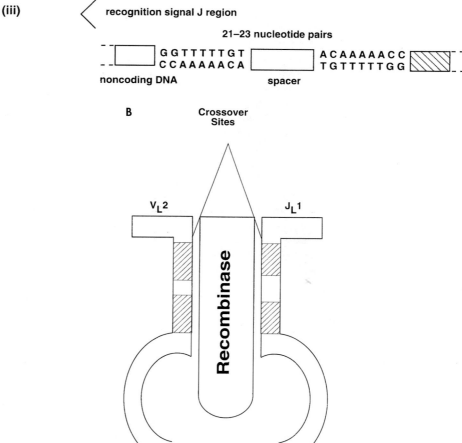

Fig. 20-5. A, (i) Diagrammatic representation of V-gene, J-gene segment (joining), D-gene segment (diversity) for light (L) and heavy (H) gene segment pools. The rejoining recognition signals for V(D)J recombination are illustrated for the V-region (ii) and the J-region (iii). The spacers of 11-12 and 21-23 nucleotide pairs are indicated. **B,** Diagrammatic representation of the pairing regions in association with the recombination enzyme that facilitates joining.

that allows for exchange between homologous sequences on homologous or nonhomologous chromosomes. The initiators or components of such a recombination process based on studies of yeast mitotic recombination are double-strand breaks and transcription proximate to sites of exchange. Additional support for this type of model comes from some studies with x-ray–sensitive cells, which are double-strand break repair mutants.[70] Two such cell lines are defective in V(D)J recombination suggesting a relationship, direct or indirect, between recombinational repair of dsb and V(D)J recombination, the former leading to enhanced cell killing. This can occur either by failure to repair or an enhance-

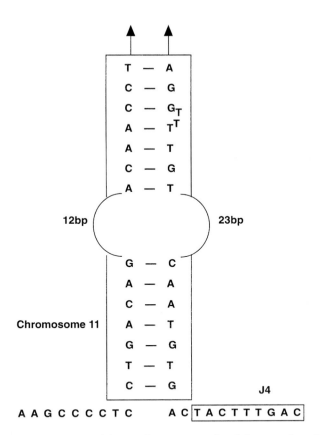

```
        T — A
        C — G
        C — G
             T
        A — T
             T
        A — T
        C — G
        A — T
12bp  (         )  23bp
        G — C
        A — A
        C — A
Chromosome 11  A — T
        G — G
        T — T
        C — G          J4

A A G C C C C T C    A C [T A C T T T G A C]
```

Fig. 20-6. A potential secondary structure involving a region of chromosome 11 and the J4 segment of an immunoglobulin gene leading to a t(11;14) translocation. Note the similarity of the paired region and spacers with those illustrated in Fig. 20-5, *A*.

ment of misrepair, an important distinction that would be worthy of further study.

The consequences of mistakes in V(D)J recombination itself or in a similar recombination system was shown by Fuscoe and colleagues.[21] They demonstrated that the majority of deletion mutants at *hprt* in fetal T lymphocytes involved breakpoint sequences that are consensus ones for V(D)J recombination. This again shows the probable involvement of a recombination process in the formation of chromosomal alterations, in this case in the absence of involvement of an immunoglobulin/T cell antigen receptor locus that has a tumor as a potential phenotype.

The molecular nature of recombination in somatic cells is being studied quite extensively, and it is important to put the derived mechanisms in the context of the formation of chromosomal aberrations under normal (background) and specific exposure (induced) conditions. Although quite a bit of the attention has been on the V(D)J recombination process, other homologous and nonhomologous recombination processes are involved in the repair (and hence misrepair) of dsb leading to mutational events and certainly can readily be involved in the production of mutations and chromo-

somal alterations during the replication process on damaged DNA templates.[12] It is also feasible that RNA splice sites in the DNA could be potential sites for increased recombination or misrepair.

Other cellular effects could be responsible for the production of specific mutational "hot spots," starting with a nonrandomness in initial DNA damage, to a propensity for repair or replication errors in specific DNA regions, and a variation in repair capability within the genome, as examples. Data are accumulating to suggest that all of these events are occurring, and subsequent research should clarify the issue. A few examples can illustrate what has been described to date.

Although at first glance it might appear that for the genome, DNA strand breaks or base alterations are randomly distributed, when one takes a closer look at the DNA sequence level, it appears that this is not the case. A heterogeneous distribution of DNA lesions has been described for x-rays, alkylating agents, and several other radiomimetic and nonradiomimetic chemicals.* Such heterogeneity seems to be related to chromatin structure so that the DNA transcribing regions are more likely to be altered, and, with some exceptions, linker DNA (histone free) being more sensitive to lesion induction than is nucleosomal DNA. DNA sequence itself can be a modifier of response. For example, the 5'-flanking region of c-Ha-*ras* is GC-rich and can be a preferred site of alkylation in vitro by nitrogen mustard.[40] Other similar examples for short sequence effects such as runs of "G" have been described. For UV-radiation, of course, there is a sequence preference for adjacent pyrimidines for induced DNA damage.

The data for demonstrating differences in the *fidelity* of DNA repair or replication[62,72] in different genomic regions is less readily obtainable. The data from Kunkel[34] have demonstrated the relative efficiency of replication on the leading and lagging strands and have shown that α-polymerase that is responsible for lagging strand synthesis is less fidelitous than δ-polymerase, which synthesizes the leading strand. Also, certain sequence motifs are prone to replication error, such as by "slipping" at sites of single or multiple base repeats. Others are prone to chemical modifications; in particular, deamination of 5 methyl cytosine to thymine at ^{mc}CpG sites results in GC→TA transversion mutations.[19] It is also likely that some mutation hot spots are a consequence of replication error hot spots caused by DNA sequence characteristics. Whether such sequence driven errors would also be a feature of nonrandom DNA repair-induced alterations is less well documented, but it would certainly be predicted that excision repair, involving relatively long regions of DNA synthesis, would follow the same general principles as for semiconservative S-phase replication. These potentially nonrandom error events are known to result in point mutations. How they might be in-

*References 3,11,16,40,63.

volved in chromosomal aberration formation has not been established, largely because of the difficulty of identifying the exact sites of such alterations at the DNA sequence level.

At the genome level, it has been established that certain regions are subject to early DNA repair; these include transcriptionally active genes, housekeeping genes, and even the transcribed strand in such genes.[24,42] This interesting story has taken on an even more fascinating twist since it has been shown that there are some functional associations between transcription and DNA repair, in part a consequence of the fact that several of the "DNA repair" genes that have been cloned and sequenced have transcriptionally related activities such as helicase action.[28,66,67] Thus, there would be expected to be, for nonradiomimetic chemicals, a chromosomal aberration, mutation pattern that would be reflective of replication errors in genomic regions not subject to rapid repair, i.e., before replication. This is the case for point mutations with, for example, a higher frequency of mutations being observed in the nontranscribed strand and/or the lagging strand.[76,81] The situation for ionizing radiation and radiomimetic chemicals has not been determined. The relative rapidity of repair of most strand breaks makes repair errors more likely than replication errors as discussed earlier.

The further identification of sites that might be frequently involved in induced chromosomal aberration and mutation induction is clearly an area of considerable importance not only for advancing the knowledge of mechanism but also for application into the risk assessment process.

SENSITIVITY AND SUSCEPTIBILITY TO THE INDUCTION OF GENETIC ALTERATIONS

The two preceding sections present a view of how background and induced chromosomal aberrations and point mutations might be produced. The similarities and differences between the mechanism of formation following exposure to ionizing radiations and radiomimetic chemicals versus nonradiomimetic chemicals and nonionizing radiations were discussed in some detail because this is important when addressing adverse health outcomes and risk. The extension of these discussions to the question of mechanisms of formation of specific alterations places the emphasis on the types of alterations that are most commonly associated with such adverse outcomes.

Enormous progress has been made during the past 5 to 10 years in the identification of specific genetic alterations associated with tumors and genetic diseases. Comprehensive catalogs of chromosomal alterations associated with (or causative of) cancer and genetic diseases can be found in Mitelman[43] and Borgaonkar.[5] Thus, individuals with genotypes that can increase sensitivity to the production of chromosomal alterations (and/or mutations) either as a background phenomenon or following exposure to physi-

cal or chemical agents have the potential to be more susceptible to the development of cancer or for the production of birth defects.

From the preceding sections, it can be discerned that sensitivity is a function of the kinetics and fidelity of DNA repair, including the relationship of repair with replication, and the kinetics and fidelity of DNA replication. As mentioned previously, the transcriptional state of cells can influence repair kinetics independently of the genotype.

In the past year or so, considerable progress has been made in the characterization of human DNA repair, based to a large extent on the availability of mutant phenotypes, such as xeroderma pigmentosum, Cockayne's syndrome, and ataxia telangiectasia, and supported by rodent and yeast mutant cell lines.[2,4,71] Although this has aided in an understanding of DNA repair processes at the molecular level and a determination, in some instances, of the repair defect itself in human "sensitivity" syndromes, it has not yet allowed for an unequivocal determination of the response in heterozygotes. This is important because it is apparent that the individuals who are homozygous recessive for these repair deficiency phenotypes are the extremes of sensitivity to exposure and manifest recognizable phenotypes. Heterozygotes could demonstrate minor increases in sensitivity in the heterozygous cells as has occasionally been claimed or, perhaps more significantly, contain clones of cells that have lost heterozygosity by one of several processes (for example, deletion of the wild-type allele, chromosome loss, mitotic recombination) and thus become homozygous or hemizygous recessive for the repair defect. Such clones would have an increased sensitivity to chromosome aberration and mutation production either as a background or an induced event. Such suggestions can take on a broader significance in light of the fact that these observed DNA repair defects might, as suggested for Cockayne's syndrome, be one manifestation of a transcriptional deficiency, thereby providing a broad range of phenotypes.[4] It has been shown that a mutation in a gene responsible for mismatch repair in human cells (equivalent to the *mut* genes in *Escherichia coli*) can give rise to a mutator phenotype that is characterized in colon tumor cell lines by an increased instability of microsatellite sequences, perhaps from an increase in replication errors.[18,36] There is an association between these mutations and the development of hereditary nonpolyposis colon cancer, which, in turn, is also associated with a high frequency of somatic mutations in colorectal tumors. It is suggested that carriers of the mutator phenotype are susceptible to the development of other tumor types. This then is a repair deficiency that can perhaps manifest itself as a DNA replication error process (slippage). Again, identifying heterozygotes would seem to be important for predicting risk from the subsequent development of homozygosity or hemizygosity. Thus, it is now singularly important to determine the DNA repair status of individuals in cancer-prone families, especially when an exogenous agent might be involved. Ideally, this would be performed at the DNA sequence level, such that genotype, rather than phenotype alone, would be diagnostic.

Similarly, over the past 3 years or so, an enormously expanded understanding of the genetic control of the cell cycle in eukaryotes has become available (see review by Murray and Hunt[44]). It is apparent that this process is quite exquisitely orchestrated with a cascade of genes being activated and repressed in sequence, generally under the control of phosphorylation and dephosphorylation. There clearly are mutations at a large number of points that can upset this orderly progression, and in the present context if the timing of DNA replication is altered, it is possible that an increased or decreased sensitivity to DNA damage could ensue, depending on the time available for repair before replication. This is such a critical process to a cell that a number of mechanisms have evolved to attempt to ensure accurate DNA replication. An alteration in such processes leads to an increased sensitivity to the production of mutations (chromosomal and point) through errors of replication on a damaged template and perhaps post-replication repair errors. These views are predicated by the demonstration that the product of the tumor suppressor gene p53 serves as a cell cycle checkpoint at the G_1/S border. This allows time for the cell to search for and repair DNA damage, particularly DNA strand breaks before DNA replication. p53 appears to act as a transcription factor that perhaps controls transcription of proteins required for S-phase initiation. It is not a singular activity because a number of other gene products are known to interact with p53 (see Pietenpol and Vogelstein[49] for a short review). Mutations in the p53 gene can result in loss of checkpoint function that leads to genomic instability.[39] Thus, sensitivity to mutation induction is, in part, a consequence of p53 status in the cell; p53 null cells are clearly hypersensitive, and p53 null animals are prone to the development of tumors early in life, although they survive to birth successfully.[14] The phenotype of p53 heterozygotes has been less well characterized, but mouse cell lines that are p53 +/− rapidly become karyotypically abnormal, perhaps owing to a propensity for conversion to a −/− or a −/0 genotype (Preston, unpublished). Also, mice that are heterozygous for a p53 gene "knockout" are susceptible to the induction of tumors by a number of different chemicals compared with p53 homozygous wild-type mice.[25] There are clearly a number of other genes that fall into the same functional category as p53—tumor suppressor or cell cycle checkpoint. The recent characterization of MTS-1 (multiple tumor suppressor) and its deletion in a wide range of tumor cell lines attest to this.[30] This simply emphasizes the potential for such genotypes to confer a susceptibility to the production of genomic alterations and probably a sensitivity, usually when heterozygous, to exogenous as well as endogenous factors. This can result, as discussed earlier, from a loss of heterozygosity to give the homozygous or hemizygous mutant genotype or from

the so-called dominant-negative phenotype. Detection and careful characterization of individuals' genotypes and phenotypes, especially for heterozygosity, will be the subject of concentrated future research. How to handle (including estimating risk from) such information on genetic susceptibility is a scientific, legal, and social issue that cannot be the subject of discussion here.

The final component of increased sensitivity is the role of DNA replication kinetics and fidelity. Several sophisticated studies by Kunkel[34] and colleagues have demonstrated that a number of factors can alter the fidelity of replication. In addition, slowing down replication can increase the frequency of sister chromatid exchanges that are a measure of errors of DNA replication.[32,48] Thus, any genetic alteration that affects the rate of replication has the potential to be hypersensitive to DNA replication errors, and similarly mutations of polymerase genes could also decrease fidelity, thereby increasing mutation and chromosomal aberration frequencies.

Current research is only beginning to scratch the surface of what controls sensitivity as well as susceptibility to mutation and chromosomal aberration induction by endogenous and exogenous factors. Understanding these processes is necessary for obtaining a true estimate of genetic and somatic risk to humans as well as for indicating approaches for intervention.

GENOTOXIC VERSUS "NONGENOTOXIC" MODES OF ACTION

As a corollary to the discussion on mechanism of formation of mutations and chromosomal alterations from background or induced DNA damage and how this impacts on sensitivity, it is necessary to consider the possible role of so-called "nongenotoxic" carcinogens in the risk assessment process[10] (see chapter 26). As an initial statement, it is more appropriate and correct to describe chemicals as DNA-reactive as opposed to non–DNA-reactive ("nongenotoxic") to put them in a mechanistic rather than an endpoint context.

It should be apparent from earlier sections that for explaining the formation of chromosomal aberrations and mutations and for understanding the relative sensitivity of their induction, the two components involved are DNA damage and the conversion of this to a genetic alteration by DNA repair or replication errors. The DNA damage can be directly induced by an exogenous agent or be endogenously produced. The cellular processes of repair and replication, however actually produce the alteration. Thus, it might be predicted that if a chemical, for example, can cause cell proliferation either as a recovery response to cytotoxicity or as a mitogenic response, genetic alterations could arise from replication errors on an endogenously damaged template or from the cell cycle of the cell involved in the compensatory proliferation being aberrant. This latter event could arise from alterations in the correct regulation of the cell cycle as a consequence of the chemical exposure or the forced entry of cells into the cycle. The ultimate response from a continued cytotoxic or mitogenic exposure and the resultant cell proliferation would be a tumor. Thus, agents that elicit such responses are described as non–DNA-reactive carcinogens. The mode of mechanism of formation of mutations and chromosomal aberrations, however, would probably be similar, if not the same as that for DNA-reactive chemicals absent the way in which the replication error is initiated. The identification of markers of abnormal cell replication might be the most practical approach for identifying non–DNA-reactive carcinogens or to look for traditional genotoxic responses after subchronic exposures of cells in vivo or in vitro.

Suffice it to say that any consideration of risk to humans to exposure from potential carcinogens that uses mechanistic data would need to incorporate considerations of both DNA reactive and nonreactive agents.

GERM CELL RESPONSES

The preceding discussions on the mechanisms of formation of chromosomal aberrations and mutations has implicated that this is what takes place in somatic cells, generally because the majority of such research has been conducted in somatic cells. Exposures to and responses in germ cells (see Chapter 33), however, have important implications for risk assessment. Such considerations cannot be exhaustively discussed within the confines of this chapter, and so some general principles are presented.

There is no reason to suppose that the mechanism of formation of chromosomal aberrations and mutations is any different from that in somatic cells, i.e., by misrepair or replication errors on a damaged template. The specificity for aberration formation via a recombination process would seem to be a likely mechanism operating in germ cells also. The major difference between somatic and germ cells is in sensitivity, particularly for agents that require DNA replication to produce the genetic alteration. The reason for this is that there are a variety of different cell cycle scenarios for germ cells. For example, differentiating spermatogonia are essentially a "somatic" cell as far as the cycle-divide-cycle is concerned, with a cell cycle duration somewhat like a typical somatic cell (approximately 24 hours). The spermatogonial stem cell has a long cell cycle (about 8 days in the mouse) with the S-phase being a small fraction of this.[46] Although the stem cell has a lifetime of many years and can thus essentially accumulate genetic alterations, it could be argued that it is relatively insensitive because of cell cycle kinetics, whereby there is the probability of repairing DNA damage before DNA replication. To some extent, however, this reduction in sensitivity might be balanced out by the fact that for chronic exposures there might well be an increased sensitivity as measured by the presence of transmissible (nonlethal) chromosomal alterations (especially reciprocal translocations) as compared to acute exposures. This is a consequence of a lower probability of inducing a lethal and nonlethal aberration in the same cell with chronic exposures in the sensitive cell population (S-phase).

In contrast, postmeiotic germ cells in the male do not undergo DNA replication until after fertilization. They are also unable to repair DNA damage, largely because of the lack of repair enzymes (no cytoplasm) and tight chromatin conformation. The sensitivity to aberration/mutation formation is determined by the extent of DNA repair between fertilization and the zygotic S-phase, i.e., how much DNA damage remains at the time of replication.[50] The postmeiotic cell is generally regarded as the most sensitive to genetic alterations induced by chemicals but based on rather few studies. This perception is further based on the fact that the majority of studies of the effects of chemicals on germ cells have been for single, acute, relatively large exposures.[56] These conditions would, in fact, bias the study toward the observation of effects in postmeiotic germ cells. The killing of sensitive cell populations (cells in the S-phase) could result in lower frequencies of transmissible chromosomal aberrations in cycling cells (spermatogonial stem cells, differentiating spermatogonia, and meiotic cells) than in postmeiotic, noncycling cells. Although the latter is subject to a reduction in induced DNA damage as a consequence of repair in the zygotic G_1 phase, it would be predicted that sufficient damage would remain for possible conversion into aberrations or mutations at the time of DNA replication. Additional studies on the extent and kinetics of DNA repair in the various germ cell stages are needed to begin to define a true genetic risk.

For the female germ cell, it is proposed that the mechanisms by which genetic alterations are produced following chemical exposure would be the same as for male germ cells and somatic cells: errors of DNA replication. However, the sensitivity of the primary oocyte, the stage present throughout the reproductive lifetime of a female, is very low.[2] The reason being that these cells have undergone an S-phase before birth, during the development of the oocyte from oogonia, and will not undergo another one until after fertilization in the zygote. The opportunity for repair before replication is thus extensive.

It should be fairly clear that a minimal consideration of mechanism can be used to understand better sensitivity to the induction/production of genetic alterations, including differences between somatic and germ cells and female and male germ cells following chemical exposure.

For radiation exposures (and radiomimetic chemical exposures), the effects in germ cells are relatively straightforward to interpret. The mutations and chromosomal aberrations are generally produced in the exposed cell as a consequence of errors of DNA repair (or replication in the genomic regions replicating at or close to the time of exposure). The types of aberrations depend on the cell cycle stage, and these differ for different germ cell types. For example, in the male, spermatogonial stem cells (largely G_1) contain chromosome-type aberrations. Postmeiotic germ cells similarly exhibit chromosome-type aberrations, because they are G_1 cells and they do not repair their induced DNA damage until the zygote. The relative sensitivities are determined to a large extent by the kinetics and fidelity of DNA repair in the different germ cell stages. Although little information is available for assessing this, Brewen and Preston[7] did discuss the concepts in a review several years ago, defining the principles behind the interpretation of the available data. The development of new detection systems, notably FISH (fluorescence in situ hybridization), in interphase as well as dividing cells should enhance the base of information and consequently improve our ability to develop estimates of genetic risk in humans from exposure to radiations and chemicals.[55]

PREDICTING RISK OR ADVERSE HEALTH EFFECTS FROM EXPOSURE TO RADIATION AND CHEMICALS

In broad terms, the purpose of gathering information on mechanisms of production and induction of genetic alterations and in parallel collecting data on the frequency of these alterations is to use them in the development of estimates of genetic and somatic risk, both qualitative and quantitative. For a number of reasons, it has been possible to develop some reasonable estimates of genetic and carcinogenetic risk from radiation exposures, particularly low LET (x-rays and gamma rays). These reasons include the ability to measure dose and calculate its tissue distribution; a knowledge of DNA damage and its relationship to dose, coupled with a database on mutation and chromosomal aberration induction in several organs; a reasonable definition and understanding of dose response relationships; and a human database, although incomplete, for the background frequencies of birth defects and cancer and radiation-induced frequencies based largely, but certainly not exclusively, on the A-bomb survivors. The nature of these data and their use in risk estimation can be found in the various sequential UNSCEAR and BEIR reports. There are data gaps and there are assumptions, and there is a continued need to provide data on the mechanisms of induction of the adverse health outcome for both birth defects and cancer that will advance the process of risk estimation, if only by determining when pragmatic extrapolation from animal data is acceptable.

The situation for chemical exposures is different; for all the reasons just given for why risk assessment for radiation is feasible, the converse is true for chemical exposure. Although it is possible to measure or estimate exposure, it is considerably more difficult to measure or calculate dose, particularly effective dose for the majority of chemicals. In brief, this is due to a paucity of knowledge, in many cases for the nature of metabolism and metabolite distribution in humans and the identification of the appropriate biomarker

for dose. Certainly the development and refinement of physiologically based pharmacokinetic (PB-PK) models has enhanced the ability to predict tissue doses in humans for some chemicals, but this still does not allow for estimate of biologically effective dose. Our knowledge of dose response relationships for genetic alterations induced by chemicals is relatively sparse, and the interpretation of these is equivocal, in part as a result of the difficulty of incorporating mechanistic data into this process. The attempts to estimate human genetic and somatic risk from chemical exposures are further compounded by the relative lack of information from human populations. This does, of course, represent a positive feature, but it is still most important to be able to provide support from human epidemiological studies for the quantitative risk assessment models that have been used for predicting human responses to low-dose chronic exposures from data obtained in animal studies. It has been argued that this process of extrapolation from species to species and from high to low dose exposures will be greatly enhanced by a better understanding of the mechanism of induction of birth defects and cancer and the genetic alterations that are known or predicted to be involved in tumor development. At this time, this seems to be a viable assumption.

Molecular and cellular genetic toxicology holds an important place in the hierarchy of information that is needed to develop and apply risk assessment models. It is certainly not sufficient to use qualitative assays; these simply provide an indication of where research effort might be best applied. Genetic toxicology studies should incorporate a mechanistic slant in design to offer assistance to risk assessment model development and application. Clearly, this section is not intended to provide a detailed description of risk prediction, but rather to identify where genetic toxicology studies can fill in some specific data gaps. The next few years will determine if indeed the provision of such information is feasible and if obtaining it does enhance the risk assessment process.

REFERENCES

1. Bakalkin G, et al: p53 binds single-stranded DNA ends and catalyzes DNA renaturation and strand transfer, *Proc Natl Acad Sci USA* 91:413, 1994.
2. Barnes DE, Lindahl T, Sedgwick B: DNA repair, *Curr Opin Cell Biol* 5:424, 1993.
3. Beckman RP et al: Assessment of preferential cleavage of an actively transcribed retroviral hybrid gene in murine cells by deoxyribonuclease I, bleomycin, neocarzinostatin, or ionizing radiation, *Biochemistry* 26:5409, 1987.
4. Bootsma D, Hoeijmakers JHJ: Engagement with transcription, *Nature* 363:114, 1993.
5. Borgaonkar DS: *Chromosomal variation in man: a catalog of chromosomal variants and anomalies,* ed 7, New York, 1993, Alan R. Liss.
6. Brewen JG, Brock RD: The exchange hypothesis and chromosome-type aberrations, *Mutation Res* 6:245, 1968.
7. Brewen JG, Preston RJ: Analysis of chromosome aberrations in mammalian germ cells. In Hollaender A, de Serres FJ, editors: *Chemical mutagens. Volume 5,* New York; 1978, Plenum Press.

8. Brewen JG, Preston RJ: Cytogenetic analysis of mammalian oocytes in mutagenicity studies. In Hsu TC, editor: *Cytogenetic assays of environmental mutagens,* Totowa, NJ, 1982, Allanheld Publishing Co.

9. Bryant PE: Use of restriction endonucleases to study relationships between DNA double-strand breaks, chromosomal aberrations and other end-points in mammalian cells; *Int J Radiat Biol* 54:869, 1988.

10. Butterworth BE: Consideration of both genotoxic and nongenotoxic mechanisms in predicting carcinogenic potential, *Mutation Res* 239:117, 1990.

11. Chiu S-M, et al: Hypersensitivity of DNA in transcriptionally active chromatin to ionizing radiation, *Biochim Biophys Acta* 699:15, 1982.

12. Derbyshire MK, et al: Nonhomologous recombination in human cells, *Mol Cell Biol* 14:156, 1994.

13. DiGiuseppe JA, Dresler SL: Bleomycin-induced repair synthesis in permeable human fibroblasts: mediation of long-patch and short-patch repair by distant DNA polymerases, *Biochemistry* 28:9515, 1989.

14. Donehower LA, et al: Mice deficient for p53 are developmentally normal but susceptible to spontaneous tumors, *Nature* 356:215, 1992.

15. Duncan AMV, Evans HJ: The exchange hypothesis for the formation of chromatid aberrations: an experimental test using bleomycin, *Mutation Res* 107:307, 1983.

16. Durante M, et al: Non-random alkylation of DNA sequences induced in vivo by chemical mutagens, *Carcinogenesis* 10:1357, 1989.

17. Evans HJ, Scott D: The induction of chromosome aberrations by nitrogen mustard and its dependence on DNA synthesis, *Proc R Soc (London) Ser B,* 173:491, 1969.

18. Fishel R et al: The human mutator gene homolog MSH 2 and its association with hereditary nonpolyposis colon cancer, *Cell* 75:1215, 1993.

19. Frederico, LA, et al: Cytosine deamination in mismatched base pairs, *Biochemistry* 32:6523, 1993.

20. Friedberg EC: *DNA repair,* New York, 1985, WH Freeman.

21. Fuscoe JC, et al: V(D)J recombinase-like activity mediates *hprt* gene deletion in human fetal T-lymphocytes, *Cancer Res* 51:6001, 1991.

22. Gajewski E, et al: Modification of DNA bases in mammalian chromatin by radiation-generated free radicals, *Biochemistry* 29:7876, 1990.

23. Groffen J, et al: Philadelphia chromosomal breakpoints are clustered within a limited region, BCR on chromosome 22, *Cell* 36:93, 1984.

24. Hanawalt PC, Mellon I: DNA repair: stranded in an active gene, *Curr Biol* 3:67, 1993.

25. Harvey M, et al: Spontaneous and carcinogen-induced tumorigenesis in p-53 deficient mice, *Nature Genet* 5:225, 1993.

26. Heartlein MW, Preston RJ: An explanation of interspecific differences in sensitivity to Xray-induced chromosome aberrations and a consideration of dose response curves, *Mutation Res* 150:299, 1985.

27. Heisterkamp N, et al: Ph-Positive leukemia. In Kirsch IR, editor: *The causes and consequences of chromosomal aberrations,* Boca Raton, Fla, 1993, CRC Press.

28. Hoeijmakers JHJ: Nucleotide excision repair II. From yeast to mammals, *Trends Genet* 9:211, 1993.

29. Iliakis G: The role of DNA double-strand breaks in ionizing radiation-induced killing of eukaryotic cells, *Bio Essays* 13:641, 1991.

30. Kamb A et al: A cell cycle regulator potentially involved in genesis of many tumor types, *Science* 264:436, 1994.

31. Kastan MB: p-53: Evolutionarily conserved and constantly evolving, *NIH Res* 5:53, 1993.

32. Kato H: Possible role of DNA synthesis in formation of sister chromatid exchanges, *Nature* 252:739, 1974.

33. Kornberg A, Baker TA: *DNA replication,* New York; 1991, WH Freeman.

34. Kunkel TA: DNA replication fidelity, *J Biol Chem* 267:18251, 1992.

35. Lane DP: p-53-guardian of the genome, *Nature* 358:15, 1992.

36. Leach FS, et al: Mutations of a *mut* S homolog in hereditary nonpolyposis colorectal cancer, *Cell* 75:1215, 1993.

37. Lewin B: *Genes V,* Oxford, 1994, Oxford University Press.

38. Lin J-J, Sancar A: A new mechanism for repairing oxidative damage to DNA: (A)BC excinuclease removes AP sites and thymine glycols from DNA, *Biochemistry* 28:7979, 1989.

39. Lu X, Lane DP: Differential induction of transcriptionally active p53 following uv or ionizing radiations: defects in chromosome instability syndromes? *Cell* 75:765, 1993.

40. Mattes WB, et al: GC-rich regions in genomes as targets for DNA alkylation, *Carcinogenesis* 9:2065, 1988.

41. McWhir J, et al: Mice with DNA repair gene (ERCC-1) deficiency have elevated levels of p53, liver nuclear abnormalities and die before weaning, *Nature Genet* 5:217, 1993.

42. Mellon I, et al: Selective removal of transcription-blocking DNA damage from the transcribed strand of the mammalian DHFR gene, *Cell* 51:241, 1987.

43. Mitelman F: *Catalog of chromosome aberrations in cancer,* ed 3, New York, 1988, Alan R. Liss.

44. Murray A, Hunt T: *The cell cycle-an introduction,* New York, 1993, WH Freeman.

45. Natarajan AT, Obe G: Molecular mechanisms involved in the production of chromosomal aberrations. III. Restriction endonucleases, *Chromosoma* 90:120, 1984.

46. Oakberg EF: Spermatogonial stem-cell renewal in the mouse, *Anat Rec* 169:515, 1971.

47. Obe G, et al: DNA double-strand breaks induced by sparsely ionizing radiation and endonucleases as critical lesions for cell death, chromosomal aberrations, mutations and oncogenic transformation, *Mutagenesis* 7:3, 1992.

48. Painter RB: A replication model for sister-chromatid exchange, *Mutat Res* 70:337, 1980.

49. Pietenpol JA, Vogelstein B: No room at the p53 inn, *Nature* 365:17, 1993.

50. Preston RJ: DNA repair and chromosome aberrations: interactive effects of radiations and chemicals. In Natarajan AT, Obe G, and Altmann H editors: *DNA repair, chromosome alterations and chromatin structure,* Amsterdam, 1982, Elsevier Biomedical Press.

51. Preston RJ: The induction of chromosome aberrations in germ cells: a discussion of factors that can influence sensitivity to chemical mutagens In *Proc 3rd Internat Conference on Environmental Mutagens, Tokyo, Japan,* Tokyo, 1982, Tokyo University Press, Alan R. Liss.

52. Preston RJ: Mechanisms of induction of specific chromosomal alterations. In Sutherland BM, Woodhead AD editors: *DNA damage and repair in human tissues,* New York, 1990, Plenum Press.

53. Preston RJ: Mechanisms of induction of chromosomal alterations and sister chromatid exchanges: presentation of a general hypothesis. In Li AP, and Heflich RH, editors: *Genetic toxicology: a treatise,* Boca Raton, Fla, 1991, CRC Press.

54. Preston RJ: A consideration of the mechanisms of induction of mutations in mammalian cells by low doses and dose rates of ionizing radiation, *Adv Radiat Biol* 16:125, 1992.

55. Preston RJ: Future of germ cell cytogenetics, *Environ Mol Mutagen* 24:54, 1994.

56. Preston RJ, Gooch PC: The induction of chromosome-type aberrations in G₁ by methyl methanesulfonate and 4-nirtoquinoline-N-oxide and the non-requirement of an S-phase for their production, *Mutation Res* 83:395, 1981.

57. Preston RJ, et al: Mammalian in vivo and in vitro cytogenetic assays: a report of the US EPA's Gene-Tox Program, *Mutation Res* 87:143, 1981.

58. Price A: The repair of ionizing radiation-induced damage to DNA, *Cancer Biol* 4:61, 1993.

59. Revell SH: Chromatid aberrations—the generalized theory. In Wolff S, editor: *Radiation-induced chromosome aberrations,* New York, 1963, Columbia University Press.

60. Revell SH: The breakage-and-reunion theory and the exchange theory for chromosomal aberrations induced by ionizing radiations: a short history, *Adv Radiat Biol* 4:367, 1974.

61. Riggins GJ, et al: CGG-repeat polymorphism of the BCR gene rules out predisposing alleles leading to the Philadelphia chromosome, *Genes Chromosomes Cancer* 9:141, 1994.

62. Roberts JD, et al: Exonucleolytic proofreading of leading and lagging strand DNA replication errors, *Proc Natl Acad Sci USA* 88:3465, 1991.

63. Ryan AJ, et al: Selective repair of methylated purines in regions of chromatin DNA, *Carcinogenesis* 7:1497, 1986.

64. Sax K: Induction by Xrays of chromosome aberrations in *Tradescantia* microspores, *Genetics* 23:494, 1938.

65. Sax K: Types and frequencies of chromosomal aberrations induced by Xrays, *Cold Spring Harbor Symp* 9:93, 1941.

66. Schaeffer L, et al: DNA repair helicase: a component of BTF2 (TFIIH) basic transcription factor, *Science* 260:58, 1993.

67. Selby CP, Sancar A: Molecular mechanism of transcription repair coupling, *Science* 260:53, 1993.

68. Showe LC, Croce CM: The role of chromosomal translocations in B- and T-cell neoplasia, *Ann Rev Immunol* 5:253, 1987.

69. Shtivelman E, et al: Fused transcript of *abl* and *bcr* genes in chronic myelogenous leukemia, *Nature* 315:550, 1985.

70. Taccioli GE, et al: Impairment of V(D)J recombination in double-strand break repair mutants, *Science* 260:207, 1993.

71. Tanaka K, Wood RD: Xeroderma pigmentosum and nucleotide excision repair of DNA, *TIBS* 19:83, 1994.

72. Thomas DC, et al: Relative probability of mutagenic translesion synthesis on the leading and lagging strands during replication of UV-irradiated DNA in human cell extract, *Biochemistry* 32:11476, 1993.

73. Troule R: Radiation-induced DNA damage and repair, *Int J Radiat Biol* 51:573, 1987.

74. Tsujimoto Y, et al: Molecular cloning of the chromosomal breakpoint on B-cell lymphomas and leukemias with the t (11;14) chromosome translocation, *Science* 224:1403, 1984.

75. Tsujimoto Y, et al: Clustering of breakpoints on chromosome 11 in human B-cell neoplasms with the t(11;14) chromosome translocation, *Nature* 315:340, 1985.

76. Vrieling H, et al: DNA strand specificity for UV-induced mutations in mammalian cells, *Mol Cell Biol* 9:1277, 1989.

77. Walker VE, Skopek TR: A mouse model for the study of *in vivo* mutational spectra: sequence specificity of ethylene oxide at the *hprt* locus, *Mutation Res* 288:151, 1993.

78. Wallace SS: The biological consequences of oxidized DNA bases, *Br J Cancer* (suppl 1) 8:118, 1987.

79. Wallace SS: AP endonucleases and DNA glycosylases that recognize oxidative DNA damage, *Environ Mol Mutagen* 12:431, 1988.

80. Ward JF: DNA damage produced by ionizing radiation in mammalian cells: mechanism of formation and reparability, *Prog Nucl Acid Res Mol Biol* 35:95, 1988.

81. Waters LC, et al: Mutations induced by ionizing radiation in a plasmid replicated in human cells, *Radiat Res* 127:190, 1991.

82. Weinert TA, Lydall D: Cell cycle checkpoints, genetic instability and cancer, *Cancer Biology* 4:129, 1993.

83. Winegar RA, et al: Spectrum of mutations produced by specific types of restriction enzyme-induced double-strand breaks, *Mutagenesis* 7:439, 1992.

84. Winegar RA, Preston RJ: The induction of chromosomal aberrations by restriction endonucleases that produce blunt-ended or cohesive-ended double-strand breaks, *Mutation Res* 197:141, 1988.

85. Zhan Q, et al: The p53-dependent γ-ray response of GADD 45, *Cancer Res* 54:2755, 1994.

Chapter 21

ACTIVE OXYGEN SPECIES

Brooke Taylor Mossman
Timothy Quinlan
Yvonne M.W. Janssen

A myriad of reports in the scientific literature implicate active oxygen species (AOS) in the pathogenesis of various diseases, including cancer, immune complex–mediated disease, ischemia-reperfusion injury, rheumatoid arthritis, and aging.[19] Many environmental agents are also potent generators of AOS either directly or after metabolism by cells. These include chemicals and particulates (e.g., ozone, hyperoxia, paraquat, mineral dusts) and ultraviolet (UV) or ionizing radiation.[46]

Mammalian cells and tissues possess a cadre of defense mechanisms in response to AOS. Thus, maintenance or adaptation to oxidative stress frequently is observed after transient or low-level exposures. These defenses, however, may be overwhelmed during extraordinary or protracted levels of exposure to oxidants, a situation resulting in cytotoxicity, cell death, compensatory hyperplasia, and ultimately disease.

Much research attention has been directed to elucidating the pathways of formation of AOS and detection of their biological effects (e.g., DNA damage, lipid peroxidation) on cells.[46] An exciting area of current pursuit is the development of biomarkers or biosensors for the prediction of oxidative stress in susceptible or highly exposed individuals.[84] Moreover, we and others are pursuing research to gain an understanding of the regulation of antioxidant enzymes and other naturally occurring antioxidants in the lung and other tissues in an effort to develop preventive and therapeutic strategies to oxidant-associated diseases.[34,86]

In this chapter, common pathways of generation of AOS and antioxidant defense mechanisms are discussed briefly. We then focus on specific oxidative stresses, the nature of exposures and pathology occurring in humans or in experimental models of disease, and mechanisms of cell and tissue injury by environmental oxidants.

PATHWAYS OF GENERATION OF ACTIVE OXYGEN SPECIES

Formation of AOS occurs normally in cellular respiration during the reduction of molecular oxygen to water. A chain of events results in the formation of superoxide (O_2^-) and hydrogen peroxide (H_2O_2), which then can be converted in the presence of iron and other cations to the reactive hydroxyl radical ($\cdot OH$) (Fig. 21-1). This reaction is known as the Haber-Weiss or modified Fenton reaction. Other metabolites of reduced oxygen may also be generated by related pathways, such as by oxidation of arginine, a process resulting in the formation of nitric oxide ($NO\cdot$). $NO\cdot$ can then react with O_2^- to form peroxynitrate ($ONOO^-$), a strong oxidant.[23]

The authors thank Laurie Sabens and Judith Kessler for valuable technical assistance. Work by Dr. Mossman's laboratory is supported by grants from the Environmental Protection Agency; National Heart, Lung and Blood Institute; and the National Institute of Environmental Health Sciences.

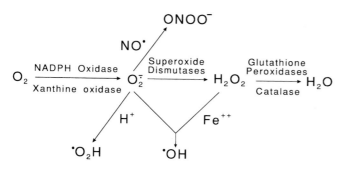

Fig. 21-1. Schematic diagram showing the formation and removal of active oxygen species (AOS). Molecular oxygen is reduced to water by the addition of four electrons. Key enzymes involved in the formation of AOS include nicotinamide-adenine dinucleotide phosphate (reduced form) *(NADPH)* oxidase and xanthine oxidase. Endogenous antioxidant enzymes involved in removal of AOS include the superoxide dismutases, glutathione peroxidase, and catalase. O_2^-, *Superoxide;* H_2O_2, hydrogen peroxide; $\cdot OH$, hydroxyl radical; $NO\cdot$, nitric oxide; $ONOO^-$, peroxynitrate.

AOS can be produced intracellularly by many enzymes, including cytochrome P-450 enzymes of the mitochondrial electron transport system and xanthine oxidase, a peroxisomal enzyme that generates O_2^- and H_2O_2 during the metabolism of xanthine to uric acid.[101] Specialized cells, such as phagocytes, also have unique enzymes, such as membrane-bound nicotinamide-adenine dinucleotide phosphate (reduced form) *(NADPH)* oxidase, which may be activated during phagocytosis to initiate a cascade of AOS (Fig. 21-1). Neutrophils also possess myeloperoxidase, which converts H_2O_2 into the relatively stable oxidant, hypochlorous acid (HOCl).

Production of AOS can occur by other endogenous mechanisms initiated by endotoxins and cytokines, such as tumor necrosis factor alpha (TNFα) and interleukin-1 (IL-1). In addition, AOS are produced exogenously by a variety of chemical and physical agents, including ozone, nitrogen and sulfur oxides, mineral dusts, phorbol esters, ionizing and UV radiation, paraquat, and hyperoxia. These pollutants, which are discussed in detail later, may foster redox reactions by acellular pathways or during their interactions with or metabolism by cells.

MECHANISMS OF ANTIOXIDANT DEFENSE

A number of elaborate defense mechanisms exist in mammalian cells that combat AOS.[32,86] Nonenzymatic antioxidants include sulfhydryl-containing molecules such as glutathione (GSH), albumin, ceruloplasmin, bilirubin, and uric acid. Vitamins A, C, and E also have antioxidant activity. Specific proteins, such as heat stress proteins, metallothionein and heme oxygenase, are also induced after oxidative stress and may act as antioxidants.[5,56]

Traditionally regarded antioxidant enzymes act at various stages in the pathway of generation of AOS, as indicated in Fig. 21-1. These include the superoxide dismutases

(SODs), catalase, and glutathione peroxidase (GPX). Mammalian cells contain three forms of superoxide dismutase, an extracellular copper-zinc-containing species (EC-SOD),[66] a copper-zinc–containing form (CuZn-SOD) occurring in both peroxisomes and the cytoplasm,[17,52] and a manganese-containing form (Mn-SOD) localized in mitochondria.[39] These enzymes appear to be independently regulated and are the product of highly conserved genes. Although the superoxide dismutases convert O_2^- to H_2O_2, questions remain as to whether or not they, in and of themselves, are protective in function. For example, H_2O_2 is toxic to cells and can be converted to the highly reactive ·OH radical (Fig. 22-1). A more plausible scenario is that superoxide dismutases act in concert with catalase and GPX to convert H_2O_2 to nontoxic byproducts.[86]

Catalase, a 240,000 molecular weight protein, occurs in peroxisomes and detoxifies H_2O_2 to oxygen and water. GPX is a smaller cytosolic protein that also eliminates H_2O_2 but has a wider range and higher affinity for substrates such as lipid peroxides. The localization, structure, and regulation of genes encoding catalase, GPX, and the superoxide dismutases are currently under investigation because they may prove to be important tools in preventive approaches and gene therapy of diseases associated with oxidative stress. The gene for CuZn-SOD is located on chromosome 21,[62] leading to some speculation that its overexpression in disease, such as Down syndrome (trisomy 21), may be contributory to the many pathological changes observed in these individuals. A controversy presently exists regarding whether Mn-SOD consists of one or two genes, but multiple messenger RNA (mRNA) species exist.[36,41] In comparison to CuZn-SOD, Mn-SOD appears to be highly inducible by a variety of oxidants.[86] The human catalase gene has been mapped to chromosome 11.[85] In contrast, genes for GPX have been mapped to chromosomes 3 and 21 and the X chromosome, but only the gene on chromosome 3 is functional.[67] Genes for several of these antioxidant enzymes have been cloned and transfected into cells or overexpressed in transgenic mice to assess their biological functions (see the section on hyperoxia).

GENERAL MECHANISMS OF CELL DAMAGE BY ACTIVE OXYGEN SPECIES

AOS production is beneficial in the metabolism of various compounds and in eradication of bacteria and other pathogens. Overproduction of AOS or malfunctioning of antioxidant defenses, however, results in deleterious effects at the cellular level that may progress to disease. Some cellular and molecular effects of AOS include lipid peroxidation, modification of proteins, and alterations in DNA, such as strand breakage or the induction of oxidative lesions.[46] Lipid peroxidation occurs in a series of reactions after interaction of AOS with polyunsaturated fatty acids primarily occurring in membranes (Fig. 21-2). This chain of re-

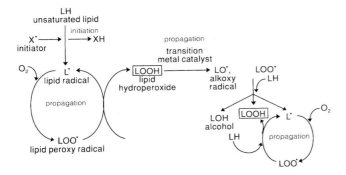

Fig. 21-2. Mechanisms of initiation and propagation of lipid peroxidation, a series of events that may be important in cell signaling, proliferation, and cytotoxicity of active oxygen species. The initiator of the reaction (X) may be a hydroxyl radical (·OH), a perhydroxy radical, or iron-dioxygen complexes. The termination of this cascade of reactions occurs when two radical species combine to form a nonradical species.

actions results in the formation of a number of AOS, such as ·OH, H_2O_2, singlet oxygen, and peroxyl and alkoxyl radicals. Because products of lipid peroxidation may be early biomarkers of cell injury and disease, sensitive techniques are being developed to localize these derivatives in situ and measure their production in lavage fluids and urine.[69,84]

AOS also can modify proteins in a way that causes their induction or inactivation. For example, guanylate cyclase is activated following sulfhydryl oxidation by H_2O_2, a process resulting in production of cyclic guanosine monophosphate (GMP).[107] Alternatively, AOS released from activated neutrophils can activate certain antioxidant enzymes, including CuZn-SOD and catalase.[8,58]

An area of intense investigation is the formation of oxidized bases and DNA lesions by AOS, particularly by ·OH. This reactive species appears to cause a spectrum of DNA alterations, such as base damage, single-strand and double-strand breakage, and DNA cross-linking.[31] One of the most widely studied types of DNA damage is the oxidative lesion, 8-hydroxyguanine (8-oxodeoxyguanine, 8-oxoG), which is associated with mutations, spontaneous cancers, and exposure to carcinogens, such as ionizing radiation and 2-nitropropane.[95] One review focuses on the critical role of DNA repair in the prevention of oxidative DNA damage and cancer development in syndromes such as xeroderma pigmentosum and ataxia telangiectasia[46] (see Chapters 19 and 26).

PATTERNS OF CELL DAMAGE AND REPAIR AFTER EXPOSURE TO ENVIRONMENTAL AGENTS INDUCING OXIDATIVE STRESS
Ozone

Ozone is formed naturally in the stratosphere and by photochemical reactions between oxygen, volatile organic compounds, nitrous oxides, and sunlight (i.e., smog).

Stratospheric ozone has a protective function in that it acts as a shield from the harmful effects of UV radiation. Decrements in lung function, however, particularly after exercise, have been observed in individuals exposed to concentrations of ozone at ambient levels approximating the current national standard.[21]

Because ozone is inhaled, the lung is the major organ affected. A number of experimental studies have documented both morphological and biochemical changes in epithelial cells at ambient concentrations of ozone.[4,13,42] In the upper airways, ozone is particularly damaging to ciliated cells, whereas destruction of type I epithelial cells and type II cell hyperplasia occurs in the peripheral lung. Progressive epithelial cell and interstitial responses occur in rats with prolonged exposures.[13]

Several investigators have also examined the effects of patterns of ozone exposure on epithelial cell injury and hyperplasia.[3,11] These experiments suggest that cell responses at low ozone concentrations are related to cumulative concentrations and not patterns of exposure. Ozone also appears to act in concert with oxidants and other pollutants in the environment to cause airway injury,[14] transformation of rodent tracheal epithelial cells,[100,112] and DNA damage in human lung cells.[59] Exposure to ozone also impairs clearance of asbestos fibers, thereby enhancing their pulmonary retention.[81]

Whether ozone causes cell injury and cell proliferation by oxidant-dependent or oxidant-independent mechanisms is a subject of debate. Kinetic analyses of reactivity suggest that ozone is short-lived and unable to react directly with cells of the lung.[82] These studies indicate that the byproducts, specifically H_2O_2 and aldehydes, of the reactions of ozone with unsaturated fatty acids and other cellular targets are possible mediators of ozone toxicity.[83]

The view that oxidants are involved in ozone-induced biological effects is also supported by in vitro studies showing partial protection after addition of antioxidants to ozone-exposed cells.[70] Ozone also causes transient depletion of GSH (reduced glutathione) stores in the lung after brief inhalation by rats.[89] Increases in gene expression and enzyme activity of antioxidant enzymes after inhalation of ozone[87] may be causally related to lung defense because rats pretreated with endotoxin, which induces Mn-SOD, do not exhibit characteristically observed lung edema.[88] Moreover, increases in GSH and GSH-dependent enzymes are observed in cells retrieved from bronchoalveolar lavage (BAL).[7] These observations and marked elevations in vitamin E content of rodent lungs after exposure to ozone suggest that vitamin E, and possibly other endogenous antioxidants, may be mobilized to the lung in response to this pollutant.[99]

Hyperoxia

Adult rats exposed to a high oxygen environment exhibit respiratory distress and eventual death. Hyperoxia-induced lung damage and oxygen therapy also are important in the development of adult respiratory distress syndrome (ARDS) and bronchopulmonary dysplasia in the newborn. Specific target cells affected in the lung include alveolar epithelial cells, vascular endothelial cells, and interstitial cells. Hyperplasia of interstitial cells coupled with proliferation of epithelial cells appears to inhibit gas exchange, although compensatory mechanisms and adaptation to hyperoxia occur in some experimental models.[18,27,96] For example, type I epithelial cells become necrotic and are replaced by rapidly dividing type II cells, which repopulate the lung and dedifferentiate into type I cells. Moreover, preexposure to hypoxia reduces the degree of hyperplasia in rats subsequently exposed to hyperoxic conditions.[96]

Subsequent tolerance to hyperoxia is also observed in rats pretreated with TNF and IL-1;[108,109] endotoxin, i.e., lipopolysaccharide (LPS);[43] cadmium;[33] or ozone.[44] These adaptive responses are attributed to the protective effects of antioxidant enzymes induced by these agents. Intratracheal instillation of red blood cells into rats also increases their survival in a high oxygen environment, presumably by potentiation of the GSH redox system involving GPX.[37]

Direct assessment of antioxidant enzymes on pathological changes associated with hyperoxia has been achieved using transgenic mice and exogenous administration of antioxidant enzymes to rodents. For example, transgenic mice overexpressing CuZn-SOD and exposed to hyperoxia show decreased mortality, particularly in younger animals, in comparison to sham controls.[110] Mice transfected with the Mn-SOD gene are also resistant, despite relatively low increases (40% above sham control values) in Mn-SOD activity in whole lung homogenates.[111] Because of their brief half-lives, antioxidant enzymes have been either incorporated into liposomes or coupled to polyethylene glycol (PEG) before their addition to cultures of lung cells or administration to animals.* These approaches, which may eventually be important clinically in the treatment of hyperoxia and other diseases associated with oxidative stress, afford significant protection from hyperoxia.

The regulation of antioxidant enzymes during initial exposure to hyperoxia and during the process of adaptation to oxidative stress appears to be complex and related to factors such as the age, species, and cell type examined. For example, rat airway epithelial cells in situ, in comparison to epithelial cells and other cell types in the peripheral lung, show intense immunolabeling for CuZn-SOD, Mn-SOD, and catalase.[12] These high endogenous levels do not appear to be increased after exposure to hyperoxia. Because hyperoxia-associated morphological and inflammatory changes are localized to the distal lung and not observed in the airways in this animal model of disease, the stores of antioxidant enzymes in tracheobronchial epithelial cells may make them more resistant to oxidative injury in comparison to peripheral epithelial cells. Reviews document alterations in gene expression, levels of immunoreactive protein, and activity of antioxidant enzymes as observed by a number of investigators after exposure of cells of the respiratory tract to hyperoxic conditions both in vivo and in vitro.[46,86] Different patterns of induction of antioxidant enzymes in many of these models reveal complex transcriptional regulation and translational/posttranslational modifications occurring during hyperoxic injury and other types of oxidative stress. Cellular responses to hyperoxia also appear to be reflected by synthesis of new proteins, which may be important in lung repair, including a tissue inhibitor of metalloproteinases (TIMP), metallothionein II, and surfactant protein A.[40]

Mineral dusts

Mineral dusts such as asbestos and silica are associated with the development of pneumoconioses in the workplace and exist at lower concentrations in the environment.[1,16,74] Both of these mineral families consist of a number of distinct mineral types with a complex physical and chemical composition. For example, six varieties of asbestos (defined as a group of crystalline hydrated silicates possessing a greater than 3:1 length-to-diameter ratio) occur in two major classes: serpentine (of which chrysotile is the only member) and amphibole (crocidolite, amosite, anthophyllite, tremolite, and actinolite).[72] Many varieties of amorphous and crystalline silica also exist, including alpha quartz and cristobalite.[1,16] These minerals, similar to asbestos, may vary both morphologically and chemically, depending on their source. Redox reactions driven by the surface chemistry of asbestos and silica as well as their iron content and composition may be important in the generation of AOS. In addition, fibers and particles may interact with cells of the immune system and target cells of the lung to generate AOS through a number of pathways.[51,75]

Occupational exposure to asbestos has been associated with the development of pulmonary fibrosis (asbestosis), bronchogenic carcinoma, and malignant mesothelioma as well as with several types of benign pleural disorders.[74] Malignant mesothelioma and possibly bronchogenic carcinomas are more prevalent in workers exposed to crocidolite, a high iron-containing, needlelike fiber that is reactive in the formation of AOS.[71] Although exposure to silica may cause nonmalignant lung disease (silicosis) in workplace settings, whether it causes lung cancers is a subject of debate and confounded by smoking influences.[15] Moreover, it is unclear whether either asbestos or silica contribute to disease at concentrations of dusts in the ambient environment, but risks appear to be small.[72,74]

AOS can be generated by several mechanisms after inhalation of fibrogenic minerals (Fig. 21-3). For example, inflammation and recruitment of alveolar macrophages to sites of dust deposition are observed in rodents after inhalation of silica or asbestos in contrast to relatively inert dusts such as titanium dioxide. Under these circumstances, AOS are elaborated by cells of the immune system.[79] One pro-

*References 6, 50, 78, 104, 105.

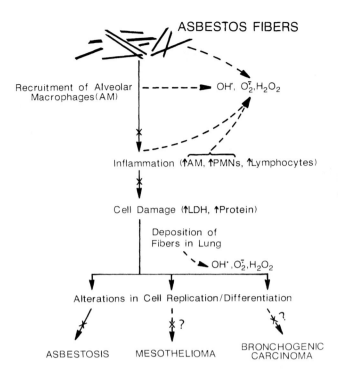

ASBESTOS FIBERS

Fig. 21-3. Possible mechanisms of oxidant injury in the respiratory tract after inhalation of asbestos fibers. Active oxygen species (AOS) may be generated from alveolar macrophages *(AM)* recruited to sites of fiber deposition as well as from other cells of the immune system involved in the localized inflammatory response to asbestos. Alternatively, AOS may be released from dying cells or after deposition of fibers in the lungs via acellular or redox reactions occurring on the fiber surface or catalyzed by iron. AOS may also mediate alterations in cell replication and differentiation associated with the development of asbestosis, malignant mesothelioma, and bronchogenic carcinoma. The X's indicate stages in the inflammatory and disease process that can be ameliorated by administration of the antioxidant enzyme, catalase, to rats. *PMN,* Polymorphonuclear neutrophils; *LDH,* lactate dehydrogenase. (From Kehrer J et al: Free radical mechanisms in chemical pathogenesis, *Tox Appl Physiol* 95:349, 1988; with permission.)

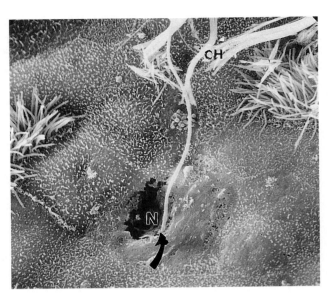

Fig. 21-4. Scanning electron micrograph showing the interaction of a long chrysotile *(CH)* asbestos fiber with the surface of a tracheobronchial epithelial cell in organ culture. Note the localized area of necrosis *(N)* at the point of fiber contact *(arrow)*. Long fibers are more cytotoxic to cells than shorter fibers, presumably because of their enhanced capacity to generate active oxygen species. (×500.)

cess that may be critical to the increased potency of long (more than 5 μ) asbestos fibers in the development of pulmonary fibrosis and mesothelioma is frustrated phagocytosis (Fig. 21-4). Because long fibers cannot be successfully encompassed by cells, they may serve as chronic stimuli for release of AOS from phagocytes. The production of cytokines such as TNF and IL-1 from alveolar macrophages and other cell types may also contribute to oxidative injury by fibrogenic minerals.[22,80]

Generation of AOS through redox reactions driven by the surface chemistry of particles or by iron on their surface, which catalyzes the Fenton reaction (see Fig. 21-1), may also be important in mineral-induced cell damage.[20,30,106,113] In this regard, it is interesting to note that the pathogenicity of various asbestos and nonasbestos types of minerals may be linked directly to their iron content[54]

or their ability to mobilize iron from cells.[63] Physicomechanical processing of minerals, such as silica by crushing, also leads to enhanced production of AOS.[20,28] As shown in Fig. 21-3, chronic generation of AOS may occur in the lung over time owing to deposition and retention of durable fibers, such as crocidolite asbestos.

The importance of antioxidant enzymes in asbestos-induced cytotoxicity, inflammation, and fibrosis is indicated by the results of a number of studies from our laboratory and others.[51,75,76] For example, the administration of PEG-coupled catalase to rats inhaling crocidolite asbestos blocks the development of inflammation, lung injury, and pulmonary fibrosis in a dosage-dependent fashion.[73] As shown in Fig. 21-3, catalase appears to act at many stages in the pathway to disease. Addition of antioxidants or iron chelators to cells of the respiratory tract in vitro also ameliorates cell injury, lipid peroxidation, and DNA damage associated with asbestos, particularly crocidolite.[29,77,94]

Increases in Mn-SOD gene expression and immunoreactive protein are striking in both lung homogenates and cells from BAL of rats exposed to crocidolite asbestos or cristobalite silica.[47] The use of Mn-SOD as a biomarker of chronic inflammation and pulmonary fibrosis may be feasible because its induction is dosage dependent and not observed after subchronic inhalation of noninflammatory dusts, such as titanium dioxide.[48] The cell type primarily responsible for increases in Mn-SOD protein in situ after exposure to fibrogenic minerals appears to be the type II epithelial cell.[39]

Human pleural mesothelial cells in vitro also show dose-dependent induction of Mn-SOD and heme oxygenase after exposure to crocidolite asbestos or the chemical generating system, xanthine and xanthine oxidase, which generates a variety of AOS.[49] Human lung fibroblasts exhibit less striking increases in mRNA levels of these enzymes, indicating that patterns of antioxidant enzyme induction may be different in various cell types. In addition to antioxidant enzymes, asbestos also causes increases in gene expression of ornithine decarboxylase (ODC) and other proliferation-specific genes, such as the protooncogenes, c-*fos*/c-*jun*, in animal inhalation models of disease and cells in vitro.[35,45] These molecular events may be linked to chronic cell proliferation and altered differentiation of cells in the lung and pleura during the pathogenesis of disease (see Fig. 21-3). Studies to determine whether elevations in gene expression by asbestos are mediated by oxidant-dependent or oxidant-independent pathways are presently under investigation.

Paraquat

Accidental or intentional ingestion of the insecticide, paraquat (1,1'-dimethyl-4,4'-bipyridinium), results in death in humans. After interaction with cells, paraquat reacts with NADPH causing cyclic, single-electron reduction of the parent molecule and generation of a paraquat radical. In the presence of molecular oxygen, O_2^- and a cascade of AOS then are released (see Fig. 21-1). Because of its AOS-generating properties, paraquat has been used as a model to study oxidant injury both in laboratory rodents and in cells in vitro.[2,9,26]

Several studies indicate that antioxidant enzymes, primarily the superoxide dismutases, are involved in paraquat-induced pathogenicity. For example, preexposure of adult rats to endotoxin or hyperoxia increases antioxidant enzyme activity in lung and prolongs survival after subsequent exposure to paraquat.[26] Moreover, human gingival fibroblasts and rodent and human type II epithelial cells in vitro show increased total superoxide dismutase activity and elevations in catalase after addition of paraquat.[93,98] Lastly, cells with increased intracellular levels of superoxide dismutase, but not catalase, exhibit less cytotoxicity after exposure to paraquat in vitro.[2] Several investigators have evaluated transfection of either CuZn-SOD or Mn-SOD genes into murine fibroblasts—approaches that have yielded increased resistance to paraquat.[53,97] Transfection of CuZn-SOD, however, also resulted in increased GPX activity, an observation supporting the premise that several antioxidant enzymes may be involved coordinately in defense from paraquat.

Tobacco smoke

Cigarette smoke contains hundreds of chemicals and particulates, which may generate oxidants by acellular reactions or during their metabolism by cells. An estimated 10^{15} radical species are created during a puff from a cigarette.

Studies on smokers indicate that levels of antioxidant enzymes are increased in alveolar macrophages from BAL[68] and in red blood cells.[102] Other naturally occurring antioxidants, such as GSH, also are elevated. If cigarette smoke is filtered to eliminate particulates, elevations in antioxidant enzyme activity are diminished in rodents.[68] Thus the bulk of oxidant activity burden appears to be in the particulate phase of smoke. Alternatively, reactions between the particulate and gaseous phases of smoke might also be critical in generation of AOS. Smoke-exposed hamsters exhibit prolonged survival in hyperoxia, an indication that antioxidant enzymes confer subsequent adaptation to other types of oxidative stress.[68]

Carcinogenesis is a multifaceted process involving initiation, promotion, and progression. Although initiators are defined as carcinogens with the capacity to interact with DNA, thus causing a heritable change in the DNA, promoters and progression factors act primarily by stimulating proliferation of initiated cells. Chronic cell proliferation then results in additional accumulation of genetic and phenotypic changes resulting in malignancy. Because components of cigarette smoke can be initiators, promoters, or complete carcinogens possessing both features, AOS may act at several stages of the carcinogenic process. For example, direct interactions of AOS with DNA occur in a number of experimental models of chemical carcinogenesis.[55,102] In addition, tumor promoters such as the phorbol esters and generating systems of AOS appear to act on target cells via common mechanisms, including the activation of protein kinase C and stimulation of cell proliferation.[10,55,103] Decreases in antioxidant enzymes also occur in many models of tumor promotion. Moreover, it is widely documented that antioxidants are anticarcinogens, which primarily exert their effects during the promotion phase of carcinogenesis.

Ultraviolet radiation (see Chapter 10)

Intense exposure to UV radiation, an environmental stress causing intracellular production of AOS, is associated with the development of skin cancer. The view that skin cancer development involves altered DNA repair of oxidative lesions is supported by study of the disease xeroderma pigmentosum, a syndrome characterized by extreme sensitivity to UV-induced DNA damage and skin cancers.[61] Patients appear to have a specific defect in a nucleotide excision pathway important in repairing DNA lesions created by the formation of thymidine dimers.[61]

UV radiation elicits a sequence of responses in mammalian cells. Initial interactions may elicit signal transduction, targeting of DNA, and more protracted cellular events. The term *UV response* refers to a collective series of genetic changes induced by UV or other DNA damaging agents involving amplification or increased expression of UV-responsive genes.[64] These alterations include the activation of transcription factors, which may promote cell replication by binding to UV-responsive genetic elements[91] or increased gene expression of ornithine decarboxylase (ODC), a rate-limiting gene in the biosynthesis of polyamines,[92] and induction of protooncogenes (c-*fos*, c-*myc*), which may be linked causally to cell proliferation, cytotoxicity, and oxidative stress.[38,90]

Another biological effect of DNA damage by UV radiation is transient inhibition of DNA synthesis and growth arrest. For example, UV radiation increases levels of p53 cellular tumor antigen, a potent transcription factor that may act as a two-edged sword by also causing arrest of the cell cycle at the G1 phase.[65] Other growth-regulatory genes induced by both UV radiation and agents (H_2O_2, methyl methanesulfonate [MMS], N-acetoxy-2-acetylaminofluorene) causing base damage to DNA are called growth *arrest* and *DNA* *d*amage inducible, i.e., gadd genes. These coordinately regulated genes appear to be critical to the control of cell growth.[24]

As illustrated previously by a number of agents inducing AOS, several genes and gene products induced by UV radiation appear to be antioxidants or important in cell defense. These include metallothionein I and II,[25] heme oxygenase,[57] and human major histocompatibility class-1 proteins, which might target altered cells for immune recognition or somatic cell selection.[60]

CONCLUSION

This chapter indicates the complexity of oxidant-induced biological effects and the considerable progress made in the understanding of molecular and cellular responses to environmental pollutants. The outcome of oxidative cell injury, which may be adaptation or the development of disease, may reflect (1) the intensity and duration of exposure, (2) endogenous stores of antioxidants or their inducibility at many levels of genetic control, (3) the balance between oxidative stress and antioxidant enzyme defense, and other factors. Several genes induced in response to various pollutants generating AOS have been identified and assessed functionally either by transfection into cells or by overexpression in transgenic animals. These molecular approaches, using genes that are linked to cell defense, may be valuable clinically in the amelioration of oxidative stress and eventually gene therapy. Other genes governing cell proliferation and aberrant differentiation of cells may serve as targets for antisense or "knock-out" methods.

REFERENCES

1. Absher MP et al: Biphasic cellular and tissue reponse of rat lungs after eight-day aerosol exposure to the silicon dioxidie cristobalite. *Am J Pathol* 134:1243, 1989.
2. Bagley A, Krall J, Lynch R: Superoxide mediates the toxicity of paraquat for Chinese hamster ovary cells. *Proc Natl Acad Sci USA* 83:3189, 1986.
3. Barr BC et al: A comparison of terminal airway remodeling in chronic daily vs. episodic ozone exposure. *Toxicol Appl Pharmacol* 106:384, 1990.
4. Barry BE, Miller FJ, Crapo JD: Effects of inhalation of 0.12 and 0.25 ppm O_3 on the proximal alveolar region of juvenile and adult rats. *Lab Invest* 53:692, 1985.
5. Bauman JW et al: Increase in metallothionein produced by chemicals that induce oxidative stress. *Toxicol Appl Pharmacol* 110:347, 1991.
6. Beckman JS et al: Superoxide dismutase and catalase conjugated to polyethylene glycol increased enzyme activity and oxidant resistance. *J Biol Chem* 263:6884, 1988.
7. Boehme DS, Hotchkiss JA, Henderson RF: Glutathione and GSH-dependent enzymes in bronchoalveolar lavage fluid cells in response to ozone. *Exp Mol Pathol* 56:37, 1992.
8. Bray RC et al: Reduction and inactivation of superoxide dismutase by hydrogen peroxide. *Biochem J* 139:43, 1974.
9. Bus JS, Gibson JE: Paraquat: Model for oxidant-initiated toxicity. *Environ Health Perspect* 55:37, 1984.
10. Cerutti PA: Pro-oxidant states and tumor promotion. *Science* 227:375, 1985.
11. Chang L et al: Alveolar epithelial cell injuries by subchronic exposure to low concentrations of ozone correlate with cumulative exposure. *Toxicol Appl Pharmacol* 109:219, 1991.
12. Chang L, Yoshino P and Crapo J: Airway respiratory epithelial cells have high antioxidant reserves and are resistant to oxidant stress. *Am Rev Respir Dis* 145:A569, 1992.
13. Chang LY et al: Epithelial injury and interstitial fibrosis in the proximal alveolar regions of rats chronically exposed to a simulated pattern of urban ambient ozone. *Toxicol Appl Pharmacol* 115:241, 1992.
14. Chen LC et al: Sulfuric acid-layered ultrafine particles potentiate ozone-induced airway injury. *J Toxicol Environ Health* 34:337, 1991.
15. Craighead JE: Do silica and asbestos cause lung cancer? *Arch Pathol Lab Med* 116:16, 1992.
16. Craighead JE et al: Diseases associated with exposure to silica and nonfibrous silicate minerals. *Arch Pathol Lab Med* 112:673, 1988.
17. Crapo JD et al: Copper-zinc superoxide dismutase is primarily a cytosolic protein in human cells. *Proc Natl Acad Sci USA* 89:10504, 1992.
18. Crapo JD et al: Pathologic changes in the lungs of oxygen-adapted rats: a morphometric analysis. *Lab Invest* 39:640, 1978.
19. Cross CE et al: Oxygen radicals and human disease. *Ann Int Med* 107:526, 1987.
20. Dalal NS, Shi X, Vallyathan V: *Potential role of silicon-oxygen radicals in acute lung injury.* In Mossman BT Begin RO, editors. *Effects of mineral dusts on cells,* Berlin, 1989, Springer-Verlag.
21. Devlin RB et al: Exposure of humans to ambient levels of ozone for 6.6 hours causes cellular and biochemical changes in the lungs. *Am J Respir Cell Mol Biol* 4:72, 1991.
22. Driscoll KE et al: Tumor necrosis factor (TNF): Evidence for the role of TNF in increased expression of manganese superoxide dismutase after inhalation of mineral dusts. *Ann Occup Hyg* 1994, (in press).
23. Floyd RA: Role of oxygen free radicals in carcinogenesis and brain ischemia. *FASEB J* 4:2587, 1990.
24. Fornace AJ Jr et al: Mammalian genes coordinately regulated by growth arrest signals and DNA-damaging agents. *Mol Cell Biol* 9:4196, 1989.
25. Fornace AJ Jr, Schalch H, Alamo I Jr.: Coordinate induction of metallothioneins I and II in rodent cells by UV irradiation. *Mol Cell Biol* 8:4716, 1988.
26. Frank L: Prolonged survival after paraquat: Role of the lung antioxidant enzyme systems. *Biochem Pharmacol* 30:2319, 1981.
27. Freeman B et al: Antioxidant enzyme activity in alveolar type II cells after exposure of rats to hyperoxia. *Exp Lung Res* 10:203, 1986.
28. Fubini B et al: *The formation of oxygen reactive radicals at the surface of the crushed quartz dusts as a possible cause of silica patho-*

genicity. In Mossman BT, Begin RO, editors. *Effects of mineral dusts on cells,* Berlin, 1989, Springer-Verlag.

29. Goodglick LA, Pietras LA, Kane AB: Evaluation of the causal relationship between crocidolite asbestos-induced lipid peroxidation and toxicity to macrophages. *Am Rev Respir Dis* 139:1265, 1989.
30. Gulumian M, Van Wyk JA: Hydroxyl radical production in the presence of fibres by a Fenton-type reaction. *Chem Biol Interact* 62:89, 1987.
31. Halliwell B, Aruoma OI: DNA damage by oxygen-derived species. Its mechanism of action and measurement in mammalian systems. *FEBS Lett* 281:9, 1991.
32. Halliwell B, Gutteridge JMC: *Free Radicals in Biology and Medicine,* Oxford, Clarendon Press, 1989.
33. Hart BA et al: Cross-tolerance to hyperoxia following cadmium aerosol pretreatment. *Toxicol Appl Pharmacol* 103:255, 1990.
34. Heffner JE, Repine JE: Pulmonary strategies of antioxidant defense. *Am Rev Respir Dis* 140:531, 1989.
35. Heintz NH, Janssen YMW, Mossman BT: Persistent induction of c-*fos* and c-*jun* proto-oncogene expression by asbestos. *Proc Natl Acad Sci USA* 90:3299, 1993.
36. Ho YS, Howard A, Crapo JD: Molecular structure of a functional rat gene for manganese-containing superoxide dismutase. *Am J Resp Cell Molec Biol* 4:278, 1991.
37. Hoidal J: Therapy with red blood cells decreases hyperoxic pulmonary injury. *Exp Lung Res* 14:977, 1988.
38. Hollander MC, Fornace AJ Jr.: Induction of *fos* RNA by DNA-damaging agents. *Cancer Res* 49:1687, 1989.
39. Holley JA et al: Increased manganese superoxide dismutase protein in Type II epithelial cells of rat lungs after inhalation of crocidolite asbestos or cristobalite silica. *Am J Pathol* 141:475, 1992.
40. Horowitz S et al: Hyperoxic exposure alters gene expression in the lung. *J Biol Chem* 264:7092, 1989.
41. Hurt J et al: Multiple mRNA species generated by alternate polyadenylation from the rat manganese superoxide dismutase gene. *Nucleic Acids Res* 20:2985, 1992.
42. Hyde DM et al: Ozone-induced acute tracheobronchial epithelial injury: relationship to granulocyte emigration in the lung. *Am J Respir Cell Molec Biol* 6:481, 1992.
43. Iqbal J et al: Endotoxin increases lung CuZn superoxide dismutase mRNA: O_2 raises enzyme synthesis. *Am J Physiol* 257:61, 1989.
44. Jackson RM, Frank L: Ozone-induced tolerance to hyperoxia in rats. *Am Rev Respir Dis* 129:425, 1984.
45. Janssen YMW et al: *Asbestos-mediated gene expression in rat lung.* In Brown RC, Hoskins JA, Johnson NF, editors. *Mechanisms in fibre carcinogenesis,* New York, 1991, Plenum Press.
46. Janssen YMW et al: Cell and tissue responses to oxidative damage. *Lab Invest,* 69:261, 1993.
47. Janssen YMW et al: Expression of antioxidant enzymes in rat lungs after inhalation of asbestos or silica. *J Biol Chem* 267:10625, 1992.
48. Janssen YWM et al: Increased expression of manganese-containing superoxide dismutase in rat lungs after inhalation of inflammatory and fibrogenic minerals. *Free Radic Biol Med ,* 16:315, 1994.
49. Janssen YWM et al: Oxidant stress responses in human mesothelial cells exposed to asbestos. *Am J Resp Crit Care Med* 149:795, 1994.
50. Jornot L, Junod AF: Response of human endothelial cell antioxidant enzymes to hyperoxia. *Am J Respir Cell Mol Biol* 6:107, 1992.
51. Kamp DW et al: The role of free radicals in asbestos induced diseases. *Free Radic Biol Med* 12:293, 1992.
52. Keller GA, et al: Cu,Zn superoxide dismutase is a peroxisomal enzyme in human fibroblasts and hepatoma cells. *Proc Natl Acad Sci USA* 88:7381, 1991.
53. Kelner M, Bagnell R: Generation of endogenous glutathione peroxidase, manganese superoxide dismutase, and glutathione transferase activity in cells transfected with a copper-zinc superoxide dismutase expression vector. *J Biol Chem* 265:10872, 1990.
54. Kennedy TP et al: Dusts causing pneumoconiosis generate ·OH and produce hemolysis by acting as Fenton catalysts. *Arch Biochem Biophys* 269:359, 1989.
55. Kensler TW, Trush MA: Role of oxygen radicals in tumor promotion. *Environ Mol Mutagen* 6:593, 1984.
56. Keyse SM et al: Oxidant stress leads to transcriptional activation of the human heme oxygenase gene in cultured skin fibroblasts. *Mol Cell Biol* 10:4967, 1990.
57. Keyse SM, Tyrrell RM: Induction of the heme-oxygenase gene in human skin fibroblasts by hydrogen peroxide and UVA (365 mn) radiation: evidence for the involvement of the hydroxyl radical. *Carcinogenesis* 11:787, 1989.
58. Kono Y, Fridovich I: Superoxide radical inhibits catalase. *J Biol Chem* 257:5751, 1982.
59. Kozumbo WJ, Agarwal S: Induction of DNA damage in cultured human long cells by tobacco smoke arylamines exposed to ambient levels of ozone. *Am J Respir Cell Mol Biol* 3:611, 1990.
60. Lambert ME et al: Enhancement of major histocompatibility class 1 protein synthesis by DNA damage in cultured human fibroblasts and keratinocytes. *Mol Cell Biol* 9:847, 1989.
61. Lehmann AR: Xeroderma pigmentosum, Cockayne syndrome and ataxia-telangiectasia: disorders relating DNA repair to carcinogenesis. *Cancer Surv* 1:93, 1982.
62. Levanon D et al: Architecture and anatomy of the chromosomal locus in human chromosome 21 encoding the Cu-Zn superoxide dismutase. *EMBO J* 4:77, 1985.
63. Lund LG, Aust AE: Iron-catalyzed reactions may be responsible for the biochemical and biological effects of asbestos. *BioFactors* 3:83, 1991.
64. Mai S et al: Mechanisms of the ultraviolet light response in mammalian cells. *J Cell Science* 94:609, 1989.
65. Maltzman W, Czyzyk L: UV irradiation stimulates levels of p53 cellular tumor antigen in nontransformed mouse cells. *Mol Cell Biol* 4:1689, 1984.
66. Marklund SL: Extracellular superoxide dismutase and other superoxide dismutase isoenzymes in tissues from nine mammalian species. *Biochem J* 222:649, 1984.
67. McBride OW et al: Gene for selenium dependent glutathione peroxidase maps to human chromosomes 3, 21 and X. *Biofactors* 1:285, 1988.
68. McKusker K, Hoidal J: Selective increase of antioxidant enzyme activity in the alveolar macrophages from cigarette smokers and smoke-exposed hamsters. *Am Rev Respir Dis* 141:676, 1990.
69. Messina MJ: Oxidative stress status and cancer: methodology applicable for human studies. *Free Radic Biol Med* 10:175, 1991.
70. Morgan DC, Wenzel DG: Free radical species mediating the toxicity of ozone for cultured rat lung fibroblasts. *Toxicology* 36:243, 1985.
71. Mossman BT: Mechanisms of asbestos-induced toxicity and carcinogenicity: the amphibole hypothesis revisited. *Br J Ind Med* 1993, (in press).
72. Mossman BT et al: Asbestos: scientific developments and implications for public policy. *Science* 247:294, 1990.
73. Mossman BT et al: Inhibition of lung injury, inflammation, and interstitial pulmonary fibrosis by polyethylene glycol-conjugated catalase in rapid inhalation model of asbestosis. *Am Rev Respir Dis* 141:1266, 1990.
74. Mossman BT, Gee JBL: Asbestos-related diseases. *N Engl J Med* 320:1721, 1989.
75. Mossman BT, Marsh JP: Evidence supporting a role for active oxygen species in asbestos-induced toxicity and lung disease. *Environ Health Perspect* 81:91, 1989.
76. Mossman BT, Marsh JP: *Role of active oxygen species in asbestos-induced cytotoxicity, cell proliferation, and carcinogenesis.* In Harris CC, Lechner JF and Brinkley BR, editors: *Cellular and molecu-*

lar aspects of fiber carcinogenesis, Cold Spring Harbor, NY, 1991, Cold Spring Harbor Press.

77. Mossman BT, Marsh JP, Shatos MA: Alteration of superoxide dismutase activity in tracheal epithelial cells by asbestos and inhibition of cytotoxicity by antioxidants. *Lab Invest* 54:204, 1986.

78. Padmanabhan RV et al: Protection against pulmonary oxygen toxicity in rats by the intratracheal administration of liposome-encapsulated superoxide dismutase or catalase. *Am Rev Respir Dis* 132:164, 1985.

79. Petruska JM et al: Brief inhalation of asbestos compromises superoxide production in cells from bronchoalveolar lavage. *Am J Respir Cell Mol Biol* 2:129, 1990.

80. Piguet PF et al: Requirement of tumour necrosis factor for the development of silica-induced pulmonary fibrosis. *Nature* 344:245, 1990.

81. Pinkerton KE et al: Exposure to low levels of ozone results in enhanced pulmonary retention of inhaled asbestos fibers. *Am Rev Respir Dis* 140:1075, 1989.

82. Pryor WA: How far does ozone penetrate into the pulmonary air/tissue boundary before it reacts? *Free Radic Biol Med* 12:83, 1992.

83. Pryor WA, Das B, Church DF: The ozonation of unsaturated fatty acids: aldehydes and hydrogen peroxide as products and possible mediators of ozone toxicity. *Chem Res Toxicol* 4:341, 1991.

84. Pryor WA, Godber SS: Noninvasive measures of oxidative stress status in humans. *Free Radic Biol Med* 10:177, 1991.

85. Quan F et al: Isolation and characterization of the human catalase gene. *Nucleic Acids Res* 14:5321, 1986.

86. Quinlan T, Spivack S, Mossman BT: Regulation of antioxidant enzymes in lung after oxidant injury. *Environ Health Perspect,* 1993 in press.

87. Rahman I, Clerch L, Massaro D: Rat lung antioxidant enzyme induction by ozone. *Am J Physiol* 260:412, 1991.

88. Rahman I, Massaro D: Endotoxin treatment protects rats against ozone-induced lung edema: with evidence for the role of manganese superoxide dismutase. *Toxicol Appl Pharmacol* 113:13, 1992.

89. Reitjers M, Van bree LV, Marra M: Glutathione pathway enzyme activities and ozone sensitivity of lung cell populations derived from O_3-exposed rats. *Toxicology* 37:205, 1985.

90. Ronai ZA, Okin E, Weinstein IB: Ultraviolet light induces the expression of oncogenes in rat fibroblast and human keratinocyte cells. *Oncogene* 2:201, 1988.

91. Ronai ZA, Weinstein IB: Identification of a UV-induced trans-acting protein that stimulates polyomavirus DNA replication. *J Virol* 62:1057, 1988.

92. Rosen CF et al: Ultraviolet B radiation induction of ornithine decarboxylase gene expression in mouse epidermis. *Biochem J* 270:565, 1990.

93. Saito K: Effects of paraquat on macromolecule synthesis in cultured pneumocytes. *Tohoku J Exp Med* 148:303, 1986.

94. Shatos MA et al: Prevention of asbestos-induced cell death in rat lung fibroblasts and alveolar macrophages by scavengers of active oxygen species. *Environ Res* 44:103, 1987.

95. Shigenaga MK, Ames BN: Assays for 8-hydroxy-2'-deoxyguanosine: a biomarker of in vivo oxidative DNA damage. *Free Radic Biol Med* 10:211, 1991.

96. Sjostrom E, Crapo J: Structural and biochemical adaptive changes in rat lung after exposure to hypoxia. *Lab Invest* 48:68, 1983.

97. St. Clair D, Oberley T, Ho YS: Overproduction of Mn-superoxide dismutase modulates paraquat-mediated toxicity in mammalian cells. *FEBS* 293:199, 1991.

98. Stevens TM et al: Induction of antioxidant enzyme activities by a phenylurea derivative, EDU. *Toxicol Appl Pharmacol* 96:33, 1988.

99. Tanswell AK, Fraher LJ, Grose EC: Circulating factors that modify lung cell DNA synthesis following exposure to inhaled oxidants. II. Effects of serum and lavage on lung pneumocytes following exposure of adult rats to 1 ppm ozone. *J Toxicol Environ Health* 29:131, 1990.

100. Thomassen DG et al: The role of ozone in tracheal cell transformation. Research report, *Health Effects Inst* 50:1, 1992.

101. Till GO, Friedl HP, Ward PA: Lung injury and complement activation: Role of neutrophils and xanthine oxidase. *Free Rad Biol Med* 10:379, 1991.

102. Toth K et al: Erythrocytes from cigarette smokers contain more glutathione and catalase and protect endothelial cells from hydrogen peroxide better than do erythrocytes from nonsmokers. *Am Rev Respir Dis* 134:281, 1986.

103. Troll W, Wiesner R: The role of oxygen radicals as a possible mechanism of tumor promotion. *Annu Rev Pharmacol Toxicol* 25:509, 1985.

104. Turrens JF, Crapo JD, Freeman BA: Protection against oxygen toxicity by intravenous injection of liposome-entrapped catalase and superoxide dismutase. *J Clin Invest* 73:87, 1984.

105. Walther FFJ et al: Mitigation of pulmonary oxygen toxicity in premature lambs with intravenous antioxidants. *Exp Lung Res* 16:177, 1990.

106. Weitzman SA, Graceffa P: Asbestos catalyzes hydroxyl and superoxide radical generation from hydrogen peroxide. *Arch Biochem Biophys* 228:373, 1984.

107. White AA et al: Activation of soluble guanylate cyclase from rat lung by incubation or by hydrogen peroxide. *J Biol Chem* 251:7304, 1976.

108. White CW et al: Cytokines increase lung antioxidant enzymes during exposure to hyperoxia. *J Appl Physiol* 66:1003, 1989.

109. White CW et al: Recombinant tumor necrosis factor/cachectin and interleukin 1 pretreatment decreases lung oxidized glutathione accumulation, lung injury, and mortality in rats exposed to hyperoxia. *J Clin Invest* 79:1868, 1987.

110. White CW et al: Transgenic mice with expression of elevated levels of copper-zinc superoxide dismutase in the lungs are resistant to pulmonary oxygen toxicity. *J Clin Invest* 87:2162, 1991.

111. Wispe JR et al: Expression of human Mn-SOD in pulmonary epithelial cells of transgenic mice confers protection from oxygen injury. *Am Rev Respir Dis* 145:A712, 1992.

112. Witschi H: Effects of oxygen and ozone on mouse lung tumorigenesis. *Exp Lung Res* 17:473, 1991.

113. Zalma R et al: Formation of oxy-radicals by oxygen reduction arising from the surface activity of asbestos. *Can J Chem* 65:2338, 1987.

Chapter 22

NITRIC OXIDE

Anne E. Huot
Miles P. Hacker

Nitric oxide (NO) has long been known to have biological activity; however, until recently, that activity was limited to toxicological reports of exposure to the gas and subsequent damage to tissue. NO is extremely reactive with atmospheric air, resulting in the immediate formation of the highly poisonous nitrogen dioxide (NO_2), nitrogen tetroxide (N_2O_4), or both. Given the insidious nature of this toxicity, gas masks and adequate ventilation are required when using even small amounts of NO or its oxidation products. Individuals exposed to as little as 100 ppm of this gas for even short periods of time can develop a mild case of pulmonary inflammation that may be unnoticed until it progresses to a life-threatening pulmonary edema several days later. The colorless gas is prepared chemically by a number of procedures, including passing air through an electrical arc, oxidation of ammonia over a platinum gauze, or the reaction of sodium nitrate ($NNaO_3$) and ferrous sulfate (FeO_4S). The gas is used in large quantities in the manufacturing of nitric acid (HNO_3) and as an inhibitor of free radical–induced decomposition of a variety of organic compounds.

For decades, nitroglycerin has been given as a treatment for heart problems and high blood pressure in the absence of an understanding of the mechanism of its action. It was discovered that nitroglycerin hydrolyzed, spontaneously or through cellular metabolism, to NO and that NO itself was involved in platelet aggregation, cell growth, and signal transduction in the brain and vessel relaxation.[157] This simple gas may potentially be one of the most potent molecules in the body. Tannenbaum is credited with the original observation that mammalian cells are capable of generating nitrates.[167] His work stemmed from the observation that humans with infectious diarrhea secreted large amounts of nitrates and that rodents fed a nitrate-controlled diet secreted more nitrates than they took in, suggesting that they were being synthesized in vivo. Evidence for the production of NO is found in other various sites, such as hepatic Kupffer cells,[18] cells of the myenteric plexus,[52] cells of the pituitary and adrenal glands,[157] and macrophages.[161] Its functions have been as varied as its origins, as investigators have linked the molecule in signal transduction and bacterial and tumoricidal activity.[83,94,158]

The biological activity of NO is mediated through a number of pathways, which include the induction of cyclic guanosine monophosphate (cGMP),[143,144] iron-sulfur cluster enzyme inactivation,[40,68] and DNA damage.[70] The enzyme nitric oxide synthase (NOS) is responsible for the production of NO. There are two types of NOS, inducible and constitutive. Both may exist in the same cell type.[90] Furthermore, the inducible form of NOS resembles cytochrome P-450 reductase in DNA sequence.[22]

Many people have now speculated that NO plays a significant role in nonspecific immunity. This is based on observations that NO is a major cytotoxic molecule to tumor cells, parasitic fungi, protozoa, helminths, and mycobacteria but not extracellular bacteria.[108] NO is able to damage healthy cells as well as the cells generating the NO.[7,42] These findings led to the speculation that NO was involved in the pathophysiology of a number of diseases, such as islet cell destruction, in which there is evidence that NO contributes to autoimmune tissue destruction.[10,97] Autoimmune tissue injury mediated by immune complex deposition has also been linked to NO.[126] Additionally, NO is known to block leukocyte adhesion,[99] and L-arginine enhances natural killer and lymphokine activated killer cell killing ability.[138] All these lines of evidence suggest an important role for NO in an immune response, both normal and aberrant.

The goal of this chapter is to discuss in some detail the biochemistry of this important gas, the physiological effects of NO, and the potential role of NO in modulating pathophysiological states such as inflammation and hypotension induced by environmental stressors.

BIOCHEMISTRY OF NITRIC OXIDE
Cellular sources and production of nitric oxide

Once thought to be the product of endothelial cells and macrophages only, NO has now been shown to be released by a vast array of cell types. The box in the first column summarizes the putative cellular sources of NO and which isoform of NOS is expressed.[20] The strength of experimental evidence supporting the various cellular sources of NO vary greatly, but what is clear from the information contained in the box in the first column is that few, if any, sites in the body are protected from NO exposure.

Regardless of the cellular source of NO, there appears to be a common biochemical pathway leading to the actual production of NO. The substrate L-arginine is metabolized to NO and citrulline by NOS. The preponderance of evidence supports the following sequence of events resulting in NO synthesis. The initial step is the hydroxylation of arginine forming N^G-OH-L-arginine, which is then followed by an oxidation of the hydroxylamine and ultimately the release of NO and citrulline.[165] A proposed pathway is shown in Fig. 22-1.[166]

NO is rapidly oxidized to NO_2 and NO_3 in the presence of O_2 and H_2O, resulting in a short half-life (3 to 6 seconds) in biological systems.[124] This is important for two reasons: (1) The biological impact of NO is limited to tissues located near the source, and (2) measurement of NO production, regardless of the source, has relied on an indirect measurement of NO oxidative products or nitrosylated by-products. Other methods employed have included the

---

Putative cellular sources of nitric oxide

Constitutive production (low output)
   Endothelial cells
   Neurons
   Neutrophils
   Platelets
   Mast cells
   Adrenal
Inducible production (high output)
   Macrophages
   Kupffer cells
   Hepatocytes
   Smooth muscle cells
   Renal mesangial cells
   Chondrocytes
   Endothelial cells
   Fibroblasts
   Pancreatic islets

From Billiar TR et al: A role for inducible nitric oxide biosynthesis in the liver in inflammation and in the allogeneic immune response; *J Lab Clin Med* 120:192, 1992.

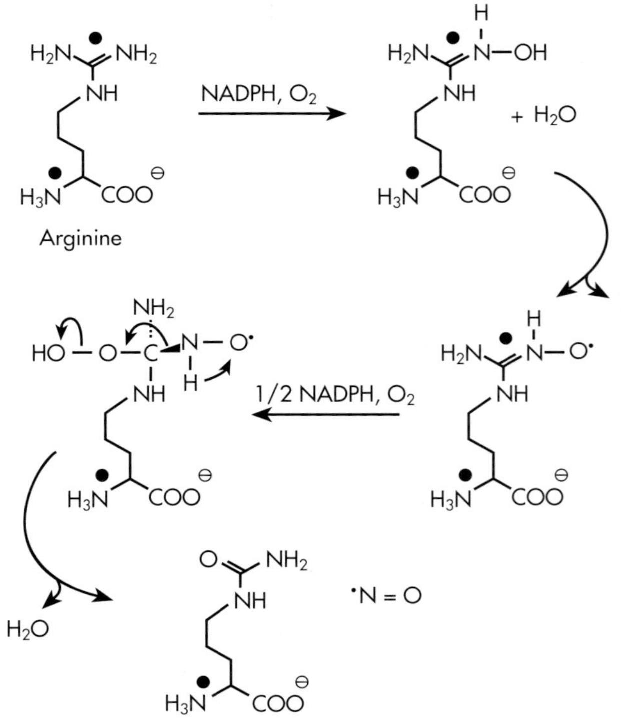

Fig. 22-1. Synthesis of nitric oxide. *NADPH,* Nicotinamide-adenine dinucleotide phosphate (reduced form). (From Stuehr DJ et al: The cytokine-induced macrophage nitric oxide synthase is a flavoprotein containing flavin adenine dinucleotide and flavin mononucleotide. In Moncada S et al, editors: *The biology of nitric oxide,* London, 1992, Portland Press.)

use of radio-labeled arginine. The technology to measure NO directly has also become available.

Nitric oxide synthase

NOS has been localized in a number of tissues and species. At present, three distinct forms of NOS, inducible (iNOS), endothelial (eNOS), and neuronal (nNOS), have been characterized, but within each class subtle differences may exist depending on the tissue origin of the enzyme. Functionally, there are two types of NOS. An inducible form, type I, is found in macrophages, hepatocytes, keratinocytes, neutrophils, endothelial cells, vascular smooth muscle cells, and myocardial cells. A constitutive form, type II, is found primarily in endothelial cells and neuronal tissue. The similarities and differences between these are summarized in Table 22-1.[48]

Type I NOS is induced within 4 to 8 hours after exposure to a number of stimulants, including cytokines, microbial products, and oxidized membrane lipoproteins. Once induced, the production of NO lasts for a prolonged period, and the concentration of NO generated is much higher than that generated by the activity of type II NOS. Furthermore, in contrast to type II NOS, which is calcium ion (Ca^{2+}) and calmodulin dependent, cell free extracts of cells containing type I NOS require no divalent cations for NO production. The constitutively expressed type II NOS is activated by calcium-calmodulin binding, and the release of NO is within seconds.[124]

To date, three isoforms of NOS (iNOS, eNOS, nNOS) have been purified and cloned.* All the isoforms have recognition sites for calmodulin, but iNOS binds calmodulin tightly even in the absence of Ca^{2+}. Therefore exogenous Ca^{2+} is not required for calmodulin binding in iNOS, making activation of this isoform Ca^{2+} independent. All display consensus binding sites for flavin adenine dinucleotide, flavin mononucleotide, and nicotinamide adenine dinucleotide phosphate (NADPH). These multiple oxidative cofactor binding sites differentiate NOS from many oxidative enzymes because the latter use one electron transfer, whereas NOS uses several.

The presence of tightly bound heme has been described for all NOS isoforms, which is of interest for several reasons. First, if the enzyme is treated with carbon monoxide, the absorbance of light at 450 nm increases, indicating that NOS shares properties with the cytochrome P-450 enzyme. Second, the heme probably serves as the ultimate electron donor in the oxidation of the guanidine moiety of arginine. Finally, the only protein with substantial sequence homology to NOS is cytochrome P-450 reductase, an enzyme responsible for donating electrons in the drug-metabolizing P-450 enzymes.[22] Hence, it is possible that NOS is a fusion between a cytochrome P-450–like enzyme and cytochrome P-450 reductase.

*References 22, 100, 111, 112, 183.

Table 22-1. Similarities and differences of nitric oxide synthase

Constitutive	Inducible
Cytosolic*	Cytosolic
NADPH dependent	NADPH dependent
Dioxygenase	Dioxygenase
Inhibited by L-arginine analogues	Inhibited by L-arginine analogues
Ca^{2+}/calmodulin dependent	Ca^{2+}/calmodulin independent
Picomoles nitric oxide released	Nanomoles nitric oxide released
Short-lasting release	Long-lasting release
Unaffected by glucocorticoids	Induction inhibited by glucocorticoids

NADPH, Nicotinamide-adenine dinucleotide phosphate (reduced form). From Forstermann U et al: Calmodulin dependent endothelium derived relaxing factor/nitric oxide synthase activity is present in the particulate and cytosolic fractions of bovine aortic endothelial cells, *Proc Natl Acad Sci USA* 88:1788, 1991.
*Evidence for a particulate form of this enzyme in the vascular endothelium has been reported by Forstermann et al in 1991.

An interesting aspect to nNOS is the fact that this enzyme and NADPH-diaphorase co-localize in neuronal tissue and may be the same moiety. This has not been established for eNOS and iNOS, but preliminary work in our laboratory indicates that alveolar macrophages activated in vivo by pulmonary inflammation are producing NO but do not express NADPH-diaphorase. Lowenstein and colleagues[111] have stated that iNOS has 50% sequence identity with nNOS; hence, this uncoupling of iNOS and NADPH-diaphorase in the macrophage seems reasonable and may well represent yet another biochemical difference between type I and type II NOS.

Mechanism(s) of action on target cells

As stated previously, NO has a short biological half-life and is rapidly converted to biologically inert nitrites and nitrates. The mechanism(s) by which NO exerts its biological effects is not fully understood, but one common denominator of NO exposure is the labilization of iron stores in the target cells. This loss of iron has been correlated with activation of guanylate cyclase[143,144] as well as inhibition of mitochondrial respiration, *cis*-aconitase, and ribonucleotide reductase.[40,68,70] Whether NO interacts directly with the target enzymes or indirectly by binding to the cell membrane, which in turn activates a signal transduction pathway, is unclear.

In many instances, the release of NO is accompanied by the release of other reactive oxygen free radicals (described in Chapter 21). It has been reported that NO and O_2 can react forming peroxynitrite free radical ($ONOO^-$), which in turn can generate two additional free radicals (·NO and ·OH).[16] The potential biological consequences of this interaction are unclear. Because NO has been shown to be a scavenger of the superoxide free radical, it is possible that NO diminishes superoxide-induced damage. Alternatively, peroxynitrite and its products are more reactive than NO and may actually enhance NO-induced biological responses. The ultimate effect of this interaction may well depend on the target and the biological effect monitored.

Nitric oxide inhibitors and generators

As is discussed in the following section, NO has been implicated in a number of homeostatic processes and in the modulation of a variety of pathophysiological states. Regulation of NOS appears to be under stringent endogenous control by either calcium-calmodulin or cytokine-receptor binding. NO production in vivo can also be affected by administration of NOS inhibitors, which are for the most part arginine analogues or inhibitors of tetrahydrobiopterin, and NO generators.

Although types I and II NOS are biochemically distinct enzymes, the development of arginine analogues with specificity for either type has met with limited success. Table 22-2 lists some of the more well-characterized NOS inhibitors and the degree of specificity attributed to these inhibitors. As can be seen, the preponderance of these analogues has altered guanido amines, the amine subject to hydroxylation by NOS, and are competitive inhibitors of NOS.[130] Given the myriad of biological functions attributed to NO, the availability of selective NOS inhibitors would prove

quite valuable. For example, the administration of a nonspecific inhibitor of NOS during an inflammatory state may well inhibit overproduction of NO by the macrophage but may simultaneously result in hypertension owing to the inhibition of eNOS. To date, this quest has met with limited success.

The use of inhibitors of tetrahydrobiopterin synthesis has potential for selectivity with respect to inhibition of type I NOS versus type II. It has been demonstrated that an initial step in up-regulation of NO production by type I NOS is increased production of tetrahydrobiopterin, a necessary cofactor for NOS.[170] Inhibition of the increased production of tetrahydrobiopterin through inhibition of guanosine triphosphate (GTP) cyclohydrolase, the enzyme responsible for initiation of biopterin synthesis, or inhibition of hydropterin reductase, the enzyme responsible for maintenance of reduced pterin pools, would therefore have greater impact on type I NOS than type II.

To date, one of the most studied inhibitors of biopterin synthesis is 2,4-diamino-6-hydroxypyrimidine (DHAP), an inhibitor of GTP cyclohydrolase.[180] The effect of GTP cyclohydrolase inhibition on NO production by activated macrophages is unclear. Schoedon and colleagues[152] reported that DHAP abolished NO production in activated murine macrophages but did not report on the biological consequences of this inhibition. Sakai and colleagues[148a] reported the 6 hours of DHAP treatment decreased tetrahydrobiopterin levels by more than 90% in RAW 264 cells, a murine

Table 22-2. Inhibitors of nitric oxide synthase

Class	Constitutive nitric oxide synthase	Inducible nitric oxide synthase
Inhibitors of action		
Substrate analogues*	N^{ω}-nitro-L-arginine	N^{ω}-amino-L-arginine
	N^{ω}-iminoethyl-L-ornithine	N^{ω}-methyl-L-arginine
	N^{ω}-amino-L-arginine	N^{ω}-nitro-L-arginine
	N^{ω}-methyl-L-arginine	
	N^{ω}-nitro-L-arginine methyl ester	
Flavoprotein binders	Diphenylene iodonium	Diphenylene iodonium
		Iodonium diphenyl
		Di-2-thienyl iodonium
Calmodulin binders	Calcineurin	None described
	Trifluoroperazine	
	N-(4-aminobutyl)-5-chloro-2-naphthalenesulfonamide	
	N-(6-aminohexyl)-1-naphthalenesulfonamide	
Heme binder	Carbon monoxide	Carbon monoxide
Depleter of tetrahydrobiopterin		2,4-Diamino-6-hydroxypyrimidine†
Inhibitors of induction	None described	Corticosteroids
		TGF-β-1, -2, -3
		Interleukin-4
		Interleukin-10
		Macrophage deactivation factor†

TGF-β, Transforming growth factor beta.

From Nathan CF: Nitric oxide as a secretory product of mammalian cells, *FASEB J* 6:3051, 1992.

*Roughly, in decreasing order of potency. The ranking is complicated by the lack of a study comparing all agents in the same system.

†Inhibits guanosine triphosphate cyclohydrolase I.

macrophage cell line, yet the effects on NO production were small. After 12 hours of treatment, biopterin levels were decreased by 95%, yet NO production decreased by only 50%. The fact that the investigators used different cellular sources of NO production may account for this apparent discrepancy in results. Therefore, the effect of biopterin modulation may highly depend on the endogenous stores of this cofactor.

A number of organic compounds that donate NO have been used as vasodilators. These include nitroglycerin, sodium nitroprusside (SNP), sydoniminies, *S*-nitroso-*N*-acetylpenicillamine, and the so-called NONOates which are complexes of NO and nucleophiles.[116] The therapeutic use of NO gas is being developed for the treatment of diseases such as adult respiratory distress syndrome (ARDS).[147,148] Further discussion of the use of inhibitors and generators of NO in the treatment of disease is included in the following sections.

FUNCTION OF NITRIC OXIDE
Nitric oxide and vessel relaxation

The realization that NO regulated blood pressure was the consequence of two simultaneous but independent observations relating to endogenous vessel relaxation and that induced by drugs. Furchgott and Zawadzki[49] observed that blood vessels required endothelium to relax in response to acetylcholine and concluded that endothelial cells released a factor responsible for smooth muscle relaxation. The factor was named endothelium-derived relaxing factor (EDRF). At the same time, it was discovered that the beneficial effects of nitroglycerin were related to its ability to release NO and NO's subsequent effect on the up-regulation of cGMP, which causes smooth muscle cells to relax.[143,144] Although there continues to be controversy as to whether NO and EDRF are identical, it is generally accepted that they are similar in nature and have the same biological properties.[80] In part, this is supported by Sakuma and colleagues[149] who showed that EDRF relaxation of vessels is prevented by N^G-mono-methyl-arginine (NMA), a competitive inhibitor of NOS, suggesting that EDRF is formed from the guanido nitrogens of an endogenous pool of arginine. The mechanism by which EDRF causes vasodilation also involves cGMP accumulation in smooth muscle cells.[127,144] Responses to EDRF and nitrovasodilators are reversible by the guanylate cyclase inhibitor methylene blue and the NO scavenger hemoglobin.[124] Furthermore, oxyhemoglobin has vasoconstrictive activity on arterial smooth muscle[179] and thus inhibits the vasodilation caused by EDRF. Methemoglobin, however, proves less effective and has a lower affinity for NO than hemoglobin.[121] Thus the role of hemoglobin in preventing vasodilation by EDRF could be important physiologically during episodes of vascular hemorrhage.

Endothelin-3 (ET-3) is an agonist of NO, and receptors for ET-3 have been found on cultured bovine endothelial cells.[43] These studies demonstrate that ET-3 receptors are functionally coupled to phosphoinositide breakdown. Furthermore, ET-3 caused a dose-dependent production of intracellular cGMP, which was ablated by NMA and methylene blue, stimulated inositol triphosphate formation, and increased calcium levels in the endothelial cells. These effects were blocked by pertussis toxin, suggesting that NO synthesis is mediated by phosphoinositide breakdown by G-proteins. This study was the first to suggest that EDRF production by endothelial cells may be mediated by ET-3.

Inhibition of platelet aggregation is important to the maintenance of vascular integrity. Not surprisingly, it has been demonstrated that NO inhibits platelet aggregation by causing an elevation of cGMP in platelets.[72] These observations, taken in conjunction with other work demonstrating that inhibitors of NOS cause an increase in blood pressure, have led to the conclusion that NO works as an endogenous regulator of blood pressure.[6,146] In blood vessel disease, it is interesting to speculate about the role of NO in the formation and maintenance of plaques. It is possible that plaques prevent NO release and result in localized areas of hypertension.

Nitric oxide and the nervous system

The discovery of the ability of selected neurons to produce NO has led to a number of speculations regarding degenerative nerve diseases, such as Alzheimer's disease and Huntington's chorea. Garthwaite and colleagues[53] made the original observation that glutamate stimulates brain tissue to make NO. The binding of glutamate to its receptor, *N*-methyl-*D*-aspartate (NMDA), on neurons causes the opening of calcium channels, which in turn activate the constitutive form of NOS leading to NO production and subsequent cGMP increases. The cGMP causes the release of more glutamate, and NO is therefore also an autocrine factor. Several cell types have been shown to produce EDRF or EDRF-like molecules. Gorsky and colleagues[57] showed that neuroblastoma cells produce an EDRF-like factor, which requires superoxide dismutase. The fact that the production of this factor is dependent on L-arginine and NADPH, yet is inhibited by NMA, strongly implicates NO as the intermediate. Deguchi and Yoshioka[36] showed that cGMP formation in brain tissue requires L-arginine. All these observations inspired Bredt and Snyder[21] to look for NOS activity in response to glutamate in brain tissue. They observed NOS activity and found that NMDA caused an increase in cGMP, which was blocked by NMA. Neurons comprise 15% of brain cells and 85% of glial cells. NOS activity was limited to a select population of neurons, which included those in the hypothalamus, the adrenal gland neurons responsible for epinephrine release, and the intestinal neurons of the myenteric plexus responsible for peristalsis. In all, only 2% of the cerebral cortex neurons have NOS activity.

As previously suggested, there has been speculation as

to the relationship of NOS and diaphorase: both require the cofactor NADPH. A phenomenon with interesting implications is that neurons that stain positive for diaphorase are selectively resistant to neurodegenerative diseases. Because nNOS and diaphorase co-localize,[74] it is interesting to speculate that NO is responsible for neuronal death in adjacent cells, but somehow the neurons that make NO are resistant. In support of this, it has been shown that the neurotoxicity of NMDA is blocked by nitroarginine and hemoglobin, and neonatal rat microglial cells have been shown to secrete nitrite in response to lipopolysaccharide (LPS) and interferon-gamma (IFN-γ).[186] These observations have led Hartung and colleagues[64] to propose that the microglial cells are activated by autoreactive T cells to secrete NO, which in turn causes damage to myelin and nearby central nervous system cells. This is supported by the fact that peripheral blood mononuclear cells and neutrophils make large amounts of NO when they are cultured with antigen-stimulated myelin basic protein reactive T cells. Thus, evidence is growing to support the notion that NO plays a pivotal role in both the development of and the resistance to neurodegenerative diseases. This too lends itself to the possibility of treatments using selective inhibitors of NOS.

Role of nitric oxide in cell growth and differentiation

The observation by Stuehr and Marletta[161] that mice with genetically deficient macrophages could make nitrates if cells were provided with endotoxin and IFN-γ has led to a vast amount of research in the area of NO and the immune system. It is now recognized that one mechanism of macrophage-induced cytostasis is L-arginine dependent[69] and that macrophages make nitrite and nitrate.[42,68,161,162] The pattern of target cell damage by the effector molecules generated through this pathway is characteristic. Damage includes intracellular iron loss and resultant mitochondrial inhibition,[40,58,67] inhibition of aconitase,[41] and inhibition of DNA synthesis.[87,96]

Hibbs and colleagues[70] first described NO as a cytotoxic effector molecule produced by activated macrophages. The proposed targets of NO damage are iron sulfur proteins, which are sensitive to Fe-NO complex formation and subsequent loss of protein function.[122,145,150,182] In these studies, it was demonstrated that the reaction of NO with non-heme iron results in a drop in intracellular adenosine triphosphate (ATP) and the resultant destruction of iron-sulfur proteins by the Fe⁻-NO complexes, which results in growth inhibition. Many enzymes involved in mitochondrial respiration have Fe⁻-S centers. In a manner similar to endothelial cell production of EDRF, activated macrophages make NO from the terminal guanidine nitrogen atom of L-arginine.[70]

Hibbs and colleagues[69] were among the first to show that specific metabolic inhibition of respiration by cytotoxic activated macrophages is amino acid dependent, specifically L-arginine dependent. They also tested several L-arginine analogues to demonstrate that, characteristic of enzyme systems, there is substrate specificity; in fact, only L-homoarginine could substitute. Also, guanido methylated derivatives of L-arginine are inhibitors of this system. When this mechanism is activated, it competes with arginase for L-arginine. Arginase may therefore be a natural regulator of the L-arginine effector mechanism. Albina and colleagues[8] provide evidence to show that high levels of arginine inhibit macrophage activity in terms of interleukin-1 (IL-1) production and oxidative burst activity. They propose that as wounds heal and arginine levels go up, macrophage function is shut down, and further tissue damage is prevented.

Stuehr and Nathan[163] defined NO as a mediator of macrophage-induced cytostasis and mitochondrial respiratory inhibition in lymphoma cells. It is known that macrophages activated by LPS and IFN-γ are capable of inhibiting growth of numerous tumors and microbial targets.[2] Several macrophage products have been implicated but frequently cannot be quantitated and are assumed not responsible for damage in many models. These include H_2O_2 tumor necrosis factor (TNF), and IL-1.[129,137,174] These investigators also established that exposures to authentic NO but neither $NaNO_3$ nor $NaNO_2$ were cytostatic to L1210 murine leukemia cells, strongly suggesting that NO played the important role. The cytostasis was measurable after 8 hours, lasted about 24 hours, and was related to inhibition of complex I and II, thus establishing the link between inhibition of mitochondrial respiration and NO production by activated macrophages.

Keller and colleagues[89] investigated whether NO production by activated mononuclear phagocytes was related to thymidine release in co-cultured target cells. They noted that the medium needed to be changed every 24 hours, probably owing to arginine depletion, and that the amount of nitrites produced correlated with the amount of thymidine released. They showed that for a variety of experimental models (meaning different macrophage activating factors), the presence of a high level of arginine enhanced activity, suggesting that arginine and its metabolites play an important role in tumor cytotoxicity.

Stuehr and colleagues[164] used a bioassay based on smooth muscle relaxation to measure NO release from murine macrophages. Ferrous heme proteins have a high affinity for NO and block vasorelaxation.[121,164,184] Macrophages release the NO compound for a longer time than endothelial cells but appear to have a limited storage capacity for arginine. Therefore, NO production may be limited by arginine availability. The fact that NO may also regulate smooth muscle tone during inflammatory or immune responses suggests that the macrophage may be the regulator of regional blood flow and might also regulate, in lymphocytes, activation of guanylate cyclase or inactivation of Fe-S enzymes and thereby contribute to immunosuppression. Lancaster and colleagues[101] have suggested that iron-sulfur clusters may be the target for immune cells in mediating various cytotoxic functions based on studies using TNF and subsequent identification of Fe-NO signals in the target cell.

Fehsel and colleagues[44] demonstrated that exposing islet cell suspensions to SNP or activated macrophages causes DNA strand breaks, which, for the macrophage, are inhibited by NMA. Strand breaks occurred within 1 hour and preceded cell lysis. The breaks were not changed by inhibitors of endogenous endonucleases; therefore it can be concluded that NO mediates DNA damage. Nicotinamide and 3-aminobenzamide suppress the cytotoxic action of chemically released NO. Both inhibit poly(ADP-ribose)polymerase and prevent nicotinamide-adenine dinucleotide (NAD) depletion during DNA repair. These results suggest that the DNA damage is direct and not mediated by the endonucleases, which have been reported to be needed for apoptosis.

POTENTIAL ROLES IN ENVIRONMENTALLY INDUCED DISEASES
Inflammation

Mediators. NO is a short-lived lipophilic molecule, which enables cells in close proximity to communicate with each other. This communication is likely to be via the second messenger cGMP. NO also increases cGMP in the cell of origin and may therefore stimulate its own production through the phosphorylation of NOS.[23,120] A number of cell types involved in both the nonspecific and the specific immune response are capable of making or responding to NO. Human neutrophils and macrophages contain guanylate cyclase which increases cGMP levels significantly in response to immune reactants. Increases in cGMP are associated with lysosomal enzyme release and phagocytosis.[82,84,156] The NO produced by one cell can elicit complementary actions in other cells via cGMP. An example of this is the concerted cell effort required for an inflammatory response.

Inflammation can be described as the process in vascular tissues in which fluid and cells accumulate in response to various stimuli. The classic observation first made by Cornelius Celsus in the first century is widely quoted today: *"Rubor et tumor cum calore et dolore"*—redness and swelling with heat and pain. All four cardinal signs can be explained by the increased vascular permeability we now recognize to be common to all inflammatory processes.

Vane and Botting[175] describe inflammation as being caused by the release of a variety of chemicals, such as prostaglandins, leukotrienes, histamine, bradykinin, platelet activating factor, and IL-1, from damaged tissues and migrating cells. A number of these and other products are made by the macrophage, which is a pivotal cell in the process of inflammation. Several of these factors are capable of inducing either cytostasis or cytolysis in target cells. Secreted products include IL-1,[155,185] arginase,[35] neutral proteases,[3] TNF,[115] reactive oxygen species,[131] metal chela-

tors,[67] and lipoxygenase derivatives.[139] The mechanisms that selectively activate the production of these agents are unknown.

The role of toxic, reactive molecules in the induction and maintenance of inflammation is an extensively pursued area of research. Reactive oxygen intermediates (ROI) and reactive nitrogen intermediates (RNI) are generated in response to various membrane stimuli and are thought to be important in host defense against tumors, microbes, carcinogens, and chronic destructive disorders. Similar to the ROI model, it has been shown that RNI are quickly detoxified. NO reacts readily with molecular oxygen to yield nitrogen dioxide, which ultimately undergoes a hydrolysis reaction to form nitrite and nitrate.[117] Ding and colleagues[38] showed that two main products of macrophage activation, ROI and RNI, are generated by independently regulated pathways. For example, NMA abolishes RNI but not ROI; casein-elicited macrophages make ROI but not RNI if triggered by LPS; LPS enhances IFN-γ induced RNI but suppresses IFN-γ induced ROI. Thus it would appear that RNI can be released in the absence of a triggering agent, whereas ROI requires that agent.

Pulmonary inflammation. Macrophages that have been stimulated have cytostatic activity against normal and transformed tissues.[88] Evidence has been presented to suggest that macrophages are injurious to lung tissue in both acute and chronic pulmonary disease, which is often manifested in response to environmental toxins. In an inflamed lung, edema develops in the alveolar space, which may play a role in alveolar macrophage (AM) activation.[55] This hypothesis is substantiated by data showing that AM taken from smokers and people with lower respiratory tract infections could be triggered by PMA to release ROI in greater amounts than similarly stimulated AM from healthy nonsmokers. The oxidants produced by pulmonary inflammatory cells may contribute to emphysema by both direct tissue toxicity from ROI and inhibition of alpha$_1$-antitrypsin, which normally protects the lung from proteolytic damage.[60]

Acute respiratory infections are the leading cause of morbidity and mortality in the very young and the very old.[106] The characteristic lesion in emphysema is respiratory bronchiolitis marked by pigmented AM, denuded epithelium, and progressive cellular influx leading to fibrosis and connective tissue deposition. This has prompted investigators to suggest a role for the macrophage in emphysema.[30,135] Hoidal and colleagues[73] suggest that the release of ROI may be responsible for initiating the lung damage.

Respiratory distress syndrome caused by hyperoxia treatment results in a major insult to the alveolar capillary endothelium. Hyperoxic pulmonary damage is characterized initially by interstitial and alveolar edema. The endothelial cell damage, which results in vascular leaking, may initiate macrophage activation.[177] Superoxide radicals, thought to be responsible for endothelial cell damage, are potent agents produced by single-electron reduction of oxygen.[31] Type I alveolar cells are destroyed, and type II cells proliferate. Destruction of type I cells is irreversible and results in protein flow into the alveolar sacs as well as hyaline membrane formation, which leads to cell death.[5,177]

The pathological features associated with ARDS are based on the disruption of normal fluid exchange in the lungs and diffuse alveolar capillary injury brought on by inflammatory cell influx, which causes interstitial and alveolar edema.[26,134] Furthermore, higher levels of fibronectin and AM derived growth factor have been demonstrated in AM taken from diseased lungs.[154]

A role for NO and NOS inhibitors has been demonstrated. Systemic administration of endotoxin to rats mimics ARDS in humans. Rats were administered endotoxin, and NOS activity was measured in the lung and liver. NOS activity peaked at 12 hours and had returned to basal levels by 24 hours, whereas myeloperoxidase activity peaked at 6 hours in the lung only and was not elevated in the liver.[1] These results suggest that NO contributes to the injury of the lung following endotoxin administration. In contrast, a pilot clinical study conducted by Rossaint and colleagues[147,148] showed that long-term inhalation of low levels of NO assisted the lung in healing and may improve treatment of patients with acute respiratory failure. These conclusions were based on the observation that inhalation of NO reduced pulmonary arterial pressure and improved blood oxygenation.

In another model, Sibille and Reynolds[154] used intratracheal instillation of immune complexes to initiate a pulmonary response and found that AM harvested from these lungs released ROI. In addition, the AM inhibited fibroblast growth and injured the matrix by releasing neutral proteases. AM obtained from the immune complex–treated animals were more in number, spontaneously released O_2^-, and made more O_2^- in response to PMA than control macrophages.[154] Johnson and colleagues[85] demonstrated that the AM from diseased lungs of smokers had secreted elastolytic and collagenolytic enzymes in significant amounts. Mulligan and colleagues[126] studied immune complex–induced injury of rat lung and dermal vasculature and found that it was L-arginine dependent and inhibitable by NMA. The protection afforded by NMA was not related to decreased recruitment of neutrophils because this number did not change. Furthermore, nitrates and nitrites were found in the bronchoalveolar lavage of animals undergoing the immune complex deposition. It has been suggested that the tissue injury associated with NO may be attributed to NO directly or its derivatives, peroxynitrite and the hydroxyl radical.[16]

Diffuse pulmonary alveolitis culminating in chronic fibrosis has been reported following exposure to a variety of agents, including paraquat, bleomycin, organic dusts, and hyperoxia.[4,14,29,62] Regardless of the nature of the initial insult, one of the first observations in the lungs is increased vascular permeability.[55] Various secretory products of activated AM have been implicated as possible mediators of pulmonary damage, including ROI,[28] TNF,[17,103,140] arginase,[35] neutral proteases[3] and NO.[9,38,70,163]

We have been using the intratracheal model for bleomycin-induced pulmonary fibrosis to study the role of the AM in this disease process. The pulmonary response to bleomycin can be separated into two distinct phases.[133,173] An acute inflammatory response occurs during which time inflammatory cells and edema are present in the alveolar space, followed by a chronic phase characterized by resolution of the acute inflammation and deposition of fibrotic tissue. Using this model, we have demonstrated that AM activated by bleomycin-induced lung damage caused cytostasis in co-cultured murine leukemia L1210 cells.[75,76] The consequences of this cytostasis included inhibition of both DNA synthesis and aconitase activity, as have been described for other target cells exposed to activated macrophages.[58,59,187] We established that the production of NO, measured as nitrite, by AM correlated with cytostatic activity.[76] Furthermore, we demonstrated that the NO was the result of an L-arginine dependent effector mechanism, which could be inhibited by the substrate-specific analogue NMA. In addition, red blood cells (RBC) in the co-culture inhibited the cytostatic activity and reduced the amount of measurable nitrite. We have also reported that the hemoglobin isolated from RBC co-cultured with AM has a significant shift in spectral characteristics suggestive of hemoglobin nitrosylation.[77] This observation is substantiated by electron pair resonance spectroscopy generated spectra, which are characteristic of hemoglobin-NO. These results indicate that the mechanism of RBC protection against AM cytostasis is through hemoglobin absorption of NO. Hence, it can be concluded that NO production is a common denominator in pulmonary inflammation resulting from a variety of agents.

Nitric oxide, inflammation, and edema. The similarities between EDRF and NO produced by activated macrophages is striking and raises many interesting questions about the link between inflammation and edema. It has long been known that EDRF is inhibitable by oxyhemoglobin and to a lesser extent by methemoglobin;[72,119,179] thus the role of hemoglobin in preventing vasodilation by EDRF could be important physiologically during hemorrhage. Similarly, there may be a role for hemoglobin in limiting damage to surrounding tissue during episodes of inflammation. One consequence of hemorrhage into an area of inflammation may be down-regulation of activated macrophages and subsequent prevention of extensive tissue damage. Furthermore, the resolution of the acute inflammatory response may be modified by the presence of blood in the area. Taken together, we hypothesize that the down-regulation of NO production by AM permits up-regulation of another process in the AM, which is important in the fibrotic phase that follows.

Ialenti et al[81] used two competitive inhibitors of NOS, L-NAME and L-NMA, on carrageenan-induced increase in vascular permeability in rat skin and in dextran and carrageenan–induced paw edema. L-NAME and NMA dose dependently inhibited increases in vascular permeability and edema, whereas L-arginine increased the inflammatory response and overcame L-NAME and NMA. Because dexamethasone-treated rats had an L-arginine-enhanced early but not late phase edema, they concluded that NO is released at the site of acute inflammation and modulates edema. Dexamethasone inhibits the inducible but not the constitutive form of NOS; therefore the constitutive form may play a relevant role in early inflammation, whereas the inducible form is important in later stages. These findings suggest that the inducible form may therefore be responsible for maintaining inflammation and thus may lead to chronic inflammation, further implicating NO as an important component of the inflammatory response.

Kubes and colleagues[99] showed that leukocyte adhesion in cat mesentery is modulated by NO. They did this by superfusing a mesenteric preparation with L-NAME or L-NMA and, finding that this caused increased leukocyte adhesion and emigration, and reduced the venular shear rate. Furthermore, the L-NMA preparation caused an up-regulation of CD11/CD18, leukocyte adhesion molecules. These results suggest that NO impairment leads to leukocyte adhesion and emigration, which is characteristic of inflammation. Because adhesion of neutrophils to the microvascular endothelium is the rate-limiting step in the initiation and maintenance of acute inflammation, the presence of constitutively expressed NO may have to be overcome for leukocyte emigration to occur. A number of investigators have shown that oxygen radicals increase adhesion[37,98,168] and that this induction of adhesion is endothelium dependent. This may suggest that superoxides inactivate endothelium-derived NO to allow adhesion. Evidence for this is provided by the fact that NO does prevent adhesion of platelets to endothelium and inhibits neutrophil aggregation in vivo.[142] These studies therefore suggest that NO production by the endothelium down-regulates acute inflammation, and therefore the presence of NO in the vasculature is a necessary normal control on inflammation.

Nitric oxide, cytokines, immune system, and wound repair. A role for NO in the induction and maintenance of inflammation is substantiated by a number of observations that demonstrate that NO is made by several cells involved in an inflammatory response, that NO has growth inhibitory effects on cells of the immune system,[78] and that production of NO appears to be influenced by a number of cytokines. Several investigators have suggested a role for NO in the regulation of lymphocyte proliferation. Hoffman and colleagues[71] have demonstrated that the addition of NMA to a con-A stimulated rat spleen cell culture results in allospecific proliferation and cytotoxic T cell induction. These studies were confirmed by Langrehr and col-

leagues[102] who suggested that NO production by the macrophage inhibited development of allosensitivity by the T cell. Interestingly, Takagi and colleagues[169] showed that T cell depletion of a con-A stimulated rat spleen cell culture resulted in inhibition of NO production. Similar results were found when they added anti-IFN-γ antibodies to the culture. They suggested that NO production depended on T cell production of IFN-γ. Several other investigators have shown that cytokines such as IFN-γ, IL-1, and TNF are capable of inducing NO production in both macrophages and endothelial cells. Taken together, these findings would suggest a feedback mechanism, whereby lymphocytes in the area would produce cytokines, which in turn would stimulate NO production by macrophages, which would prevent allospecific proliferation by lymphocytes. This may be one of the mechanisms by which the macrophage controls the response to acute damage. During an acute inflammatory response, considerable damage occurs to normal tissue in the local environment. It is possible that secretion of NO by macrophages recruited to the site inhibits clonal expansion to prevent a response to neoantigens. Concurrently the lymphocyte is still able to produce cytokines, which in the local environment augment NO production by the macrophage. Because these cytokines are hormonal in nature, it would seem logical that they would also have effects distal to the site of damage, such as being signals for tissue remodeling when the acute inflammation subsides.

Langrehr and colleagues[102] reported that NO may regulate the in vivo response to allograft by initiating a response and then limiting proliferation. They further speculate that the accessory cell function of the macrophage may be altered in these circumstances. We have reported that macrophages taken from inflamed lungs secrete NO and have increased expression of the Ia antigen known to be important in presentation of processed antigen to lymphocytes.[92] We therefore speculate that NO serves not to suppress the immune response but rather to limit that response by controlling clonal expansion at the site of initiation. This may be a physiological mechanism by which the host protects normal tissue.

The influence of cytokines on the expression of NO is a well-documented phenomenon. Forstermann and colleagues[47] used the murine, macrophage-like cell line, RAW 262.7, to show that LPS and IFN-γ induced NOS whereas transforming growth factor beta 1 (TGF-β) inhibited the induction of NOS. Assoian and colleagues[12] showed that macrophages secrete TGF-β when they are activated. TGF-β is made by platelets, macrophages, and lymphocytes, all of which are involved in inflammation and repair.[12,25,86] TGF-β stimulates collagen and fibronectin,[134] suggesting that it may be the endogenous mediator of repair. Support for this is that TGF-β has effects on proliferation of smooth muscle cells[11] and in other proliferative diseases.[159]

Another murine macrophage-like cell line, J774, makes

NO and NOS in response to IFN-γ and LPS.[33] This is inhibited by interleukin-10 (IL-10) if IL-10 was used as a pretreatment. Simultaneous treatment with IL-10 or adding it after the stimulators had no effect. This suggests that IL-10, from helper T lymphocyte 2 (Th-2), antagonizes IFN-γ, a product of helper T lymphocyte 1 (Th-1). Th-1 make interleukin-2 (IL-2) and IFN-γ, whereas Th-2 make interleukins 4, 5, and 10 (IL-4, IL-5, IL-10).[125] These subsets of T lymphocytes work as antagonists to balance the immune response to infectious and autoimmune diseases.[107,110,141] An example of this is leishmaniasis, in which Th-1 cells are host protective and Th-2 are disease promoting.[66,153] IFN-γ inhibits proliferation of Th-2 cells,[51] and IL-4 and IL-10 inhibit IFN-γ production by Th-1.[46,50] IL-4 inhibits murine and human macrophage activation by IFN-γ.[104] IL-4 inhibits NOS.[109] Other functions of IL-10 include enhancement of mast cell growth in combination with IL-3 or IL-4,[172] support of growth of thymocytes with IL-2 and IL-4,[114] increased major histocompatibility complex (MHC) class II expression, and viability of B cells.[56] It may be concluded from these studies that IFN-γ promotes expression of NO, and IL-4, and IL-10 prevent expression of NO.

Heck and colleagues[65] showed that primary human keratinocytes and a mouse keratinocyte cell line make NO and hydrogen peroxide in response to IFN-γ and LPS or TNF-α. These mediators also caused growth inhibition of keratinocytes, which was reversible by NMA. Epidermal growth factor (EGF) promotes wound healing by stimulating cell proliferation and antagonizes NO and hydrogen peroxide production by keratinocytes. NO may therefore control cellular proliferation during wound healing, and EGF may regulate production of these radicals to facilitate resolution of inflammation following wounding. These findings suggest that NO is proinflammatory at the site of inflammation, and for the inflammation to resolve, NO must be downregulated. Potentially, these complex interactions are regulated by cytokines. EGF could down-regulate NOS by phosphorylating the tyrosine on the NOS, causing downregulation, or inhibiting induction of NOS.[39,136] The localized release of growth factors by macrophages at the site of tissue injury stimulates regeneration of damaged tissue.[105]

Evidence is mounting to suggest that inflammation of liver is also mediated, in part, by NO. Altered hepatic function occurs during trauma, infection, and exposure to some environmental toxins. A widely reported alteration is the expression of the hepatic acute phase proteins.[93] Severe liver damage or failure happens if the underlying cause is not treated;[24] however, the mechanisms of liver failure induction are not well understood. A number of investigators have proposed that Kupffer cells exposed to inflammatory stimuli in the portal circulation mediate alterations in the function of adjacent hepatocytes. Hepatocytes make NO, and this is associated with a decrease in protein synthe-sis.[160] The results suggest that inhibition of protein synthesis was unrelated to mitochondrial respiration inhibition and therefore may not be related to NO. Geller and colleagues[54] measured NOS messenger RNA (mRNA) in rat hepatocytes (single band at 4.5 kb) and saw maximal up-regulation with a combination of TNF, IL-1, IFN-γ, and LPS, which peaked at 6 to 8 hours poststimulation with a 25% decline by 24 hours. TNF and IL-1 were able to induce message by themselves, but there is significant synergy with the combination of TNF, IL-1, and IFN-γ. Increased message correlated with NO release and cGMP release into the supernate. Dexamethasone and cycloheximide inhibited induction in a dose-dependent fashion, suggesting the inducible form of the enzyme was responsible for the production of NO. They also demonstrated that NMA had no effect on mRNA but did inhibit NO release and that hepatocytes produce NO in vivo during chronic inflammation. Billiar and colleagues[20] showed that NO causes a decrease in protein synthesis in hepatocytes that is not related to cGMP. They hypothesize that NO protects liver from damage via interaction with platelets or with superoxide molecules.

Nitric oxide and inflammation of the gut. Chronic inflammation of the gut is the end result of a number of gastroenteric diseases. A number of these diseases are autoimmune in nature, and a cause for their initiation remains speculative. Several lines of investigation point to a role for NO in the initiation and maintenance of chronic inflammatory bowel disorders. Grisham and colleagues[61] showed that neutrophils in the gut make NO. In ulcerative colitis, infiltration of a large number of neutrophils into the mucosal interstitium is a hallmark. NOS is induced in neutrophils during extravasation therefore the control mechanism is different than that of macrophages. Miller and colleagues[123] used luminal lavages from rabbits, piglets, and guinea pigs with normal and injured small intestine. Nitrite, protein, and granulocyte infiltration were measured. In both acute and chronic ileitis, nitrite levels were increased as were protein levels and myeloperoxidase activity. L-NAME reversed the epithelial permeability, so nitrites are a useful indicator of gut injury, and NO may contribute to functional repair of the epithelial barrier under acute conditions. Nitrite levels are up in chronic intestinal inflammation in all species and models studied; therefore an increase in NO is a common response to gut injury. NO levels paralleled well-accepted indices of intestinal inflammation, protein, and myeloperoxidase activity. MacNaughton and colleagues[113] showed that NO (provided by SNP) protected rat gastric mucosa from ethanol damage. Endothelin-1, an antagonist of NO, is a vasoconstrictor and has been shown to be ulcerogenic to the gastric mucosa.[176] Maintenance of gastric mucosal blood flow is crucial to determining mucosal integrity. Severe, chronic inflammation of the colon is associated with increased risk of colon cancer.[27,95,178] Nitrosamines have been shown to activate oncogenes and may therefore give rise to tumors.[15] The by-products of NO, the nitrogen dioxides and tetraoxides, are known to have the ability to nitrosate amines and may therefore act as a cancer-promoting agent in chronic inflammation of the gut.[118] Hence the investigation of the clinical use of NO inhibitors in the treatment of chronic inflammatory disease of the bowel is warranted.

Hypotension

Endotoxemia. Sepsis is a consequence of maladies such as surgery, injury, and immune deficiency. The resulting systemic bacterial infection causes a heterogeneous pattern of vasodilation or vasoconstriction depending on the organ under study. The cumulative effect is systemic hypotension due to a fall in total peripheral vascular resistance and a concomitant regional maldistribution of blood flow and localized tissue hypoxia. It has been known for some time that LPS produced by gram-negative bacteria is an important component in this disease state. Exactly how LPS induces this vascular response remains obscure, but reports have implicated NO as an important mediator of LPS-induced loss of vascular tone.[181] Supporting evidence includes the findings that urinary nitrates are elevated in endotoxemia, endotoxin has been shown to induce NOS in a number of tissues, and NOS inhibitors can block endotoxin-induced hypotension.[171] Further evidence supporting the role of NO in this disease process is the fact that cytokines known to be induced by LPS, including IL-1 and TNF, have also been shown to induce NOS synthesis either alone or in combination with LPS.

The actual role of NO in determining the ultimate outcome of endotoxic shock is a point of debate. Inhibition of NOS by arginine analogues reverses much, but not necessarily all, of the loss of peripheral resistance associated with endotoxemia. Whether this is a therapeutic advantage, however, is controversial. Such intervention has been shown to increase the lethality, increase endothelium-dependent vasoconstriction, and enhance damage to other tissues, such as liver and intestine.[19,34,79] Hence, although there is reversal of systemic hypotension, the disease process is not necessarily altered.

There are several possible explanations for the apparent increase in endotoxemic damage following NOS inhibition. Parker and Adams[138a] have shown that NAME unmasks a thromboxane A_2–mediated vasoconstrictor action of adenosine diphosphate (ADP), which could in effect increase localized tissue hypoxia. Harbrecht and colleagues[63] reported that NOS inhibition promoted intrahepatic thrombosis and enhanced oxygen radical–mediated liver damage. They suggested that NO was important in preventing thrombosis and serving as a free radical scavenging agent, which would therefore actually be protective in endotoxemia. An interesting study reported by Nava and colleagues[132] demonstrated that although 10 mg/kg NMA given in conjunction with LPS prevented the LPS-induced hypotension and elevated levels of alanine aminotransferase, 300 mg/kg NMA

exacerbated LPS toxicity. These results indicate that the difference between a beneficial and adverse effect of NOS inhibitors may well be related to the degree of enzyme inhibition. NO is clearly an important component in endotoxemia, but whether it plays a beneficial or detrimental role (or perhaps both) has yet to be conclusively established.

Cytokine-induced hypotension. There has been interest in the use of biological response modifiers for the treatment of cancer. Treatments have included the use of IFN-γ and IL-2. Determining the efficacy of these treatments, however, has been hampered by the life-threatening toxicity of hypotension. A number of investigators have been exploring the use of NOS inhibitors to counter the hypotension and, it is hoped, enhance the therapeutic effects of cytokine therapy by allowing higher doses to be administered. It has been demonstrated that NOS inhibitors are capable of reversing the hypotensive problems associated with septic shock and cytokine immunotherapies.[91,151] Kilbourn and Belloni[90] showed that IFN-γ in combination with TNF, IL-1, or endotoxin induced murine brain endothelial cells to secrete nitrites dependent on L-arginine and blocked by NMA. Endothelial cells can produce NO in response to immunomodulators and may play a role in development of hypotension in patients treated with TNF or interleukins. Therefore the use of NMA in immunotherapies may be to enhance the antitumor effects by allowing the administration of higher doses. The use of NOS modulators in the treatment of vessel disease is thus quite promising.

Organophosphate and carbamate insecticide poisoning. The organophosphates and carbamates serve an important role in controlling insect infestation in agribusiness as well as urban pest control. Both classes of insecticides act through inhibition of acetylcholinesterase enzymes resulting in increased synaptic residency times of acetylcholine. This causes overactivity of the cholinergic components of the autonomic nervous system, inhibition of myoneural junctions in skeletal muscle, and interference of central nervous system synapse transmission.[128] The manifestations of toxicity are related to acetylcholine buildup and include meiosis, blurred vision, chest tightness, increased bronchial secretion, wheezing, and pulmonary edema.[13] Because acetylcholine is a stimulant of constitutively expressed NOS, it is likely that NO plays a role in mediating some of the symptoms.[45] Thus a role for NOS inhibitors in the management of acute poisoning may have therapeutic advantage.

SUMMARY

NO has been extensively studied during the last decade, as evidenced by the number of publications related to this molecule.[32] The use of molecular biology techniques has led to a rapid understanding of the regulatory mechanisms involved in the expression of NO. This in turn has given rise to an explosion in the development of NOS modifiers and NO producers. The promise of these drugs in the treatment and management of an array of physiological disorders is staggering. Yet the physiological role of NO remains an intense area of controversy. As discussed throughout this chapter, there are few sites in the body devoid of NO-producing capability, and a number of homeostatic mechanisms, such as maintenance of vessel tone, neuronal signaling, and immune system functioning, appear to be intimately linked to the presence and absence of this molecule. In all cases, NO seems to have both advantageous and deleterious effects. The outcome may be attributed to the dose of NO and the cell types involved. For example, although NO appears to be a novel signal molecule in neurotransmission, overstimulation may result in destruction of nerve cells, leading to neurodegenerative diseases. Similarly, basal expression of NO is required for the maintenance of blood vessel tone and too much or too little lead to hypotension or hypertension. A number of environmental toxins can lead to acute or chronic inflammation and blood vessel disease. Presumably, NO plays a role in the outcomes of environmental poisoning; however, it is unclear as to whether this is positive or negative. Does the activation of NO production give rise to the physiological symptoms associated with some environmental toxins, or is the activation crucial to the host's ability to survive the consequences of environmental toxins? Much remains unresolved about this highly reactive, tiny, yet powerful molecule.

REFERENCES

1. Abate JA, Albina JE: *Temporal expression of nitric oxide synthase in post-endotoxin rat lung.* In Moncada S et al, editors: *Biology of nitric oxide,* vol 2, London, 1992, Portland Press, pp 197-199.
2. Adams DO, Hamilton TA: The cell biology of macrophage activation, *Annu Rev Immunol* 2:283, 1984.
3. Adams DO et al: Effector mechanisms of cytolytically activated macrophages. II. Secretion of a cytolytic factor by activated macrophages and its relationship to secreted neutral proteases, *J Immunol* 124:293, 1980.
4. Adamson IYR: Drug-induced pulmonary fibrosis, *Environ Health Perspect* 55:25, 1984.
5. Adamson IYR, Bowden DH, Wyatt JP: Oxygen poisoning in mice: ultrastructural and surfactant studies during exposure and recovery, *Arch Pathol* 90:463, 1970.
6. Aisaka K et al: N^G-Methylarginine, an inhibitor of endothelium-derived nitric oxide synthesis, is a potent pressor agent in the guinea pig: does nitric oxide regulate blood pressure in vivo? *Biochem Biophys Res Commun* 160:881, 1989.
7. Albina JE et al: Regulation of macrophage functions by L-arginine, *J Exp Med* 169:1021, 1989.
8. Albina JE et al: Regulation of macrophage physiology by L-arginine: role of the oxidative L-arginine deiminase pathway, *J Immunol,* 143:3641, 1989.
9. Amber IJ et al: The L-arginine dependent effector mechanism is induced in murine adenocarcinoma cells by culture supernatant from cytotoxic activate macrophages, *J Leukocyte Biol* 43:187, 1988.
10. Appels B et al: Spontaneous cytotoxic of macrophage against pancreatic islet cells, *J Immunol* 142:3803, 1989.
11. Assoian RK, Sporn MB: Type beta transforming growth factor in human platelets: release during platelet degranulation and action on vascular smooth muscle cells, *J Cell Biol* 102:1217, 1986.
12. Assoian RK et al: Transforming growth factor beta in human plate

13. lets. Identification of a major storage site, purification and characterization, *J Biol Chem* 258:7155, 1983.
14. Baker EL et al: Epidemic malathon poisoning in Pakestan malaria workers, *Lancet* 1:31, 1978.
15. Barry BE, Crapo JD: Patterns of accumulation of platelets and neutrophils in rat lungs during exposure to 100% and 85% oxygen, *Am Rev Respir Dis* 132:548, 1985.
16. Bartsch HE, Hietanen E, Malaveille C: Carcinogenic nitrosamines: free radical aspects of their action, *Free Radic Biol Med* 7:637, 1989.
17. Beckman JS et al: Apparent hydroxyl radical production by peroxynitrite: implications for endothelial injury from nitric oxide and superoxide, *Proc Natl Acad Sci USA* 87:1620, 1990.
18. Beutler B, Cerami A: Tumor necrosis cachexia, shock and inflammation: a common mediator, *Ann Rev Biochem* 57:505, 1988.
19. Billiar TR et al: An L-arginine dependent mechanism mediates Kupffer cell influences on hepatocyte protein synthesis in vitro, *J Exp Med* 169:1467, 1989.
20. Billiar TR et al: *Inhibition of L-arginine metabolism by N^G-monomethyl-L-arginine in vivo promotes hepatic damage in response to lipopolysaccharide.* In Moncada S, Higgs EA, editors: *Nitric oxide from L-arginine: a bioregulatory system,* Amsterdam, 1990, Elsevier.
21. Billiar TR et al: A role for inducible nitric oxide biosynthesis in the liver in inflammation and in the allogeneic immune response, *J Lab Clin Med* 120:192, 1992.
22. Bredt DS, Snyder SH: Nitric oxide: A novel neuronal messenger, *Neuron* 8:8, 1992.
23. Bredt DS et al: Cloned and expressed nitric oxide synthase structurally resembles cytochrome P450 reductase, *Nature* 351:714, 1991.
24. Brotherton AFA: Induction of prostacyclin biosynthesis is closely associated with increased guanosine 3',5'-cyclic monophosphate accumulation in cultured human endothelium, *J Clin Invest* 78:1253, 1986.
25. Cerra FB: Hypermetabolism, organ failure and metabolic support, *Surgery* 101:1, 1987.
26. Childs CB et al: Serum contains a platelet-derived transforming growth factor, *Proc Natl Acad Sci USA,* 79:5312, 1982.
27. Christner P et al: Collagenase in the lower respiratory tract of patients with adult respiratory distress syndrome, *Am Rev Respir Dis* 131:690, 1985.
28. Collins RH, Feldman M, Fordtran JS: Colon cancer, dysplasia and surveillance in patients with ulcerative colitis: a critical review, *N Engl J Med* 316:1654, 1987.
29. Conkey NS et al: Bleomycin increases superoxide anion generation by pig peripheral alveolar macrophages, *Mol Pharmacol* 30:48, 1986.
30. Cooper JAD Jr, Zitnik RJ, Matthay RA: Mechanisms of drug-induced pulmonary disease, *Ann Rev Med* 39:395, 1988.
31. Cosio M et al: The relationship between structural changes in small airways and pulmonary function tests, *N Engl J Med* 298:1277, 1977.
32. Crapo JD, Tierney DF: Superoxide dismutase and pulmonary oxygen toxicity, *Am J Physiol* 226:1401, 1974.
33. Culotta E, Koshland DE Jr: NO news is good news, *Science,* 258:1862, 1992.
34. Cunha FQ, Moncada S, Liew FY: Interleukin-10 inhibits the induction of nitric oxide synthase by interferon-γ in murine macrophages, *Biochem Biophys Res Commun* 182:1155, 1992.
35. Curran RD et al: Hepatocytes produce nitrogen oxides from L-arginine in response to inflammatory products from Kupffer cells, *J Exp Med* 170:1769, 1989.
36. Currie GA: Activated macrophages kill tumor cells by releasing arginase, *Nature* 273:758, 1978.
37. Deguchi T, Yoshioka M: L-arginine identified as an endogenous activator for soluble guanylate cyclase from neuroblastoma cells, *J Biol Chem* 257:10147, 1982.

37. Del Maestro RF, Planker M, Arfors KE: Evidence for the participation of superoxide anion radical in altering the adhesive interaction between granulocytes and endothelium, in vivo, *Int J Microcirc Clin Exp* 1:105, 1982.

38. Ding AH, Nathan CF, Stuehr DJ: Release of reactive nitrogen intermediates and reactive oxygen intermediates from mouse peritoneal macrophages, *J Immunol* 141:2407, 1988.

39. Ding AH et al: Macrophage deactivating factor and transforming growth factors-beta 1, -beta 2 and -beta 3 inhibit induction of macrophage nitrogen oxide synthesis by interferon-gamma, *J Immunol* 145:940, 1990.

40. Drapier J-C, Hibbs JB Jr: Injury of neoplastic cells by murine macrophages leads to inhibition of mitochondrial respiration, *J Clin Invest* 65:357, 1980.

41. Drapier J-C, Hibbs JB Jr: Murine cytotoxic activated macrophages inhibit aconitase in tumor cells, *J Clin Invest* 78:790, 1986.

42. Drapier J-C, Hibbs JB Jr: Differentiation of murine macrophages to express nonspecific cytotoxicity for tumor cells results in L-arginine dependent inhibition of mitochondrial iron-sulfur enzymes in the macrophage effector cells, *J Clin Invest* 140:2829, 1988.

43. Emori T et al: Endothelin-3 stimulates production of endothelium-derived nitric oxide via phosphoinositide breakdown, *Biochem Biophys Res Commun* 174:228, 1990.

44. Fehsel K et al: Islet cell DNA is a traget of inflammatory attack by nitric oxide, *Diabetes* 42:496, 1993.

45. Ferreira SH, Duarte ID, Lorenzetti BB: Molecular basis of acetylcholine and morphine analgesia, *Agents Actions* 32:101, 1991.

46. Fiorentino DF, Bond MW, Mosmann TR: Two types of mouse T helper cell. IV. Th2 clones secrete a factor that inhibits cytokine production by Th1 clones, *J Exp Med* 170:2081, 1989.

47. Forstermann U et al: Induced RAW 264.7 macrophages express soluble and particulate nitric oxide synthase:inhibition by transforming growth factor-B, *Eur J Pharmacol* 225:161, 1992.

48. Forstermann U et al: Calmodulin dependent endothelium derived relaxing factor/nitric oxide synthase activity is present in the particulate and cytosolic fractions of bovine aortic endothelial cells, *Proc Natl Acad Sci USA* 88:1788, 1991.

49. Furchgott RF, Zawadzki JV: The obligatory role of endothelial cells in the relaxation of arterial smooth muscle by acetylcholine, *Nature* 288:373, 1980.

50. Gajewski TF, Fitch FW: Differential activation of murine Th1 and Th2 clones, *Immunol Rev* 142:19, 1991.

51. Gajewski TF et al: Regulation of T-cell activation: differences among T-cell subsets, *Immunol Rev* 111:79, 1989.

52. Garthwaite J: Glutamate, nitric oxide, and cell-cell signaling in the nervous system, *Trends Neurosci* 14:60, 1991.

53. Garthwaite J, Charles SL, Chess-Williams R: Endothelium-derived relaxing factor release on activation of NMDA receptors suggests role as intracellular messenger in the brain, *Nature* 336:385, 1988.

54. Geller DA et al: Cytokines, endotoxin and glucocorticoids regulate the expression of inducible nitric oxide synthase in hepatocytes, *Proc Natl Acad Sci USA* 90:522, 1993.

55. Gerberick GF et al: Relationships between pulmonary inflammation, plasma transudation and oxygen metabolite secretion by alveolar macrophages, *J Immunol* 137:114, 1986.

56. Go NF et al: Interleukin-10, a novel B cell stimulatory factor, *J Exp Med* 172:1625, 1990.

57. Gorsky LD et al: Production of an EDRF-like activity in the cytosol of N1E-115 neuroblastoma cells, *FASEB J* 4:1494, 1990.

58. Granger DL, Lehninger AL: Sites of inhibition of mitochondrial electron transport in macrophage injured neoplastic cells, *J Cell Biol* 95:527, 1982.

59. Granger DL et al: Injury to neoplastic cells by murine macrophages leads to inhibition of mitochondrial respiration, *J Clin Invest* 65:357, 1980.

60. Greening AP, Lowrie DB: Extracellular release of hydrogen perox-

61. Grisham MB et al: Neutrophil-mediated nitrosamine formation: role of nitric oxide in rats, *Gastroenterology* 103:1260, 1992.

62. Hampson ECGM, Pond SM: Ultrastructure of canine lung during the proliferative phase of paraquat therapy, *Br J Exp Pathol* 69:57, 1988.

63. Harbrecht BG, Billiar TR, Stadler J: Nitric oxide synthase serves to reduce hepatic damage during acute murine endotoxemia, *Crit Care Med* 20:1568, 1992.

64. Hartung HP et al: Inflammatory mediators in demyelinating disorders of the CNS and PNS, *J Neuroimmunol* 40:197, 1992.

65. Heck DE et al: Epidermal growth factor suppresses nitric oxide and hydrogen peroxide production by keratinocytes, *J Biol Chem* 267:21277, 1992.

66. Heinzel FP et al: Reciprocal expression of interferon gamma or interleukin 4 during the resolution or progression of murine leishmaniasis. Evidence for expansion of distinct helper T cell subsets, *J Exp Med* 169:59, 1989.

67. Hibbs JB Jr, Taintor RR, Vavrin Z: Iron-depletion: possible cause of tumor cell cytotoxicity induced by activated macrophages, *Biochem Biophys Res Commun* 123:716, 1984.

68. Hibbs JB Jr, Taintor RR, Vavrin Z: Iron-depletion: possible cause of tumor cell cytotoxicity induced by activated macrophages, *Biochem Biophys Res Commun* 123:716, 1987.

69. Hibbs JB Jr, Vavrin Z, Taintor RR: L-arginine is required for expression of the activated macrophage effector mechanism causing selective metabolic inhibition in target cells, *J Immunol* 138:550, 1987.

70. Hibbs JB Jr et al: Nitric oxide: a cytotoxic activated macrophage effector molecule, *Biochem Biophys Res Commun* 157:87, 1988.

71. Hoffman RA et al: Alloantigen-induced activation of rat splenocytes is regulated by the oxidative metabolism of L-arginine, *J Immunol* 145:2220, 1990.

72. Hogan JC, Lewis MJ, Henderson AH: In vivo EDRF activity influences platelet function, *Br J Pharmacol* 94:1020, 1988.

73. Hoidal JR et al: Altered oxidative metabolic responses in vitro of alveolar macrophages from asymptomatic cigarette smokers, *Am Rev Respir Dis* 123:85, 1981.

74. Hope BT et al: Neuronal NADPH diaphorase is a nitric oxide synthase, *Proc Natl Acad Sci USA* 88:2811, 1991.

75. Huot AE, Gundel RM, Hacker MP: Effect of erythrocytes on alveolar macrophage cytostatic activity induced by bleomycin lung damage in the rat, *Cancer Res* 50:2351, 1990.

76. Huot AE, Hacker MP: The role of reactive nitrogen intermediate production in alveolar macrophage cytostatic activity induced by bleomycin lung damage, *Cancer Res* 50:7863, 1990.

77. Huot AE et al: Formation of nitric oxide hemoglobin in erythrocytes co-cultured with alveolar macrophages taken from bleomycin treated rats, *Biochem Biophys Res Commun* 182:151, 1992.

78. Huot AE et al: Nitric oxide modulates lymphocyte proliferation but not secretion of IL-2, *Immunol Invest* 22:319, 1993.

79. Hutcheson IR, Whittle BJR, Boughton-Smith NK: Role of nitric oxide in maintaining vascular integrity in endotoxin-induced acute intestinal damage in the rat, *Br J Pharmacol* 101:815, 1990.

80. Hutchinson PJA, Palmer RMJ, Moncada S: Comparative pharmacology of EDRF and nitric oxide on vascular strips, *Eur J Pharmacol* 141:445, 1987.

81. Ialenti A et al: Modulation of acute inflammation by endogenous nitric oxide, *Eur J Pharmacol* 211:177, 1992.

82. Ignarro LJ: *Regulation of PMN leukocyte, macrophage and platelet function*. In Hadden JW, Coffey BG, Spreafico F, editors: *Immunopharmacology*, New York, 1977, Plenum, pp. 61-86.

83. Ignarro LJ: Nitric oxide: a novel signal transduction mechanism for transcellular communication, *Hypertension* 16:477, 1990.

84. Ignarro LJ, George WJ: Hormonal control of lysosomal enzyme re-

lease from human neutrophils: elevation of cyclic nucleotides by autonomic neurohormones, *Proc Natl Acad Sci USA* 71:2022, 1974.

85. Johnson KJ et al: Mediators of IgA induced lung injury in the rat. Role of macrophages and reactive oxygen products, *Lab Invest* 54:499, 1986.

86. Kehrl JH et al: Production of transforming growth factor beta by human T lymphocytes and its potential role in the regulation of T cell growth, *J Exp Med* 163:1037, 1986.

87. Keller R: Cytostatice elimination of syngeneic rat tumor cells in vitro by nonspecifically activated macrophages, *J Exp Med* 138:625, 1973.

88. Keller R: Susceptibility of normal and transformed cell lines to cytostatic and cytocidal effects exerted by macrophages, *J Natl Cancer Inst* 56:369, 1976.

89. Keller R, Geiges M, Keist R: L-arginine-dependent reactive nitrogen intermediates as mediators of tumor cell killing by activated macrophages, *Cancer Res* 50:1421, 1990.

90. Kilbourn RG, Belloni R: Endothelial cell production of nitrogen oxides in response to interferon-γ in combination with tumor necrosis factor, interleukin-1, or endotoxin, *J Natl Cancer Inst* 82:772, 1990.

91. Kilbourn RG et al: N^G-methyl-L-arginine inhibits tumor necrosis factor-induced hypotension: implications for the involvement of nitric oxide, *Proc Natl Acad Sci USA* 87:3629, 1990.

92. Kimberly PJ, Huot AE, Hacker MP: Enhanced IA expression by alveolar macrophages following intratracheal administration of bleomycin to rats, *Immunol Invest* 21:169, 1992.

93. Koj A: Biological functions of acute phase proteins. In Gordon AH, Koj A, editors: *The acute phase response to injury and infection,* New York, 1985, Elsevier, pp. 145-160.

94. Kolb H, Kolb-Bachofen V: Nitric oxide: a pathogenic factor in autoimmunity, *Immunol Today* 13:157, 1992.

95. Korelitz BI: Carcinoma of the intestinal tract in Crohn's disease: results of a survey conducted by the National Foundation for Illeitis and Colitis, *Am J Gastroenterol* 78:44, 1983.

96. Krahenbuhl JL, Remington JS: The role of activated macrophages in specific and non-specific cytostasis of tumor cells, *J Immunol* 113:507, 1974.

97. Kroncke K-D et al: Activated macrophages kill pancreatic syngeneic islet cells via arginine-dependent nitric oxide generation, *Biochem Biophys Res Commun* 175:752, 1991.

98. Kubes P, Suzuki M, Granger DN: Modulation of PAF-induced leukocyte adherence and increased microvascular permeability, *Am J Physiol* 259:G859, 1990.

99. Kubes P, Suzuki M, Granger DN: Nitric oxide: an endogenous modulator of leukocyte adhesion, *Proc Natl Acad Sci USA* 88:4651, 1991.

100. Lamas S et al: Endothelial nitric oxide synthase: molecular cloning and characterization of a distinct constitutive enzyme isoform, *Proc Natl Acad Sci USA* 89:6348, 1992.

101. Lancaster JB Jr et al: Iron-sulfer center destruction by nitric oxide production in immune cytotoxicity, *FASEB J* 4:A1917, 1990.

102. Langrehr JM et al: Nitric oxide synthesis in the in vivo allograft response: a possible regulatory role, *Surgery* 110:335, 1991.

103. Lee J, Vilcek J: Tumor necrosis factor and interleukin 1: Cytokines with multiple, overlapping biological activities, *Lab Invest* 56:234, 1987.

104. Lehn M et al: IL-4 inhibits H2O2 production and antileishmanial capacity of human cultured monocytes mediated by IFN-gamma, *J Immunol* 143:3020, 1989.

105. Leibovich SJ et al: Macrophage-induced angiogenesis is mediated by tumour necrosis factor-alpha, *Nature* 329:630, 1987.

106. Leowski J: Mortality from acute respiratory infections in children under 5 years of age. Global estimate, *World Health Stat Q* 39:138, 1986.

107. Liew FY: Functional heterogeneity of CD4+ T cells in leishamniasis, *Immunol Today* 10:40, 1989.

108. Liew FY, Cox FEG: Nonspecific defence mechanism: The role of nitric oxide, *Immunol Today* 12:A17, 1991.

109. Liew FY et al: A possible novel pathway of regulation by murine T helper type 2 (Th2) cells of a Th1 cell activity via the modulation of the induction of nitric oxide synthase on macrophages, *Eur J Immunol* 21:2489, 1991.

110. Locksley RM et al: Induction of Th1 and Th2 CD4+ subsets during murine Leishmania major infection, *Res Immunol* 142:28, 1991.

111. Lowenstein CJ et al: Cloned and expressed nitric oxide synthase contrasts with brain enzyme, *Proc Natl Acad Sci USA* 89:6711, 1992.

112. Lyons CR, Orloff GJ, Cunningham JM: Molecular cloning and functional expression of an inducible nitric oxide synthase from a murine macrophage cell line, *J Biol Chem* 267:6370, 1992.

113. MacNaughton WK, Cirino G, Wallace JL: Endothelium-derived relaxing factor (nitric oxide) has protective actions in the stomach, *Life Sci* 45:1869, 1989.

114. MacNeil IA et al: IL-10, a novel growth cofactor for mature and immature T cells, *J Immunol* 145:4167, 1990.

115. Mannel DN, Moore RN, Mergenhagen SE: Macrophages as a source of tumoricidal activity (tumor necrotizing factor), *Infect Immun* 30:523, 1980.

116. Maragos CM et al: Complexes of NO with nucleophiles as agents for the controlled release of nitric oxide. Vasorelaxant effects, *J Med Chem* 34:3242, 1991.

117. Marletta MA: Nitric oxide: biosynthesis and biological significance, *TIBS* 14:488, 1989.

118. Marletta MA: Mammalian synthesis of nitrite, nitrate and N-nitrosating agents, *Chem Res Toxicol* 1:249, 1988.

119. Martin W, Smith JA, White DG: The mechanisms by which heamoglobin inhibtis the relaxation of rabbit aorta induced nitrovasodilations, nitric oxide or bovine retractor penis inhibitory factor, *Br J Pharmacol* 89:563, 1986.

120. Martin W, White DG, Henderson AH: Endothelium-derived relaxing factor and atriopeptin II elevate cyclic GMP levels in pig aortic endothelial cells, *Br J Pharmacol* 93:229, 1988.

121. Martin W et al: Selective blockade of endothelium-dependent and glyceral trinitrate-induced relaxation by hemoglobin and methylene blue in the rabbit aorta, *J Pharmacol Exp Ther* 232:708, 1985.

122. Meyer J: Comparison of carbon monoxide, nitric oxide and nitrite as inhibitors of nitrogenase from *Clostridium pasteurianum, Arch Biochem Biophys* 210:246, 1981.

123. Miller MJS et al: Nitric oxide release in response to gut injury, *Scand J Gastroenterol* 28:149, 1993.

124. Moncada S, Palmer RMJ, Higgs EA: Nitric oxide: physiology, pathophysiology and pharmacology, *Pharmacol Rev* 43:109, 1991.

125. Mosmann TR, Coffman RL: TH1 and TH2 cells: different patterns of lymphokine secretion lead to different functional properties, *Annu Rev Immunol* 7:145, 1989.

126. Mulligan MS et al: Tissue injury caused by deposition of immune complexes is L-arginine dependent, *Proc Natl Acad Sci USA* 88:6338, 1991.

127. Murad F: Cyclic guanosine monophosphate as a mediator of vasodilation, *J Clin Invest* 78:1, 1986.

128. Namba T, Nolte CP, Jackerel J: Poisoning due to organophosphate insecticides: acute and chronic manifestations, *Am J Med* 50:475, 1971.

129. Nathan CF: Secretion of oxygen intermediates: role in effector functions of activated macrophages, *FASEB J* 41:2206, 1982.

130. Nathan CF: Nitric oxide as a secretory product of mammalian cells, *FASEB J* 6:3051, 1992.

131. Nathan CF, Murray HW, Cohn ZA: The macrophage as an effector cell, *N Engl J Med* 303:622, 1980.

132. Nava E, Palmer RM, Moncada S: The role of nitric oxide in endotoxic shock: effects of N^G-monomethyl-L-arginine, *J Cardiovasc Pharmacol* 20:S132, 1992.

133. Newman RA et al: Assessment of bleomycin, tallysomycin and

polyamine-mediated acute lung toxicity by pulmonary lavage angiotensin converting enzyme activity, *Toxicol Appl Pharmacol* 61:469, 1981.

134. Niederman MS et al: Demonstration of a free elastolytic metalloenzyme in human lavage fluid and its relationship to alpha-1-antiprotease, *Am Rev Respir Dis* 129:943, 1984.

135. Niewoehner DE, Kleinerman J, Rice DB: Pathologic changes in the peripheral airways of young cigarette smokers, *N Engl J Med* 291:755, 1974.

136. O'Dell TJ, Kandel ER, Grant SGN: Long-term potentiation in the hippocampus is blocked by tyrosine kinase inhibitors, *Nature* 353:558, 1991.

137. Onozaki K et al: Role of interleukin-1 in promoting human monocyte-mediated tumor cytotoxicity, *J Immunol* 135:314, 1985.

138. Park KGM et al: Stimulation of lymphocyte natural cytotoxicity by L-arginine, *Lancet* i, 337:645-646, 1991.

138a. Parker JL, Adams HR: Selective inhibition of endothelium dependent vasodilator capacity by *Escherichia coli* endotoxemia. *Circ Res*, 72:539-551, 1993.

139. Perret GI, Lemaire C: Dexamethasone inhibits antitumor potential of activated macrophages by a receptor mediated action, *Biochem Biophys Res Commun* 136:130, 1986.

140. Piguet PF et al: Tumor necrosis factor/cachectin plays a key role in bleomycin-induced pneumopathy and fibrosis, *J Exp Med* 170:655, 1989.

141. Powrie F, Mason D: OX-22 high CD4+ T cells induce wasting disease with multiple organ pathology: prevention by the OK-22 low subset, *J Exp Med* 172:1701, 1990.

142. Radomski MW, Palmer RMJ, Moncada S: An L-arginine/nitric oxide pathway present in human platelets regulates aggregation, *Proc Natl Acad Sci USA* 87:5193, 1990.

143. Rapport RM, Draznin MB, Murad F: Endothelium-dependent relaxation of aorta may be mediated through cyclic GMP-dependent protein phosphorylation, *Nature* 306:174, 1983.

144. Rapport RM, Murad F: Agonist-induced endothelial dependent relaxation in rat thoracic aorta may be mediated through cGMP, *Circ Res* 52:352, 1983.

145. Reddy D, Lancaster JR Jr, Cornforth DP: Nitrite inhibition of *Clostridium botulinum:* electron spin resonance detection of iron-nitric oxide complexes, *Science* 221:769, 1983.

146. Rees DD, Palmer RMJ, Moncada S: Role of endothelium-derived nitric oxide in the regulation of blood pressure, *Proc Natl Acad Sci USA* 86:3375, 1989.

147. Rossaint R et al: *Successful treatment of severe adult respiratory distress syndrome with inhaled nitric oxide—a pilot clinical study.* In Moncada S et al, editors: *The biology of nitric oxide,* vol 1, London, 1992, Portland Press, pp. 334-336.

148. Rossaint R et al: *Inhaled nitric oxide improves arterial oxygenation in severe ARDS—a preliminary case report,* In Moncada S et al, editors: *The biology of nitric oxide,* vol 1, London, 1992, Portland Press, pp. 364-367.

148a. Sakai N, Kaufman S, Milstein S: Tetrahydrobiopterin is required for cytokine-induced nitric oxide production in a murine macrophage cell line (RAW 264), *Molecular Pharm* 43:6-10, 1993.

149. Sakuma I et al: Identification of arginine as a precursor of endothelium-derived relaxing factor, *Proc Natl Acad Sci USA* 85:8664, 1988.

150. Salerno JC et al: Tetranuclear and binuclear iron-sulfer clusters in succinate dehydrogenase: a method of iron quantitation by formation of paramagnetic complexes, *Biochem Biophys Res Commun* 73:833, 1976.

151. Salvemini D et al: Nitric oxide activates cyclooxygenase enzymes, *Proc Natl Acad Sci USA* 90:7240, 1993.

152. Schoedon G et al: Regulation of the L-arginine-dependent andtetrahydrobiopterin-dependent biosynthesis of nitric oxide in murine macrophages, *Eur J Biochem* 213:833, 1993.

153. Scott P et al: Immunoregulation of cutaneous leishmaniasis. T cell lines that transfer protective immunity or exacerbation belong to different T helper subsets and respond to distinct parasite antigens, *J Exp Med* 168:1675, 1988.

154. Sibille Y, Reynolds HY: Macrophages and polymorphonuclear neutrophils in lung defense and injury, *Am Rev Respir Dis* 141:471, 1989.

155. Simon PC, Willoughby WF: The role of subcellular factors in pulmonary immune function: physiochemical characterization of two distinct species of lymphocyte-activating factor produced by rabbit alveolar macrophages, *J Immunol* 126:1534, 1981.

156. Smith RJ, Ignarro LJ: Bioregulation of lysosomal enzyme secretion from human neutrophils: roles of cyclic GMP and calcium is stimulus-secretion coupling, *Proc Natl Acad Sci USA* 72:108, 1975.

157. Snyder SH, Bredt DS: Nitric oxide as a neuronal messanger, *Trends Pharmacol Sci* 12:125, 1991.

158. Snyder SH, Bredt DS: Biological roles of nitric oxide, *Sci Am* 266:68, 1992.

159. Sporn MB, Harris ED Jr: Proliferative diseases, *Am J Med* 70:1231, 1981.

160. Stadler J et al: Effect of endogenous nitric oxide on mitochondrial respiration of rat hepatocytes in vitro and in vivo, *Arch Surg* 126:186,1991.

161. Stuehr DJ, Marletta MA: Mammalian nitrate biosynthesis: mouse macrophages produce nitrite and nitrate in response to *Escherichia coli* lipopolysaccharide, *Proc Natl Acad Sci USA* 82:7738, 1985.

162. Stuehr DJ, Marletta MA: Synthesis of nitrite and nitrate in murine macrophage cell lines, *Cancer Res* 47:5590, 1987.

163. Stuehr DJ, Nathan CF: Nitric oxide: a macrophage product responsible for cytostasis and respiratory inhibition in tumor target cells, *J Exp Med* 169:1543, 1989.

164. Stuehr DJ et al: Activated murine macrophages secrete a metabolite of arginine with the bioactivity of endothelium-derived relaxing factor and the chemical reactivity of nitric oxide, *J Exp Med* 169:1011, 1989.

165. Stuehr D et al: N^G-hydroxy-L-arginine is an intermediate in the biosynthesis of nitric oxide from L-arginine, *J Biol Chem* 266:6259, 1991.

166. Stuehr DJ et al: *The cytokine-induced macrophage nitric oxide synthase is a flavoprotein containing flavin adenine dinucleotide and flavin mononucleotide.* In Moncada S et al, editors: *The biology of nitric oxide,* London, 1992, Portland Press.

167. Suzuki M et al: *Endogenous formation of N-nitroso compounds: a current perspective.* In Bartsch H, O'Neill IK, Schulte-Herman R, editors: *Relevance of N-nitroso compounds to human cancer: exposures and mechanisms,* Lyon, France, 1987, IARC Scientific Publishers, pp. 292-296.

168. Suzuki M et al: Superoxide mediates reperfusion-induced leukocyte-endothelial cell interactions, *Am J Physiol* 257:H1740, 1989.

169. Takagi K et al: Induction of nitrite production in mouse spleen cells by immunization, *Biochim Biophys Acta* 1092:15, 1991.

170. Tayeh MA, Marletta MA: Macrophage oxidation of L-arginine to nitric oxide, nitrite and nitrate. Tetrahydrobiopterin is required as a cofactor, *J Biol Chem* 264:19654, 1989.

171. Thiemermann C, Vane J: Inhibition of nitric oxide synthesis reduces the hypotension induced by bacterial lipopolysaccharides in the rat in vivo, *Eur J Pharmacol* 182:591, 1990.

172. Thompson-Snipes LA et al: Interleukin-10: a novel stimulatory factor for mast cells and their progenitors, *J Exp Med* 173:507, 1991.

173. Thrall RS et al: Bleomycin induced pulmonary fibrosis in the rat: inhibition by indomethacin, *Am J Pathol* 95:117, 1979.

174. Urban JL et al: Tumor necrosis factor: a potent effector molecule for tumor cell killing by activated macrophages, *Proc Natl Acad Sci USA* 83:5233, 1986.

175. Vane J, Botting R: Inflammation and the mechanism of action of inflammatory drugs, *FASEB J* 1:89, 1987.

176. Wallace JL et al: Endothelin has potent ulcerogenic and vasoconstrictor actions in the stomach, *Am J Physiol* 256:G661, 1989.

177. Weibel ER: Oxygen effect on lung cells, *Arch Intern Med* 128:54, 1971.

178. Weitzman SA, Gordon LI: Inflammation and cancer: role of phagocytic-generated oxidants in carcinogenesis, *Blood* 76:655, 1990.

179. Wellum GR, Irvine TW Jr, Zervas NT: Dose response of cerebral arteries of the dog, rabbit and man to human hemoglobin in vitro, *J Neurosurg* 53:486, 1980.

180. Werner-Felmayer G et al: Tetrahydrobiopterin dependent fromation of nitrate and nitrite in murine fibroblasts, *J Exp Med* 172:1599, 1990.

181. Westenberger U et al: Formation of free radicals and nitric oxide derivative of hemoglobin in rats during shock syndrome, *Free Radic Res Commun* 11:167, 1990.

182. Woods LFJ, Woods JM, Gibbs PA: The involvement of nitric oxide in the inhibition of the phosphoroclasitic system in *Clostridium sporogenes* by sodium nitrite, *J Gen Microbiol* 125:399, 1981.

183. Xie QW et al: Cloning and characterization of inducible nitric oxide synthase from mouse macrophages, *Science* 256:225, 1992.

184. Yonetani T et al: Electromagnetic properties of hemoproteins, *J Biol Chem* 247:2447, 1972.

185. Zawalich WS, Diaz VA: Interleukin-1 inhibits insulin secretion from isolated perfused rat islets, *Diabetes* 35:1119, 1986.

186. Zielasek J et al: Production of nitrite by neonatal rat microglial cells/ brain macrophages, *Cell Immunol* 141:111, 1992.

187. Zwilling BS, Campolito LB: Destruction of tumor cells by BCG activated alveolar macrophages, *J Immunol* 119:838, 1977.

Chapter 23

ENERGY-PRODUCING METABOLIC PATHWAYS

Robert C. Woodworth

Glycolysis
Pentose phosphate pathway
Fat oxidation
Catabolism of amino acids and nitrogen disposal
Tricarboxylic acid cycle
Mitochondrial electron transport and oxidative phosphorylation
Enzymes involved in heme synthesis and energy transduction
Impact of vitamin deficiency on energy metabolism

This chapter considers the derivation of metabolic energy from the main catabolic pathways of carbohydrates, fats, and amino acids and the inhibition of enzymes of these pathways by toxic agents. Anabolic reactions leading to storage of energy sources are not considered, although they are important to the overall function and survival of living systems. Metabolic pathways are exquisitely controlled by various feedback and feed ahead loops in which end products and precursors are able to modulate the activities of specific enzymes. Because the focus here is on toxic substances, these normal activation/suppression mechanisms are beyond the purview of this chapter. Furthermore, because the details and mechanisms of action of most inhibitors have been worked out with purified or partly purified enzymes, the precise mode of the physiological action of these substances in the intact body is frequently not clear.

Fig. 23-1 gives a broad outline of energy flow from the three main fuel sources of metabolic energy—carbohydrates, fats and amino acids—to adenosine triphosphate *(ATP)*, the "common currency" of metabolic energy utili-

zation in living systems. ATP is then the common energy source for various physiological functions, e.g., active transport of many substances across cell membranes, muscular contraction, synthesis of functional biomacromolecules. The fuel sources contain carbon in a relatively reduced state; i.e., carbon atoms are covalently bonded to other carbon atoms and to one or more hydrogen atoms. During metabolic processing, the carbon atoms eventuate in carbon dioxide (CO_2) and the hydrogen atoms in H_2O. That is to say, carbon and hydrogen are oxidized maximally. The reducing equivalents, i.e, electrons, given up during these oxidations are captured initially by enzymatic reduction of nicotinamide-adenine dinucleotide (phosphate) [$NAD(P)^+$] to nicotinamide-adenine dinucleotide (phosphate) (reduced form) [NAD(P)H]. These reduced cofactors pass the electrons on to the electron transport system of mitochondria, wherein electron flow through an ordered series of electron transport proteins results, via chemiosmotic coupling, in the production of ATP from adenosine diphosphate (ADP) and inorganic phosphate (P_i).

Figure 23-2 presents in considerably more detail an integrated view of (1) glycolysis, (2) the pentose phosphate pathway, (3) β-oxidation of long-chain fatty acids, (4) transamination of amino acids and the urea cycle for disposal of nitrogen, and (5) the tricarboxylic acid cycle. Enzymes of the various pathways are numbered and coded to Table 23-1, which lists the common name of each enzyme and its cofactors and inhibitors, if any. References to compendia of metabolic inhibitors are also given so the reader may readily access the original literature.

Metabolic inhibitors are of different kinds in terms of specificity, point of attack, and mechanism. Thus the "b"

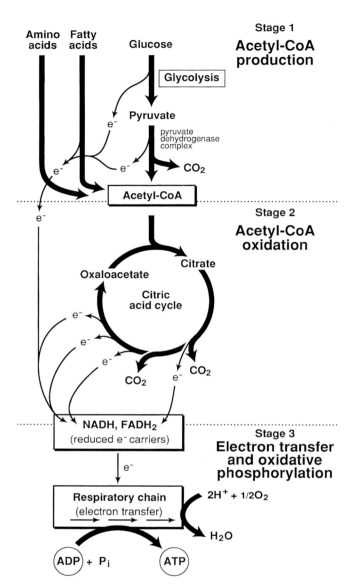

Fig. 23-1. General outline of energy-producing metabolic pathways. Stage 1 involves the conversion of amino acids, fatty acids, and sugars into acetyl coenzyme A *(CoA)*, the immediate fuel source for the tricarboxylic acid cycle. Sugars pass through glycolysis at this stage, yielding "anaerobic" energy as adenosine triphosphate *(ATP)* and nicotinamide-adenine dinucleotide (reduced form) (NADH). Stage 2 involves the gradual oxidation of two carbons derived from acetyl CoA, yielding two CO_2, production of reducing equivalents as nicotinamide-adenine dinucleotide *(NADH)* for fueling the electron transport system and some ATP. Stage 3 involves the transfer of electrons to gradually more positive oxidation-reduction values and the eventual reduction of O_2 to H_2O. Coupled to this electron flow is the pumping of protons out of the mitochondrial matrix. Return of these protons through a structure containing an ATPase allows the synthesis of ATP. $FADH_2$, Flavin adenine dinucleotide (reduced form); *ADP*, adenine diphosphate.

class (soft) metals and metallo-organics thereof tend to react selectively with enzymes bearing free SH (sulfhydryl) groups.[2] Organic alkylating reagents, e.g., iodoacetate (IA), iodoacetamide (IAM), *N*-ethylmaleimide (NEM), also attack free SH groups. The specificities of these reagents for various enzymes are highly variable, however, so that a given enzyme may be inhibited by one or a few sulfhydryl reagents but not others.

Another type of inhibition is caused by highly specific substances, which either react covalently with the substrate binding site or active site of the enzyme or bind so tightly as not to be readily displaced by the natural substrate. Examples are fluoroacetate and fluorocitrate.

Then again some inhibitors act by binding to or replacing a cofactor essential for the function of a given enzyme. Examples are fluoride and arsenate ions. Clearly a dietary lack of a vitamin required for the synthesis of an essential cofactor has a similar result.

GLYCOLYSIS

The utilization of carbohydrates for the production of metabolic energy begins with the stepwise breakdown of glucose derived from absorption of hydrolyzed polysaccharides from the intestine; the depolymerization of glycogen in the tissues, primarily liver and muscle; or gluconeogenesis from pyruvate recycled from anaerobic glycolysis in muscle tissue or from the catabolism of glucogenic amino acids in the liver. The action of glycogen phosphorylase [1] involves the splitting off of single glucose units as glucose-1-phosphate (G-1-P) by the introduction of P_i. Organic mercurials, e.g., *p*-chloromercuribenzoate (PCMB), can inhibit this enzyme. The isomerization of G-1-P to glucose-6-phosphate (G-6-P) by phosphoglucomutase [2] requires G-1,6-diP as a cofactor and can be inhibited by F^- or organic mercurials. Fluoride is an example of an agent that reacts with and thereby makes unavailable an essential cofactor, e.g., Mg^{2+}. Hexokinase [4] requires ATP as cofactor and can be inhibited by organic arsenicals, by organic mercurials, implying essentiality of sulfhydryl groups for enzyme function, and by 2-deoxyglucose-6-phosphate. The latter substance readily enters cells in the nonphosphorylated form via the glucose transporter and is phosphorylated by hexokinase to give the phosphorylated form, which, similar to G-6-P, inhibits the enzyme, but in contrast to G-6-P, cannot be metabolized further.[3] Phosphoglucoisomerase [5] converts G-6-P to fructose-6-phosphate (F-6-P), which is then phosphorylated by 6-phosphofructo-1-kinase [6] with ATP as cofactor. The latter enzyme serves a pivotal role in control of glycolysis and is under exquisite hormonal control.[3]

At this point, two ATPs have been used to activate glucose, and one ATP has been used to activate one glucose subunit from glycogen. It should be borne in mind, however, that each glucose originally incorporated into glycogen required the cleavage of *two* ATPs. Aldolase [7]

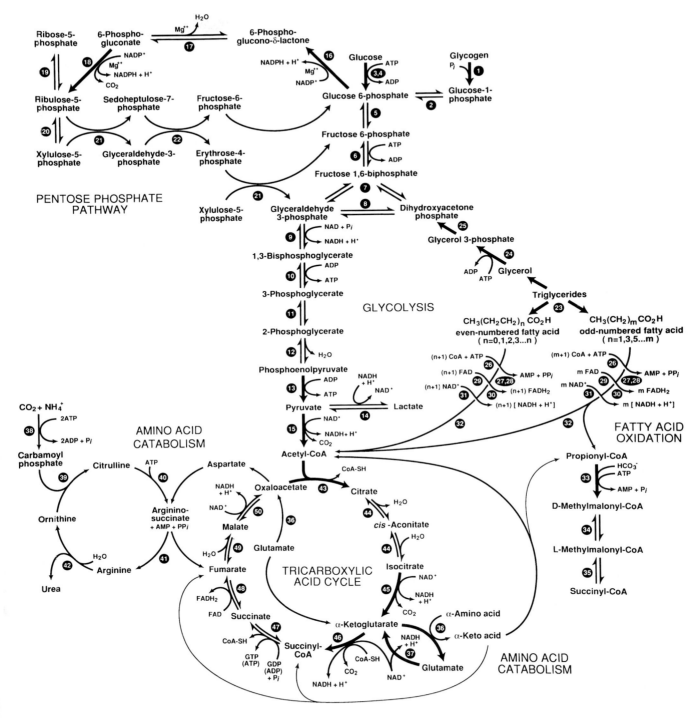

Fig. 23-2. Integrated scheme for the catabolism of amino acids, fats, and carbohydrates. Each enzyme is numbered and keyed to its name, cofactors, and toxic inhibitors listed in Table 23-1.

cleaves fructose-1,6-bisphosphate into two three-carbon sugar phosphates, glyceraldehyde-3-phosphate (G-3-P) and dihydroxyacetone phosphate (DHP), and is inhibited by various SH reagents, e.g., Ag^+ (silver ion), organic mercury and arsenic compounds. Triose phosphate isomerase [8] readily interconverts G-3-P and DHP. The action of

glyceraldehyde-3-phosphate dehydrogenase [9] results in the first capture of energy in the glycolytic pathway by incorporating P_i and transferring two reducing equivalents to nicotinamide-adenine dinucleotide (NAD^+) to give nicotinamide-adenine dinucleotide (reduced form) (NADH). Oxidation of the aldehyde carbon of G-3-P oc-

Table 23-1. Enzymes involved in energy production, coded to Figs. 23-2 through 23-4

Enzyme No./name	Cofactor	Toxic inhibitor	Ref,vol,page
Enzymes of the glycolytic pathway			
[1] Glycogen phosphorylase	P_i	Org. Hg	4, II, 138ff
[2] Phosphoglucomutase	Glucose 1,6-diphosphate	F^-, org. Hg	4, II, 401 9, II, 780
[3] Glucokinase	ATP		
[4] Hexokinase	ATP	2-Deoxyglucose(-6-phosphate), org. As, org. Hg	9, II, 782
[5] Phosphoglucoisomerase			
[6] 6-Phosphofructo-1-kinase	ATP		
[7] Aldolase		Org. Hg, Ag^+	9, II, 780
[8] Triose phosphate isomerase			
[9] Glyceraldehyde-3-phosphate dehydrogenase	NAD^+, P_i	AsO_4^{2-}, org. As, org. Hg, Ag^+ IA, IAM	4, II, 103 4, II, 136 9, II, 783 9, III, 19
[10] Phosphoglycerate kinase	ADP		
[11] Phosphoglycerate mutase	2,3-DPG		
[12] Enolase	Mg^{2+}, P_i	F^-	4, II, 401
[13] Pyruvate kinase	ADP, K^+		
[14] Lactate dehydrogenase	NADH		
[15] Pyruvate decarboxylase (pyruvate dehydrogenase)	TPP, Lip, CoASH, FAD, NAD^+	Hg compounds, AsO_3^{2-}, org. As, IA, ISBZ	9, II, 783 4, II, 110 10, 813
Enzymes of the pentose phosphate pathway			
[16] Glucose-6-phosphate dehydrogenase	$NADP^+$	Org. Hg, ISBZ, IAM, primaquine	4, II, 104 10, 805 9, II, 781
[17] Glucose lactonase		Hg^{2+}	9, II, 845
[18] 6-Phosphogluconate dehydrogenase	Mg^{2+}, $NADP^+$	Org. Hg, Hg^{2+}, IA	4, II, 104
[19] Phosphopentose isomerase			
[20] Phosphopentose epimerase			
[21] Transketolase	TPP, Mg^{2+}	Org. Hg, Hg^{2+}	4, II, 857 10, 815
[22] Transaldolase			
Enzymes of fat oxidation			
[23] Lipase		Antilipolytic drugs, org. As and Hg, ISBZ	4, IV, 312ff 10, 808
[24] Glycerol kinase	ATP		
[25] Glycerol phosphate dehydrogenase	NAD^+	IA, NEM, org. AS, org. Hg	10, 805
[26] Acyl CoA synthetase	ATP, Mg^{2+}, CoASH	F^-, atractyloside, hypoglycin, 4-pentenoate	4, IV, 315 4, IV, 316
[27] Carnitine palmitoyl transferase I	⎱ Carnitine	⎰ 3 (+)-acylcarnitines, 2-bromocarnitines, sulfhydryl reagents	4, IV, 320
[28] Carnitine palmitoyl transferase II	⎰	⎱	4, IV, 317ff
[29] Acyl CoA dehydrogenase	FAD	Org. Hg?	
[30] Enoyl CoA hydratase			
[31] L-β-Hydroxyacyl CoA dehydrogenase	NAD^+		
[32] β-Ketothiolase	CoASH		
[33] Propionyl CoA carboxylase	ATP, biotin	Org. Hg, NEM, IAM	10, 811
[34] Methylmalonyl CoA racemase			
[35] Methylmalonyl CoA mutase	B_{12}		

Table 23-1. Enzymes involved in energy production, coded to Figs. 23-2 through 23-4—cont'd

Enzyme No./name		Cofactor	Toxic inhibitor	Ref,vol,page	

Enzymes of amino acid catabolism and the urea cycle

[36]	Transaminases	PLP	Org. Hg, NEM, IAM	10,	815
[37]	Glutamate dehydrogenase	NAD(P)$^+$	Org. As, org. Hg, IAM	9, II,	104
				10,	805
[38]	Carbamoyl phosphate synthetase I	ATP, Mg^{2+}, N-acetylglutamate			
[39]	Ornithine transcarbamoylase				
[40]	Argininosuccinate synthetase	ATP, Mg^{2+}			
[41]	Argininosuccinase				
[42]	Arginase	Mn^{2+}	Hg^{2+}	4, II, 374	

Enzymes of the tricarboxylic acid cycle

[43]	Citrate synthetase		Fluoroacetate (substrate)	4, II, 405	
[44]	Aconitase	FeS	Fluorocitrate, Hg^{2+}	4, II, 491	
[45]	Isocitrate dehydrogenase	NAD(P)$^+$,Mg^{2+}	Org. Hg,	9, II, 782	
			org. As, IA, IAM	10,	807
[46]	α-Ketoglutarate dehydrogenase	TPP, Lip, CoASH, FAD, NAD$^+$	Org. As and Hg, AsO$_3^{2-}$, IA, IAM	4, II, 110	
				10,	807
[47]	Succinyl CoA synthetase	GDP, P$_i$			
[48]	Succinate dehydrogenase (succinate-CoQ reductase)	FAD, FeS	Malonate, alloxan, AsO$_3^{2-}$, org. As and Hg F$^-$+P$_i$, ethyl-IA, quinones, I$_2$	4, II, 475	
				4, II, 103	
				4, II, 153, 403, 481ff	
				10,	815
[49]	Fumarase		Org. Hg, fluorooxaloacetate	9, II, 780	
[50]	Malate dehydrogenase	NAD$^+$	F- and F$_2$-oxaloacetate	4, II, 490	

Mitochondrial electron transporters and enzymes of ATP and heme synthesis

[51]	NADH dehydrogenase (NADH-CoQ reductase)	NAD$^+$, FMN	Quinones, org. Hg, IAM	4, II, 153	
				10,	809
[52]	FeS center	CoQ	Rotenone, amytal, piericidin A, Fe(CN)$_6^{3-}$	1, XIII, 203ff	
[53]	Cytochromes b$_{562}$, b$_{566}$	Heme	Antimycin A	5,	549
[54]	Cytochrome c$_1$	Heme			
[55]	Cytochrome c	Heme	CN$^-$	4, II, 418	
[56]	Cytochrome a	Heme			
[57]	Cytochrome a$_3$	Heme, O$_2$	HCN, CO, HN$_3$, HS$^-$, F$^-$	4, II, 387, 404, 406	
[58]	ATP synthase	ADP, P$_i$	Oligomycin, DCCD, venturicidin	4, II, 512	
				5	552
[59]	Proton gradient		Dicoumarol, nitrophenols, phenylhydrazone, carbonyl cyanide, dinitrophenol, vanilomycin	4, II, 507, 510	
				5,	552

Enzymes of heme synthesis and energy transfer; hemoglobin

[60]	ALA synthase		Pb^{2+} increases	8,	65-67
[61]	ALA dehydratase		Pb^{2+} inhibits, Org. Hg, IAM	8,	65-67
[62]	Uroporphyrinogen III decarboxylase		Org. Hg	9, II, 859	
[63]	Ferrochelatase		Pb^{2+} inhibits	8,	65-67
[64]	Hb + O$_2$ ⇄ HbO$_2$	Heme	CO, SH$^-$	4, II, 540	
[65]	Hb(Fe^{2+}) → Hb(Fe^{3+})	Heme	Amylnitrite (NO$_2^-$)	4, II, 550	
[66]	NADH/NADPH oxidoreductase	NAD$^+$, NADP$^+$	Org. Hg, Hg^{2+}, AsO$_3^{2-}$, ISBZ	10,	809
[67]	Creatine kinase	ATP, ADP	Org. Hg, ISBZ	10,	803
[68]	ATP-ADP translocase	ATP, ADP	Atractyloside, bongkrekic acid	5,	552

P_i, Inorganic phosphate; *org. Hg*, organic mercury compounds, e.g., methylmercury, p-chloromercury benzoate; *ATP*, adenosine 5'-triphosphate; *org. As*, organic arsenic compounds, e.g., cacodylate, Lewisite, phenylarsenoxide; Ag^+, silver ion; *NAD$^+$*, nicotinamide adenine dinucleotide; AsO_4^{2-}, arsenate; AsO_3^{2-}, arsenite; *IA*, iodoacetate; *IAM*, iodoacetamide; *ADP*, adenosine 5'-diphosphate; *2,3-DPG*, 2,3-diphosphoglycerate; Mg^{2+}, magnesium ion; K^+, potassium ion; F^-, fluoride ion; *NADH*, nicotinamide-adenine dinucleiotide (reduced form); *TPP*, thiamine pyrophosphate; *Lip*, lipoic acid, *CoASH*, coenzyme A; *FAD*, flavin adenine dinucleotide; *ISBZ*, o-iodosobenzoate; *NADP$^+$*, nicotinamide-adenine dinucleotide phosphate; Hg^{2+}, mercuric ion; *NEM*, N-ethylmaleimide; *B$_{12}$*, vitamin B$_{12}$, cobalamin; *PLP*, pyridoxal phosphate; *FMN*, flavin mononucleotide; *CoQ*, coenzyme Q, ubiquinone; CN^-, cyanide ion; *O$_2$*, oxygen; *HCN*, hydrogen cyanide; *CO*, carbon monoxide; *HN$_3$*, hydrazoic acid; *HS$^-$*, hydrosulfide ion; *DCCD*, dicyclohexylcarbodiimide; *ALA*, aminolevulinic acid; Pb^{2+}, lead ion; *SH*, sulfhydryl group; Mn^{2+}, manganous ion; *FeS*, iron-sulfur center; *GDP*, guanosine 5'-diphosphate; I$_2$, iodine.

curs in thiohemiacetal linkage to a cysteine of the enzyme, thus creating a high-energy thioester. This energy is captured by phosphorolysis of the thioester to regenerate the cysteinyl SH and a molecule of 1,3-diphosphoglycerate (1,3-DPG). As might be expected, this enzyme is inhibited by various sulfhydryl reagents, e.g., Ag^+, organic mercurials, IA, IAM. Another inhibitor is arsenate (AsO_4^{2-}), which is not a sulfhydryl reagent but mimics P_i in some reactions. The product, rather than 1,3-DPG in this case, is 1-arsenato-3-phosphoglycerate, which spontaneously hydrolyzes to 3-phosphoglycerate and AsO_4^{2-}, thus wasting the high-energy bond. In the normal course of events, the high-energy phosphate of 1,3-DPG is transferred to an ADP through the action of phosphoglycerate kinase [10] to yield ATP and 3-phosphoglycerate (3-PG). This is the first instance of substrate level phosphorylation in the glycolytic pathway. Phosphoglycerate mutase [11] rearranges 3-PG to 2-phosphoglycerate (2-PG) with 2,3-diphosphoglycerate as an essential cofactor.[3] Enolase [12] then dehydrates 2-PG to give phosphoenolpyruvate (PEP) with Mg^{2+} (magnesium ion) and P_i as cofactors. Fluoride inhibits enolase by complexing with the Mg^{2+}.

The next step of substrate level phosphorylation occurs as pyruvate kinase [13] transfers the high-energy phosphate from PEP to ADP to give ATP and pyruvate. Potassium is required as a cofactor, as is ADP. At this point, in anaerobic glycolysis, lactate dehydrogenase [14] uses the NADH produced by the action of G-3-P dehydrogenase to reduce pyruvate to lactate. Under aerobic conditions, however, the reducing equivalents of NADH are transferred into mitochondria via one of two pathways, the glycerol phosphate or the malate-aspartate shuttle, where via the electron transport system they drive oxidative phosphorylation. The pyruvate from glycolysis then enters the tricarboxylic acid (TCA) cycle through the action of a multienzyme complex called pyruvate decarboxylase [15], which requires as cofactors thiamine pyrophosphate (TPP), lipoic acid (Lip), coenzyme A (CoASH), flavine-adenine dinucleotide (FAD), and NAD^+. The final products are CO_2, acetyl-CoA, and NADH. This step results in the first release of a fully oxidized carbon, two reducing equivalents to drive mitochondrial oxidative phosphorylation and acetyl-CoA to feed into the TCA cycle. If entry into the TCA cycle is blocked, so that only anaerobic glycolysis occurs, one mole of glucose results in the net production of two moles of ATP; however, one mole of glucose that has passed through glycogen synthesis and breakdown results in the net synthesis of but one mole of ATP.

PENTOSE PHOSPHATE PATHWAY

A parallel cycle to glycolysis is the pentose phosphate pathway (hexose monophosphate shunt, 6-phosphogluconate pathway), the main functions of which are not the direct production of energy, but of NADPH and pentose intermediates for biosynthesis of lipids and nucleic acids. The relative roles of glycolysis and the pentose phosphate pathway depend on the tissue, the former being of greater importance in muscle and the latter in adipose tissue, e.g., lactating mammary gland. The transfer of reducing equivalents between NADH and NADPH, however, can be mediated via NADH/NADPH oxidoreductase [66], which is inhibitable by organic mercurials. Three of the enzymes of the pentose phosphate pathway inhibitable by sulfhydryl reagents are glucose-6-phosphate dehydrogenase [16], 6-phosphogluconate dehydrogenase [18], and transketolase [21], with somewhat different specificities (Table 23-1). The first two of these three enzymes require $NADP^+$ as cofactor, the latter two require Mg^{2+}, and the third requires TPP. Six turns of this pathway result in the net conversion of 1 mole of G-6-P into 6 moles of CO_2 and the production of 6 moles of NADPH.

FAT OXIDATION

The oxidation of long-chain triglycerides begins with hydrolysis to fatty acids and glycerol via the action of lipase(s) [23]. These enzymes are inhibited by antilipolytic drugs, organic arsenic and mercury compounds and o-iodosobenzoate (ISBZ). Glycerol kinase [24] with ATP phosphorylates glycerol to glycerol-3-phosphate, which is oxidized to G-3-P by glycerol phosphate dehydrogenase [25] with transfer of two reducing equivalents to NAD^+. The latter enzyme is inhibited by IA, NEM, organic arsenic, and mercury compounds. The G-3-P then enters the glycolytic pathway. The long-chain fatty acids are activated to acyl CoAs by acyl CoA synthetase [26], which requires ATP, Mg^{2+}, and CoASH as cofactors. This enzyme can be inhibited by F^-, atractyloside, hypoglycin, and 4-pentenoate. The acyl group of acyl CoA is then transferred to carnitine by the action of, for instance, carnitine palmitoyl tranferase I [27], enters the mitochondrial matrix as acyl carnitine, is transferred to CoASH by carnitine palmitoyl transferase II [28], and enters the β-oxidation helical pathway. The carnitine transferases may be inhibited by (+)-acyl carnitines, 2-bromocarnitine, or sulfhydryl reagents. Acyl CoA dehydrogenase [29] transfers two reducing equivalents to an FAD-protein on the inside of the inner mitochondrial membrane, where they can enter the electron transport system at coenzyme Q (CoQ, ubiquinone) and can therefore result in the production of two ATP at most. The double bond now residing between the α- and β-carbons of the acyl CoA is hydrated through the action of enoyl CoA hydratase [30], and two reducing equivalents are transferred to NAD^+ by L-β-hydroxyacyl CoA dehydrogenase [31] to give the corresponding β-keto acid and NADH, which can donate two reducing equivalents to the electron transport system for the production of 3 ATP. Addition of CoASH by β-ketothiolase [32] eventuates in the production of one acetyl CoA and an acyl CoA foreshortened by two carbons. This shorter acyl CoA then reenters the β-oxidation path, and the spiral repeats until all carbons have been converted to acetyl CoA, which then enters the TCA cycle. In the event that the original fatty acid was odd-numbered, the final piece from the cycle will be propionyl CoA. With ATP and biotin as cofactors, propionyl CoA carboxylase [33] adds a CO_2 to propionyl CoA to yield D-methylmalonyl CoA. This product is equilibrated to the L-isomer by methylmalonyl CoA racemase [34]. Finally, methylmalonyl CoA mutase [35] with B_{12} as cofactor converts L-methylmalonyl CoA to succinyl CoA, which can enter the TCA cycle. As an example, the complete β-oxidation of palmitoyl CoA yields eight acetyl CoA, seven $FADH_2$, and seven NADH. Unsaturated fatty acids sometimes require relocation of the double bond, accomplished through the action of enoyl CoA isomerase. Sometimes an initial α-oxidation is required to deal with shorter chain or methylated fatty acids.

CATABOLISM OF AMINO ACIDS AND NITROGEN DISPOSAL

Generally the first step in catabolism of amino acids is the removal of amino groups, usually by transamination to α-ketoglutarate to give glutamate and the corresponding α-keto acid. The transaminases [36] comprise a set of enzymes with different amino acid specificities, each requiring pyridoxal phosphate (PLP) as cofactor. They are often inhibitable by sulfhydryl reagents. Certain amino acids, e.g., serine and threonine, can release the amino group through the action of PLP-dependent dehydratases. The keto acids then enter the TCA cycle at various points, dependent on the structure. Branched-chain keto acids finally result in a residue of propionyl CoA, which is handled as described under the oxidation of odd-numbered fatty acids. The amino group is removed from glutamate by a specific enzyme, glutamate dehydrogenase [37], with $NAD(P)^+$ as cofactor to yield α-ketoglutarate and NH_3. Organic arsenic and mercury compounds and IAM can act as inhibitors. Waste nitrogen enters the urea cycle as NH_3 to form carbamoyl phosphate and as aspartate, via transamination of oxaloacetate with glutamate. Carbamoyl phosphate synthetase I [38] is located in high concentration in the matrix of liver mitochondria and requires ATP and Mg^{2+} as cofactors. This synthetic step requires one HCO_3^-, one NH_3, and two ATP and is tightly regulated by N-acetylglutamate, which is required for activation of the enzyme. The level of this effector is regulated in turn by the level of arginine in the liver cells.

Condensation of carbamoyl phosphate with ornithine forms citrulline via ornithine transcarbamoylase [39] to which carbamoyl phosphate is tightly bound. Argininosuccinate synthetase [40] with ATP and Mg^{2+} as cofactors condenses citrulline with aspartate. In this reaction, one ATP is cleaved to AMP and PP_i. The PP_i is then cleaved to P_i by pyrophosphatase, rendering the entire reaction sequence irreversible. Argininosuccinase [41] cleaves its substrate to arginine and fumarate, which reenters the tricarboxylic acid

cycle from whence its carbon skeleton was derived as oxaloacetate. Thus each turn of the urea cycle requires an intersection with the last two steps of the TCA cycle. Arginine is cleaved to urea and citrulline by arginase [42] with Mn^{2+} (manganese ion) as cofactor, thus completing the cycle. Note that the production of each urea, containing two nitrogens, requires the energy equivalent of four ATPs. The required fumarate-to-oxaloacetate segment of the TCA cycle and glutamate dehydrogenase reaction, however, result in the production of two NADH and, via oxidative phosphorylation, six ATP. Disposal of nitrogen is then an energy-producing catabolic process, with a net yield of one ATP per nitrogen disposed of as urea.

THE TRICARBOXYLIC ACID CYCLE

The final oxidative steps of acetate to CO_2 and H_2O occur in the Krebs TCA cycle or citric acid cycle. As in glycolysis, this stepwise process leads to the complete oxidation of carbon, the passage of reducing equivalents to NAD^+ or FAD, and substrate level phosphorylation. In the first step, acetyl CoA combines with oxaloacetate through the action of citrate synthetase [43] to yield citroyl CoA as a transient intermediate. Spontaneous hydrolysis of citroyl CoA with its large $-\Delta G$ produces CoASH plus citrate in an essentially irreversible step. Fluoroacetate, naturally found in a South African plant, *Dichapetalum cymosum*,[6] is one of the most potent inhibitors of the TCA cycle. Metabolically, it is converted to fluoroacetyl CoA, which serves as a substrate for citrate synthetase. The product of this reaction, fluorocitrate, is a potent inhibitor of aconitase [44], the next enzyme in the sequence. Although by definition not a suicide substrate, fluoroacetate might be called a "suicide inhibitor" of the TCA cycle. Aconitase, tightly bound to fluorocitrate, is unable to bind and process its natural substrate, citrate, which accumulates. Aconitase is also inhibited by Hg^{2+}. This inhibition could be a consequence of the fact that the enzyme contains as a cofactor a Fe_4S_4 (four iron–four sulfur) cluster. Studies have shown that aconitase is capable of losing reversibly one iron and that the iron may be replaced by other metals. Such substitutions may offer a control mechanism for this enzyme.[7] The product of the action of aconitase, isocitrate, is acted on by isocitrate dehydrogenase [45] with $NAD(P)^+$ and Mg^{2+} as cofactors to give α-ketoglutarate, CO_2, and NAD(P)H.

At this step, the first of two maximally oxidized carbons is lost. Note that the two carbons lost as CO_2 in the TCA cycle derive from the oxaloacetate, not the acetyl group, incorporated into citrate. The acetyl carbons become part of the oxaloacetate produced at the end of the first turn of the cycle. This enzyme is inhibited by organic mercury compounds. The other product, α-ketoglutarate, can branch to other pathways, e.g., transaminases [36], or glutamate dehydrogenase [37], or continue via α-ketoglutarate dehydrogenase [46] to succinyl CoA and CO_2. The cofactors required are TPP, lipoic acid, CoASH, FAD, and NAD^+, and inhibitors include organic mercury and arsenic compounds, arsenite (AsO_3^{2-}), IA, and IAM. In these respects, the enzyme mimics pyruvate decarboxylase. Succinyl CoA can branch into porphyrin synthesis or continue in the TCA cycle. Succinyl CoA synthetase [47] captures the high energy of the thioester by coupling its hydrolysis to the synthesis of GTP from GDP plus P_i. This is the only instance of substrate-level phosphorylation in the TCA cycle. The high-energy phosphate can be transferred from GTP to ADP to yield GDP plus ATP by the action of diphosphokinase. Succinate, another product of the cycle reaction, is acted on by succinate dehydrogenase [48] with FAD and an iron-sulfur protein [52] as cofactors, which are bound to the inner mitochondrial membrane. The two reducing equivalents from succinate pass to CoQ in the ETS and can therefore result in the production of two ATP at most. Succinate dehydrogenase is inhibited by malonate, which competes competitively with succinate for the enzyme, by alloxan, AsO_3^{2-}, organic mercury and arsenic compounds, ethyliodoacetate (ethyl-IA), and F^- plus P_i. The last inhibition is unique inasmuch as fluoride plus phosphate form a tight complex with the enzyme. The product of succinate dehydrogenase, fumarate, is hydrated to L-malate by fumarase [49], which is inhibited by organic mercury compounds and fluorooxaloacetate. Malate dehydrogenase [50] removes the final reducing equivalents in the TCA cycle by transferring them to its cofactor NAD^+ and producing oxaloacetate to begin the cycle once again. This enzyme is inhibited by monofluorooxaloacetate and difluorooxaloacetate.

MITOCHONDRIAL ELECTRON TRANSPORT AND OXIDATIVE PHOSPHORYLATION

Oxidative phosphorylation is driven by the electron transport system in the inner mitochondrial membrane as depicted in Fig. 23-3. This system operates by a stepwise passage of electrons from NADH or $FADH_2$, produced during glycolysis, β-oxidation of fatty acids, and operation of the TCA cycle, through a series of electron acceptor/donor complexes. The active species in these complexes are arranged generally in the order of increasing standard oxidation-reduction potentials, E_0', as listed in Table 23-2. Because the relationship between the standard free energy change and the standard electrode potential for these reactions is given by the relationship

$$\Delta G^{0\prime} = -nF\Delta E_0'$$

it follows that as the electrons pass from lower to higher oxidation potentials, the free energy changes are negative, i.e., the electron flow is in the thermodynamically favored direction.

The components of the electron transport system (ETS) are clustered in three complexes as shown in Fig. 23-3, *A*. Complex I accepts electrons from NADH, which in flowing to the lipophilic coenzyme Q (CoQ), pump protons,

Table 23-2. Sequential electron transfer steps of the inner mitochondrial membrane and associated standard reduction potentials at pH 7.0

Reduction half-reaction	E_0' (V)
$NAD^+ + H^+ + 2e^- \longrightarrow NADH$	−0.320
$NADP^+ + H^+ + 2e^- \longrightarrow NADPH$	−0.324
$FMN + 2H^+ + 2e^- \longrightarrow FMNH_2$ (complex I)	−0.30
$Ubiquinone + 2H^+ + 2e^- \longrightarrow ubiquinol$	0.045
Cytochrome b (Fe^{3+}) + $e^- \longrightarrow$ cytochrome b (Fe^{2+})	0.077
Cytochrome c_1 (Fe^{3+}) + $e^- \longrightarrow$ cytochrome c_1 (Fe^2)	0.22
Cytochrome c (Fe^{3+}) + $e^- \longrightarrow$ cytochrome c (Fe^{2+})	0.254
Cytochrome a (Fe^{3+}) + $e^- \longrightarrow$ cytochrome a (Fe^{2+})	0.29
Cytochrome a_3 (Fe^{3+}) + $e^- \longrightarrow$ cytochrome a_3 (Fe^{2+})	0.55
$\frac{1}{2}O_2 + 2H^+ + 2e^- \longrightarrow H_2O$	0.816

NADH, Nicotinamide-adenine dinucleotide (reduced form); *NADPH,* nicotinamide-adenine dinucleotide phosphate (reduced form); *FMN,* flavin mononucleotide; *$FMNH_2$,* reduced flavin mononucleotide.

H^+, out of the mitochondrial matrix into the intermembrane space. Succinate and the β-oxidation helix pass electrons via complex II without proton pumping to CoQ. Reduced CoQ then passes these electrons on to complex III, which again couples electron flow to proton pumping. The electrons pass from complex III to cytochrome c and thence to complex IV. Again electron flow in complex IV is coupled to proton pumping. The electrons are passed from complex IV to O_2, which is reduced to two H_2O by four electrons originally from two NADH or two $FADH_2$. The proton gradient set up across the mitochondrial inner membrane, in addition to the inherent charge polarization of this membrane, tends to drive the protons from the inner membrane space back into the matrix. The flow of protons, however, is most readily accommodated by complex V, consisting of a transmembrane proton channel coupled to an ATPase on the inner surface of this membrane. Because the entire system is completely reversible, the thermodynamically favored flow of protons from the intermembrane space into the matrix can drive the nonthermodynamically favored synthesis of ATP from ADP and P_i by the ATPase. This scheme is the so-called chemiosmotic coupling mechanism of oxidative phosphorylation (Fig. 23-3, *B*). Note that even though the ΔG of each of the three electron transport complexes is sufficient to drive the synthesis of one ATP per pair of electrons transported, the coupling, according to the chemiosmotic mechanism, is via the general proton gradient. The passage of electrons from NADH provides more than sufficient free energy for the synthesis of three ATP, whereas the passage of two electrons from $FADH_2$ (from succinate or β-oxidation of fatty acids) provides sufficient free energy for the synthesis of two, but not three, ATP.

Complex I contains NADH dehydrogenase (NADH-CoQ reductase) [51], which contains flavin mononucleotide (FMN) and an iron-sulfur center [52] as cofactors and is

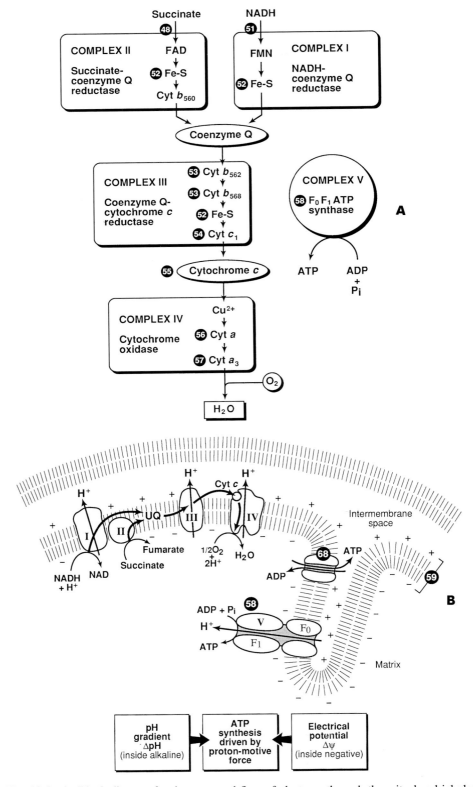

Fig. 23-3. A, Block diagram for the entry and flow of electrons through the mitochondrial electron transport system. Electron transporters and adenosine triphosphate *(ATP)* synthase are keyed to Table 23-1. **B,** Possible schematic representation for the arrangement of electron carriers and the ATP synthesizing complex in the inner mitochondrial membrane. The basis for the chemiosmotic hypothesis of coupling of electron flow to ATP synthesis is represented in this diagram.

inhibited by quinones, organic mercury compounds, rotenone, amytal, piericidin A, and ferricyanide ($Fe(CN)_6^{3-}$), which accepts electrons, thus diverting them from CoQ. Recall that NADH reducing equivalents produced in the cytoplasm enter the mitochondria via the malate or glycerol-3-phosphate shuttles. The malate shuttle delivers these electrons to NAD^+ in the matrix, so they can then enter at complex I and result in the synthesis of three ATP. The glycerol-3-P shuttle delivers its electrons to complex II, so the maximum yield is two ATP. Complex II contains succinate dehydrogenase (succinate-CoQ reductase) [48], which contains FAD and an FeS center as cofactors and is inhibited as described under the TCA cycle. Complex III contains cytochromes b_{562} and b_{566} [53], an iron-sulfur center, and cytochrome c_1 [54]. Electron flow from cytochromes b to c_1 is inhibited by antimycin A. Complex III passes electrons to cytochrome c [55], thence to complex IV. Cytochrome c can be locked in the Fe^{3+} state by CN^-, thus inhibiting its activity. Complex IV contains cytochromes a [56] and a_3 [57]. All of the cytochromes contain heme as a cofactor. In addition, cytochrome a_3 contains copper, which shuttles between cuprous and cupric oxidation states during electron transport. The passage of electrons to O_2 from cytochrome a_3 is blocked by reagents that coordinate tightly to its heme iron in one oxidation state or the other, e.g., HCN (hydrogen cyanide), CO (carbon monoxide), HN_3 (hydrazoic acid), HS^- (hydrosulfide ion), F^- (fluoride ion). Complex V contains a membrane-spanning portion, F_0, made up of several subunit proteins; an F_1 inhibitor stalk of a few subunits, which controls proton flow; and a peripheral F_1 headpiece of five different subunits, which make up the ATP synthesizing complex [58]. Complex V is inhibited by oligomycin, venturicidin, and dicyclohexylcarbodiimide (DCCD). Finally, electron transport can be uncoupled from ATP synthesis by lipophilic compounds, which reversibly bind protons or act as transmembrane ionophores, e.g., carbonyl cyanide, phenylhydrazone, dinitrophenol, and vanilomycin, and effectively discharge the proton gradient [59] or membrane polarization required to drive ATP synthesis.

ENZYMES INVOLVED IN HEME SYNTHESIS AND ENERGY TRANSDUCTION

The inclusion of the pathway for heme synthesis (Fig. 23-4) is appropriate to this chapter inasmuch as the delivery of oxygen to the tissues as the ultimate electron acceptor for the mitochondrial electron transport system depends on hemoglobin in the erythrocytes. The major fraction of hemoglobin synthesis occurs in the erythron of the red bone marrow. The first cellular form to appear in the blood, the reticulocyte, contains about 90% of the hemoglobin of the mature erythrocyte and continues to synthesize the remaining 10% during the few days required for its maturation. Various stages of heme synthesis are particularly susceptible to inhibition by lead. Lead is a "b" class (soft) metal[2]

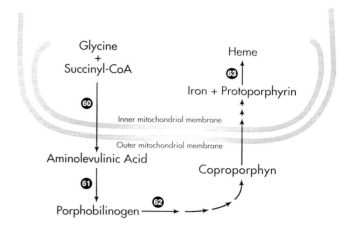

Fig. 23-4. Outline of cellular heme synthesis. Selected enzymes are keyed to Table 23-1.

and elicits profound deleterious effects on the development of the central nervous system.[8] As Pb^{2+}, it has a rather high affinity for sulfhydryl groups but does not appear to be a significant inhibitor of various SH enzymes of the energy-producing pathways. In the developing red cell, however, it appears to increase the synthesis of aminolevulinic acid (ALA) [60] from succinyl CoA and glycine, perhaps by removing a natural control, and to inhibit ALA dehydratase [61] and ferrochelatase [63]. The net result is a reduction in the rate of heme synthesis and an overproduction of ALA, which along with spontaneous condensation products, appears in the urine.

Other sulfhydryl reagents inhibit enzymes of the heme synthesis pathway. ALA dehydratase [61] is inhibited by organic mercury compounds and IAM, and uroporphyrinogen III decarboxylase [62] is inhibited by organic mercury compounds. Hemoglobin [64] itself can be functionally inhibited by agents that bind tightly in place of O_2, carbon monoxide being the prime example, or oxidize the heme iron to the ferric state [65], e.g., NO_2^- (nitrite ion) and amylnitrite. Occupancy of only 25% of the hemoglobin binding sites by CO is sufficient to block oxygen transport by hemoglobin. This level of binding effectively shifts the normal sigmoidal binding curve for O_2 to the left into a nearly hyperbolic binding curve. As a result, the O_2 carried by hemoglobin is not readily released to the tissues. The formation of sulf-hemoglobin from incorporation of sulfur of SH^- or certain drugs into the porphyrin ring can have an opposite effect to CO on the O_2-binding curve but in sufficient amounts blocks the O_2-binding sites. The appropriate dose of an oxidizing agent, e.g., amylnitrite, can be used to prevent the lethal results of cyanide poisoning. The chemical basis for this therapy is to provide a sink for CN^- (cyanide ion), which will leave its binding site on cytochrome oxidase to bind the much larger pool of methemoglobin induced by the amylnitrite. The cyanide can then be metabolically removed by giving thiosulfate, which, through the action of the enzyme rhodanese, converts CN^- plus $S_2O_3^{2-}$ (thiosulfate ion) into SO_3^{2-} (sulfite ion) and SCN^- (thiocyanate ion), which can be excreted. Heme iron spontaneously oxidizes to metheme in red blood cells at about 1% per day. The cell contains a methemoglobin reductase to reverse this trend with NADH as cofactor. As with other cells, the erythrocyte is protected against the ravages of active oxygen species by, among other enzymes, glutathione peroxidase. This selenium-containing enzyme converts H_2O_2 (hydrogen peroxide) into H_2O and glutathione (GSH) into oxidized glutathione (GSSG). To maintain the oxidation-reduction potential of the cell and the protective effect of GSH, GSSG is reduced back to GSH by glutathione reductase with NADPH as cofactor. A genetic lack or modification of glucose-6-phosphate dehydrogenase [16] can eventuate in certain chemicals or drugs, e.g., primaquine and other antimalarials, analgesics, and sulfonamides, overwhelming the reductive capacity of the erythrocyte and lead to intravascular hemolysis.

Finally, enzymes that interconvert ultimate energy forms must be mentioned. In muscle tissue, in particular, energy charge levels are buffered by a significant store of creatine phosphate, which contains a high-energy phosphate but cannot be used directly. Rather, as ATP levels drop during muscle contraction, high-energy phosphate is transferred from creatine phosphate to ADP to restore ATP levels through the action of creatine kinase [67], and the sequence reverses in muscle at rest. The enzyme is inhibited by organic mercury compounds and O-iodosobenzoate (ISBZ). For the ATP produced during oxidative phosphorylation to be used in the cytoplasm, it exits the mitochondrial matrix via an ATP-ADP translocase [68], a dimeric protein transmitting the inner mitochondrial membrane. This antiporter thereby allows ADP to enter the matrix as a substrate for ATP synthesis. It is specifically inhibited by atractyloside and bongkrekic acid.

IMPACT OF VITAMIN DEFICIENCY ON ENERGY METABOLISM

Tissue deficiencies of vitamins can result in general physiological effects or in highly specific effects dependent on the enzymic cofactor nature of a given vitamin or derivative thereof. Lack of vitamin A can lead to impaired intestinal iron absorption and thus to iron deficiency anemia and reduced O_2 transport by the blood. Vitamin E deficiency can lead to increased red blood cell fragility and decreased survival time. This effect may be related to the antioxidant and free radical–destroying abilities of vitamin E. Thiamine (vitamin B_1) is rapidly converted to thiamine pyrophosphate (TPP), an essential cofactor for pyruvate decarboxylase and α-ketoglutarate dehydrogenase. Lack of this vitamin therefore leads to a severe diminution of energy metabolism in tissues. The transketolase of the pentose phosphate pathway also requires TPP. Thus thiamine deficiency can lead to a reduced capacity to synthesize the ribose required for the synthesis of RNA, DNA, $NAD(P)^+$, FMN, FAD, PRPP, and so forth. Beriberi is a disease of severe thiamine deficiency. Riboflavin (vitamin B_2) is an essential component of the enzyme cofactors FMN and FAD required for certain electron transfer steps leading to energy production via oxidative phosphorylation. Although rare, riboflavin deficiency is most likely to occur in alcoholics. Niacin is only partially required as a vitamin because humans are able to synthesize it from tryptophan, albeit inefficiently, and then only after all other bodily requirements for tryptophan have been met. This synthesis also depends on adequate amounts of thiamine, pyridoxine, and riboflavin; therefore, deficits in these vitamins increase the dietary requirement for niacin. Nicotinamide is a component of $NAD(P)^+$ and is therefore essential for all stages of energy metabolism. Pellagra is the disease associated with severe niacin deficiency. Pyridoxine (vitamin B_6) is converted in tissues to pyridoxal phosphate (PLP), an essential cofactor for transaminases, dehydratases, and decarboxylases. Therefore it is necessary for the synthesis of all nonessential amino acids, for the catabolism of all amino acids, and for the synthesis of various neurotransmitters from amino acid precursors. PLP is also a cofactor for glycogen phosphorylase. Deficiencies in humans are rare but can be induced by the antituberculosis drug, isoniazid, with which it forms a covalent compound.

Pantothenic acid is a component of coenzyme A and of phosphopantetheine required for fatty acid synthesis. Thus it is essential for the metabolism of all foodstuffs. This member of the vitamin B complex is so widely distributed in foodstuffs that deficiencies are rarely documented. Biotin (vitamin H) serves as a cofactor for carboxylase enzymes, e.g., pyruvate and acetyl CoA carboxylases, and thus is an essential factor for energy metabolism. Deficiencies are unlikely because biotin is synthesized by the intestinal flora. A diet containing extraordinary amounts of egg white (30% of all calories) can cause biotin deficiency by the tight binding of the vitamin to avidin.[3] Folate (vitamin Bc) is an essential cofactor for C-1 metabolism. In terms of energy metabolism, creatine is synthesized from arginine, glycine, and S-adenosylmethionine. The "active methyl" of the last substance is primarily derived from the C-1 pool via tetrahydrofolate intermediates. (See Chapter 9.) Also, folate deficiency can lead to a megaloblastic anemia and thereby to reduced transport of O_2 to the tissues. Cobalamine (vitamin B_{12}) is an essential cofactor for the rearrangement of carbon skeletons, e.g., methylmalonyl CoA mutase [35], and for the transfer of the methyl groups from N^5-methyltetrahydrofolate to homoserine for the resynthesis of methionine, a precursor of S-adenosylmethionine. Therefore, a deficit in B_{12} can result in a blockade in this arm of the C-1 cycle and lead to a megaloblastic anemia similar to that seen in folate deficiency. Although the anemia is reversible, neurological changes in the central nervous system, resulting from B_{12}

deficiency, are not readily reversed. Ascorbic acid (vitamin C) is an important antioxidant and reductant with a variety of roles. In the diet, it aids the absorption of iron by reducing ferric to ferrous forms. It may help "spare" other antioxidant vitamins, A and E, as well as some B vitamins. The vitamin C deficiency disease, scurvy, is associated with poor healing of wounds, hemorrhaging, and resultant anemia.

REFERENCES

1. Boyer PD, editor: *The enzymes,* vol. XIII, New York, 1976, Academic Press.
2. da Silva JJRF, Williams RJP: *The biological chemistry of the elements,* Oxford, 1991, Clarendon Press.
3. Devlin TM: *Textbook of biochemistry with clinical correlations,* ed 2, New York, 1986, John Wiley & Sons.
4. Hochster RM, Quastel JH, editors: *Metabolic inhibitors,* vols I, II, New York, 1963, Academic Press; Hochster RM, Kates M, Quastel JH, editors: *Metabolic inhibitors,* vols III, IV, New York, 1972-73, Academic Press.
5. Lehninger AB, Nelson DL, Cox MM: *Principles of biochemistry,* ed 2, New York, 1993, Worth Publishers.
6. *The Merck index,* ed 10, Rahway, NJ, 1983, Merck & Co.
7. Thomson AJ: Iron-sulfur clusters with labile metal ions, *J Inorg Biochem* 47:197, 1992.
8. *Toxicological profile for lead,* Agency for Toxic Substances and Disease Registry, US Public Health Service and US Environmental Protection Agency, prepared by Syracuse Research Corporation and Oak Ridge National Laboratory, 1990 Oak Ridge, Tenn.
9. Webb JL: *Enzyme and metabolic inhibitors,* vol 2, 3, New York, 1963-66, Academic Press.
10. Zollner H: *Handbook of enzyme inhibitors,* New York, 1990, VCH Publishers.

Chapter 24

MEDIATORS OF INFLAMMATION

Steven L. Kunkel
Kevin Driscoll
Peter A. Ward
Brian J. Nickoloff
Robert M. Strieter

The pathogenesis of inflammation after exposure to either occupational or environmental agent(s) is dependent on complex cellular and humoral mediator interactions. Although the precise mechanisms that orchestrate the initiation, resolution, or maintenance of this inflammation remain to be fully elucidated, it is evident that the cause of a variety of lung diseases can be attributed to an environmental exposure while at work or in the home. The inflammatory response in the lung is stereotypical and can be classified as either acute or chronic, depending on both the duration of the inflammatory response and the specific cellular infiltration of the lesion. An acute inflammatory response can result on inhalation of either a noxious agent or immunogen in a previously unsensitized or sensitized host. In the lung, this response is often clinically manifested as airway inflammation that possesses the characteristics of asthma, including neutrophil and eosinophil infiltrates, edema, and smooth muscle contraction. These pathologi-

cal events result in hyperreactivity and narrowing of the airways. Other inhaled irritants may cause an acute inflammatory response in the distal lung, as exemplified by the predominant recruitment of neutrophils, release of proteolytic enzymes, generation of arachidonic acid metabolites and reactive oxygen species, and activation of complement within the lung parenchyma. For example, this response could be a consequence of exposure to aerosolized cutting oil or cotton dust (byssinosis) containing lipopolysaccharide (LPS). The pathophysiology associated with inhaled LPS shares salient features with that in patients afflicted with acute bacterial pneumonia, including infiltration of neutrophils, fibrin deposition, and activation of a variety of humoral mediators. Usually the resolution of this initial exposure is rapid and not associated with progression to fibrosis and end-stage lung disease. Repeated exposures to these agents, however, cause recurrence of pulmonary inflammation, ultimately compromising lung function owing to irreversible pathological changes in the lung.

There is no doubt that acute occupational or environmental exposures culminating in an acute inflammatory response are important sources of debilitating pulmonary disease. More insidious occupational or environmental exposures, however, as a consequence of long-term, low-level exposure, are contributing factors to chronic pulmonary and skin inflammation that is associated with a variety of occupational exposures. Usually, these chronic lesions are manifestations of intense cell-mediated reactions that often result in destruction of normal lung tissue architecture and end-stage fibrosis. Chronic cell-mediated inflammatory reactions (granulomatous inflammation), interstitial pulmonary fibrosis, and cancer may be manifestations of chronic exposure to various occupational or environmental agents. Clinically, chronic diseases related to environmental or occupational exposure are often difficult to treat. Intervention requires both removal of the patient from the offending agent and the use of immunosuppressive pharmaceutical agents. The few treatment protocols available to manage these patients underscore our limited understanding of the cellular and molecular mechanisms that propagate these diseases.

An increased awareness of the deleterious effects of exposure to various agents in the environment has had a positive influence in lowering the incidence of certain occupational diseases. Nevertheless, the lung and skin remain vulnerable to the development of both acute and chronic inflammation owing to their unknown and potentially unprotected exposure. This chapter focuses on the basic mechanisms responsible for the initiation, resolution, and maintenance of pulmonary and skin inflammation associated with occupational and environmental diseases.

MEDIATORS OF INFLAMMATION

The response to inhalation of an environmental or occupational agent depends on the orchestration of a number of molecular and cellular events that are mediated by an elaborate signaling network.[48] The pathogenesis of inflammation in response to an environmental agent is the manifestation of multiple and redundant systems that interact in a cascade manner. This ultimately ensures the successful elicitation and activation of various inflammatory cells at the site of tissue injury.[3,43,54,59] During leukocyte recruitment-activation, a number of physiological alterations occur owing to the release of soluble mediators. These inflammatory mediators may not only be important in modulating local tissue injury, but also may be released into the circulation and have deleterious systemic effects. These events are due to the autocrine, paracrine, and endocrine nature of many of these mediators generated in the context of an inflammatory response. A partial listing of potentially important inflammatory mediators is found in the box at top. Exposure to various occupational agents can lead to the generation of inflammatory mediators, activation of leukocytes, and pathological changes not dissimilar to a number of nonoccupationally related lung diseases. Although the etiological agents of occupational and nonoccupational diseases are different, a number of stereotypical mechanisms appear to be involved in mediating the pathology of these disorders.[10,19,69] For example, reactive oxygen and lipid metabolites, split products of complement, proteases, adhesion molecules, and cytokines are all important contrib-

---

Chemical mediators of inflammation
Cytokines
Platelet activating factor
Complement activation
Prostaglandins
Nitric oxide
Oxygen radicals
Leukotrienes
Clotting Cascade
Vasoactive amines
Thromboxane

The various protein mediators that constitute the cytokine family
Tumor necrosis factors
Colony stimulating factors
Migration inhibitory factors
Chemotactic factors
Interleukins
Growth factors
Interferons

utors to the initiation, resolution, or maintenance of environmentally and occupationally related diseases.

CYTOKINES

One of the major advances in the area of inflammation research in the last decade has been the increased appreciation of the role of cytokines in health and disease. Historically, these proteins were termed *lymphokines* or *monokines* as a means to denote a nonantibody protein mediator produced by lymphocytes or monocytes. Several investigations have demonstrated that cells other than immune cells, such as fibroblasts, epithelial cells, neutrophils, and endothelial cells, can participate in the inflammatory response through the production of these same protein mediators of inflammation.* Thus, the term *cytokine* is now used to describe a large number of protein mediators that serve as communication networks between cells and tissue during the evolution of an inflammatory response. Although the interleukins are the largest members of the group of cytokines, other cytokines include the tumor necrosis factors, interferons, growth factors, and colony stimulating factors (see second box above). Interestingly, each cytokine was originally named according to a defined biological activity; however, many of these cytokines possess pleiotropic and overlapping biological activities.[50] The multifunctional activities of these protein mediators are not restricted to inflammation, as many cytokines exert their actions under ho-

---

*References 13, 24, 32, 80, 81, 84.

meostatic conditions. For example, the circadian rhythm of body temperature, changes in appetite, and patterns of sleep is influenced by fluctuations in low levels of certain cytokines. The increased production of cytokines in response to inflammation, however, can lead to significant alterations in the physiology of the host.[14,18,78] This pathophysiology is often manifested by systemic signs and symptoms of disease, such as fever, alterations in heart rate and blood pressure, lethargy, and loss of appetite. Thus, the biological effects of cytokines can be related to the magnitude of their production. At low concentrations, cytokines are often involved in homeostasis, whereas during acute inflammation on the local level, the production of low levels of cytokines is important in mediating the inflammatory event. As the concentrations of these protein mediators are further increased (e.g., during initiation and maintenance of chronic inflammation), however, both local and systemic effects of these cytokines can be demonstrated as alterations in the physiology of the host. Ultimately, exaggerated and perhaps dysregulated expression of cytokines is associated with life-threatening diseases, such as septic shock and multiple organ failure. Thus, the concentration-dependent bioactivities of these cytokines appear to be instrumental in transforming the host's physiology from that of homeostasis to the extreme of severe pathophysiology with life-threatening consequences.

Cytokines in general are glycosylated proteins with an average molecular weight of 30 Kd. These mediators regulate cellular differentiation, proliferation, and activation.[5] Not only do they induce the differentiation of bone marrow–derived hematopoietic progenitor cells, but they also regulate lymphocyte, macrophage, neutrophil, basophil, eosinophil, and mast cell activation, differentiation, and proliferation. Moreover, cytokines can stimulate a variety of nonimmune cells via specific cytokine cell surface receptors, which are found on essentially all nucleated cells of the body. This finding supports their role in the cellular signaling necessary for cellular communication. For example, receptors for both interleukin-1 (IL-1) and tumor necrosis factor (TNF) have been identified on circulating inflammatory cells and cells from all tissue compartments. Studies directed at isolating, cloning, and understanding cytokine receptors would allow improved means to regulate the cellular response to cytokines by the generation of specific cytokine receptor antagonists.

Although cytokines exhibit pleiotropic bioactivities that influence a variety of systems in vivo, perhaps the greatest advance in the appreciation of cytokine biology has been made in the field of immunity and inflammation. Functionally, cytokines can be classified based on their role in immunological-inflammatory recognition, recruitment, removal, and repair.

Recognition cytokines are classified as early response mediators, which are induced and expressed rapidly during the initiation of an immunological-inflammatory response.

Diverse biological activities of interleukin-1

Lymphocyte activation
Increase interleukin-2R expression
Endothelial cell activation
β islet cell cytotoxicity
Amino acid turnover
Suppression of cytochrome P-450
Osteoblast activation
Neutrophil priming
Hyperlipidemia
Fever
Collagenase synthesis
Cytokine induction

The prototypical cytokines that belong to this group are IL-1 and TNF-α. Although IL-1 and TNF-α are the products of different genes, they possess overlapping pleiotropic effects in a number of biological systems.[15] Originally, IL-1 was isolated, purified, and cloned based on its function as a lymphocyte-activating factor (LAF), whereas TNF-α was isolated based on its biological effect in mediating the necrosis of certain solid animal tumors. Although these early defined activities for IL-1 and TNF-α are still under intense scientific investigation, it is widely accepted that both IL-1 and TNF-α exert multiple activities related to both acute and chronic inflammatory processes.[52] A partial listing of the diverse biological effects of IL-1 is provided in the box above. These two early response cytokines are potentially associated with all initiation, resolution, or maintenance events common to inflammation. Accumulating evidence supports the hypothesis that IL-1 and TNF-α are pivotal protein mediators of inflammation. For example, the early expression and production of these cytokines set in motion a cascade of events leading to the development of cytokine networks important in orchestrating an inflammatory response.[24,81] IL-1 and TNF-α not only network with different leukocyte populations/subpopulations, leading to the increase in production of other distally produced cytokines, but also induce the expression of a variety of cytokines from nonimmune cells, such as fibroblasts, smooth muscle cells, epithelial cells, and endothelial cells.[24,81-83] The ability of IL-1 and TNF-α to stimulate the production of different cytokines from a variety of cellular sources is due to the presence of specific receptors for these cytokines on all somatic cells.

Increasing evidence supports the notion of networking between early response cytokines such as IL-1 and TNF-α, and more distal cytokines, such as interleukin-8 (IL-8) and monocyte chemotactic protein-1 (MCP-1).[81,80] In the context of the lung, alveolar and interstitial macrophages can respond to various stimuli by producing IL-1 and TNF-α. Rapidly synthesized IL-1 and TNF-α then interact in an autocrine or paracrine manner with contiguous resident cells in the alveolar-capillary wall (ACW), including epithelial cells, fibroblasts, endothelial cells, and other resident immune cells. This leads to the production of other cytokines from the resident cells of the lung. The subsequent cytokine cascade induced by IL-1 and TNF-α appears to be especially important in leukocyte recruitment because many of the resident nonimmune cells of the lung can generate leukocyte chemotactic factors IL-8 and MCP-1 in response to these early response cytokines. This event underscores the important role of resident cells as inflammatory effector cells necessary to localize and maintain the signals essential for the emigration of leukocytes. Cytokine networks between immune and nonimmune cells are conceivably initiated by exposure to a number of environmental and occupational hazards. For example, mineral dust inhalation has been found to be a triggering agent for the generation of cytokine networks leading to leukocyte recruitment. Both silica and titanium dioxide (TiO$_2$) exposure have been found to be potent, efficacious agents for the expression of chemotactic cytokines via a TNF-dependent cascade.

Recruitment cytokines are chemotactic cytokines usually generated in response to TNF-α or IL-1. There appears to be a high degree of redundancy built into the system in regard to the signals involved in the elicitation of leukocytes. A diverse group of lipids, oligopeptides, and protein mediators have been determined to possess chemotactic activity for leukocytes. Many of these chemotactic mediators, such as leukotrienes (LTB$_4$), platelet-activating factor (PAF), f-met-leu-phe (fMLP), and C5$_a$, lack specificity for the recruitment of individual populations of leukocytes. Yet inflammatory diseases are characterized by the elicitation and accumulation of rather specific populations and subpopulations of leukocytes. This phenomenon has been at least partially clarified with the discovery of a supergene family of chemotactic cytokines, known as chemokines, which possess a high degree of cellular specificity for the recruitment of leukocyte populations to an area of inflammation.[4,56,57] These chemokines share homology based on four conserved cysteine amino acid residues. They can be further subdivided on the basis of the position of the first two cysteine amino acid residues of the primary structure. The C-X-C chemokine family is characterized by the separation of the first two cysteine amino acid residues by one amino acid (X), whereas the C-C chemokine family is characterized by the first pair of cysteine amino acid residues in juxtaposition. IL-8 and MCP-1 are the most well-characterized and studied members of the C-X-C and C-C family of chemokines. The two disulfide bonds that are formed between the first and third and the second and fourth cysteine amino acid residues are important for the highly stable biological activity of these chemokines. The box above lists representative members of these chemokine families. In general, the C-X-C chemokines possess specific chemotactic activity for neutrophils and the C-C chemokines for monocytes and subpopulations of lymphocytes.

Partial listing of members of the C-C and C-X-C chemokine supergene family

C-C

Monocyte chemotactic protein-1
Rantes
Macrophage inflammatory protein-1

C-X-C

Interleukin-8
Neutrophil-activating protein-2 (NAP-2)
Epithelial cell–derived neutrophil-activating factor-78 (ENA-78)

Removal cytokines are essential to the maintenance of an inflammatory response and are necessary to the full activation of leukocyte function. Gamma-interferon (IFN-γ) is a pivotal cytokine required to maintain an immunological-inflammatory response.[30] This cytokine was originally defined as a protein mediator that protected cells from viral infection. It is now known, however, that this multifunctional cytokine can activate and differentiate monocytes into macrophages. This IFN-γ–dependent event results in the increased ability of macrophages to phagocytize, destroy, and remove an initiating agent or antigen. Additional cytokines are intricately involved in the removal process of inciting agents. Many of these cytokines are involved in leukocyte activation that leads to their continued participation in the inflammatory response. In addition to IFN-γ, other cytokines that belong to this group include colony-stimulating factors IL-2, IL-4, IL-5, and IL-6.

Repair cytokines, lastly, are important to the normal healing or resolution phase of inflammation. These cytokines are important in the orchestration of tissue remodeling, neovascularization, and fibrosis. Several of the repair cytokines belong to a large group of proteins that are potent growth factors, including platelet-derived growth factor (PDGF), fibroblast growth factor (FGF), and transforming growth factor (TGF). These growth factors are instrumental in directing the proliferation of specific resident cells needed to reestablish normal tissue structure after injury.[86] A number of pulmonary diseases, however, are associated with an exuberant repair process characterized by altered fibroblast activation and uncontrolled collagen deposition, culminating in fibrosis and end-stage lung disease. The mechanism(s) whereby repair cytokines are overexpressed and participate in the mediation of pathological fibrosis remain to be fully elucidated. Many environmentally and occupationally related pulmonary diseases exhibit an exuberant fibrotic component, especially pulmonary diseases related to pneumoconiosis. These diseases, once established, are dominated by an overwhelming fibrosis and are extremely difficult to treat, resulting in a high degree of morbidity and mortality. These findings underscore our limited knowledge regarding the mechanism(s) responsible for the process of end-stage fibrosis.

LIPID MEDIATORS

One of the fascinating aspects of inflammatory mediators is their wide degree of heterogeneity. The products of phospholipid metabolism represent an additional group of lipid inflammatory mediators important in the initiation, resolution, and maintenance of lung inflammation.[65] Reactive lipid mediators are derived from membrane phospholipids that are cleaved by specific phospholipases and further metabolized to active endproducts. These lipid mediators are not stored but are generated de novo on cellular activation. Once generated and released, they can exert both an autocrine and paracrine effect on surrounding target cells. Under certain conditions, these lipid mediators can cause additive or synergistic effects during the inflammatory response. Two of the most prominent groups of lipid mediators are the metabolites of arachidonic acid and PAF.[12,58] These lipid mediators are derived from the oxidative metabolism of membrane-released arachidonic acid and lysophosphatidylcholine. Products derived from the metabolism of arachidonic acid include lipoxygenase-derived leukotrienes and cyclooxygenase-derived prostaglandins, prostacyclin, and thromboxane.

PAF is known to be a product of a variety of immune and nonimmune cells, including platelets, neutrophils, macrophages, and endothelial cells.[41] Although originally recognized for its platelet aggregation and activation function, it can also serve as a potent stimulus for the activation and chemotaxis of phagocytic cells. In the context of the lung, PAF has been implicated in a variety of disease states. The role of PAF appears to be related to its ability to mediate the pathophysiology of hypersensitivity reactions. The release of PAF following an antigenic challenge results in immediate changes in pulmonary vascular permeability, smooth muscle contraction, and the recruitment of leukocytes. The consequence of these effects results in airway narrowing and bronchial hyperreactivity. Thus, PAF may play a major role in mediating airway hyperresponsiveness associated with exacerbations of asthma or environmentally or occupationally related lung disorders.

Although PAF has been associated with acute hypersensitivity type of inflammatory reactions, products of arachidonic acid metabolism appear to have bioactivities associated with other acute and chronic inflammatory disorders. Interestingly, cells of the lung appear to possess specificity with regard to the expression of arachidonic acid–derived mediators. For example, when challenged with a phagocytic stimulus, alveolar macrophages and neutrophils synthesize predominately leukotriene B_4 (LTB_4) and prostaglandin E_2 (PGE_2), whereas antigen-challenged mast cells generate predominantly prostaglandin D_2; PGE_2; and leukotrienes C_4, D_4, and E_4. The exaggerated release of arachidonic acid–derived lipid mediators can cause the following: alterations in lung mechanics, pulmonary hypertension, hypoxemia, and loss of the hypoxic vasoconstriction response. Arachidonic acid–derived mediators in vivo may cause either additive or synergistic effects. For example, the administration in vivo of LTB_4 leads to augmented recruitment of leukocytes in the presence of additional PGE_2.[11,34] The mechanism for this phenomenon appears to be the enhancing effect of PGE_2 on vascular permeability. Thus, the change in permeability, in combination with a leukocyte chemotactic factor, results in the synergistic recruitment of leukocytes to a site of inflammation.

The information just given demonstrates that many diverse inflammatory mediators are important in the initiation, resolution, and maintenance of an inflammatory response. Many studies have addressed the expression, production, and regulation of these mediators in vitro and have suggested analogous events in vivo. Although this scientific approach has generated useful information, it provides only evidence for an association without fulfilling Koch's postulate as related to their role in mediating environmentally or occupationally related lung disorders. This limitation has been addressed, in part, by the use of specific animal models of occupational lung disease. The following section provides additional perspective on the in vivo role of specific inflammatory mediators in the pathogenesis of occupational diseases.

ROLE OF CYTOKINES AND LIPID MEDIATORS IN LUNG INFLAMMATION (see Chapter 28)

Evidence demonstrates that mineral dusts, such as the various forms of silica (e.g., α-quartz, cristobalite) and asbestos (e.g., crocidolite, chrysotile) that cause pulmonary inflammation and fibrosis in humans, are potent stimuli for production of a variety of inflammatory mediators. In contrast, relatively innocuous dusts, such as titanium dioxide and aluminum oxide, appear to be, at best, weak stimuli for inflammatory mediator production.[19,22,24,27] This differential effect of mineral dusts on generation of inflammatory mediators is illustrated in Figs. 24-1 and 24-2. Rat alveolar macropohages challenged in vitro with either silica or asbestos responded with dose-dependent increases in TNFα production; in contrast, titanium dioxide and aluminum oxide did not induce the release of TNF-α. A similar pattern of response is observed for macrophage production of the proinflammatory lipid, LTB_4 (Fig. 24-2). Importantly, studies with human macrophages in vitro have shown that they respond in a manner similar to rodent alveolar macrophages.[38,92] These studies suggest that the inflammatory activity of silica and asbestos in vivo results, at least in part, from their ability to directly stimulate production of potent mediators of inflammatory cell recruitment and activation. Although the precise mechanism(s) by which "inflammatory mineral dusts" can increase the expression of TNF-α are not entirely clear, preliminary stud-

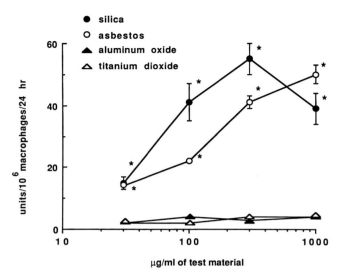

Fig. 24-1. Release of tumor necrosis factor by rat alveolar macrophages exposed for 24 hours in vitro to silica, asbestos, aluminum oxide, or titanium dioxide particles. Values represent the X ± SE; N=3 experiments. The asterisk denotes a statistically significant difference from the nonexposed control group; P < 0.05. Silica and asbestos, but not the relatively innocuous dusts titanium dioxide and aluminum oxide, activate production of tumor necrosis factor. (From Hanahan DJ: Platelet activating factor: a biologically active phosphoglyceride, *Ann Rev Biochem* 55: 483, 1986; with permission.)

ies have shown that the molecular mechanism(s) are, at least in part, at the transcriptional level. Using a myelomonocytic cell line transfected with a TNF-α CAT reporter construct, investigators have demonstrated that in vitro exposure to silica can double the chloramphenicol acetyltransferase (CAT) activity as compared with non−silica-treated cells.[75]

Animal models of silica-induced lung inflammation have greatly expanded knowledge gained from in vitro systems and have provided further insights into the role of inflammatory mediators in occupational lung diseases.[17,26,27,74] Early investigations demonstrated that animals such as rats, mice, or guinea pigs given intratracheal instillation or inhalation exposure to silica developed granulomatous inflammation and a progressive fibrotic reaction. The lung response to silica exposure in animals exhibits a number of characteristics of silicosis in humans, supporting the use of well-characterized animal models for investigating mechanisms of silica toxicity and developing therapeutic interventions to treat silicosis.[17,26,27,74,76] Studies using animal models of silicosis to investigate the contribution of various inflammatory cytokines have demonstrated that silica increases expression of TNF-α mRNA (messenger RNA) in the lung as well as production of TNF-α protein by alveolar macrophages,[63,71] findings consistent with the in vitro observations described previously. In addition, although there is a paucity of information on TNF-α production in lungs of humans with silicosis, studies with alveolar macrophages obtained by bronchoalveolar lavage of asbestosis or coal worker's pneumoconiosis patients demonstrated that these cells were activated to release increased amounts of TNF-α.[51,92]

Studies using a murine model of silicosis have provided compelling evidence that increased TNF-α production plays an essential role in the lung's fibrotic response to silica.[71] In these experiments, mice were passively immunized with an anti-TNF-α antibody or a nonimmune antibody and then intratracheally instilled with 2 mg of silica. Control mice that received the nonimmune antibody developed silicosis characterized by the presence of fibrotic nodules and increased lung hydroxyproline (a biochemical marker of lung collagen). In contrast, in mice passively immunized with neutralizing anti-TNF-α antibody, the silica-induced fibrosis was prevented. Using a similar experimental approach, passive immunization of mice with anti-TNF-α antibody also has been shown to attenuate pulmonary fibrosis in a bleomycin model of interstitial lung disease.[72] Overall, these findings support a cause-and-effect relationship between increased TNF-α production and fibrosis resulting from silica as well as other pneumotoxic agents. It is noteworthy in the studies described here, however, that intraperitoneal perfusion of mice with recombinant TNF-α alone did not affect lung collagen content, whereas perfusion of TNF-α combined with silica exposure produced a fibrotic response greater than that produced by silica alone. These latter observations indicate that although TNF-α is a key mediator of silica fibrosis, other factors also are essential to this disease process. Although the mechanism by which TNF-α influences the fibrotic response is not fully understood, several studies indicate this cytokine may act indirectly to stimulate fibroblast proliferation and synthesis of extracellular matrix proteins.[31,40,68] For example, TNF-α can induce secretion of PDGF by endothelial cells as well as augment the expression of epidermal growth factor (EGF) receptors by fibroblasts. Therefore, increased production of TNF-α at sites of tissue injury may result in an expansion of the local population of collagen-synthesizing cells. To date, a direct relationship between TNF and the subsequent development of fibrosis in human silicosis has not been established. It is likely, however, that further research will provide evidence that cytokines play a significant role in this disease process.

The elicitation of leukocytes to sites of inflammation appears to be a key factor in the pathogenesis of many occupational lung diseases. This observation is particularly true with regard to the initiation and maintenance of silica-induced lung disease. Studies using animal models of silicosis have demonstrated that leukocyte depletion before silica exposure or blocking inflammatory cell recruitment with anti-CD11 antibody significantly attenuates silica toxicity.[42,70] Thus, inflammation and the mediators that regulate the recruitment and activation of inflammatory cells

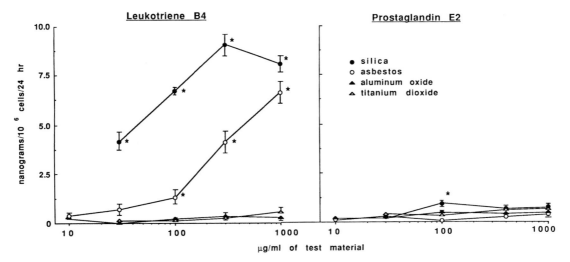

Fig. 24-2. Release of leukotriene B_4 and prostaglandin E_2 by rat alveolar macrophages exposed for 24 hours in vitro to silica, asbestos, aluminum oxide, or titanium dioxide particles. Values represent the X ± SE; $N=3$ experiments. The asterisk denotes a statistically significant difference from the nonexposed control group; $P < 0.05$. Silica and asbestos, but not the relatively innocuous dusts titanium dioxide and aluminum oxide, activate production of leukotriene B_4. (From Hanahan DJ: Platelet activating factor: a biologically active phosphoglyceride, *Ann Rev Biochem* 55: 483, 1986; with permission.)

play a key role in silicosis. As described in the previous section on inflammatory mediators, TNF-α appears to be able to establish a cytokine network, resulting in the expression of chemokines that are the proximate mediators of cell recruitment. Using various animal models, the role of TNF-α and associated cytokine networks in silica inflammation have been investigated. Studies in mineral dust–exposed rats have demonstrated a positive correlation between silica-induced increases in pulmonary inflammatory cell numbers and the activation of macrophage TNF-α production.[27] More recently, it has been shown that passive immunization of rats with antibodies to TNF-α markedly attenuates the recruitment of neutrophils to the respiratory air spaces after mineral dust exposure.[21] The central role of TNF-α in eliciting leukocytes to the lungs after challenge with mineral dust is also supported by the increased expression of TNF-inducible chemotactic cytokines in the lungs of dust-exposed animals.[24] As shown in Fig. 24-3, intratracheal instillation of rats with inflammatory doses of silica or TiO_2 increased steady-state levels of mRNA for the TNF-α-inducible chemokines, macrophage inflammatory proteins 1 and 2 *(MIP-1α, MIP-2)*, and *MCP-1* mRNA.

Increasing evidence supports the theory that cytokines and cytokine networks are active in mineral dust–induced lung disease. These types of occupational diseases, however, are not the only ones in which cytokines have a potential pathological role. Occupational exposure to cadmium aerosols can result in pulmonary functional changes indicative of restrictive lung disease.[79] Animal models of cadmium-induced lung disease have been described in which intratracheal instillation of cadmium chloride into rat

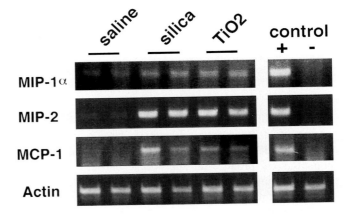

Fig. 24-3. Ethidium bromide stained gels showing macrophage inflammatory proteins 1α and 2 *(MIP-1α, MIP-2)*, monocyte chemotactic protein-1 *(MCP-1)* and β-actin polymerase chain reaction products ($N=2$ rats) amplified from 1 μg RNA from the lungs of rats 6 hours after intratracheal instillation of 10 mg/kg body weight silica (α quartz) or titanium dioxide *(TiO₂)* particles. (+) and (−) controls represent total lung RNA from lipopolysaccharide-instilled (+) and normal (−) rats. Mineral dust exposure increased levels of the tumor necrosis factor–inducible chemotactic cytokines MIP-1α, MIP-2, and MCP-1 mRNA (messenger RNA) expression in lung tissue. No changes in β-actin mRNA expression were detected.

lungs produced lung injury and acute inflammation within 24 hours of exposure followed by a rapid progression to a fibrotic reaction within 7 days of exposure.[23,28,36,66] Characterization of cytokine expression in this lung disease model has demonstrated increased levels of TNF-α mRNA by 12 hours after cadmium instillation into rat lungs, a response accompanied by an increase in the expression of the chemokine, MIP-2. Thus, similar to inflammatory cell recruitment following mineral dust exposure, the response to cadmium-induced injury likely also involves TNF-α and TNF-inducible chemotactic cytokines.

Finally, studies indicate that oxidant stress may be an important stimulus for chemokine-mediated inflammatory cell recruitment. The irritant gas, ozone, is an important environmental pollutant. Acute exposure of humans or animals to near-ambient levels of ozone results in reversible changes in lung function as well as pulmonary inflammation characterized by increased numbers of neutrophils.[20,47,77] Neutrophils may contribute to tissue injury through release of tissue-damaging oxidants and proteases and thus may represent an important component of ozone lung toxicity. Studies using ozone-exposed mice have demonstrated that this pollutant increases expression of MIP-2 in lung, a response associated with the recruitment of neutrophils to the respiratory air spaces and suggesting that MIP-2 plays a role in oxidant-induced inflammation.[25] Interestingly, direct in vitro exposure of alveolar macrophages to hydrogen peroxide has been shown to stimulate dose-related increases in MIP-2 expression.[25] Overall, these observations imply that up-regulation of MIP-2 may be a general mechanism for inflammatory cell recruitment following exposure to agents that result in increased oxidant stress within the lung or other tissues.

PATHOBIOLOGY OF OCCUPATIONAL SKIN DISEASES (see Chapter 27)

Because of its location, the skin, similar to the lung, is an important organ that is frequently bombarded by a diverse array of environmental agents. Not only must the skin constitutively produce an appropriate barrier to minimize any environmental perturbations, but should the insult be of sufficient magnitude to breach this barrier, the skin must also be capable of rapidly and effectively responding to change in order to maintain internal homeostasis. One of the principal mechanisms by which the skin can subserve this "environmental protection" assignment is by producing cytokines that can mediate the inflammatory and immunological reactions that occur following injury and restore the structure and function of the integument. Besides the overt toxic effects of various chemicals, irradiation from various sources, solvents, allergens, and irritants, the two most frequent occupationally related disorders affecting the skin are irritant dermatitis and allergic contact dermatitis.[1]

Based on both in vitro and in vivo data, we postulated several years ago that the key resident skin cell responsible for ensuring a rapid response to epicutaneously derived stimuli was the keratinocyte.[6] The central focus for this novel proposition was the recognition of the remarkable capability of keratinocytes to serve as "signal transducers" that could convert a wide variety of environmental cues,

such as ultraviolet irradiation, tumor promoters, allergens, and irritants, into the production of soluble mediators (i.e., cytokines) such as IL-1 and TNF-α. Subsequent to this proposal, at least 11 publications have appeared demonstrating that keratinocytes can produce IL-1 or TNF-α rapidly (within minutes to hours) following several different stimuli.* Thus, it is becoming clear that, in addition to assisting the skin to function as a protective coat (resulting from keratinocyte production of keratins and lipids that accumulate in the stratum corneum), these cells, which occupy more than 95% of the epidermal mass, also actively participate in the genesis and propagation of various cutaneous responses to injury. Once these cytokines are produced by keratinocytes, they can subsequently induce adhesion molecules and chemotactic polypeptides on other adjacent cell types, including endothelial cells.

When the endothelial cells become activated, they express various adhesion molecules, thereby promoting the influx of mononuclear cells into the skin. These immunocompetent cells are directed toward the surface because keratinocytes also produce appropriate directional signals via IL-8 and monocyte chemotactic and activating factor (MCAF) secretion.[8,9] Once T lymphocytes are juxtaposed to cytokine-activated keratinocytes (which can now express human lymphocyte antigen-DR [HLA-DR] and intercellular adhesion molecule-1 [ICAM-1]), the keratinocytes can also serve an accessory cell role and mediate T-cell proliferation and the production of additional cytokines such as IFN-γ.[62] IFN-γ and TNF-α can synergistically amplify these signals because they greatly enhance coordinate production of keratinocyte adhesion molecule and chemotactic factors.[7] This newly appreciated immunological role for keratinocytes has led us to propose that these cells are key immunocytes of the skin.[61]

As one can begin to appreciate, cytokine networks are established that start in the epidermis but involve crosstalk from both sides of the basement membrane zone, including important contributions from dermal cell types. For psoriasis, a common skin disease that can be exacerbated by various environmental perturbations, it appears that dermal dendrocyte TNF-α production is important in the overall TH-1 type cytokine network that maintains this disorder.[63,85] In other conditions, mast cells may be recruited into the skin secondary to keratinocyte-derived mast cell growth factor production.[53] At least one lymphoproliferative disease that involves the skin (i.e., mycosis fungoides) has been linked to chronic environmental or occupational exposure, and this disease also is characterized by a TH-1 type of cytokine network.[35,90] Not all T-cell–mediated skin diseases are of the TH-1 type, as it has been observed that atopic dermatitis and the early phases of allergic contact dermatitis are more closely linked to a TH-2 type of immune response.[46] The specific

---

*References 2, 33, 37, 39, 44, 49, 60, 64, 67, 73, 91.

molecular basis for determination of a TH-1 versus a TH-2 type of response is unclear but probably involves the nature of the antigenic stimulus, the type of antigen-presenting cell, and the influx of specific subsets of memory T lymphocytes.

Finally, it should be clear that, because of its accessibility, many new insights into the inflammatory and immunological basis for diseases can be gained by studies of the skin. As a growing appreciation for the full immunological repertoire of the keratinocyte emerges, it is likely that epithelial cells in other organs—particularly the lung—will be subjected to greater scrutiny. Such new insights may provide therapeutic opportunities to better prevent or treat those diseases that arise from environmental and occupational exposures.

SUMMARY

The major pathological changes observed during the initiation and maintenance of occupational lung diseases are consistent with the induction of an inflammatory response in the host. Although the mechanism(s) that initially activate the inflammatory system during exposure to an occupational or environmental challenge may be unique, the subsequent reactivity is stereotypical of the inflammatory response. A strict requirement for the establishment of an inflammatory response, independent of the initial activation step, is the elicitation of leukocytes to the involved tissue. Advances in this area have demonstrated a redundant system involving lipid products, oligopeptides, and protein mediators of inflammation. There is no doubt that the large number of different mediators that may be expressed in vivo underscores the importance of the recruitment process to the full expression of inflammation. The discovery of chemokines has further focused on this aspect of inflammation because these chemokines demonstrate a degree of specificity for the recruitment of individual leukocyte populations to an area of inflammation. Continued research in this area will have a high likelihood of not only providing an understanding of these enigmatic disease processes, but also developing therapeutic strategies and reagents useful in treating these disorders.

REFERENCES

1. Adams RM: Medicolegal aspects of occupational skin diseases, *Dermatol Clin* 6:121, 1988.
2. Ansel JC, Luger TA, Green I: Effect of in-vitro and in-vivo UV irradiation on the production of ETAF activity by human and murine keratinocytes, *J Invest Dermatol* 81:519, 1983.
3. Arnaout MA: Structure and function of the leukocyte adhesion molecules CD11/CD18, *Blood* 75:1037, 1990.
4. Baggiolini M, Walz A, Kunkel SL: Neutrophil activating peptide-1/interleukin-8, a novel cytokine that activates neutrophils, *J Clin Invest* 84:1045, 1989.
5. Balkwill FR, Burke F: The cytokine network, *Immunol Today* 10:299, 1989.
6. Barker JNWN et al: Keratinocytes as initiators of inflammation, *Lancet* 1 337:211, 1991.
7. Barker JNWN et al: Marked synergism between tumor necrosis factor-alpha and interferon-gamma in regulation of keratinocyte derived chemotaxic and adhesion molecules, *J Clin Invest* 85:605, 1990.
8. Barker JNWN et al: Modulation of keratinocyte derived interleukin-8 which is chemotactic for neutrophils and T lymphocytes, *Am J Pathol* 139:869, 1991.
9. Barker JNWN et al: Regulation of keratinocyte derived monocyte chemotaxis and activity factor by interferon gamma, *J Immunol* 146:1192, 1991.
10. Bitterman PR, Rennard SI, Crystal RG: *Environmental lung disease and the interstitium. Clinics in chest medicine.* In Brooks SM, Lockey JE, Harper P, editors: *Occupational lung disease,* ed 2, New York, 1981, Marcel Dekker.
11. Bray MA, Cunningham FM, Ford-Hutchinson A: Leukotriene B4: a mediator of vascular permeability, *Br J Pharmacol* 72:483, 1981.
12. Brigham KL, Duke SS: Prostaglandins in lung disease, *Semin Respir Med* 7:11, 1985.
13. Brown Z et al: Cytokine activated human mesangial cells generate the neutrophil chemoattractant interleukin-8, *Kidney Int* 40:86, 1991.
14. Cerami A: Inflammatory cytokines, *Clin Immunol Immunopathol* 62:S3, 1992.
15. Clark BD et al: Genomic sequence for human prointerleukin 1 beta: possible evolution from a reverse transcribed prointerleukin-1 alpha gene, *Nucleic Acids Res* 14:868, 1986.
16. Cochrane CG, Spragg R, Revak SD: Pathogenesis of the adult respiratory distrtess syndrome: evidence of oxidant activity in bronchoalveolar lavage fluid, *J Clin Invest* 71:754, 1983.
17. Dauber JH et al: Experimental silicosis. Morphologic and biochemical abnormalities produced by intratracheal instillation of quartz into guinea pig lungs, *Am J Pathol* 101:595, 1980.
18. Dinarello CA: Interleukin-1 and its biologically related cytokines, *Adv Immunol* 44:153, 1989.
19. Driscoll KE, Maurer JK: Cytokine and growth factor release by alveolar macrophages: potential biomarkers of pulmonary toxicity, *Toxicol Pathol* 19:938, 1991.
20. Driscoll KE, Vollmuth T, Schlesinger RB: Acute and subchronic ozone inhalation in the rabbit: response of alveolar macrophages, *J Toxicol Environ Health* 21:37, 1987.
21. Driscoll KE et al: *Contribution of macrophage-derived cytokines and cytokine networks to mineral dust-induced lung inflammation.* In *Proc. 4th International Inhalation Symposium on "toxic and carcinogenic effects of solid particles in the respiratory tract,* Hannover, Germany, 1994, in press.
22. Driscoll KE et al: Differential effects of mineral dusts on the in vitro activation of alveolar macrophage eicosanoid and cytokine release, *Toxicol In Vitro* 4:284, 1990.
23. Driscoll KE et al: Expression of TNF-α and MIP-2 in rat lung after cadmium chloride-induced lung injury, *Am Rev Respir Dis* 145:A695, 1992.
24. Driscoll KE et al: Macrophage inflammatory proteins 1 and 2: expression by rat alveolar macrophages, fibroblasts, and epithelial cells in rat lung after mineral dust exposure, *Am J Respir Cell Mol Biol* 8:311, 1993.
25. Driscoll KE et al: Ozone inhalation stimulates expression of a neutrophil chemotactic protein, macrophage inflammatory protein-2, *Toxicol Appl Pharmacol* 119:306, 1993.
26. Driscoll KE et al: Pulmonary response to inhaled silica or titanium dioxide, *Toxicol Appl Pharmacol* 111:210, 1991.
27. Driscoll KE et al: Pulmonary response to silica or titanium dioxide: inflammatory cells, alveolar macrophage-derived cytokines, and histopathology, *Am J Respir Cell Mol Biol* 2:381, 1990.
28. Driscoll KE et al: Stimulation of rat alveolar macrophage fibronectin release in a cadmium model of lung injury and fibrosis, *Toxicol Appl Pharmacol* 116:30, 1992.
29. DuBois CM, Bissonnette E, Rola-Pleszcynski: Asbestos fibers and sil-

ica particles stimulate rat alveolar macrophages to release tumor necrosis factor, *Am Rev Respir Dis* 139:1257, 1989.

30. Dumonde DC et al: "Lymphokines": non-antibody mediators of cellular immunity generated by lymphocyte activation, *Nature* 224:38, 1969.

31. Elias JA et al: Regulation of human lung fibroblast collagen production by recombinant interleukin-1, tumor necrosis factor, and gamma interferon, *Ann NY Acad Sci* 580:233, 1990.

32. Elner VM et al: Neutrophil chemotactic factor (IL-8) expression by cytokine treated retinal pigmented epithelial cells, *Am J Pathol* 136:745, 1990.

33. Enk AE, Katz SI: Early molecular events in the induction of contact sensitivity, *Proc Natl Acad Sci (USA)* 89:1398, 1992.

34. Fels AOS, Pawalowski NA, Cramer EB: Human alveolar macrophage produce leukotriene B4, *Proc Natl Acad Sci (USA)* 79:7866, 1982.

35. Fivenson DP et al: Cytokine mRNA profiles in CTCL: mycosis fungoides is TH-1 and Sezary syndrome is TH-2, *J Invest Dermatol* 100:556, 1993 (abstract).

36. Frankel FR et al: Induction of unilateral pulmonary fibrosis in the rat by cadmium chloride, *Am J Respir Cell Mol Biol* 5:385, 1991.

37. Gatto H et al: Study of immune-associated antigens (IL-1 and ICAM-1) in normal human keratinocytes treated by sodium lauryl sulphate, *Arch Dermatol Res* 284:186, 1992.

38. Gosset P et al: Production of tumor necrosis factor and interleukin-6 by human alveolar macrophages exposed in vitro to coal mine dust, *Am J Respir Cell Mol Biol* 5:431, 1991.

39. Griffiths CEM et al: Modulation of leukocyte adhesion molecules, a T-cell chemotaxin (IL-8) and a regulatory cytokine (TNF-a) in allergic contact dermatitis (rhus dermatitis), *Br J Dermatol* 124:519, 1992.

40. Hajjar KA et al: Tumor necrosis factor-mediated release of platelet derived growth factor from cultured endothelial cells, *J Exp Med* 166:235, 1991.

41. Hanahan DJ: Platelet activating factor: a biologically active phosphoglyceride, *Ann Rev Biochem* 55:483, 1986.

42. Henderson RF et al: Effect of blood leukocyte depletion on the inflammatory response of the lung to quartz, *Toxicol Appl Pharmacol* 109:127, 1991.

43. Hogg N: The leukocyte integrins, *Immunol Today* 10:111, 1989.

44. Hunziker T et al: Increased levels of inflammatory cytokines in human skin lymph derived from sodium lauryl sulphate-induced contact dermatitis, *Br J Dermatol* 127:254, 1992.

45. Jenkinson SG: Free radical effects on lung metabolism, *Clin Chest Med* 10:37, 1989.

46. Kay AB et al: Messenger RNA expression of the cytokine gene cluster IL-3, IL-4, IL-5 and GM-CSF in allergen late-phase cutaneous reactions in atopic subjects, *J Exp Med* 173:775, 1991.

47. Koren HS et al: Ozone-induced inflammation in the lower airways of human subjects, *Am Rev Respir Dis* 139:407, 1989.

48. Kunkel SL, Strieter RM: Cytokine networks in lung inflammation, *Hosp Pract* 25:63, 1990.

49. Kurimoto J, Streilein JW: Deleterious effects of cis-urocanic acid and UVB radiation on Langerhans cells and on induction of contact hypersensitivity are mediated by tumor necrosis factor-alpha, *J Invest Dermatol* 99:695, 1992.

50. Larrick JW, Kunkel SL: The role of tumor necrosis factor and interleukin-1 in the immunoinflammatory response, *Pharmacol Res* 5:129, 1988.

51. Lassalle P et al: Abnormal secretion of interleukin-1 and tumor necrosis factor a by alveolar macrophages in coal worker's pneumoconiosis: comparison between pneumoconiosis and progressive massive fibrosis, *Exp Lung Res* 16:73, 1990.

52. Le J, Vilcek J: TNF-α and IL-1: cytokines with multiple overlapping biological activities, *Lab Invest* 56:234, 1987.

53. Longley BJ et al: Altered metabolism of mast cell growth factor (c-kit ligand) in cutaneous mastocytosis, *N Engl J Med* 328:1302, 1993.

54. Lukacs NW et al: The role of macrophage inflammatory protein-1 alpha in Schistosoma mansoni egg-induced granulomatous inflammation, *J Exp Med* 177:1551, 1993.

55. Matheson NR, Wong PS, Pravis J: Enzymatic inactivation of human alpha-1-proteinase inhibitor by neutrophil myeloperoxidase, *Biochem Biophys Res Comm* 88:402, 1979.

56. Matsushima K, Oppenheim JJ: Interleukin-8 and MCAF: novel inflammatory cytokines inducible by IL-1 and TNF-α, *Cytokine* 1:2, 1989.

57. Matsushima K et al: Molecular cloning of a human monocyte-derived neutrophil chemotactic factor (MDNCF) and the induction of MDNCF mRNA by interleukin-1 and tumor necrosis factor, *J Exp Med* 167:1883, 1988.

58. McManus LM, Deavers SI: Platelet activating factor in pulmonary pathobiology, *Clin Chest Med* 10:107, 1989.

59. Mulligan MS et al: Roles of beta-2 integrins of rat neutrophils in complement and oxygen radical-mediated acute inflammatory injury, *J Immunol* 148:1847, 1992.

60. Nickoloff BJ, Naidu Y: Perturbation of epidermal barrier function by repeated tape stripping correlates with initiation of cytokine cascade, *Clin Res* 41:255, 1993.

61. Nickoloff BJ, Turka LA: Keratinocytes: key immunocytes of the integument, *Am J Pathol* 143:325, 1993.

62. Nickoloff BJ et al: Accessory cell function of keratinocytes for superantigens: dependence on LFA-1/ICAM-1 interactions, *J Immunol* 150:2148, 1993.

63. Nickoloff BJ et al: Cellular localization of interleukin-8 and its inducer-tumor necrosis factor-alpha in psoriasis, *Am J Pathol* 138:129, 1991.

64. Norris P et al: The expression of endothelial leukocyte adhesion molecule-1, intercellular adhesion molecule-1, and vascular cell adhesion molecule-1 in experimental cutaneous inflammation: a comparison of ultraviolet B erythema and delayed hypersensitivity, *J Invest Dermatol* 96:763, 1991.

65. O'Flaherty JT: Lipid mediators of inflammation and allergy, *Lab Invest* 47:314, 1982.

66. Ohno I et al: Sequential expression of cytokine in lung tissues exposed to cadmium chloride, *Am Rev Respir Dis* 147:A734, 1993.

67. Oxholm A et al: Immunohistochemical detection of interleukin-like molecules and tumor necrosis factor in human epidermis before and after UVB irradiation in-vivo, *Br J Dermatol* 118:369, 1988.

68. Palombella VJ et al: Tumor necrosis factor increases the number of epidermal growth factor receptors on human fibroblasts, *J Biol Chem* 262:1950, 1987.

69. Piquet PF: Is "tumor necrosis factor" the major effector of pulmonary fibrosis, *Eur Cytokine Net* 1:257, 1990.

70. Piquet PF et al: Antibody to the leukocyte integrins CD11a or b prevent or cure pulmonary fibrosis elicited in mice by bleomycin or silica, *Am Rev Respir Dis* 145:A190, 1992.

71. Piquet PF et al: Requirement for tumour necrosis factor for development of silica-induced pulmonary fibrosis, *Nature* 344:345, 1990.

72. Piquet PF et al: Tumor necrosis factor/cachectin play a key role in bleomycin-induced pneumopathy and fibrosis, *J Exp Med* 170:655, 1989.

73. Piquet PF et al: Tumor necrosis factor is a critical mediator in hapten-induced irritant and contact hypersensitivity reactions, *J Exp Med* 173:673, 1991.

74. Reiser KM et al: Experimental silicosis. I. Acute effects of intratracheally instilled quartz on collagen metabolism and morphology of rat lungs, *Am J Pathol* 110:30, 1982.

75. Savici D et al: Silica increases release of tumor necrosis factor from-mononuclear phagocytes, in part, by increasing expression of the tumor necrosis factor (TNF) gene, *Clin Res* 40:186A, 1992.

76. Seaton A: *Silicosis.* In Morgan W, Seaton A, editors: *Occupational lung disease,* ed 2, Philadelphia, 1989, WB Saunders.

77. Seltzer J et al: Ozone-induced change in bronchial reactivity to methacholine and airway inflammation in humans, *J Appl Physiol* 60:1321, 1986.

78. Sherry B, Cerami A: Cachectin/tumor necrosis factor exerts endocrine, paracrine, and autocrine control of inflammatory responses, *J Cell Biol* 107:1269, 1988.

79. Smith TJ et al: Pulmonary effects of chronic exposure to airborne cadmium, *Am Rev Respir Dis* 114:161, 1976.

80. Standiford TJ et al: Alveolar macrophage-derived cytokines induce monocyte chemoattractant protein-1 expression from human pulmonary type II-like epithelial cells, *J Biol Chem* 266:9912, 1991.

81. Standiford TJ et al: Interleukin-8 expression by pulmonary epithelial cells: a model for cytokine networks in the lung, *J Clin Invest* 86:1945, 1990.

82. Strieter RM et al: Endothelial cell gene expression of a neutrophil chemotactic factor by TNF, LPS and IL-1, *Science* 243:1467, 1989.

83. Strieter RM et al: Monokine-induced neutrophil chemotactic factor gene expression in human fibroblasts, *J Biol Chem* 264:10621, 1989.

84. Thornton AJ et al: Cytokine-induced gene expression of a neutrophil chemotactic factor/interleukin-8 in tumor hepatocytes, *J Immunol* 144:2609, 1990.

85. Uyemura K et al: The cytokine network in psoriasis is characterized by a T-helper type 1 cell mediated response, *J Invest Dermatol* 101:685, 1993.

86. Wahl SM et al: Transforming growth factor beta induces monocyte chemotaxis and growth factor production, *Proc Natl Acad Sci (USA)* 84:5788, 1987.

87. Ward PA: Mechanism of endothelial cell killing by hydrogen peroxide or products of activated neutrophils, *Am J Med* 91:89S, 1991.

88. Ward PA, Varani J: Mechanisms of neutrophil-mediated killing of endothelial cells, *J Leukoc Biol* 48:97, 1990.

89. Weiss SJ: Tissue destruction by neutrophils, *N Engl J Med* 320:365, 1989.

90. Whittemore AS et al: Mycosis fungoides in relation to environmental exposures and immune response: a case control study, *J Natl Cancer Inst* 47:1560, 1989.

91. Wood LC et al: Cutaneous barrier perturbation stimulates cytokine production in the epidermis of mice, *J Clin Invest* 90:482, 1992.

92. Zhang Y et al: Enhanced interleukin-1 and tumor necrosis factor release and messenger RNA expression in macrophages from idiopathic pulmonary fibrosis or after asbestos exposure, *J Immunol* 150:4188, 1993.

Chapter 25

IMMUNOPATHOLOGY

Sally A. Huber

The immune system is designed to combat infections and protect the individual. The same responses that can protect the body from infection, however, can also cause tissue injury and disease. One of the clearest examples of the harmful aspects of immunity is hay fever, an aggressive response of the body to an innocuous pollen. Interestingly the mechanisms of immune sensitization and response are identical in both beneficial and injurious forms of immunity. What determines the nature of the response is the initiating agent and the efficacy of the regulatory systems for immunity (i.e., whether the immune response can be shut off). This chapter discusses the basic precepts in immunity and how these apply to diseases associated with environmental toxins.

THE NATURE OF ANTIGENS

Antigens are compounds that are able both to stimulate an immune response and to react with the components of that response (i.e., antibodies or lymphocytes). Generally, antigens require a minimal size of several thousand daltons.[107] Other factors influencing the antigenicity of a compound include its molecular composition, shape, and ability to be catabolized.[67,107] Generally, inorganic compounds cannot function as antigens. Among organic material, the most effective antigens are proteins or polypeptides followed by polysaccharides, lipids, and nucleic acids. Increasing the complexity of the chemical composition of a compound usually makes it a better antigen. For example, polypeptides made up of a single amino acid are not antigenic, but copolymers of two amino acids can be antigenic in some species. Polypeptides made up of more than five or six types of amino acids are likely to be antigenic in most species.[67]

Some compounds that are not antigenic can still be important immunologically. These compounds can function as haptens. Haptens are molecules that cannot induce an immune response but can react with the products of immunity.[67,107] For example, dinitrophenol (DNP) is too small to act as an antigen, but when DNP is conjugated to a larger molecule, called a carrier, immunity to DNP can be induced. Once antibodies to DNP have been obtained, these can bind directly to the DNP molecule. The carrier molecule provides the size and framework needed for the hapten to be processed for antigenic presentation to the immune system. Importantly, even self-molecules can be used as carriers. Thus, individuals develop sensitivity to penicillin, a small organic molecule that acts as a hapten, when the antibiotic attaches to cells or protein "carriers" in the body.[62,71] Similarly, inorganic compounds such as nickel cannot function as independent antigens but can stimulate immune responses as haptens attached to other organic carrier molecules.

ANTIGEN PROCESSING AND IMMUNE SENSITIZATION

The initiation of an immune response usually starts with processing of the antigen by a group of cells called "antigen presenting cells" (APC). These are usually macrophages, B lymphocytes, or members of the reticuloendothelial system, but other specialized cells, such as keratinocytes in the skin, can also perform this function.* The antigen is internalized through phagocytosis or pinocytosis into vesicles within the cytoplasm. Lysosomes fuse with these vesicles, and the proteases released from the lysosomes degrade the antigen into peptides. Normally, this phagocytic process would be an innate form of host defense because infectious organisms undergoing proteolysis would be destroyed. At the same time that the antigen is being degraded, a population of cellular proteins, called major histocompatibility complex (MHC) molecules, is synthesized. These MHC molecules come in two forms: class I and class II proteins. Class I MHC molecules consist of a single polypeptide chain coded by the MHC gene and a β_2 microglobulin chain, which is identical for all class I MHC molecules. The class II protein consists of an α and β polypeptide chain coded by two separate genes in the MHC locus. Although the polypeptides composing the class I and class II MHC molecules are different, the tertiary structures of these two types of MHC molecules are quite similar. The most notable characteristic of the MHC molecules is a deep groove, which is used to bind small peptides of about 9 to 16 amino acids in size.[12,15] The MHC is a polyallelic system. This means that there are many different possible types of MHC proteins in the population. The important genetic differences defining a particular MHC type appear to be centered in the groove. Because the groove is the antigen-binding portion of the MHC molecule and each MHC molecule binds a different antigenic peptide, the fine specificity of the immune response to any particular antigen can vary substantially within the whole population.[59] That is, although all individuals experiencing an influenza viral infection would produce "anti-influenza" immune T cells, the actual peptide epitope of the influenza virus recognized by each individual would differ in accordance with their MHC haplotype.

The diversity in how individuals react to specific antigens is usually beneficial. Infectious agents frequently mutate, and there is always the possibility that individual T-cell epitopes could be altered or lost in the mutant microbe. Because each individual has multiple different MHC antigens (in humans, there are at least three class I antigens and three class II antigens coded by each chromosome, resulting in a potential of 12 different MHC antigens expressed codominantly on that person's APC), however, it is highly unlikely that all of the epitopes binding to each of these MHC molecules will be changed simultaneously. In certain situations,

the MHC haplotype may be inadvertently responsible for disease. In these cases, individuals with particular MHC antigens may be more likely to develop pathogenic immunity to environmental agents because their MHC molecules bind and present these antigens, whereas the MHC molecules of other individuals do not.*

The MHC molecules are synthesized in the endoplasmic reticulum and are glycosylated in the Golgi complex. As with other cell membrane proteins, the MHC molecules are inserted into the membranes of endosomes, which pinch off from the Golgi and are transported to the plasma membrane. Here the endosome and plasma membranes fuse, resulting in the addition of a new segment of membrane to the cell surface with the transmembrane proteins already in place. During this process of synthesis and transport of the MHC molecules, the antigenic peptides must enter the groove. The class I and class II molecules bind the foreign peptides in different compartments of the cytoplasm.[49,59] Basically, class II molecules bind and present exogenous peptides, whereas the class I molecules bind endogenously made peptides. When class II molecules are made, the groove is covered with an "invariant chain" or I chain peptide. This prevents the groove from binding any of the peptides present in the endoplasmic reticulum or Golgi. During the transport of the class II molecules to the cell surface, however, the endosomes may fuse with the phagosomes containing the proteolytically digested foreign peptides. The fusion of the endosome and phagosome decreases the pH of the endosome. The lowered pH causes the I chain to dissociate from the groove. Any peptides present in the vesicle may now bind to the MHC molecule and are transported to the cell surface. In contrast, for class I antigen presentation, the relevant peptides must be transported to the endoplasmic reticulum, where the class I molecules fold around them as the MHC molecules are synthesized. As with the class II molecules, the class I proteins with their associated antigenic peptide are ultimately transported to the cell membrane.

The APC display their MHC molecules primed with foreign peptides to passing T lymphocytes. The T cells have specific structures on their surfaces called "T-cell receptor," or TcR, molecules.[4,32,79] Two types of TcR have been identified. One consists of an α and a β chain, which combined have a tertiary structure to complement a particular MHC-peptide complex. The effect is much like a key in a lock. Any particular TcR should ideally fit only one MHC-peptide complex. The T cell would then respond to only that antigenic peptide. The second type of TcR consists of a γ and a δ chain. T cells expressing the $\gamma\delta+$ TcR are found in limited numbers in the blood and peripheral lymphoid organs, but the frequency of these T cells in the epithelia of the gut, skin, or uterus can be quite high. Much remains unknown about the $\gamma\delta+$ T cell. The antigenic diversity of

*References 3, 6, 49, 59, 68, 80, 116.

*References 17, 41, 51, 65, 99.

this population appears to be restricted compared with αβ+ TcR cells, and antigen presentation of peptides to γδ+ T cells differs from presentation to αβ+ T cells using either different cell surface molecules or nonvariable regions of the MHC molecule. A large proportion of γδ+ T cells react to a population of molecules called heat shock proteins (hsp).[123] hsp represent a family of highly conserved molecules that are important in cell function and protein transport in the phylogenetic range of species from microbes to humans. The conserved nature of the hsp in microbes may provide early protection from these infectious agents before the induction of antigen-specific αβ+ T cells. Lymphocytes expressing the γδ+ TcR could be maintained in specific locations, such as the epithelium of the intestines, by the normal microbial flora present. These cells would be immediately available to combat pathogenic organisms introduced into the gut, whereas stimulation of antigen-specific αβ+ T cells usually requires up to 7 days. Thus the γδ+ T cells would act as the first line of defense before highly antigen-specific αβ+ T cells become available. Lymphocytes belonging to the γδ+ T cell population have been shown to accumulate in the skin lesions of patients with the tuberculous form of leprosy and with cutaneous leishmaniasis.

Hsp are not exclusively present in microbes. In cells, certain hsp are constitutively produced, whereas others are present only during periods of stress.[123] Various types of cellular injury can cause hsp induction, including inhibition of cellular metabolism and production of oxygen free radicals. Antibiotics, including adriamycin[58] and bleomycin,[81] activate hsp production in exposed cells, and T lymphocytes, reactive to hsp, may participate in tissue injury associated with these drugs. Other hsp correspond to proteins made by cellular oncogenes and accumulate during transformation.[123] Activated γδ+ T cells are cytolytic to many types of tumor cells, and lines of these lymphocytes have been established from tumor infiltrating lymphocytes isolated from Wilms tumors, melanomas, and sarcomas. Although direct proof is lacking, circumstantial evidence implies that γδ+ T cells might be involved in immune surveillance against cancers.[123]

PROLIFERATION OF αβ+ T LYMPHOCYTES

The binding of the αβ TcR to the MHC-peptide complex is only the first step in the T-cell activation process. Other signals (co-stimulatory factors) are additionally required for lymphocyte activation.[43,46,59] The T cell expresses a protein called CD28 on its surface. This must interact with a protein called B7 on the macrophage surface for lymphocyte activation to occur. Binding of the lymphocyte to the APC through the TcR-MHC-peptide bridge without also binding through the CD28-B7 complex would inactivate the T cell rather than stimulate it.[8,73] With B-T lymphocyte interactions, a similar complex must form between the CD40 molecule on the B cell and the CD40 ligand on the T lymphocyte.[92] Once the appropriate signal is transmitted through these cell surface associations, kinases in the greater TcR complex are activated and transmit the signal for proliferation to the T-cell nucleus.

T cells are divided into different categories based either on their function or on the expression of specific cell surface markers. The major division is based on the expression of either CD4 or CD8 molecules on the lymphocyte surface.[93] CD8 T cells are known as "killer" T cells because these lymphocytes are often involved in T cell–mediated lysis of target cells, such as cells infected with viruses or bacteria. Thus, the CD8+ T cell is primarily an effector lymphocyte, which is directly responsible for elimination of infectious agents through the destruction of the invaded host cells before new microbes can be made and released. CD4 T cells are "helper" cells. These lymphocytes generally direct other cells toward some action through the release of specific proteins called lymphokines. The helper cells are crucial for both T and B lymphocyte proliferation responses and cell differentiation into efficient effector cells.[11,29,43,59] Mostly, CD8+ T cells respond to antigen presented in class I MHC molecules, whereas CD4+ T cells respond to antigen presented in class II molecules.[93] Nearly all cells in the body express class I MHC molecules. Therefore, any tissue that can be infected can also be subjected to CD8+ T cell–mediated lysis.

In contrast, distribution of the class II MHC proteins is usually restricted to the population of cells in the body with APC activity. Limiting the interaction of helper cells to a specific population of APC acts as a control mechanism on the initiation of immune responses. Specifically, this restriction will prevent proliferation of lymphocytes to normal tissue antigens, which helps limit the potential for induction of autoimmunity. Once T cells are activated, however, they release cytokines, which can recruit additional antigen-presenting function from tissues not usually involved with that function. For example, keratinocytes normally express little class II MHC antigen and other accessory molecules such as the B7/BB-1 or ICAM-1 adhesion molecules, which are necessary for antigen presenting activity.[34,46] Coculture of lymphocytes with these resting keratinocytes results in tolerization or anergy of the lymphocyte response rather than sensitization.[8] Thus, under normal circumstances, keratinocytes would not be effective APCs. When the keratinocytes are activated, however, expression of class II MHC and adhesion molecules is substantially increased, and these cells acquire antigen presenting activity for CD4+ cells.* Murine studies indicate that various chemical irritants, including oxazalone, picryl chloride and 2,4-dinitrochlorobenzene, cause enhanced class II MHC antigen expression on keratinocytes but only in animals with competent T lymphocytes.[114] Cytokines, such as interferon-γ (IFN-γ), are needed to activate the kerati-

*References 18, 34, 84, 87, 109, 114.

nocytes for antigen presentation function, and these cytokines are usually produced by sensitized lymphocytes (see Chapter 24). Thus, keratinocytes are unlikely to initiate T cell sensitization to toxic agents in the skin. Once an immune reaction has begun, however, keratinocytes can be recruited as additional antigen presenting cells to extend and influence the later phases of the immune reaction. Increased MHC antigen and adhesion molecule expression has been noted in a number of skin diseases, including acute urticaria, lichen planus, psoriasis vulgaris, mycosis fungoides, and purpura pigmentosa chronica.[9,13,109] Presumably, in these patients, keratinocytes are functioning in the disease process.

Two major subpopulations of helper cells have been distinguished among the CD4+ T lymphocytes based on their requirements for stimulation, their biological activities, and the lymphokines that they produce.[43,82] These are designated Th1 and Th2 cells. Th1 cells produce a specific set of lymphokines, including interleukin-2 (IL-2), IFN-γ, and tumor necrosis factor-β (TNF-β). Th1 cells are involved in the inflammatory cell responses of delayed hypersensitivity reactions and immunoglobulin G_{2a} (IgG_{2a}) antibody responses. Th2 cells produce IL-4, IL-5, IL-6, and IL-10 and are involved in IgG_1, IgE, and IgA antibody responses.

Most likely, Th1 and Th2 cells are derived from a common precursor helper cell, and factors present during the activation and differentiation of the precursor population determine whether the "mature" helper cell will have the characteristics of either the Th1 or Th2 subset.[96,98,115] In murine cutaneous leishmaniasis, Th1 and Th2 cell clones have been isolated that share identical Vα8-JαA72,Vβ4 heterodimers, indicating that both Th cell populations react to the same antigenic epitope and presumably could have a common cellular precursor.[96] Various factors could determine whether antigenic stimulation results in Th1 or Th2 cell responses. Most likely, different APCs are involved in activating the two Th subpopulations.[43,47] Generally, splenic adherent cells and hepatic nonparenchymal cells (possibly Kupffer cells) preferentially activate the Th1 cell response, whereas B lymphocytes are similarly more effective in proliferation of Th2 rather than Th1 cells. Keratinocytes have also been reported to stimulate Th1-like cells. In contrast to splenic adherent cells and Kupffer cells, peritoneal macrophages have been reported to stimulate both Th1 and Th2 cells. This observation indicates that all macrophage-like cells do not have equivalent APC function. What determines whether an APC stimulates preferentially Th1 or Th2 phenotypic responses is not clear. The effect does not appear to be related to antigen processing or peptide interaction with the MHC because Th1 and Th2 cells can react to identical epitopes in class II MHC molecules. Rather the deciding factors may relate to the accessory antigens expressed by the APCs and the different TcR-associated signaling pathways used for Th1 and Th2 cell proliferation.

Th1 and Th2 cells also regulate each other.[43] IFN-γ produced by the Th1 cell inhibits IL-4 production by Th2 cells and suppresses antibody responses. IL-10 released by Th2 cells indirectly inhibits Th1 cell responses by acting on the macrophage, suppressing cytokine production needed for proliferation of this T cell subset. The network of lymphokines is probably responsible for most aspects of immunoregulation. Indeed, many investigators now believe that the old concept of "suppressor T lymphocytes" may actually describe the differential regulatory effects of the various T-cell populations on each other through the lymphokines they produce. When differential activation of T-cell populations occurs, this can substantially affect the pathogenesis of specific diseases. An excellent example of this process is demonstrated by the model of murine cutaneous leishmaniasis.[55] Balb/c mice, which develop a progressive disease, give a predominant Th2 cell response to infection. C57Bl/6 mice, which develop localized lesions that ultimately resolve, give a predominant Th1 cell response. Elimination of the pathogen in this disease depends on IFN-γ, a lymphokine produced by the Th1 cell subpopulation. Thus, individuals giving predominant Th1 cell responses would release more of this lymphokine than animals giving a predominant Th2 cell response.

REGULATION OF HUMORAL IMMUNITY AND IMMUNOGLOBULIN ISOTYPE SWITCHING

Antibodies are glycoproteins produced by B lymphocytes and plasma cells. The basic antibody structure consists of two "light" polypeptide chains of approximately 25 kd and two "heavy" polypeptide chains of approximately 50 kd. Each chain can be further divided into a variable region, which binds to the antigen (antigen-binding region or F_{ab} region) and is therefore unique for different antigen-specific antibodies, and a constant region, which is identical for each antibody in a particular isotype.[59] A functional heavy chain variable region is obtained by rearrangement of the DNA coding for different "variable (V)," "diversity (D)," and "joining (J)" genes during B lymphocyte ontogeny.[39,106] Similar rearrangements occur in variable region genes of the light chain, although only V_L and J_L genes are involved in this chain's rearrangement. The particular interaction of the light and heavy chain variable regions gives the final antigen specificity of the antibody.

The constant region of the antibody is not involved in determining antigen specificity but is important in antibody function. Different antibody isotypes vary significantly in their ability to agglutinate antigen, fix complement, cross basal membranes, and interact with Fc receptors on different cells in transmembrane signaling events. The heavy chain determines the antibody isotype. There are eight mouse antibody isotypes and nine human isotypes, and they correspond to the use of different constant genes. The major isotypes are IgM, IgG, IgD, IgE, and IgA with subclasses existing for IgG (IgG1, IgG2, IgG3, and IgG4) and

IgA (IgA1 and IgA2). Individual genes coding for these constant regions are clustered at the 3' end of the immunoglobulin heavy chain locus. Synthesis of the immunoglobulin heavy chain occurs first in pre-B cells and involves interaction of a successfully rearranged V_HDJ_H gene with the $C\mu$ gene. No immunoglobulin is expressed on the B cell surface, however, until the light chain has been produced. The initial class switching event occurs in the naive B lymphocyte and results in cells simultaneously expressing both surface IgM and IgD. This is an antigen-independent event and most likely indicates that the B lymphocyte is ready to respond to antigen stimulation.

On antigen stimulation, the IgM-producing B lymphocytes can proliferate and differentiate into IgM-producing plasma cells. During the primary response to most antigens, there is class switching of antibody production to IgG, IgE, or IgA isotypes. This class switching can occur only during cell division and involves recombination of the V_HDJ_H gene to a switch region immediately preceding one of the $C\gamma$, $C\alpha$ or $C\epsilon$ genes. This isotype switch is controlled by specific lymphokines produced by Th cell subsets. IL-4, the lymphokine produced by Th_2 cells, is required for the selective switch to IgE antibody production and is also necessary to maintain ongoing IgE responses. IL-4 also promotes isotype switching to the IgG1 antibody class. IFN-γ inhibits IL-4–dependent isotype responses but increases expression of IgG2a antibodies. Transforming growth factor-β (TGF-β) is most likely the switch signal for IgA production. The ability of different cytokines to activate distinct isotype switches can be important in pathogenic conditions because the various antibody subclasses have different functions. For example, IgE antibodies trigger mast cell degranulation during allergic reactions. Thus, immune responses provoking preferential Th_2 cell responses would aggravate allergic reactions through the IL-4 these T cells produce, whereas preferential activation of Th_1 cell responses would suppress allergies through the production of IFN-γ. The compartmentalization of active lymphokines in certain parts of the body may additionally explain why certain antibody isotypes are more prevalent in specific locations in the body. For example, although TGF-β is produced widely in the body, it must undergo proteolytic cleavage to be active. The presence of large amounts of proteases in the gut may result in greater TGF-β activation in this location than in other parts of the body and therefore explain the predominance of IgA-secreting cells in this organ.[39,92,106]

HYPERSENSITIVITY REACTIONS

Distinct types of immunopathogenic mechanisms causing disease were first described by Gell and Coombs in 1963.[48] These were categorized as type I (atopic or anaphylactic), type II (cytotoxic), type III (immune complex), and type IV (delayed hypersensitivity) reactions. Since then, Roitt in 1971[100] and Sell in 1972[107] have added two

more mechanisms: stimulatory or inactivation/activation and granulomatous. Which type occurs in a particular immunopathogenic disease depends largely on the characteristics of the antibody or sensitized lymphoid cells induced and the nature or location of the antigen (Table 25-1).

Activation/inactivation

This type of pathogenic response occurs when antibodies react with biologically reactive molecules and alter their function.[24,107,110] Examples include pernicious anemia, polyendocrinopathy, and myasthenia gravis. In pernicious anemia, antibodies either to intrinsic factor or parietal cells in the stomach that make this factor prevent proper adsorption of vitamin B_{12}. In myasthenia gravis, autoantibodies to the acetylcholine receptor interfere with impulse transmission from nerve to muscle. This form of hypersensitivity reaction can also occur in certain drug hypersensitivity reactions.[110] Specifically, antibodies to drugs, such as insulin or digoxin, can prevent binding of these molecules to their relevant tissue receptors. Generally, this form of immunopathogenicity is not involved in environmental diseases but is more likely to occur in autoimmunity.

Type I: atopic or anaphylactic response

Allergies are a major health problem that affects 20% of the U.S. population. Asthma, a result of chronic allergy, costs an estimated $3.6 billion in 1990, or approximately 1% of the total health care costs of the United States alone.[70,77] The immunological mechanisms involved in allergies resemble the responses against parasites.[70] That is, both induce high levels of IgE, whereas immunity to other microbes such as bacteria or viruses involves other immunoglobulin isotypes. Presumably, this allergic response would be beneficial to individuals residing in areas of high parasite exposure. Over many generations, selective pressures most likely would have increased the proportion of the population with potent allergic responses. When the parasites were eliminated from the environment, however, the immune responses that developed as a protective defense mechanism might have been diverted toward responding to other substances. Thus the low incidences of parasitic infections in the developed countries may be, in part, responsible for the high allergy rates seen in these populations.[70]

The manifestations of allergy differ in different parts of the body. Reactions occurring in the upper respiratory tract result in allergic rhinitis involving sneezing and nasal congestion. In the lower respiratory tract, the same responses cause constriction and obstruction of the bronchi, symptoms involved in asthma. Systemic responses result in anaphylaxis, a potentially lethal condition. Regardless of the location, the basic mechanisms and steps in the allergic response are the same.[64,65,70,89,103] During the sensitization phase, an individual is exposed to the foreign substance designated as an allergen. This allergen is phagocytized by the

Table 25-1. Hypersensitivity reactions to environmental factors

Reaction type	Immediate mediators	Time required for appearance of reaction	Disease manifestations	Etiological agent
Type I	IgE, mast cells or basophiles	0.5-4 hours	Bronchial asthma, anaphylactic shock, urticaria, edema	Ragweed, dust mites, bacterial products, food allergy (milk, eggs, nuts, fish), insect venom, and drug allergies (penicillin, aspirin)
Type II	IgG, IgM complement	0.5-4 hours	Thrombocytopenia, agranulocytosis, hemolytic anemia	Penicillin, quinine
Type III	IgG, IgA (IgE) (usually) complement, polymorphonuclear cells	0.5-4 hours	Glomerulonephritis, vasculitis, SLE and lupuslike reactions, enteropathy	Mercury, group A streptococcal infections, gluten
Type IV	T lymphocytes, macrophages (dentritic cells)	>4-6 hours, peak 24-48 hours	Erythema, vesicle and microabscess formation, psoriasis, contact dermatitis	Poison ivy, metals (nickel, silver, copper), viruses, inflammatory reactions
Granuloma	Either antibody (IgG, IgM) or T lymphocytes, macrophages	Chronic reaction (weeks, months or years) to insoluble antigen	Granulomas, hypersensitivity pneumonitis	Chronic silicosis and berylliosis, zerconium, organic dusts, bacterial, fungal and parasitic infections

APC and activates the relevant population of antigen-specific T cells.

T lymphocytes clearly play a critical role in allergic responses. Antigen-specific T cells to a number of environmental agents, including grass pollen,[16] ragweed,[37] house dust mites,[95] and metals,[5] have been identified in allergic individuals (see Chapters 6 and 28). Interestingly, T-cell responses to allergens can be demonstrated in both allergic and nonallergic individuals.[21] The specific epitopes (those portions of the antigen that bind in the MHC groove and stimulate T-cell response) recognized by lymphocytes from allergic and nonallergic individuals differ.[41] Thus, although nearly all individuals recognize a particular allergen such as ragweed pollen, only those individuals having specific genes give immunopathogenic reactions.*

The importance of the T lymphocytes in allergic reactions depends on the cytokines they produce. IL-4, the lymphokine elaborated by the sensitized Th2 cells, is especially important in allergy because it encourages the B lymphocytes to convert to IgE production.[39,42,70,90] IFN-γ, the lymphokine produced by Th1 cells, inhibits IgE production.[33] Once initiated, IgE production can persist for months or years after the initial antigenic exposure. The IgE binds through the Fc portion of the molecule to specific receptors on either mast cells or basophils. The mast cell is derived from bone marrow cells but migrates to peripheral

tissues, where it most often is located close to blood vessels and in the epithelium. The basophils, also of bone marrow origin, circulate in the blood. As with IgE production, Th2 cell cytokines (IL-3, GM-CSF [granulocyte-macrophage—colony-stimulating factor], and IL-4) increase the growth and differentiation of mast cells, whereas Th1 cell cytokines (IFN-γ) are inhibitors (see Chapter 24).[85,117] Thus the T helper cells have an impact on allergic responses at multiple levels. Once mast cells or basophils become "armed" with the bound IgE molecules, subsequent exposure of the individual to the antigen initiates the allergic response. The antigen binds to the Fab portions of two IgE molecules, causing the receptors bound by these immunoglobulin molecules to be cross-linked. This activates a cascade of enzymes within the plasma membrane of the mast cell, including tyrosine kinase; phospholipases A2, C, and D; and protein kinase C.[70] The immediate result is the opening of the calcium channels in the membrane with a substantial influx of ions into the cell. The ions cause polarization of the cytoplasm, migration of the granules within the cytoplasm to the plasma membrane, fusion of the granule and cellular membranes, and release of the granule contents into the extracellular space. The granules are rich in histamine, serotonin, and platelet-activating factor. The phospholipase A2 breaks down phospholipids into arachidonic acid and ultimately into prostaglandins and leukotrienes.[70,74,107]

Histamine, one of the most potent of the chemicals re-

*References 17, 28, 51, 56, 99.

leased during allergic reactions, primarily acts on the blood vessels, smooth muscles, and exocrine glands.[107] Histamine-releasing factors, which were initially found in monocytes, are now known to be produced by a number of different cell types. These factors greatly enhance the amount of IgE-dependent histamine-released from mast cells. IL-8 most likely acts as a histamine releasing factor.[72,89,122] The effects of histamine can vary. For example, large blood vessels and arterioles usually constrict with histamine exposure, whereas the capillaries and small blood vessels dilate. Two types of receptors, designated H1 and H2, have been identified on different cells for histamine and may be largely responsible for the observed differences in histamine responses.[107] Interestingly, drugs used as antihistamines are not usually effective against both H1 and H2 receptor mediated histamine events. The classic antihistamines work against H1 receptor mediated responses, whereas the thiourea derivatives, burimamide and metiamide, act on H2 receptor mediated response. Other effects of histamine release include increased mucus production, increased permeability of small blood vessels, stimulation of nerve endings resulting in itching or pain, and constriction of bronchial airways.

The aforementioned actions represent the acute phase of the allergic response and occur within minutes to hours of antigen exposure. The late phase or chronic allergic reaction involves recruitment of other immune cells from the circulation into the affected region.[45,64,65] These include basophils and eosinophils as well as lymphocytes and macrophages. Platelet activating factors (PAFs), leukotrienes, and perhaps other chemicals released from the activated mast cells diffuse into adjacent blood vessels and increase the expression of adhesion molecules on both the endothelial cells and the circulating white blood cells. This results in attachment of the white blood cells to the vessel wall near the reaction site with subsequent migration of the cells into the affected tissue. The type of cytokines released in an allergic reaction influences the type of cells migrating into the area. For example, IL-3 and IL-5, which are lymphokines made by Th2 cells, enhance eosinophil and basophil accumulation in tissues.[104] The invasion of the initial area of allergic reaction with the white blood cells can prolong the immune reaction and extend tissue injury.

IgE-dependent mechanisms may not be the only methods for mast cell degranulation. Many of the chemical mediators in allergic reactions, including leukotrienes, histamine, bradykinin, PAF, and C5a, are produced in response to cold temperature.[91] During exposure to cold, a sufficient amount of these mediators may be released to cause vasodilation, bronchospasm, and edema. The chronic eczematous skin lesions that are present in some atopic individuals may be exacerbated by cold because these lesions usually are restricted to exposed skin and are more severe in the winter than in the summer (see Chapter 27).[91] Chronic irritation can also result in reactions that closely resemble

allergic reactions. For example, the cellular infiltrates in irritant and allergic contact dermatitis are similar. Both conditions result in lesions containing increased numbers of CD4+ T cells and enhanced MHC class II antigen expression on Langerhans cells and keratinocytes.[7] The irritants can directly stimulate prostaglandin, histamine, or lysosomal enzyme beta-G release from mast cells, which is primarily responsible for the inflammatory lesions.[94] There is evidence, however, that although lipoxygenesis is enhanced during irritant dermatitis resulting in increased leukotriene production, lipoxygenesis is inhibited during allergic reactions. Similarly, PAF is elevated in allergic but not irritant dermatitis.[101,102] Examples of irritants include acids, alkalis, solvents, epoxy resins, metallic oxides, wool, and cement dust.

The Langerhans cell may be important in allergic reactions. Langerhans cells represent a population of dendritic cells that are derived from the bone marrow and are a form of monocyte.[63,120] Similar dendritic cells are present in the gastrointestinal mucosa,[75,121] bronchial epithelium,[57] and many other tissues[112] and probably share identical functional characteristics with Langerhans cells in the skin. One of the best-known functions of Langerhans-like cells is antigen presentation. Basically, allergens and small compounds, which act as haptens and combine with tissue proteins, are taken up by Langerhans-like cells. These cells then migrate from the peripheral tissue to the paracortical (T-cell dependent) areas of the draining lymph node. Here the dendritic cell may act as the initial APC.[44,112,113] The dendritic cells are substantially more potent APC than macrophage or B lymphocytes because approximately 30 to 100 times fewer of these cells than spleen cells are required for T-cell activation.[44,112,113] Emigration of the Langerhans cells from the skin is not T-cell dependent, but these cells fail to localize in the spleens or lymph nodes of congenital athymic animals, suggesting that T cells or lymphokines are necessary for the Langerhans cell to home to lymphoid tissue. Indeed, naive Langerhans cells may lack APC function despite expressing high levels of MHC antigens. Only after treatment with cytokines such as GM-CSF do Langerhans cells attain full antigen presenting activity (see Chapter 24).[112] Activated Langerhans cells produce various cytokines, including IFN-γ. In the skin, these cytokines may be essential in promoting migration of activated T lymphocytes from the circulation into the tissue.[2,36]

Langerhans-like cells participate at several levels in allergic reactions. First, because of their potent APC function, they support the T-cell activation needed for IgE production. Additionally, Langerhans cells bind IgE through the antibody F_c fragment. These IgE-armed Langerhans cells are not only more effective APCs for specific allergens to T lymphocytes, but also may interact with and activate mast cells.[44]

Many environmental agents cause allergic reactions. These include reactions to molds, bacteria, pollens, insect venom, metals (including diisocyanates, cobalt chloride, nickel, copper, and silver), drugs (including penicillin and aspirin), dyes, coal tar, and foods (including nuts, fish, milk, eggs, and watermelon)* (see Chapters 27 and 28). Allergic reactions to foods can be deceiving because in some cases, the reaction may be to food additives or even to penicillin or fungicides used on the food source.[107]

Type II: cytotoxic reactions

Cytotoxic reactions occur when an antibody attaches to either a foreign molecule passively attached to a cell or to the cell itself. The antibody causes the lysis of the cell by activation of complement or phagocytosis of the cell through interaction with the Fc or C3b receptors on phagocytic cells.[19,107] Antibodies mediating cytotoxic reaction belong primarily to the IgM, IgG3, and IgG1 isotypes because these classes are most effective in binding complement. The cells usually affected in immunopathogenic diseases associated with cytotoxic reactions include erythrocytes (hemolytic anemia), leukocytes (agranulocytosis), platelets (thrombocytopenia), and vascular endothelial cells (vascular purpura). An excellent example of a cytotoxic reaction is hemolytic anemia owing to penicillin, such as might occur in a pharmaceutical manufacturer. Penicillin covalently binds to the erythrocyte membrane allowing antibody to the drug to attach to the cell. Bound antibody can be demonstrated by the direct Coombs test, and when extracted from the cells, the antibody reacts only with other cells treated with penicillin.[71] A similar phenomenon occurs in some individuals treated with hydralazine.[53] Undoubtedly, many other substances in our environment can similarly trigger type II reactions, but to a large extent, the possibilities have not been explored.

A second example of cytolytic reactions associated with environmental factors is the cutaneous lesions associated with exposure to sunlight in systemic lupus erythematosus (SLE) patients (see Chapter 10). SLE patients have circulating autoantibodies to Ro/SSA antigen. In normal keratinocytes, this antigen is not available for antibody interaction. With subsequent to exposure to ultraviolet irradiation, however, keratinocytes show enhanced antigen expression and increased ability to bind the autoantibodies.[50,61,108] Once bound, the autoantibodies activate complement and ultimately lyse the epidermal cells. This reaction may be primarily responsible for initiating the cutaneous lesions of SLE.

Ultraviolet irradiation can affect immunity in other ways. Langerhans cells and keratinocytes exposed to ultraviolet irradiation show decreased ability to present antigen to the T lymphocytes involved in delayed hypersensitivity reactions.[97] This suppressive effect is mediated by IL-10 produced by the keratinocytes, and IL-10 is highly effective in inhibiting Th1 cells responses.[43] Ultraviolet irradia-

*References 2, 40, 54, 66, 105, 107, 111.

tion can additionally affect natural killer cell function.[88] Delayed hypersensitivity reactions and natural killer cells are the key elements in immune surveillance. Immune surveillance has been proposed as an important mechanism for eliminating transformed cells. Thus, ultraviolet irradiation may promote cancer formation both by its ability to damage DNA directly leading to cell transformation and by its ability to prevent the body's defense system to eliminate the damaged or transformed cells.

Although ultraviolet light can suppress immunity, other forms of light may have the opposite effect. Studies by McGrath and colleagues[78] have suggested that fluorescent light suppresses autoimmunity and enhances antigen-specific immune response in experimental animals. As yet, the mechanism of immunomodulation by this light source is not known.

Type III: immune complex reactions

Immune complex reactions occur when antibodies react with antigen, causing precipitates of antigen-antibody complexes to deposit in tissue and activate complement.[107] The type of disease associated with this immunopathogenic mechanism depends on the location of the lesion. Damage to the elastic lamina or arteries occurs during serum sickness. Soluble complexes that precipitate in the glomerulus result in glomerulonephritis. Damage occurring in the walls of small blood vessels is known as an Arthus reaction, and lesions in the articular cartilage of joints results in arthritis.

Serum sickness was initially a disease that occurred in individuals given large amounts of horse antitetanus toxin serum as a form of passive immunization.[107] Within a week of injection of the serum, antibodies to the foreign proteins would begin. Initially the high antigen-to-antibody ratios would prevent precipitate formation (antigen excess), and few lesions would occur. As the concentration of antibody increases and the concentration of circulating antigen decreases, the number of complexes increases because the divalent binding sites on the antibody molecule are likely to interact with epitopes on different antigen molecules, causing cross-linking of these molecules. These precipitates deposit in the wall of arteries and in the renal glomerulus and initiate the complement cascade. Activation of complement requires two antibody molecules bound to antigen and in close proximity to each other. A single IgG molecule bound to antigen cannot activate complement. Thus, antigen-antibody complexes in either high antigen or high antibody excess and that fail to form precipitates are less likely to activate complement or cause tissue damage.[26,52,107] Although binding of the initial components of complement occurs directly on the Fc portion of the antibody molecules, C3 and later complement components attach to adjacent cellular membranes. Thus, complement activated by the immune complexes precipitated onto vascular cells inadvertently causes destruction of the cells. Further damage is caused by the release of C3a and C5a fragments during complement activation, which are chemotactic factors for neutrophils. Neutrophils accumulating in the glomeruli or vessel walls release lysozymes and oxygen metabolites, further damaging the vessels through the release of lysosomal enzymes and oxygen free radicals. Indeed, superoxide dismutase, catalase, and other free radical scavengers block much of the damage induced during immune complex–mediated injury* (see Chapter 21).

Arthus reactions are classically used to describe a dermal inflammatory response caused by the precipitation of antigen-antibody complexes in the skin, which can result in edema, erythema, and hemorrhage between 2 and 5 hours after antigen exposure. The steps in this process are first the localization of the antigen in the dermis and subsequent diffusion of the antigen into the small blood vessels. Circulating antibody precipitates the antigen onto the vessel walls, and these complexes activate the complement cascade. Release of C3a and C5a results in constriction and separation of the endothelial cells. C5a and C5a des-Arg chemotactic factors also attract neutrophils, causing these cells to release their lysosomal enzymes. The enzymes digest the vascular wall producing fibrinoid necrosis.[25,27,83,107]

Two examples of Arthus-like reactions are erythema multiforme and gluten-sensitive enteropathy. Generally, erythema multiforme occurs as a reaction to a drug. The lesions that begin in the dermal vessels result in large accumulations of lymphocytes, edema, separation of the dermis and epidermis, and ultimate necrosis of the epithelial cells. In gluten-sensitive enteropathy, gluten, a gelatinous protein in wheat and other grains, is adsorbed through the gut. Apparently, IgA that is reactive to gluten and that is produced in the gut epithelium is also adsorbed into the circulation with the antigen. Deposition of the gluten-IgA complexes in the small blood vessels in the skin ultimately activates complement.[107]

Immune complex disease of the skin and kidney are common secondary complications of infections caused by group A, beta-hemolytic streptococcal hepatitis B and *Neisseria meningitidis*. They also occur in those with SLE.

Type IV: delayed hypersensitivity

Delayed hypersensitivity reactions are primarily mediated by activated T lymphocytes and macrophages and the cytokines they produce. In contrast to the type I, type II, and type III reactions described previously, which usually are observed within minutes or hours of antigen exposure, delayed hypersensitivity responses develop over a period of several days.† In the skin, delayed hypersensitivity reactions are primarily responsible for the lesions associated with contact dermatitis (e.g., poison ivy, dinitrochlorobenzene [DNCB]).[119] Similar responses are probably involved

*References 10, 20, 22, 25, 27, 30, 83, 86, 107.
†References 2, 31, 60, 76, 107.

in beryllium-associated fibrotic disease of the lung and may play a role in the development of the nodular lesions of silicosis (see Chapter 28).[31,69] The antigen is taken up by the dendritic cells, which then migrate to the draining lymph node. Much of the sensitization of T cells occurs in the lymph node as described earlier. The sensitized T cells subsequently leave the node through the efferent lymph to the reaction site.

An important question in delayed hypersensitivity reactions relates to the mechanism whereby sensitized T cells "home" (i.e., focus on) a particular reaction site. Most likely, interaction of the inducing agent with the resident macrophages or dendritic cells results in production of TNF-α and IL-1. Both factors can stimulate adhesion molecule (intercellular adhesion molecule [ICAM-1], endothelial leukocyte adhesion molecule [ELAM-1]) expression on vascular endothelial cells and keratinocytes in the immediate region of the allergen.[119] These adhesion molecules act as "homing" signals for circulating lymphocytes to attach to the endothelial cells and migrate out into the tissue. Once there, the sensitized T cells recognize antigen presented on dendritic cells and produce an array of lymphokines IFN-γ, TGF-β, migration inhibition factor, macrophage activating factor, and GM-CSF involved in accumulating and activating macrophage and other leukocyte cells (eosinophils, neutrophils, basophils and mast cells)[35] in the reaction site. Activated macrophages produce toxic oxygen (O_2^- and hydrogen peroxide [H_2O_2]) or nitrogen metabolites (NO_2), which have potent antibacterial and antiparasitic activities but are also damaging to tissues, especially under conditions of chronic exposure.[31] Tumor necrosis factor (TNF), which is produced primarily by macrophage-monocytes and lymphocytes, mast cells, polymorphonuclear leukocytes, and keratinocytes, may be a pivotal cytokine in developed hypersensitivity reactions.[31,119]

Two forms of TNF are known. TNF-α (cachectin) and TNF-β (lymphotoxin) are encoded by adjacent genes and have similar activities but share only about 30% peptide sequence homology. These cytokines activate prolonged viability of macrophages, stimulate IL-2 receptor expression on T lymphocytes, promote coagulation, and enhance expression of MHC class I and adhesion molecules on surrounding cells.[119] Once activated, macrophages damage adjacent tissue through the superoxide and L-arginine–dependent nitric oxide pathways as well as by the release of enzymes, including elastase collagenase and neutral proteases.[31] In addition, release of insulin-like growth factor, platelet-derived growth factor, IL-1, and TNF-α promotes proliferation of fibroblasts and an increase in production of collagen, leading to fibrosis of the tissue. The importance of TNF in delayed hypersensitivity responses is illustrated in the experimental model of contact dermatitis owing to DNCB.[119] Exposure to DNCB on the skin of previously sensitized animals results in immediate degranulation of mast cells (1 hour after exposure) probably through IgE-mediated mechanisms. Within 2 hours, there is an increased expression of ELAM-1 on dermal postcapillary venules. Within 4 hours, CD4+ memory T cells accumulate in situ, which subsequently results in increased TNF, messenger RNA (mRNA), and ICAM-1 expression in keratinocytes. Treatment of the animals with antibody to TNF-α before DNCB exposure effectively prevents the edema, lymphocytic infiltration, and epidermal necrosis. This indicates that, at least in this example of contact dermatitis, TNF-α is essential for the initiation or maintenance of the reaction. Generally, antigen-specific T cells constitute only a small percentage of the total inflammatory cell population in contact dermatitis or inflammatory reactions in the lungs owing to silica and organic dust exposure.

Thus, one must ask whether or not T lymphocytes are essential to the disease process. Certainly, in more classic forms of delayed hypersensitivity reactions such as graft rejection or reactions to tuberculin antigens, the T lymphocyte is vital because immunosuppression of this cell population substantially inhibits the immune reaction. Additionally, patients with many inflammatory lung diseases such as hypersensitivity pneumonitis[60] and berylliosis[69] have antigen-specific T lymphocyte responses that correlate with symptomatic disease (see Chapter 28). Most likely, only limited numbers of activated T cells are needed in pathological reactions because the major effectors of tissue injury are the macrophage and leukocytes. The cytokines released from small numbers of lymphocytes could aggregate and activate large numbers of these effector cells in an inflammatory lesion.

Granulomatous reactions

Granulomas arise as cellular reactions to either chronic irritants (nonimmunological) or poorly cleared antigens (immunological). (Table 25-1).[1,23,107,118] In nonimmunological granulomas, aggregates of macrophage often form around foreign bodies in an attempt to eliminate them. The most common form of this type of granuloma occurs around insoluble sutures. Immunological granulomas can form in tissues as cellular responses to a number of agents, including organic or inorganic dusts, bacteria, or molds. Generally the antigen must be either insoluble or poorly soluble, making clearance of the antigen during the immune reaction unlikely. Initiation of the lesions involves interaction of sensitized lymphocytes and phagocytes with antigen resulting in release of various cytokines. Macrophages are activated in situ by either cytokines released from T lymphocytes or by antibody complexing with the insoluble antigen, which results in precipitation of the complexes in the tissue. The insoluble immune complexes either activate complement directly or enhance phagocytosis of the complexes by macrophages (by binding to these cells through either the Fc or the C3 receptors). Macrophages can produce substantial tissue injury through production of cytokines and lysosomal enzymes and release of superoxide rad-

icals. The importance of superoxide radical formation in granulomas is demonstrated in chronic granulomatous disease. This is an inherited disorder involving genetic defects in a phagocyte-specific nicotinamide-adenine dinucleotide phosphate (reduced form) (NADPH)–oxidase complex, resulting in persistent production of superoxide radicals.

The main difference between the immune response resulting in granulomatous disease and other forms of delayed hypersensitivity responses is that the inability of the tissue to eliminate the insoluble antigens results in chronic stimulation of the immune system. The activated macrophages differentiate into epithelioid cells, which have a prominent amorphous cytoplasm and a large nucleus. Other macrophages or epithelioid cells may fuse into multinucleate giant cells. The lesions evolve over extended periods of time into spherical masses of predominantly mononuclear cells having a laminated appearance. In later-stage lesions, there can be substantial fibrosis. Cellular infiltrates may be decreased, and macrophages present in the lesions may contain pigments or lipidic inclusions. The centers of some granulomas may undergo necrosis, depending on the degree of hypersensitivity.

The granulomatous response is most likely a defense mechanism designed to isolate and contain invading agents, such as parasites, bacteria, and molds. Health problems occur when the growing granulomas either displace or constrict normal tissues, preventing them from functioning normally. Granulomas can be found in many different tissues but often occur in the lungs in response to a wide variety of inhaled materials, including silica, beryllium, smoke particulates, and biphasic fungi, such as *Histoplasma capsulatum* (see Chapter 28).

AUTOIMMUNITY

Toxic injury to tissues may result in the induction of autoimmunity. This is clearly documented in animals exposed to mercury which causes the induction of autoantibodies to myeloperoxidase.[14,38] The mechanisms by which environmental toxin exposure could initiate autoimmunity are probably quite similar to those involved in autoimmunity induced by virus infections.[29] First, many environmental agents must haptenize "self"-proteins to induce immunity to the toxin. The haptenization of the self-molecule may actually confer an appearance of "foreignness" to self-protein. For example, injection of a small number of membrane-altered erythrocytes into the erythrocyte donor can result not only in destruction of the modified red blood cells, but also in normal cells, leading to generalized hemolytic anemia. In other cases, the increased expression of MHC and adhesion molecules on tissue cells during inflammatory reactions to environmental agents may lead to the inadvertent presentation of self-molecules to the immune system that are not normally available for appropriate antigen presentation. Self-antigens presented by MHC molecules in the absence of the appropriate secondary signal (co-stimulatory molecules on the APC such as B7) would normally induce anergy rather than immune sensitization. During the reaction to the environmental toxin, however, lymphokines released in situ such as IFN-γ could induce de novo expression of the co-stimulatory molecules on tissue cells. This could lead to effective antigen presentation of the "self"-antigens and autoimmunity.

The significance of the induction of autoimmunity in environmental disease is twofold. First, because the autoimmune response attacks normal as well as abnormal cells, the damage can be more extensive and persist longer than would be expected from hypersensitivity reactions to the environmental toxin alone. Indeed, even if the environmental toxin were removed, the autoreactivity might continue. Second, the presence of a pathogenic autoimmune reaction may obscure the initiating environmental exposure, which may have been transient. Moreover, the toxin might not persist in the tissue. Yet the autoreactivity that results from the exposure may become a chronic condition lasting many years.

REFERENCES

1. Adams DO: The granulomatous inflammatory response, *Am J Pathol* 84:164, 1976.
2. Adams RM: *Allergic contact dermatitis*. In Adams RM, editor: *Occupational skin disease*, Philadelphia, 1990, WB Saunders, p. 26.
3. Allen PM, Unanue ER: Differential requirements for antigen processing by macrophages for lysozyme-specific T cell hybridomas, *J Immunol* 132:1077, 1984.
4. Allison JP, Havran WL: The immunobiology of T cells with invariant γδ antigen receptors, *Ann Rev Immunol* 9:679, 1991.
5. Al-Tawil NC, Marensson JN, Moller E: HLA-class II restriction of the proliferative T lymphocyte responses to nickel, cobalt and chromium compounds, *Tiss Antigens* 25:163, 1985.
6. Augustin M et al: Phorbol-12-myristate 13 acetate treated human keratinocytes express B7-like molecules that serve a co-stimulatory role in T-cell activation, *J Invest Dermatol* 100:275, 1993.
7. Avnstorp C, Ralfkiaer E, Jorgensen J: Sequential immunophenotypic study of lymphoid infiltrates in allergic and irritant reactions, *Contact Derma* 16:239, 1987.
8. Bal V et al: Antigen presentation by keratinocytes induces tolerance in human T cells, *Eur J Immunol* 20:1893, 1990.
9. Barker JN: Role of keratinocytes in allergic contact dermatitis, *Contact Derm* 26:145, 1992.
10. Bedi TR, Pinkus H: Histopathologic spectrum of erythema multiforme, *Br J Dermatol* 95:243, 1976.
11. Benjamin DC et al: The antigenic structure of proteins, *Ann Rev Immunol* 2:67, 1984.
12. Berzofsky JA: Intrinsic and extrinsic factors in protein antigenic structure, *Science* 229:932, 1985.
13. Bieber T et al: Keratinocytes in lesional skin of atopic eczema bear HLA-DR, CD1a and IgE molecules, *Clin Exp Derm* 14:35, 1989.
14. Bigazzi PE: Lessons from animal models: the scope of mercury-induced autoimmunity, *Clin Immunol Immunopathol* 65:81, 1992.
15. Bjorkman PJ et al: The foreign antigen binding site and T cell recognition regions of class I histocompatibility antigens, *Nature* 329:512, 1987.
16. Black PL, Marsh DG: Correlation between lymphocyte responses and immediate hypersensitivity to purified allergens, *J Allergy Clin Immunol* 59:394, 1980.
17. Blumenthal M, Mendell N, Yunis E: Immunogenetics of atopic diseases, *J Allergy Clin Immunol* 65:403, 1980.
18. Boehncke WH et al: Differential expression of adhesion molecules on infiltrating cells in inflammatory dermatoses, *J Am Acad Dermatol* 26:907, 1992.
19. Boyle MDP, Borsos T: The terminal stages of immune hemolysis: a brief review, *Mol Immunol* 17:425, 1980.
20. Brentjens JR et al: Experimental immune complex disease of the lung, *J Exp Med* 140:105, 1974.
21. Buckley RH et al: Lymphocyte responses to purified allergens in vitro. *J Allergy Clin Immunol* 59:70, 1977.
22. Cavenish A: A case of dermatitis from 9-bromofluorene and peculiar reaction to a patch test, *Br J Dermatol* 52:155, 1940.
23. Chambers TJ, Spector WG: Inflammatory giant cells, *Immunobiology* 161:283, 1982.
24. Cinader B, editor: *Antibodies to biologically active molecules*, New York, 1967, Pergamon Press.
25. Cochrane CG: Mediators of the arthus and related reactions, *Progr Allergy* 11:1, 1967.
26. Cochrane CG: The role of immune complexes and complement in tissue injury, *J Allergy* 42:113, 1968.
27. Cochrane CG, Koffler D: Immune complex disease in experimental animals and in man, *Adv Immunol* 16:185, 1973.
28. Cookson WO et al: Linkage between immunoglobulin E responses underlying asthma and rhinitis and chromosome 11q, *Lancet* 1:1295, 1989.
29. Craighead JE, Huber SA, Sriram S: Animal models of picornavirus-induced autoimmune disease, *Lab Invest* 63:432, 1990.
30. Daniele RP, editor: Symposium on immune complex injury of the lung, *Am Rev Respir Dis* 124:738, 1981.
31. Davis CS, Calhoun WJ: *Occupational and environmental causes of interstitial lung disease*. In Schwarz MI, King TE Jr, editors: *Interstitial lung disease*, ed 2. St. Louis, 1993, Mosby.
32. Davis MM, Bjorkman PJ: T-cell antigen receptor genes and T-cell recognition, *Nature* 334:395, 1988.
33. Del Prete G et al: IL-4 is an essential factor for the IgE synthesis induced in vitro by human T cell clones and their supernatants, *J Immunol* 140:4193, 1988.
34. DePanfilis G et al: Adhesion molecules on the plasma membrane of epidermal cells, *Regional Immunol* 4:19, 1992.
35. Dovarak HF, Dvorak AM: *Basophilic leukocytes in delayed-type hypersensitivity reactions in animals and man*. In Jankovic BD, Isakovic K, editors: *Microenvironmental aspects of immunity*, New York, 1973, Plenum, p. 573.
36. Dustin ML, Springer TA: Role of lymphocyte adhesion receptors in transient interaction and cell locomotion, *Ann Rev Immunol* 9:27, 1991.
37. Eisenbrey AB et al: Seasonal variation of in vitro lymphocyte proliferative response to ragweed antigen E, *J Allergy Clin Immunol* 75:84, 1985.
38. Esnault VLM et al: Autoantibodies to myeloperoxidase in brown Norway rats treated with mercuric chloride, *Lab Invest* 67:114, 1992.
39. Esser C, Radbruch A: Immunoglobulin class switching: molecular and cellular analysis, *Ann Rev Immunol* 8:717, 1990.
40. Evans R 3rd, Kim K, Mahr TA: Current concepts in allergy: drug reactions, *Curr Prob Pediatr* 21:185, 1991.
41. Ferguson TA et al: Immunoregulatory properties of antigenic fragments from bovine serum albumin, *Cell Immunol* 78:1, 1983.
42. Finkelman FD et al: Lymphokine control of in vivo immunoglobulin isotype selection, *Ann Rev Immunol* 8:303, 1990.
43. Fitch FW et al: Differential regulation of murine T lymphocyte subsets, *Ann Rev Immunol* 11:29, 1993.
44. Fokkens WJ et al: The Langerhans cell: an understimated cell in atopic disease, *Clin Exp Allergy* 20:627, 1990.
45. Frew AJ, Kay AB: Eosinophils and T-lymphocyte in late-phase allergic reactions, *J Allergy Clin Immunol* 85:533, 1990.
46. Gaspari AA et al: Accessory and alloantigen-presenting cell func-

tions of A431 keratinocytes that stably express the B7 antigen, *Cell Immunol* 149:291, 1993.

47. Gajewski TF et al: Murine TH1 and TH2 clones proliferate optimally in response to distinct antigen presenting cell populations, *J Immunol* 146:1750, 1991.

48. Gell PGH, Coombs RRA: *Clinical aspects of immunology,* Oxford, 1963, Blackwell.

49. Germain RN: Immunology: the ins and outs of antigen processing and presentation, *Nature (Lond)* 322:687, 1986.

50. Golan TD et al: Enhanced membrane binding of autoantibodies to cultured keratinocytes of systemic lupus erythematosis patients after ultraviolet B/ultraviolet A irradiation, *J Clin Invest* 90:1067, 1992.

51. Goodfriend L et al: Ra5G, a homologue of Ra5 in grant ragweed pollen: isolation, HLA-DR associated activity and amino acid sequence, *Mol Immunol* 22:899, 1985.

52. Griswold WR, Brams M, McNeal R: The rapidly changing nature of acute immune complex disease, *J Lab Clin Med* 96:57, 1980.

53. Hahn BH et al: Immune responses to hydralazine and nuclear antigens in hydralazine-induced lupus erythematosus, *Ann Intern Med* 16:365, 1972.

54. Hanifin JM: Atopic dermatitis, *J Allergy Clin Immunol* 73:211, 1984.

55. Heinzel FP et al: Reciprocal expression of interferon γ or interleukin 4 during the resolution or progression of murine leishmaniasis, *J Exp Med* 169:59, 1989.

56. Holt PG, Leivers S: Tolerance induction via antigen inhalation: isotype specificity, stability and involvement of suppressor T cells, *Int Arch Allergy Appl Immunol* 67:155, 1982.

57. Holt PG et al: Ia-positive dendritic cells form a tightly meshed network within the human airway epithelium, *Clin Exp Allergy* 19:597, 1989.

58. Huber SA: Heat-shock protein induction in adriamycin and picornavirus-infected cardiocytes, *Lab Invest* 67:218, 1992.

59. Janeway CA Jr: How the immune system recognizes invaders, *Sci Am* 269:72, 1993.

60. Johnson KJ, Chapman WE, Ward PA: Immunopathology of the lung, *Am J Pathol* 95:794, 1979.

61. Jones SK: Ultraviolet radiation (UVR) induces cell surface R_o/SSA antigen expression by human keratinocytes in vitro: a possible mechanism for the UVR induction of cutaneous lupus lesions, *Br J Dermatol* 126:546, 1992.

62. Katz SI: The role of Langerhans cells in immunity, *Arch Dermatol* 116:1361, 1980.

63. Katz S, Tamaki K, Sachs D: Epidermal Langerhans cells are derived from cells originating in the bone marrow, *Nature* 282:324, 1979.

64. Kay AB: *Mechanisms in allergic and chronic asthma which involve eosinophils, neutrophils, lymphocytes and other inflammatory cells.* In Kay AB, editor: *The allergic basis of asthma,* London, 1988, Balliere & Tindall.

65. Kay AB, Durham SR: T-lymphocytes, allergy and asthma, *Clin Exp Allergy* 21:17, 1991.

66. Kim K, Evans R 3rd, Mahr TA: Drug allergy, *Allergy Proc* 11:299, 1990.

67. Klein J: *Immunology: the science of self-nonself discrimination,* New York, 1982, John Wiley & Sons.

68. Kouralsky P, Claverie JM: The peptide self-model, *An Inst Pasteur/Immunol* 137:3, 1986.

69. Kreiss K et al: Epidemiology of beryllium sensitization and disease in nuclear workers, *Am Rev Respir Dis* 148:985, 1993.

70. Lichtenstein LM: Allergy and the immune system, *Sci Am* 269:116, 1993.

71. Lin RY: A perspective on penicillin allergy, *Arch Intern Med* 152:930, 1992.

72. MacDonald SM et al: Studies of IgE-dependent histamine releasing factors, *J Immunol* 139:506, 1987.

73. Marrack P, Kappler JW: How the immune system recognizes the body, *Sci Am* 269:81, 1993.

74. Marx JL: The leukotrienes in allergy and inflammation, *Science* 215:1380, 1982.

75. Mayrhofer G, Holt PG, Papadimutriou JM: Functional characteristics of the veiled cells in afferent lymph from the rat intestine, *Immunology* 58:379, 1986.

76. McCombs RT: Diseases due to immunologic reactions in the lungs, *N Engl J Med* 286:1245, 1972.

77. McFadden ER Jr, Gilbert IA: Asthma, *N Engl J Med* 327:1928, 1992.

78. McGrath H Jr, et al: Fluorescent light decreases autoimmunity and improves immunity in B/W mice, *J Clin Lab Immunol* 32:113, 1990.

79. Meuer SC et al: The human T-cell receptor, *Ann Rev Immunol* 2:23, 1984.

80. Morrison LA et al: Differences in antigen presentation to MHC class I and class II-restricted influenza virus specific cytolytic T lymphocyte clones, *J Exp Med* 163:903, 1986.

81. Moseley PL, York SJ, York J: Bleomycin induces the hsp 70 heat shock promoter in cultured cells, *Am J Respir Cell Mol Biol* 1:89, 1989.

82. Mosmann TR, Coffman RL: TH1 and TH2 cells: different patterns of lymphokine secretion lead to different functional properties, *Ann Rev Immunol* 7:145, 1989.

83. Movat HZ: Pathways to allergic inflammation: the sequelae of antibody-antigen complex formation, *Fed Proc* 35:2435, 1976.

84. Mutis T et al: HLA class II+ human keratinocytes present Mycobacterium lepral antigens to CD4+ TH1-like cells, *Scand J Immunol* 37:43, 1993.

85. Nafziger J et al: Specific high-affinity receptors for interferon-γ on mouse bone marrow-derived mast cells, *Eur J Immunol* 20:113, 1990.

86. Nagai T et al: IgE deposits in glomeruli with membrane nephropathy and marked asthmatic predisposition in humans, *Jpn Circ J* 37:1227, 1973.

87. Nickoloff BJ: Role of interferon-γ in cutaneous trafficking of lymphocytes with emphasis on molecular and cellular adhesion events, *Arch Dermatol* 124:1835, 1988.

88. Nived O, Johansson I, Sturfelt G: Effects of ultraviolet irradiation on natural killer cell function in systemic lupus erythematosis, *Ann Rheum Dis* 51:726, 1992.

89. O'Hehir RE et al: The specificity and regulation of T cell responsiveness to allergens, *Ann Rev Immunol* 9:67, 1991.

90. Okumura K, Tada T: Regulation of homocytotropic antibody formation in the rat, *J Immunol* 106:1012, 1971.

91. Parker CW: Environmental stress and immunity. Possible implications for IgE-mediated allergy, *Persp Biol Med* 34:197, 1991.

92. Parker DC: T cell-dependent B cell activation, *Ann Rev Immunol* 11:331, 1993.

93. Parnes JR: Molecular biology and function of CD4 and CD8, *Adv Immunol* 44:265, 1989.

94. Patrick E, Burkhalter A, Maibach HI: Recent investigations of mechanisms of chemically-induced skin irritation in laboratory mice, *J Invest Dermatol* 88:245, 1987.

95. Rawle FC, Mitchell EB, Platts-Mills TAE: T cell responses to the major allergen from the house dust mite, *Dermatophagoides pteromyssinus* antigen P1, *J Immunol* 133:195, 1984.

96. Reiner SL et al: Th_1 and Th_2 cell antigen receptors in experimental Leishmaniasis, *Science* 259:1457, 1993.

97. Rivas JM, Ullrich SE: Systemic suppression of delayed-typed hypersensitivity by supernatants from UV-irradiated keratinocytes. An essential role for keratinocyte derived IL-10, *J Immunol* 149:3865, 1992.

98. Röckin M, Saurat J-H, Hauser C: A common precursor for CD4+ T cells producing IL-2 or IL-4, *J Immunol* 148:1031, 1992.

99. Rocklin RE et al: Generation of antigen-specific suppressor cells during allergy desensitization, *N Engl J Med* 302:1213, 1980.

100. Roitt IM: *Essential immunology,* Oxford, 1971, Blackwell.

101. Rosenbach T, Csato M, Czarnetzki BM: Studies on the role of leukotrienes in murine allergic and irritant contact dermatitis, *Br J Dermatol* 118:1, 1988.

102. Ruzicka T, Printz MP: Arachidonic acid metabolism in skin: experimental contact dermatitis in guinea pigs, *Int Arch Allergy Appl Immunol* 69:347, 1982.

103. Ryan GB, Majno G: Acute inflammation. A review, *Am J Pathol* 86:247, 1977.

104. Saito H et al: Selective differentiation and proliferation of hematopoietic cells induced by recombinant human interleukins, *Proc Natl Acad Sci (USA)* 85:2288, 1988.

105. Sampson HA, Mendelson L, Rosen JP: Fatal and near fatal anaphylactic reactions to food in children and adolescents, *N Engl J Med* 327:380, 1992.

106. Schatz DG, Oettinger MA, Schlissel MS: V(D)J recombination: molecular biology and regulation, *Ann Rev Immunol* 10:359, 1992.

107. Sell S: *Immunology, immunopathology and immunity,* ed 4, New York, 1987, Elsevier.

108. Sequi J, Leigh I, Isenberg DA: Relationship between antinuclear antibodies and the autoimmune rheumatic diseases and disease type and activity in systemic lupus erythematosis using a variety of cultured cell lines, *Ann Rheum Dis* 50:167, 1991.

109. Simon M Jr, Hunvadi J, Dobozu A: Expression of beta-2-integrin molecules on human keratinocytes in cytokine-mediated skin disease, *Acta Dermato-Venereol* 72:169, 1992.

110. Smolarz A, Roesch E, Lenz E: Digoxin specific antibody (Fab) fragments in 34 cases of severe digitalis intoxication, *Clin Toxicol* 23:327, 1985.

111. Sontheimer RD, Gilliam JN: Immunologically mediated epidermal cell injury, *Semin Immunopathol* 4:1, 1981.

112. Steinman RM: The dendritic cell system and its role in immunogenicity. *Ann Rev Immunol* 9:271, 1991.

113. Stingl G et al: The functional role of Langerhans cells, *J Invest Dermatol* 74:315, 1980.

114. Stringer CP, Hicks R, Botham PA: The expression of MHC class II (Ia) antigens on mouse keratinocytes following epicutaneous application of contact sensitizers and irritants, *Br J Dermatol* 125:521, 1991.

115. Swain SL et al: Helper T cell subsets, *Immunol Rev* 123:115, 1991.

116. Townsend ARM et al: Cytotoxic T lymphocytes recognize influenza haemagglutinin that lacks a signal sequence, *Nature (Lond)* 324:575, 1986.

117. Tsuji K et al: Effects of interleukin-3 and interleukin-4 on development of "connective tissue-type" mast cells, *Blood* 75:421, 1988.

118. Turk JL: The role of delayed hypersensitivity in granuloma formation, *Res Monogr Immunol* 1:275, 1980.

119. Vassalli P: The pathophysiology of tumor necrosis factors, *Ann Rev Immunol* 10:411, 1992.

120. Volc-Platzer B et al: Cytogenetic identification of allogeneic epidermal Langerhans cells in a bone marrow graft recipient, *N Engl J Med* 310:1123, 1984.

121. Wilders MM et al: Large mononuclear Ia-positive veiled cells in Peyer's patches. Isolation and characterization in rat, guinea pig and pig, *Immunology* 48:453, 1983.

122. Willems J et al: Human granulocyte chemotactic peptide (IL-8) as a specific neutrophil degranulation, *Immunology* 67:540, 1989.

123. Young RA: Stress proteins and immunity, *Ann Rev Immunol* 8:401, 1990.

Chapter 26

CARCINOGENESIS

John E. Craighead

Cancer is a complex, multistage process. It occurs when a clonal population of cells evolves that is not responsive to normal growth control mechanisms and exhibits a degree of autonomy. Some cancers result from either a single intragenic mutation or a chromosomal alteration, but the majority reflect the outcome of a series of cumulative changes in the cell's genetic apparatus associated with ongoing clonal selection. Although the initiating factors and the host susceptibility influences, as well as the myriad of cellular events that occur in carcinogenesis, currently defy definition, the process in the simplest of terms can be considered a disorder of cell transduction.

The initial interaction of a carcinogen or its metabolites with the DNA of a replicating cell results in a genetic alteration, should the damage not be repaired (see Chapter 19). The event is known as *initiation* if it has the potential for contributing to a carcinogenic transformation in the cell or its progeny. Changes in DNA can be a consequence of an interaction with endogenous mutational factors, such as oxygen free radicals, or of the countless exposures to exogenous carcinogens that humankind experience from the embryonic stages of life. There is good reason to believe that healthy adults acquire a large but undefined number of initiated (but not cancerous) cells during a lifetime. The timing of the initiating mutational events no doubt is critical, for those occurring during embryogenesis could lead to mosaic populations of cells in the developing fetus, whereas the later events usually affect only one type of cell.

In their seminal study, Berenblum and Shubik[7] elucidated a second significant series of events during carcinogenesis termed *promotion*.[22] Promotion has a functional definition. Concisely and classically stated, promoter substances are not genotoxic but act to transform initiated cells by shortening the latency period for tumor development or by increasing the susceptibility of cells to genetic injury when the exposure to an initiator alone is insufficient to cause cancer. These effects are generally considered to be epigenetic, but some promoters may also possess the ability to serve as initiators. In the initial studies, a phorbol ester (a croton plant extract) was the promoter, and a polycyclic aromatic hydrocarbon was the initiator. Phorbol esters appear to act through a receptor to stimulate protein kinase activity and thus play a significant role in signal transduction.[9] In recent years, a wide variety of physical and chemical substances has been found to act as promoters in carcinogenesis. The mode of action of these substances (which range in complexity from estrogens to asbestos) in carcinogenesis is not well defined.

Transformation is the process whereby cells develop a degree of autonomy consequent to a genetic alteration. The biologic characteristics of the transformed cell in various tissues differ. It is unclear whether the transformed state is stable and for how long, but the evidence suggests that transformation is followed by *progression*. This is a dynamic state during which tumor cells acquire new biologic characteristics through mutation, at least some of which alter the expression of the cellular proto-oncogenes and regulatory genes (including suppressor genes). Chromosomal instability also characterizes this process and may contribute to aneuploidy. Ultimately, these clones of transformed cells produce some of the more devastating characteristics of clinical cancer (unrelenting growth, invasiveness, and metastasis).

This chapter is concerned with the molecular and cellular events of initiation, promotion, transformation, and progression as they relate to environmental carcinogenesis. In this context, I consider various chemical and physical insults that humans experience in the context of dosages that exceed thresholds, because little is known regarding cellular events resulting from exposure to many of these agents in apparent subthreshold amounts. Carcinogens of contemporary importance are emphasized, whereas those of historical relevance (such as azo compounds and vinyl chloride) are not considered (see Chapter 5).

GENOTOXIC AND NONGENOTOXIC CARCINOGENS

The somatic mutation theory initially advanced by Boveri in 1914 serves as the basis for our modern concept of carcinogenesis.[11] It links with contemporary thought regarding the mutational role of environmental factors such as chemicals (see Chapters 4, 5, 8, and 13) and radiation (see Chapters 10-12) in the pathogenesis of many human cancers. The mechanisms of genotoxic injury are considered in detail in Chapters 10 and 20 and are not discussed further here. However, abundant experimental evidence now indicates that many chemicals and some foreign bodies can initiate neoplastic transformation by their direct effect on the rate of cell multiplication rather than by genotoxic mechanisms.[52,54] If fidelity of DNA replication is inherently imperfect, then errors in the DNA of the gene accumulate in rough proportion to the replication rate of the cells. Exogenously or endogenously derived mutagens appear to act more efficiently on cells in a rapid replicative state, for there is an increased probability that transcription will be affected during a mitogenic event. The p53 suppressor gene serves as a regulator of the cell cycle and, in its absence or when the gene is mutated, cells pass more readily from the G_1 phase to the S phase of the cell cycle. Under this circumstance, there is insufficient time for the normal repair of DNA damage.

These concepts have broad ramifications with respect to the potential impact of multiple carcinogenic exposures to nongenotoxic chemicals at relatively low concentrations in the human environment. A diversity of environmental agents can induce cell multiplication. Sodium saccharin, a sugar substitute, was rejected as a food additive by the Food and Drug Administration when it was found to have carcinogenic effects in rats. In the urinary bladder epithelium of

adult rats, cell multiplication is increased fivefold to tenfold, either after systemic or topical administration of saccharin. Cigarette smoke and asbestos have a direct effect on the multiplication rate of mucosal cells of the lower respiratory tract. Several carcinogenic agents may act by this mechanism. Of these, dioxan has proved to be one of the most potent of carcinogens in animal toxicity studies, despite the lack of a direct mutagenic effect on the cell. Foreign bodies (glass, stainless steel, cholesterol, and wax), when introduced subcutaneously or in the lower urinary tract, cause inflammatory and proliferative cell responses that ultimately can result in cancer. Cytotoxic agents also stimulate cell multiplication, presumably as a response to injury and inflammation, most probably as a result of the local elaboration and release of mitogenic free radicals and growth factors. Carbon tetrachloride, alcohol, and hepatitis B virus infections are recognized carcinogenic stimuli that appear to act by this means. A third, recently elucidated but unproven mechanism of carcinogenesis is the result of exposures to estrogenic substances of relative low potency in the environment.

ONCOGENE AND SUPPRESSOR GENE MUTATIONS POTENTIALLY RELATED TO ENVIRONMENTAL EXPOSURES

Oncogenes and suppressor genes have been the subject of countless publications during the past decade, for they play a key role in neoplastic transformation and tumor progression. In recent years, abundant evidence has accumulated to suggest that molecular specificity of the mutations of the oncogene, ras, and the tumor suppressor gene, p53, may provide insight into the causes of neoplastic transformation and, presumably, the biology of the resulting tumors. Of the many genes characterized as oncogenes or suppressor genes, thus far, ras and p53 appear to be intrinsic to consideration of environmental carcinogenesis.[33]

ras oncogenes

The ras proto-oncogene superfamily is comprised of four extensively characterized, highly conserved genes (Ha-ras, K-ras [A and B], and N-ras) that encode highly homologous monomeric GTP-binding proteins.[26] The ras gene products, 21kd proteins, play an intrinsic role in signal transduction at the internal aspect of the cell membrane, where ras proteins exist in an activated form when bound to GTP. By interacting with the raf-1 protein kinase, they initiate the cytoplasmic MAP kinase cascade (Fig. 26-1). Point mutations at codon 12, 13, or 61 convert the ras gene into an oncogene. The GTPase activity of the ras protein product of mutant genes appears to function less efficiently than the normal gene product and is not stimulated by GDP. As a result, the level of ras:GTP increases in the cell, and its various kinase-mediated activities are enhanced.

The potential role of ras proteins in malignant transformation first became apparent when DNA from a diversity

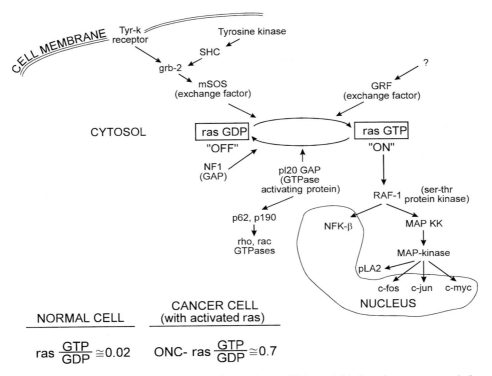

ras $\dfrac{GTP}{GDP} \cong 0.02$ ONC- ras $\dfrac{GTP}{GDP} \cong 0.7$

Fig. 26-1. Current model of the ras signaling pathway. This model is based on recent work from numerous laboratories. Tyrosine kinase *(Tyr-k)* receptors autophosphorylate upon ligand occupation and dimerization. The adaptor protein grb-2, which consists of two SH3 and one SH3 domains, binds to phosphorylated tyrosine residues on the receptors (or on the kinase substrate SHC, in some cases). The SH3 domains or grb-2 bind to mSOS, which is a ras-specific guanine nucleotide exchange factor. Binding occurs through a proline-rich sequence in mSOS. The translocation of SOS to the membrane activates nucleotide exchange on ras, converting it to the GTP-bound state. In this state, ras can associate with the RAF protein kinase. Translocation of RAF to the membrane activates it, perhaps through interaction with lipids or another protein; RAF can then phosphorylate and activate the MAP kinase, which in turn can phosphorylate and activate MAP kinase. The MAP kinase is phosphorylated on both Tyr and Thr residues. The full complement of substrates for MAPKK is not known, but it can phosphorylate and activate phospholipase A2 (pLA2) and phosphorylate several transcription factors. MAPKK translocates to the nucleus. Another transcription factor, NFK-B, is a substrate for RAF. Ras is switched off by the hydrolysis of the bound GTP. This reaction is catalyzed by GAPs (GTPase activating proteins), which include p120 and neurofibromin, the product of the neurofibromatosis type 1 (NF1) gene. The p120 GAP may also have effector functions. It interacts with at least two proteins, p62 and p190, which is a GAP for two other small GTPases, rac and rho, which control cell morphology and motility. The p62 may regulate RNA processing. Oncogenic mutants of ras do not interact with GAP and possess low intrinsic GTPase activities. They are, therefore, constitutively trapped in the GTP-bound state. (Prepared by Ian Macara, PhD, University of Vermont.)

of cancers was transfected into cultured fibroblasts. These cells, thereafter, exhibited morphological features of malignancy in vitro as exemplified by a loss in density-dependent inhibition. The transforming genes and their products were subsequently found to be similar to the previously characterized Ha-ras and K-ras genes of the Harvey and Kirsten sarcoma viruses, which had incorporated them as proto-oncogenes during intracellular replication. Although it is difficult to establish in human cancers, mutations leading to the activation of ras are believed to be early events in carcinogenesis, rather than a reflection of later tu-

mor progression. In part, the evidence relates to the demonstration of characteristic gene lesions associated with specific exposures and evidence of oncogene expression in premalignant lesions and chemically injured, but nonneoplastic cells in experimentally exposed animals.[47]

Codon 12 K-ras mutations are consistently found in adenocarcinomas of the pancreatic parenchyma, a cancer that has been associated with cigarette smoking in some epidemiological studies. Roughly 40% to 50% of colorectal cancers and a similar number of small (<1 cm) tubular adenomas of the colon have similar mutations.[10,24,25] Codon 12 mutations occur commonly in bronchogenic adenocarcinomas developing in smokers and former smokers but are rarely detected in adenocarcinomas of an apparent spontaneous nature and in cigarette smoke–related lung cancers of other morphological types (Fig. 26-2).[51,66] Interestingly, benzo[a]pyrene, the highly carcinogenic constituent of tobacco smoke, induces smilar K-ras mutations in cultured cells. The predominant mutations related to tobacco smoke exposure are G:C→T:A transversions. A relatively small number of human tumors of diverse type exhibit Ha-ras mutations, but this mutant gene is commonly found in invasive human carcinoma of mammary origin.[82]

p53 suppressor gene

Tumor suppressor genes are believed to play an intrinsic role in either the development or progression of a neoplasm. The concept of a suppressor gene is an outgrowth of the elegant work of Harris,[35] in which cultured tumor cells were fused with normal cells in vitro. In his experimental studies, the characteristics of the cancer cells occasionally were found to revert to those of the normal cells, an observation consistent with the acquisition of growth-limiting (i.e., suppressor) factors from the normal cells. During the past decade, a number of well-characterized and candidate suppressor genes have been described as an outgrowth of studies of unique heritable cancer syndromes in which loss of heterogeneity results in a predisposition to

tumor development (Table 26-1). Although the absence of these genes through chromosomal deletions, or mutational germline variants of these genes, appears to contribute to the pathogenesis of specific types of tumors, only the p53 mutant genes thus far have been found to play a contributory role (albeit undefined) in a broad spectrum of human cancers. Indeed, mutant suppressor p53 genes are the most common of the many genetic alterations discovered thus far in human cancers.[34]

Located on chromosome 17 at p13, the p53 gene codes a well-characterized 393 amino acid, phosphoprotein, which interacts with cyclin-dependent kinases, thus regulating cyclin activity and cell growth. Mutations of p53 lead to the elaboration of an altered protein with a longer half-life than the native "wild" protein, but nonetheless, a protein that is less effective in regulating the cell cycle. As a result, cells move more rapidly from the G_1 growth phase to the S phase, an effect that is thought to compromise the ability of normal DNA repair mechanisms to eliminate and replace damaged DNA segments.[46] This appears to increase the likelihood that mutations will accumulate in certain cells consequent to either endogenous mutagens or exposure to exogenous carcinogens.

Several types of specific mutations of the p53 gene have been described in human cancers.[40] Transversions, characterized by missense mutational substitution of amino acids into the evolutionary highly conserved regions of the gene, regularly are found in esophageal carcinomas and hepatocarcinomas. Specifically, G:C→T:A transversions at residue 249 are frequently detected in hepatomas developing in residents of geographically endemic areas where aflatoxin B is believed to be the predominant liver carcinogen.[15,42,43,59] Similarly, transversions occur in benzo[a]pyrene-exposed cells in vitro and in the non–small cell lung cancers of smokers (Table 26-2).[88] By contrast, in colorectal cancers, CpG dinucleotides prove to be hot spots for G:C→A:T mutations resulting from the deamination of 5-methylcytosine.[12,61] This alternate mechanism of mutation is an exceedingly common event in these lower in-

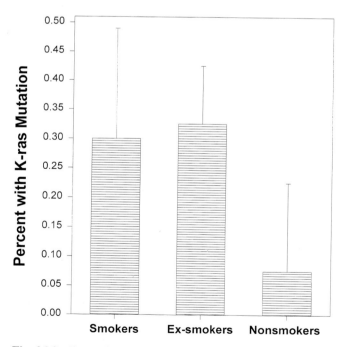

Fig. 26-2. Comparison of frequencies of K-ras mutations in bronchogenic adenocarcinoma among smokers, ex-smokers, and nonsmokers. (Adapted from Westra WH, et al: K-ras oncogene activation in lung adenocarcinomas from former smokers, *Cancer* 72:432, 1993; with permission.)

Table 26-1. Features of candidate human tumor suppressor genes

Product location	Mode of action	Hereditary syndrome
Membrane	Receptor tyrosine kinase	Multiple endocrine neoplasia type 2
Cytoplasm	GTPase-activator	Neurofibromatosis type 1
Inner membrane?	Links membrane to cytoskeleton?	Neurofibromatosis type 2
Nucleus	Transcription factor	Li-Fraumeni syndrome
Nucleus	Transcription factor	Retinoblastoma
Nucleus	Transcription factor	Wilms tumor

Adapted from *Science* 261:1385, 1993.

testinal tumors, although the specific carcinogen(s) involved is not known. The p53 mutations are only one of several altered genetic elements in the cells of adenocarcinomas of colonic and rectal tissues.

Much of our information on human tumors is based on studies of clinically advanced lesions or cell cultures derived from these cancers.[4,12] It is currently unclear whether the high prevalence of p53 mutations in these neoplasms is a reflection of changes that develop during tumor progression (or in culture) or whether the prevalence represents early events that occur during the initiation stages of carcinogenesis (or both).[34,40,51]

CHEMICAL CARCINOGENESIS[33]

In 1761, John Hill described cancer of the nasal mucosa in two users of snuff,[38] a product of the tobacco leaf adulterated by various chemical additives. Thus, he may have been the father of chemical carcinogenesis. Some 14 years later, the perceptive epidemiological observations of Percival Pott, an accomplished English surgeon, established a relationship between exposure to coal tar and the development of cancer.[60] Pott was struck by the prevalence of warty growths on the scrota of boys and young men who were regularly exposed to soot in their work as chimney sweeps. Because of their social status, these men bathed irregularly or not at all. By introducing the elementary hygienic step of bathing, the prevalence of these lesions was reduced and a causative association established. Twenty years later, the role of tobacco smoke in respiratory carcinogenesis was first suggested.[79]

The carcinogenicity of coal tar was demonstrated experimentally almost a century and a half later. In 1895, an exceptional prevalence of urinary bladder cancers in workers exposed to azo dye was first noted. Subsequently, investigations ultimately led to the removal of these dyes and azo compounds from commerce. Hutchison, in 1888, described hyperkeratosis of the skin of patients with dermatitides treated with arsenicals. Later, studies of workers in metal refineries and several other industries confirmed the role of

arsenic in cancer uniquely localized to the scrotum, nipples, and both the palmar and plantar surfaces of the hands and feet. In the mid-1930s, cancer of the nasal cavities was associated with the refining of chromium and nickel ores. These initial observations were followed by epidemiological studies that demonstrated a role for several different metals in the causation of lung cancer. The pathfinding contributions summarized here ushered in an era of epidemiological and fundamental biologic research of extraordinary proportions that continues to the present.

The publication of *Silent Spring* by Rachael Carson in 1962 proved to be a turning point in public attitudes regarding the adverse health potential of chemicals in the human environment. Vivid photographs of earth from orbiting spacecraft emphasized to the general public humankind's isolation on earth. Public concerns culminated in an outburst of environmental awareness and activism on Earth Day, 1969. The atmosphere fostered congressional action during the 1970s, including the Clean Air Act (1970) and Clean Water Act (1972), the Federal Insecticide, Fungicide and Rodenticide Act of 1972 (FIFRA), the Resource Conservation and Recovery Act (RCRA-1974), and the Toxic Substances Control Act (TOSCA) of 1976. As a result, the National Toxicological Program evolved, first under the auspices of the National Cancer Institute and later under the National Institute of Environmental Health Sciences. This milestone program, for the first time, brought under strict federal control the scientific assaying and monitoring of potential carcinogenic agents, using animals and the screening of a wide variety of chemicals by mutagenic assays. These programs, complemented by an international effort under the auspices of the International Agency for Cancer Research, have provided the fundamental data upon which much of our knowledge of the biologic effects of toxic substances is based. Although our current methods for evaluating and regulating products of industry with potentially carcinogenic effects have significant limitations (and are the subject of considerable criticism), we currently lack more insightful, prospective approaches for assessing the human health risks of chemicals.

Table 26-2. p53 mutations in selected human cancers

| | | Number of mutations | | | Number of nucleotide changes | | |
| | | | | | Transitions | | |
Type of cancer	Total	Amino acid substitution	Other substitutions	Microdeletions and/or microinsertions	At CpG	Non-CPG	Transversions
Breast	32	29	0	3	2	11	15
Colon	35	33	2	0	25	8	2
Lung	35	29	2	4	1	4	26
Hepatoma	13	12	0	1	0	0	12
Esophagus	9	7	1	1	1	4	3

Adapted from Sommer SS, et al: Pattern of p53 gene mutations in breast cancers of women of the midwestern United States, *J Natl Cancer Inst* 84:246, 1992.

Rodent bioassays of potential carcinogens

The development of the National Toxicological Program and the increasing public concern regarding environmental carcinogenesis and food safety (Delaney Act; see Chapter 9) forced regulatory agencies to rely on small animal bioassays for the evaluation of chemicals and manufactured products. Although in vitro assays for mutagenesis in bacteria and yeast are now well accepted as screening tests of mutagenesis, three fundamental questions have plagued regulators in their efforts to interpret the results of these tests in the context of the human experience. (1) Are all mutagenic substances carcinogenic? Alternatively (2), are all carcinogens mutagenic? (3) To what extent can the results obtained in in vitro experimental systems suffice to answer complex questions regarding events that occur in animals and humans? Industry and government have increasingly turned to screening bioassays, employing rodents as surrogates for humans. However, the appropriateness of these animal tests is vigorously debated.[28] Many scientists consider the results sufficiently reliable to extrapolate them into calculations that assess the risks for humans. A recent editorial in *Science* voiced a quite contrary view[1]:

The principal method of determining potential carcinogenicity of substances is based on studies of daily administration of huge doses of chemicals to inbred rodents for a lifetime. Then, by questionable models, which include large safety factors, the results are extrapolated to effects of minuscule dosages in humans. Resultant stringent regulations and attendant frightening publicity have led to public anxiety and chemophobia. If current ill-based regulatory levels continue to be imposed, the cost of cleaning up phantom hazards will be in the hundreds of billions of dollars with minimal benefit to human health. In the meantime, real hazards are not receiving adequate attention . . . the standard carcinogen tests that use rodents are an obsolescent relic of the ignorance of past decades.

Regardless of these well-founded criticisms, alternative, reliable scientific approaches are lacking for the screening of the well over 3000 new chemicals that are introduced from industrial and research laboratories each year. All of the chemicals known to cause cancer in humans also cause cancer in laboratory animals, but the inverse is infrequently true.

Because of the large number of potential carcinogenic substances available for bioassay and the complexities and expense of these studies, only a fraction of the many candidates are selected for detailed evaluation, largely based on (1) their chemical structure and thus the predictability of carcinogenicity, (2) the outcome of in vitro mutagenesis assays, or (3) the results of epidemiological studies in human populations, and (4) their widespread use in food or in commerce.

The complexities and limitations of the bioassays conducted by industry and the National Toxicological Program are beyond the scope of this discussion. For practical purposes, these assays are generally conducted by administering to laboratory rodents the maximum tolerable dosages of the unknown substance (which can be defined as the largest amount that can be administered without resulting in significant toxicity and weight loss). The relevance of the dosage and schedule of administration with regard to human exposures at much lower levels is a key question from the perspective of extrapolation across species gaps and dosage ranges. For example, at the high, maximally tolerated dosages used, the potential for subtle cell injury, that is, cytotoxicity, exists, and metabolic pathways of degradation of the agent may be altered or overwhelmed. The complexity of the genetic differences among strains of rodents is another issue of major concern.

More than 100 chemicals are listed among the substances identified by the National Toxicological Program as "known" or "may reasonably be anticipated to be" carcinogens. Many of these substances prove to be medicinals or agents used in research and, thus, have limited general environmental importance. They are not considered further here. Many of the remaining substances are known or suspected to be genotoxic, although some are nongenotoxic (saccharin and dioxin). The discussion that follows focuses on selected classes of chemicals of compelling importance.

Conversion of procarcinogens to ultimate carcinogens

The seminal studies of Miller and Miller,[56] a husband-and-wife team, in the 1970s showed that various diverse types of chemical carcinogens are metabolized by animal tissues and activated in vivo to reactive electron-deficient compounds. These so-called electrophiles develop by a variety of metabolic steps to become the ultimate carcinogens that have the ability to react with a variety of electron donors in the cells, including the hydrogen-binding sites of the constituent bases of DNA. Adducts of the electrophile to DNA are the basis for mutations, because DNA covalently bound to these toxic intermediaries often evades repair.

Microsomal monooxygenase enzymes in the p450 superfamily metabolize a wide variety of biologically active, naturally occurring compounds (see Chapters 5 and 17).[29,31,58] They also facilitate the oxidation of countless therapeutic agents and environmental pollutants, including chemical carcinogens. Thus, these enzymes play an intrinsic role in the activation of inert lipophilic carcinogens within the cells. Numerous genetically distinct p450 enzyme systems exist in tissues. The type, concentration, and activity of the members of this superfamily in different tissues are variable and, in part, are influenced by previous chemical and drug exposure (see box).[31,33,58] Differences among species, tissues, sexes, and age groups further affect the ability of the enzymes to activate chemical carcinogens in specific organs. Genetically programmed variability in the activity of these enzymes among humans most probably is an additional factor dictating individual susceptibility.[50] Monooxygenases are not the only enzymes activating carcinogens in cells, but they seem to play a major role.

A number of different conjugation reactions participate in the deactivation of electrophiles (Fig. 26-3). Conjugation detoxifies the compounds and increases their water solubility, thus facilitating elimination. The balance between the intracellular interaction of reactive electrophiles with macromolecules and excretion influences the carcinogenicity of an agent. These broad generalizations serve as the basic unifying concept for the induction of cellular transformation by a diversity of environmental chemicals. We now consider individual classes of agents.

Polycyclic aromatic hydrocarbons (PAHs)

Polycyclic aromatic hydrocarbons are ubiquitous in the modern human environment (Fig. 26-4). They are found in various concentrations and combinations in coal, petroleum, and plant materials and are formulated during incin-

eration. Most effluents and products of industry and energy generation contain PAHs in variable concentrations, along with a complex mélange of other chemicals and metals (Table 26-3). For example, emissions from coke ovens are composed of complex mixtures of benzene, naphthylamine, cadmium, arsenic, beryllium, nickel, and chromium, as well as various vapors and gases. Because of their ubiquity and relatively low concentrations in ambient air, it is difficult to evaluate the specific role of PAHs in disease. They constitute approximately 2% to 3% of the particulates in coke oven emissions and 3% to 6% of the benzene-soluble fraction. Coal and wood soots, pitch, and tars contain similar mixtures. More than 400 compounds have been identified in coal tars and many more are, doubtless, present. Only a few of these are PAHs, but they make up roughly 75% of the mass of creosote, a distillation product of coal tar. The complex montage of incineration products in cigarette smoke is discussed in Chapter 13.

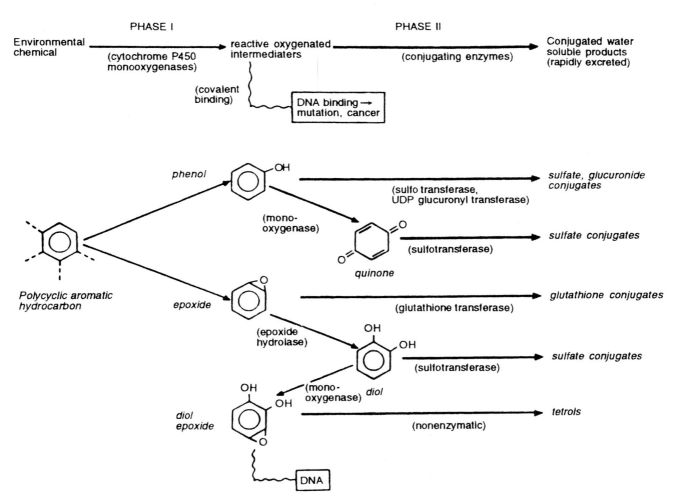

Fig. 26-3. Phase 1 oxygenation mediated by p450 monooxygenase converts polycyclic hydrocarbons to compounds that are water soluble or are subsequently conjugated with endogenous compounds such as glucuronic acid, sulfate and glutathione. (From Law MR: Genetic predisposition to lung cancer, *Br J Cancer* 61:195, 1990; with permission.)

Examples of common inducers of p450 mixed function oxidases

Drugs	Barbiturates
	Phenytoin
	Rifampicin
	Clofibrate
Alcohols	Ethanol
Flavones	5,6-Benzoflavone
Food additives and anutrients	Butylated hydroxyanisole (BHA)
	Butylated hydroxytoluene (BHT)
Halogenated hydrocarbons	2,3,7,8-Tetrachlorodibenzo-*p*-dioxin (TCDD)
	3,3',4,4'-Tetrachlorobiphenyl
	3,3',4,4',5,5'-Hexabromobiphenyl
Insecticides	DDT (dichlorodiphenyltrichloroethane)
	Chlordecone (Kepone)
	Piperonyl butoxide
Polycyclic aromatic hydrocarbons	3-methylcholanthrene
	1,2-benzanthracene, phenanthrene, and benzo[*a*]pyrene
Solvents	Toluene and xylenes

Numerous case reports and epidemiological studies have provided compelling circumstantial evidence implicating PAHs in the causation of cancer of the skin and cancer of the aerodigestive tracts. Because of the many confounding factors involved in the assessment of risk, on the one hand, concrete epidemiological evidence implicating PAHs in human cancer resulting from environmental exposure is lacking. On the other hand, countless experimental studies have established the intrinsic role of PAHs in the inductive pathogenesis of a wide variety of animal neoplasms after systemic, aerosol, and topical administration. Environmental PAHs are water insoluble and require oxidative, enzymatic activation by cellular p450 mixed-function oxidases to become the "ultimate" high-energy electrophile carcinogens capable of DNA adduct formation (Fig. 26-5).[5,56] Although details are lacking in studies of humans, the great variability in the outcome of PAH exposures most probably are dictated by differences in p450 monooxygenase concentrations and types in various tissues and among individuals. As noted previously, the state of activation of the p450 enzymes is influenced by prior chemical exposure (see the box to the left) and genetic factors unique to the host. Because metabolic activation is required for the elimination of PAHs

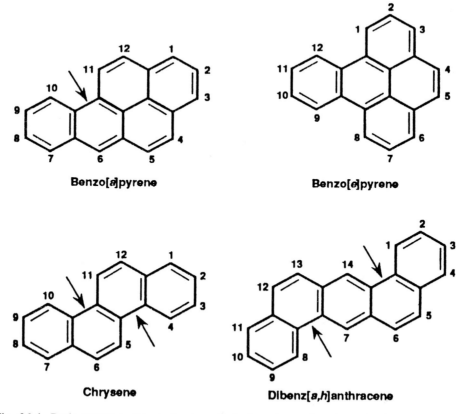

Fig. 26-4. Basic structure of typical polycyclic hydrocarbons of environmental importance. The arrow indicates the so-called Bay region. Electrophiles are hypothesized to be more reactive when diol epoxides form at the Bay region of the compound.

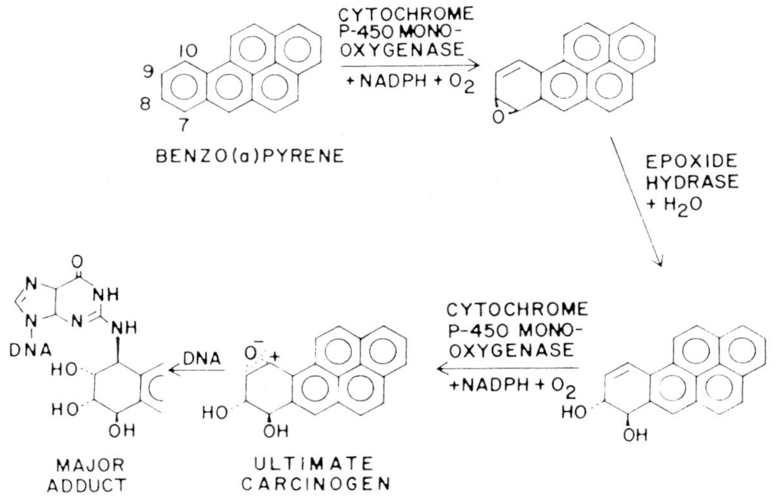

Fig. 26-5. A major route for the metabolic activation of benzo[a]pyrene to a diol epoxide electrophile and the formation of a DNA adduct. (From Miller EC, Miller JA: Searches for ultimate chemical carcinogens and their reactions with cellular macromolecules, *Cancer* 47:2327, 1981; with permission.)

Table 26-3. Polycyclic aromatic hydrocarbon air pollutants by source

Compounds	Mainstream smoke (ng per cigarette)	Woodstove emission factor (ng/kg)	Urban air (ng/m^3)
Benzanthracene	2-70	1.8×10^4	1-70
Benzofluoranthene	16-55	1.4×10^4	—
Benzo[a]pyrene	20-40	9×10^3	1-50
Chrysene	40-60	5×10^3	—
Dibenz[a,h]anthracene	4	1×10^3	—
Dibenz[a,i]pyrene	1.7-3.2	—	—
Indeno[1,2,3-c,d]pyrene	4-20	—	—
5-Methylchrysene	0.6	—	—

Data derived from JM Samet, editor: *Epidemiology of lung cancer.* New York, 1994, Marcel Dekker.

and secondary conjugates, the functional carcinogenic implications of exposure of specific target tissues to the electrophiles must invariably be balanced against the rate and the mechanism of excretion (Fig. 26-3).[50]

N-nitroso compounds

Experimentally, more than 300 different nitrosamides and nitrosamine compounds are carcinogenic in animals (Table 26-4), but the etiologic role of these substances in specific human cancers has not been established.[57] Nitrosamides are "direct-acting" carcinogens and, thus, do not require metabolic activation to initiate cell transformation; whereas nitrosamines must be hydrolyzed in a reaction requiring p450 monooxygenase enzymes in order to produce neoplasia. Humans are exposed to N-nitroso compounds in foods and tobacco smoke (Table 26-5).[39,44] On a more limited basis, exposure to nitrosamines occurs among workers in the rubber and chemical industry and among those employed in tanneries and steel mills. The estimated intake by smokers of some 17 µg/day of nitrosamines is several

Table 26-4. Localization of tumors induced by N-nitroso compounds in rats

Target organ	Number of N-nitroso compounds affecting target organ	
	N-nitrosamines	N-nitrosamides
Liver	35	2
Esophagus-pharynx	32	3
Nasal cavities	18	—
Respiratory tract	10	1
Kidney	8	9
Bladder	4	1
Central and peripheral nervous systems	2	9
Mammary glands	1	2
Glandular stomach	—	6
Skin	—	3
Hemopoietic system	—	2

Adapted from Montesano R, Bartsch H: Mutagenic and carcinogenic N-nitroso compounds: possible environmental hazards, *Mutat Res* 32:179, 1976.

Table 26-5. Estimated exposure of United States residents to nitrosamines

Source	Nitrosamines	Primary exposure route	Daily intake (μg/person)
Beer	NDMA	Ingestion	0.34
Cosmetics	NDELA	Dermal absorption	0.41
Cured meat; cooked bacon	NPYR	Ingestion	0.17
Scotch whiskey	NDMA	Ingestion	0.03
Cigarette smoking	VNA	Inhalation	0.3
	NDELA	Inhalation	0.5
	NNN	Inhalation	6.1
	NNK	Inhalation	2.9-16.2
	NAT and NAB	Inhalation	7.2
Snuff dipping	VNA	Ingestion	3.1
	NDELA	Ingestion	6.6
	NNN	Ingestion	75.0
	NNK	Ingestion	16.1-164.5
	NAT and NAB	Ingestion	73.4

NDMA, N-nitrosodimethylamine; *NDELA,* N-nitrosodiethanolamine; *NPYR,* N-nitrosopyrrolidine; *VNA,* Volatile nitrosamines; *NNN,* N'-nitrosonornicotine; *NNK,* 4-(methylnitrosamino)-1-(3-pyridyl)-1-butanone; *NAT,* N'-nitrosoanatabine; *NAB,* N'-nitroanabasine.
Adapted from Hoffmann D, Hecht SS: Nicotine-derived N-nitrosamines and tobacco-related cancer: current status and future directions, *Cancer Res* 45:935, 1985.)

orders of magnitude greater than that found in an average helping of meat that has been smoked or cured by modern methods.[44]

N-nitroso compounds are also formed in the digestive tract of humans from nitrates and nitrites in potable water and in foods. Nitrates are derived largely from vegetables, whereas nitrites are found in cured meat. However, nitrates are converted by bacteria to nitrites in the stomach, where nitrosation occurs with various food-derived "primary" and "secondary" amine precursors. Tobacco-specific nitrosamines result from the nitrosation of tobacco alkaloids during curing and processing of the leaf (about 25% to 45%) and the remainder form as a result of pyrosynthesis during incineration as a result of the reaction of nitrogen oxides (NO_x) with the alkaloids.[39] Tobacco-specific nitrosamines also appear to form endogenously because of the action of oropharyngeal bacteria on the nitrogen-containing compounds and tobacco alkaloids in smoke and smokeless tobacco products (Fig. 26-6).

Nitrosamides react at neutral pH with water or thiol compounds to form electrophiles that, in turn, react directly with tissues at the site of administration. After ingestion, it is likely that nitrosamides form at stomach pH from amides and nitrites in food. The repeated interaction of these compounds with the stomach mucosa is a likely cause of cancer in this organ. The substantial body of evidence supporting this concept is reviewed in Chapter 9.

In animals, nitrosamines often produce tumors in organs distant from the site of administration. Organ tropism seems to relate largely to the chemical structure of the nitroso compound and may depend on the enzymatic activation capability of different organs. Figure 26-7 depicts a p450-dependent, metabolic bioactivation sequence envisioned by Archer.[5] Because the active metabolites are highly unstable, direct verification of the chemistry in the tissues of the intact animal is impossible. A variety of guanine adducts are believed to form, but the spectrum of adducts developing in vivo is incompletely documented. Although the body of experimental information on nitrosamine mutagenesis and carcinogenicity in experimental animals is vast, our knowledge of the uptake and metabolism of nitrosamines in humans is limited. Moreover, no demonstrable relationship between exposure and the development of specific neoplasms has been established, even though humans regularly are exposed to these substances.

Aflatoxins

A compelling body of epidemiological studies has established a geographical association of hepatocellular carcinoma with the ingestion of aflatoxins as food contaminants.[91] In concert, experimental studies in various species of rodents, birds, fish, and subhuman primates have documented both the hepatotoxicity and the liver carcinogenicity of aflatoxins, particularly aflatoxin B_1, the most potent analogue. However, animals vary substantially in susceptibility to the carcinogenic effects of these mycotoxins. As little as 20 ppb in the food was found to produce liver tumors in trout. As discussed in detail in Chapter 29, the role of the hepatitis B virus in the pathogenesis of hepatocellular carcinoma in humans remains to be clarified, for it is

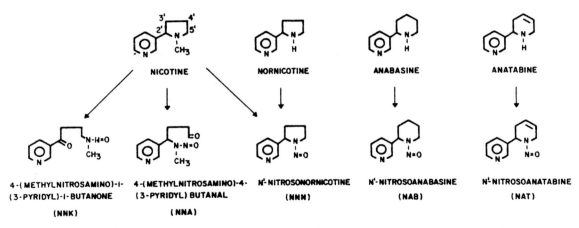

Fig. 26-6. Nitrosamine compounds derived as a result of the incineration of the nicotine in tobacco smokers. (From Hoffmann D, Hecht SS: Nicotine-derived *N*-nitrosamines and tobacco-related cancer, *Cancer Res* 45:935, 1985; with permission.)

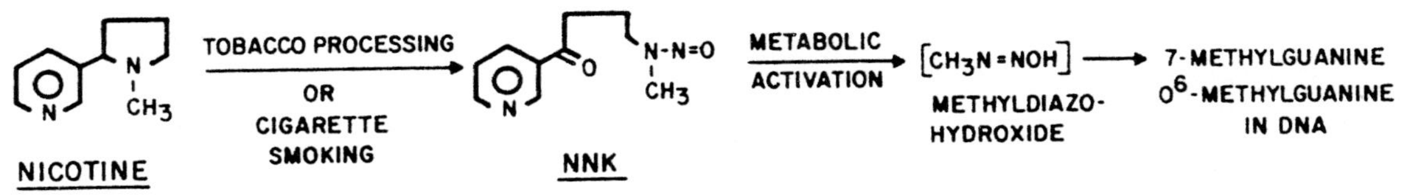

Fig. 26-7. Hypothetical schema for the bioactivation of a typical nitrosamine and the resulting adduct formation. (From Hoffmann D, Hecht SS: Nicotine-derived *N*-nitrosamines and tobacco-related cancer, *Cancer Res* 45:935, 1985; with permission.)

an exceedingly common, perinatally acquired chronic infection in those parts of Africa and Asia where this cancer occurs commonly.

Aflatoxins and their toxic metabolites are recovered from cultures of *Aspergillus flavus* and *A. parasiticus,* as well as from grains and ground nuts (peanuts) contaminated with these same fungi. The amounts in food vary widely, but concentrations of as high as 1.2×10^4 ppb have been reported. Aflatoxins comprise a family of bifurano-coumarin compounds with an unstable lactone ring.[73] Metabolized by p450 monooxygenases in the liver, the resulting highly reactive epoxides form electrophile adducts with cellular and serum proteins, RNA, and DNA, the last of which presumably leads to genetic change and carcinogenesis. Several groups of workers have searched for the expression of ras and myc gene expression in human primary liver cancers with mixed results, but a pattern of gene mutation has not been described. Thus, expression of both *c*-myc and *n*-ras was demonstrated in the majority of liver tumors studied by Gu and associates,[30] but the results of others conflict with this finding. A specific mutagenic pattern of the p53 suppressor gene in liver cancer cells has been found in highly endemic areas of sub-Saharan Africa and Southeast Asia where aflatoxin is a likely contributor to the development of the disease. As noted previously, point mutations are predominantly found at the third-base position of codon 249 with either a G:T or a G:C transversion.[42,43] This picture contrasts with observations in nonendemic regions (such as Europe and North America), where comparable mutations customarily are not found in hepatomas occurring in those with alcoholic cirrhosis.

The evidence, although incomplete, supports the notion that aflatoxins may be an important class of carcinogens in high-prevalence areas where they are commonly found in food, whereas alcoholic cirrhosis is the key risk factor in the Western world.[91] Several questions naturally evolve from these findings. Are p53 mutations a reflection of tumor progression, or are they involved in the initiation of the lesion? Are other mutations related to aflatoxins or other carcinogens important in the initiation event? Does chronic active hepatitis, resulting from hepatitis B infection in early life, promote the development of the neoplasm by stimulating liver cell multiplication?[76] These questions are considered further in Chapter 29.

Benzene and other organic solvents[84]

Shortly before the turn of the century, Santesson reported several cases of fatal aplastic anemia occurring among workers in a tire factory.[71] Some 30 years later, a case of acute lymphoblastic leukemia attributable to benzene exposure was described.[20] The clinical and epidemiological association of bone marrow depression followed after variable periods of latency by acute leukemia consequent to benzene exposure is now well established. In the major-

Table 26-6. Leukemia types in two benzene-exposed industrial groups

	Percent	
Type of leukemia	Goguel (1967)	Aksoy (1985)
Preleukemia	11	13
Acute mylogenous	36	71
Acute lymphogenous	4	9
Chronic myelogenous	30	6
Chronic lymphocytic	18	0

Adapted from Aksoy M: Benzene as a leukemogenic and carcinogenic agent, *Am J Ind Med* 8:9, 1985.

ity of cases, the leukemia is of the acute myelogenous type and occurs with a latency period from 5 to 20 years after exposure (Table 26-6).

Benzene (C_6H_6) is one of several aromatic hydrocarbons found in crude and refined petroleum products.[84,87] It is extensively used as an intermediary in bulk and specialty chemical production and as an industrial solvent. In low concentrations, benzene is present in fruit and vegetable products and in cigarette smoke. Thus, it is universally found in our modern industrialized environment and is an exceedingly common indoor contaminant to which most of us are exposed chronically. However, overt toxicity (such as aplastic anemia) is not demonstrable at the exceedingly low ambient concentrations experienced by the great majority of those who are exposed environmentally.

Epidemiological investigations to assess the hematological effects of benzene have been difficult to conduct because of the sporadic and infrequent occurrence of leukemia among those who experience long-term, relatively heavy exposures in industry.[16] In a recently reported study, air concentrations of 1 to 5 ppm over a period of 40 years (40 to 200 ppm-years) yielded a standardized mortality rate (SMR) of 322, whereas a 400 ppm-year exposure was found to result in an SMR of 6637![65] Regulatory efforts have had a substantial effect on the benzene concentrations now found in most occupational settings and current regulations restrict the amounts in ambient air to no greater than 1 ppm. However, exposure to aromatic hydrocarbons other than benzene in various industries is an ongoing concern because of the difficulties of accessing possible risks to hematopoietic tissues.[41] For example, butadiene is a major constituent of the elastomeres used in manufacturing synthetic rubber products, nylons, and plastics. Although carcinogenic in mice, it has not yet been clearly demonstrated in epidemiological studies to be leukemogenic in those exposed occupationally.[49]

Benzene is rapidly absorbed from the respiratory and digestive tracts. Acutely, it appears to concentrate in the liver

*References 2, 3, 15, 65, 85.

and bone marrow, where it is metabolized by mixed-function oxidases to phenol and to hydroxylated compounds such as hydroquinones, semiquinones, catechols, and 1,2,4-trihydroxybenzene. Although the mechanisms are unclear, in hematopoietic tissue the benzene metabolites appear to bind to various cellular macromolecules, including DNA. The resulting, poorly understood toxic effects are believed to account for the carcinogenicity of benzene. It is not clear to what extent toxicity results in DNA point mutations, but chromosomal aberrations have been described in the hematopoietic cells of workers in industries where chronic benzene exposure occurs.

Nongenotoxic promotional environmental carcinogens[53]

As previously discussed, the concept of multistage carcinogenesis implies that cells sustain superimposed mutational events and clonal selection in the process of transformation. Thus, the likelihood that an initiated cell will ultimately develop into a malignant neoplasm is dependent on clonal expansion and the probability that additional mutations will be superimposed upon the progeny. Cells proliferate in response to either cytotoxic injury or mitogenic stimulation. Cytotoxicity leads to cellular regeneration as influenced by various transcriptional influences. In this context, there is good reason to believe that leukemogenesis consequent to bone marrow irradiation or benzene exposure could, in whole or in part, be a reflection of endogenous mutagenic events occurring during regeneration of the marrow elements under the influence of hematopoietic growth factors.

Nevertheless, mitogenesis resulting from chemical exposures can be a receptor-mediated event, acting through secondary messengers that ultimately regulate the events of cell replication. Because all chemicals prove cytotoxic at some dosage, albeit it unphysiologic, the influence of dosage, uptake, transport, and metabolic activation are key considerations in assessing the cytotoxicity of an environmental chemical as a promoter of carcinogenesis in humans. Ethanol, when consumed in excess (see Chapter 14), and carbon tetrachloride (see Chapter 5) resulting from chronic occupational exposure are examples of hepatotoxic chemicals that stimulate cell multiplication in the liver and may promote carcinogenesis by this mechanism. Hepatitis B infection is another specific agent that potentially contributes to neoplastic transformation of the liver as a result of chronic cytotoxic damage to this organ.

Several mitogenic chemicals of considerable environmental importance have been found to be highly carcinogenic in rodent assays but are not metabolized to carcinogens in vivo and lack the ability to bind DNA covalently. Of these, 2,3,7,8-tetrachlorodibenzo-*p*-dioxin (TCDD) is the most notable and toxic member of a group of structurally similar compounds that includes numerous different dioxins, biphenyls, and furans and many other isomers too numerous and too chemically complex to summarize here (Fig. 26-8). The ubiquitous nonbiodegradable environmental contaminant TCDD is a by-product of the manufacturing and use of halogenated aromatic compounds such as the phenoxy herbicide 2,4,5-trichlorophenoxy acetic acid (Agent Orange) (see Chapter 8). In contrast, polychlorinated biphenyls were widely produced in industrialized countries for use as a fluid insulator and fire retardant until they were banned by governmental action in 1977.

Human bioavailability from the many potential environmental sources (primarily air and foods) is poorly defined, but storage in body adipose tissue is inevitable because of the lipid solubility of these compounds. The biologic half-life of TCDD in human tissue is uncertain but is variously estimated to be from 3 to 8 years.[74] All of us have within our adipose tissue low concentrations of a variety of chlorinated hydrocarbons, and those who have been exposed to these chemicals occupationally have substantially greater concentrations in their body fat (Figs. 26-9 and 26-10).[74,75]

TCDD binds reversibly with the high-affinity (Kd 10^{-10}M) Ah (aryl hydrocarbon) receptor that is widely distributed in the cytosol of cells of most animal tissues. The receptor is similar, but not identical, to the glucocorticoid receptors that interact with physiological steroids. However, it does not bind these naturally occurring hormones. Polychlorinated biphenyls (PCBs) and polychlorinated dibenzofurans (PCDs) also bind the Ah receptor and induce biochemical responses similar to those of TCDD. Through a complex but poorly understood series of intracellular events, the TCDD-Ah ligand interacts with specific nuclear regulatory genes in the cell, thereby inducing cell growth and multiplication.[53,77,90]

The hepatic carcinogenicity of TCDD and related compounds in experimentally exposed female rodents has been clearly demonstrated, although there are marked species and strain differences. These appear to relate, at least in part, to heritable differences in the affinity of the Ah receptors for the compounds. Endogenous estrogens play a key role in the ultimate outcome; male rodents and female castrates are resistant to tumor development. Experimental studies in laboratory rodents indicate that a wide variety of epithelial cells undergo nonneoplastic proliferative responses to TCDD treatment. Because dioxin is not mutagenic, the effects of these compounds would appear to be promotional. Although concern is voiced repeatedly regarding the potential carcinogenicity of the large family of chlorinated hydrocarbons, as of yet, epidemiological evidence has not accumulated, demonstrating an increased prevalence of cancer in environmentally exposed humans.

The induction of p450 mixed-function oxidase expression in animals and humans exposed to a wide variety of environmental chemicals and pharmacological agents was noted before. The chlorinated hydrocarbons have a similar transcriptional effect after binding with the Ah receptor of the cells. The implications of this observation with regard

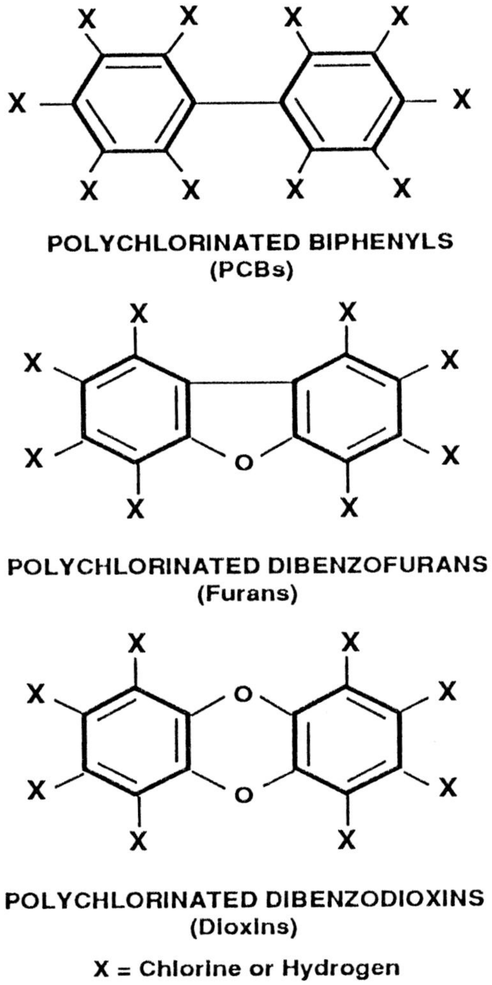

POLYCHLORINATED BIPHENYLS (PCBs)

POLYCHLORINATED DIBENZOFURANS (Furans)

POLYCHLORINATED DIBENZODIOXINS (Dioxins)

X = Chlorine or Hydrogen

Fig. 26-8. Basic chemical structure of halogenated hydrocarbons found ubiquitously in the human environment.

to human susceptibility to mutagenic chemical carcinogens and therapeutic agents is, at present, uncertain.

An enormous body of epidemiological and experimental evidence has established a role for estrogens in the pathogenesis of cancer of the female breast and the endometrium.[36] In addition, synthetic exogenous estrogen administration during pregnancy is strongly associated with the development of vaginal adenocarcinoma in female offspring[37] and possibly germ cell tumors of the testes.[21] Estrogens play a key role in the replication of cells of the mammary gland and counteract the effects of progestational hormones in the endometrium. Thus, by stimulating cell growth in target tissues, these compounds could enhance susceptibility to exogenous and endogenous carcinogens or increase the likelihood of replicative errors in the DNA of these estrogen-sensitive tissues.

A wide variety of xenobiotic compounds manifest properties that mimic the estrogenic effects of hormonal estrogens when evaluated in a variety of animal species. The

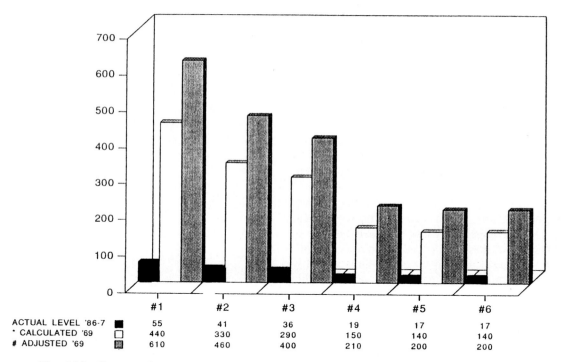

		#1	#2	#3	#4	#5	#6
ACTUAL LEVEL '86-7	■	55	41	36	19	17	17
* CALCULATED '69	☐	440	330	290	150	140	140
# ADJUSTED '69	▨	610	460	400	210	200	200

Fig. 26-9. Concentrations (parts/trillion) of 2,3,7,8-tetrachlorodibenzo-*p*-dioxin (TCDD) in adipose tissue of U.S. military personnel exposed to Agent Orange defoliant between 1962 and 1970 in Vietnam. The calculated concentration for 1969 is based on a 3- to 6-year half-life and adjusted for changes in body adipose tissue. The data are from six applicators of Agent Orange, a phenoxy-herbicide mixture of equal amounts of butyl ester of 2,4-dichlorophenoxyacetic acid (2,4-D) and butyl ester of 2,4,5-trichlorphenoxyacetic acid (2,4,5-T) contaminated with approximately 2 to 3 ppm TCDD. (From Schecter A, et al: Chlorinated and bromiated dixoins and dibenzofurans in human tissue following exposure, *Environ Health Perspect* 102(suppl 1):135, 1994.)

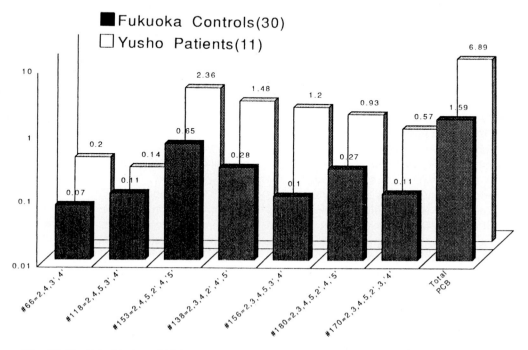

Fig. 26-10. Polychlorinated biphenyl (PCB) ppb in the blood serum of "sick" Japanese residents *(open bars)* 21 years after consuming contaminated rice oils used for domestic cooking. The solid bar represents data from matched controls from the general population. The cause of the illness is uncertain, but the persistence of the PCB in the body is evident. (From Schecter A, et al: Polychlorinated biphenyl levels in the tissues of exposed and non-exposed humans, *Environ Health Perspect* 102(suppl 1):149, 1994.)

potency of these compounds is quite variable but, in general, estradiol exhibits $1 \cdot 10^3$ to $1 \cdot 10^4$ more in vivo estrogenic activity than do these various chemicals. However, because the substances persist in body fat for indefinite periods, their effects may be manifest in a sustained fashion for much of the lifetime of the animal (or human). Critical analysis of the research data is difficult because of large gaps in the available literature and because "field-grade" compounds are variable in potency and contaminated with extraneous chemical substances that, in themselves, may have estrogenic effects. The bulk of the critical information is based on studies with dichlorodiphenyltrichloroethane (DDT) and its analogues, but methoxychlor, chlordecone (Kepone), mirex, and various PCBs (Aroclor series 1221 through 1268) have also been studied.[17]

The estrogenic effects of these compounds generally are demonstrable in ovarectomized and adrenalectomized adult female rats or in immature males. Uterine enlargement and vaginal cytologic changes develop in the castrated females, whereas decreases in testicular, seminal vesicular, and prostatic weight are observed in males. Based on these findings, it is generally concluded that the various compounds (or their metabolites) act directly on hormone-sensitive tissue. However, an indirect action at the neuroendocrine level also has been hypothesized. In general, high doses and prolonged administration of DDT and its analogues are required to evoke an indirect effect on the endocrine system of the animal. Estrogenic effects of the type described experimentally have not been observed in humans exposed inadvertently to high concentrations of the various xenobiotic compounds.

Halogenated hydrocarbons with estrogenic activity are common environmental pollutants that are found in soils and water, and in lake, river, and stream sediments.[17,23,67,68] As a result, they also enter the food chain of humans. Several investigators have demonstrated PCBs in the milk of lactating women, and two studies now have documented the presence of increased concentrations of halogenated hydrocarbons in the adipose tissue and serum of women with breast cancer. Falck and colleagues[23] conducted a study of patients with breast cancer in which the breast adipose concentrations were compared with the amount found in comparable tissue from noncancer patients. Both dichlorodiphenyl/dichloroethane (DDE) and PCB concentrations were increased significantly. Only 20 patients and 20 control subjects were included in this study. In an ongoing study, Wolff and colleagues[92] analyzed the blood serum of 58 women with a recent diagnosis of breast cancer and 171 matched control, noncancer subjects from the same study group. A fourfold increase in relative risk for breast cancer was found when serum concentrations exceeded 2 ng/ml. Efforts were made in this study to address confounding influences affecting the development of the disease. Additional studies failed to demonstrate an association with PCBs.

Abundant survey data acquired in studies of various human populations worldwide have documented the almost universal presence of a wide variety of environmental chemicals in body adipose tissue and serum lipids.[74,75] Although the concentrations of these substances are generally low and their estrogenic activity relatively modest, it is not unreasonable to hypothesize that these chemicals chronically stimulate estrogen-sensitive tissues of the fetus and persons of all ages. Although the possible role of these chemicals in human carcinogenesis remains to be established, the evidence thus far accumulated serves as a basis for concern.

Metal carcinogenesis

Although the oncogenic properties of various salts of heavy metals have long been recognized, the pathogenic mechanisms involved in carcinogenesis are incompletely understood. The subject proves exceedingly complex, in part because of the many significant gaps in the epidemiological and experimental information. However, confusion also relates to the different forms of these metals found in our environment and variables in human exposure to the various chemical analogues of the metals.

As previously noted, Hutchison described the development of skin cancers among patients being treated with arsenical compounds for various dermatological conditions in 1888. Subsequently, similar lesions of the skin were noted to occur among members of certain occupational groups exposed to arsenic either by direct skin contact or by the respiratory route, or after ingestion of therapeutic agents.[80] For unknown reasons, these lesions exhibited a unique and pathognomonic distribution pattern on the palmar and plantar surfaces, the scrotum, and the nipple. In the early 1900s, cases of lung cancer attributable to industrial exposure to chromium and arsenical compounds were first described. Later, epidemiological investigations established an association between employment in the metal smelting industry and respiratory tract cancer. The specificity of the link between lung cancer and smelter effluents has been obscured by the chemical complexities of these by-products of smelting and the commonality of cigarette smoking among the exposed blue-collar workers.

Table 26-7 provides a summary of the vast body of experimental and epidemiological data that has accumulated associating the heavy metals (arsenic, nickel, and chromium) with the development of cancer in humans. As noted before, epidemiological studies have implicated each of the three metals as salts in the initiation of bronchogenic and nasal (chromium and nickel) carcinomas. However, models documenting respiratory carcinogenesis in animals with these same metals have not been established, although intramuscular inoculation of the metal salts produces sarcomas at the injection site (see Chapter 4). In cell culture systems, nickel salts (sulfides and chlorides) have been shown to enter the nucleus and form DNA-protein complexes re-

Table 26-7. Summary of properties of carcinogenic metals

	Chromium	Nickel	Arsenic	Cadmium
Human carcinogen (epi)	+++	+++	++	+
Cancer(s)	lung	lung	lung, skin	lung (prostate)
Animal carcinogen	++	+	±	++
Point mutations—bacterial	++	+	—	—
Point mutations—mammalian	++	+	—	—
Sister chromatid exchange	++	+	+	±
Chromosomal aberrations	++	+	+	±
Cell transformation	+++	++	++	+
Gene amp/recombinations/deletions	+	++	+	+
Teratogen	+	+	++	++
Mechanism?	genetic (DNA damage)	genetic (DNA damage)	epigenetic? (gene amplification)	epigenetic? (oxygen radicals)

Summary provided through the courtesy of Dr. Joshua Hamilton, Dartmouth College.
+, Relative strength of data; ±, uncertain.

sulting in single-strand DNA breaks. Chromium (VI) is the only readily available salt of this metal that enters the cell, but it is reduced intracellularly to a more active form (chromium III). As a result of the formation of chromium (III) DNA adducts, DNA-interstrand crosslinks occur. Chromosomal breaks and gaps and aneuploidy result, but point mutations have not been described. Although these events are mutagenic, they lack specificity, and the ultimate mechanisms involved in carcinogenesis remains obscure. Nonetheless, as an endpoint, cells treated in vitro with metal salts exhibit typical features of transformation (i.e., a loss of density inhibition and anchorage independence). In contrast to many common chemical carcinogens, the metals are not enzymatically transformed to activated compounds in biologic systems.[27,48,89]

Arsenic salts do not bind to the DNA of cells, and reproducible models of animal carcinogenicity have not been established. Accordingly, arsenic is not believed to be genotoxic but may act in an epigenetic fashion. The basis for the unique distribution of skin tumors in humans is unknown (Fig. 26-11).

The carcinogenicity of cadmium in experimental animals is well established, although the mechanisms are obscure. Tumors develop in the lungs after respiratory exposure and at the subcutaneous and intramuscular injection sites. Testosterone-dependent models of prostatic and testicular carcinoma in rats exposed to cadmium have also been described. Despite evidence demonstrating multiorgan carcinogenicity in animals, the role of cadmium in neoplasia in humans is uncertain.

Evidence for carcinogenicity of a variety of other metals (cobalt, zinc, magnesium, manganese, and calcium) found in the human environment is lacking. However, Fe^{2+} and Cu^{1+}, two catalytic agents involved in the generation of activated oxygen species by the Fenton reaction, are mutagenic, and their possible role in human carcinogenicity is a consideration (see Chapter 21).

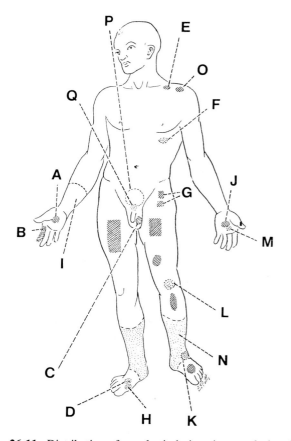

Fig. 26-11. Distribution of neoplastic lesions in a steel plant inspector who was administered an unknown amount of Fowler's solution (potassium arsenite) from age 26 through 38 as treatment for enlarged lymph nodes. At age 43, an epidermoid carcinoma developed on the right palm *(A);* 2 years later, the right forefinger was amputated because of a similar lesion *(B).* Thereafter, scrotal *(C),* foot *(D),* shoulder *(E),* and chest (Bowen's disease) *(F)* lesions developed. Additional skin carcinomas developed over the ensuing years *(F-O).* Finally, a lower urinary tract *(P)* and prostatic carcinomas *(Q)* appeared in later life. (Adapted from Sommers SC and McManus RG: Multiple arsenical cancers of skin and internal organs, *Cancer* 6:347, 1953; with permission.)

RADIANT ENERGY CARCINOGENESIS

Chapters 10, 11, and 12 consider, respectively, ionizing, nonionizing, and electromagnetic energy and review various aspects of their biologic effects. Accordingly, this section more specifically addresses carcinogenesis from the perspective of humans resulting from environmental exposure. The reader is referred to these previous chapters for specific technical considerations regarding the characteristics of the various types of radiant energy.

Ionizing radiation is a universal carcinogen having the potential to induce cancer in a great diversity of human tissues. The effects are dose-dependent and are critically influenced by the mode of exposure as well as the type and quality of the radiation. A considerable body of information has accumulated on the effects of therapeutic and diagnostic dosages of radiation, but these observations are beyond the scope of this discussion. More importantly, we are concerned here with long-term, relatively low-energy environmental and occupational exposures to humans. Aside from cosmic radiation, the most common source of ionizing energy exposure for members of the general population today is radon from terrestrial sources, a topic discussed in Chapter 3. Alternatively, the major occupational sources of exposure are in the nuclear energy industry and among health care personnel and biomedical scientists. Because the use of radiation in these industries has been carefully regulated for decades, little meaningful epidemiological information on human carcinogenicity related to chronic, low-energy radiation exposure has accumulated.

The history of radiation carcinogenesis is replete with anecdotal, nonquantitative observations concerned with the occurrence of radiation dermatitis, skin cancer, and leukemia in early radiologists who experienced heavy, but undocumented, exposures. The development of aseptic necrosis of bone and osteosarcomas among watch dial workers resulting from the oral uptake of radium and its deposition in bone has been described repeatedly (see Chapter 31). Presumably, episodes of this type will not recur as a result of misadventure and ignorance, but they do emphasize the potential carcinogenicity of ionizing radiation.

The most thoroughly documented prospective studies of radiation effects on human populations are those conducted on survivors of the Hiroshima and Nagasaki atomic bomb explosions in 1945 (Fig. 26-12). Since that time, some 2.4×10^3 Japanese victims have died of various causes, with roughly 400 cancer deaths among them being attributed to radiation. Although surveillance and analysis of exposure data have been exhaustive, the specific types and dosages of radiation experienced by the individual victims are far from satisfactorily documented. Moreover, the quality of the radiation in the two cities differed. In Nagasaki, x-rays, but relatively few neutrons, were released; in Hiroshima, victims were exposed to a mixture of x-rays and neutrons. The relevance of a transient, albeit intense, exposure to our understanding of chronic, low-energy expo-

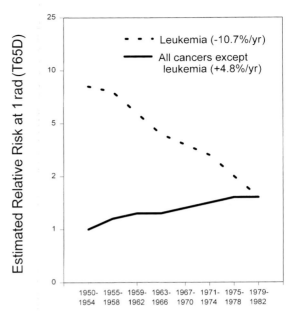

Fig. 26-12. Occurrence of leukemia among Hiroshima and Nagasaki atomic bomb survivors (1945) of both sexes *(broken line)* in comparison to occurrence of all other types of cancer in this population *(solid line)*. Leukemia proved to be a relatively early event, whereas the common cancers of other organs occurred within the customary range for these types of cancers. (Adapted from Beir V, editor: *Health effects of exposure to low levels of ionizing radiation,* Washington, DC, 1990, National Academy Press.)

sures is far from clear and, in fact, may not provide useful information. There is ample experimental evidence to indicate that exposures of this type are not applicable to the assessment of risk among those exposed to low-energy radiation on a continous basis over long periods of time.

Certain types of atomic explosions have yielded high concentrations of radioactive iodine in the fallout. The Bikini atoll test bomb catastrophe of 1956 was one such case (Fig. 26-13). As events developed, native populations in the other, nearby islands of the Marshall chain were exposed to heavy fallout of radioactive isotopes of iodine. Specifically, metabolized by the thyroid, the iodine isotope (a beta-ray emitter) had devastating carcinogenic effects on this tissue, as illustrated in Table 26-8.

The mechanisms involved in the genetic injury that ultimately results in neoplastic transformation are incompletely defined but reflect both chromosomal damage (see Chapter 20) and point mutations (see Chapter 19).[15] The effect on chromosome structure depends on dosage and radiation type, with neutrons and alpha particles being more injurious than x-rays (Fig. 26-14). As a result, breaks, translocations, rearrangements, and deletions in chromosomes occur in proportion to the square of the dosage. It is likely that these clastogenic manifestations of irradiation account for the leukemogenic outcomes of exposures because

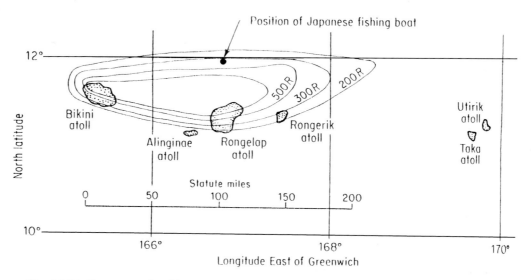

Fig. 26-13. Exposures of residents of the Marshall islands to radioactive fallout from an atomic bomb trial at the Bikini atoll on March 1, 1954. Data on the subsequent occurrence of thyroid disease among residents of the nearby Ronglop atoll are recorded in Table 26-8. (From Beir V, editor: *Health effects of exposure to low levels of ionizing radiation,* Washington, DC, 1990, National Academy Press.)

Table 26-8. Prevalence of thyroid abnormalities among Marshall Islanders (Ronglop atoll) 27 years after exposure to fallout from a thermonuclear device detonated 100 miles away on Bikini island

Age at time of exposure (yrs)	Dose (rad)	Hypothyroid	Nodule	Cancer
Exposed				
1	≥15	83	67	0
2-9	8-15	25	81	6
≥10	3-8	9	13	7
Control				
<10	—	0.4	2.6	0.9
≥10	—	0.3	7.8	0.8

Adapted from Beir V: *Health effects of exposure to low levels of ionizing radiation,* Washington, DC, 1990, National Academy Press.

cytogenetic alterations are so common in this group of the diseases.[69,70] It is noteworthy, however, that ras and p53 point mutations also are identified in granulocytic cells in many (but not all) cases of myelogenous leukemia. Thus, point mutations most probably also play a role in some cases.

Whereas considerable fundamental information exists to account for damage to atoms in the chemicals comprising DNA (caused by energy transfer from the photon), a sizable body of evidence indicates that interactions of the radiation particle with intracellular water results in the generation of free radicals in irradiated cells. As a consequence, hydroxyl adducts could interact with bases, glyco-

side bonds might be broken from the DNA, and single- or double-strand breaks would be expected to occur in the sugar phosphate backbone of the molecule. Experimentally, antioxidants serve to protect cells from the clastogenic and carcinogenic effects of irradiation (Fig. 26-14).

Aside from the absolute influence of dosage, irradiation-induced neoplastic transformation of individual cells and tissues is influenced by (1) the linear energy transfer (LET) to the target DNA, which differs with the various types of irradiation (Fig. 26-15); (2) the exposure schedule, that is, a single exposure in contrast to repeated low-energy exposures (Fig. 26-16); and (3) the anatomic type of cell and, more specifically, the replicative state of the cells and their possible exposure to a promoter substance (Fig. 26-17). The promotional effects of estrogens no doubt influence the differential susceptibility of women of various age groups to the development of mammary cancer after irradiation (Fig. 26-18).

Mutations in oncogenes and suppressor genes are likely explanations for certain aspects of transformation, but the effects may be exceedingly complex and may be influenced by individual host factors. The unusual susceptibility of cells carrying the ataxic telangiectasia gene (AT) (Fig. 26-19), which is found in approximately 10% of our population, and the influences of nutritional antioxidants (see Chapter 21) cannot be currently appraised, but they may be critical determinants of the outcome in humans.

FOREIGN BODY (SOLID STATE) CARCINOGENESIS

In 1941, Turner described the development of sarcomas in rats adjacent to subcutaneously implanted bakelite

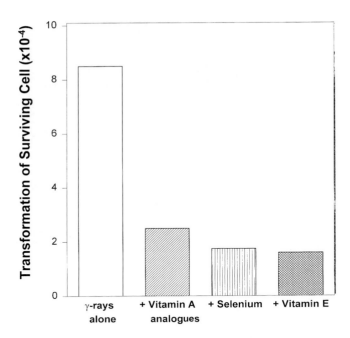

Fig. 26-14. The protective effects of classic antioxidants on transformation in vitro by 3 rad of gamma irradiation. (Adapted from Beir V, editor: *Health effects of exposure to low levels of ionizing radiation,* Washington, DC, 1990, National Academy Press.)

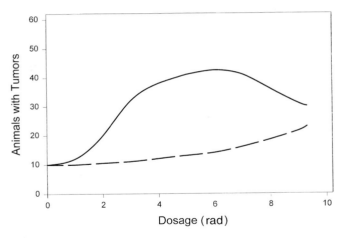

Fig. 26-16. Induction of tumors in mice exposed to different dosages of ionizing whole-body low-LET radiation. The solid curve represents the effects of a single exposure, whereas the broken line shows the effect of 1 rad/day, resulting in the same total dosage. (Adapted from Rauth AM, *Radiation Carcinogenesis.* In Tannock IF, Hill RP, editors: *The basic science of oncology,* New York, 1992, McGraw-Hill, pp 119-132.)

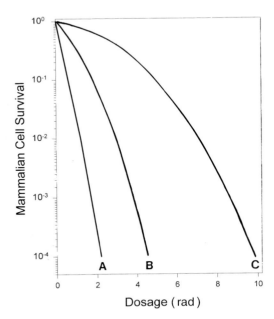

Fig. 26-15. Cell injury is dictated by the type of irradiation and dosage. At relatively high dosages, the effect is roughly comparable with the three types of radiation illustrated, whereas at lower dosages, alpha particles *(A)* and neutrons *(B)* are more injurious than x-rays *(C)*. These observations are a reflection of the linear energy transfer (LET), which is an indication of the energy loss from radiation along the route of the particle in a cell. (Adapted from Rauth AM: *Radiation carcinogenesis.* In Tannock IF, Hill RP, editors: *The basic science of oncology,* New York, 1992, McGraw-Hill, pp 119-132.)

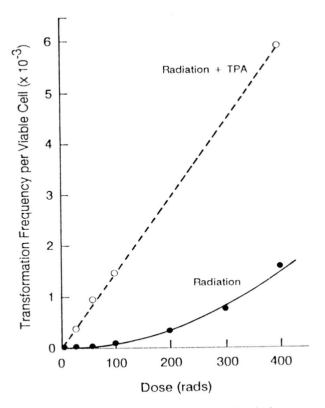

Fig. 26-17. The enhancing effect of the classical promoter tetradecanoyl-phorbol-acetate *(TPA)* on the transformation of mammalian cells. The response to x-ray becomes linear in the presence of TPA. A similar effect is observed in the animal. (From Beir V, editor: *Health effects of exposure to low levels of ionizing radiation,* Washington, DC, 1990, National Academy Press.)

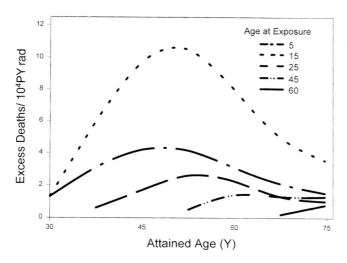

Fig. 26-18. Effect of age at time of exposure on the occurrence of breast cancer among female Hiroshima and Nagasaki atomic bomb survivors. (Adapted from Beir V, editor: *Health effects of exposure to low levels of ionizing radiation,* Washington, DC, 1990, National Academy Press.)

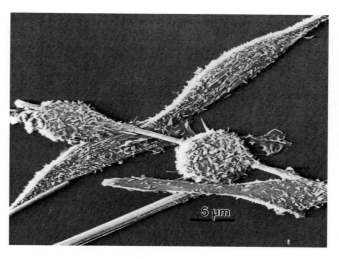

Fig. 26-20. Scanning electron micrograph of long fibers (>10 μm) of crocidolite asbestos in association with alveolar macrophages lavaged from the lungs of rats. In this in vitro experiment, the macrophages attempt unsuccessfully to envelop the fibers, releasing large amounts of oxygen free radicals into the fluid environment.

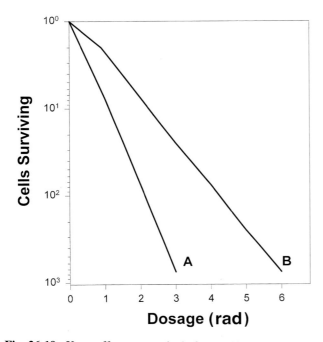

Fig. 26-19. X-ray effects on survival of normal human fibroblasts *(B)* and fibroblasts grown from a patient with ataxic telangiectasia *(A)*. The basis for the increase in susceptibility of the latter cells has not been established. (Adapted from Hall EJ: *Radiobiology for the radiologist,* Philadelphia, 1987, JB Lippincott; with permission.)

disks.[83] Since that time, implants of a wide variety of foreign materials have been shown to cause neoplasms experimentally. In addition, rare, anecdotal examples of tumors developing in humans associated with cosmetic or therapeutic implants have been reported. The experimental studies

have yielded descriptive observations, but information providing insights into the pathogenesis of this unique phenomenon has yet to accrue.[8]

To a large extent, the experimental work has been conducted in rats and mice. Differences have been found between the two species, and convincing evidence of a strain predisposition (or resistance) to the development of neoplasms is now evident. For cancers to develop, the shape and size of the implant proves critical, but the surface must be smooth and unabraded. Large, single bodies are most carcinogenic, but the same material, as a homogenate, does not produce a cancer. There is no evidence to suggest that the chemical makeup of the foreign body is critical because inert implants are highly pathogenic.[14] Histologically, a dense accumulation of macrophages accumulates around the implant, followed by the gradual development of a thick, fibrous capsule.[45] This observation suggests that the macrophages play a key pathogenic role. Could it be that the surface of the foreign body attracts macrophages, resulting in the activation of these cells and the release of oxygen radicals having mutagenic potential for the adjacent mesenchymal cells? Although tumor development requires a long latency period, the studies of Brand and his colleagues[13] indicate that chromosomal alterations and transformed clones of cells develop in the fibrous capsule relatively soon after implantation.[62,64] These events occur long before sarcomas become evident. The relevance of these experimental studies with regard to human disease is obscure, but several examples of possible foreign body carcinogenesis, in fact, may commonly occur in humans, as discussed next.

Malignant mesotheliomas occasionally develop sponta-

HYPOTHETICAL MECHANISM OF MESOTHELIOMA FORMATION

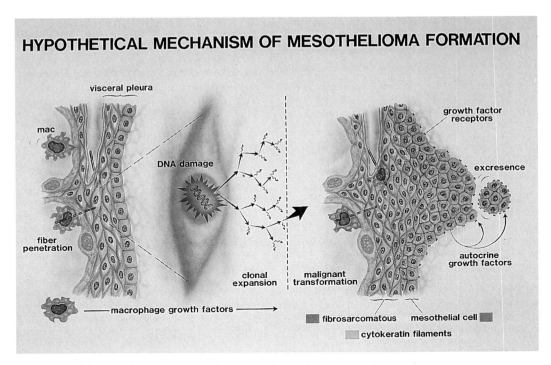

Fig. 26-21. Hypothetical schema whereby the interaction of macrophages with amphibole asbestos in the subpleural space in the generation of oxygen free radicals and macrophage growth factors. The DNA damage is hypothesized to occur in mesothelial progenitor cells thereafter, with the outgrowth of mutant clones being stimulated by the growth factor. This process, occurring on a continuous basis, is believed to result in the neoplasm. (From Craighead JE, Kane AB: *The pathogenesis of malignant and nonmaligtnant serosal lesions in body cavities consequent to asbestos exposure.* In Jaurand MC, Bignon J, editors: *The mesothelial cell and mesothelioma,* New York, 1994, Marcel Dekker; with permission.)

neously, but most cases result from prolonged exposure to amphibole asbestos in the workplace (see Chapter 28). Long (≥8 μm) and thin (<0.25 μm) fibers are believed to be highly pathogenic, based on the experimental studies of Stanton and colleagues.[19,32,81,86] Because these particles have a relatively large surface area in relationship to mass and persist in the lung tissue indefinitely after inhalation, extensive reactive surfaces exist for interactions with macrophages (Fig. 26-20). The chemical makeup of the particle appears to be of limited importance, because fiberglass produces mesotheliomas in experimental animals when introduced into body cavities, and fibrous zeolite (specifically, an aluminum silicate known as eronite) produces tumors when injected into the body cavities of rats and in humans after natural environmental exposure.[6,72] A hypothetical schema for the development of the malignant mesothelioma is shown in Figure 26-21. It is based on the notion that foreign bodies stimulate the generation of oxygen radicals from activated macrophages at the surface of the foreign body. Injury to the genetic material of the progenitor cell of the mesothelioma ultimately results in the development of the neoplasm over the long periods of time required for these cancers to develop in the experimental animal and in humans.

Circumstantial clinical and pathological evidence suggests that the flukes *(Fasciola hepatica)* and *Clonorchis sinensis* account, at least in part, for the increase in prevalence of biliary tract carcinoma occurring in the endemic areas of these two parasites in Southeast Asia.[55] However, a cause-and-effect relationship has not been established epidemiologically. Both organisms invade and chronically lodge in the lumen of the biliary tract of infected humans, where they provoke an adenomatous hyperplasia of the lining of the epithelium and neoformation of biliary ducts.[55] Is this, then, an example of foreign body carcinogenicity? Alternatively, one might ask whether the parasites play a promotional role under these circumstances, enhancing the effects of yet to be identified soluble carcinogens in the biliary tract secretions. Nitrosamines have been suggested as one such carcinogen.

A somewhat similar sequence of events has been hypothesized to occur in endemic areas of Africa where infection with *Schistosoma haematobium* occurs. The fertilized female of this schistosome migrates in the veins of the wall of the urinary bladder, where they implant in the submucosa and ovulate. Accumulation of eggs in the submucosa of the bladder follows and results in a persistent granulomatous and chronic inflammatory response. Repeated infestations of the bladder wall with the recurrent inflammatory events result in extensive scarring and contraction of the bladder wall. Squamous metaplasia is associated with these changes. The epithelial proliferative response might well be expected to increase susceptibility to urinary tract carcinogens, resulting in the high prevalence of squamous carcinoma of the bladder in endemic areas of the world.[18]

REFERENCES

1. Abelson PH: Testing for carcinogens with rodents, *Science* 249:1357, 1990.
2. Aksoy M: Benzene as a leukemogenic and carcinogenic agent, *Am J Ind Med* 8:9, 1985.
3. Aksoy M: Hematotoxicity and carcinogenicity of benzene, *Environ Health Perspect* 82:193, 1989.
4. Andreassen A, et al: p53 abnormalities in different subtypes of human sarcomas, *Cancer Res* 53:468, 1993.
5. Archer MC: *Chemical carcinogenesis,* In Tannodz IF, Hill RP, editors: *The basic science of oncology,* pp. 102-118.
6. Baris YI, et al: Malignant mesothelioma and radiological chest abnormalities in two villages in Central Turkey, *Lancet*:984, 1981.
7. Berenblum I, Shubik P: A new quantitative approach to the study of the stages of chemical carcinogenesis in the mouse's skin, *Br J Cancer* 1:384, 1947.
8. Bischoff F, Bryson G: *Carcinogenesis through solid state surfaces,* In Homburger F, editor: Progr exp tumor res, vol 5, Basel/New York, 1964, Karger, pp 85-133.
9. Blumberg PM: Protein kinase C as the receptor for the phorbol ester tumor promoters: sixth Rhoads Memorial award lecture, *Cancer Res* 48:1, 1988.
10. Bos JL, et al: Prevalence of ras gene mutations in human colorectal cancers, *Nature* 327:293, 1987.
11. Boveri T: *Zur trage der entstehung maligner tumoren,* Jena, Germany, 1914, G. Fisher.
12. Brambilla E, et al: Immunohistochemical study of p53 in human lung carcinomas, *Am J Pathol* 143:199, 1993.
13. Brand KG, et al: Etiological factors, stages, and the role of the foreign body in foreign body tumorigenesis: a review, *Cancer Res* 35:279, 1975.
14. Brandt L: Exposure to organic solvents and risk of haematological malignancies, *Leuk Res* 16:67, 1992.
15. Bressac B, et al: Selective G to T mutations of p53 gene in hepatocellular carcinoma from southern Africa, *Nature* 350:429, 1991.
16. Brett SM, Rodricks JV, Chinchilli VM: Review and update of leukemia risk potentially associated with occupational exposure to benzene, *Environ Health Perspect* 82:267, 1989.
17. Bulger WH, Kupfer D: *Estrogenic activity of pesticides and other xenobiotics on the uterus and male reproductive tract.* In Thomas JA, et al, editors: *Endocrine toxicology,* New York, 1985, Raven Press, pp 1-33.
18. Cheever AW: Schistosomiasis and neoplasia, *J Natl Cancer Inst* 61:13, 1978.
19. Davis JMG, et al: The pathogenicity of long versus short fibre samples of amosite asbestos administered to rats by inhalation and intraperitoneal injection, *J Exp Pathol* 67:415, 1986.
20. Delore P, Borgamano J: Leucemie aique en cours d'intoxication benzenique, *J Med Lyon* 9:227, 1928.
21. Depue RH, Pike MC, Henderson BE: Estrogen exposure during gestation and risk of testicular cancer, *J Natl Cancer Inst* 71:1151, 1983.
22. Diamond L: Tumor promoters and cell transformation, *Pharmacol Ther* 26:89, 1984.
23. Falck F Jr, et al: Pesticides and polychlorinated biphenyl residues in human breast lipids and their relation to breast cancer, *Arch Environ Health* 47:143, 1992.
24. Fearon ER, Vogelstein B: A genetic model for colorectal tumorigenesis, *Cell* 61:759, 1990.
25. Forrester K, et al: Detection of high incidence of K-ras oncogenes during human colon tumorigenesis, *Nature* 327:298, 1987.
26. Fox TR, Goldsworthy TL: Molecular analysis of the H-ras gene: an understanding of mouse liver tumor development, *CIIT Activities* 13:1, 1993.
27. Furst A: Toward mechanisms of metal carcinogenesis, genotoxic or carcinogenic metals. In Fishbein A, Furst A, Mehlman M, editors: Environmental and occupational occurrence and exposure, Princeton, NJ, 1987, Princeton Scientific Publishing.
28. Gold LS, et al: Rodent carcinogens: setting priorities, *Science* 258:261, 1992.
29. Gonzalez FJ, Crespi CL, Gelboin HV: cDNA-expressed human cytochrome P450s: a new age of molecular toxicology and human risk assessment, *Mutat Res* 247:113, 1991.
30. Gu J-R, et al: Oncogenes in primary hepatic cancer, *J Cell Physiol Suppl* 4:13, 1986.
31. Guengerich FP: Roles of cytochrome p450 enzymes in chemical carcinogenesis and cancer chemotherapy, *Cancer Res* 48:2946, 1988.
32. Harington JS: Fiber carcinogenesis: epidemiologic observations and the Stanton hypothesis, *J Natl Cancer Inst* 67:977, 1981 (editorial).
33. Harris CC: Chemical and physical carcinogenesis: advances and perspectives for the 1990s, *Cancer Res* 51(suppl):5023, 1991.
34. Harris CC, Hollstein M: Clinical implications of the p53 tumor-suppressor gene, *N Engl J Med* 329:1318, 1993.
35. Harris H: Cell fusion and the analysis of malignancy, *J Natl Cancer Inst* 48:851, 1972.
36. Henderson BE, Ross R, Bernstein L: Estrogens as a cause of human cancer: the Richard and Hinda Rosenthal Foundation award lecture, *Cancer Res* 48:246, 1988.
37. Herbst AL, et al: Epidemiologic aspects and factors related to survival in 384 registry cases of clear cell adenocarcinoma of the vagina and cervix, *Am J Obstet Gynecol* 135:876, 1979.
38. Hill J: *Cautions against the immoderate use of snuff.* London, 1761, R Baldwin.
39. Hoffmann D, Hecht SS: Nicotine-derived *N*-nitrosamines and tobacco-related cancer: current status and future directions, *Cancer Res* 45:935, 1985.
40. Hollstein M, et al: p53 mutations in human cancers, *Science* 253:49, 1991.
41. Hricko A: Rings of controversy around benzene, *Environ Health Perspect* 102:276, 1994.
42. Hsia CC, et al: Mutations of p53 gene in hepatocellular carcinoma, *Natl Cancer Instit* 84:1638, 1992.
43. Hsu IC, et al: Mutational hotspot in the p53 gene in human hepatocellular carcinomas, *Nature* 350:427, 1991.
44. Institute of Food Technologists' Expert Panel on Food Safety & Nutrition: Potential mechanisms for food-related carcinogens and anticarcinogens, *Food Technology* (47):105, 1993.
45. Johnson KH, et al: Light-microscopic morphology of cell types cultured during preneoplasia from foreign body-reactive tissues and films. *Cancer Res* 37:3228, 1977.
46. Kastan MB, et al: Participation of p53 protein in the cellular response to DNA damage, *Cancer Res* 51:6304, 1991.
47. Kumar R, Sukumar S, Barbacid M: Activtion of ras oncogenes preceding the onset of neoplasia, *Science* 248:1101, 1990.
48. Landolph JR: *Neoplastic transformation of mammalian cells by carcinogenic metal compounds: cellular and molecular mechanisms.* In Foulkes EG, editor: *Biological effects of toxic metals,* 1990, CRC Press.
49. Lang L: Baffling butadiene, *Environ Health Perspect* 102:282, 1994.
50. Law MR: Genetic predisposition to lung cancer, *Br J Cancer* 61:195, 1990.
51. Li Z-H, et al: c-K-ras and p53 mutations occur very early in adenocarcinoma of the lung, *Am J Pathol* 144:303, 1994.

52. Loeb LA: Endogenous carcinogenesis: molecular oncology into the twenty-first century, presidential address, *Cancer Res* 49:5489, 1989.

53. Lucier GW: *Receptor-mediated carcinogenesis.* In Vainio H, et al, editors: *Mechanisms of carcinogenesis in risk identification,* Lyon, 1992, International Agency for Research on Cancer, pp 87-112.

54. Lutz WK: Endogenous genotoxic agents and processes as a basis of spontaneous carcinogenesis, *Mutat Res* 238:287, 1990.

55. Marcial-Rojas RA, editor: *Pathology of protozoal and helminthic diseases,* Baltimore, 1971, Williams & Wilkins.

56. Miller EC, Miller JA: Searches for ultimate chemical carcinogens and their reactions with cellular macromolecules, *Cancer* 47:2327, 1981.

57. Montesano R, Bartsch H: Mutagenic and carcinogenic *N*-nitroso compounds: possible environmental hazards, *Mutat Res* 32:179, 1976.

58. Nebert DW, Gonzalez FJ: p450 genes: structure, evolution, and regulation, *Annu Rev Biochem* 56:945, 1987.

59. Ozturk M, et al: p53 mutation in hepatocellular carcinoma after aflatoxin exposure, *Lancet* 338:1356, 1991.

60. Pott Sir P: Chirurgical observations relative to . . . the cancer of the scrotum [etc], Chirurgical Works of Percivall Pott, F.R.S. and Surgeon to St. Bartholomew's Hospital. London, 1775, pp 734-736.

61. Purdie CA, et al: p53 expression in colorectal tumors, *Am J Pathol* 138:807, 1991.

62. Rachko D, Brand KG: Chromosomal aberrations in foreign body tumorigenesis of mice, *Proc Soc Exp Biol Med* 172:382, 1983.

63. Rauth AM: *Radiation carcinogenesis.* In Tannock IF, Hill RP, editors: *The basic science of oncology,* New York, 1992, McGraw-Hill, pp 119-135.

64. Reddy AL, Fialkow PJ: Probable clonal development of foreign-body–induced murine sarcomas, *J Natl Cancer Inst* 72:467, 1984.

65. Rinsky RA: Benzene and leukemia: an epidemiologic risk assessment, *Environ Health Perspect* 82:189, 1989.

66. Rodenhuis S, Slebos RJC: Clinical significance of ras oncogene activation in human lung cancer, *Cancer Res* 52(suppl):2665, 1992.

67. Rogan WJ, Bagniewska A, Damstra T: Pollutants in breast milk, *N Engl J Med* 302:1450, 1980.

68. Rogan WJ, et al: Polychlorinated biphenyls (PCBs) and dichlorodiphenyl dichloroethane (DDE) in human milk: effects on growth, morbidity and duration of lactation, *Am J Public Health* 77:1294, 1987.

69. Rowley JD: Molecular cytogenetics: Rosetta stone for understanding cancer, twenty-ninth GHA Clowes Memorial award lecture, *Cancer Res* 50:3816, 1990.

70. Rowley JD: The Philadelphia chromosome translocation: a paradigm for understanding leukemia, *Cancer* 65:2178, 1990.

71. Santesson GG: Uber chroische Vergiftungen mit Steinkohlen benzin, *Vier Todesfälle Arch Hyg* 31:336, 1897.

72. Saracci R, et al: The age-mortality curve of endemic pleural mesothelioma in Karain, Central Turkey, *Br J Cancer* 45:147, 1982.

73. Scarpelli DG: *Human liver carcinogenesis: a complex problem.* In Scarpelli DG, Craighead JE, Kaufman N, editors: *The pathologist and the environment,* Baltimore, 1985, Williams & Wilkins, pp 168-189.

74. Schecter A, et al: Chlorinated and bromiated dixoins and dibenzofurans in human tissue following exposure, *Environ Health Perspect* 102(suppl 1):135, 1994.

75. Schecter A, et al: Polychlorinated biphenyl levels in the tissues of exposed and non-exposed humans, *Environ Health Perspect* 102 (Suppl)1:149, 1994.

76. Sell S, et al: Synergy between hepatitis B virus expression and chemical hepatocarcinogen transgenic mice, *Cancer Res* 51:1278, 1991.

77. Silbergeld EK, Gasiewicz TA: Dioxins and the Ah receptor, *Am J Ind Med* 16:455, 1989.

78. Sommer SS, et al: Pattern of p53 gene mutations in breast cancers of women in midwestern United States, *J Natl Cancer Inst* 84:246, 1992.

79. Sommering ST: *De morbis vasorum absorbentium corporis humani. Trajectinae ad moenum, varrentrappii et wenneri,* 1795.

80. Sommers SC, McManus RG: Multiple arsenical cancers of skin and internal organs, *Cancer* 6:347, 1953.

81. Stanton MF, Wrench C: Mechanisms of mesothelioma induction with asbestos and fibrous glass, *J Natl Cancer Inst* 48:797, 1972.

82. Thor A, et al: ras gene alterations and enhanced levels of ras p21 expression in a spectrum of benign and malignant human mammary tissues, *Lab Invest* 55:603, 1986.

83. Turner FC: Sarcomas at sites of subcutaneously implanted bakelite disks in rats, *J Natl Cancer Inst* 2:81, 1941.

84. US Department of Health and Human Services, Agency for Toxic Substances and Disease Registry: *Case studies in environmental medicine: benzene toxicity,* Washington, DC, 1992, Government Printing Office.

85. Vigliani EC, Saita G: Benzene and leukemia, *N Engl J Med* 271:872, 1964.

86. Wagner JC, Griffiths DM, Hill RJ: The effect of fibre size on the in vivo activity of UICC crocidolite, *Br J Cancer* 49:453, 1984.

87. Wallace LA: Major sources of benzene exposure, *Environ Health Perspect* 82:165, 1989.

88. Westra WH, et al: K-ras oncogene activation in lung adenocarcinomas from former smokers, *Cancer* 72:432, 1993.

89. Wetterhahn KE, et al: Metal carcinogenesis: a chemical pathology study section workshop, workshop report from the Division of Research Grants, National Institutes of Health, *Cancer Res* 52:4058, 1992.

90. Whitlock JP Jr: Genetic and molecular aspects of 2,3,7,8-tetrachlorodibenzo-*p*-dioxin action, *Annu Rev Pharmacol Toxicol* 30:251, 1990.

91. Wogan GN: Aflatoxins as risk factors for hepatocellular carcinoma in humans, *Cancer Res* 52(suppl):2114, 1992.

92. Wolff MS, et al: Blood levels of organochlorine residue and breast cancer, *J Natl Cancer Inst* 85:648, 1993.

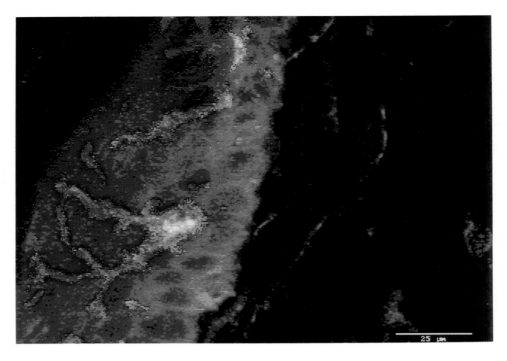

Color Plate 1. Langerhans cell detected by confocal scanning laser microscopy and immuno-fluorescence to CD1a antigen. Note elaborate branching dendrites *(orange)* extending toward the epidermal surface (*green layer,* epidermis; *underlying unstained layer,* dermis). (Acknowledgment: Brett Telegan provided critical assistance in the production of this figure.)

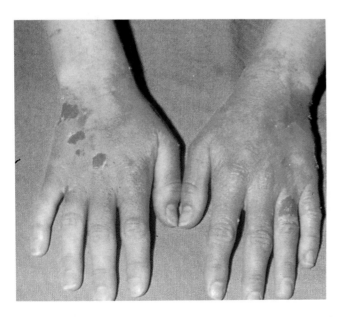

Color Plate 2. Photosensitivity contact dermatitis. Many chemicals need light to activate and produce the complete phototoxin or photoallergen. Psoralens in limes produced this vesicular phototoxic dermatitis in a bartender who squeezed limes all afternoon in direct sun.

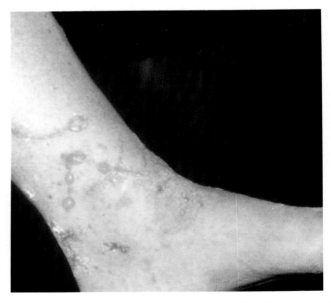

Color Plate 3. Poison ivy contact dermatitis. The *Rhus* genus of plants includes poison ivy, poison oak, and poison sumac. Poison ivy dermatitis may be acquired from direct contact with the plant or from the smoke of burning poison ivy plants.

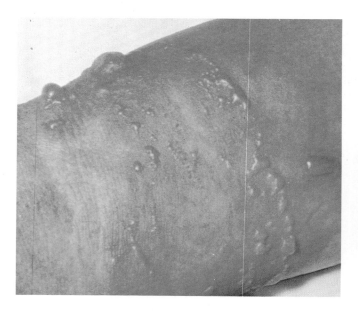

Color Plate 4. Acute irritant contact dermatitis. Exposure to a strong irritant, ethylene oxide, produced this markedly swollen arm and an acute vesiculobullous dermatitis. A similar pattern may be seen with contact allergy.

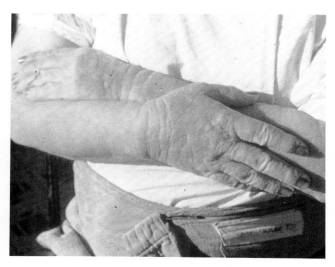

Color Plate 6. Chronic irritant contact dermatitis. The hands, wrists, and forearms are the most common sites of involvement in cases of industrial contact dermatitis. The hands and wrists of this worker show the effect of long-term exposure to a solvent, kerosene, which he used to clean his skin. The skin is markedly thickened, hyperpigmented, dry, and fissured. Itching is usually a major symptom.

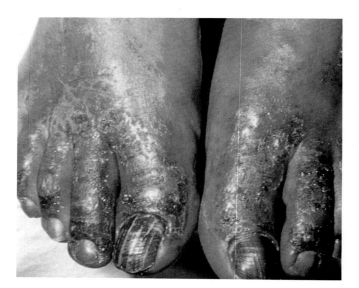

Color Plate 5. Subacute irritant contact dermatitis. This patient developed a bilateral and symmetric subacute dermatitis from the rubber accelerator, mercaptobenzothiazole, which was leached from the rubber portion of his work shoe when his foot perspired. Some edema and erythema with an eczematous eruption can be noted.

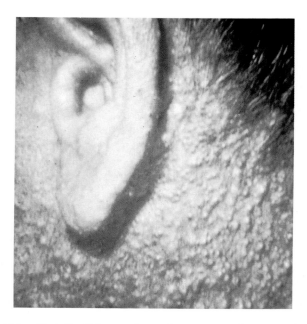

Color Plate 7. Chloracne is a refractory type of acne caused by certain halogenated aromatic chemical compounds; it can be accompanied by systemic toxicity. Chloracne in this herbicide production worker involved almost every follicular orifice on his face and neck, producing comedones, papules, and cystlike lesions.

Part **III**

ORGAN PATHOLOGY OF ENVIRONMENTAL AND OCCUPATIONAL DISEASE

Chapter 27

SKIN

George F. Murphy

The skin is the primary interface between the internal and external environment. In contrast to the hairy covering of most mammals, Homo sapiens must make their way in the world as "naked apes," and their skin has therefore adapted to become the most sophisticated organ in the body. For example, the epidermal layer consists predominantly of keratinocytes, which produce a resilient protective scale of keratin protein, minute membranous organelles ("Odland bodies") that assist in establishing a permeability barrier to the external milieu, and cytokines (e.g., interleukin-1[IL1]) with pleiotropic implications in inflammation and wound healing. The epidermis also contains melanocytes, which produce melanin pigment and transfer it evenly to keratinocytes, resulting in an endogenous screen to ultraviolet (UV) irradiation. Midepidermal Langerhans cells take up, process, and present environmental antigens so as to effect specific T-cell responses, putatively against microbes and neoantigens expressed by tumor cells. The underlying dermis also contains a rich array of cells with functions designed to maintain epidermal integrity, to promote inflammatory cell homing, and to transmit neurogenic signals important in avoidance of noxious stimuli.

It is therefore little wonder that many (if not most) of the skin diseases encountered by dermatologists and pathologists are environmentally related. Such conditions occur either when normal protective mechanisms malfunction (e.g., in the setting of albinism, xeroderma pigmentosum, or systemic immunosuppression) or when environmental exposure overcomes the limits of protection. UV irradiation accounts for much of the dermatological disease that affects humans. This is ironic because radiant energy from the sun has been responsible for the evolution and continuation of life-forms on this planet and also because most cutaneous injury from UV light is avoidable. Chemical agents, producing both immunologically specific and non-specific forms of dermatitis, also produce skin lesions that are commonly encountered in dermatological practice and are the primary cause of occupational dermatitis. The effects of microbial infestation and infection of skin are no longer considered trivial in light of evidence demonstrating human immunodeficiency virus (HIV) harbored within epidermal cells.[35] For dermatopathologists, understanding of environmentally induced skin diseases accounts for a significant portion of their practices. Recognition of environmental linkages to such lesions provides a critical feedback loop to clinicians and epidemiologists, who will define the impact of such disorders on patient morbidity, medical economics, and attempts at prevention. It is likely that, at present, the impact is grossly underestimated.

SOLAR RADIATION

The acute and chronic effects of solar radiation are discussed in this section. See Chapter 10 for more information on solar radiation.

Acute effects

The clinical effect of acute overexposure to UV irradiation is sunburn. Sunburn is heralded by a sensation of tingling and vague edema minutes to several hours after a minimal erythemagenic dose is reached and by erythema that develops approximately 24 hours after exposure. This biphasic response may be related to early events affecting dermal mast cells and later events involving local recruitment of circulating leukocytes. The histology of the sunburn reaction is characteristic, although not entirely specific (Fig. 27-1, *A*). There is focal dyskeratosis of the basal cell layer of the epidermis, papillary dermal edema, and evidence of mast cell degranulation. The dyskeratotic epidermal cells have dense, eosinophilic cytoplasm, pyknotic nuclei, and cell contours that are attenuated along the vertical axis (so-called streak dyskeratosis). There has been interest in the possibility that the ability of UV light to degranulate mast cells and provoke dermal inflammation may also be related to a less common form of acute solar injury, photodermatitis.[11] Photodermatitis is a name applied to a diverse group of disorders that clinically and histologically fall into the following categories: phototoxic dermatitis, photoallergic dermatitis, polymorphous light eruption, and photoexacerbated dermatitis (Fig. 27-1, *B*). All have in common the recruitment of inflammatory cells to superficial dermal venues. Table 27-1 summarizes the salient aspects of various forms of acute solar injury to the skin.

Pathophysiology. The pathogenesis of acute ultraviolet B (UVB)–mediated injury to the skin is still not completely understood. As described in Chapter 10, UVB results in depletion of the skin's ability to present antigenic signals to T cells, probably initially via depletion of relevant glycoproteins in Langerhans cells, and eventually by the destruction of Langerhans cells. Also, alterations in melanogenesis and melanin transfer occur. The sunburn reaction, however, is in large part an inflammatory process initially mediated by transient erythema and increased vascular permeability followed by more persistent erythema delayed in onset by 4 to 24 hours and correlated with a superficial perivascular inflammatory infiltrate.[30] These clinical and histological observations have resulted in speculation that primary cutaneous targets of UVB radiation include the endothelium and associated cells that reside in the perivascular space. We have found, for example, that short-term exposure of human skin to UVB (290 to 320 nm wavelength), even in suberythemagenic doses, induces in dermal vessels

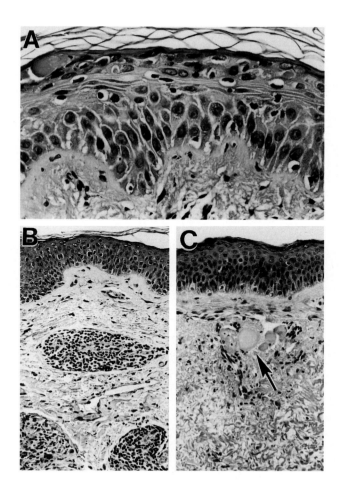

Fig. 27-1. Acute and chronic effects of ultraviolet (UV) light. **A,** Resolving acute sunburn reaction. Note the pulse of necrotic keratinocytes in the upper third of the epidermal layer as well as the mild, residual vacuolization of basal cells. **B,** Polymorphous light eruption. A brisk, perivascular lymphocytic infiltrate is induced after acute UV light exposure. **C,** Solar elastosis owing to chronic exposure to sunlight. Normal papillary dermal collagen is replaced by amorphous nodular aggregates of elastin *(arrow)*.

endothelial leukocyte adhesion molecule-1 (also known as E-selectin, a glycoprotein that is involved in leukocyte adhesion during early inflammation.[3,6,23,25] These events are associated with degranulation of mast cells and release of the cytokine tumor necrosis factor-α (TNF-α), a known inducer of E-selectin that is contained within mast cells as a preformed mediator.[18,39,40,43] Exposure to long-wave ultraviolet (320 to 400 nm, UVA) or infrared (> 400 nm) radiation does not induce E-selectin. Such observations suggest that early molecular events potentially contributory to inflammation in sunburn or photo-induced forms of dermatitis may be elicited by highly specific environmental stimuli: in this case a specific region of the electromagnetic spectrum.

The effects of acute exposure of UV light on skin are paradoxical, in that they may induce immunosuppressive as well as proinflammatory alteration. Exposure of rodent skin

Table 27-1. Acute solar injury to skin

Condition	Clinical features	Histological features	Cause (s)
Sunburn	Delayed erythema; vesicles; sloughing	Mast cell degranulation; dermal edema; basal cell layer dyskeratosis	Unprotected sunbathing
Phototoxic	Same as sunburn, but often more florid	Same as sunburn; epidermal necrosis often pronounced	Photosensitizing drugs (e.g., psoralens) (Color Plate 2)
Photoallergic	Poison ivy–like course of erythema, vesicles, scaling	Superficial perivascular T-cell infiltrate with intercellular edema within epidermal layer	Drug-induced: topical—paraaminobenzoic acid; systemic—thiazides
Polymorphous light eruption	Erythematous plaques and papules	Superficial and sometimes deep perivascular lymphocytic infiltrate; papillary dermal edema	Unknown
Photoexacerbated dermatitis	Malar erythema; development of new lesions in sun	Superficial dermal lymphocytic infiltrate; vacuolar degeneration of basal cells associated with infiltrate; dermal mucin deposits	Lupus erythematosus

to UVB is known to produce both local and systemic suppression of contact delayed hypersensitivity.[7,20,27] Local suppression results from effects of UVB on antigen presenting cells, such as epidermal Langerhans cells, which on exposure shed class II major histocompatibility complex (MHC) molecules requisite for their functional interaction with T–helper cell recipients of antigenic signals.[1] In addition, in rodents Thy-1+ and I-J+ dendritic epidermal cells, which may present antigens preferentially to T suppressor cells, are relatively resistant to UVB, potentially favoring the induction of antigen-specific suppressor pathways.[19] Systemic suppression results from higher doses and appears to be unrelated to local alterations in antigen-presenting pathways. Although the role of local and systemic immunosuppression by sunlight is best understood in animal models, extrapolation to humans would suggest that acute exposure to UVB could render defective immunosurveillance pathways critical to elimination of neoplastic clones of epithelial cells and melanocytes. Such clones may then go on to produce clinically evident tumors.

Chronic effects

Photoaging. The term *photoaging* was developed to convey a form of cutaneous degeneration that superficially resembled an accelerated version of the normal aging process.[22] Skin exposed repeatedly to excessive sunlight becomes prematurely furrowed and erythematous, assuming the clinical phenotype of advanced chronological aging. Histologically, however, photoaged skin is quite distinctive. Although skin from elderly individuals without excessive sun exposure shows diffuse epidermal and dermal atrophy, photoaged skin has the additional feature of abnormal deposition of dermal elastin (Fig. 27-1, *C*). This presumed product of actinically damaged fibroblasts replaces normal elastic fibers in the papillary dermis, which tether the epidermal layer to the underlying connective tissue.

Loss in normal elasticity produces wrinkles and contributes to dilated and plugged follicular ostia, which may be associated with hyperplastic sebaceous lobules. Interestingly, photoaged skin also often has a superficial perivascular lymphocytic infiltrate, leading to speculation that some of the abnormalities in dermal matrix may also be attributable to a form of low-grade, chronic photodermatitis,[24] with associated elaboration of cytokines that may influence normal fibroblast homeostasis.

Neoplasia. In addition to photoaging, chronic exposure to UV light has a number of effects that result in abnormal proliferation and metabolic activity of epidermal cells. For example, low-grade, repeated exposure to the sun results in increased pigment synthesis and melanin transfer by melanocytes. Over time, however, melanocytes themselves may become focally hyperplastic, resulting in uniform or variegated brown macules, termed solar lentigines (Fig. 27-2, *A*). Langerhans cells acutely lose the ability to synthesize and express class II MHC antigens (integral to their immunological function). Eventually, chronic sun exposure may result in profound depletion of this important immunosurveillance cell. Keratinocytes typically express abnormalities consisting of hypoproliferation and hyperproliferation, variable dysplasia, and, in some instances, progression to frank malignancy. Focal abnormalities in sun-damaged keratinocytes, characterized clinically by abnormal scale and histologically by variable dysplasia of the lowermost epidermal layers, are termed *actinic or solar keratoses* (Fig. 27-2, *C*). Although not all of these lesions evolve into carcinoma, some become basal and squamous cell cancers (Figs. 27-2, *D* and 27-3). Cup-shaped benign to locally destructive tumors of keratinocytes, termed keratoacanthomas (Fig. 27-2, *B*), may also arise in skin exposed to chronic sun. In areas of vitiligo or in albinism, where endogenous pigmentation is absent, somatic cells undergo mutation at a higher rate than normal. The

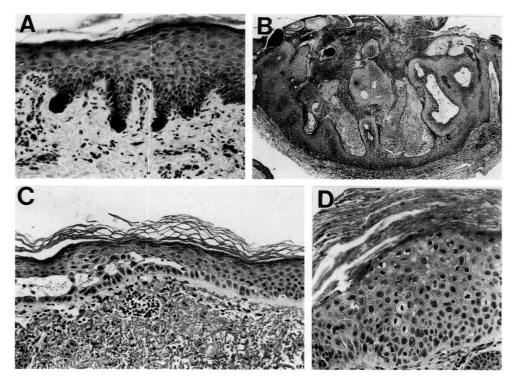

Fig. 27-2. Pigmentary and proliferative epidermal lesions after chronic ultraviolet (UV) light exposure. **A,** An actinic lentigo, characterized by hyperpigmentation and downward elongation of rete ridges in association with melanocytic hyperplasia occurred in this patient receiving chronic PUVA (photosensitizing psoralen plus ultraviolet light A) treatments for psoriasis. **B,** Keratoacanthoma, consisting of cup-shaped endophytic proliferation of chronically sun-damaged keratinocytes. **C,** Actinic keratosis. Note the atypia and dyshesive growth of the lowermost epidermal layers *(left)*. The dermis is almost completely replaced by abnormal elastic tissue. **D,** Squamous cell carcinoma, in situ. There is full-thickness atypia, with midepidermal mitoses and abnormal surface scale.

inability of cells to repair all of the damaged DNA would result in increased numbers of actinic keratoses and related skin cancers.[28]

Basal cell carcinoma may be associated with preexisting actinic keratosis or may arise in diffusely actinically damaged skin. Typical tumors are composed of islands and strands of small tumor cells with oval, basophilic nuclei, inconspicuous cytoplasm, and inconspicuous nucleoli (Fig. 27-3, *A–C*). There is a characteristic palisade formed by a single layer of basal cells about the perimeter of lobules, and the associated dermis is often fibrotic and contains abundant mucopolysaccharide. This stroma typically retracts from the epithelial elements of the tumor on fixation, producing "separation artifact" helpful in histological diagnosis. In contrast, squamous cell carcinoma is composed of larger, polyhedral cells with abundant, often eosinophilic cytoplasm interconnected along adjacent cell membranes by intercellular "bridges" representing desmosome-containing attachment plaques. Nuclei are large, and nucleoli are often conspicuous. In situ lesions are confined to the epidermal layer; in contrast to actinic keratoses, in which dysplasia is confined to the lower epidermal layers, in situ carcinoma shows dysplasia that extends to the level of the stratum corneum. Invasive squamous cell carcinoma extends into the dermis as irregular tongues of malignant cells embedded within a desmoplastic stroma (Figs 27-3, *D, E*).

Most skin cancers derived from keratinocytes do not metastasize, although locally aggressive courses generally supervene when lesions remain untreated. This is not the case for malignant melanoma, which progresses inexorably over time from surgically curable to incurable stages characterized by widespread systemic dissemination.[9] Those at greatest risk for development of malignant melanoma are lightly pigmented individuals who burn rather than tan on exposure to the sun. These patients often have a history of antecedent blistering sunburns and frequently are covered with sun-related lentigines and benign melanocytic nevi. Although the precise role of sun exposure in initiating the molecular and cellular changes that result in melanoma has not as yet been defined, a form of malignant melanoma called lentigo maligna melanoma provides an important paradigm for the role of the sun in the provocation of this po-

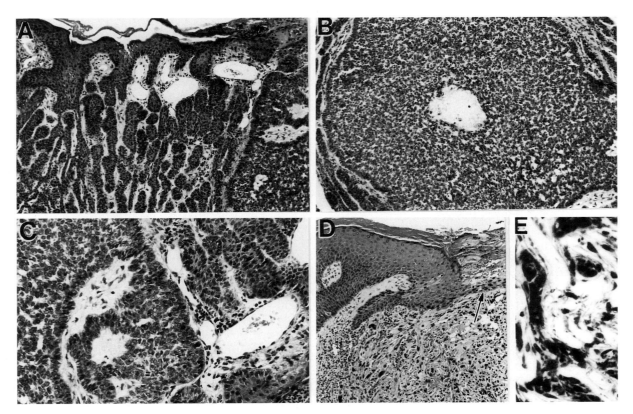

Fig. 27-3. Ultraviolet (UV) light-induced carcinogenesis—epidermal cancers. **A-C,** Basal cell carcinoma. The tumor grows into the dermis as organoid strands and nodules of cells with deeply stained nuclei and scant cytoplasm. At the periphery of tumor islands and cords, cells palisade against a loose, mucinous stroma containing telangiectatic blood vessels (**B** and **C**). **D** and **E,** Invasive squamous cell carcinoma. **D,** This tumor originates from an epidermal layer showing in situ dysplasia *(arrow)* and grows downward as anaplastic, nonkeratinizing cells with abundant eosinophilic cytoplasm. **E,** In desmoplastic spindle cell variants of invasive squamous cell carcinoma, immunohistochemical detection of cytokeratin (darkly stained cords of cells) may be necessary to differentiate tumor cells from reactive mesenchymal elements or from other types of spindle cell malignancy.

tentially lethal tumor.[5] Lentigo maligna, the precursor form of this form of melanoma, begins as a localized proliferation of dysplastic melanocytes along the lowermost epidermal layers of chronically sun-exposed skin. Although this proliferation may persist for many years without dermal invasion, eventually melanoma cells acquire the ability to transgress the basement membrane that separates the epidermal and dermal layers. Once dermal invasion occurs, progressive growth into deeper dermal layers is associated with increasing tendency for metastatic spread.

In general, melanomas are classified according to four groups based on the presence and related morphology of intraepidermal growth: superficial spreading, lentigo maligna, acral-mucosal lentiginous, and nodular (inconspicuous intraepidermal growth) (Figs. 27-4, *A, B*). Typically, melanomas grow radically within the epidermis and as single cells within the papillary dermis (radial growth) for variable periods of time before they grow as nodules within the

dermis (vertical growth). The ability to metastasize develops with the onset of the vertical growth phase and increases progressively with depth of melanoma cell penetration into the deeper dermal layers and the subcutaneous fat. Cytologically, melanoma cells tend to be epithelioid; contain large vesicular nuclei with prominent, eosinophilic nucleoli; and may express dusty melanin granules within their cytoplasm. Many melanomas, however, show spindle cell differentiation; show small, dense nuclei; and are amelanotic. Detection of melanocyte-associated S-100 protein of melanoma cell–associated HMB-45 antigen may facilitate diagnosis in such instances.

In addition to skin neoplasms derived from keratinocytes and melanocytes, chronic exposure to UV light is associated with the genesis of several other commonly encountered tumors. Many keratoacanthomas, for example, occur in chronically sun-damaged skin. Atypical fibroxanthoma, a mesenchymal proliferation of highly pleomorphic fibro-

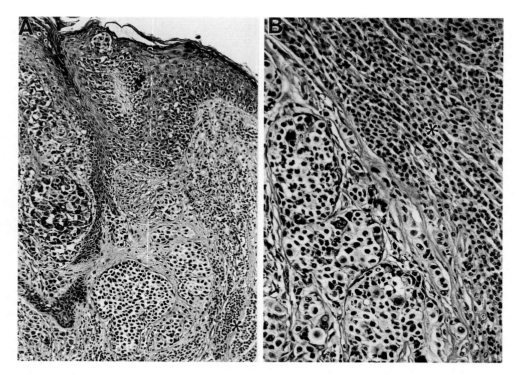

Fig. 27-4. Ultraviolet (UV) light-induced carcinogenesis—malignant melanoma. **A** and **B,** Vertical growth stage of malignant melanoma is characterized by variably pigmented nodules of malignant cells within the superficial and deep dermis in association with residual pagetoid intraepidermal growth (radial growth). The asterisk in each panel denotes a population of smaller, nevus cells, possibly representing a precursor lesion. Acquired melanocytic nevi also occur at a high incidence in chronically sun-exposed skin in patients predisposed to develop these tumors.

blasts and histiocytes, regularly affects facial skin with significant elastin deposition within the adjacent dermis. Although the ability of UV light to induce errors in the DNA replication to promote activation of proto-oncogenes may explain its association with these histogenetically diversified tumors, it should be emphasized that sunlight alone is but one of a number of factors that are likely to foster the development of these lesions. This is particularly true in the case of melanoma, in which genetic factors, local immunity, and provocative environmental agents may collaborate to produce specific neoplasms.

IONIZING RADIATION

The effects of acute and chronic exposure to ionizing radiation have a number of similarities and differences from those induced by UV irradiation (Table 27-2). Briefly, acute effects of gamma or x-irradiation produce inflammatory lesions typified by degeneration and necrosis within the epidermal layer and related adnexal structures. The inflammatory infiltrate is more florid than that of the sunburn reaction, and epidermal changes are generally more pronounced. Chronic radiation dermatitis shows a characteristic histological picture consisting of sclerosis of dermal connective tissue associated with enlarged fibroblasts and endothelial cells, which often appear to be atypical owing to nuclear prominence and hyperchromasia (Fig. 27-5, *A*). This change differs from the effects of chronic exposure to UV irradiation, which results in superficial dermal elastin deposition (Fig. 27-1, *C*), and from the effects of repeated local exposure to infrared irradiation (erythema ab igne), which produces loss of epidermal melanin pigment into the underlying dermis (Fig. 27-5, *B*). See Chapter 11.

CHEMICAL AND MECHANICAL HAZARDS
Allergic contact dermatitis

Exposure of skin to environmental antigens or haptens often results in sensitization, which causes immunologically specific recall on rechallenge. This recall phenomenon may be mediated primarily by memory T lymphocytes,[38] as in type IV delayed hypersensitivity reactions, or by immunoglobulin E (IgE) cross-linking on the surface of mast cells, as in type I immediate hypersensitivity responses. A listing of the environmental causes of allergic contact dermatitis could fill the pages of this entire book. More commonly implicated agents include certain heavy metals (nickel and gold in jewelry); chemical products of perfumes, soaps, and

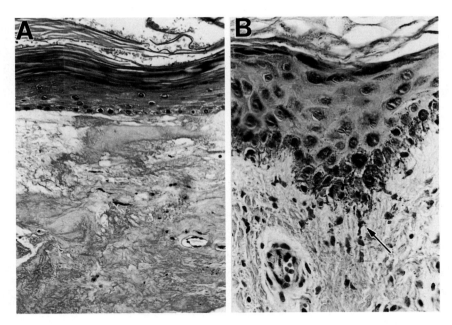

Fig. 27-5. Cutaneous effects of chronic ionizing and infrared irradiation. **A,** Chronic radiation dermatitis. There is marked sclerosis of the superficial dermis, epidermal atrophy, and hyperkeratosis. Rare mesenchymal cells in the altered dermal matrix exhibit characteristic nuclear enlargement and hyperchromasia. **B,** Chronic exposure to infrared irradiation (erythema ab igne). Note the ongoing loss of particulate epidermal melanin into the underlying dermal matrix *(arrow)*.

Table 27-2. Acute and chronic effects of ionizing irradiation

	Acute	Chronic
Clinical appearance	Erythema, edema, vesiculation, ulceration	Atrophy, telangiectasia, induration due to fibrosis, mottled hyperpigmentation and hypopigmentation
Epidermal changes	Epidermal and adnexal vacuolization and necrosis	Hyperkeratosis, atrophy with focal hyperplasia; adnexal loss
Dermal changes	Dermal edema, vascular ectasia, microthrombosis; mixed perivascular inflammatory infiltrate	Thickened, homogenized collagen bundles; enlarged stellate fibroblasts and plump endothelial cells with hyperchromatic nuclei; vessel ectasia
Subcutaneous changes	Minimal or absent	Fibrosis may be present

cosmetics; and naturally occurring substances from plants (rhus in the poison ivy leaf) (Color Plate 3.). Photoeczematous dermatitis, described earlier, most likely represents photoactivation of an antigen, or photoinduced provocation of inflammatory signals at sites of antigen challenge. (See Chapter 25.)

Contact urticaria (type I reaction) is characterized clinically by the development of an urticarial wheal and flare response at the site of antigen contact within minutes of exposure. These lesions may be intensely pruritic. Histologically, there is mast cell degranulation, superficial dermal edema, lymphatic ectasia, and a sparse superficial perivascular mixed lymphocytic and neutrophilic infiltrate (Fig. 27-6, *A*). Such lesions regress spontaneously within 24 hours of antigen withdrawal. Contact dermatitis of the eczematous type begins as an ill-defined zone of urticaria, which, within 24 to 96 hours, evolves into an erythematous, pruritic plaque, often studded with microvesicles. If antigenic challenge is chronic, a scaling plaque develops at this site. Histologically, allergic contract dermatitis shows defined stages of temporal evolution consisting of urticarial (> 24 hours), spongiotic (24 to 96 hours),

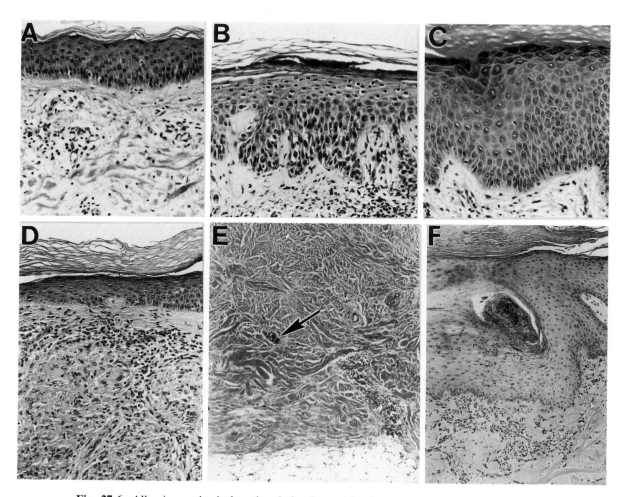

Fig. 27-6. Allergic, mechanical, and toxic insults to skin. **A,** Contact urticaria (type I reaction). Collagen fibers in the superficial dermis are widely spaced as a result of fluid transudation across venules cuffed by sparse collection of lymphocytes and neutrophils. **B,** Allergic contact dermatitis (type IV reaction). The epidermis is characterized by spongiosis (widened intercellular spaces owing to edema) and abnormal scale formation. The dermis contains a superficial angiocentric infiltrate of lymphocytes and eosinophils. **C,** Primary irritant dermatitis. The epidermal layer is hyperplastic, and the stratum granulosum and stratum corneum are thickened. The dermis contains a sparse infiltrate of lymphocytes. **D,** Granulomatous dermatitis due to inorganic particulates (silica). The dermis is essentially replaced by noncaseating granulomas. **E,** Deep dermal sclerosis due to polyvinyl chloride exposure. An atrophic remnant of an eccrine coil (*arrow*) demarcates the normal interface between reticular dermis and subcutaneous fat. All of the underlying hyalinized collagen is therefore abnormal; the pattern is precisely that observed in scleroderma. **F,** Acneiform follicular injury subsequent to dioxin exposure. The follicular infundibulum is hyperplastic, dilated, and plugged by cornified material containing inflammatory debris. The perifollicular adventitia contains a chronic lymphocytic infiltrate.

eczematous (1 or more weeks), and lichenified (many weeks to months) stages. The urticarial phase is indistinguishable clinically from the changes seen in type I reactions. The spongiotic phase is the most typical (Fig. 27-6, *B*), consisting of a superficial perivascular lymphocytic infiltrate often with eosinophils, along with intercellular edema within the epidermal layer (spongiosis). This edema results in microvesiculation, which develops into

the clinically observed fluid-filled blisters typical at this stage. The eczematous phase consists of residual spongiosis coupled with epidermal hyperplasia and excess scale production. With chronicity, "lichenified" plaques develop, in which epidermal hyperplasia and excessive scale production become the preponderant findings, resulting in clinical lesions that resemble lichen that grows on the bark of a tree.

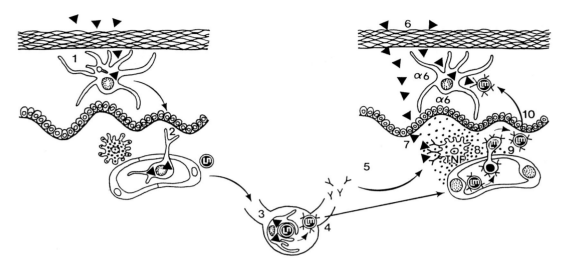

Fig. 27-7. Schematic diagram of immunological hypersensitivity stimulated by environmental antigens. Haptens or intact protein antigens (triangles) come into contact with the epidermal surface, are taken up by Langerhans cells *(1)*, and are transported to draining lymph nodes via dermal lymphatics *(2)*. Within the nodes *(3)*, processed antigen is presented to naive T lymphocytes (Ln), which acquire specific immunological memory for the antigen (memory T cells, Lm) *(4)*. Some cells at this juncture may also be stimulated to produce antigen-specific IgE–like molecules capable of binding to the surfaces of mast cells *(5)*. On reexposure to the sensitizing hapten or antigen *(6)*, mast cells are induced to degranulate by putative cross-linking of membrane-bound antibody formed in steps 4 and 5. Degranulation releases vasoactive substances capable of activating endothelial cells *(8)* to display adhesive proteins for leukocytes and rendering antigen-containing Langerhans cells immobile within the epidermal layer. Mast cell–activated endothelial cells express E-selectin, an adhesive ligand for Lm *(9)*. Resultant Lm binding and entry into the dermis and epidermis leads to antigen presentation by Langerhans cells *(10)*. Lm so stimulated then releases a potent array of cytokines that recruit antigen-nonspecific lymphocytes and monocytes, resulting in clinical erythema and induration. (Illustration courtesy of Dr. Michael Ioffreda.)

Because contact allergy may resemble primary irritant dermatitis (see later) and other types of dermatitis unrelated to environmental or industrial exposure, careful history is necessary in formulating a clinical-pathological assessment. In the case of household exposure, information concerning changes in cosmetics and detergents is important. In industrial agriculture, one must consider airborne as well as direct forms of contact. Specific occupations (e.g., hairdressers) are particularly prone to contact dermatitis involving the hands. Once a complete history has been obtained, a therapeutic trial of avoidance of suspected agents may be implemented. In some situations, patch testing may be helpful in specifically identifying the offending chemical.

Pathophysiology. The pathogenesis of allergic contact dermatitis involves remarkable cellular interactions initiated by the most peripheral outpost of the body's immune system, Langerhans cells within the epidermal layer (see Color Plate 1). The schema in Fig. 27-7 illustrates the cellular pathways set into motion on topical exposure to an environmental antigen or hapten. Contact of antigen to the skin surface via direct application (e.g., poison ivy), aerosolization (e.g., pollen), waterborne mechanisms (e.g., laundry detergent in clothing plus perspiration), or photoactivation (inert protein plus sunlight-producing antigen) results in uptake by Langerhans cells *(1)*. These highly dendritic cells are situated in the midepidermis, where they extend delicate dendrites upward toward the skin surface. Once internalized within the Langerhans cell, protein antigens are partially degraded into a form that may be easily presented to T lymphocytes. Although T cells pass throughout the skin in low numbers normally, in order to present the processed antigen most efficiently, the Langerhans cell migrates from the epidermis into the superficial dermis and subsequently into lymphatic channels *(2)*, where it travels to draining lymph nodes. In the lymph node *(3)*, the antigenic peptides are presented to naive T cells via precise membrane-membrane interaction involving class II proteins and the T-cell receptor complex.[13] Once the antigenic signal is so communicated, the now *sensitized* T cells are capable of recalling the antigen on reexposure, and they are therefore referred to as a T memory cells.

Antigenic recall by previously sensitized T cells is referred to as the *challenge* reaction and is an example of a delayed hypersensitivity of type IV immune response. On topical reexposure to the sensitizing antigen (6), the Langerhans cell again takes up the peptide and processes it internally. However, it no longer has the need to migrate to an environment rich in naive T cells. Rather, the charge of the Langerhans cell is now to present the processed antigen to a T memory cell locally at the site of antigen exposure. Through mechanisms not entirely understood, T memory cells show increased homing to the challenge site via dermal microvessels. One possible mechanism is antigen-induced mast cell degranulation.[2] In rodents, for example, it has been shown that antigen sensitization (4) is also associated with the production of a non-IgE antigen-specific molecule that binds to the membrane of perivascular dermal mast cells (5). Exposure to the sensitizing antigen causes cross-linking of the membrane-bound molecule (7) in a manner similar to IgE cross-linking implicit in type I immune reactions. The result is mast cell degranulation, an event known to result in TNF-α release from mast cell granules and adhesion molecule induction (8) in membranes of adjacent endothelial cells. Waldorf and co-workers[38] and Picker and colleagues[31] have shown that this event is associated with specifically increased binding of T memory cells to endothelium (9), providing an explanation for the increased homing to the challenge site. Only one T memory cell is required to receive antigenic signals locally from the Langerhans cell (10). Such T memory cells result in secondary elaboration of cytokines, which recruit additional antigen-nonspecific T cells and monocytes to the region. Note that the Langerhans cell in the challenge reaction remains fixed in the epidermis, enabling the local antigen presentation required for the challenge reaction to transpire. The inhibition of Langerhans cell motility (in contrast to sensitization) may also reside in local release of TNF-α by degranulating mast cells,[12,36] an event that induces cell membrane adhesive integrins, such the α6 subunit. The clinical result, which is fully initiated within 24 hours of challenge, is the dermal and epidermal inflammatory process that characterizes contact hypersensitivity. Once inflammatory cells are present, they, along with epidermal keratinocytes, produce a number of provocative cytokines, including IL-1, TNF-α, and immune interferon,[21,29] which further develop and perpetuate the inflammatory reaction (see Chapter 24).

Primary irritant dermatitis

Mechanical. Irritant dermatitis is a nonspecific term that conveys the protective reactions of skin to nonimmunological stimuli, such as mechanical or chemical injury. Because some of the clinical and histological alterations observed in primary irritant dermatitis superficially resemble those of allergic contact dermatitis, confusion exists regarding potential ambiguities between these two entities. In the case of contact allergy, however, sensitized, antigen-specific immune cells are the effectors of the resultant dermatitis, whereas in primary irritant dermatitis, inflammation does not involve antigen-specific memory. An example of primary irritant dermatitis of the mechanical type is the cutaneous response to chronic rubbing. Clinical examples of such changes may be seen in musicians (fiddler's neck) and athletes at sites of repeated mechanical trauma. Histologically, although a nonspecific superficial perivascular mononuclear cell infiltrate and spongiosis may be observed in acute phases, most lesions are predominated by irregular epidermal hyperplasia with little or no spongiosis (Fig. 27-6, C). With chronicity, the underlying dermal collagen typically shows vertically oriented fibrosis within dermal papillae. These histological changes are often described as lichen simplex chronicus in the setting of a clinical plaque and as prurigo nodularis in association with a localized papule or nodule. Such lesions may have variable increases in scale, and at some anatomical sites (sole and palm), scale may be the most prominent histological feature (callous or clavus).

Chemical. There is an extensive list of environmental chemicals that may provoke skin inflammation and epidermal hyperplasia in the absence of evidence of antigen-specific induction of memory T-cell pathways. (Color Plates 4, 5, and 6.) Local pathways involving cytokines and skin adhesion molecules that are potentially responsible for this phenomenon are addressed elsewhere in this book (see Chapter 24). It is important, however, to emphasize that many chemicals appear to be both primary irritants as well as immunological sensitizers of varying potency. It is also clear that many seemingly innocuous substances may be classified as chemical irritants. For example, surfactants, such as sodium laurel sulfate, are known to possess significant primary irritant capability.[41] Such effects are believed to be in part the result of the ability of surfactants to remove stratum corneum lipids, extract amino acids and proteins, and alter the water barrier within the upper epidermal layers, resulting in increased transepidermal water loss.

The histological alteration induced by chemical irritants may mimic low-grade allergic contact dermatitis, although epidermal hyperplasia and scale abnormalities generally predominate over spongiosis and dermal inflammation in early evolutionary stages. Clinical distinction between chemical irritants and true contact sensitizers may not be possible. Prevention requires identification of putative environmental factors prone to causing chemical irritation, and avoidance of these putative offending agents. In the case of irritant dermatitis induced by surfactants, the use of lipid-containing emollients may assist in restoring the compromised water barrier at the skin surface.

Pathophysiology. Although significant information has accumulated with respect to mechanisms of antigen-mediated skin inflammation, relatively little is known concerning the pathogenesis of irritant dermatitis. The epidermis is replete with a potent array of preformed proinflammatory cytokines, such as IL-1,[21] and during wound healing, spillage or release by other mechanisms of these mediators into the dermis is believed to provoke inflammatory cell influx. It is therefore likely that chronic, subtle injury to keratinocytes could stimulate similar pathways, resulting in epidermal proliferation and dermal fibroplasia. Partitioning of biologically active cytokines is likely to occur normally within the epidermis, and any agent, mechanical or chemical, capable of perturbing this normal equilibrium could result in induction of proinflammatory pathways without invoking involvement of antigen-presenting cells.

Toxic dermatitis

Inorganic particulates. Although most chemical irritants produce effects via contact with the cytokine-rich epidermal layer, others appear to provoke changes of inflammation and fibrosis via direct toxic interaction with dermal cells. Occupational scleroderma,[10] for example, is the result of exposure to a seemingly diverse array of environmental agents, which include polyvinyl chloride and silica. Silica introduced directly into the dermis provokes granulomatous dermatitis with associated fibrosis (Fig. 27-6, *D*). Occupational exposure to silica dust results in inhalation as well as direct cutaneous exposure. It remains unclear as to how silica produces scleroderma-like changes in skin. Such alterations typically involve deep dermal sclerosis, adnexal atrophy, and fibrous replacement of subcutaneous fat and thus are indistinguishable for morphea or progressive systemic sclerosis not associated with industrial agents (Fig. 27-6, *E*).

Follicular toxicity. The hair follicle is an often overlooked site of environmental and industrial injury to the skin. It has already been mentioned that chronic UV exposure may result in dilated follicular ostia in regions of abnormal superficial dermal elastin deposition. In allergic contact dermatitis, the epithelium that surrounds hair follicles may be preferentially involved (e.g., follicular eczema owing to nickel contact). Acneiform lesions, characterized by plugging of follicles by keratotic material and variable associated follicular inflammation, may result from iatrogenic administration of steroids or from topical exposure of occlusive compounds, such as petrolatum or engine grease (mechanic's acne). A significant industrial accident occurred at a chemical plant in Seveso, Italy.[17] As a result, 2,3,7,8-tetrachlorodibenzo-*p*-dioxin (TCDD) spread as a toxic cloud over a populated area, resulting in inhalation and ingestion of this substance by thousands of adults and children. One to two months after the incident, acneiform lesions (chloracne) developed in a significant number of individuals exposed to the TCDD cloud. (Color Plate 7.) The majority of affected individuals were children and adolescents. Comedones and cystic lesions were present on facial skin, and some patients also showed involvement of extremity skin (Fig. 27-6, *F*). Similar lesions have also been described after military exposure to the defoliant known as "agent orange."

Chemical carcinogenesis

The most widely recognized chemical carcinogen affecting the skin is arsenic,[33] used in the past as part of a therapeutic regimen for psoriasis in the form of orally administered Fowler's solution. Many of these patients have developed atypical keratoses of the palms and soles along with associated squamous cell carcinomas. Arsenic toxicity, however, is not germane to modern environmental pathology of the skin. Rather, focus has shifted to potential industrial carcinogens as well as agents in therapeutic preparations. Of the latter, coal tar and its derivatives may contribute to the genesis of cancer in a number of ways, including pathways involving complete carcinogens (benzo[*a*]pyrene), tumor promoters (phenols), and enhancement of the carcinogenic effects of UV light. Tar has been responsible for a significant number of skin cancers related to industrial exposure, although as a therapeutic agent, it is generally both safe and effective. Nitrogen mustards, used in the topical treatment of cutaneous T-cell lymphoma, are also full carcinogens, causing breaks and cross-links in DNA molecules in skin cells. In one study, 27% of patients treated with topical nitrogen mustard for cutaneous T-cell lymphoma developed premalignant and malignant nonmelanocytic skin cancers.[37] Psoralen, a photosensitizing agent used in combination with UVA, has been shown both to initiate and promote cutaneous cancers in experimental animals.

The histology of nonmelanocytic skin cancers induced by chemicals is essentially that of ordinary squamous and basal cell carcinomas, described previously. Without careful environmental and industrial history, the potential linkage between exposure to environmental chemicals and common forms of skin cancer may go unappreciated.

MICROBIAL HAZARDS
Bacteria

There has been concern that trends in global warming and the "greenhouse effect" may produce an environment conductive to human infection by certain bacteria and fungi that normally flourish in warm, humid climates. Bacterial infections of skin, such as that caused by β-hemolytic *Streptococcus pyogenes,* are plentiful in conditions of high ambient temperature and humidity. Even when bacteria are abundant, compromise in host defenses is generally required for infection to occur, although highly virulent strains of streptococcus causing extensive skin necrosis have recently come to public attention. Vulnerabilites that predispose to bacterial infection themselves may be environmentally determined. For example, chronic alterations in the water permeability barrier function owing to the surfactant effects of soaps and detergents may result in fissuring of the skin surface, providing a portal of entry for bacterial infection. Similar cracking of the skin surface may be a complication of allergic contact or primary irritant dermatitis, providing sites for colonization of bacteria such as *Staphylococcus aureus.*

Bacterial colonization at the epidermal surface, usually at sites of serum extravasation into stratum corneum (scale-crust), is often referred to as impetiginization (Fig. 27-8, *A*). Bacterial colonies, admixed neutrophils and cellular debris, serum components, and abnormal scale combine to produce yellow-tan granular material resembling the "honey-colored crust" of true impetigo. Bacterial infection of the underlying dermis, termed pyoderma, is characterized by diffuse or aggregated permeation by neutrophils, dermal edema, and relative absence of vascular injury. True

bacterial abscess may occur in the setting of pyoderma or as a result of localized rupture of an infected cyst or adnexal structure.

Fungi

In immunologically normal hosts, the most common fungal infection is dermatophytosis. Ubiquitous in the environment and carried by domesticated animals, dermatophytes flourish in humid, warm environments and have a predilection for infection of macerated intertriginous skin. The numerous strains of dermatophytes show preferences for regional anatomical sites, such as feet (tinea cruris). Histologically, hyphal forms exist exclusively in the stratum corneum, where presumed release of antigens provokes a mild

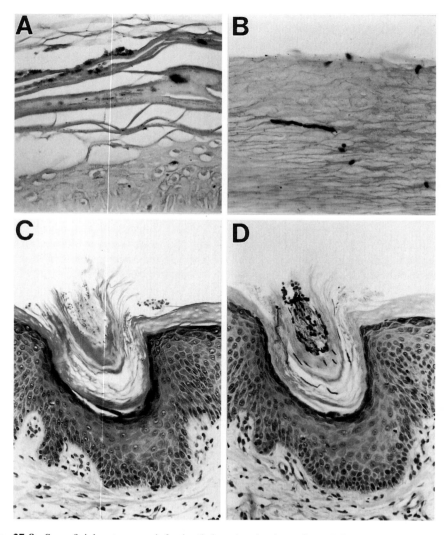

Fig. 27-8. Superficial cutaneous infection/infestation by bacteria and fungi. **A,** Aggregates of gram-positive cocci are present in the stratum corneum of this impetiginized epidermal layer (tissue Gram stain). **B,** Dermatophyte hyphae within the stratum corneum are usually difficult to observe without the assistance of a periodic acid–Schiff (PAS) stain. This is also true when follicular shafts are infested by hyphae in the setting of fungal alopecia: **C,** routine hematoxylin and eosin stain; **D,** adjacent section stained with PAS reagent.

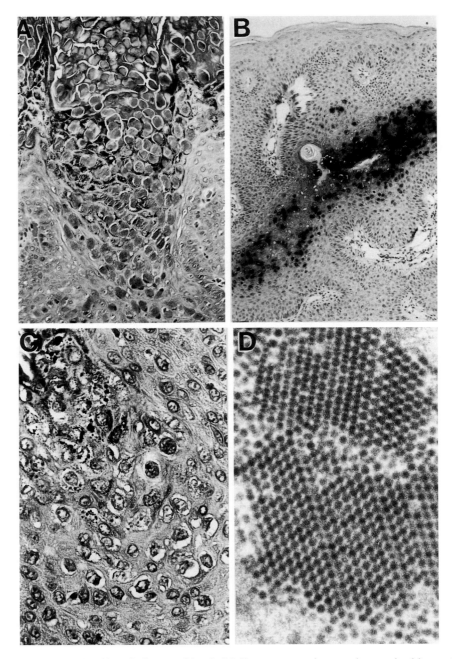

Fig. 27-9. Viral alterations in human skin. **A,** Molluscum contagiosum, characterized by marked hyperplasia of infected keratinocytes containing rounded cytoplasmic bodies composed of viral particles. **B,** Human papillomavirus protein, demonstrated by immunohistochemistry, is present in the proliferative epithelial lesion known as condyloma acuminatum. **C,** Higher magnification of human papillomavirus viral cytopathic effect; note the cytoplasmic lucency ("koilocytosis") and the nuclear pallor that corresponds to sites of viral infection. **D,** Electron micrograph of human papillomavirus virons within an infected keratinocyte nucleus. Viral replication occurs only in more differentiated, superficial epithelial layers, which interface most directly with the external environment. Viral genome, however, is detected within basal cells.

contact hypersensitivity reaction characterized by a superficial perivascular lymphocytic infiltrate, mild epidermal hyperplasia and spongiosis, and focal scale abnormalities (parakeratosis) (Fig. 27-8, *B–D*). The clinical result of these events is an annular, erythematous, slightly elevated plaque with central clearing and a trailing collarette of scale. Follicular involvement may result in localized alopecia.

Viruses

The viral infections that commonly affect the skin all may be considered hazards of the environment. Human papillomavirus (HPV), the cause of common warts and condylomata; molluscum contagiosum (Fig. 27-9, *A*); herpes viruses resulting in shingles, herpes simplex, chickenpox, and venereal-transmitted herpetic ulcerations; and less cosmopolitan viruses, such as those causing orf and milker's nodules, all result in diverse lesions too numerous to describe fully in this chapter. The primary alterations, however, are those of keratinocyte hyperproliferation, as is seen in HPV-induced lesions (Fig. 27-9, *B–D*), and blister formation owing to viral cytopathic effects of the viruses belonging to the herpes family. Because certain subtypes of HPV confer oncogenic potential, possibly by inactivation of tumor suppressor genes, these environmental threats are of particular concern, especially in immunocompromised individuals.[26] Other viruses are more protean in the manner in which they infect and potentially affect skin cells. Human immunodeficiency virus (HIV), for example, has been shown to be harbored within epidermal Langerhans cells, where they may serve as a reservoir for systemic dissemination or spread to adjacent tissues.[15] Moreover, it has been hypothesized that the local immunocompromise that is seen in skin of patients with acquired immunodeficiency syndrome (AIDS) could also be in part the result of immune cell targeting of HIV-infected Langerhans cells.[32]

Infestations and stings

Certain cutaneous infestations, such as the presence of the ubiquitous hair mite, *Demodex folliculorum,* within the infundibular keratin of pilosebaceous units of facial skin, are of little or no pathological significance. Other infestations, such as scabies or cutaneous larva migrans, may cause considerable patient discomfort and morbidity. Stings from injected venom of bees, wasps, mosquitoes, spiders, and aquatic invertebrates may produce a wide range of tissue responses, from urticarial reactions to necrotizing lesions. Global warming theoretically may contribute to increased incidence of certain infestations and infections of skin, such as dermatophytosis, streptococcal pyoderma, and scabies.[34]

The cutaneous pathology of infestations and stings is varied. Most dermatophytes colonize the stratum corneum and provoke only a mild delayed hypersensitivity reaction consisting of spongiosis, abnormal scale production, and a sparse superficial perivascular lymphocytic infiltrate. Scabies mites also track within the interface between stratum corneum and stratum granulosum (Fig. 27-10, *A*) and gen-

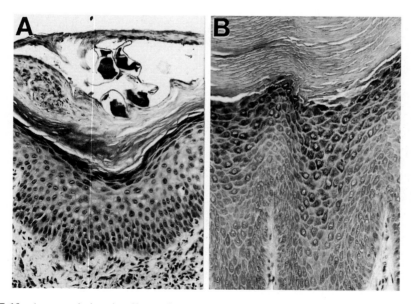

Fig. 27-10. Acute and chronic effects of cutaneous infestation with scabies mite. **A,** The organism (dark bodies in scale) is detected within and directly beneath the stratum corneum. **B,** Intense pruritus resulting from host response to mite antigens results in excoriation and secondary chronic irritant dermatitis (lichen simplex chronicus). As a result, the epidermal layer shows thickening of the stratum corneum, stratum granulosum, and stratum spinosum. Evidence of intact mites is not present in this field.

erally produce only a dermal lymphoeosinophilic infiltrate consistent with a type IV delayed hypersensitivity response. Marked inflammation and epidermal hyperplasia may occur, however, in certain individuals. This is particularly the case in those afflicted with Norwegian scabies, or in those who chronically excoriate lesions producing lichen simplex chronicus owing to superimposed mechanical insult (Fig. 27-10, *B*). Arthropod bites may elicit granulomatous dermal reactions to retained mouth parts, type I and type IV reactions to injected antigens, or necrotizing responses to injected toxins and enzymes. Similar tissue reactions may be produced by coelenterate stings, echinoderm punctures, and the bites of certain fish. "Swimmer's itch" is characterized by urticarial wheals resulting form destruction by a vigorous immune response within hours after exposure to cercariae of acquatic schistosomes in the human epidermis.

CONCLUDING REMARKS

The disorders discussed in this chapter represent a mere sampling of the multiplicity of complex cutaneous reactions provoked by the environment. Table 27-3 below summarizes some of these lesions and supplements them with additional environmental and industrial insults. Although some are transient or of only cosmetic concern, others have far-reaching implications for human environmental pathology. In particular, the pleiotropic effects of ultraviolet irradiation with respect to immunosuppression and carcinogenesis deserve special consideration in view of growing evidence of depletion of protective atmospheric ozone by environmental pollutants. In terms of cost-to-benefit ratio, it becomes obvious that an enormous number of skin conditions encountered by dermatologists are environmentally related. Accordingly, heightened public and professional awareness of environmental threats to the skin seems to be

Table 27-3. Representative examples of environmental and industrial skin disease

Category	Example (s)	Effect(s) on skin structure and function
Contact dermatitis	Urushiol (rhus antigen)	Acute vesicular dermatitis (eczema); delayed hypersensitivity
	Foods, industrial chemicals (resins)	Contact urticaria, type I hypersensitivity reaction
Irritant dermatitis	Fiberglass	Pruritic irritant dermatitis; inflammation and epidermal hyperplasia
	Fiddler's neck	Lichen simplex chronicus (epidermal hyperplasia)
Physical skin injury	Pounding (basketball)	"Black heel," epidermal hyperplasia, and dermal hemorrhage
	Chemical burns (e.g., acids)	Ulcers, saponification of subcutaneous fat
	Cold (frostbite)	Dermal vascular injury; blisters and ischemic necrosis
	Water immersion (trench foot)	Inflammation, swelling, necrosis; secondary infection
Biological skin diseases	Animal industry (e.g., anthrax)	Hemorrhagic vesicles; necrosis
	Viral (e.g., orf, cat scratch)	Inflammation, epidermal hyperplasia (depends on cause)
	Viral (retrovirus; HIV)	Langerhans cells and dermal dendritic cells infected; local immunity decreased; possible link to Kaposi's sarcoma
Chemical carcinogens	Polycyclic aromatic hydrocarbons (e.g., tar)	Squamous cell carcinoma
	Arsenic	Squamous cell carcinoma
Irradiation	Ionizing (x-rays)	Squamous and basal cell carcinomas; atrophic dermatitis
	Ultraviolet light	Squamous and basal cell carcinomas, melanoma; matrix abnormalities—wrinkles
Substances affecting pigment	Alkyl phenols	Localized leukoderma due to melanocyte injury
Acneogenic substances	Dioxins ("agent orange")	Chloracne
Substances inducing connective tissue disorders	Quartz dust	Sclerodermalike syndrome
Percutaneous systemic toxicity	Aniline dyes	Dermatitis; methemoglobinemia; liver and genitourinary disease

a reasonable focus for efforts to promote cutaneous health, both from a therapeutic and a preventive perspective.

It also should be noted that surprisingly little is presently known of the detailed pathogenesis of most forms of environmentally related skin disease. This may be in part related to the fact that research efforts have only begun to focus on this issue in an organized and vigorous manner. Importantly, there have been relatively few in vitro assays or animal models relevant to human skin. Skin of mammalian species intended by nature to bear a protective pelage has important differences when compared with the relatively hairless human integument with respect to thickness, transepidermal water loss and permeation, complement of immune cells, and patterns of cellular reactivity. An important stride, however, has been made with regard to an in vivo model of human environmentally determined cutaneous toxicity. Long-term human skin xenografts may now be effectively maintained on mice inbred for severe combined immunodeficiency mutation.[42] These animals show profound impairment in differentiation of T and B lymphocytes because of alterations in the DNA recombinase system that is responsible for rearranging the variable diversity joint of immunoglobulin and T-cell receptors.[4,8] Human skin so engrafted demonstrates normal microanatomy, antigenicity, and cellular inductive function for months after xenotransplantation.[42] Moreover, it develops certain skin diseases typical of humans after reconstitution with human effector lymphocytes,[15] supports the growth and differentiation of human melanoma cells,[14] and demonstrates normal reparative responses at cellular and molecular levels after wounding.[16] Development of such models holds promise for further studies that will enable investigators to test and study the effects of potentially deleterious environmental agents on intact living human skin.

REFERENCES

1. Aberer W et al: UV light depletes surface markers of Langerhans cells, *J Invest Dermatol* 76:202, 1981.
2. Askenase PW et al: T cell dependent mast cell degranulation and release of serotonin in murine delayed-type hypersensitivity, *J Exp Med* 152:1358, 1980.
3. Bevilacqua MP et al: Endothelial leukocyte adhesion molecule 1: an inducible receptor for neutrophils related to complement regulatory proteins and lectins, *Science* 243:1160, 1989.
4. Bosma GC, Custer RP, Bosma MJ: A severe combined immunodeficiency mutation in the mouse, *Nature (Lond)* 301:527, 1983.
5. Clark WH Jr, Mihm MC Jr: Lentigo maligna and lentigo maligna melanoma, *Am J Pathol* 55:39, 1969.
6. Cotran RS et al: Induction and detection of a human endothelial activation antigen in vivo, *J Exp Med* 164:661, 1986.
7. Cruz PD, Bergstresser PR: The low-dose model of UVB-induced immunosuppression, *Photodermatology* 5:151, 1988.
8. Dorshkind K, Pollack SB, Bosma MJ: Severe combined immunodeficiency (SCID) in the mouse: pathology, reconstitution, neoplasms, *Am J Pathol* 120:464, 1985.
9. Elder DE, Murphy GF: *Atlas of tumor pathology: melanocytic tumors of the skin,* Washington, DC, 1990, Armed Forces Institute of Pathology.
10. Haustein UF, Ziegler V: Environmentally induced systemic sclerosis-like disorders, *Int J Dermatol* 24:147, 1985.
11. Hawk JLM: *Ultraviolet radiation and the photosensitivity disorders.* In Marks R, Plewig G, editors: *The environmental threat to the skin,* United Kingdom, 1992, Martin Dunitz.
12. Ioffreda MD, Whitaker D, Murphy GF: Mast cell degranulation upregulates α6 integrins on epidermal Langerhans cells, *J Invest Dermatol* 101:150, 1993.
13. Janeway CA: How the immune system recognizes invaders. *Sci Amer* 269:73, 1993.
14. Juhasz I et al: Growth and invasion of human melanomas in human skin grafted to immunodeficient mice, *Am J Pathol* 143:528, 1993.
15. Juhasz I et al: Development of pemphigus vulgaris–like lesions in severe combined immunodeficiency disease mice reconstituted with lymphocytes from patients, *J Clin Invest* 92:2401, 1993.
16. Juhasz I et al: Regulation of extracellular matrix proteins and integrin cell substratum adhesion receptors on epithelium during cutaneous human wound healing in vivo, *Am J Pathol* 143:1458, 1993.
17. Kaputo R: *Cutaneous manifestations of tetrachlorodibenzo-p—dioxin* in children and adolescents. In Marks R, Plewig G, editors: *The environmental threat to the skin,* United Kingdom, 1992, Martin Duntz.
18. Klein LM et al: Degranulation of human mast cells induces an endothelial antigen central to leukocyte adhesion, *Proc Natl Acad Sci (USA)* 86:8972, 1989.
19. Kripke M, McClendon E: Studies of the role of antigen-presenting cells in the systemic suppression of contact hypersensitivity by UVB radiation, *J Immunol* 137:443, 1986.
20. Krutman J, Elmets CA: Recent studies on mechanisms in photoimmunology, *Photochem Photobiol* 48:787, 1988.
21. Kupper TS: The activated keratinocyte: a model for inducible cytokine production by non-bone marrow-derived cells in cutaneous inflammatory and immune responses, *J Invest Dermatol* 94:146S, 1990.
22. Lavker RM: Structural alterations in exposed and unexposed aged skin, *J Invest Dermatol* 90:325, 1988.
23. Lavker RM, Kaminer MS, Murphy GF: *Mast cell degranulation results in endothelial activation after acute exposure of human skin to ultraviolet irradiation.* In Marks R, Plewig G, editors: *The environmental threat to the skin,* United Kingdom, 1992, Martin Dunitz.
24. Lavker RM, Kligman AM: Chronic heliodermatitis: a morphologic evaluation of chronic actinic dermal damage with emphasis on the role of mast cells, *J Invest Dermatol* 90:325, 1988.
25. Messadi DV et al: Induction of an activation antigen on post-capillary venular endothelium in human skin organ culture, *J Immunol* 139:1557, 1987.
26. Milburn PB et al: Disseminated warts and evolving squamous cell carcinoma in a patient with acquired immunodeficiency syndrome, *J Invest Acad Dermatol* 19:401, 1988.
27. Morison WL: Effects of ultraviolet radiation on the immune system in humans, *Photobiol* 50:515, 1989.
28. Murphy GF, Elder DE: *Atlas of tumor pathology: non-melanocytic tumors of the skin,* Washington, DC, 1990, Armed Forces Institute of Pathology.
29. Nickoloff BJ. Role of interferon-γ in cutaneous trafficking of lymphocytes with emphasis on molecular and cellular adhesion events, *Arch Dermatol* 124:1835, 1988.
30. Parrish JA: *Responses of the skin to visible and ultraviolet radiation.* In Goldsmith LA, editor: *Biochemistry and physiology of the skin,* New York, 1983, Oxford University Press.
31. Picker LJ et al: ELAM-1 is an adhesion molecule for ski-homing T cells, *Nature* 349:796, 1991.
32. Ringler DJ, Murphy GF: Transmucosal passage of lentiviruses and the epinodal hypothesis: relevance to the pathogenesis of AIDS, *Mod Pathol* 1:135, 1988.
33. Roberston WO: *Arsenic and other heavy metals.* In Haddad LM, Winchester JF, editors: Clinical management of poisoning and drug overdose, Philadelphia, 1983, WB Saunders.

34. Taplan D et al: *The effects of global warming on skin infections and infestations.* In Marks R, Plewing G, editors: *The environmental threat to the skin,* United Kingdom, 1992, Martin Dunitz.

35. Tschachler E et al: Epidermal Langherans cells: a target for HTLV-III/LAV infection, *J Invest Dermatol* 88:233, 1987.

36. Vermeer M, Streilein JW: Ultraviolet B light-induced alterations in epidermal Langerhans cells are mediated in part by tumor necrosis factor-alpha, *Photodermatol Photoimmunol Photomed* 7:258, 1990.

37. Vonderheid EC, VanScott EJ, Johnson WC: Topical chemotherapy and immunotherapy of mycosis fungoides, *Arch Dermatol* 113:454; 1977.

38. Waldorf HA et al: Early cellular events in evolving cutaneous delayed hypersensitivity in humans, *Am J Pathol* 138:477, 1991.

39. Walsh LJ, Lavker RM, Murphy GF: Determinants of immune cell trafficking in the skin, *Lab Invest* 63:592, 1990.

40. Walsh LJ et al: Human dermal mast cells contain and release tumor necrosis factor-α which induces endothelial leukocyte adhesion molecule-1, *Proc Natl Acad Sci (USA)* 88:4220, 1991.

41. Willis CM, Stephens CJM, Wilkinson JD: Epidermal damage induced by irritants in man: a light and electron microscopic study, *J Invest Dermatol* 93:695, 1989.

42. Yan Horng-Chin et al: Human/severe combined immunodeficient mouse chimeras. An experimental in vivo model system to study the regulation of human endothelial cell-leukocyte adhesion molecules, *J Clin Invest* 91:986, 1993.

43. Young JD et al: Identification, purification, and characterization of a mast cell-associated cytolytic factor related to tumor necrosis factor, *Proc Natl Acad Sci (USA)* 84:9175, 1987.

Chapter 28

AIRWAYS AND LUNG

John E. Craighead

The adult respiratory tract exchanges roughly 5×10^3 to 15×10^3 L of air daily, depending on physical activity. Countless organic and inorganic particles are suspended in the air we breathe. Indoor and outdoor air contains variable amounts of gaseous pollutants, predominantly ozone, nitrogen oxides, and sulfur dioxide (see Chapters 2 and 3); pollen and other forms of organic debris; inorganic dusts; and traces of a vast number of aliphatic and aromatic hydrocarbons, largely of industrial origin. Thus, the normal, healthy respiratory tract transports and clears an enormous mass of foreign material on a continuous basis. Acute and chronic pulmonary diseases and environmental toxin exposures tend to alter clearance and facilitate the uptake of foreign gases and particulates into and through the walls of the lower respiratory tract.[51]

The nares, with their complex of turbinates, serve as an effective barrier for a substantial proportion of the larger, more complex particulates. The internal nares remove a substantial proportion of the particulates we breathe, depending on their size. The tracheobronchial tree transports gases and particulates by the kinetics of laminar flow through a branching series of tubular structures of decreasingly smaller size. Inhaled dust tends to accumulate on the walls of the airways because of electrostatic attraction and by impaction, particularly on the roughly 20 to 23 bifurcations of the bronchial tree (Fig. 28-1). The depth of transport of foreign particles into the lung depends on their aerodynamic diameters and electrostatic charge. Only particles with a diameter of less than 5 μm reach the distal unit of the airways, which is composed of the respiratory bronchioles, alveolar ducts, and alveoli (i.e., the acinus) (Fig. 28-2).

The nasal and lower airway mucosa from the larynx to the respiratory bronchioles is lined by a mucociliary epithelium that effectively eliminates roughly 80% of the dust

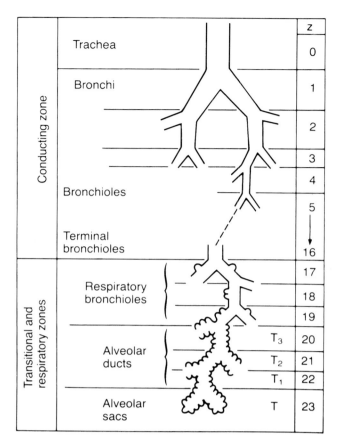

Fig. 28-1. Diagrammatic outline of airways of human lung demonstrating the branching complexity. (From Murray JF: *The normal lung: the basis for diagnosis and treatment of pulmonary disease,* Philadelphia, 1976, WB Saunders; with permission.)

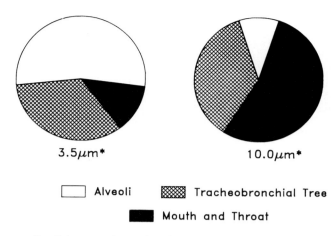

Fig. 28-2. Regional distribution of particles in the respiratory tract by size.

that transits beyond the nares (Fig. 28-3). In severe chronic respiratory disease, this mucosa undergoes both mucinous and squamous metaplasia, changes that alter particle transport (Fig. 28-4, *A, B*).[11] The distal segments of the airways (i.e., the membranous and respiratory bronchioles) are lined by simple cuboidal or flat epithelial cell layers in the healthy individual. These cells undergo structural and functional changes in the cigarette smoker and those exposed to excessive concentrations of toxic gases and airborne particulates.[24,147,245] The velocity of airflow in the respiratory bronchioles and acini approximates zero, and for this reason, they are the major anatomic site of particulate deposition and gas diffusion. The inhalation of toxic gases and foreign particulates provokes the influx and accumulation of pulmonary alveolar macrophages and (depending on the material) variable numbers of neutrophils, which generate cytokines, proteases, and oxygen species.[106,141,142,149] This response alters the permeability of the mucosa and influences particle and gas uptake by the tissue.

Most foreign particulates that accumulate in the nares and oropharynx are expectorated or swallowed. Particulates

that penetrate deeper in the lungs are cleared by the mucociliary escalator system and macrophages or are flushed into the lymphatic system that invests the lungs. Clearance is a two-phase process. The half-life for elimination of the bulk of the lung's burden of foreign material is 20 to 30 days, whereas much of the remainder is removed over the ensuing year. Although our understanding of the kinetics of lymphatic clearance is poor, the lymphatic system undoubtedly serves as an important conduit for foreign particulates. Disease caused by silica and silicate dust inhalation develops from fine dust particulates transported by, and deposited adjacent to, intrapulmonary lymphatics.[51,54]

AIRWAY DISEASE

Few subjects in pulmonary medicine are as confusing to physicians as the complex of disorders affecting airflow in the distal airways of the lung. Aside from respiratory infections, these conditions often, but not invariably, result from exposure to one or more of a vast variety of organic and inorganic inhalants in the outside environment, workplace, and home. Cigarette smoke is, of course, the most pervasive, and its effects often confound the assessment of the role of other types of inhalants in respiratory disease. Meteorological conditions, individual susceptibility, and immunological responsivity are also critical but difficult to define variables. Finally, pathophysiological responses are superimposed on pathological changes in the airway to a variable and unpredictable extent. In this chapter, the morphological features of the pulmonary conditions are stressed, and key examples of the types of environmental agents involved are provided.

Chronic bronchitis

In past decades, chronic bronchitis owing to cigarette smoking and the concomitant exposure to urban gaseous

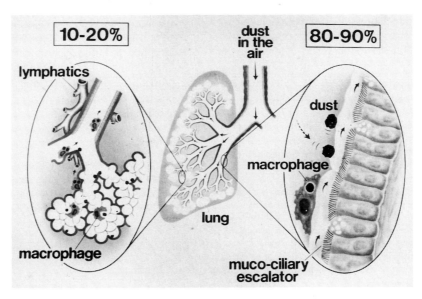

Fig. 28-3. Clearance mechanism in lung airways. Roughly 80% of dust particulates are eliminated by the mucociliary escalator system, whereas the remainder are either phagocytized or move out of the lung through its sewer system, the lymphatics. A small fraction of the inhaled dust particulates are retained in the lung tissue. This is in part influenced by cigarette smoking (see Table 28-3).

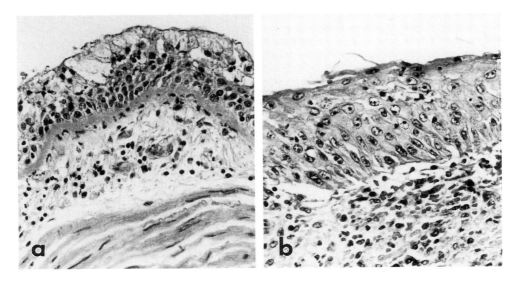

Fig. 28-4. A, Mucinous metaplasia in the bronchial tree of a chronic smoker with emphysema. **B,** Squamous metaplasia in the bronchial tree of a smoker with asbestosis.

and particulate pollutants was a common respiratory problem in developed countries.[168,183] Tending to occur in the humid, cool setting of winter, the direct effects of the irritants and allergens on the mucosa were compounded by noninvasive bacterial infections of the upper respiratory tract, particularly with nonencapsulated *Haemophilus* species, which resulted in chronic inflammation of the tracheobronchial tree. The "coughing and spitting" of this syndrome can largely be attributed to mucous and squamous

cell metaplasia and hyperreactivity of the airway epithelium and, to a lesser extent, hypertrophy of the mucous gland and squamous metaplasia of the tracheobronchial mucosa.[11] Reid[183] quantitated morphometrically the structural changes that develop in the submucosal glands of the major airways (Fig. 28-5) and established the widely recognized but infrequently used Reid index of mucous gland enlargement. The results of a quantitative analysis of the anatomical changes in chronic bronchitis are summarized in Table

28-1. Additional investigators have characterized changes in the rheology and biochemistry of the mucus produced in this disease condition. With the reduction in cigarette use among members of the population (see Chapter 13) and the overall amelioration of indoor and outdoor air pollution, the syndrome occurs much less commonly in developed coun-

tries. It continues to be an important problem, however, in industrialized urban areas elsewhere in the world where smoking and pollution abatement have yet to be realized. It is important to differentiate this condition, which affects the bronchial branches proximal to the bronchioles, from the obstructive functional disease of the smaller airways, discussed later.

Bronchial asthma

The common asthma syndrome affects roughly 5% of the world's population.[153] It usually results from exposure to common allergens in the environment, although ancil-

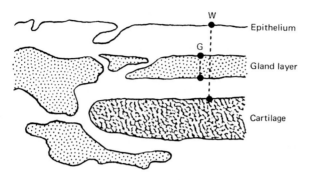

Fig. 28-5. Diagrammatic representation of gland-to-wall (G/W) ratio. At a site where epithelium is parallel to cartilage, gland thickness *(G)* is measured; at the same point, the wall thickness, i.e., the distance from epithelium to perichondrium *(W)* also is measured. This is the Reid index. Table 28-1 provides numerical data documenting changes associated with airway disease. (From Fishman AP, editor: *Pulmonary diseases and disorders*, ed 2, New York, 1991, McGraw-Hill; with permission.)

Table 28-1. Measurements of gland and bronchial wall thickness*

	Wall	Gland	Mean ratio	Range	Acini
Normal	4.4	1.2	0.26	0.14-0.36	24
Bronchitis	7.4	4.4	0.59	0.41-0.79	14
Emphysema	5.4	2.1	0.37	0.28-0.49	22

Adapted from Reid L: *Pathology of bronchial asthma.* In Orie NGM, Sluiter HJ, editors: *Bronchitis,* Assen, Netherlands, 1961, Charles C Thomas.
*Expressed as graticule units.

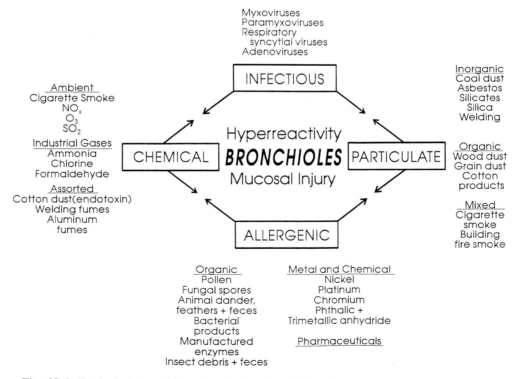

Fig. 28-6. Extrinsic factors influencing the function of the pulmonary bronchioles, resulting in inflammatory and bronchospastic disease, accompanied by obstructive pulmonary phenomenology. Rarely do these factors act in isolation, one from another.

lary cofactors (infection, cold temperature, chemicals, and particulates) often trigger an attack in an individual with hyperresponsiveness of the small airways.[153] Asthma almost invariably occurs in genetically predisposed, atopic individuals, many of whom manifest multiple allergies to a diversity of indoor and outdoor pollutants and foods (see Chapter 25). The importance of cofactors in the pathogenesis of asthma nonetheless cannot be underestimated in the context of the initiating mechanisms and the environmental influences that predispose to chronicity (Fig. 28-6).[32,237] A study from central Europe, however, claimed that the prevalence of asthma among children was comparable in two communities that differed substantially in the level of air pollutants.[233] The demonstration of acute inflammation in the airways of ozone-exposed humans suggests the possibility of a synergistic effect on the initiation of an asthmatic attack.[8]

The pathological features of bronchial asthma are in a dynamic state of reevaluation, based on systematic investigations of fatal cases and a limited number of transbronchial biopsy specimens. Morphometric studies demonstrate thickening of the small airway walls owing to increases in the volumes of all of the anatomical components (i.e., submucosa, musculature, and adventitia).[132,139] The submucosa exhibits inflammation and edema associated with variable degrees of fibrosis and increases in small blood vessel number and size. Customarily the smooth muscle mass is increased twofold to threefold. For reasons that are unclear, the mucosa often is denuded (Fig. 28-7). Studies of autopsied cases have documented heterogeneity in the cellular responses of the submucosal tissue. Although eosinophilic infiltrates traditionally have been thought to characterize the airway lesion of asthma, these cells frequently are not found in pronounced numbers. Further investigations have shown that the number of eosinophils in the airway submucosa directly correlates with the duration of acute symptoms (Fig. 28-8).[222] Indeed, in those with sudden-onset, fatal attacks accompanied by asphyxia, neutrophils, but not eosinophils, are often found in increased numbers in the submucosa. The inflammation mediators associated with these tissue responses have been the subject of numerous reviews (see Chapter 24).[55]

Industrial or occupational asthma is caused largely or in part by chemical and allergenic agents and particulate exposure in the workplace and has a general temporal relationship to the exposure but does not necessarily occur concomitantly.[35,125,193,238] For example, symptoms may develop only after months or years of contact with the agent in question. On a daily basis, detectable physiological changes often develop at the end of the workday or during off hours. The nonspecific environmental influences depicted in Fig. 28-6 are also contributory factors. Table 28-2 lists the relative frequency of compensation claims in the United Kingdom for the agents accepted for recognition by that government. Similar information from other countries

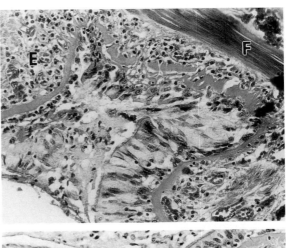
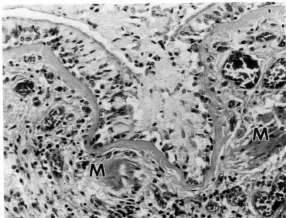
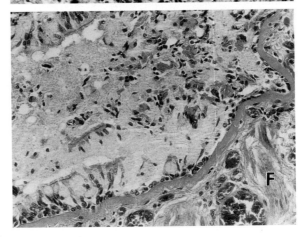

Fig. 28-7. Selected samples of the walls of the bronchi in the lungs of a middle-aged man dying with acute asthma. Note the mixed inflammatory cell infiltrate including eosinophils *(E),* "basement membrane" thickening, fibrosis *(F),* and smooth muscle hyperplasia *(M)* in the submucosa, and the mucous secretions and sloughed respiratory epithelium in the bronchial lumina.

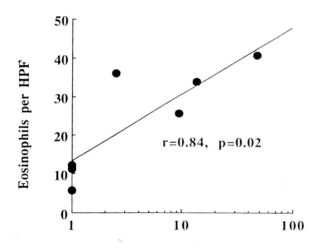

Fig. 28-8. Correlation of time interval between onset of attack of asthma and death and the numbers of eosinophils in the airway submucosa. *HPF,* High-power field (of magnification). (From Sar S, et al: Sudden onset fatal asthma, *Am Rev Respir Dis* 148:713, 1993; with permission.)

no doubt would demonstrate a different list of causes. For example, in central Europe, flour exposure in bakers predominates, whereas in Norway, the most common cause is the aerosolized products of aluminum smelting. Soya flour is the common allergen in Asia. Although information on the causes of occupational asthma in developed countries has gradually accumulated, the causes of this syndrome elsewhere in the world remain to be defined. Given these considerations, it is not surprising that few histopathological studies have been carried out on the respiratory tract tissue of affected workers.[193]

Small airway disease

This term nominally refers to both acute and chronic disorders of the membranous and respiratory bronchioles characterized to a variable extent by obstructive pulmonary functional manifestations.[225] The acute phenomenology relates largely to bronchospastic responses to irritation that commonly, but not invariably, occur in atopic persons. Fig. 28-6 depicts the interrelationship of the various types of injurious insults to this clinical syndrome and lists foreign influences that are commonly responsible. These interactive effects are manifest acutely and may have chronic effects over the life of the individual. For example, exposure of infants in the home to sidestream cigarette smoke results in an increased prevalence of infectious respiratory disease and asthmatic symptoms concomitantly and bronchiolar hyperresponsivity later in life.[79,123,195,250] Nonallergic chemical and particulate interactions with the small airways can result in fibrotic changes in the walls of both the membranous and the respiratory bronchioles.[245] For a variety of ob-

Table 28-2. Major causes of compensable occupational asthma in the United Kingdom

Agent	Percentage of total 1987-1989
Isocyanates	29
Flour and grain	19
Antibiotics	6
Soldering flux	12
Epoxy resin hardeners	11
Wood dusts	11
Platinum salts	4
Animals and insects	4
Proteolytic enzymes	2
Azodicarbonamide	2

Adapted from Sherwood Burge P: *Occupational and environmental asthma.* In Clark TJH, Godfrey S, Lee TH, editors: In *Asthma* New York, 1992, Chapman & Hall Medical.

vious reasons, the prevalence of these changes in the lung parenchyma has not been determined, and the contribution of the various factors potentially involved is difficult to assess. Cigarette smoke effects on the bronchioles have been the most thoroughly evaluated.[165] These begin with an inflammatory response in the walls of the airways (smokers' bronchiolitis) (Fig. 28-9, *A*),[4,165] occurring within months or years of the time of the onset of smoking. The lesion appears to evolve into fibrosis and chronic inflammation of the walls of the membranous and respiratory bronchioles with the passage of years (Fig. 28-9, *B*). Similar responses seem to occur in workers chronically exposed to asbestos, nonfibrous silicates, and silica.[43,97,125,167] The concomitant exposure to inorganic dust and cigarette smoke has been found to affect the severity and extent of the lesions. As reported by Wright and colleagues,[245] severe fibrosis was observed in 16% of the membranous bronchioles of cigarette smokers who were not exposed to dust, in 37% of those inhaling nonasbestos dust, and in 51% of smokers exposed to asbestos. The pathogenesis of these lesions has not been critically examined, although inflammation and the cytokine products of the inflammatory response doubtless play a key role (see Chapter 24).

The fibrotic thickening of the walls of the bronchioles described previously appears to result from the deposition of dust in, and the direct effects of chemicals on, the distal airway mucosa. The term constrictive bronchiolitis has been applied to this lesion to contrast it with the better characterized proliferative bronchiolitis obliterans.[131] Although the latter results from persistent insults to the distal airways, resulting in chronic inflammation with the fibrotic organization of intra-air space exudates, the former is a chronic inflammatory lesion predominantly of the membranous and respiratory bronchioles, accompanied to a variable degree by a progressive concentric submucosal chronic inflammation and fibrosis.[4]

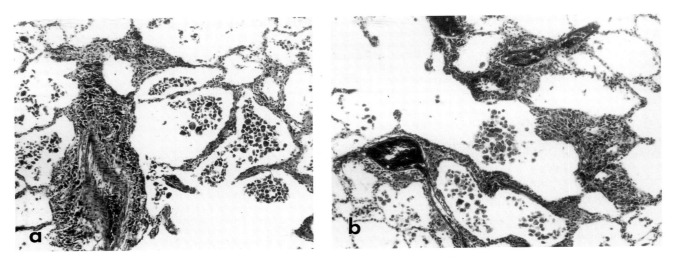

Fig. 28-9. A, Smoker's bronchiolitis. Note the prominent mononuclear inflammatory response in the respiratory bronchioles associated with the accumulation of macrophages in the air spaces. Many of these cells contain an ochre-colored pigment that is characteristic of the cigarette smoker. **B,** Fibrotic changes in the walls of the respiratory bronchioles and adjacent alveolar ducts in the lung of a middle-aged, long-term smoker. The inflammatory response is still evident but less prominent than in **A.**

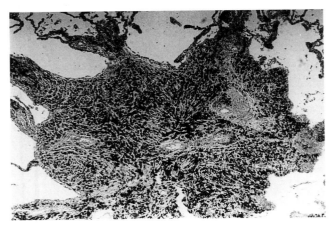

Fig. 28-10. Dust macule in the lung of a 90-year-old smoker with a 55-year history of underground mining. (Courtesy of V. Vallyathan, National Institute for Occupational Safety and Health.)

The dust macule is a unique, second type of lesion affecting the bronchiole but attributable to the deposition of free dust and macrophages heavily laden with particles at the confluence of lymphatics (Fig. 28-10). These lesions are seen in the lungs of workers in a variety of trades where exposure to nonfibrogenic dust occurs. They are, however, most prominent in coal miners, in whom the carbon-labeled macules are pathagonomonic of coal dust exposure.

Carbon dust accumulations in the lungs at autopsy have long intrigued pathologists by their variability. Microscopically, one observes these deposits in the region of the respiratory bronchioles and in proximity to lymphatics or in the walls of emphysematous lesions. In the majority, the particulates are finely granular, whereas in foundry workers and others employed in "dusty" trades, the particles often are crude and variable in dimension. Pratt and Kilburn[178] developed a morphometric approach for quantitating accumulations of dust in whole sections of lung. The resulting studies on rural and urban Americans are summarized in Table 28-3. The data clearly demonstrate the prevailing influence of cigarette smoke and, in particular, its effect on environmental dust accumulations in the lungs of urban inhabitants. In these studies, considerable individual variability was observed, presumably an indication of differences among individuals in the efficiency of clearance, regardless of smoking.

Organic dust syndromes of uncertain etiology

In 1713, Ramazzini, the father of occupational medicine, noted the respiratory irritant effects of organic dusts among grain workers in his classic, *De morbis artificum diatriba*. Over the ensuing centuries, respiratory problems attributable to a myriad of organic dusts have been described, but to date our understanding of the pathogenesis of these syndromes has remained limited. The variability of the clinical disease is compounded by the extraordinary diversity of organic materials implicated. Byssinosis attributable to exposure to cotton, flax, or hemp dust clearly is the best-defined syndrome of this type. Although affecting airway function, it exhibits a distinct clinical pattern of response that differentiates it from bronchial asthma and hypersensitivity pneumonitis. Although the decrements in respiratory function appear to be greater in those with atopy, symptoms develop regardless of an immunological predisposition in those exposed to high concentrations of dust in the

Table 28-3. Morphometric determinations and comparisons of pigmented area in whole lung sections from routine autopsies on urban and rural residents

Residential/ smoking status	Percentage of pigmented area	Residential/ smoking status	Percentage of pigmented area
Smokers	6.7	Nonsmokers	2.6
City smokers	7.4	Country smokers	5.4
City nonsmokers	2.7	Country nonsmokers	3.2

Modified from Pratt PC, Kilburn KH: *Extent of pulmonary pigmentation as an indicator of particulate environmental air pollution.* In Davies DN, editor: *Third International Symposium on Inhaled Particles,* vol 2, London, 1971, Pergamon Press.

workplace.[113] Postmortem studies have failed to find small airway lesions comparable to the changes observed in asthmatics (although mucous gland hyperplasia and goblet cell hyperplasia are commonly present in larger airways).[72,73,177,179]

Byssinosis would appear to be attributable to the inhalation of bracts of the seed pod of the cotton boll. The origin of other organic dust-related syndromes is less clear because many extraneous contaminants, including insect and microorganism debris, are found in these dusts (see Chapter 6).[146] Episodes of fever are a common feature accompanying respiratory symptoms, possibly because endotoxin is frequently found in contaminated organic material. As might be expected, this so-called organic toxic dust syndrome is frequently observed in agricultural workers.[214,232]

PARENCHYMAL LUNG DISEASE
Emphysema

The American Thoracic Society defines emphysema as "a condition of the lungs characterized by abnormal, permanent enlargement of airspaces distal to the terminal bronchiole, accompanied by the destruction of their walls, and without obvious fibrosis."[216] Cigarette smoking is well recognized as the major cause of the centrilobular form of emphysema,[218] but for unknown reasons, the lesion occurs in only a minority of those who smoke.[85,98] Thus, the symptoms and physiological changes of chronic obstructive pulmonary disease, more often than not, are attributable to bronchospasm, rather than to major anatomical structural changes in the acini of the lungs. Yet lung function does not return to normal in those who cease smoking.[12,247]

The pathogenesis of the common centrilobular and much less frequently occurring panlobular emphysema has been the subject of countless investigations. Cigarette smoke constituents appear to act by two mechanisms to result in lung injury focused on the walls of the respiratory bronchioles. The first relates to the capacity of cigarette smoke to elicit a brisk but persistent inflammatory response in the acini even after termination of smoking.* As a consequence, oxygen radicals and acid proteases are released at

*References 4, 68, 106, 108, 149.

the local site.[106,141] The balance between the effects of these agents and the counteracting neutralizing influences of antioxidants and antiproteases appears to determine the extent of injury. Tissues adapt to environmental exposures by up-regulating enzymatically acting antioxidants (superoxide dismutases and catalase) (see Chapter 21). Thus, adaptation to environmental oxidant stress is an important determinant of ultimate tissue injury. Nutritional factors influencing the generation of oxidants in the Haber-Weiss reaction (iron) and antioxidants (vitamin E, carotenes) appear to be important, as do genetic influences on antiprotease elaboration and breakdown (see Chapter 28), but other unquantitated factors affect the severity of tissue injury.

The pathological features of emphysema have been presented in numerous excellent books and monographs.[68,225] A key but unresolved question relates to the fibrosis in the walls of the bronchioles that is observed in the lungs of many smokers in the absence of emphysematous dilation of the airway.[4,240] How does one resolve this inconsistency, i.e., the development of centrilobular emphysema in some smokers and bronchiolar fibrosis (with or without emphysema) in others? Although the answer is not readily apparent, cofactors influencing the continuity of the wall of the respiratory bronchiole may be of critical importance. For example, experimental exposure of rodents to cadmium chloride results in pulmonary fibrosis, whereas administration of the cadmium compound with a lathyritic agent, β-aminoproprionitrile furmurate produces emphysema.[106,164] Presumably the structural alterations in lung collagen resulting from the administration of this lysyl oxidase inhibitor determine the outcome of toxic injury to the lung. Chronic exposure to cadmium fumes in the workplace has been associated with the development of diffuse emphysema.[215]

As noted elsewhere in this chapter, coal dust macules and silicotic nodules are associated with localized emphysematous lesions, presumably owing to the retraction of lung parenchyma into the developing lesion. These lesions frequently are termed scar emphysema (see later).

Silica-associated disease

Silicosis is a chronic, progressive disease of the pulmonary parenchyma caused by exposure to crystalline silica.[42,54,133,249] The history of silicosis parallels the industrialization of society. Although exposure to silica dust is common in many industries and under a variety of environmental conditions, clinical silicosis occurs rarely today. This is largely due to an increased awareness of the risk, with the consequent use of respiratory protective equipment and government regulations that reduce air dust concentrations in the workplace. Nonetheless, sporadic new cases do appear, often in industrial settings where the exposure is cryptic and limited to a few workers in specialty trades. For example, in the last year, I have seen silicosis in a worker in an abrasives factory and in a dental prosthesis technician. Silicosis rarely develops as a result of nonindustrial exposure, although it has been described in Bedouins inhabiting the Sahara desert, where fine particles of silica are aerosolized during sand storms.[224A,15A,176A]

Silica is amalgamated into a variety of geological deposits and is often a minor component of some igneous rock, such as granite. Often the associated mineral particulates are found in addition to silica in the lung tissue of exposed workers (see Chapter 6). Silicosis usually occurs consequent to exposure to alpha quartz, although the more pathogenic crystallographic variants, cristobalite and tridymite, are occasionally responsible (such as in foundry and steel mill workers exposed to fire brick dust in blast furnaces or among those working with diatomaceous earth). Particle size is a critical factor, for only those less than 5 μ in diameter can be inhaled deep into the acini. Silica particles 1 μ or less in size are most pathogenic, and recently fractured particles prove to be more pathogenic than those with "weathered" crystal facets.[127] Dosage considerations obviously are important because most inhaled particulates are removed in the nasal turbinates and by the mucociliary escalator system of the airways. Thus, a threshold must be exceeded before the concentrations of dust are sufficient to accumulate in the airspaces. Here the particles are phagocytized or are either transported into lymphatics or carried to the oropharynx by the mucociliary escalator. Repeated daily exposures to concentrations of silica that exceed this threshold usually are required for disease to develop.[54,58]

Lymphatic flow from the periphery of the lung is routed to the pleura before it is carried centrally through lymphatics in the pulmonary septae to the hilar and mediastinal lymph nodes. The initial sites of silica dust deposition are at confluence points in the lymphatic network of the pleura, the deeper lymphatics in the lung parenchyma, and the hilar lymph nodes. Often the only evidence of silica exposure is the nodules on the pleural surface (candlewax lesions) (Fig. 28-11) or in the hilar lymph nodes.

Acute and accelerated silicosis. Acute and accelerated forms of silicosis occur in those exposed industrially to massive amounts of silica dust.[15,28,38,84] The clinical picture of acute silicosis resembles the adult respiratory distress syndrome with diffuse alveolar damage and proteinaceous exudation into airspaces as its morphological fea

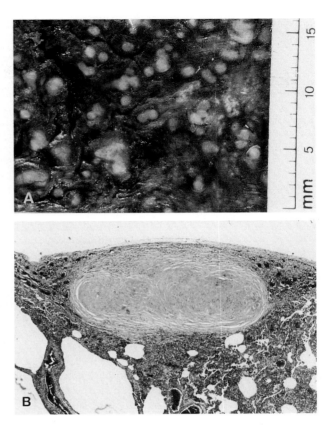

Fig. 28-11. Candlewax lesions in the pleura of a silicotic foundry worker. **A,** The features of the lesions on the intact pleura. **B,** Microscopic section of a typical silicotic nodule located subjacent to the pleura in proximity to lymphatics. Often, these are the only lesions observed in individuals exposed to silica dusts in amounts insufficient to cause the diffuse lung disease, silicosis. (From Craighead JE, et al: Diseases associated with exposure to silica and nonfibrous silicate minerals, *Arch Pathol Lab Med* 112:673, 1988. Copyright 1988, American Medical Association; with permission.)

tures.[47] Although this potentially fatal condition should not occur with contemporary industrial standards and regulations, outbreaks and sporadic cases continue to occur due to unrecognized exposures. Accelerated silicosis is less well defined pathologically and clinically, but the disease assumes a somewhat more protracted course and rudimentary silicotic nodules are scattered in the lung, often accompanied by focal lesions of acute silicosis.

Chronic silicosis. Silicotic nodules composed of whorled bundles of hyalinized collagen are the typical lesions of chronic silicosis (Fig. 28-12, *A, B*).[86,102] They have within them focal accumulations of silica particles that exhibit birefringence of low refractivity. The pathogenesis of the silicotic nodule is at present incompletely defined. The generation of reactive oxygen species by macrophages is a central event in the development of lesions. Presumably, cytokine growth factors originating in macrophages contribute to the formation of the fibrotic nodule. Autoim

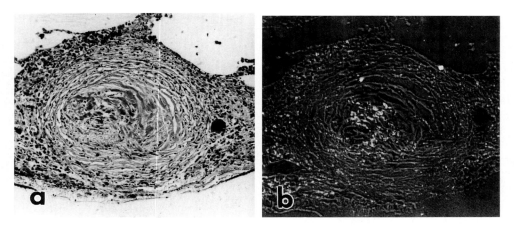

Fig. 28-12. A, Typical silicotic nodule composed of whorled bundles of collagenous tissue with a hyalinized central core and accumulation of mononuclear inflammatory cells at the periphery. These lesions usually are located adjacent to blood vessels, where they originate from the lymphatic channels of the lung. **B,** Back-scatter spectrometric electron microscopic illustration of silica particles in a silicotic nodule. These fine particles exhibit a low degree of birefringence and are frequently difficult to observe unless conditions for polarization microscopy are ideal. (From Craighead JE, et al: Diseases associated with exposure to silica and nonfibrous silicate minerals, *Arch Pathol Lab Med* 112:673, 1988. Copyright 1988, American Medical Association; with permission.)

mune mechanisms are hypothesized to play a contributory role. These discrete nodules increase in size with time, encompassing more of the adjacent lung substance.

The number of nodules and their size is variable and roughly correlates with the severity and duration of exposure (simple silicosis). Characteristically, they predominate in the upper lung lobes. As noted earlier, the distorted lung parenchyma adjacent to the nodules often contracts to form irregular emphysematous spaces (Fig. 28-13). In cases of long duration, the nodules become confluent (conglomerate silicosis) (Fig. 28-14). Rarely, confluent nodules coalesce to form the typical lesions of progressive massive fibrosis. These conglomerates of silicotic nodules frequently exhibit areas of necrosis because of compromised blood flow (the so-called vasculitis of silicosis) or mycobacterial infections. The various stages of this disease are fully illustrated in a recently published monograph.[54]

Extrapulmonary silica lesions. It is common in industrial workers today to find silicotic nodules in hilar or mediastinal lymph nodes in the absence of lung parenchymal lesions. These lesions should not be considered silicosis for compensation purposes. I prefer to restrict this term to disease involving the lung parenchyma. Lesions sporadically are found in cervical and abdominal lymph nodes and in the spleen and liver (Fig. 28-15).[210] They appear to result from lymphatic transport of dust particulates from the lungs to these organs.

Parasilicotic syndromes. Clinical case reports document the development of acute glomerulonephritis in persons with acute and accelerated silicosis (see Chapter 32). In some cases, the renal disease is fulminating; it occurs as a result of exceedingly heavy exposure to dust, but the

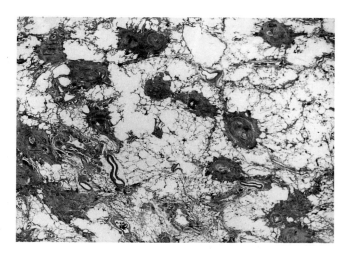

Fig. 28-13. Silicotic nodules in a case of simple silicosis. Note the scar emphysematous lesions resulting from the contraction of the fibrous tissue in the nodule. (From Craighead JE, et al: Diseases associated with exposure to silica and nonfibrous silicate minerals, *Arch Pathol Lab Med* 112:673, 1988. Copyright 1988, American Medical Association; with permission.)

mechanism is obscure.[14,23,88] Because chronic kidney disease in those exposed to silica dust occurs sporadically, a fully satisfactory cause-and-effect relationship has not been established. Scleroderma develops sporadically but with an unusually high frequency in workers heavily exposed to silica, both in the presence and in the absence of radiological silicosis (see Chapter 27).[48,76,211] In silica workers with rheumatoid arthritis, the lesions of silicosis seem to progress more rapidly, and progressive massive fibrosis occurs more commonly.[213] The immunological mechanisms

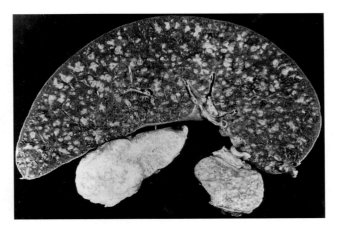

Fig. 28-15. Silicotic nodules in the liver and hilar lymph nodes of an individual with advanced pulmonary silicosis. Silica particles are disseminated by lymphatics and can produce miliary lesions of this type in the various abdominal organs. (From Slavin KE, et al: Extrapulmonary silicosis: A clinical, morphologic, and ultrastructural study, *Hum Pathol* 16:393, 1985; with permission.)

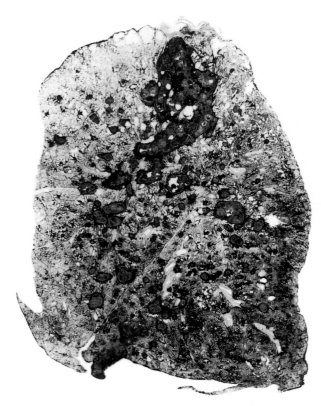

Fig. 28-14. Conglomerate silicosis with the lesion of progressive massive fibrosis in the upper lung lobe. These massive lesions frequently undergo necrosis as a result of the vasculitis that accompanies the silicotic lesion. In the past, sites such as this were the nidus of tuberculosis, which later disseminated in individuals with advanced silicosis. (From Craighead JE, et al: Diseases associated with exposure to silica and nonfibrous silicate minerals, *Arch Pathol Lab Med* 112:673, 1988. Copyright 1988, American Medical Association; with permission.)

involved in these disorders are obscure but may involve haptenization of tissue proteins by silica particles, resulting in an autoimmune response.

Asbestos-associated disease

No subject in the field of environmental and occupational medicine has provoked as much controversy as the role of asbestos in disease.[42,53,188] Although asbestos is ubiquitous in the contemporary environment, asbestosis almost universally occurs in those who are heavily exposed to asbestos in their occupation(s). Many different types of cancer have been attributed to asbestos exposure, but the epidemiological evidence establishes only a pathogenic role for asbestos in bronchogenic carcinoma and mesothelioma. As discussed in Chapter 6, asbestos is not one but a family of silicate minerals having a fibrous composition but strikingly different physical features. This is an important consideration because not all types of asbestos have the same potential for causing disease.

Asbestosis. Asbestosis is a chronic, fibrotic disease of

the lungs attributable to long-term exposure to high concentrations of aerosolized asbestos over periods of 15 to 20 years. The dosage and duration of exposure required to induce the disease are uncertain because of the many variables involved. Amphibole asbestos generally is considered more pathogenic than chrysotile, and long fibers of asbestos appear to be responsible for much of the pulmonary damage.[3,93] For clinically relevant lesions to develop, the exposure must be sufficiently heavy to overcome the defense mechanisms of the lung on a regular, if not daily, basis (Fig. 28-16, *A, B*). With continuous and repeated exposures, cumulative injuries to the lung ultimately lead to development of clinically apparent disease.

Clinical criteria for diagnosis of asbestosis have been established and are widely accepted.[159] In addition to an appropriate history of exposure, these include two or more of the following features in an individual patient: (1) the presence of a typical radiological picture, (2) restrictive pulmonary function, and (3) the occurrence of dry crackling expiratory rales. Obviously, these criteria are descriptive and imprecise and may lead to incorrect clinical diagnoses in some cases because exposure to asbestos is difficult to document, and the radiological features of the fibrotic pulmonary disease are not specific. Although a pathological evaluation of the lung often would be useful, rarely is lung biopsy warranted to establish the diagnosis.

Unfortunately, pathologists often disagree with regard to the histological criteria required for the diagnosis of asbestosis when the disease is limited in severity and extent. Asbestos bodies (fibers of asbestos encased in accumulations of an iron-containing protein) in the lung tissue are the hallmark of exposure. Although typical asbestos bodies (see Fig. 6-27) have a characteristic microscopic appearance, the

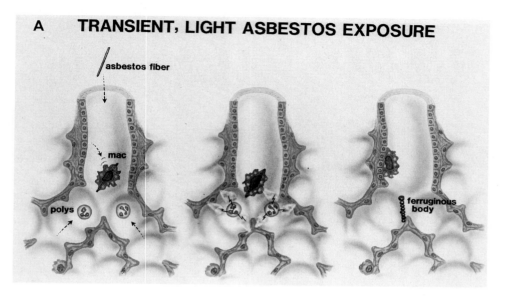

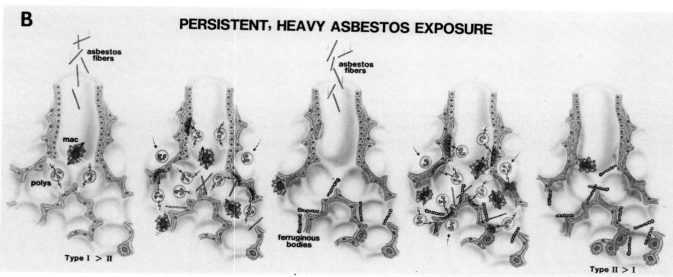

Fig. 28-16. Pathogenic construct of the interaction of the lungs with inhaled asbestos. **A,** Transient, light asbestos exposure in which asbestosis does not develop. Inhalation of fibers provokes an inflammatory process, but destructive and fibrotic changes do not occur in the lungs because the proteases and oxygen radicals released by the macrophages and leukocytes are inactivated by enzyme systems and antioxidants generated in the wall of the airways. Nonetheless, ferruginous bodies gradually accumulate and are a marker of exposure. **B,** Events that are hypothesized to occur in a heavy asbestos exposure sustained over a period of many years. In this circumstance, the exposure is persistent, and the inflammatory response damages the walls of the airways, resulting in focal deposits of scar tissue in the airway walls. This is the earliest stage in the development of asbestosis. With repeated exposures, the scar tissue becomes more extensive in the respiratory bronchioles and then in the alveolar ducts, until the lungs are distorted by fibrous tissue. Asbestosis results from exposure to amounts of asbestos that exceed the threshold of the lung and its ability to modulate the inflammatory response. As a result, fibrosis occurs.

Table 28-4. Asbestos in lung tissue by patient category, measured by various techniques

	Asbestos bodies	Uncoated asbestos fiber	
	LM	SEM ($\times$ 10^6)	TEM ($\times$ 10^6)
Control subjects	0.04 to 0.3 $\times$ 10^2	0.03-0.25	0.6-1.3
Mesothelioma patients	0.3 to 1.8 $\times$ 10^4	0.3	5-238
Asbestosis patients	1.2 to 3.8 $\times$ 10^5	3.3	—

LM, Light microscope; *SEM,* scanning electron microscope; *TEM,* transmission electron microscope.
Adapted from Roggli VL, Greenberg SD, Pratt PC, editors: *Pathology of asbestos-associated diseases,* Boston, 1992, Little, Brown.

features are quite variable. Moreover, a wide variety of organic and inorganic particles in the lungs can become coated with a similar iron/protein menstruum and thus superficially resemble asbestos bodies (Fig. 28-17, *A, B*). These particles in the lung are termed ferruginous bodies to emphasize their important difference from true asbestos bodies. Asbestos bodies usually represent only a small proportion of the fibrous asbestos in the lung tissue and thus are only a crude measure of exposure (Table 28-4). The majority of asbestos bodies contain amphibole asbestos fiber cores; only rarely do chrysotile fibers form asbestos bodies.

Criteria for the pathological diagnosis and assessment of severity of asbestosis have been established and are described in detail elsewhere (Fig. 28-18).[53] Because variable degrees of fibrosis are present in the lungs of many older individuals, particularly cigarette smokers, the pathologist must be cautious in attributing localized and possibly insignificant degrees of pulmonary fibrosis to asbestos. Asbestos bodies are found occasionally in histological sections of the lungs of many urban residents (Table 28-5). Thus, their presence alone is not diagnostic of asbestosis.

The early pathological changes of asbestosis are not discernable by traditional chest x-ray techniques; however, high-resolution radiological approaches and computed tomography are increasingly improving our ability to diagnose the disease. Characteristically the fibrotic disease process is most prominent in the lower lobes of the lung, often in association with pleural thickening and pleural plaques. Advanced asbestosis is an increasingly uncommon disease in developed countries owing to rigorous regulation of dust exposure in the workplace during the past several decades.

It is commonly stated that the lesions of asbestosis progress, becoming more prominent with the passage of time in the absence of asbestos exposure. Indeed, roughly 15% to 25% of patients with asbestosis seem to exhibit features suggestive of disease progression radiologically or by pulmonary functional parameters.[17,119] Definitive proof supporting the concept of progression is lacking, however, and intercurrent disease processes or physiological changes unrelated to asbestos exposure could account for the clinical observations. Morphological studies fail to define an active pathological process consistent with progression.

Table 28-5. Asbestos bodies in human lungs

Location	Percentage of lungs positive
Cape Town	26
Miami	27
Pittsburgh	41
Johannesburg	39
Finland	58
Montreal	48
San Francisco	42

Adapted from Lynch JR: Brake lining decomposition products, *J Air Pollut Cont Assoc* 18:824, 1968.

Cigarette smoking appears to accentuate the radiological features of asbestosis.[22,190,240] It is unclear whether this reflects the influence of tobacco smoke on the accumulation of particulates in the lung or a superimposition of the lesions of asbestosis on the fibrotic changes in the respiratory bronchioles attributed to cigarette smoking. A synergistic interaction also is possible.

Commercial asbestos comprises particles of variable dimensions. The relatively long fibers (i.e., longer than 5 μ) appear to play a key role in the pathogenesis of asbestosis at the primary site of disease in the respiratory bronchioles.[3,93] This is a critical point because the bulk of an industrial product is composed of much shorter fibers. Moreover, asbestos breaks down chemically and physically during some of its applications. For example, the dust from worn brake shoes contains relatively few fibers, and the majority of these are short and nonpathogenic. After inhalation, the long particles are phagocytized by alveolar macrophages, resulting in the generation of cytokines, which attract polymorphonuclear neutrophils to the scene (see Chapter 24). The active oxygen species and hydrolases generated by the inflammatory cells have the potential for damaging tissue when they overcome the neutralizing effects of locally elaborated superoxide dismutase, catalases, and other proteases should the exposure be heavy (see Chapter 21). Macrophages also elaborate fibrogenic growth factors after phagocytosis of asbestos fibers. Fibrosis begins in the walls of the respiratory bronchioles. With continued expo-

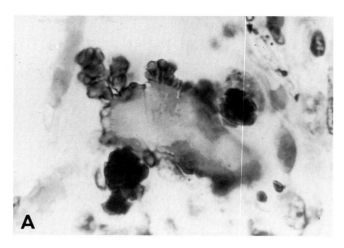

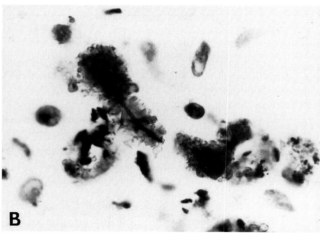

Fig. 28-17. A, A ferruginous body developing on a platy particle of talc. **B,** A ferruginous body developing on a graphite fiber. A variety of inorganic and organic particulates in the lung can serve as the nidus for the formation of ferruginous bodies. The asbestos body has a fiber core and thus should not be readily confused with other types of ferruginous bodies. (From Craighead JE, et al: Diseases associated with exposure to silica and nonfibrous silicate minerals, *Arch Pathol Lab Med* 112:673, 1988. Copyright 1988, American Medical Association; with permission.)

sure, the acini are involved, and fibrotic bridging between individual respiratory units occurs.

Numerous investigators have attempted to relate quantitatively the asbestos fiber content of the lung to the extent and severity of the fibrotic disease. Although there is a general correlation (Fig. 28-19), the diagnosis cannot be accomplished by determining the numbers of asbestos fibers and bodies in the tissue. Relatively high airborne concentrations of asbestos and long durations of exposure are required for the scarring of the lung to become sufficiently severe to result in clinically apparent disease.

Asbestos pleural disease

Plaques. Distinctive circumscribed plaques of dense, fibrous tissue deposited at specific sites in the parietal pleura

are a unique and sensitive marker of asbestos exposure (Fig. 28-20). The exposure threshold for plaque development is relatively low. Thus, plaques frequently are found in the absence of radiological and pathological evidence of asbestosis. The duration of exposure required for the development of plaques is not known, but they become increasingly evident in chest films with the passage of time (Fig. 28-21).[75] Little observational and experimental information exists on the mechanism whereby plaques develop. It is hypothesized that fibers entering the pleural cavity after inhalation into the lungs accumulate at the stomata of lymphatics on the parietal pleura. An inflammatory and scarring process follows, ultimately resulting in plaque development (Fig. 28-22).

Visceral pleural fibrosis. To a variable extent, a dense layer of hyalinized, relatively avascular fibrous tissue develops on the visceral pleural surface of the lungs of some workers exposed to asbestos, both in the presence and in the absence of asbestosis.[234] The pathogenesis of this unique asbestos-associated pleural fibrosis is obscure. Rarely, this "rind" of dense, fibrous tissue folds inwardly into the lung to form a dense, complex meshwork, which radiologically can resemble a neoplasm (so-called rounded atelectasis or Blesovsky's syndrome).[148]

Malignant mesothelioma. This rare cancer of the pleural, peritoneal, and pericardial cavity has been known as a curiosity to pathologists for more than a century. In 1960, its etiological association with amphibole asbestos was established.[234] Countless cases have occurred since then in developed countries among men and women exposed to asbestos in the workplace, particularly during and after World War II. Much less frequently, these tumors occur in persons who come into contact with asbestos avocationally and in the home. Roughly 20% to 40% of patients with malignant mesotheliomas have experienced no recognized asbestos exposure, and the disease is believed to be spontaneous.[9,104]

The commercial amphibole asbestos types, amosite and crocidolite, have been established as the major cause of malignant mesothelioma in numerous epidemiological studies conducted in North America and Europe. The role of chrysotile asbestos in the cause of this cancer is controversial, particularly because chrysotile often is contaminated with small amounts of the noncommercial asbestos, tremolite, a recognized cause of mesothelioma. It is universally agreed that chrysotile is relatively nonpathogenic, although it may be responsible for a few mesotheliomas when exposure to chrysotile is heavy and prolonged. In these cases, tremolite contaminants may be the causative factor in the disease.[5,41,182,239] I believe that chrysotile has no carcinogenic potential once it is processed for commercial use and the bulk of fibrous tremolite contaminants removed.

The carcinogenic mechanisms involved are not known, but it is believed that deposits of the durable long, thin fibers of amphibole asbestos accumulate in or immediately

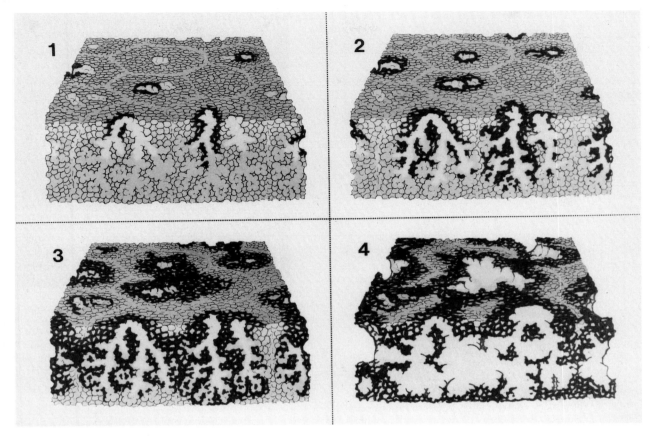

Fig. 28-18. Stages in the development of asbestosis. Initially the lesions develop in the walls of the respiratory bronchioles (stage 1). As the lesion progresses, bridging occurs between individual respiratory units, and the alveolar walls are involved (stages 2 and 3). With the progression of the disease, more respiratory units are involved. Destruction of the parenchyma by the contraction of scars occurs in stage 4. The "honeycomb" lung, which is characteristic of advanced disease, results from the contraction of fibrotic scars.

subjacent to the pleura, resulting in transformation of the mesothelial cell or its progenitor.[49] Oxygen free radicals generated by phagocytic interaction of macrophages with amphibole fibers may result in cumulative injury to the DNA of the mesothelial progenitor cells (see Chapter 21). This multistage series of events ultimately results in the selection of malignant tumor cell clones over periods of 20 or more years. The process is relatively inefficient because fewer than 20% of a population of heavily exposed persons develop the neoplasm.

Malignant mesothelioma enjoys a well-deserved reputation as a diagnostic challenge. The tumors exhibit an enormous diversity of morphological features and frequently are composed of both fibrosarcomatous and carcinomatous elements intermixed in a complex montage of configurations (Figs. 28-23 and 28-24). Histochemical, immunochemical, and ultrastructural studies often are required to establish the diagnosis and differentiate the tumor from metastatic adenocarcinomas and sarcomas.

The pathological features and diagnosis of malignant

mesothelioma have been the subject of countless excellent publications in recent years.* Accordingly the details are not considered here.

SILICATOSIS

Humans are exposed to a variety of airborne granular and platelike silicate particulates, both in the course of their daily lives and occupationally (see Chapter 6).[29,42,54] These ubiquitous mineral particles originate in soil and street dust and are found to a variable extent in the lungs of all of us. They are mined and quarried for the manufacture of countless consumer products and building materials. After inhalation, the nasal cavities and pulmonary clearance mechanisms effectively eliminate particulates at low concentrations in the ambient air (Fig. 28-3). Thus, silicates pose a potential health problem only when exposure is heavy and prolonged, such as in the so-called dusty trades. Workers who quarry shales[201] and slate[54]

*References 18, 117, 130, 150, 188, 205, 235.

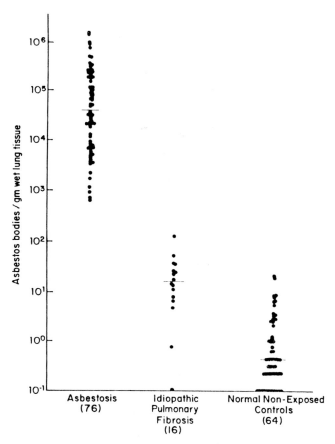

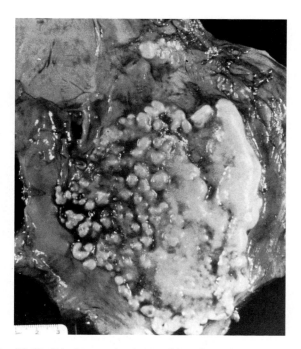

Fig. 28-20. Diaphragmatic plaques. Note the well-circumscribed margins of these elevated bosselated and nodular masses, which exhibit the appearance of ivory. Adhesions are not present. As these lesions advance, they often become calcified. (From Craighead JE, et al: The pathology of asbestos-associated diseases of the lungs and pleural cavities: diagnostic criteria and proposed grading schema, *Arch Pathol Lab Med* 106:544, 1982. Copyright 1982, American Medical Association; with permission.)

Fig. 28-19. Asbestos body concentrations as determined by scanning electron microscopy in the lungs of patients with asbestosis and idiopathic pulmonary fibrosis and a normal, unexposed control group. Asbestos is found in the lungs of the majority of the subjects, with a high concentration of bodies in those with asbestosis. The accumulation of modest amounts of asbestos in the lungs of those with idiopathic pulmonary fibrosis is most probably compatible with impeded lung clearance in this disease process. Note the lack of an overlap with the asbestotic group. (From Roggli VL, Greenberg SD, Pratt PC, editors: *Pathology of asbestos-associated diseases, Boston, 1992, Little, Brown; with permission.*)

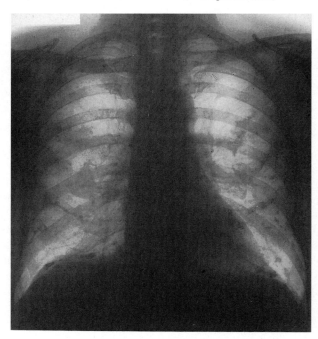

Fig. 28-21. Chest x-ray film of a chrysotile miner with extensive pleural plaquing. Note the shieldlike structures in the intercostal spaces bilaterally. Extensive plaques of this type can develop in the absence of significant pulmonary insufficiency. (From Craighead JE, et al: The pathology of asbestos-associated diseases of the lungs and pleural cavities: diagnostic criteria and proposed grading schema, *Arch Pathol Lab Med* 106:544, 1982. Copyright 1982, American Medical Association; with permission.)

and those engaged in the mining and milling of kaolinite,[134,157] talc,[87,229] and mica[56,173] are affected, as are those exposed to several other less well-known silicates.* Under the circumstances of unusually heavy exposure, the clearance threshold is regularly exceeded, and particulates gradually accumulate in the lungs (Fig. 28-25). In turn, they are transported by lymphatics to the centrally located lymph nodes in the hilus of the lung and mediastinum. For reasons that are not clear, silicate particles accumulate preferentially adjacent to the peribronchial and perivascular lymphatics of the lung, where, over time,

*References 34, 90, 111, 194, 226.

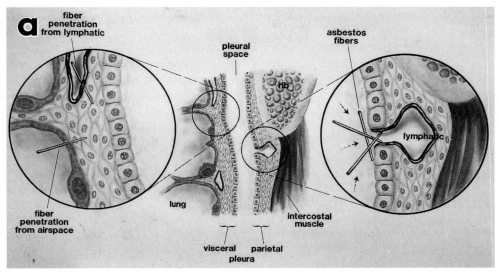

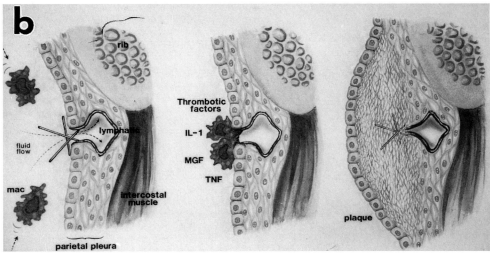

Fig. 28-22. Hypothetical construct for plaque development. **A,** During periods of exposure, asbestos fibers move through the pleural linings of the lungs by direct passage or through lymphatics to enter the pleural space. Fluids in this pleural space are cleared through the stomata of the lymphatics, which line the parietal pleura and are located subjacent to ribs. Because of the size of fibers, they tend to accumulate at this point without entering the lymphatics. **B,** The presence of fibers attracts macrophages, which elicit an inflammatory response accompanied by the generation of cytokines and mediators. As a result, fibrosis occurs in a localized, relatively circumscribed manner. This schema is consistent with the limited information that is available on this process. *IL-1,* Interleukin-1; *MGF,* macrophage growth factor; *TNF,* tumor necrosis factor. (From Craighead JE, Kane AB: *The pathogenesis of malignant and non-malignant serosal lesions in body cavities consequent to asbestos exposure.* In Jaurand M-C, Bignon J, editors: *The mesothelial cell and mesothelioma,* New York, 1994, Marcel Dekker; with permission.)

they elicit a fibrotic reaction (Fig. 28-26). Although the lesions of silicosis are nodular and tend to occur at confluence points in the lymphatic system, those produced by the silicates are more diffusely distributed along the course of these channels. In advanced stages of the disease, the lungs are extensively involved by massive deposits of the dust associated with fibrous tissue (Table 28-6).

COALWORKERS' PNEUMOCONIOSIS

Coalworkers' pneumoconiosis (CWP) is defined simply as the accumulation of coal dust in the lungs and the tissue reaction to its presence.[42,129] The term, however, is ambiguous because it is used to describe either the anatomical lesions or the radiological picture, features of disease that do not necessarily correlate. The term black lung first was used medically in the United Kingdom in reference to the

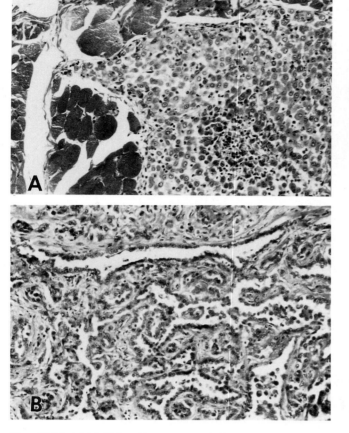

Fig. 28-23. Epithelial malignant mesothelioma. A, This tumor consists of sheets of neoplastic mesothelial cells. It is invading striated muscle of the thorax. Note the central area of necrosis. B, A glandular and papillary lesion.

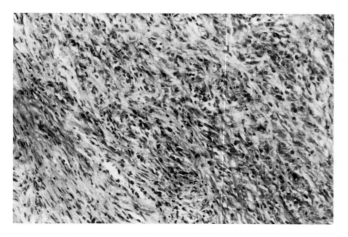

Fig. 28-24. A fibrosarcomatous mesothelioma exhibiting variable pleomorphism of the tumor cells.

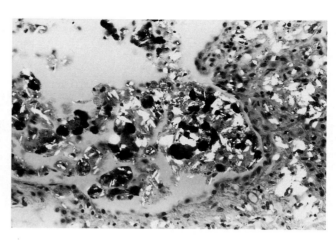

Fig. 28-25. Silicates of a platy or possibly fibrous composition in alveolar macrophages and interstitium of a worker with mica lung disease. The platy particles, when prepared in histologic sections, exhibit a lancet-shaped configuration. Note the variability in size of the particulates and their distribution. The silicates exhibit a high degree of birefringence in contrast to silica (see Fig. 6-28). (From Craighead JE, et al: Diseases associated with exposure to silica and nonfibrous silicate minerals, *Arch Pathol Lab Med* 112:673, 1988. Copyright 1988, American Medical Association; with permission.)

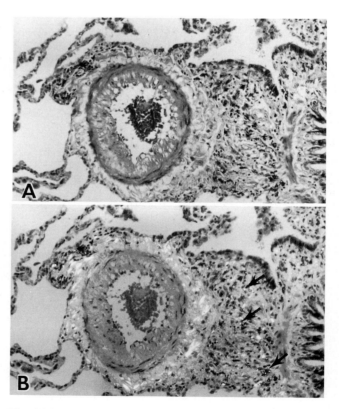

Fig. 28-26. Talc pneumoconiosis. A, Light microscopy exhibits interstitial fibrosis particularly in peribronchial and perivascular space. B, Polarization microscopy features of this lesion. Note the silicate particles in the interstitium *(arrow)*. The collagen in the vessel wall is also birefringent. (From Craighead JE, et al: Diseases associated with exposure to silica and nonfibrous silicate minerals, *Arch Pathol Lab Med* 112:673, 1988. Copyright 1988, American Medical Association; with permission.)

Table 28-6. Characteristics of common occupational airborne particles

	Character of dust particle silicates		
Fibrogenicity	**Granular**	**Platy**	**Fibrous**
4+	Sandstone Silica flour Diatomaceous earth		Crocidolite asbestos Amosite asbestos
3+	Granite		Chrysotile asbestos
2+	Slate	Talc	Talc
+	Feldspar Shale	Kaolinite Vermiculite Mica	Sepolite Woolastonite Attapullgite

+, Mild; 2+, moderate; 3+, moderately severe; 4+ severe.

black-tinged sputum and pigmented lungs of coal miners. It now has acquired a legal connotation because a diagnosis of "black lung" entitles one in the United States to receive compensation under the program established by the U.S. Congress for "any respiratory or pulmonary impairment arising out of employment in or around coal mines." Considerable controversy centers around the potential pathogenic role of coal dust in the lung and its contribution to respiratory insufficiency. The question is compounded by the superimposed effects of cigarette smoking, a common habituation of underground coal miners. Questions also arise regarding the possible pathogenic role of silica dust in coal mine dust and thus the concomitant occurrence of silicotic lesions with those attributable to coal dust.[59] An additional issue is the contribution of coal dust to bronchial hyperresponsivity, so-called industrial asthma. These issues are considered in more detail subsequently.

The mineralogical properties of coal of various types (anthracite, bituminous, sub-bituminous and lignite) are considered in Chapter 6. In brief, coal is a carbonaceous plant residue containing varying amounts of nonfibrous silicates and silica dust (so-called ash) and various elemental and hydrocarbon contaminants at low concentrations (benzene, phenols, naphthalene, and aromatic hydrocarbons). The hydrocarbons of plant origin in the noncombusted state have no recognized carcinogenic properties, in contrast to the highly carcinogenic aromatic hydrocarbon effluents from coal-derived, partially incinerated coal (coke), which is used in steel production and smelting.

As with other pneumoconioses, the extent and severity of pulmonary disease are changing as increasingly restrictive regulations on coal dust in the underground workplace are promulgated. CWP is clearly a dose-related and time-related disease, but its development is influenced by the "rank" of the coal (see Fig. 6-31).[110,114] With present mining practices and the use of personal respiratory protective apparatus, the severe degrees of CWP seen in the past by pathologists are no longer occurring. In addition, an increasing proportion of the coal mined worldwide is from open pits and strip mines, where dust concentrations are insufficient to cause disease. Thus, the lesions of CWP are not presented exhaustively here. The reader is referred to several excellent publications that consider its pathology in detail.[42,45,60,129]

After periods of exposure of 10 or more years, the macules of CWP gradually become evident on microscopic examination of the lung. They predominate in the upper lobes of the lung adjacent to lymphatics and are located at branches of the respiratory bronchioles. The macules of CWP are palpable and obvious to the naked eye in lung tissue but customarily are less than 1 cm in diameter. They represent a confluence of coal particle–laden alveolar macrophages that accumulate in the lymphatics that parallel the branches of the respiratory bronchioles (Figs. 28-10 and 28-27). Macules contain sparse deposits of collagen and reticulum, and they may be more transient lesions, evolving by confluence over time into nodules. Associated with these focal lesions are enlarged air spaces, which represent a form of emphysema consequent to localized dust-induced damage to the lung parenchyma; i.e., the so-called scar emphysema.[191,200] To a variable extent, coal dust accumulations in the lung contain silica and silicate particulates, and occasionally silicotic nodules are found.

Nodules yield a radiological picture identical to silicosis (Fig. 28-28). As with silicosis, localized lesions that compromise only limited proportions of the lung parenchyma yield few, if any, symptoms and signs of respiratory insufficiency. Based on numerous clinical and epidemiological studies, one concludes that many of the symptoms of coal workers are due to cigarette smoking (rather than coal dust), compounded to a variable extent by the bronchospastic effects of dust on the smaller airways of the lung.

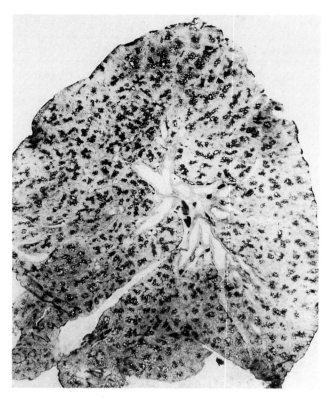

Fig. 28-27. Whole lung (Goff-Wentworth) section exhibiting macules of coalworker's pneumoconiosis in the lungs of a miner with 18 years of underground experience. He also smoked 1.5 packs of cigarettes per day over a 21-year period. Note the association of the macules with the vasculature and the related "scar" emphysema. (Courtesy of V. Vallyathan, National Institute for Occupational Safety and Health.)

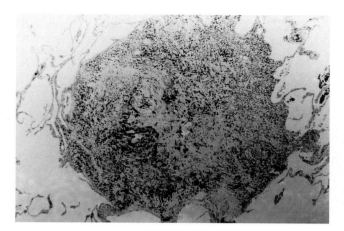

Fig. 28-28. A fibrotic anthrocotic nodule in the lung of a coal miner. The nodule contains silica particles as well as coal dust. These are more advanced changes than the macule demonstrated in Fig. 28-10.

Progressive massive fibrosis is a rare, advanced stage of CWP (Fig. 28-29). It typically develops in the upper lung lobes and comprises a confluence of dust-laden nodules into a mass that radiologically can simulate a neoplasm. Progressive massive fibrosis lesions contain variable amounts of collagen as well as silica and silicate particles in association with coal dust. Typically, foci of liquefaction necrosis are found within these lesions. This change results from localized vascular insufficiency and, occasionally, superimposed mycobacterial infections.

Caplan's lesions are concentrically defined nodules found occasionally in the lungs of those with CWP and silicosis.[31,94] They characteristically occur in patients with active rheumatoid arthritis.[32] The lesions exhibit the palisading histiocytes and coagulative necrosis seen in typical rheumatoid granulomas (Fig. 28-30).

Mixed dust lesions

Dusts of a wide variety of types are commonly seen in the lungs of workers employed in steel mills and foundries, and in mining.[37,161,192] Welders commonly have "dirty" lungs, which contain, in addition to the aforemen-

tioned dusts, metal particulates unique to their trade and the so-called welder's granules. Coal and hematite miners and quarriers of shales and slates often have silica nodules in their lungs mixed with deposits of carbon and silicates. Some talc miners have asbestosis owing to contaminants of the mineral, and foundry workers often have pulmonary deposits of iron, asbestos and silica particles, along with massive amounts of carbon. Many of these foreign materials are relatively nonpathogenic. McLaughlin and Harding[154] described a specific lesion that microscopically exhibits a stellate "Medusa-head" configuration (Fig. 28-31). It typically is comprised of a central region of hyalinized collagen surrounded by radially arrayed, flamelike extensions composed of fibrous tissue and exhibiting a mixture of dust particulates.

Siderosis

Arc welders, steel mill workers, and iron miners often accumulate relatively large amounts of iron and iron oxides in their lungs.[7,156] This nonfibrogenic material elicits a prominent macrophage response that at times becomes sufficiently abundant to result in parenchymal shadows in x-ray films of the lungs.[171] Microscopically, these deposits can superficially resemble asbestos bodies.

Aluminum pneumoconiosis

Fine metallic aluminum powder as well as aluminum oxide in fumes and fine particulates in sufficient concentration cause diffuse pulmonary fibrosis.* Aluminum is used commonly and in many forms in industry, but aluminum lung occurs only rarely. The particle size and biological reactivity of the aluminum appears to be a critical determinant of the outcome of an exposure (Fig. 28-32).

*References 116, 120, 160, 204, 230.

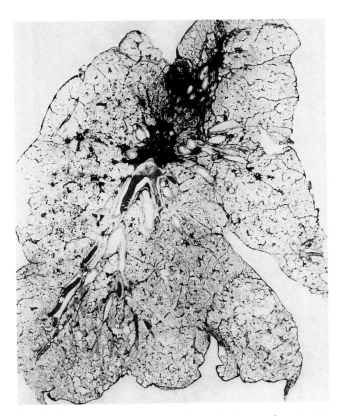

Fig. 28-29. Progressive massive fibrosis in the emphysematous lung of a 72-year-old coal miner who worked underground for 39 years. A massive upper lobe lesion is apparent. Note the macules scattered nearby in the upper lobes. The diffuse panlobular emphysema is, no doubt, secondary to the long history of cigarette smoking. (Courtesy of V. Vallyathan, National Institute for Occupational Safety and Health.)

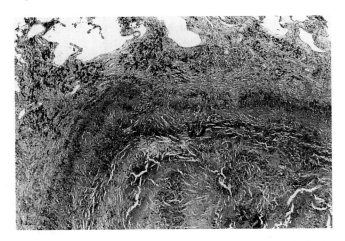

Fig. 28-30. A Caplan's lesion (rheumatoid pneumoconiosis) in the lung of a 65-year-old coal miner with extensive pneumoconiosis and rheumatoid arthritis. Note the palisading of the fibroblasts in a geographical pattern around the central area of necrosis. At the periphery of the lesion is interstitial fibrosis associated with dust deposits. (From Craighead JE, et al: Diseases associated with exposure to silica and nonfibrous silicate minerals, *Arch Pathol Lab Med* 112:673, 1988. Copyright 1988, American Medical Association; with permission.)

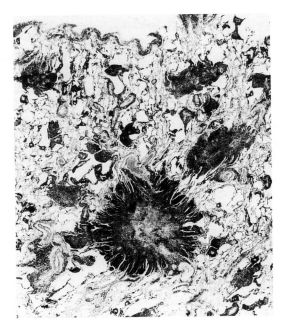

Fig. 28-31. A so-called medusa head lesion of mixed dust exposure in the lung of a foundry worker. This lesion contains silica particles, silicates, and carbonacous dust. (From Craighead JE, et al: Diseases associated with exposure to silica and nonfibrous silicate minerals, *Arch Pathol Lab Med* 112:673, 1988. Copyright 1988, American Medical Association; with permission.)

HYPERSENSITIVITY DISEASES CHARACTERIZED BY MULTINUCLEATE GIANT CELL AND GRANULOMA FORMATION

Several uncommon, sporadically occurring pulmonary disorders having a presumptive immunological pathogenesis are considered here (see Chapter 25).[147] The diagnosis and establishment of an etiological basis for these conditions characteristically require the correlation of epidemiological and clinical information as well as careful pathological evaluation. Giant cells in this context include fused macrophages or epithelial cells and range morphologically from the traditional foreign body giant cell to vaguely defined multicellular structures in the loosely arrayed granulomas of hypersensitivity pneumonitis. Histological evidence of immunological reactivity is presumptive and variable, for it depends on the stage of the disease in relation to the time of exposure. Often, it consists of noncaseating granulomas or interstitial infiltrates of lymphocytes or both. All of these diseases are characterized by interstitial fibrosis and, to a variable extent, intra-airspace organizing exudates and bronchiolitis obliterans.

Hypersensitivity pneumonitis

The term extrinsic allergic alveolitis is a commonly used synonym for this sporadically occurring pulmonary response to inhaled organic particulates of a diversity of types (Table 28-7). Clinical observations establish the immuno-

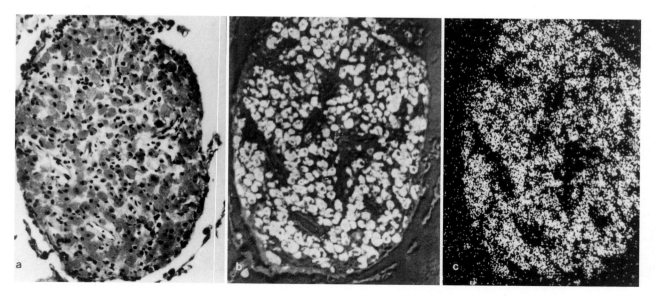

Fig. 28-32. Aluminum deposits in the lung of a 35-year-old aluminum arc welder who developed radiological opacities in the lung. He was a smoker who worked in confined spaces aboard ships. **A,** Photomicrograph of a focal pulmonary lesion with pasty aluminum pigmented alveolar macrophages. **B,** A back-scatter spectrometry electron micrograph of this same lesion. **C,** X-ray mapping for aluminum, as illustrated by the dots. (From Vallyathan NV, et al: Pulmonary fibrosis in an aluminum arc welder, *Chest* 81:34, 1982; with permission.)

logical basis for a syndrome characterized by the onset of symptoms shortly after exposure either in the natural setting or by experimental antigenic challenge in the laboratory. Despite the demonstration of circulating immunoglobulin G (IgG) against the antigen in question in the blood of many (but not all) of those who are affected, the mechanism involved in the hypersensitivity response is unclear. A combination of several immunological pathways seems most probable in many cases.[186,227] Perhaps different patterns of expression reflect the antigen, means of sensitization, and individual susceptibility.

Farmers' lung, a condition resulting from the inhalation of spores of thermophilic actinomyces in rotting hay, is the prototype syndrome. It occurs sporadically in rural communities and is a disappearing disease as farmers acquire understanding of its causation. Of more contemporary interest in urban communities is air conditioner lung[13] and disease caused by home humidifiers[30,207,223] resulting from exposure to the spores of fungi growing in the moist nooks and crannies of air conditioners in offices and homes. Because it occurs sporadically and in only a small proportion of those at risk, the milder forms of the disease frequently are not recognized by physicians and pathologists. Countless other environmental exposures are implicated in occasional cases or outbreaks of disease, but often only circumstantial evidence supports the claims of causation.[29,138,231] One recent report notes that pigeon fancier's lung is the most common cause of pulmonary fibrosis in Mexico City.[174]

Hypersensitivity pneumonitis is characterized by acute episodes during which fluid and mononuclear cell exudates accumulate interstitially and in airspaces, resulting in shortness of breath.[199] Usually the acute episode resolves uneventfully even with continued exposure to antigen, a process best considered to be analogous to desensitization. This lesion is rarely documented pathologically. Recurrent episodes of exudative pneumonia are ultimately followed by the development of the chronic stage of the disease when interstitial fibrosis and mononuclear cell accumulations are observed microscopically, accompanied by varying degrees of bronchiolitis obliterans (Fig. 28-33). At this stage, variable numbers of loosely arrayed granulomas are evident in the interstitium. The pathogenesis of the granulomas and the composition of the vaguely described inclusions often seen within them are ill-defined. One might speculate that they represent a response to plant products in the inhalant. Doubtless in many cases of hypersensitivity pneumonitis, bronchiolar hyperreactivity and thus occupational asthma are components of the acute disease. In the late stages, after many recurrent episodes of acute disease, bronchiolitis obliterans contributes to respiratory insufficiency, resulting in severe disability or even death. The details of the pathological features of hypersensitivity pneumonitis are well described in several publications.[185,199]

Berylliosis

Berylliosis is a systemic granulomatous disease that results from the inhalation of a variety of beryllium-

Table 28-7. Common etiological (or suspected) agents of hypersensitivity pneumonitis

Agent	Disease	Exposure
Definitive causative agents		
Thermophilic actinomycetes		
Micropolyspora faeni	Farmer's lung	Moldy hay
Thermoactinomyces viridis	Farmer's lung	Moldy hay
Thermoactinomyces vulgaris	Mushroom worker's lung	Moldy compost
Thermoactinomyces sacharii	Bagassosis	Moldy sugar cane
Thermoactinomyces candidus	Ventilator pneumonitis	Contaminated forced air system
Fungi		
Cryptostroma corticale	Maple bark stripper's disease	Moldy maple bark
Aspergillus clavatus	Malt worker's lung	Moldy malt
Penicillium frequentans	Suberosis	Moldy cork dust
Penicillium caseii	Cheese worker's lung	Cheese mold
Alternaria sp.	Woodworker's lung	Moldy wood chips
(*Cryptostroma corticale*)		
Pullularia sp.	Sequoiosis	Moldy redwood dust
(*Aureobasdium* sp.)		
Mucor sp.	Paprika splitter's lung	Paprika dust
Lycoperdon	Mushroom picker's lung	Puffballs
Arthropods		
Sitophilus granarius	Wheat weevil disease	Infested wheat
Animal proteins		
Avian proteins	Bird breeder's lung	Avian droppings
Animal fur	Furrier's lung	
	Pituitary snufftaker's lung	Dessicated pituitary dust
Chemicals		
Phthalic anhydride	Epoxy resin worker's lung	Epoxy resin
Toluene diisocyanate	Porcelain refinisher's lung	Paint catalyst
Probable causative agents		
Amoeba	Ventilator pneumonitis	Contaminated systems
Various fungi		
Bacillus subtilis	Enzyme worker's lung	Detergent enzymes
Hair dust	Furrier's lung	Animal proteins
Coffee dust	Coffee worker's lung	?
Trimellitic anhydride	TMA disease	Trimellitic anhydride
Possible causative agents		
Altered humidifier water	Humidifier lung	Humidifier water
Various saprophytic fungi	Hypersensitivity pneumonitis	Contaminated environments

Adapted from Fink J: *Hypersensitivity pneumonitis.* In Merchant J, editor: *Occupational respiratory disease,* Publication No 86-102, Washington, DC, 1981, US Public Health Service, Department of Health and Human Services.

containing materials (the ore, oxides, and alloys of beryllium and various finished products) in particulate, aerosolized form. It occurs in roughly 1% to 10% of those who are exposed, an observation that suggests a role for genetic influences and hypersensitivity in its pathogenicity.[219] Beryllium is one of the wonder metals of the twentieth century; it is used in a variety of manufactured products ranging from high-performance steel to nuclear generation and the space program. A disease of significant environmental and occupational proportions in past decades, occurrence of berylliosis now is limited by regulation of dust in the workplace. Yet because of the diversity of industries using beryllium-containing products, effective control sometimes is difficult to establish. Also reports suggest that federal reg-

ulations may be insufficiently rigorous to prevent the occurrence of disease in some people. Boeck's sarcoid and berylliosis are inseparably linked as pathological lesions because of their common features. Both are associated with aberrations of immunological responsivity, but they exhibit different clinical pictures. A detailed evaluation of the pathology of berylliosis, using cases in the national registry established some years ago, has been published.[83]

Boeck's sarcoidosis

Sarcoidosis is a systemic disease manifest by granulomatous involvement of the skin, eyes, salivary glands, and lymph nodes as well as the lungs. The lungs and hilar lymph nodes are involved in the majority of cases, and the dis-

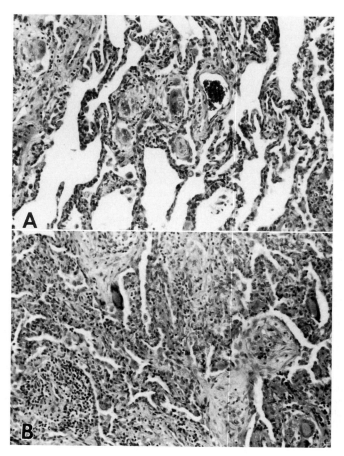

Fig. 28-33. Hypersensitivity pneumonitis in a young farmer with severe progressive respiratory insufficiency. Numerous multinucleate giant cells are seen in the interstitium and in air spaces of the lungs (**A**). An organizing exudative process (bronchiolitis obliterans) is seen in this same case (**B**). Note the multinucleate giant cells.

ease is said to be limited to pulmonary tissue in 25% to 30% of cases. It is difficult to estimate the prevalence of pulmonary sarcoidosis because many cases most probably are not recognized medically, and a substantial number regress spontaneously without treatment. Both epidemiological and pathological evidence suggest the possibility that sarcoidosis is caused by extrinsic factors, either microbial or particulate. The demonstration of recurrent lesions developing in the lung allografts of four of five sarcoid patients, however, provides a compelling argument for a systemic disease process independent of external influences.[115]

Of great interest are the dramatic differences in prevalence of sarcoidosis in various geographical areas worldwide and its almost exclusive occurrence in young and middle-aged adults. Although Sweden, with an exclusively white population, has the world's highest prevalence, in the United States, pulmonary sarcoidosis is eightfold more common in blacks than in whites. Yet the cause remains

obscure. Arguments for a mycobacterial cause remain unsubstantiated, and the proposed relationship to inhaled conifer pollen goes unproven. It is possible that the so-called sarcoidlike granuloma is a nonspecific response to a variety of environmental or infectious agents.

Fig. 28-34 diagrammatically depicts the hypothetical pathogenetic mechanisms involved in granuloma formation in both berylliosis and sarcoidosis.[109] Activated T cells clearly play a key role in both disease processes and are an intrinsic component of the lesions. Sensitization of T cells to beryllium salts now can be demonstrated in members of occupationally exposed groups.

Hard metal disease

The unique lesions of giant cell interstitial pneumonia, first described by Liebow[136] (Fig. 28-35), characterize this rare, sporadically occurring disease of workers in industries using hard metal or diamond bits for cutting or polishing metal or diamonds.* Whether or not all cases of giant cell interstitial pneumonia are due to hard metal dust exposure is unclear, but it seems unlikely. Hard metal bits are fabricated by fusing fine particulates of tungsten and tantalum carbides at high temperature with a salt of cobalt. The resulting bit is polished and subsequently used in a variety of industrial applications in which bits of a hardness approaching that of industrial diamonds are required. The disease occurs among workers employed in all stages of the manufacturing process and in users of hard metal bits involved in either wet or dry cutting of metal. It is believed to be caused by inhalation of particulates of solubilized salts of cobalt. This is controversial, however, because the hard metal particulates may serve as carriers for the cobalt in lung tissue and could contribute to giant cell formation. Overt giant cell interstitial pneumonia is uncommon in workers and may occur only in persons with inordinate susceptibility. Chronic disease appears to occur more commonly but is confused clinically with other forms of pulmonary disease. An immunological hypersensitivity response may be a critical step in the pathogenesis of the disorder, but this concept is unproved. An immunological basis for the condition is supported by the occurrence of airway and skin hypersensitivity in workers in the involved industries.

EOSINOPHILIC PNEUMONIA SYNDROMES

A group of incompletely defined, subacute and chronic pulmonary eosinophilic inflammatory diseases with variable amounts of interstitial fibrosis are termed eosinophilic pneumonia.[137] Worldwide the conditions are most commonly attributed to intestinal parasitism resulting either from the migration of larvae of intestinal parasites through the lungs (*Ascaris lumbricoides, Ancylostoma duodenale, Strongyloides stercoralis*) or the incomplete maturation of migrat-

*References 1, 44, 62, 63, 80, 163.

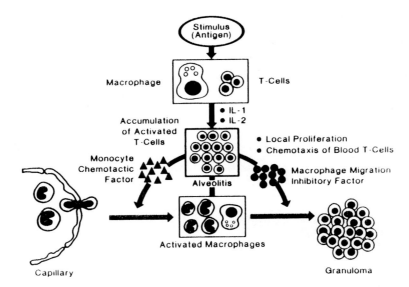

Fig. 28-34. Pathogenesis of granuloma formation. A stimulus (which may be an antigen) activates alveolar macrophages to release interleukin-1 *(IL-1)* and lung T cells to release interleukin-2 *(IL-2)*. The release of these mediators results in an accumulation of activated T cells in the lung, both by stimulating lung T cells to proliferate locally and by functioning as chemoattractants that recruit additional blood T cells to the lung. The activated T cells that are present in the lung regulate granuloma formation by secreting other lymphokines, such as monocyte chemotactic factor, which attracts blood monocytes to the lung. Once monocytes are present in the lung, other T cell–derived lymphokines, such as macrophage migration inhibitory factor and immune interferon, stimulate the differentiation of these cells into activated macrophages, which form the compact structure utlimately recognized as a granuloma. (From Thomas PD, Hunninghake GW: Current concepts of the pathogenesis of sarcodosis, *Am Rev Respir Dis* 135:747, 1987; with permission.)

ing filarial nematodes (*Wuchereria* species) in the lung. The clinical syndrome, which often is accompanied by asthma and peripheral blood eosinophilia, was known as Loeffler's syndrome (tropical eosinophilic lung) in the past.

The acute bronchospastic features of allergic sensitization in eosinophilic pneumonia are believed to result from the release of cytokines by the eosinophilic cell accumulations in the lung tissue. Documentation of the long-term effects of this syndrome in residents of the tropics and other underdeveloped lands is lacking. Studies of U.S. troops in the Pacific Islands during the World War II, however, indicate that the condition is relatively transient.

Sporadic cases of eosinophilic pneumonia frequently are attributed to pharmacological agents. Nickel exposure was reported as the cause of an outbreak of evanescent, radiologically demonstrated pulmonary infiltrates accompanied by eosinophilia. A similar outbreak was reported among workers in a rubber product plant.[16] Because the causes of many cases of pulmonary eosinophilia are unknown, chemical exposure is an appropriate consideration for future investigation.

In the United States, eosinophilic pneumonia accompanied by asthma occasionally has been associated with non-invasive *Aspergillus* species infections of the airways. Bronchocentric granulomatosis, accompanied by, or in the absence of, eosinophilic pulmonary infiltrates and asthma,

also has been attributed to an allergic reaction to *Aspergillus species,* but the association is unproven.[124]

TOXIC GAS AND FUME EFFECTS ON THE RESPIRATORY TRACT

Sporadically, and usually by accident, humans are exposed to toxic gases in concentrations that result in acute, occasionally fatal, respiratory insufficiency. Because these lethal episodes occur uncommonly, much of the available pathological and physiological information is found in reports of individual autopsy cases. As demonstrated in a population-based study using hospital emergency room data, symptomatic, nonfatal episodes of acute irritant exposures occur commonly among residents of urban communities.[21] The long-term pathophysiological outcomes of these less severe exposures are uncertain, although in some cases they could account for the nonspecific pulmonary fibrosis and bronchiolitis obliterans that is sporadically found in the lungs of members of the general population at autopsy.

Acute exposures to toxic gases are also now recognized as a major contributing factor to the so-called reactive airway dysfunction syndrome.[25] This condition is characterized by persistent respiratory symptoms and continued airway hyperreactivity to air pollutants and cigarette smoke for variable periods of time after the incident.

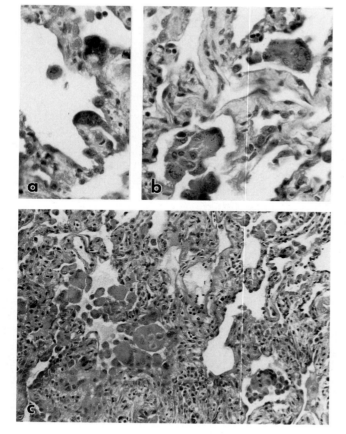

Fig. 28-35. Hard metal disease in a young mill worker. The severity of the pulmonary insufficiency necessitated lung transplantation. **A,** Multinucleate cells forming from alveolar lining cells. **B,** Giant cells have within their cytoplasms fine granules of tungsten carbide as demonstrated by X-ray spectrometry. **C,** Diffuse interstitial fibrosis and multinucleate cells formed from coalescent alveolar macrophages. Focal bronchiolitis obliterans were also observed in this lung.

The box at right lists volatile chemicals that have been associated with acute, sometimes fatal occurrences of acute pulmonary disease characterized by diffuse alveolar damage.[36] Exposures to high concentrations of ammonia,[82,105,217] chlorine,[198] formaldehyde, sulfur dioxide (SO_2)[36,77,242] and a variety of other volatile chemicals* have customarily occurred as a result of accidents in the chemical industries or when chemicals are transported. Less severe exposures have been described among end users of these products in countless workplaces. Custodial personnel have been found to be at particular risk as a result of exposure to mixtures of cleaning fluids in poorly ventilated circumstances. Chlorine is produced by the addition of acid cleaning fluids to the sodium hypochlorite (Clorox®), and monochloramine and dichloramine are generated by mixtures of ammonia and sodium hypochlorite.[39,184] Exposure

*References 19, 61, 95, 96, 118, 121, 126, 172, 246.

Gases having the potential for significant acute pulmonary toxicity with diffuse alveolar damage, after accidental exposure

Ammonia
Chlorine
Formaldehyde
Ammonia-sodium hypochloride mixtures
Glacial acetic acids
Methyl isocyanite
Phosgene
NO, NO_2, N_2O_4
Carbon tetrachloride
Cadmium fumes
Polyurethane

NO, Nitric oxide; *NO_2,* nitrogen dioxide; *N_2O_4,* nitrogen tetroxide.

to nitric oxide (NO) (and more frequently, its oxidation products, nitrogen dioxide [NO_2] and nitrogen tetroxide [N_2O_4]) occurs in a variety of settings among workers in the chemical industry, in agriculture (silo filler's disease and in manure pits)[77,158,181] (Fig. 28-36), among those who use or manufacture explosives, arc welders, and firemen.* A classic outbreak of NO_2 toxicity resulted in more than 100 deaths as a consequence of the burning of x-ray films made with nitrocellulose.

Water-soluble chemicals, such as SO_2 and formaldehyde, produce major symptomatic upper respiratory effects owing to direct toxicity to mucous membranes, whereas insoluble gaseous chemicals and fumes tend to manifest their effects on the lower airways. It is at this location that some of the major short-term and long-term effects are manifest as bronchospasms and bronchiolitis, the severity of which is an expression of the type of chemical and its concentration as well as the presence of preexisting airway disease. Sloughing of the mucosa of the lower respiratory tract often is associated with small airway hyperresponsivity and obstructive phenomenology long after mucosal regeneration has occurred. Acute toxicity to the lower airways results in an exudative pneumonitis, which may be followed by fatal pulmonary edema or by the development of bronchiolitis obliterans among those who survive. The pathological features of these classes of exposures were first recognized among those who were fatally gassed with phosgene during World War I. The tragedy in Bophol, India, which killed or severely damaged the lungs of thousands, illustrates the acute and long-term effects of methylisocyanate, a commonly used intermediate chemical of industry.[155]

More than 300 different types of welding and allied industrial processes are currently in use. As a result, workers in these trades are exposed to a variety of fumes related to the constituents of the electrode coating and the metal be-

*References 69, 100, 140, 180, 206.

Chapter 28 Airways and lung **481**

fer thermal burns that require medical care and more than 1×10^5 are hospitalized. Toxic gas inhalation is experienced by many of these persons, but the number is uncertain because the respiratory problems of burn victims often go unreported. The occurrence of thermal injury to the respiratory epithelium and toxic fume inhalation among firefighters is common. The toxicology of gasses emanating from fires is exceedingly complex because it is so dependent on the fuel load and the character of the fire. Moreover, fires in closed spaces consume oxygen, reducing the oxygen concentrations of the ambient air to 10% to 15%, leading to hypoxia of the victims. This obviously can be compounded by CO and by hydrogen cyanide (HCN) generated by fires consuming urethanes, polyacrylamides, certain plastics, nylon, and the natural fibers wool and silk. Water-soluble gases from rubber and plastic (such as acrylics and poly(vinyl chloride) fires can contain chlorine, ammonia, SO_2 and hydrogen sulfide (H_2S), which react with water in the respiratory tract to yield strong bases and acids. Lipid-soluble nitrogen oxides (NO_x), acrolein, various aldehydes, and other aromatic hydrocarbons are transported across pulmonary membranes. Particles of carbon and other contaminants also deposit in the respiratory tract and at high concentrations serve as irritants. Among firefighters, evidence of an acute bronchospastic response to smoke often occurs in those who have preexisting bronchial hyperresponsivity.

RESPIRATORY INFECTIONS ACQUIRED BY ENVIRONMENTAL AEROSOL EXPOSURE

A variety of organisms infect the respiratory tract consequent to dissemination by airborne routes (Table 6-9). Commonly, these organisms replicate independently of humans in unique but hospitable circumstances, but with some the origin is zoonotic. Individually and as a group, these various organisms have ecological niches into which humans enter and become infected. Because the organisms are not well-adapted human pathogens transmitted by person-to-person contact, they often are highly pathogenic for humans and cause fulminating disease, once infection occurs. Details of the epidemiology, pathogenesis, and pathology are beyond the scope of this chapter.

CANCER OF THE UPPER AERODIGESTIVE TRACT

Rare neoplasms of the nasal cavities are believed to have an environmental basis. Several studies have claimed a relationship of nasal adenocarcinomas with woodworking and exposure to processed and unprocessed hardwood dust.[2] Exposure to nickel fumes also is believed to be associated with carcinomas at this site.[66] Squamous cell carcinomas of the nasal cavity have been induced in rats experimentally by chronic inhalation exposure to formaldehyde vapor.[224] This observation has provoked considerable concern because of the widespread use of formaldehyde in the chem-

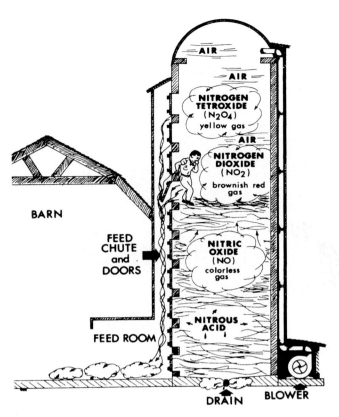

Fig. 28-36. Silo filler's disease. Diagrammatic illustration demonstrating the generation of nitric oxide from silage. Nitric oxide *(NO)* is rapidly oxidized to nitrogen dioxide *(NO₂)*, and nitrogen tetroxide *(N₂O₄)*, the more toxic elements of this series. A worker entering a silo immediately inhales high concentrations of these oxides of nitrogen in the absence of oxygen. Although the affect may be acute, it is often delayed for 24 to 48 hours (for unknown reasons). (From Ramirez RJ, Dowell AR: Silo fillers disease: nitrogen dioxide—induced lung injury, *Ann Inter Med* 74:569, 1971; with permission.)

ing welded. The processes also generate carbon monoxide (CO) and carbon dioxide (CO_2) as well as the various oxides of nitrogen and ozone. Fine particulates (the majority of which are less than 1 μ in diameter) (see under siderosis, previously) are also found in the air of the work environment. It is difficult to generalize regarding the health relevance of these exposures because working conditions are so variable. Metal fume fever sporadically develops in welders who are exposed to zinc-containing fumes, but fumes of other types of metals have been implicated as causes of the syndrome. It is a relatively transient condition characterized by "flu-like" symptoms of fever and chills, fatigue, headache, muscle aches, and digestive tract symptoms. Although chronic bronchitis seems to occur with increased frequency in welders, no compelling information has accumulated to suggest that the long-term exposure to welding fumes results in significant pulmonary parenchymal disease and cancer.

Roughly 2×10^6 people in the United States alone suf-

Pounds per Adult

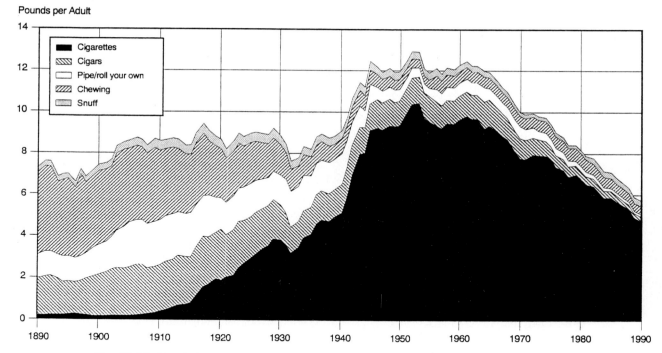

Fig. 28-37. Trends in tobacco use in the United States since the turn of the century. (From *Smokeless tobacco and health,* Publication No 93-3461, Washington, DC, 1993, US Department of Health and Human Services, National Institutes of Health.)

ical and manufacturing industries. In humans, an association of formaldehyde exposure with disease has not been demonstrated, despite efforts to explore this possibility.[145]

In North America, approximately 4% of the primary epithelial neoplasms of men and 2% of those in women originate in the oropharynx and larynx. Environmental factors play a key role in the development of these tumors, the vast majority of which are squamous cell carcinomas. Alcoholic beverage consumption imposes a substantial risk ($\times$ 4) on the occurrence of disease with a striking dosage relationship. Smoking also is a significant risk factor ($\times$ 10) at all sites.

Before 1940, consumption of smokeless tobacco was common worldwide (Fig. 28-37). Promoted by intense advertising, cigarette use mushroomed during and after World War II. The use of smokeless tobacco in the form of snuff and chewing tobacco is currently the most rapidly growing detrimental lifestyle change in the United States.[162] Snuff is a finely ground tobacco adulterated with sugar, licorice, and other additives. It is commonly used in the mandibular labial groove, although some users sniff it. Chewing tobacco is sold in the form of loose leaf, plugs, or twists and is held as a quid in the cheek. It, too, contains additives, which generally are trade secrets. Young males are the predominant users, and professional athletes such as baseball players seem to be habituated because of a tradition of the game. Surveys conducted

throughout North America in the 1980s indicate that about 8% to 10% of boys between ages 7 and 19 consume smokeless tobacco products. Worldwide usage is variable. With the exception of Sweden, the habit is not prevalent in Europe. In India and some southeastern Asian countries, plant product extracts (for example, betel nuts) mixed with lime and tobacco are used by up to 50% of both men and women in certain regions.

Chronic use of oral smokeless tobacco is followed by periodontal gingival recession, leukoplakia, and, on rare occasions, squamous cell carcinoma. Epidemiological survey data, however, are limited because of the somewhat subjective nature of the nonneoplastic lesions. The development of cancer would appear to require long-term, continuous usage, as is seen among residents of the Indian subcontinent and among an interesting subset of elderly white women in the southeastern United States who have chronically used dry snuff.[243] In the latter group, 81% of those with mouth cancer had a consumption history of 40 or more years. They consistently developed the lesion in the buccal and gingival areas where the quid customarily is held; oral squamous carcinomas are usually found at the base of the tongue or the floor of the mouth.

The effect of cigarette smoking is most pronounced in the intrinsic larynx, where the influence of alcohol consumption appears to be least. These two risk factors appear to interact in a multiplicative fashion, indicating that syn-

Table 28-8. Original early studies establishing the relative risk (RR) dose-response relationship of bronchogenic carcinoma with tobacco smoking in males.*

	Nonsmokers	Smokers	Number of cigarettes/day			
			1-9	10-20	21-39	>40
US veterans[122]	1	12	6	10	17	24
American Cancer Society volunteers[99]	1	10	5	9	15	19
British physicians[65]	1	18	8	20	32	—

*Table provides the RR of death related to cigarette use by number/day.

Table 28-9. Occurrence of five major types of lung cancer at Mayo Clinic and percentage not associated with smoking, by sex

Cancer type	Male		Female		Total cases
	No. of cases	% Nonsmokers	No of cases	% Nonsmokers	
Epidermoid	899	<1	93	16	992
Small cell	537	<1	103	3	640
Large cell	405	4	61	24	466
Adenocarcinoma	531	8	229	44	760
Bronchoalveolar	39	10	29	55	68
Total cases	2411	<0.01	515	28	2926

From Rosenow EC III, Carr DT: Bronchogenic carcinoma, *CA* 29:233, 1979.

ergistic, but poorly understood, mechanisms are involved.[74,228]

Several attempts have been made to associate laryngeal cancer epidemiologically with occupation.[26,248] Metal processors, machinists, and chemical workers consistently have been found to be at increased risk. In recent years, an association of laryngeal cancer with asbestos exposure has been claimed, but epidemiological studies have failed to establish a causative relationship.[71,188]

BRONCHOGENIC CARCINOMA

The role of tobacco combustion effluents in the causation of lung cancer in smokers and those in their immediate environment (sidestream smoke) is discussed in Chapter 13. Recently published data from a multicenter study provides additional new evidence emphasizing the importance of spousal smoking as a risk factor for bronchogenic carcinoma.[82a] Table 28-8 summarizes data from the landmark studies that established the association of lung cancer with tobacco use. A careful analysis of the data, however, shows that lung cancers do develop in nonsmokers (Table 28-9) although the pathogenesis of these infrequently occurring lesions is unknown. Accumulating evidence suggests that ill-defined heritable influences and dietary factors play a contributing role (see Chapter 9).[6,152,203] The age of first usage and thus the duration of consumption,[176] appears

to be more critical than packs per day consumption and cigarette tar content. Although lung cancer is still a disease that predominantly occurs among white men in the United States, changing patterns now strongly suggest that women and blacks may be unusually susceptible.[187]

In this section, other environmental exposures that increase the likelihood that cancer will occur in those who do not smoke are considered (Table 28-9). Although lung cancer is increasing in incidence in nonsmoking members of the world's population, the factors responsible for this change are not well-defined, largely because the question is difficult to address epidemiologically.

In 1981, Doll and Peto[67] suggested that 15% of lung cancers in the United States may be due to occupational exposure. More recent analyses provide support for this view. The number of cancers attributable to general environmental pollutants (such as radon) defies accurate calculation, although estimates have been advanced (see Chapters 2 and 3).[99]

Pathologists have focused considerable effort on attempts to associate specific histological types of bronchogenic carcinoma with various environmental exposures. The problem is complex because of potential sampling errors related to different diagnostic approaches, variability in the classification of tumors, and the importance of age and cigarette smoke dosage in influencing the development of different morphological types of cancer. As a generalization, the types of cancer commonly occurring in autopsied patients differ from the types found in patients undergoing surgery or among those diagnosed by cytological means. For example, squamous cell carcinoma tends to occur in older individuals, whereas small cell and adenocarcinoma develop more frequently in the young. An exhaustive analysis of this question was published by Ives and colleagues.[112] These authors concluded that the available data do not allow one to associate a specific histological tumor type with an exposure to recognized environmental respiratory carcinogens.

Ionizing radiation exposure (see Chapters 11 and 26)

An increase in lung cancer incidence among those exposed acutely to atomic bomb radiation in Japan has been reported. Before World War II, however, the likely role of radon and its daughter products in the causation of lung cancer among miners in central Europe was recognized. The risks again became evident when both smoking and nonsmoking uranium miners in the United States were found to develop lung cancer with an unusually high frequency.[135] In the smoker, the effect would appear to be additive, an indication of the genotoxic effects of the predominantly alpha particle radiation emanating from radon. During the past 10 years, household surveys in the United States have suggested that some individuals are chronically exposed to relatively high concentrations of radon. Calculations based on extrapolations from much heavier exposures suggest that significant numbers of the population may be at risk of developing bronchogenic cancer.

Low-level environmental exposure occurs at scattered sites worldwide where deposits of radioactive materials are found (see Chapter 3). In central Florida, uranium-238 is found in the naturally occurring phosphate deposits which are widely used for fertilizer. A twofold increase in lung cancer was observed among nonsmoking male residents of this area but not in females.[220] These findings require confirmation.

Silica dust exposure

Considerable controversy centers around the question — does silica cause bronchogenic cancer? There are no simple answers. In rats (but not in mice and hamsters), lifetime exposure to silica is clearly associated with an increase in the numbers of lung adenomas and adenocarcinomas. Because smoking is so common in blue-collar workers, it has been difficult to conduct critical epidemiological studies that could clearly establish an independent carcinogenic effect of silica in exposed workers. In addition, hard rock miners are exposed to radon, and industrial workers come in contact with pyrolysis products to a variable extent. These confounding factors thus far have prohibited the accumulation of definitive information on the role of silica in lung cancer, but my analysis of the enormous literature on

this topic leads me to conclude that heavily exposed individuals who smoke cigarettes may have a slightly increased likelihood of developing lung cancer.* Under these circumstances, chronic silica dust exposure may serve as a promoter, enhancing the effects of cigarette smoke (see Chapter 26). Published studies do not link silica exposure to a specific morphological type of cancer.

Asbestos dust exposure

In the mid-1930s, the occurrence of bronchogenic carcinoma in persons with asbestosis was first reported by pathologists.[89,143] Subsequently a statistical relationship was established.[64] In 1968, Selikoff and colleagues[202] noted a severalfold increase in lung cancer among asbestos workers who smoked. Cancer also was said to develop in nonsmoking asbestos workers, an observation suggesting that asbestos is a carcinogen in the airways. In recent years, the evidence supporting an independent role for asbestos in the pathogenesis of bronchogenic carcinoma has dwindled. Abundant documentation now indicates that asbestos serves as a promoter (see Chapter 26) in the pathogenesis of bronchogenic cancer in cigarette smokers when and if the exposure to the mineral is of sufficient duration and intensity to cause asbestosis.† Under these circumstances, asbestosis appears only to be an indicator of prolonged, heavy exposure to asbestos, although the possibility of "scar" carcinogenesis has been advanced by some pathologists.

Early literature suggested that adenocarcinomas occur commonly in those who are exposed to asbestos. Tumors also appeared to develop more frequently in the lower lobes of the lung than might be expected.[10,241] These observations may have been correct decades ago when asbestosis was common, but there is little evidence to support such a conclusion today. Indeed, epidemiological studies have clearly shown that cancers developing in asbestos workers are comparable in type and location to those occurring in the nonexposed population.

Heavy metal exposure

Exposure to salts of heavy metals (arsenic [As], mercury [Hg], nickel [Ni], Chromium [Cr])‡ in industrial aerosols has been linked epidemiologically to the occurrence of bronchogenic carcinoma among persons who are exposed for long periods of time. Case-control studies, however, have not been carried out, and experimental models in which cancer has been induced by aerosol exposure do not exist. The mechanisms whereby heavy metals cause neoplastic transformation in humans are obscure, despite considerable contemporary research (see Chapters 4 and 26). In addition, threshold considerations cannot be addressed because the epidemiological evidence is so sparse.

---

*References 54, 92, 103, 151, 169, 209.
†References 27, 40, 50, 70, 107, 128, 212.
‡References 57, 66, 91, 101, 166, 175, 196, 221, 226.

Bischloromethyl ether exposure

Chloromethyl ethers are a group of highly reactive alkylating agents that were widely used as chemical manufacturing intermediaries in the past (see Chapter 5). Exposure has been associated with the development of lung cancer in several epidemiological studies.[46] Paradoxically, exposed workers who smoke are at a substantially lower risk than nonsmokers, epidemiological observation that remains unexplained. Because of the recognized risk to industrial workers, use of these compounds has been eliminated or reduced to presumptively nontoxic levels in the workplace.

REFERENCES

1. Abraham JL: Lung pathology in 22 cases of giant cell interstitial pneumonia (GIP) suggests GIP is pathognomonic of cobalt (hard metal) disease, 3rd Internat. Conference on Environmental Lung Disease, Montreal, 1986.
2. Acheson ED, et al: Is nasal adenocarcinoma in the Buckinghamshire furniture industry declining? *Nature* 299:263, 1982.
3. Adamson IYR, Bowden DH: Pulmonary reaction to long and short asbestos fibers is independent of fibroblast growth factor production by alveolar macrophages. *Am J Pathol* 137:523, 1990.
4. Adesina AM, et al: Bronchiolar inflammation and fibrosis associated with smoking: a morphological cross-sectional population analysis, *Am Rev Respir Dis* 143:144, 1991.
5. Amandus HE, et al: Mortality of vermiculite miners exposed to tremolite, *Ann Occup Hyg* 32:459, 1988.
6. Ambrosone CB, et al: Lung cancer histologic types and family history of cancer, *Cancer* 72:1192, 1993.
7. Angervall L, Hansson G, Rockert H: Pulmonary siderosis in electrial welder: a note on pathological appearances, *Acta Pathol Microbiol* 49:373, 1960.
8. Aris RM, et al: Ozone-induced airway inflammation in human subjects as determined by airway lavage and biopsy, *Am Rev Respir Dis* 148:1363, 1993.
9. Arul KJ, Holt PF: Mesothelioma possibly due to environmental exposure to asbestos in childhood, *Int Arch Occup Environ Health* 40:141, 1977.
10. Auerbach O, et al: Histologic type of lung cancer and asbestos exposure, *Cancer* 54:3017, 1984.
11. Auerbach O, et al: Changes in bronchial epithelium in relation to cigarette smoking and in relation to lung cancer, *N Engl J Med* 265:253, 1961.
12. Auerbach O, et al: Smoking habits and age in relation to pulmonary changes. Rupture of alveolar septums, fibrosis and thickening of walls of small arteries and arterioles, *N Engl J Med* 269:1045, 1963.
13. Banaszak EF, Thiede WH, Fink JN: Hypersensitivity pneumonitis due to contamination of an air conditioner, *N Engl J Med* 283:271, 1970.
14. Banks DE, et al: Silicon nephropathy mimicking Fabry's disease, *Am J Nephrol* 3:279, 1983.
15. Banks DE, et al: Silicosis in silica flour workers, *Am Rev Respir Dis* 124:445, 1981.
15A. Bar-Ziv J, Goldberg GM: Simple siliceous pneumocmiosis in Negev bedouins *Arch Snv Health* 29:121, 1974.
16. Bascom R, et al: Eosinophilia, respiratory symptoms and pulmonary infiltrates in rubber workers, *Chest* 93:154, 1988.
17. Becklake MR, et al: Radiological changes after withdrawal from asbestos exposure, *Br J Ind Med* 36:23, 1979.
18. Bedrossian CWM, Bonsin S, Moran C: Differential diagnosis between mesothelioma and adenocarcinoma: a multimodal approach based on ultrastructure and immunocytochemistry, *Semin Diagn Pathol* 9:124, 1992.
19. Beton DC: Acute cadmium fume poisoning. Five cases with one death from renal necrosis, *Br J Ind Med* 23:292, 1966.
20. Bignon J, editor: *Health related effects of phyllosilicates,* NATO ASI Series, v G 21, Berlin, 1990, Springer-Verlag.
21. Blanc PD, et al: Morbidity following acute irritant inhalation in a population-based study, *JAMA* 266:664, 1991.
22. Blanc PD, et al: Asbestos exposure-cigarette smoking interactions among shipyard workers, *JAMA* 259:370, 1988.
23. Bolton WK, Suratt PN, Sturgill BC: Rapidly progressive silicon nephropathy, *Am J Med* 71:823, 1981.
24. Boucher RC, et al: The effect of cigarette smoke on the permeability of guinea pig airways, *Lab Invest* 43:95, 1980.
25. Brooks SM, Weiss MA, Bernstein IL: Reactive airways dysfunction syndrome (RADS): persistent asthma syndrome after high level irritant exposures, *Chest* 88:376, 1985.
26. Brown LM, et al: Occupational risk factors for laryngeal cancer on the Texas Gulf coast, *Cancer Res* 48:1960, 1988.
27. Browne K: Is asbestos or asbestosis the cause of the increased risk of lung cancer in asbestos workers? (editorial), *Br J Ind Med* 43:145, 1986.
28. Buechner HA, Ansari A: Acute silicoproteinosis: pathologic variant of acute silicosis in sandblasters, characterized by histologic features resembling alveolar proteinosis, *Chest* 55:274, 1969.
29. Buechner HA, et al: Bagassosis. A review, with further historical data, studies of pulmonary function, and results of adrenal steroid therapy, *Am J Med* 25:234, 1958.
30. Burke GW, et al: Allergic alveolitis caused by home humidifiers, *JAMA* 238:2705, 1977.
31. Caplan A, Cowen EDH, Gough J: Rhematoid pneumoconiosis in a foundry worker, *Thorax* 13:181, 1958.
32. Caplan A, Payne RB, Withley JL: A broader concept of Caplan's syndrome related to rheumatoid factors, *Thorax* 17:205, 1962.
33. Carroll N, et al: The structure of large and small airways in nonfatal and fatal asthma, *Am Rev Respir Dis* 147:405, 1993.
34. Casey KR, et al: Zeolite exposure and associated pneumoconiosis, *Chest* 6:837, 1985.
35. Chan-Yeung M, Lam S: Occupational asthma, *Am Rev Respir Dis* 133:686, 1986.
36. Charan N, et al: Pulmonary injuries associated with acute sulfur inhalation, *Am Rev Respir Dis* 119:555, 1979.
37. Chen W-J, et al: Aluminum induced pulmonary granulomatosis, *Hum Pathol* 9:705, 1978.
38. Cherniack M: *The Hawk's Nest incident: America's worst industrial disaster.* New Haven, 1986, Yale University Press.
39. Chlorine gas toxicity from mixture of bleach with other cleaning products—California, *JAMA* 266:2529, 1991.
40. Churg A: Asbestos, asbestosis, and lung cancer (editorial), *Mod Pathol* 6:509, l993.
41. Churg A: Chrysotile, tremolite, and malignant mesothelioma in man, *Chest* 93:621, 1988.
42. Churg A, Green FHY, editors: *Pathology of occupational lung disease,* New York, 1988, Igaku-Shoin Medical Publishers.
43. Churg A, et al: Small airways disease and mineral dust exposure, *Am Rev Respir Dis* 131:139, 1985.
44. Coates EO, Watson JHL: Pathology of the lung in tungsten carbide workers using light and electron microscopy, *J Occup Med* 15:280, 1973.
45. Cockcroft A, et al: Postmortem study of emphysema in coal workers and noncoal workers, *Lancet* 2:600, 1982.
46. Collingwood KW, Pasternack BS, Shore RE: An industry-wide study of respiratory cancer in chemical workers exposed to chloromethyl ethers, *J Natl Cancer Inst* 78:1127, 1987.

47. Corrin B, King E: Pathogenesis of experimental pulmonary alveolar proteinosis, *Thorax* 25:230, 1970.

48. Cowie RL: Silica-dust-exposed mine workers with scleroderma (systemic sclerosis), *Chest* 92:260, 1987.

49. Craighead JE: Current pathogenetic concepts of diffuse malignant mesothelioma, *Hum Pathol* 18:544, 1987.

50. Craighead JE: Do silica and asbestos cause lung cancer? *Arch Pathol Lab Med* 116:16, 1992.

51. Craighead JE: *Inorganic mineral particulates in the lung.* In Corn M, editor: *Selected topics in hazardous materials,* San Diego, 1993, Academic Press.

52. Craighead JE, Emerson RJ, Stanley DE: Slateworkers' pneumoconiosis, *Hum Pathol* 23:1098, 1992.

53. Craighead JE, et al: The pathology of asbestos-associated diseases of the lungs and pleural cavities: diagnostic criteria and proposed grading schema, *Arch Pathol Lab Med* 106:544, 1982.

54. Craighead JE, et al: Diseases associated with exposure to silica and nonfibrous silicate minerals, *Arch Pathol Lab Med* 112:673, 1988.

55. Crapo J, et al: Environmental lung diseases: relationship between acute inflammatory responses to air pollutants and chronic lung disease, *Am Rev Respir Dis* 145:1506, 1992.

56. Davies D, Cotton R: Mica pneumoconiosis, *Br J Ind Med* 40:22, 1983.

57. Davies JM: Lung cancer mortality among workers making lead chromate and zinc chromate pigments at three English factories, *Br J Ind Med* 41:158, 1984.

58. Davis GS: The pathogenesis of silicosis, *Chest* 89:166, 1986.

59. Davis JMG, et al: *Further studies on the importance of quartz in the development of coalworkers' pneumoconiosis,* Edinburgh, 1991, Institute of Occupational Medicine.

60. Davis JMG, et al: Variations in the histological patterns of the lesions of coal workers' pneumoconiosis in Britain and their relationship to lung dust content, *Am Rev Respir Dis* 128:118, 1983.

61. Davison AG, et al: Cadmium fume inhalation and emphysema, *Lancet* 1:663, 1988.

62. Davison AG, et al: Interstitial lung disease and asthma in hard-metal workers: bronchoalveolar lavage, ultrastructural, and analytical findings and results of bronchial provocation tests, *Thorax* 38:119, 1983.

63. Demedts M, et al: Cobalt lung in diamond polishers, *Am Rev Respir Dis* 130:130, 1984.

64. Doll R: Mortality from lung cancer in asbestos workers, *Br J Ind Med* 12:81, 1955.

65. Doll R, Hill AB: Mortality in relation to smoking: ten years' of observations of British doctors, *Br Med J* 1:1399, 1964.

66. Doll R, Mathews JD, Morgan LG: Cancers of the lung and nasal sinuses in nickel workers, *Br J Ind Med* 34:102, 1977.

67. Doll R, Peto R: The causes of cancer: quantitative estimates of avoidable risks of cancer in the United States, *J Natl Cancer Inst* 66:1191, 1981.

68. Dong W, et al: Centrilobular and panlobular emphysema in smokers: two distinct morphologic and functional entities, *Am Rev Respir Dis* 144:1385, 1991.

69. Dyer RF, Esch VH: Polyvinyl chloride toxicity in fires, *JAMA* 235:393, 1976.

70. Edelman DA: Does asbestosis increase the risk of lung cancer? *Int Arch Occup Environ Health* 62:345, 1990.

71. Edelman DA: Laryngeal cancer and occupational exposure to asbestos, *Int Arch Occup Environ Health* 61:223, 1989.

72. Edwards C, Carlile A, Rooke G: The larger bronchi in byssinosis: a morphometric study, *J Clin Pathol* 37:20, 1984.

73. Edwards C, et al: The pathology of the lung in byssinosis, *Thorax* 30:612, 1975.

74. Elwood JM, et al: Alcohol, smoking, social and occupational factors in the aetiology of cancer of the oral cavity, pharynx and larynx, *Int J Cancer* 34:603, 1984.

75. Epler GR, McLoud TC, Gaensler EA: Prevalence of asbestos pleural effusion in a working population, *JAMA* 247:617, 1982.

76. Erasmus LD: Scleroderma in goldminers on the Witwatersrand with particular reference to pulmonary manifestations, *S Afr J Lab Clin Med* 3:209, 1957.

77. Fatalities attributed to entering manure waste pits—Minnesota, 1992, *JAMA* 269:3098, 1993.

78. Fink J: *Hypersensitivity pneumonitis.* In Merchant J, editor: *Occupational respiratory disease,* Publication No 86-102, Washington, DC, 1981, US Public Health Service, Department of Health and Human Services.

79. Finklea JF, et al: Cigarette smoking and acute non-influenzal respiratory disease in military cadets, *Am J Epidemiol* 93:457, 1971.

80. Fischbein A, et al: Clinical findings among hard metal workers, *Br J Ind Med* 49:17, 1992.

81. Fishman AP, editor: *Pulmonary diseases and disorders,* ed 2, New York, 1991, McGraw-Hill.

82. Flury KE, et al: Airway obstruction due to inhalation of ammonia. *Mayo Clin Proc* 58:389, 1983.

82A. Fontham ETH, Correa P, Reynolds P: Environmental tobacco smoke and lung cancer in nonsmoking women. *J Am Med Soc* 271:1752, 1994.

83. Frieman DG, Hardy HL: Beryllium disease. The relation of pulmonary pathology to clinical course and prognosis based on a study of 130 cases from the U.S. Beryllium Case Registry, *Hum Pathol* 1:25, 1970.

84. Gardner LU: Pathology of so-called acute silicosis, *Am J Public Health* 23:1240, 1933.

85. Gelb AF, et al: Limited contribution of emphysema in advanced chronic obstructive pulmonary disease, *Am Rev Respir Dis* 147:1157, 1993.

86. Gibbs AR, Wagner JC: *Diseases due to silica.* In Churg A, Green FHY, editors, *Pathology of occupational lung disease,* New York, 1988, Igaku Shoin.

87. Gibbs AR, et al: Talc pneumoconiosis: a pathologic and mineralogic study, *Hum Pathol* 23:1344, 1992.

88. Giles RD, et al: Massive proteinuria and acute renal failure in a patient with acute silicoproteinosis, *Am J Med* 64:336, 1978.

89. Gloyne SR: Two cases of squamous carcinoma of the lung occurring in asbestosis, *Tubercle* 17:5, 1935.

90. Gloyne SR, Marshall G, Hoyle C: Pneumoconiosis due to graphite dust, *Thorax* 4:31:1949.

91. Goldberg M, et al: Epidemiology of respiratory cancers related to nickel mining and refining in New Caledonia (1978-1984), *Int J Cancer* 40:300, 1987.

92. Goldsmith DF, Guidotti TL, Johnston DR: Does occupational exposure to silica cause lung cancer? *Am J Ind Med* 3:423, 1982.

93. Goodglick LA, Kane AB: Cytotoxicity of long and short crocidolite asbestos fibers in vitro and in vivo, *Cancer Res* 50:5153, 1990.

94. Gough J, Rivers D, Seal RME: Pathological studies of modified pneumoconiosis in coal miners with rheumatoid arthritis (Caplan's syndrome), *Thorax* 10:9, 1955.

95. Gould VE, Smuckler EA: Alveolar injury in acute carbon tetrachloride intoxication, *Arch Intern Med* 128:109, 1971.

96. Greenberg SD, et al: Alveolar epithelial cells following exposure to nitric acid, *Arch Environ Health* 22:655, 1971.

97. Griffith DE, et al: Airflow obstruction in nonsmoking, asbestos- and mixed dust-exposed workers, *Lung* 171:213, 1993.

98. Hale KA, et al: Lung disease in long-term cigarette smokers with and without chronic air-flow obstruction, *Am Rev Respir Dis* 130:716, 1984.

99. Hammond ED: *Smoking habits and air pollution in relation to lung cancer.* In Lee DHK, editor: *Environmental factors in respiratory disease,* New York, 1972, Academic Press.

100. Haselton PS, McWilliam L, Haboubi NY: The lung parenchyma in burns, *Histopathology* 7:333, 1983.

101. Hayes RB: Review of occupational epidemiology of chromium chemicals and respiratory cancer, *Sci Total Environ* 71:331, 1988.

102. Heppleston AG: Silica and asbestos: contrasts in tissue response, *Ann NY Acad Sci* 330:725, 1979.

103. Heppleston AG: Silica, pneumoconiosis and carcinoma of the lung, *Am J Ind Med* 7:285, 1985.

104. Hillerdal G: Malignant mesothelioma 1982: review of 4710 published cases, *Br J Dis Chest* 77:321, 1983.

105. Hoeffler HB, Schweppe I, Greenberg SD: Bronchiectasis following pulmonary ammonia burn, *Arch Pathol Lab Med* 106:686, 1982.

106. Hoidal JR, Niewoehner DE: Lung phagocyte recruitment and metabolic alterations induced by cigarette smoke in humans and in hamsters, *Am Rev Respir Dis* 126:548, 1982.

107. Hughes JM, Weill H: Asbestosis as a precursor of asbestos related lung cancer: results of a prospective mortality study, *Br J Ind Med* 48:229, 1991.

108. Hunninghake GW, Crystal RG: Cigarette smoking and lung destruction, *Am Rev Respir Dis* 128:833, 1983.

109. Hunninghake GW, et al: Pathogenesis of the granulomatous lung diseases, *Am Rev Respir Dis* 130:476, 1984.

110. Hurley JF, et al: Coalworkers' simple pneumoconiosis and exposure to dust at ten British coalmines, *Br J Ind Med* 39:120, 1982.

111. Huuskanen MS, et al: Woolastonite exposure and lung fibrosis, *Environ Res* 30:29, 1983.

112. Ives JC, Buffler PA, Greenberg SD: Environmental associations and histopathologic patterns of carcinoma of the lung: the challenge and dilemma in epidemiologic studies, *Am Rev Respir Dis* 128:195, 1983.

113. Jacobs RR, et al: Bronchial reactivity, atopy, and airway response to cotton dust, *Am Rev Respir Dis* 148:19, 1993.

114. Jacobsen M, et al: *The relation between pneumoconiosis and dust exposure in British coalmines.* In Walton WH, editor: *Inhaled particles III,* Old Woking, Surrey, 1971, Unwin Bros.

115. Johnson BA, et al: Recurrence of sarcoidosis in pulmonary allograft recipients, *Am Rev Respir Dis* 148:1373, 1993.

116. Jederlinic PJ, et al: Pulmonary fibrosis in aluminum oxide workers, *Am Rev Respir Dis* 142:1179, 1990.

117. Jones JSP, editor: *Pathology of the mesothelium,* Berlin, 1987, Springer-Verlag.

118. Jones RN, et al: Abnormal lung function in polyurethane foam producers, *Am Rev Respir Dis* 146:871, 1992.

119. Jones RN, et al: Progression of asbestos effects: a prospective longitudinal study of chest radiographs and lung function, *Br J Ind Med* 46:97, 1989.

120. Jordan JW: Pulmonary fibrosis in a worker using an aluminium powder, *Br J Ind Med* 18:21, 1961.

121. Kaelin RM, Kapanci Y, Tschopp JM: Diffuse interstitial lung disease associated with hydrogen peroxide inhalation in a dairy worker, *Am Rev Respir Dis* 137:1233, 1988.

122. Kahn HA: *The Dorn Study of Smoking and Mortality among U.S. Veterans: Report on 8 1/2 Years of Observation,* National Cancer Institute Monograph 19, Washington, DC, 1966, US Government Printing Office.

123. Kark JD, Lebiush M, Rannon L: Cigarette smoking as a risk factor for epidemic A(H$_1$N$_1$) influenza in young men, *N Engl J Med* 307:1042, 1982.

124. Katzenstein A-L, Liebow AA, Friedman PJ: Bronchocentric granulomatosis, mucoid impaction, and hypersensitivity reactions to fungi, *Am Rev Respir Dis* 111:497, 1975.

125. Kauffman F, et al: Occupational exposure and 12-year spirometric changes among Paris area workers, *Br J Ind Med* 39:221, 1982.

126. Kern DG: Outbreak of the reactive airways dysfunction syndrome after a spill of glacial acetic acid, *Am Rev Respir Dis* 144:1058, 1991.

127. King EJ, et al: The action of different forms of pure silica on the lungs of rats, *Br J Ind Med* 10:9, 1953.

128. Kipen HM, et al: Pulmonary fibrosis in asbestos insulation workers with lung cancer: a radiological and histopathological evaluation, *Br J Ind Med* 44:96, 1987.

129. Kleinerman J, et al: Pathology standards for coal workers' pneumoconiosis, *Arch Pathol Lab Med* 103:373, 1979.

130. Koss M, et al: Pseudomesotheliomatous adenocarcinoma: a reappraisal, *Semin Diagn Pathol* 9:117, 1992.

131. Kraft M, et al: Cryptogenic constrictive bronchiolitis. A clinicopathologic study, *Am Rev Respir Dis* 248:1093, 1993.

132. Kuwano K, et al: Small airways dimensions in asthma and in chronic obstructive pulmonary disease, *Am Rev Respir Dis* 148:1220, 1993.

133. Lanza AJ, editor: *Silicosis and asbestosis,* New York, 1938, Oxford University Press.

134. Lapenas D, et al: Kaolin pneumoconiosis: radiologic, pathologic and mineralogic findings, *Am Rev Respir Dis* 4:282, 1983.

135. Lerchen ML, Wiggins CL, Samet JM: Lung cancer and occupation in New Mexico, *J Natl Cancer Inst* 79:639, 1987.

136. Liebow AA: *New concepts and entities in pulmonary disease.* In Liebow AA, editor: *The lung,* Baltimore, 1968, Williams & Wilkins.

137. Liebow AA, Carrington CB: The eosinophilic pneumonias, *Medicine* 48:251, 1969.

138. Liippo KK, et al: Hypersensitivity pneumonitis and exposure to zirconium silicate in a young ceramic tile worker, *Am Rev Respir Dis* 248:1089, 1993.

139. Linden M, et al: Airway inflammation in smokers with nonobstructive and obstructive chronic bronchitis, *Am Rev Respir Dis* 148:1226, 1993.

140. Liu D, et al: The effect of smoke inhalation on lung function and airway responsiveness in wildland fire fighters, *Am Rev Respir Dis* 146:1469, 1992.

141. Ludwig PW, Hoidal JR: Alterations in leukocyte oxidative metabolism in cigarette smokers, *Am Rev Respir Dis* 126:977, 1982.

142. Ludwig PW, et al: Cigarette smoking causes accumulation of polymorphonuclear leukocytes in alveolar septum, *Am Rev Respir Dis* 131:828, 1985.

143. Lynch JM, Smith WA: Pulmonary asbestosis: carcinoma of the lung in asbesto-silicosis, *Am J Cancer* 24:56, 1935.

144. Lynch JR: Brake lining decomposition products, *J Air Pollut Cont Assoc* 18:824, 1968.

145. Marsh GM, Stone RA, Henderson VL: A reanalysis of the National Cancer Institute Study on lung cancer mortality among industrial workers exposed to formaldehyde, *J Occup Med* 34:42, 1992.

146. Marx JJ, et al: Inhaled aeroallergen and storage mite reactivity in a Wisconsin farmer nested case-control study, *Am Rev Respir Dis* 147:354, 1993.

147. Mason GR: Alterations of pulmonary epithelial permeability caused by smoking and other injuries to the lungs, *Chest* 88:484, 1985.

148. Matthews JI, et al: Rounded atelectasis: a new criterion for benignancy, *South Med J* 79:767, 1986.

149. Matulionis DH, Traurig HH: In situ response of lung macrophages and hydrolase activities to cigarette smoke, *Lab Invest* 37:314, 1977.

150. McCaughey WTE, Kannerstein M, Churg J: *Tumors and pseudotumors of the serous membranes,* Atlas of Tumor Pathology, Fascicle 20, Washington, DC, 1985, Armed Forces Institute of Pathology.

151. McDonald JC: Silica, silicosis and lung cancer, *Br J Ind Med* 46:289, 1989.

152. McDuffie HH: Clustering of cancer in families of patients with primary lung cancer, *J Clin Epidemiol* 44:69, 1991.

153. McFadden ER Jr, Gilbert IA: Asthma, *N Engl J Med* 327:1928, 1992.

154. McLaughlin AIG, Harding HE: Pneumoconiosis and other causes of

death in iron and steel foundry workers, *Arch Ind Health* 14:350, 1956.

155. Misra NP: Effect of toxic gas inhalation on respiratory system in Bhopal gas victims, 7th Internat. Pneumoconioses Conference, 1988, Pittsburgh, Pa (abstract).

156. Morgan WKC, Kerr HD: Pathologic and physiologic studies of welders' siderosis, *Ann Int Med* 58:293, 1963.

157. Morgan WKC, et al: The effects of kaolin on the lung, *Am Rev Respir Dis* 138:813, 1988.

158. Morrissey WL, et al: Silo-filler's disease, *Respiration* 32:81, 1975.

159. Murphy RL, et al: The diagnosis of nonmalignant diseases related to asbestos, *Am Rev Respir Dis* 134:363, 1986.

160. Musk AW, Greville HW, Tribe AE: Pulmonary disease from occupational exposure to an artifactual aluminum silicate used for cat litter, *Br J Ind Med* 37:367, 1980.

161. Nagelschmidt G: The relation between lung dust and lung pathology in pneumoconiosis, *Br J Ind Med* 17:247, 1960.

162. National Cancer Institute: *Smokeless tobacco or health. An international perspective,* National Institute of Health, Publication No 93-3461, Washington, DC, 1992, US Department of Health and Human Services Public Health Service, National Institutes of Health.

163. Nemery B, et al: Rapidly fatal progression of cobalt lung in a diamond polisher, *Am Rev Respir Dis* 141:1373, 1990.

164. Niewoehner DE, Hoidal JR: Lung fibrosis and emphysema: divergent responses to a common injury? *Science* 217:359, 1982.

165. Niewoehner DE, Kleinerman J, Rice DB: Pathologic changes in the peripheral airways of young cigarette smokers, *N Engl J Med* 291:755, 1974.

166. Norseth T: The carcinogenicity of chromium and its salts, *Br J Ind Med* 43:649, 1986.

167. Oxman AD, et al: Occupational dust exposure and chronic obstructive pulmonary disease, *Am Rev Respir Dis* 148:38, 1993.

168. Orie NGM, Sluiter HJ, editors: *Bronchitis,* Assen, Netherlands, 1961, Charles C. Thomas.

169. Pairon JC, et al: Silica and lung cancer: a controversial issue, *Eur Respir J* 4:730, 1991.

170. Parker CW: Various roles of lipids and lipid metabolizing enzymes in inflammatory processes and their possible implications for therapy, *Am Rev Respir Dis* 135:S22, 1987.

171. Parkes WR: *Occupational lung disorders,* ed 2, London, 1982, Butterworth.

172. Patwardhan JR, Finckh ES: Fatal cadmium-fume pneumonitis, *Med J Aust* 1:962, 1976.

173. Pementel JC, Menezes AP: Pulmonary and hepatic granulomatous disorders due to the inhalation of mica dusts, *Thorax* 33:219, 1978.

174. Perez-Padilla R, et al: Mortality in Mexican patients with chronic pigeon breeder's lung compared with those with usual interstitial pneumonia, *Am Rev Respir Dis* 148:49, 1993.

175. Pershagen G: Lung cancer mortality among men living near an arsenic-emitting smelter, *Am J Epidemiol* 122:684, 1985.

176. Peto R: *There is no such thing as ageing, and cancer is not related to it.* In Likhachev A, Anisimov V, Montesano R, editors: *Age-related factors in carcinogenesis* (IARC Scientific Publications No 58), Lyon, 1985, International Agency for Research on Cancer.

176A. Policart A, Collet A: Deposition of siliceous dust in the lungs of inhabitants of the Saharian region, *Arch Ind Hyg Occup Med* 5:527, 1982.

177. Pratt PC: A rationale for evaluation of byssinosis, *N Carolina Med J* 51:447, 1990.

178. Pratt PC, Kilburn KH: *Extent of pulmonary pigmentation as an indicator of particulate environmental air pollution.* In Davies DN, editor: *Third international symposium on inhaled particles,* vol 2, London, 1971, Pergamon Press.

179. Pratt PC, Vollmer RT, Miller JA: Epidemiology of pulmonary le-

sions in nontextile and cotton textile workers: a retrospective autopsy analysis, *Arch Environ Health* 35:133, 1980.

180. Ramage JE Jr, et al: Interstitial lung disease and domestic wood burning, *Am Rev Respir Dis* 137:1229, 1988.

181. Ramirez RJ, Dowell AR: Silo-fillers disease: nitrogen dioxide-induced lung injury, *Ann Intern Med* 74:569, 1971.

182. Reger R, Morgan WKC: On talc, tremolite, and tergiversation, *Br J Ind Med* 47:505, 1990.

183. Reid L McA: Pathology of chronic bronchitis, *Lancet* 1:275, 1954.

184. Reisz GR, Gammon RS: Toxic pneumonitis from mixing household cleaners, *Chest* 89:49, 1986.

185. Reyes CN, et al: Pulmonary pathology of farmer's lung disease, *Chest* 81:142, 1982.

186. Richardson HB: Hypersensitivity pneumonitis—pathology and pathogenesis, *Clin Rev Allergy* 1:469, 1983.

187. Risch HA, et al: Are female smokers at higher risk for lung cancer than male smokers? A case-control analysis by histologic type, *Am J Epidemiol* 138:281, 1993.

188. Roggli VL, Greenberg SD, Pratt PC, editors: *Pathology of asbestos-associated diseases,* Boston, 1992, Little, Brown.

189. Rosenow EC III, Carr DT: Bronchogenic carcinoma, *CA* 29:233, 1979.

190. Rosenstock L: The relation among pulmonary function chest roentgenographic abnormalities, and smoking status in an asbestos-exposed cohort, *Am Rev Respir Dis* 138:272, 1988.

191. Ruckley VA, et al: Emphysema and dust exposure in a group of coal workers, *Am Rev Respir Dis* 129:528, 1984.

192. Ruettner JR: Foundry workers pneumoconiosis, *Arch Ind Hyg Occup Med* 9:297, 1954.

193. Saetta M, et al: Airway mucosal inflammation in occupational asthma induced by toluene diisocyanate, *Am Rev Respir Dis* 145:160, 1992.

194. Sakula A: Pneumoconiosis due to Fuller's earth, *Thorax* 16:176, 1961.

195. Samet JM, Tager IB, Speizer FE: The relationship between respiratory illness in childhood and chronic air-flow obstruction in adulthood, *Am Rev Respir Dis* 127:508, 1983.

196. Sawyer HJ: *Chromium and its compounds.* In Zenz C, editor: *Occupational medicine, principles and practical applications,* Chicago, 1988, Year Book Medical Publishers.

197. Schatz M, Patterson R, Fink J: Immunologic lung disease, *N Engl J Med* 300:1310, 1979.

198. Schwartz DA, Smith DD, Lakshminarayan S: The pulmonary sequelae associated with accidental inhalation of chlorine gas, *Chest* 97:820, 1990.

199. Seal RME, et al: The pathology of the acute and chronic stages of farmer's lung, *Thorax* 23:469, 1958.

200. Seaton A: Coal mining, emphysema, and compensation, *Br J Ind Med* 47:433, 1990.

201. Seaton A, et al: Pneumoconiosis of shale miners, *Thorax* 36:412, 1981.

202. Selikoff IJ, Hammond EC, Churg J: Asbestos exposure, smoking and neoplasia, *JAMA* 204:106, 1968.

203. Sellers TA, et al: Evidence for Mendelian inheritance in the pathogenesis of lung cancer, *J Natl Cancer Inst* 82:1272, 1990.

204. Shaver CG, Riddell AR: Lung changes associated with the manufacture of alumina abrasives, *J Ind Hyg Toxicol* 29:145, 1947.

205. Sheibani K, et al: Immunopathologic and molecular studies as an aid to the diagnosis of malignant mesothelioma, *Hum Pathol* 23:107, 1992.

206. Sheppard D, et al: Acute effects of routine firefighting on lung function, *Am J Ind Med* 9:333, 1986.

207. Sherwood Burge P: *Humidifier fever.* In Brewis RAL, Gibson GJ, Geddes DM, editors, *Respiratory Medicine,* London, 1990, Balliere Tindall.

208. Sherwood Burge P: *Occupational and environmental asthma.* In Clark TJH, Godfrey S, Lee TH, editors: *Asthma,* New York, 1992, Chapman & Hall Medical.

209. Simonato L, Saracci R: *Epidemiological aspects of the relationship between exposure to silica dust and cancer.* In Simonato L, Fletcher AC, Saracci R, Thomas TL, editors, *Occupational exposure to silica and cancer risk,* Lyon, France, 1990, International Agency for Research on Cancer.

210. Slavin RE, et al: Extrapulmonary silicosis: A clinical, morphologic, and ultrastructural study, *Hum Pathol* 16:393, 1985.

211. Sluis-Kremer GK: Silica, silicosis and progressive systemic sclerosis, *Br J Ind Med* 41:838, 1987.

212. Sluis-Kremer GK, Bezuidenhout BN: Relationship between asbestosis and bronchial cancer in amphibole asbestos miners, *Br J Ind Med* 46:537, 1989.

213. Sluis-Kremer GK, et al: Relationship between silicosis and rheumatoid arthritis, *Thorax* 41:596, 1986.

214. Smid T, et al: Dust- and endotoxin-related respiratory effects in the animal feed industry, *Am Rev Respir Dis* 146:1474, 1992.

215. Smith JP, Smith JC, McCall AJ: Chronic poisoning from cadmium fume, *J Pathol Bact* 80:287, 1960.

216. Snider GL, et al: The definition of emphysema, *Am Rev Respir Dis* 132:182, 1985.

217. Sobonya R: Fatal anhydrous ammonia inhalation, *Hum Pathol* 8:293, 1977.

218. Spain DM, Siegel H, Bradess VA: Emphysema in apparently healthy adults, *JAMA* 224:322, 1973.

219. Sprince NL, et al: Reversible respiratory disease in beryllium workers, *Am Rev Respir Dis* 117:1011, 1978.

220. Stockwell HG, et al: Lung cancer in Florida. Risks associated with residence in the Central Florida phosphate mining region, *Am J Epidemiol* 128:78, 1988.

221. Sunderman Jr FW: Recent advances in metal carcinogenesis, *Ann Clin Lab Sci* 14:93, 1984.

222. Sur S, et al: Sudden-onset fatal asthma. A distinct entity with few eosinophils and relatively more neutrophils in the airway submucosa? *Am Rev Respir Dis* 148:713, 1993.

223. Sweet LC, et al: Hypersensitivity pneumonitis related to a home furnace humidifier, *J Allergy Clin Immunol* 48:171, 1971.

224. Swenberg JA, et al: Induction of squamous cell carcinomas of the rat nasal cavity by inhalation exposure to formaldehyde vapor, *Cancer Res* 40:3398, 1980.

224A. Tapp E, et al: Sand pneumoconiosis in an Egyptian mummy, *Brit Med J* 2:276, 1975.

225. Thurlbeck WM: *Chronic airflow obstruction in lung disease,* Philadelphia, 1976, WB Saunders.

226. Tonning HO: Pneumoconiosis from Fuller's earth, *J Ind Hyg Toxicol* 31:41, 1949.

227. Trentin L, et al: Longitudinal study of alveolitis in hypersensitivity pneumonitis patients: an immunological evaluation, *J Allergy Clin Immunol* 83:577, 1988.

228. Tuyns AJ, et al: Cancer of the larynx/hypopharynx, tobacco and alcohol: IARC International case-control study in Turin and Varese (Italy), Zaragoza and Navarra (Spain), Geneva (Switzerland) and Calvados (France), *Int J Cancer* 41:483, 1988.

229. Vallyathan NV, Craighead JE: Pulmonary pathology in workers exposed to nonasbestiform talc, *Hum Pathol* 12:28, 1981.

230. Vallyathan NV, et al: Pulmonary fibrosis in an aluminum arc welder, *Chest* 81:372, 1982.

231. Vandenplas O, et al: Hypersensitivity pneumonitis-like reaction among workers exposed to piphenylmethane diisocyanate (MDI), *Am Rev Respir Dis* 147:338, 1993.

232. Von Essen S, et al: Organic dust toxic syndrome: an acute febrile reaction to organic dust exposure distinct from hypersensitivity pneumonitis, *J Toxicol Clin Toxicol* 28:389, 1990.

233. von Mutius E, et al: Prevalence of asthma and allergic disorders among children in united Germany: a descriptive comparison, *Br Med J* 305:1395, 1992.

234. Wagner JC: The sequelae of exposure to asbestos dust, *Ann NY Acad Sci* 132:691, 1965.

235. Warhol MJ, Hickey WF, Corson JM: Malignant mesothelioma. Ultrastructural distinction from adenocarcinoma, *Am J Surg Pathol* 6:307, 1982.

236. Warren CPW: *Overview of repiratory health risks in agriculture.* In Dosman JA, Cockcroft DW, editors: *Principles of health and safety in agriculture,* Boca Raton, Fla, 1989, CRC Press.

237. Weidemann HP, et al: Acute effects of passive smoking on lung function and airway reactivity in asthmatic subjects, *Chest* 89:180, 1986.

238. Weill H, Waddell LC, Ziskind M: A study of workers exposed to detergent enzymes, *JAMA* 217:425, 1971.

239. Weill H, et al: Health effects of tremolite, *Am Rev Respir Dis* 142:1453, 1990.

240. Weiss W: Cigarette smoke, asbestos, and small irregular opacities, *Am Rev Respir Dis* 130:293, 1984.

241. Whitwell F, Newhouse M, Bennett DR: A study of the histological cell types of lung cancer in workers suffering from asbestosis in the United Kingdom, *Br J Ind Med* 31:298, 1974.

242. Williams MK: Sickness, absence and ventilatory capacity of workers exposed to sulfuric acid mist, *Br J Ind Med* 27:61, 1970.

243. Winn DM, et al: Snuff dipping and oral cancer among women in the southern United States, *N Engl J Med* 304:745, 1981.

244. Wolbot GL: *Health effects of environmental pollutants,* St. Louis, 1973, CV Mosby.

245. Wright JL, et al: Diseases of the small airways, *Am Rev Respir Dis* 146:240, 1992.

246. Wyatt JP, Riddell ACR: The morphology of bauxite-fume pneumoconiosis, *Am J Pathol* 25:447, 1949.

247. Xu X, et al: Effects of cigarette smoking on rate of loss of pulmonary function in adults: a longitudinal assessment, *Am Rev Respir Dis* 146:1345, 1992.

248. Zagraniski RT, Kelsey JL, Walter SD: Occupational risk factors for laryngeal carcinoma: Connecticut, 1975-1980, *Am J Epidemiol* 124:67, 1986.

249. Ziskind M, Jones RN, Weill H: Silicosis, *Am Rev Respir Dis* 113:634, 1976.

250. Zwick H, et al: Effects of ozone on the respiratory health, allergic sensitization, and cellular immune system in children, *Am Rev Respir Dis* 144:1075, 1991.

Chapter 29

LIVER

J. W. Grisham

The liver is the first of the body's "lines of defenses" from potentially toxic environmental chemicals that are ingested;

The author is grateful to Theo Cantwell for editorial assistance and for her continuing help during the many revisions of this chapter. Dr. William B. Coleman kindly read and made trenchant comments on a near-final version.

through the splanchnic circulation, it receives the venous blood from virtually the entire gastrointestinal tract, which constitutes about two thirds of the total hepatic blood flow. Additionally, because it has a double source of blood, receiving arterial blood that constitutes about one third of its total blood supply from the systemic circulation, the liver also quickly encounters environmental pollutants that enter the body through the skin and lungs, the other major portals of entry of chemicals encountered in the environment. Because it is a major site of metabolism of chemicals, it is reasonable to assume that the liver may frequently be the site of lesions resulting from chemical toxicity. Numerous chemicals are hepatotoxic, as indicated by studies in experimental animals and case reports of exposed humans. Humans in many environments are exposed to generally low levels of polluting chemicals that clearly have hepatotoxic potential at high exposure dose.

The data reviewed here suggest that synthetic chemicals, at levels that currently pollute the environment, are not alone responsible for causing major liver diseases in humans. However, hepatocellular carcinoma, the liver disease that has received perhaps the most detailed etiological study, both in human populations and in experimental animals, is caused by multiple agents. In human populations, hepatocellular carcinoma may be caused by complex mixtures of agents, which may include polluting chemicals as components. Although the hepatic metabolism of chemicals and the pathogenesis of hepatocellular carcinoma in humans and rodents share general features, there are sufficient differences to cast doubt on the sensitivity and specificity of mice and rats as human surrogates for identifying specific hepatotoxic and hepatocarcinogenic agents that pose a risk to humans.

General aspects of the hepatotoxicity of environmental chemicals, emphasizing pathological lesions induced by chemicals in livers of experimental animals used as surrogates for humans exposed to similar chemicals, have been well presented already.[100,107,156] Instead of such a presentation of potential human diseases by interspecies analogy, this chapter focuses on hepatic toxicity and liver diseases and lesions as they have been documented to occur in humans in response to exposure to chemical pollutants in the environment. Chemical hepatotoxins in the environment are discussed in context with the major infectious and genetic causes of liver disease in humans, and the natural history and molecular pathogenesis of hepatocellular carcinoma in humans and rodents are compared.

STRUCTURAL PLAN OF THE LIVER

From the standpoints of blood supply and tissue perfusion pathways, cytological composition, and cellular properties, the liver is well structured to extract from the blood, metabolize, and excrete the plethora of chemicals that it receives. The structure of the hepatic parenchyma in humans resembles a sponge formed of hepatocytes organized into plates one cell thick. The sponge-work of hepatic plates is tunneled by unique capillary vessels (sinusoids) whose walls are fenestrated and lack a basal lamina separating blood and hepatocytes and through which blood flows at low pressure and low resistance. Each hepatocyte touches a sinusoid on at least two surface facets whose area is expanded by the presence of numerous short microvilli. This arrangement of blood vessels and hepatocytes, combined with the unusual structure of the sinusoids, permits intimate contact between the plasmatic components of the blood and the receptor-rich surfaces of hepatocytes. As a consequence, hepatocytes avidly extract solutes from the sinusoidal blood. Hepatocytes, which are equipped with the body's richest repertory of cytochrome P-450 enzymes (more than 20 types),[49,50] metabolize the chemicals extracted from the perfusing blood and excrete the metabolic products into blood, lymph, or bile. Bile is formed by the hepatocytes and excreted into the biliary canaliculi, which are intracellular channels formed by the modification of the membranes of the nonsinusoidal surfaces of two adjacent hepatocytes. Canaliculi connect with the bile ducts in portal tracts, which ultimately empty into the intestine. In addition to hepatocytes, the hepatic parenchyma contains several other types of cells, including sinusoidal endothelial cells, macrophages (Kupffer cells) located in the lumina of sinusoids, and fat-storing (Ito) cells located in the tissue space between sinusoids and hepatocytes. Each of these types of cells participates importantly in hepatic function.

Portal tracts contain the major connective tissue components of the liver as well as the larger branches of the afferent vessels, intrahepatic branches of bile ducts, lymphatic vessels, and nerves. Hepatic veins, the efferent vessels that drain blood from the liver, are lightly invested with connective tissue also. The parenchyma of the normal human liver is continuous throughout, lacking defined lobules

that can be dissected along connective tissue planes. Tissue patterns resembling lobulation are conferred by the courses taken by blood flowing between branches of afferent vessels (terminal branches of the hepatic artery and portal vein located in microscopic portal tracts), which supply blood to sinusoids, and the efferent vessels (terminal or centrolobular hepatic veins), which drain blood from sinusoids; microscopic portal tracts and terminal hepatic veins interdigitate in a regular pattern throughout the hepatic parenchyma. Hepatocytes are disposed in hepatic plates between the smallest portal and hepatic veins, and they are exposed to different microenvironments, depending on their location in hepatic plates relative to inflow and outflow of blood. Hepatocytes express different activities of several enzymes, including the enzymes that metabolize exogenous chemicals—the cytochrome P-450 enzymes and conjugating enzymes—related to their locations in hepatic plates.[41,69] The relative level of oxygen in the blood also varies significantly from afferent to efferent ends of sinusoids.[136] The heterogeneity of their structural and functional properties causes the hepatocytes in different parts of the hepatic plates to differ in their susceptibility to chemically induced toxicity.[105,106]

HEPATIC METABOLISM OF CHEMICALS

Chemicals are metabolized in the liver and other tissues by a generally biphasic process in which oxidation of the chemical substrates by cytochrome P-450 enzymes (phase I) is coupled with hydrolysis of epoxides and conjugation of polar groups to glucuronic acid, glutathione, or other compounds (phase II).[44] These metabolic pathways convert the highly lipophilic environmental chemicals to more hydrophilic forms that can be excreted. In phase I, the parental chemicals are converted to chemically reactive forms, many of which have increased toxic potential, and these reactive species are further modified in phase II by enzymatic introduction of groups that increase their water solubility and generally reduce their toxicity. The liver contains a rich repertory of cytochrome P-450 enzymes; more than 20 distinct cDNAs (complementary DNA) representing gene sequences from at least 7 subfamilies have been isolated from human liver cDNA libraries.[49,50] Substrate specificities of the enzymes coded by these cDNAs have been studied in detail, as have the levels of constitutive and induced expression of those forms represented in the liver. Four cytochrome P-450 enzymes, CYP1A2, CYP2A6, CYP2E1, and CYP3A4 (Table 29-1), appear to be responsible for the metabolism of the majority of the exogenous chemicals encountered by the human liver.[45] Enzymes of the CYP3 group, including CYP3A4, compose the major constitutively expressed enzymes in human livers.[45] The activities of other major hepatic forms of cytochrome P-450 are appreciably increased when induced, and the inducers themselves may be exogenous compounds, including environmental pollutants.[45,49,50] Furthermore, the genes for many

Table 29-1. Major features of the most important human cytochrome P-450 enzymes

CYP-450 type	Selected substrates	Selected inducers
1A2	Arylamines and heterocyclic arylamides, aflatoxin B1, acetaminophen, caffeine	Cigarette smoking, polycyclic aromatic hydrocarbons
2A6	Aflatoxin B1, N-nitrosodiethylamine	Polycyclic aromatic hydrocarbons
2E1	At least 15 promutagens and procarcinogens, including carbon tetrachloride, methylene chloride, vinyl chloride	Ethanol
3A4	Aflatoxin B1, pyrrolidine alkaloids, polycyclic aromatic hydrocarbons, numerous drugs	Barbituate drugs

From Guengerich FP, Shimada, T: Oxidation of toxic and carcinogenic chemicals by human cytochrome P-450 enzymes, *Chem Res Toxicol* 4: 391, 1991; with permission.

cytochrome P-450 enzymes show polymorphisms that affect their activities and inducibilities, which leads to marked heterogeneity in the capabilities of individual humans to metabolize xenobiotic chemicals.[25,45] The hepatic enzymes that are responsible for further modifying oxidized metabolites in phase II reactions include epoxide hydrolases, glutathione S-transferases, uridine diphosphate (UDP)-glucuronyl transferase, acetyltransferase, and sulfotransferase.[44] Activities of these enzymes also are affected by polymorphic variations that affect many individuals[25] (see Chapters 17 and 26).

MECHANISMS OF CHEMICAL HEPATOTOXICITY

The liver is vulnerable to toxic effects of exogenous chemicals largely from the action of metabolic products that are produced as the fat-soluble xenobiotic chemicals are modified so that they become soluble in water and can be excreted.[44] Even though most metabolites with toxic potential are contained without damage to the cells of the liver, the metabolic processes involved are multifaceted, complex, and finely balanced. During phase I, the oxidation of chemicals typically activates their toxic potentials, as highly reactive metabolites are produced for further metabolism in phase II reactions. Imbalance between phases of metabolism, including the increase in the activities of phase I enzymes or the depletion of substrates used for conjugation during phase II, can lead to the accumulation of toxic metabolites beyond the ability of the cell to cope with them, with the outcome that vulnerable components of the cell are

damaged and the cell may become pathologically deranged. Occurrence of polymorphisms in the activities of both phase I and phase II enzymes can cause some human individuals to be either more or less susceptible to the cellular damage caused by some chemicals.[25] Although the toxic potential of most metabolites resulting from phase I oxidations is reduced by phase II modifications, a few chemicals may be further activated to toxic or carcinogenic forms by phase II metabolism (Table 29-2). A few chemicals are metabolized partially or completely by enzymes other than the P-450 cytochromes, however, this monooxygenase system accounts for the metabolism of the majority of xenobiotic chemicals.

Mechanisms by which metabolic products may damage cell membranes and other vital cellular components include free radical attacks on lipid membrane components, covalent modification of integral membrane proteins and of DNA by chemical metabolites, and trapping of essential substrates.[104,120] In general, the intermediate metabolites that are formed during the biphasic metabolism of xenobiotic chemicals are strong electrophilic reactants,[44] which can form irreversible bonds with nucleophilic sites on cellular macromolecules. Modifications of tissue macromolecules by electrophilic attack lead to their malfunction and may result in cellular damage and death or neoplastic transformation.

CHEMICAL POLLUTION OF THE ENVIRONMENT

Many areas of the environment are polluted by chemicals, including some chemicals that are known to have hepatotoxic potential when either experimental animals or humans are exposed to high doses. Pesticides (the term is used to include fungicides, insecticides, herbicides, and rodenticides) and fertilizers that may produce liver injury are applied extensively to agricultural fields, gardens, forests, lawns, and golf courses. A wide variety of organic and inorganic chemicals, often in complex mixtures, are located in numerous underground chemical waste disposal sites, some of which were constructed without proper barriers to reduce leakage and allow chemicals to leach into the surrounding soil and underground water. Numerous subterranean storage tanks have leaked petroleum products into soil and water. Products of incomplete fuel combustion from automobiles, trucks, and airplanes and chemicals released from factories have led to further pollution of air, water, and soil with organic and inorganic chemicals that have hepatotoxic potential. Both soilborne and airborne chemical pollutants eventually find their way into surface water and groundwater.[48] Some drinking water sources now contain detectable levels of certain chemicals that have hepatotoxic potential.[117] Many foods are also contaminated with pesticide residues.[40] Residues of some chemicals that pollute the environment can be found in body tissues and secretions of human inhabitants of polluted areas,[68,85] indicating that significant exposures of humans occur.

Table 29-2. Inactivation and activation of protoxic and procarcinogenic chemicals by phase II enzymes

Enzymes	Inactivation	Activation
Epoxide hydrolases	*Majority* Butadiene, vinyl chloride Many herbicides, insecticides, and drugs	Benzo[a]pyrene-7,8-oxide
Glutathione S-transferase	*Majority* Benzene epoxide, aflatoxin B1-8,9-oxide Benzo[a]pyrene-7,8-dihydrodiol-9,10-oxide	Ethylene dibromide or ethylene chloride
UDP-glucuronyl transferases	*Majority* Phenols, dihydrodiols, guanines, and quinols of many chemicals, such as benzene, chlorinated benzenes, and benzo[a]pyrene	N-hydroxy metabolites of heterocyclic amines
Acetylation (Enzymatic-acetyl transferase or nonenzymatic)	Arylamines and hydrazines	Aromatic amines and food pyrolysates, including benzidine, 2-aminofluorene, 4-aminobiphenyl, and β-naphthylamine 2-acetylaminofluorene
Sulfotransferases	*Majority* Hydroxyl and amino group of many chemicals	

From Goldstein JA, Faletto MB: Advances in mechanisms of activation and deactivation of environmental chemicals, *Env Health Persp* 100:169, 1993; with permission.

Not all potentially hepatotoxic chemical pollutants in the environment are synthetic, however. Naturally occurring toxic chemicals are found in numerous plants used for food.[1] Mushroom toxins[150] and pyrrolizidine alkaloids,[82] from plants of the *Senecio* and related species, pose significant risks for hepatic toxicity in humans. Naturally occurring aflatoxins (from the fungi *Aspergillus flavus* and *Aspergillus parasiticus*) contaminate many food grains and the food products derived from animals that are fed contaminated grains.[65] Polycyclic aromatic hydrocarbons and heterocyclic amines may be produced during the cooking of meats at high temperature.[67,74] High levels of arsenic occur naturally in the groundwater in some parts of the world, associated with its accumulation in the tissues of water consumers.[147] Human populations are exposed to numerous environmental chemicals, either synthetic or natural, that have hepatotoxic potential.

LIVER LESIONS AND DISEASES ASSOCIATED WITH HEPATOTOXIC CHEMICALS

The major hepatic lesions and diseases, including those that are associated with exposure to hepatotoxic chemicals, are outlined in the box on the next page. Acute lesions evolve soon after exposure to a hepatotoxic agent and may develop after a single high-dose exposure. Chronic lesions generally evolve from acute lesions, as the result of repeated exposures to the same agent, or from the entrainment of a tissue process that evolves more or less autonomously over time following a single initiating exposure (such as the necrosis of hepatocytes and the subsequent replacement of necrotic parenchyma by collagenous connective tissue or the prolonged, multistep process of carcinogenesis). Exposure dose is important in determining tissue response. Heavy exposure to hepatotoxic chemicals may produce massive necrosis of virtually the entire population of hepatocytes, a situation that results in rapid functional failure of the liver and death of the affected person. Hepatocellular necrosis of a lesser extent may also lead to life-threatening chronic lesions, particularly if the necrosis recurs following repeated exposure to a toxic chemical. Acute hepatocellular deficits resulting from necrosis caused by chemical exposure are usually repaired rapidly by the healthy livers of all animals, humans included. In contrast, repeated hepatocellular necrosis, even of a relatively minor extent, may lead to the loss of hepatocytes at rates faster than new cells are produced; where dead hepatocytes have permanently "dropped out" of the tissue fabric, the supporting stroma collapses and aggregates, and additional collagen may be formed. The end result is a permanent collagenous scar that replaces the preceding area of hepatocellular necrosis.

Unless exposure to a hepatotoxic chemical is intense and results in massive necrosis, necrosis tends to occur selectively in hepatocytes located in areas of the relatively most vulnerable parenchyma.[105,106] An area that is particularly susceptible to the toxic potential of many chemicals is located in the vicinity of the terminal (centrolobular) hepatic veins and extends from centrolobular areas around the outsides of acinar units towards the adjacent portal tracts.[105,106] Hepatocytes in these areas share tissue microenvironments (including relatively poorer oxygen-

---

Some major hepatic lesions

Acute

Fatty liver

Hepatitis, with or without hepatocellular necrosis
    Scattered single cells
    Focal confluent
        Periportal or acinar zone 1
        Centrolobular or acinar zone 3
        Massive confluent

Porphyria
Cholestasis
    Canalicular
    Ductal
Biliary duct necrosis

Chronic

Fatty liver
Porphyria
Cholestasis
Hepatic enlargement
    Hypertrophy
    Nodular regenerative hyperplasia
    Focal nodular hyperplasia
Hepatitis
    Chronic persistent
    Chronic active
Hepatic fibrosis, with or without inflammation
    Portal
    Centrolobular
    Perisinusoidal
Vasculitis with subendothelial proliferation (veno-occlusive disease)
Cirrhosis
Neoplasms
    Epithelial
        Benign
            Hepatocellular, adenoma
            Biliary duct, adenoma
        Malignant
            Hepatocellular carcinoma
            Hepatoblastoma
            Cholangiocarcinoma
    Mesenchymal
        Benign
            Hemangioma
        Malignant
            Hemangiosarcoma

---

ation)[136] and cellular biochemical characteristics (including relatively lower cellular levels of reduced glutathione[125] and relatively higher levels of cytochrome P-450 Cyp 2E1[95,143]) that probably cause them to be most susceptible to the toxic effects of many chemicals. Such relatively vulnerable areas of liver parenchyma are repeated in each of the millions of microscopic vascular units (acini or lobules) throughout the organ. Persistently recurring focal areas of confluent necrosis, repeated in every microvascular unit in the entire organ, are replaced by bands of collagen that lead to fibrosis deposited uniformly in microvascular units throughout the liver.[98,105,106] Severe fibrosis dispersed throughout the liver segregates residual hepatocytes into parenchymal nodules, resulting in the condition termed cirrhosis.[98,106] Cirrhosis of the liver eventuates when the fibrosis is of such an extent and location that it obstructs the flow of blood through the liver, leading to the diversion of sinusoidal blood, hypertension in the portal venous system, and progressively increasing deficits in hepatocellular functions.

Hepatocellular cancers appear to evolve slowly from hepatic cells that bear the consequences of unrepaired genomic lesions by repeated clonal evolutions of populations of ever more abnormal cells.[91] Populations of altered cells that precede the development of hepatocellular cancer are especially prominent in rodents' livers, and include oval cells,[32,75,116] foci and areas of phenotypically altered hepatocytes, and benign hepatocellular adenomas.[7,79] Some or all of these aberrant populations of cells are thought to evolve sequentially to hepatocellular carcinoma.[7] Preneoplastic alterations in human livers are less well studied than are those in rodent livers, but they may include similar foci of phenotypically altered hepatocytes,[35] atypical hepatocytes,[3] and macroregenerative nodules (adenomatous hyperplasia).[34,140] Cirrhosis is a common accompaniment of hepatocellular carcinoma in humans[23,98] but not in mice,[144] and it is less common in rats than in humans.[6,130] Although most of the chemicals that cause hepatocellular carcinomas in experimental animals or humans can also cause acute and chronic hepatocellular necrosis, the chemical dose required for hepatocarcinogenesis in laboratory animals is typically much lower than is the dose required for hepatocellular necrosis and death of the animal.[81] Consequently, acute necrosis, chronic hepatitis, and cirrhosis are not seen often in rodents undergoing carcinogenesis tests.[57] Hepatocellular cancer, therefore, may occur in rodents and possibly in humans in the absence of cirrhosis if the carcinogen dose is in a critical, relatively nontoxic range.

Every type of cell in the liver tissue is susceptible to injury from the action of some toxic chemicals. It is beyond the scope of this chapter to present a comprehensive discussion of the effects of toxic chemicals on various types of liver cells. Two lesions—occlusive sclerosis of the smaller branches of the hepatic veins and angiosarcoma (a malignant tumor of sinusoidal endothelial cells)—that are caused by exposures to environmental chemicals illustrate toxic effects on cells other than hepatocytes. Sclerotic narrowing of small branches of hepatic veins (veno-occlusive disease) appears to arise from prior damage to the subendothelial tissues of these small vessels, especially by chemicals such as pyrrolizidine alkaloids.[12,82] Angiosarcomas are derived from endothelial cells of the hepatic sinusoids that have incurred genomic damage from exposure to certain chemical agents, such as vinyl chloride, arsenic, and radioactive thorium dioxide.[33,103] Experimental studies have shown that some types of chemicals exert high degrees of cell specificity in their hepatotoxic effects, producing, for example, numerous genomic lesions in certain types of cells in the liver while leaving other cells relatively unaffected.[72] The biochemical basis for this cell specificity of hepatotoxic action of chemical agents probably depends on the varying abilities of different types of liver cells metabolically to activate chemicals and to repair the lesions they produce, coupled with the transfer of toxic metabolites from one type of hepatic cell to another type.[132]

ASSESSMENT OF HEPATIC DAMAGE

Damage to the liver can be assessed indirectly by the measurement of analytes in the blood, including enzymes that leak from damaged hepatocytes, serum proteins (including coagulation factors) that are synthesized by hepatocytes, and bilirubin and other metabolic products that are secreted by hepatocytes into blood or bile (Table 29-3). The sensitive serum transaminase enzymes are found in several types of cells in addition to hepatocytes, and they leak into the serum when any of these cells are damaged or killed. Thus, measurement of transaminases unfortunately lacks the specificity required to detect liver damage per se. Biochemical tests of liver damage are most useful for assessing the evolution of liver disease in patients after the diagnosis has been established by a combination of clinical and laboratory studies, and disease in other tissues has been excluded.

Liver damage can also be assessed by examination of cells and tissue removed from the liver by transcutaneous biopsy. Although more expensive and cumbersome than measurement of serum analytes, cytological and histological analyses, including histochemical, immunohistochemical, and molecular methods of analyses, afford both fairly sensitive and specific methods to assess hepatic damage. Accumulation of water (cell swelling) or lipids (fatty change) in hepatocytes, interruption of bile flow (cholestasis), and presence of dead hepatocytes (either apoptotic or necrotic), with or without accumulations of inflammatory cells, afford incontrovertible evidence of hepatic damage. In addition, histological examination can demonstrate fibrosis (cirrhosis) and identify malignant cells. Application of immunohistochemical and molecular biological assays to cytological and histological preparations can provide information on the involvement of certain etiological agents and on the occurrence of lesions in specific macromolecules.

Table 29-3. Biochemical tests on blood used to assess hepatic damage

Test	Damage	Liver Specific	Sensitive
Biosynthetic activity			
Albumin level	Reflect chronic injury and diminished function	Yes	No
Prothrombin time			
Serum enzyme activity			
Aspartate aminotransferase	Reflect acute injury to hepatocytes	No	Yes
Alanine aminotransferase		Somewhat	Yes
Alkaline phosphatase	Reflect acute/chronic injury to hepatocytes and bile ducts	No	Yes
Gamma glutamyl transferase		No	Yes
Excretory products			
Bilirubin level	Reflects obstruction to bile flow and/or increased erythrocyte destruction or inability of hepatocyte to metabolize heme	Yes	Yes

EVIDENCE OF HUMAN RISK OF LIVER DAMAGE AND DISEASES FROM EXPOSURE TO ENVIRONMENTAL CHEMICALS

There is considerable evidence that certain chemicals that pollute the environment have the *potential* to produce hepatic damage in humans, when exposures occur in sufficiently high doses. This evidence comes from three types of observation: studies to evaluate the hepatotoxicity of chemicals in experimental animals, case reports of hepatotoxicity in individual or small groups of humans that have been exposed to chemicals, and epidemiological studies of populations of humans thought to be at risk from chemical exposure.

Experimental studies

Many synthetic chemicals and a few naturally occurring chemicals have been tested for their toxicities in experimental animals. For example, in the United States, the potential toxicity of many synthetic chemicals must be evaluated experimentally in studies required for registering a chemical product for agricultural or other environmental applications by the U.S. Environmental Protection Agency or for evaluating the potential toxicity of drugs and chemical additives or contaminants in foods by the U.S. Food and Drug Administration. Studies conducted by the U.S. National Toxicology Program (NTP), designed to test the carcinogenic potential of selected pure chemicals in lifetime studies in mice and rats, also include acute and chronic studies on target organ toxicities.[20] The NTP studies[61] and other studies reviewed and evaluated by the International Agency for Research on Cancer (IARC)[151] show that many of the tested chemicals are hepatotoxic or hepatocarcinogenic in these animals. In fact, the liver is the most common site of tumors induced in rats and mice by chronic exposure to chemicals at high doses.[151]

Uncertainties impair the confidence that animal studies performed at high exposure doses accurately identify chemicals that may damage the liver in humans exposed to low doses. Animal studies are typically performed at high exposure doses because the economics of toxicity testing precludes the use of the thousands of animals that would be required for studies at the generally low levels of exposure characteristic of exposures of humans in polluted environments. Exposure dose is an essential determinant of chemically induced hepatotoxicity, in terms of both cell necrosis and neoplastic transformation. High doses used in many experimental studies may saturate metabolic systems and perturb the metabolism of the chemicals being tested, possibly causing either more or less of the potentially toxic or carcinogenic metabolites to be produced.[132] For chemicals whose toxicity depends on metabolites, saturation of phase I enzymes may limit the production of toxic metabolites and therefore underestimate toxic potential, whereas saturation of phase II enzymes may lead to overproduction of toxic

metabolites and an overestimation of toxic potential. Uncertainty about the true relationship at low-exposure doses between chemical dose and toxic endpoint, either cell necrosis or cancer, makes equally uncertain the extrapolation of data from studies on toxicity of a chemical tested at high dose in experimental animals to determine the risk to humans from exposure to the same chemical at much lower dose. For virtually any chemical, the relationship of dose and toxic endpoint is ambiguous at low doses in any animal species. As a result of this dilemma, current methods used to extrapolate risk of chemical toxicity from high-dose studies on experimental animals may either overestimate or underestimate the true level of risk for humans exposed to the much lower levels of chemicals that are usually present in polluted environments.

A second area of uncertainty concerns the validity of extrapolating risk of chemical toxicity from that detected in laboratory animals to humans. Mice, rats, and humans differ in important pharmacokinetic aspects of chemical absorption and distribution[126] as well as in the details of specific metabolic pathways; some classes of cytochrome P-450s mainly involved in metabolism of exogenous chemicals in human livers have no exact counterparts in livers of mice and rats.[50] Although analyses of data from the NTP[61] and from the IARC reviews[151] show that the majority (but not all) of the chemicals that are proven human carcinogens are also carcinogenic for mice or rats (although not necessarily in the same tissues), other reviews have found only limited concordance between the hepatotoxicity per se of the same chemicals in experimental animals and in humans.[107,156] For the majority of the chemicals reviewed, although hepatotoxicity was readily detectable in experimental animals, it was often ambiguous in humans, possibly because data on human susceptibility to chemicals come mainly from case reports of unplanned, single-dose exposures. In addition to possible false-positive assignment of chemical risk to humans, animal studies may sometimes underestimate the risk to humans, by not detecting chemicals that are toxic to humans but not to the test animals (false-negative assignment).

A major difference between laboratory studies of chemical toxicity in experimental animals and real-life situations of chemical exposure in human populations pertains to the fact that most laboratory studies involve the exposure of highly inbred, genetically homogeneous strains of experimental animals to a single purified chemical, whereas most human environmental exposures are to complex mixtures of multiple chemicals, and the exposed human populations contain individuals of widely varying genetic backgrounds and susceptibilities to chemical toxicity. Few laboratory studies have been attempted on mixtures of chemicals, and the results of these studies demonstrate that the outcome is complex.[18,86] Mixtures of two or more chemicals of known individual toxic potential may show increased, decreased, or unchanged toxicity as compared with a single chemical, and increased toxicity may be additive or synergistic.[18] The ability to predict the toxicity of chemical mixtures from knowledge of the toxicity of the individual chemical components in the mixture is poor.[86]

Despite the difficulty of accurately delineating the risk of development of liver disease in humans from exposure to environmental chemicals by extrapolating from high-dose studies in laboratory animals, positive studies in experimental animals clearly indicate a general, if not precise, level of risk in humans. The ambiguity inherent in extrapolating animal studies to predict the risk to humans of exposure to environmental chemicals does not allay concern about potential human risk, especially if the animal studies yield a significant number of false assignments (either positive or negative) of chemical risk to humans, as seems possible.

Case reports of hepatotoxicity in humans

Reports of exposures of individual humans or groups of humans usually to high doses of selected chemicals resulting from consumption of foods that are heavily contaminated, from exposures in the workplace and during industrial accidents, and from ingestion accidentally or associated with suicidal or homicidal attempts corroborate the opinion that chemicals of types that are found in the general environment can damage the human liver when exposure doses are high. Although case reports of human exposure and toxicity are necessarily anecdotal and often lack important information, such as precise exposure data or adequate comparison with unexposed controls, they indicate, at least, the types of chemical hepatotoxins to which some humans are susceptible and the forms of hepatic pathological responses that may ensue.

Several excellent reviews of reports of hepatotoxicity occurring in human groups or individuals exposed to specific chemicals have been published.[43,100,107,156] Because no new edifying principles are evident from a perusal of these reports, they are not reviewed again here. The previous reviews may be consulted for the lists of hepatotoxic chemicals and the types of liver lesions associated with chemical exposures. Suffice it here to say that these reports of hepatotoxic events indicate that chemicals representing virtually every chemical class, including chemicals that pollute the environment, are potentially hepatotoxic at some dose in some individual humans. Furthermore, exposure to chemicals at high doses is associated with virtually every known type of acute and chronic liver lesion and disease in affected humans (see box on p. 495). However, because of the unplanned nature of most of these episodes of chemical exposure, and the consequent lack of many important data, the results do not contribute greatly to understanding the relative susceptibilities of humans (as compared with rodents) to the various chemical agents involved.

Therapeutic drugs are chemicals of various types that have medical utility. Hepatic metabolism of drugs involves the same pathways used to metabolize environmental chemicals, and drug-induced hepatotoxicity encompasses the entire spectrum of acute and chronic lesions of the liver listed in the box on p. 495. Furthermore, the dose of drug administered is usually well controlled, facilitating the analysis of dose dependency of drug-induced hepatoxicity. Because therapeutic drugs are not considered as environmental pollutants, however, a discussion of drug-induced hepatotoxicity is not included here. Excellent reviews of drug-induced hepatotoxicity are available.[131,156]

Epidemiological studies

Epidemiological studies of human populations are useful to identify agents and conditions that are associated with diseases in humans. Although human populations are clearly exposed to polluting chemicals with hepatotoxic potential, there has been little clear evidence from epidemiological studies of the occurrence of hepatotoxicity in human populations from synthetic chemical pollutants at levels encountered environmentally. Except in rare instances of exposure of a group of people to chemicals through consumption of well water grossly contaminated with chemicals leached from a chemical waste disposal site[16,145] or through consumption of grossly contaminated food,[19,70] there has been little clear evidence from epidemiological studies of the occurrence of hepatotoxicity in human populations from exposure to synthetic chemicals in the environment. The difficulty of detecting chemical-related toxicity in human populations and of firmly ascribing a toxic response to chemical exposure is illustrated by the general inability to detect toxic reactions, including hepatotoxicity, in groups of people living near leaking disposal sites for toxic waste chemicals.[16,48,145] For example, in the vicinity of a chemical waste site that contained 300,000 barrels of liquid and solid waste from a pesticide plant, water wells were found to contain up to 1900 μg/L of various chemicals, including carbon tetrachloride, hexachloropentadiene, and several other toxic chlorinated compounds.[27] A cross-sectional study of 49 local residents exposed to the pesticide-contaminated well water showed only mild hepatomegaly and mild, transient elevations in serum enzyme levels as compared with 59 unexposed controls. The extent of water use by individual affected residents or presence of chemicals in their tissues, however, was not ascertained (reviewed in Upton, Kneip, and Tonsolo[145]). Similar problems have affected other attempts to detect the hepatotoxicity of polluting chemicals.[16,48,145]

Failure to detect hepatotoxicity by epidemiological studies of populations thought to be exposed to hepatotoxic chemicals in the environment may have any of several possible explanations. Epidemiological studies may be handicapped by a lack of sufficient "power" to detect low levels of adverse health effects from exposure to environmental chemicals. Detection of diseases related to low levels of environmental pollution may be limited by study groups that are too small, by lack of data on exposures to chemicals of each individual in the populations studied, by insensitivity in the detection of acute hepatotoxic lesions or liver diseases, and by use of inappropriate or inadequate control populations. Furthermore, the complexity of the total environment in which humans live, including presence of infectious biotic agents and the variations in the personal habits of the members of the population under study that may also affect the incidence of liver diseases, can confound the interpretation of results and prevent the assignment of causality to specific environmental agents. Misattribution of exposures can readily confuse the interpretation of epidemiological studies. Indirect measures of exposure, such as the inclusion of all persons living within a certain distance from a potential source of exposure, must often be used in epidemiological studies whether or not all of these individuals had actually been exposed equivalently. New methods to measure exposure from the presence of chemicals or their metabolic products or from the molecular lesions they produce in target tissues ("molecular dosimetry") promise to improve the assessment of individual exposure. Detection and quantification of chemical adducts in albumin or hemoglobin, in genomic DNA, and in nucleosides from damaged DNA that are excreted in the urine appear to offer relatively specific and sensitive measures of recent chemical exposure and molecular injury.[62]

Although liver damage may occur in individuals exposed to environmental chemicals, such damage may not be of enough severity to be detected by the performance of laboratory tests for assessing acute hepatic damage, or an increased level of acute or chronic liver disease in the exposed population may not be differentiable from the background level of the same disease in the population under study. Unfortunately, none of the biochemical tests widely used in clinical medical practice to assess hepatic damage (Table 29-3) has sufficient specificity to detect subtle levels of liver injury per se (as opposed to injury to other tissue or to normal individual biochemical variations in serum enzyme levels) to enable their use to screen populations for hepatotoxicity resulting from chemical exposure. Even with a hypothetical test that is 95% sensitive and 95% specific for detecting liver damage, in a population in which liver damage occurs with the low frequency expected to be produced by low levels of environmental contamination, most of the "positive" test results are false positives.[38]

Cytological and histological methods to detect hepatic damage are sensitive but require invasive procedures of cell sampling and tissue biopsy that carry a small but appreciable risk to injure the subject. This situation and the fact that the techniques for analysis of cells and tissues are technically cumbersome and expensive preclude their use for screening for liver diseases in populations of chemically exposed individuals. These sensitive methods to assess liver damage, however, are appropriate for evaluating individual patients or small groups of patients who show clinical

and biochemical evidence of liver disease after having been exposed to known or potential hepatotoxic chemicals. Cytological and histological evaluation of liver tissue, in combination with biochemical tests, provides a sound basis for predicting the future condition of the damaged liver (prognosis) and for guiding and assessing the efficacy of treatment.

Even when microscopic evaluation of liver cells or tissue is feasible, the lack of specificity of the pathological response of the liver to different toxic agents poses a major handicap to the correct attribution of causality in studies of either individuals or populations. Environmental chemicals as a group do not produce hepatic pathologies that are distinct from those produced by other categories of causal agents, including viruses and radiation, and it is usually impossible from the examination of the pathological specimen alone to infer chemical-related causality. Low levels of hepatotoxicity and liver disease attributable to environmental pollution may occur in a population at risk but may be obscured because the slight increase in prevalence cannot be distinguished from the background level of liver diseases that are due to other causes but share identical expressions.

Perhaps reflecting the difficulty of detecting chemically induced hepatoxicity in human populations exposed to low levels of polluting chemicals, results of epidemiological studies on human populations have been judged by IARC to show conclusive evidence of hepatocarcinogenicity in humans by exposure to only three chemicals or chemical mixtures (aflatoxins, combined formulations of estrogenic steroid oral contraceptive mixtures, and vinyl chloride).[151] Evidence of chemically induced hepatocarcinogenicity in humans contrasts starkly with the studies at high dose in animals, which have incriminated hundreds of chemicals as rodent carcinogens and shown that the liver is the most frequent site of cancer development.[61,151] Certain identification of the three designated chemicals as human hepatocarcinogens was aided by features of their exposure or by the characteristics of the liver tumors that they produced. The populations of people exposed to estrogenic steroids in combined formulation and vinyl chloride monomer were easily identified and the levels of exposure were readily evaluated because the steroid combination was a prescription drug given to a limited population, and vinyl chloride monomer is an industrial chemical used in a small number of plants. Furthermore, both of these chemicals were associated with uncommon hepatic neoplasms (vinyl chloride monomer with angiosarcoma and contraceptive steroids with hepatocellular adenoma), which made their detection in the background of liver diseases in the general population relatively easy.[103] Identification of aflatoxin as a human carcinogen was aided no doubt by the high potency of this chemical as a hepatotoxin-hepatocarcinogen,[65] which increased the sensitivity of epidemiological studies to detect effects from exposure to relatively low levels of this chemical.

POSSIBLE CONTRIBUTIONS OF ENVIRONMENTAL CHEMICAL POLLUTANTS TO THE RISK OF HEPATOCELLULAR CANCER IN HUMANS

The most detailed knowledge of the worldwide prevalence of any liver disease in humans pertains to hepatocellular carcinoma. Hepatocellular carcinoma is one of the major causes of death from cancer in the entire world population; in 1985, about 300,000 cases of primary liver cancer occurred worldwide.[96] The incidence of hepatocellular carcinoma and the mortality from this disease vary dramatically from one area of the world to another; age-adjusted incidence rates for hepatocellular carcinoma among native male inhabitants of the United States and the countries of western Europe range from about 1.5 to 4 per 100,000 population, whereas similar rates in southeast Asia and southern Africa range from 11 to 113 per 100,000 population.[64] Such observations suggest that the variations in incidence of hepatocellular carcinoma reflect differences in exposure to hepatocarcinogenic agents in different regions. The possibility that chemical or biological (infectious) agents that contaminate the environment are responsible for this geographical variation in incidence has long attracted the attention of investigators. Although individual synthetic chemicals have not been shown to cause liver diseases in humans except at high dose, it is possible that environmental chemicals at low ambient levels may contribute to the risk of hepatocellular carcinoma in humans as components of multifactorial mixtures. Consideration of this possibility requires a brief review of the other well-established risk factors for this tumor in humans and of the evidence for its multifactorial etiology.

Chronic infection with hepatitis B virus

Chronic infection with hepatitis B virus, a human DNA virus of the hepadnavirus group, signaled by presence of hepatitis B surface antigen (HBsAg) in the serum, is strongly and specifically associated with the risk of hepatocellular carcinoma in humans (reviewed in the IARC monograph on hepatitis viruses[66]). Numerous retrospective case-control and prospective cohort epidemiological studies show that the relative risk of hepatocellular carcinoma from HBsAg-associated chronic liver disease is up to 200 times that for individuals who are HBsAg negative, when corrected for other confounding factors. Naturally occurring infections with hepadnaviruses related to hepatitis B virus in other animal species support the association between hepatitis B virus and hepatocellular carcinoma in humans. Infection of woodchucks in the eastern United States with woodchuck hepatitis virus and of Beechey ground squirrels in the western United States with ground squirrel hepatitis virus is closely associated with the development of hepatocellular carcinoma in these species.[77,78,101,102]

Chronic infection with hepatitis C virus

Hepatitis C virus (formerly known as nonA, nonB agent), an RNA virus distantly related to both pestiviruses and flaviviruses, is associated with acute and chronic liver diseases similar to those caused by hepatitis B virus (reviewed in the IARC monograph on hepatitis viruses[66]). Prevalence of infection by this agent, as measured by antibodies in the serum of patients, is strongly associated with the risk of developing hepatocellular carcinoma. Numerous case-control studies have shown that the relative risk for development of hepatocellular carcinoma was increased up to 134-fold in individuals who were positive for hepatitis C virus antibodies as compared with individuals lacking such antibodies.

Exposure to aflatoxins

Aflatoxin B_1 (AFB$_1$), the most potent of the aflatoxins, is a powerful hepatocarcinogen in many species, ranging from fish to humans (reviewed in the IARC monograph on aflatoxins[65]). Several epidemiological studies have shown a strong association between the estimated level of AFB in the diet and incidence of hepatocellular carcinoma in a population.[65] For example, a cohort study in which dietary AFB was estimated showed a seventeenfold increase in relative risk of hepatocellular carcinoma among individuals whose diet was estimated to be heavily contaminated and an increased relative risk of fourteenfold for individuals whose diet was estimated to be moderately contaminated as compared with individuals whose diet was lightly contaminated.[17] Until recently, epidemiological study of AFB hepatocarcinogenicity in humans has been hampered by a lack of methods to assess exposure of individuals in the populations evaluated. A prospective cohort study using the urinary excretion of AFB-N7-guanine adducts as a marker of exposure confirms the role of AFB$_1$ in hepatocellular carcinoma in humans,[111] with a relative risk of 7.8-fold. Studies also suggest that AFB exposure is associated with a specific mutation at codon 249 of the p53 tumor suppressor gene[14,60] (see Chapter 26).

Consumption of ethanol

Numerous epidemiological studies of the risk of hepatocellular carcinoma from ethanol consumption demonstrate significant associations. Relative risks of hepatocellular carcinoma in ethanol drinkers range up to fiftyfold compared with nondrinkers or drinkers of moderate amounts of ethanol (reviewed in Duffy and Sharples[30] and in the IARC monograph on alcohol drinking[64]).

Use of tobacco products

Epidemiological studies have shown an equivocal association of tobacco smoking with hepatocellular carcinoma. Cohort studies in which residual risk of tobacco use was determined after excluding the effects of other risk factors, such as hepatitis B virus infection and ethanol consumption, suggest a relative risk to development of hepatocellular carcinoma of 2.4-fold to 7.3-fold for persons smoking more than 30 cigarettes per day as compared with nonsmokers.[138] Other case-control studies, however, have not shown an association between tobacco smoking and hepatocellular carcinoma.[4]

Chemical pollutants in the environment

Epidemiological studies designed to detect a role for environmental chemical pollutants in the development of hepatocellular carcinoma have yielded equivocal results. Case-control studies have shown weakly positive or negative associations between jobs involving farming, highway construction, and usage of organic solvents, presumed to reflect exposure to pesticides, chemicals in paving materials, and various organic solvents, with odds ratios that range generally below twofold as compared with matched controls when corrected for other risk factors.[5,51,129] An elevated risk for the development of hepatocellular cancer (odds ratio increased 4.7-fold) was found in Vietnamese farmers, who said that they had used more than 30 L per year of organochlorine or organophosphorus pesticides before 1970.[22] Furthermore, this same study also associated residence in South Vietnam, in areas sprayed with Agent Orange, for more than 10 years with an increased risk of hepatocellular cancer (odds ratio increased 8.8-fold).[22] Although chronic infection with hepatitis B virus and consumption of ethanol were taken into account in this study, the possible confounding effect of dietary exposure to aflatoxin was not excluded. Furthermore, no association between service in South Vietnam and hepatocellular cancer has been found among American veterans.[115]

Cirrhosis

Cirrhosis appears to some investigators to be a risk factor for hepatocellular carcinoma in humans,[23] because this neoplasm usually occurs in the cirrhotic liver. This association, however, may reflect the fact that most of the agents that increase the risk of hepatocellular carcinoma in humans also cause acute and chronic lesions that eventuate in cirrhosis. Although this relationship between hepatotoxicity and hepatocarcinogenicity also obtains for mice and rats exposed to chemical agents, the carcinogenic dose for rodents is usually much smaller than is the toxic dose, allowing hepatocellular carcinoma to occur in the absence of cirrhosis at certain chemical exposures.[81] Although the relative susceptibility of humans to hepatotoxic and hepatocarcinogenic effects of various agents is not known, cirrhosis clearly is not an obligate precursor to hepatocellular carcinoma in humans; 10% to 40% of all hepatocellular carcinomas occur in otherwise normal livers, and in most instances, cirrhosis is not accompanied by liver cancer.[23] Cirrhosis is relatively common in human populations in all parts of the world, affecting from about 5% to 10% of most human population groups.[23] However, the frequency with which cirrhosis is complicated by hepatocellular carcinoma varies geographically,[23] possibly reflecting variations in the cause of this tumor. Hepatocellular carcinoma occurs most frequently (more than 15%) in cirrhosis caused by hepatitis B (and probably hepatitis C) virus infection and hemochromatosis, less frequently (5% to 15%) in cirrhosis caused by chronic alcoholism, and least frequently (less than 5%) in cirrhosis caused by Wilson's disease, chronic passive congestion, autoimmune hepatitis, and primary biliary cirrhosis.[23] Cirrhosis may promote the development of hepatocellular carcinoma indirectly because of the generally elevated rate of hepatocytic proliferation in regenerative nodules.

Multifactorial etiology of hepatocellular carcinoma

Development of hepatocellular carcinoma in humans may result from the combined action of more than one causative agent. A multifactorial cause of hepatocellular cancer was suggested by the demonstration that certain populations affected by a high incidence of hepatocellular carcinoma were characterized both by high levels of exposure to AFB_1 in the diet and by a high incidence of chronic infection by the hepatitis B virus.[97] In an epidemiological study in which it was possible to evaluate simultaneously AFB exposure and chronic infection with hepatitis B virus, both were shown to confer independent risk, and the combined risk appeared to be multiplicative.[153] Prospective studies, in which AFB_1 exposure was assessed by urinary AFB-N7-guanine adducts, corroborated these findings; HBsAg-positive, AFB-negative subjects showed an increased relative risk of 7.8-fold, whereas the relative risks for HBsAg-negative, AFB-positive subjects was 1.9-fold and that of HBsAg-positive, AFB-positive subjects was 60-fold.[111] Populations have been studied in which individuals are chronically infected by both hepatitis viruses B and C.[66] Analysis of several epidemiological studies for evidence of the separate effects of chronic infection with each virus showed that each infection conferred independent risk of hepatocellular carcinoma (antihepatitis C virus alone, relative risk increased up to 43.4-fold; and HBsAg alone, relative risk increased up to 17.7-fold) and suggested the possibility that conjoint infection with both viruses might multiply the risk of hepatocellular carcinoma (antihepatitis C virus and HBsAg combined, relative risk increased up to 517-fold) (see Tables 2.4.1 and 2.4.2 in the IARC monograph on hepatitis viruses[66]). The combined effects of the two viruses remain tentative, however, because of the small number of cases and controls that have been studied.[66]

Ethanol consumption may increase the risk of hepatocellular carcinoma from AFB exposure or from chronic infection with either hepatitis B or C. In an epidemiological study in which both AFB intake and ethanol consumption were estimated, heavy exposure to both agents was associated with a doubled risk of hepatocellular carcinoma as compared with the risk from heavy exposure to AFB alone (relative risk = thirty-five-fold versus seventeenfold, respectively).[17] Hepatocellular carcinoma occurring in livers of chronic alcoholics with cirrhosis has been shown to contain hepatitis B virus DNA integrated into the genomic DNA of tumor cells even in the absence of HBsAg positivity,[13] suggesting that hepatitis B virus had a role in the development of hepatocellular carcinoma in alcoholic cirrhosis. Epidemiological studies have also disclosed an association between excess ethanol consumption and hepatocellular carcinoma in patients infected chronically with either hepatitis B virus[93,94] or hepatitis C virus.[133] In some studies of other risk factors, tobacco smoking appears to confer moderately increased risk of hepatocellular carcinoma in individuals chronically infected with hepatitis B virus,[138,154] but other studies have not disclosed such an association.[4]

Taken together, these observations raise the possibility that risk to development of hepatocellular carcinoma in humans is predicated by a multifactorial mixture of etiological agents and that the components of the etiological mixture may vary in different parts of the world. Exposure to synthetic chemicals that pollute the environment may play an important role in the multifactorial etiology of hepatocellular carcinoma in humans. In recent years, the incidence of hepatocellular carcinoma has increased dramatically in Japan.[66,90] This increase in hepatocellular carcinoma is now attributed mainly to hepatitis C virus infection,[66,92] but some investigators speculate that other risk factors, including chemicals that pollute the environment, are involved.[92] An epidemiological study from Vietnam was interpreted to show that chronic infection with hepatitis B virus interacted with residence in South Vietnam for greater than 10 years (putatively reflecting exposure to chemical residues from Agent Orange) to strengthen the association with hepatocellular carcinoma.[22] No direct measure of chemical exposure was provided, however, and other potentially confounding factors were not excluded in this study. Further studies are needed to assess the potential involvement of environmental chemical pollutants in determining risk of hepatocellular carcinoma in human populations.

Additional risk factors for hepatocellular carcinoma

Additional risk factors may also interact with those already mentioned to form complex multifactorial mixtures that pose a risk for development of hepatocellular carcinoma in humans. Nutrition has been posited to account for up to 30% of the excess risk of cancer at all sites.[27] It was long suspected that nutritional deficiencies, especially protein-calorie malnutrition, were associated with various acute and chronic liver diseases, including fatty liver (kwashiorkor), cirrhosis, and hepatocellular carcinoma in sub-Saharan Africa[139] (see Chapter 9). As a reflection, early research on experimental production of hepatocellular carcinoma in rodents focused on nutritional deficiencies.[53,135] Despite the early incrimination of malnutrition as a cause of chronic liver disease in tropical countries, subsequent

studies have yielded a less clear picture. Much of the confusion has arisen because the geographical areas in which protein-calorie malnutrition is a problem often coincide with those in which foods are heavily contaminated with aflatoxins and in which the populations at risk show a high incidence of markers of past or current infection with hepatitis viruses B or C, or both. Specific epidemiological studies designed to evaluate a relationship between development of hepatocellular carcinoma and malnutrition in human populations have apparently not been performed. Studies in rats, however, in which effects of diet and of specific hepatotoxins-carcinogens can be readily analyzed, show that diets deficient in protein *reduce* the production of acute hepatotoxic necrosis as well as the development of hepatocellular carcinoma.[87] The mechanism by which dietary factors and chemical hepatocarcinogens may interact are numerous, but one of the more obvious is through the biphasic metabolism of protoxic, procarcinogenic chemicals. Both phases of chemical metabolism are markedly affected by dietary manipulations, especially by protein content and quality, as well as by the content of lipotropic factors and certain vitamins.[2,8] For example, hepatic levels of both cytochrome P-450 and glutathione are reduced by dietary protein deficiency.[2,8] Protein deficiency impairs the metabolism of most protoxic, procarcinogenic chemicals and therefore reduces their carcinogenic potential.[87] In contrast, deficiency of dietary methyl donors is hepatocarcinogenic in rats,[76] and markedly accelerates development of liver cancer from other agents in rats and possibly in humans.[87] Further nutritional studies are needed in human populations to assess fully the association of nutritional deficits and risk of chronic liver diseases, including hepatocellular carcinoma.

Other risk factors for chronic liver disease and hepatocellular carcinoma in humans include several inborn metabolic abnormalities, including hemochromatosis[11,88] and α_1-antitrypsin deficiency.[31] Although these inborn conditions each occur in only a small fraction of the general population, each confers increased susceptibility to development of hepatocellular carcinoma, estimated to range from 20-fold to 200-fold.[29] Chronic exposure to certain steroids, including contraceptive steroid formulations containing 17α-ethinylestradiol[110] and anabolic steroids,[10] confers increased risk for the development of benign hepatocellular adenoma and possibly for hepatocellular carcinoma. Polymorphic expression of hepatic enzymes that metabolize chemicals may also affect the susceptibility of the liver to chemically induced damage and therefore to hepatocellular carcinoma arising in affected patients. Abnormalities in the function of tumor suppressor genes involved in hepatocellular carcinoma development, such as the p53 gene, may also play a role. The p53 gene appears to be involved in hepatocellular carcinoma in humans resulting from AFB exposure[14,60] but not in hepatocellular carcinomas that are caused by other agents.[58] Individuals who suffer from the

Li-Fraumeni syndrome, however, which results from a germ-line mutation in one allele of the p53 gene, are apparently not known to be more susceptible to the development of hepatocellular carcinoma.[73]

Possible mechanisms of causal interactions

The mechanisms by which multiple risk factors for hepatocellular carcinoma, including chemicals, may interact are not known. It is not entirely clear whether the conjoint exposure to any two agents confers additive or multiplicative risk. Separate analysis of the effects of individual risk factors among combinations of risk factors is difficult to perform with conventional epidemiological studies. Not only is the precise measurement of exposure to multiple agents in each individual required, but also large at-risk and control populations are necessary to provide sufficient power for multivariate analysis. A plausible mechanistic point of interaction of multiple agents involves the hepatic cytochrome P-450 enzymes and the phase I oxidation and activation of chemical substrates. Aflatoxins, ethanol, tobacco smoking, and numerous environmental chemicals share the characteristic attribute of being able to induce the activities of specific cytochrome P-450 enzymes that are involved in the metabolism of these or other protoxic/procarcinogenic chemicals.[45,50] Ethanol, for example, is known to sensitize the liver to the hepatotoxic effects of a variety of chemicals through the mechanism of ethanol-induction of cytochrome P-450 2E1.[50] Evidence suggests that chronic infection with the hepatitis B virus is also associated with induction of certain P-450 enzymes and the ability of the liver to metabolize certain exogenous chemicals.[42] Generalized or specific induction of hepatic cytochrome P-450 enzymes could sensitize the liver to other agents that are metabolically activated by these enzymes.

Action through a common metabolic pathway (rather than the addition of the effects of two agents that confer risk by independent cellular pathways) offers a plausible mechanism for determining risk of hepatocellular cancer from multifactorial exposures. The metabolic activation and inactivation of potential hepatocarcinogens by hepatic phase I and phase II enzymes could represent such a common mechanistic pathway. Supporting this mechanism of multifactorial interaction, mathematical analysis of hepatocarcinogenesis data from areas of low and high incidence in human populations by the clonal emergence model suggests that acceleration of mutation frequencies in hepatic cells in high-incidence areas provides a good fit for the model.[128] Increased mutation frequencies in affected cells would be a plausible outcome of increased production of toxic metabolites from procarcinogens. The exploration of this possibility must proceed through future research studies, which now appear feasible, although not easy. Continuing studies, using more precise and sensitive means to measure exposures to multiple agents and hepatotoxic effects and including at-risk and control populations of sufficient size to detect multiple risk factors, are necessary to shed further light on the possible role of environmental chemicals in the causation of hepatocellular carcinoma as well as of other acute and chronic liver diseases in humans.

COMPARISON OF HEPATOCELLULAR CARCINOMA IN HUMANS AND RODENTS

Despite the fact that hepatocellular carcinoma is a common neoplasm both in humans and in rodents used to test chemicals for their carcinogenicity, and although chemicals that pollute the environment are potent hepatocarcinogens in mice and rats, the evidence that synthetic chemicals that pollute the environment are a major cause of hepatocellular carcinoma in humans is scant. This section considers this striking contradiction by comparing features of hepatocellular carcinoma and of the molecular mechanisms of hepatocarcinogenesis in humans and rodents. Both general similarities and major differences typify the development and expression of hepatocellular carcinoma in these three species (Table 29-4).

The histopathology of hepatocellular carcinomas of humans and rodents is strikingly similar,[24,63,114] although tumors in mouse livers tend to be better differentiated than are their counterparts in rats and humans. This feature makes it difficult to distinguish benign from malignant hepatic neoplasms in mice by histological criteria.* Aside from the close morphological similarities, there are major differences in the nonneoplastic lesions that precede hepatocellular carcinoma as well as in genetic and molecular alterations in the neoplastic cells in each species. The clinical course of hepatocellular cancer appears to differ substantially in humans and rodents. For example, in keeping with its relatively benign appearance, hepatocellular carcinoma in mice is a slowly progressive disease that does not appreciably shorten the life span of the affected animal,[114,144] whereas in humans, it is rapidly progressive and uniformly fatal.[24,99] As a corollary to the morphology and clinical course, hepatocellular carcinoma in mice rarely metastasizes[144] whereas metastases are common in humans and rats.[24]

Liver lesions that precede hepatocellular carcinoma

Humans and rodents differ considerably in the described lesions that precede hepatocellular carcinoma. In humans, development of hepatocellular cancer is usually preceded by recurring episodes of acute and chronic hepatocellular necrosis and inflammation.[23,99,103] Chronic hepatitis and cirrhosis occur in about 80% of humans who have hepatocellular carcinoma.[23,24,99,103] In contrast, cirrhosis rarely accompanies hepatocellular carcinoma in mice,[144] and this lesion is less common in rats than in humans.[6,114,130] The relative paucity of cirrhosis in mice and rats with hepatocellular carcinoma may reflect the fact that many hepato-

---

*References 6, 63, 99, 114, 130, 144.

Table 29-4. Comparison of hepatocellular carcinoma and hepatocarcinogenesis in humans and rodents

Feature	Humans	Rats	Mice
Clinical course	Rapid, fatal outcome	Rapid	Slow, life span normal
Morphology	Well-differentiated to poorly differentiated hepatocytes in trabeculae and pseudoglands	Same	Well-differentiated
Metastasis	Common	Occurs	Rare
Preceding/accompanying lesions			
Foci and nodules of phenotypically altered hepatocytes	Rare	Common	Common
Adenomas	Uncommon	Common	Common
Acute/chronic necrosis	Common	Occurs	Rare
Chronic inflammation	Common	Occurs	Rare
Cirrhosis	Common	Occurs	Rare
Atypical hepatocytes	Occur	Not recognized	Not recognized
Chromosomal lesions			
Nonrandom alterations	Yes	Yes	Unknown
Locus deletions	Yes	Unknown	Unknown
Tumor suppressor/loss/mutation			
p53	Yes	Yes	No
Other	Probable	Unknown	Unknown
Mutation of protooncogenes	No	Rare	Common in susceptible strains; uncommon in resistant strains

See text for literature citations.

carcinogenic chemicals are not highly hepatotoxic for these animals at doses that are carcinogenic.[57,81] The relative hepatotoxicity and hepatocarcinogenicity of various agents in humans is not known. In rats, hepatic reactions to some carcinogens are characterized by the florid proliferation of oval or ductular cells, which emerge from portal areas and spread throughout the lobular parenchyma.[75] Some investigators believe that oval cells are stem cell–like progenitors of hepatocytes and constitute the cell of origin of some hepatocellular carcinomas in the rat.[32] Cells morphologically and phenotypically similar to oval cells also may be related to the development of hepatocellular carcinoma in humans.[59]

A distinct group of lesions that involve hepatocytes has been described in mice and rats on carcinogenic regimens, and these lesions have been inferred to be precursors of hepatocellular carcinomas.[7] These lesions, which consist of focal proliferations of hepatocytes that express altered phenotypic properties (foci of phenotypically altered hepatocytes), hyperplastic foci, and adenomatous nodules,[7,79] are thought to represent hepatocytes that are progressing to cancer.[7] Foci of phenotypically altered hepatocytes are rarely recognized in livers of humans.[35] Although benign adenomas do occur in noncirrhotic livers of humans, these le-

sions are usually found in individuals exposed to certain steroid drugs and appear to confer only a modest risk to the ultimate development of cancer.[103] A lesion in cirrhotic livers, termed the macroregenerative nodule[34] or, alternatively, adenomatous hyperplasia,[140] has been posited to represent a precancerous lesion in human livers. This lesion may sometimes contain small foci of hepatocellular carcinoma,[140] suggesting that it is a precursor of this tumor. The relationship between macroregenerative nodules of cirrhotic livers and adenomas of noncirrhotic livers in humans is not clear, although they share common morphological features.[34] Although hepatocellular carcinomas sometimes develop in a setting of macroregenerative nodules in humans,[140] this sequence does not appear to be obligatory.[34] So-called atypical hepatocytes, containing hyperchromatic, polyploid nuclei, are also considered by some investigators to be a preneoplastic change in livers of humans.[3]

Chromosomal lesions

Cells from hepatocellular carcinomas in humans, rats, and mice all show genomic aberrations. Cells from liver cancers in humans contain structural abnormalities (rearrangements and translocations) in chromosomes as well as nonrandom losses of chromosomes or parts of chromosomes or of specific alleles. Human chromosomes 1, 5, 6, 7, 9, 17, 22, and X are involved in visible structural translocations and rearrangements,* whereas all or parts of chromosomes 1, 4, 5, 10, 11, 13, 16, 17, and 22 may be lost.† Most of these same chromosomal loci are also sites of integration of hepatitis B virus DNA, suggesting that integration of the viral DNA may have a causal role in some chromosomal aberrations.[80,121] Cells from liver cancers of rats also show recurring nonrandom structural abnormalities in chromosomes 1, 2, 3, 4, 6, 7, 8, 10, and 11.‡ Crossbreeding studies indicate that loci on mouse chromosomes 7, 8, and 12 may determine the relative susceptibility of various mouse strains to develop hepatocellular carcinoma.[39,46] Mouse chromosome 7, rat chromosome 1q, and human chromosome 11p contain a syntenic gene locus cluster[71] that appears to contain a gene or genes involved in the development of hepatocellular carcinoma in each species. Some of the other chromosomal sites nonrandomly affected in cells of hepatocellular carcinomas from humans, mice, and rats are also homologs that contain clusters of syntenically conserved gene loci.[71] These observations suggest the possibility that some of the same genes may be involved in the pathogenesis of hepatocellular carcinoma in these species. Studies to evaluate the deletion of specific alleles in hepatocellular carcinoma in rats have not been reported. Specific chromosomal structural abnormalities and locus deletions in hepatocellular carcinomas of mice have apparently not been reported.

Tumor suppressor gene loss/mutation

Some hepatocellular carcinomas in humans contain mutations in or deletions of the p53 gene, apparently reflecting the result of exposure to AFB_1.[14,60,64] The p53 gene, however, is not frequently affected in hepatocellular carcinomas resulting from chronic infection with the hepatitis B virus.[58] Some altered hepatocellular foci in rats have also been found to contain abnormal p53 protein.[122] Hepatocellular carcinomas produced in rats by some carcinogenic regimens contain mutations in the p53 gene,[123] whereas similar tumors produced in rats by other carcinogens do not contain p53 mutations.[124] In contrast, abnormalities in the p53 gene have not been identified in hepatocellular carcinomas of mice.[47]

Mutations of proto-oncogenes

Nearly all of the hepatocellular carcinomas in strains of mice highly susceptible to this neoplasm (C3H and CBA strains and their crosses[29]) contain mutations in the H-*ras* proto-oncogene§ in sharp contrast to cells from similar tumors in mice of resistant strains (A, DBA, BALB, and others) and in rats and humans. Only sporadic mutations in

K-*ras* and H-*ras* genes have been described in hepatocellular carcinomas from mouse strains resistant to this tumor,[28] or from similar tumors in rats[83] and humans.[141] The rarity of mutated *ras* genes in hepatocellular cancers of resistant mice, rats, and humans indicates that these mutated genes do not play an essential role in the pathogenesis of hepatocellular carcinoma in these species (see Chapter 26).

Comparing rodents and humans

This brief comparison of features of the natural history and molecular pathogenesis of hepatocellular carcinoma in humans and in rodents used for evaluating the carcinogenicity of chemicals shows that liver cancers in the three species are morphologically similar. It also discloses differences in the patterns of development and clinical progression and in the molecular pathogenesis of hepatocellular carcinoma among these species, extending earlier reviews of this topic.[29,99,114] Hepatocellular carcinomas in humans, rats, and resistant mice appear to share some genetic features, but the molecular pathogenesis of hepatocellular carcinoma in genetically susceptible mice appears to differ distinctly from that in the other species. Susceptible mice are also atypical in the relative benignity of liver cancer and in the almost total lack of preceding hepatocellular necrosis and accompanying cirrhosis. When coupled with the fact that livers of humans and rodents contain carcinogen-activating enzymes that differ in their metabolic specificities and metabolic products, the possibility that the three species may vary markedly in their susceptibilities to different carcinogenic chemicals seems likely. There appears to be little reason, therefore, to expect precise concordance between the chemicals that are carcinogenic for the livers of rodents and of humans. Nevertheless, it is likely that the reason that so many synthetic chemicals are proved hepatocarcinogens for mice and rats, and so few for humans, is that rats and mice are exposed to vastly higher doses in carcinogenicity studies than are the environmental levels to which humans are exposed.

REFERENCES

1. Ames B: Dietary carcinogens and anticarcinogens. Oxygen radicals and degenerative diseases, *Science* 221:1256, 1983.
2. Anderson KE, Kappus A: Dietary regulation of cytochrome P450, *Ann Rev Nutr* 11:141, 1991.
3. Anthony PP: Precursor lesions of liver cancer in man, *Cancer Res* 36:2579, 1976.
4. Austin H et al: A case-control study of hepatocellular carcinoma and hepatitis B virus, cigarette smoking, and alcohol consumption, *Cancer Res* 46:962, 1986.
5. Austin H et al: Case-control study of hepatocellular carcinoma, occupation and chemical exposure, *J Occup Med* 29:665, 1987.
6. Bannasch P, Zerban H: *Tumors of the liver*. In Turusov VS, Mohr U, editors: *Pathology of Tumors in Laboratory Animals*, ed 2, vol 1, *Tumors in the Rat*, Lyon, 1990, International Agency for Research on Cancer.
7. Bannasch P, Zerban H: *Predictive value of hepatic preneoplastic lesions as indicators in carcinogenic response*. In Vainio H, Magee PN, McGregor DB, McMichael AJ, editors: *Mechanisms of Carci-*

---

*References 56, 84, 119, 137.

†References 9, 24, 37, 89, 112, 118, 134, 142, 146, 148, 149, 155.

‡References 55, 113, 127.

§References 15, 28, 36, 46, 54, 108, 109, 152.

nogenesis in Risk Identification, IARC Scientific Publications No. 116, Lyon, 1992, International Agency for Research on Cancer.

8. Beutler E: Nutritional and metabolic aspects of glutathione, *Ann Rev Nutr* 9:287, 1989.

9. Beutow KH et al: Loss of heterozygosity suggests tumor suppressor gene responsible for primary hepatocellular carcinoma, *Proc Natl Acad Sci USA* 86:8852, 1989.

10. Boyd PR, Mark GJ: Multiple adenomas and a hepatocellular carcinoma in a man on oral methyltestosterone for eleven years, *Cancer* 40:1765, 1977.

11. Bradbear RA et al: Cohort study of internal malignancy in genetic hemachromatosis and other chronic non-alcoholic liver disease, *J Natl Cancer Inst* 75:81, 1985.

12. Bras G, Hill KD: Veno-occlusive disease of the liver: essential pathology, *Lancet* 1:960, 1957.

13. Brechot C et al: Evidence that hepatitis B virus has a role in liver cell carcinoma in alcoholic liver disease, *N Engl J Med* 306:1384, 1982.

14. Bressac B et al: Selective G to T mutations of p53 gene in hepatocellular carcinoma from southern Africa, *Nature* 350:429, 1991.

15. Buchmann A et al: Mutational activation of the c-Ha-ras gene in liver tumors of different rodent strains, correlation with susceptibility to hepatocarcinogenesis, *Proc Natl Acad Sci USA* 88:911, 1991.

16. Buffler PA, Crane M, Key MM: Possibility of detecting health effects by studies of populations exposed to chemicals from waste disposal sites, *Environ Health Perspect* 62:423, 1985.

17. Butalao-Jayme J et al.: A case-control dietary study of primary liver cancer risk from aflatoxin exposure, *Int J Epidemiol* 11:112, 1982.

18. Calabrese EJ: *Multiple Chemical Interactions,* Chelsea, Mich., 1991, Lewis Publishers.

19. Cam C, Nigosyan G: Acquired toxic porphyria cutanea tarda due to hexachlorobenzene: report on 438 cases caused by this fungicide, *JAMA* 183:88, 1963.

20. Chhabra RS et al: An overview of prechronic and chronic toxicity/carcinogenicity experimental study designs and criteria used by the National Toxicology Program, *Environ Health Res* 86:313, 1990.

21. Clark CS et al: An environmental health survey of drinking water contamination by leachate from a pesticide waste dump in Hardeman County, Tennessee, *Arch Environ Health* 37:9, 1982.

22. Cordier S et al: Viral infection and chemical exposures as risk factors for hepatocellular carcinoma in Vietnam, *Int J Cancer* 55:196, 1993.

23. Craig JR, Klatt EC, Yu M: *Role of cirrhosis in the development of HCC. Evidence from histologic studies in large populations.* In Tabor E, DiBisceglie AM, Purcell RH, editors: *Etiology, Pathology, and Treatment of Hepatocellular Carcinoma in North America,* Houston and London, 1991, Gulf Publishing.

24. Craig JR, Peters RL, Edmondson HA: *Tumors of the Liver and Intrahepatic Ducts, Atlas of Tumor Pathology,* 2nd series, fascicle 26, Washington DC, 1989, Armed Forces Institute of Pathology.

25. Daly AK et al: Metabolic polymorphisms, *Pharmac Ther* 57:129, 1993.

26. Ding SF et al: Loss of heterozygosity on chromosome 5q in hepatocellular carcinoma without cirrhosis, *Br J Cancer* 64:1083, 1991.

27. Doll R, Peto R: *The Causes of Cancer,* Oxford and New York, 1981, Oxford University Press.

28. Dragani TA et al: Incidence of mutations in codon 61 of the H-*ras* gene in liver tumors of mice genetically susceptible and resistant to hepatocarcinogenesis, *Oncogene* 6:333, 1991.

29. Dragani TA et al: *Genetics of hepatocarcinogenesis in mouse and man.* In Zervos C, editor: *Oncogene and Transgenics Correlates of Cancer Risk Assessments,* New York, 1992, Plenum Press.

30. Duffy SW, Sharples LD: *Alcohol and cancer risk.* In Duff JC, editor: *Alcohol and Cancer Risk,* Edinburgh, 1992, Edinburgh University Press.

31. Ericksson S, Carlson J, Velez R: Risk of cirrhosis and primary liver cancer in α_1-AT deficiency, *N Engl J Med* 314:736, 1986.

32. Evarts R: A precursor-product relationship between oval cells and hepatocytes in rat liver, *Carcinogenesis* 8:1737, 1987.

33. Falk H et al: Epidemiology of hepatic angiosarcoma in the United States: 1964-1974, *Environ Health Perspect* 41:107, 1981.

34. Ferrell L et al: Incidence and diagnostic significance of macroregenerative nodules vs. small hepatocellular carcinomas in cirrhotic livers, *Hepatology* 16:1372, 1992.

35. Fischer G et al: Histochemical and immunochemical detection of putative preneoplastic liver foci in women after long-term use of oral contraceptives, *Virchows Arch Cell Pathol* 50:321, 1986.

36. Fox TR et al: Mutational analysis of the H-*ras* oncogene in spontaneous C57BL/6 × C3H/He mouse liver tumors and tumors induced with genotoxic and nongenotoxic hepatocarcinogens, *Cancer Res* 50:4014, 1990.

37. Fumimori M et al: Allelotype study of primary hepatocellular carcinoma, *Cancer Res* 51:89, 1991.

38. Galen RS, Gambino SR: *Beyond Normality: The Predictive Value and Efficiency of Medical Diagnosis,* New York, 1975, John Wiley & Sons.

39. Garabaldi M et al: Chromosome mapping of murine susceptibility loci to liver carcinogenesis, *Cancer Res* 53:209, 1993.

40. Gartrell MD et al: Pesticides, selected elements and other chemicals in adult total diet samples, *J Assoc Official Anal Chem* 68:862, 1985.

41. Gebhardt R: Metabolic zonation of the liver: regulation and implications for liver function, *Pharmac Ther* 53:275, 1992.

42. Geubel AP et al: Increased Cyt P-450 dependent function in healthy HBsAg carriers, *Pharmac Ther* 33:193, 1987.

43. Gitlin N: *Clinical aspects of liver diseases caused by industrial and environmental toxins.* In Zakin D, Boyer TD, editors: *Hepatology. A Textbook of Liver Disease,* ed 2, vol II, Philadelphia, 1990, WB Saunders.

44. Goldstein JA, Faletto MB: Advances in mechanisms of activation and deactivation of environmental chemicals, *Environ Health Perspect* 100:169, 1993.

45. Gonzalez FJ: *Cytochrome P450 in humans.* In Shenkman JB, Greim H, editors: *Cytochrome P450,* vol 105, Born GV, Cuatrecasas P, Hellam H, editorial board, *Handbook of Experimental Pharmacology,* Berlin, Heidelberg, New York, 1993, Springer-Verlag.

46. Goodrow TL et al: Activation of K-*ras* by codon 13 mutations in C57BL/6 × C3HF$_1$ mouse tumors by exposure to 1,3-butadiene, *Cancer Res* 50:4818, 1990.

47. Goodrow TL et al: Murine p53 intron sequences 5-8 and their use in polymerase chain reaction/direct sequencing analysis of p53 mutations in CD-1 mouse liver and lung tumors, *Mol Carcinogen* 5:9, 1992.

48. Grisham JW, editor: *Health Aspects of the Disposal of Waste Chemicals,* New York, 1986, Pergamon Press.

49. Guengerich FP: Characterization of human cytochrome P450 enzymes, *FASEB J* 6:745, 1992.

50. Guengerich FP, Shimada T: Oxidation of toxic and carcinogenic chemicals by human cytochrome P-450 enzymes, *Chem Res Toxicol* 4:391, 1991.

51. Hardell L et al: Aetiological aspects of primary liver cancer with special regard to alcohol, organic solvents, and acute intermittent porphyria—an epidemiological investigation, *Br J Cancer* 50:389, 1984.

52. Harris RH et al: Adverse health effects of a Tennessee hazardous waste disposal site, *Hazardous Waste* 1:183, 1984.

53. Hartroft WS: Hepatic cancer. Nutritional factors and the production by dietary choline deficiency of cancer de novo in mice, *Gastroenterology* 37:669, 1957.

54. Heg ME et al: Analysis of activated protooncogenes in B6C3F$_1$

mouse liver tumors induced by ciprofibrate, a potent peroxisome proliferator, *Carcinogenesis* 14:145, 1993.

55. Hevens C et al: Cytogenetic changes in hepatocarcinomas from rats treated with chronic exposure to diethylnitrosamine, *Cytogenet Cell Genet* 60:45, 1992.
56. Hino C, Shows R, Rogler CE: Hepatitis B virus integration site in hepatocellular carcinoma at chromosome 17:18 translocation, *Cytogenet Cell Genet* 48:72, 1988.
57. Hoel DG et al: The impact of toxicity on carcinogenicity studies: implications for carcinogenesis risk assessment, *Carcinogenesis* 9:2045, 1988.
58. Hosono S et al: Infrequent mutation of p53 gene in hepatitis B virus positive primary hepatocellular carcinoma, *Oncogene* 8:491, 1993.
59. Hsia CC et al: Occurrence of oval-type cells in hepatitis B virus-associated human hepatocellular carcinogenesis, *Hepatology* 16:1327, 1992.
60. Hsu IC et al: Mutational hotspot in the p53 gene in human hepatocellular carcinoma, *Nature* 350:427, 1991.
61. Huff JE et al: Carcinogenesis studies. Results from 398 experiments on 104 chemicals from the US National Toxicology Program, *Ann NY Acad Sci* 534:1, 1988.
62. Hulka BS, Wilcosky TC, Griffith JD: *Biological Markers in Epidemiology,* London 1990, Oxford University Press.
63. Institute of Laboratory Animal Resources, NRC/NAS, Histologic typing of liver tumors in the rat, *J Natl Cancer Inst* 64:177, 1980.
64. International Agency for Research on Cancer, *IARC Monographs on the Evaluation of Carcinogenic Risks to Humans,* vol 44, *Alcohol Drinking,* Lyon, 1988, International Agency for Research on Cancer.
65. International Agency for Research on Cancer, *IARC Monographs on the Evaluation of Carcinogenic Risks to Humans,* vol 58, *Aflatoxins,* Lyon, 1994, International Agency for Research on Cancer.
66. International Agency for Research on Cancer, *IARC Monographs on the Evaluation of Carcinogenic Risks to Humans,* vol 59, *Hepatitis Viruses,* Lyon, 1994, International Agency for Research on Cancer.
67. Ito N et al: A new colon and mammary carcinogen in cooked food, 2-amino-1-methyl-6-phenyl-imadazo(4,5-g)pyridine (PhIP), *Carcinogenesis* 12:1503, 1991.
68. Jensen AA: Chemical contaminants in human milk, *Residue Rev* 89:1, 1983.
69. Jungermann K, Katz N: Functional specialization of different hepatocyte populations, *Physiol Rev* 69:708, 1989.
70. Koppelman H et al: The Epping jaundice, *Brit Med J* 1:514, 1966.
71. Levan G et al: The gene map of the Norway Rat *(Rattus norvegicus)* and comparative mapping with mouse and man, *Genomics* 10:699, 1991.
72. Lewis JG, Swenberg JA: DNA alkylation repair and replication in hepatocytes, Kuppfer cells and sinusoidal endothelial cells in rat liver during continuous exposure to 1,2-dimethylhydrazine, *Cancer Res* 43:4382, 1983.
73. Li FP et al: A cancer family syndrome in twenty-four kindreds, *Cancer Res* 48:5358, 1988.
74. Lijinsky W, Shubik P: Benzo(a)pyrenes and other polynuclear hydrocarbons in charcoal-broiled meat, *Science* 145:53, 1964.
75. Lombardi B: On the nature, properties and significance of oval cells, *Recent Trends Chem Carcinogen* 1:37, 1982.
76. Lombardi B, Chandcar N, Locker J: Nutritional model of hepatocarcinogenesis: rats fed a choline-devoid diet, *Dig Dis Sci* 36:979, 1991.
77. Marion PL et al: Hepatocellular carcinoma in ground squirrels persistently infected with ground squirrel hepatitis virus, *Proc Natl Acad Sci USA* 83:4543, 1986.
78. Marion PL et al: *Ground squirrel hepatitis virus and hepatocellular carcinoma.* In Koike K, Robinson W, Will H, editors: *Hepadna Vi-*

ruses (UCLA Symposia on Molecular and Cellular Biology, vol 70), New York, 1987, Alan R. Liss.

79. Maronpot RR et al: National toxicology program nomenclature for hepatoproliferative lesions in rats, *Toxicol Pathol* 14:263, 1986.
80. Matsubara K, Tokino T: Integration of hepatitis B virus DNA and its implication for hepatocarcinogenesis, *Mol Biol Med* 7:243, 1990.
81. McGregor DB: *Chemicals classified by IARC: Their potency in tests for carcinogenicity in rodents and their genotoxicity and acute toxicity.* In Vainio H, Mapee PN, McGregor DB, McMichael AJ, editors: *Mechanisms of Carcinogenesis in Risk Identification,* IARC Scientific Publications No. 116, Lyon, 1992, International Agency for Research on Cancer.
82. McLean EK: The toxic actions of pyrrolizidine (Senecio) alkaloids, *Pharmacol Rev* 22:429, 1970.
83. McMahon G et al: Characterization of c-Ki-*ras* and N-*ras* oncogenes in aflatoxin B1-induced rat liver tumors, *Proc Natl Acad Sci USA* 87:1104, 1990.
84. Meyer M et al: A chromosome 17:7 translocation is associated with a hepatitis B virus integration site in hepatocellular carcinoma DNA, *Hepatology* 15:665, 1992.
85. Murphy RS, Kutz KW, Strassman SC: Selected pesticide residues or metabolites in blood and urine. Specimens from a general population survey, *Environ Health Perspect* 48:81, 1983.
86. Nelson N: Perspectives in testing for toxic agents, *Environ Health Perspect* 75:97, 1987.
87. Newberne PM, Rogers AM: Labile methyl groups and the promotion of cancer, *Ann Rev Nutr* 6:407, 1986.
88. Niederau C et al: Survival and causes of death in cirrhotic and in noncirrhotic patients with primary hemochromatosis, *N Engl J Med* 313:1256, 1985.
89. Nishida N et al: Accumulation of allelic loss on arms of chromosomes 13q, 16q, and 17p in advanced stages of human hepatocellular carcinoma, *Int J Cancer* 51:862, 1992.
90. Nishioka K et al: A high prevalence of antibody to hepatitis C virus in patients with hepatocellular carcinoma in Japan, *Cancer* 67:429, 1991.
91. Nowell PC: The clonal evolution of tumor cell populations, *Science,* 194:23, 1976.
92. Okuda K, Kojiro M, Okuda M: *Neoplasms of the liver.* In Schiff L, Schiff ER, editors: *Diseases of the Liver,* ed 7, vol 2, Philadelphia, 1993, JB Lippincott.
93. Onishi K et al: The effect of chronic ethanol intake or development of liver cirrhosis and hepatocellular carcinoma: relation to hepatitis B surface antigen carriage, *Cancer* 49:672, 1982.
94. Oshima A et al: Follow up study of HBs Ag-positive blood donors with special reference to effect of drinking and smoking on development of liver cancer, *Int J Cancer* 34:775, 1984.
95. Palmer CNA et al: Localization of cytochrome P-450 gene expression in normal and diseased human livers by in situ hybridization of wax-embedded archival material, *Hepatology* 16:682, 1992.
96. Parkin DM, Pisani P, Ferlay J: Estimates of the world wide incidence of eighteen major cancers in 1985, *Int J Cancer* 54:594, 1993.
97. Peers RG et al: Aflatoxin exposure, hepatitis B virus infection and liver cancer in Swaziland, *Int J Cancer* 34:545, 1987.
98. Popper H: Pathologic aspects of cirrhosis. A review, *Am J Pathol* 87:228, 1977.
99. Popper H: Hepatic cancer in man: quantitative perspectives, *Environ Res* 19:482, 1979.
100. Popper H et al: Environmental hepatic injury in man, *Prog Liver Dis* 6:605, 1977.
101. Popper H et al: Woodchuck hepatitis and hepatocellular carcinoma: correlation of histologic with virologic observations, *Hepatology* 1:91, 1981.

102. Popper H et al: Hepatocarcinogenicity of the woodchuck hepatitis virus. *Proc Natl Acad Sci USA* 84:866, 1987.

103. Popper H et al: *Comparison of neoplastic hepatic lesions in man and experimental animals*. In Hiatt HH, Watson JD, Winston JA, editors: *Origins of Human Cancer, Book C, Human Risk Assessment*, vol 4, Cold Spring Harbor, NY, 1977, Cold Spring Harbor Press.

104. Potten CS, editor: *Perspectives on Cell Death*, Oxford, 1987, Oxford University Press.

105. Rappaport AM: The microcirculatory acinar concept of normal and pathological hepatic structure, *Beitr Pathol* 157:215, 1976.

106. Rappaport AM et al: The scarring of the liver acini (cirrhosis): tridimensional and microcirculatory considerations, *Virchows Arch Path Anat [A]* 402:107, 1983.

107. Reynolds ES, Moslen MT: *Liver and biliary tree*. In Mottet NK, editor: *Environmental Pathology*, New York, 1985, Oxford University Press.

108. Reynolds SH et al: Activated oncogenes in B6C3F$_1$ mouse liver tumors. Implications for risk assessment, *Science* 237:1309, 1987.

109. Richardson KK et al: Temporal changes in the mutant frequency and mutational spectra of the 61st codon of the H-*ras* oncogene following exposure of B6C3F$_1$ mice to *N*-nitrosodiethylamine (DEN), *Carcinogenesis* 9:271, 1988.

110. Rooks JB et al: Epidemiology of hepatocellular adenoma. The role of contraceptive use, *JAMA* 242:644, 1979.

111. Ross RK et al: Urinary aflatoxin biomarkers and risk of hepatocellular carcinoma, *Lancet* 339:943, 1992.

112. Sakai K et al: Loss of heterozygosity on chromosome 16 in hepatocellular carcinoma, *J Gastroenterol Hepatol* 7:288, 1992.

113. Sargent LM et al: Ploidy and specific karyotypic changes during promotion with phenobarbital 2,5,2′,5′-tetrachlorobiphenyl, and/or 3,4,3′,4′-tetrachlorobiphenyl in rat liver, *Cancer Res* 52:955, 1992.

114. Scarpelli DG: Comparative histopathology of the development of selected neoplasms of the liver, pancreas and urinary bladder in rodents, *Environ Health Perspect* 64:177, 1980.

115. Selected Cancers Cooperative Study Group: The association of selected cancers with service in the US Military in Vietnam. III. Hodgkin's disease, nasal cancer, nasopharylgeal cancer and primary liver cancer, *Arch Intern Med* 150:2495, 1990.

116. Sell S: The role of determined stem-cells in the cellular lineage of hepatocellular carcinoma, *Int J Dev Biol* 37:189, 1993.

117. Shy CM: Chemical contamination of the water supply, *Environ Health Perspect* 62:339, 1985.

118. Simon D, Knowles BB, Werth A: Abnormalities in chromosome 1 and loss of heterozygosity on 1p in primary hepatomas, *Oncogene* 6:765, 1991.

119. Simon D et al: Chromosomal rearrangements in a primary hepatocellular carcinoma, *Cancer Genet Cytogenet* 45:255, 1990.

120. Singer B, Grunberger D: *Molecular Biology of Mutagens and Carcinogens*, New York, 1983, Plenum Press.

121. Slagle BL, Zhou YZ, Butel JS: Hepatitis B virus integration site in human chromosome 17p near the p53 gene identifies the region of the chromosome commonly deleted in virus-positive hepatocellular carcinoma, *Cancer Res* 51:49, 1991.

122. Smith ML et al: Expression of mutant protein(s) in diethylnitrosamine-induced foci of enzyme altered hepatocytes in male Fischer 344 rats, *Carcinogenesis* 12:1137, 1991.

123. Smith ML et al: p53 mutations in hepatocellular carcinoma induced by a choline-devoid diet in male Fischer 344 rats, *Carcinogenesis* 14:503, 1993.

124. Smith ML et al: Lack of mutation of p53 tumor suppressor gene in hepatocellular carcinoma induced in rats by a peroxisome proliferator, *Mol Carcinogen* 7:89, 1993.

125. Smith MT et al: The distribution of glutathione in the rat liver lobule, *Biochem J* 182:1103, 1979.

126. Standaert FG: Absorption and distribution of xenobiotics, *Environ Health Perspect* 77:63, 1988.

127. Steadman JS et al: DNA contents and chromosomes of transformed rat liver epithelial cells and cells from their derived tumors, *Carcinogenesis*, 1994, in press.

128. Stein WD: Analysis of cancer incidence data on the basis of multistage and clonal models, *Adv Cancer Res* 56:161, 1991.

129. Stemhagen A et al: Occupational risk factors and liver cancer. A retrospective case-control study of primary liver cancer in New Jersey, *Am J Epidemiol* 117:443, 1983.

130. Stewart HL: *Comparative aspects of certain cancers*. In Becker FF, editor: *Cancer, A Comprehensive Treatise, vol 4, Biology of Tumors*, New York and London, 1975, Plenum Press.

131. Stricker BHCH: *Drug-induced Hepatic Injury*, ed 2, Amsterdam, 1992, Elsevier.

132. Swenberg JA et al: *Relationship between carcinogen exposure, DNA adducts and carcinogenesis*. In Clayson DB et al, editors: *Progress in Predictive Toxicology*, Amsterdam, 1990, Elsevier Science Publishers.

133. Takada A, Takase S, Tsutsumi M: *Alcohol and hepatic carcinogenesis*. In Yirmiya R, Taylor AM, editors: *Alcohol, Immunity, and Cancer*, Boca Raton, Fla, 1993, CRC Press.

134. Takahashi T et al: Frequent loss of heterozygosity on chromsome 22 in hepatocellular carcinoma, *Hepatology* 17:794, 1993.

135. Tannenbaum A: Nutritional factors in the formation of hepatic cancer, *Acta Unio Contra Cancrum* 13:847, 1957.

136. Thurman RG, Ji S, LeMasters JJ: *Lobular oxygen gradients: possible role in alcohol-induced hepatotoxicity*. In Thurman RG, Kauffman FC, Jungerman K, editors: *Regulation of Hepatic Metabolism*, New York, 1986, Plenum Press.

137. Tokino T et al: Chromosome translocation and inverted duplication associated with integrated hepatitis B virus in hepatocellular carcinoma, *J Virol* 61:3848, 1987.

138. Trichopoulos D et al: Smoking and hepatitis B-negative hepatocellular carcinoma, *J Natl Cancer Inst* 65:111, 1980.

139. Trowell HC et al: Definition of Kwashiorkor and its relationship to cirrhosis and primary carcinoma of the liver, *Acta Unio Contra Cancrum* 13:543, 1957.

140. Tsuda H et al: Clonal origin of atypical adenomatous hyperplasia of the liver and clonal identity with hepatocellular carcinoma, *Gastroenterology* 95:1664, 1988.

141. Tsuda H et al: Low incidence of point mutations of c-Ki-*ras* and N-*ras* oncogenes in human hepatocellular carcinoma, *Jpn J Cancer Res* 80:196, 1989.

142. Tsuda H et al: Allele loss on chromosome 16 associate with progression of human hepatocellular carcinoma, *Proc Natl Acad Sci USA* 87:6791, 1990.

143. Tsutsumi M et al: The intralobular distribution of ethanol inducible P450IIE1 in rat and human liver, *Hepatology* 10:437, 1989.

144. Turusov VS, Takayama S: *Tumors of the liver*. In Turusov VS, editor: *Pathology of Tumors in the Laboratory Mouse*, vol II, Lyon, 1979, International Agency for Cancer Research.

145. Upton AC, Kneip T, Tonsolo P: Public health aspects of toxic chemical disposal sites, *Ann Rev Public Health* 10:1, 1989.

146. Urano Y et al: Interstitial chromosomal deletion within 4q11-q13 in a human hepatoma cell line, *Cancer Res* 51:1460, 1991.

147. Valentine JL, Kavy HK, Spivey G: Arsenic levels in human blood, urine and hair in response to exposure via drinking water, *Environ Res* 20:24, 1979.

148. Walker GJ et al: Loss of heterozygosity in hepatocellular carcinoma, *Cancer Res* 51:4367, 1991.

149. Wang HP, Rogler CE: Deletions in human chromosome arms 11p and 13q in primary hepatocellular carcinoma, *Cytogenet Cell Genet* 48:72, 1988.

150. Wieland T: Poisonous principles of mushrooms of the genus *Amanita, Science* 159:945, 1968.

151. Wilbourn J et al: Response of experimental animals to carcinogens: an analysis based upon the IARC Monographs Programme, *Carcinogenesis* 7:1853, 1986.

152. Wiseman RW et al: Activating mutations of the c-Ha-*ras* protooncogene in chemically induced hepatomas of the male B6C3F$_1$ mouse, *Proc Natl Acad Sci USA* 80:5822, 1986.

153. Yeh FS, Mo C-S, Yen RC: Risk factors for hepatocellular cancer in Guangxi, People's Republic of China, *Natl Cancer Inst Monogr* 69:47, 1985.

154. Yu MC et al: Hepatitis, alcohol consumption, and hepatocellular carcinoma in Los Angeles, *Cancer Res* 43:6077, 1983.

155. Zhang W et al: Frequent loss of heterozygosity on chromosome 16 and 4 in human hepatocellular carcinoma, *Jpn. J Cancer Res* 81:108, 1990.

156. Zimmerman HJ: *Hepatotoxicity,* New York, 1978, Appleton-Century-Crofts.

Chapter 30

CENTRAL AND PERIPHERAL NERVOUS SYSTEMS

Thomas J. Montine
William M. Valentine
Doyle G. Graham

The history of neurotoxicology is strewn with episodes of egregious occupational and environmental "accidents" that have yielded a tremendous quantity of preventable human disease and death. In the 1930s, tens of thousands of people were poisoned with tri-*o*-cresyl-phosphate (TOCP) in

The reader is referred to Chapters 4, 5, 14, and 15 for specific information about many of the substances referred to in this chapter.

  This work was supported by the National Institutes of Health under grants F32 ES05625 (TJM), F32 ES05559 and RO1 ES06387 (WMV), and R37 ES02611 (DGG).

  The authors wish to thank Mrs. B. Lynch for her help in preparing this manuscript.

the United States, Europe, and South Africa. In the 1940s, the neurological effects of occupational exposure to tetraethyl lead were recognized in Great Britain. In the 1950s, industrial waste containing mercury contaminated Minamata Bay in Japan and led to what is perhaps the most infamous episode of environmental contamination with a neurotoxicant. The 1950s also saw outbreaks of human neurotoxicant diseases from organotin compounds and manganese, along with another episode of TOCP intoxication in Morocco. In the 1960s and 1970s, methyl mercury exposure was responsible for four more outbreaks of human neurotoxic disease. Also in the 1970s, hexachlorophene, *n*-hexane, methyl *n*-butyl ketone, and chlordecone were accidentally discovered to be neurotoxicants in humans. Parkinsonism secondary to 1-methyl-4-phenyl-1,2,3,6-tetrahydropyridine (MPTP) injection, toxic oil syndrome in Spain, domic acid intoxication in Canada, and still another episode of TOCP exposure in India all occurred in the 1980s. It would be incorrect to conclude that neurotoxicant-induced disease in humans has been limited to isolated "epidemics"; occupational carbon disulfide (CS_2) poisoning has been repeatedly reported for more than a century. The lessons from this ongoing tragedy are that neurotoxic compounds continue to be created and released into the environment and that even to this day, humans continue to serve as the sentinel species for neurotoxicants. In contrast to these high-dose exposure events, chronic low-dose exposures that produce subclinical dysfunction, now beginning to be explored, will probably win the ignominious struggle for causing the greatest amount of human suffering.

Despite the large number of symptomatically intoxicated patients and a tremendous volume of clinical and experimental studies, relatively little has been reported on the pathological changes that are induced in humans by neurotoxicant exposure, and even less is known about pathogenetic mechanisms. The goals of this chapter are (1) to recast this large body of information from the perspective of tissue manifestation in humans and (2) to outline selected pathogenetic mechanisms that have been delineated more clearly. Before embarking on this task, however, a discussion of germane neurotoxicological and neuropathological principles is required.

NEUROPATHOLOGY OF TOXICOLOGY
Basic concepts in neurotoxicology

Nervous systems have as their essence excitability and impulse conduction. In higher animals and humans, a remarkable cellular specialization has evolved to accomplish these fundamental functions. The underlying biochemical processes are well-known: generation and maintenance of electrochemical gradients, intracellular transport systems, myelination, and synaptic neurotransmission. Nervous system specialization, however, has come at a price. Terminally differentiated neurons have lost the capacity to replicate, axons of the central nervous system (CNS) have an extremely limited capacity to regenerate or to be remyelinated, neurons are exquisitely dependent on aerobic respiration and are metabolically reliant on glia, and neurons need to transport molecules and organelles over comparatively vast distances. In addition, a different set of processes is essential to the developing nervous system: proliferation, migration, synapse formation, and myelination. The primary defense of the nervous system is the blood-brain and blood-nerve barriers that present an anatomical boundary to many xenobiotics. The combination of unique molecular targets and protective structures in the nervous system is thought to underlie the selective vulnerability of nervous tissue to certain environmental toxicants.

Neuropathological manifestations of toxicant exposure

The macroscopic patterns of tissue damage in both the central and the peripheral nervous systems that are produced by neurotoxicants can be broadly conceptualized as either symmetrical or asymmetrical. Symmetrical tissue damage is seen most commonly following systemic exposure to toxicants that directly injure some element of the nervous system or that result in cardiopulmonary collapse with secondary lesions in the nervous system. Prime histopathological features of the former are maintenance of basic tissue architecture and only mild inflammatory infiltrates. The central/peripheral distal axonopathies are examples of this type of lesion. In contrast, symmetrical tissue damage secondary to global hypoxia/ischemia is characterized microscopically by parenchymal necrosis with or without hemorrhage and the typical procession of inflammatory and phagocytic

cells. Delayed manifestations of carbon monoxide poisoning are an example of this class of insult. Finally, asymmetrical lesions are usually vascular-based pathological processes that demonstrate histopathological changes indistinguishable from their non–neurotoxicant-induced counterparts. Cocaine-induced intracerebral hemorrhage is an example. Of course, there are exceptions to this general outline, especially when toxicant exposure is superimposed on underlying disease. In addition, some toxicants can produce both types of tissue damage; ethanol may produce cerebellar granular cell degeneration as well as intracerebral hemorrhages.

These general pathological changes that are observed following neurotoxicant exposure apply to the central and peripheral nervous systems and provide a framework to help distinguish neurotoxic diseases from other disease processes. Although a given neurotoxicant may produce a characteristic constellation of pathological changes, it must be stressed that we are aware of no pathognomonic feature for any neurotoxicant-induced disease. It should be obvious that neurotoxic diseases share many features with primary degenerative diseases of the nervous system. Indeed, this pathological equivalence has fostered several hypotheses of a neurotoxicant basis for primary neurodegenerative diseases, e.g., aluminum in Alzheimer's disease, MPTP and related compounds in idiopathic Parkinson's disease, and nitriles in motor neuron disease.

Central nervous system. Diffuse edema is the most prevalent and striking macroscopic finding in acute toxic encephalopathies (Fig. 30-1). The brain is heavy, swollen, and boggy, even after fixation, with broadened cortical gyri and obliterated sulci. In severe cases, transtentorial and even cerebellar tonsilar herniations may occur with fatal flattening of the brain stem. Despite the diffuse nature of

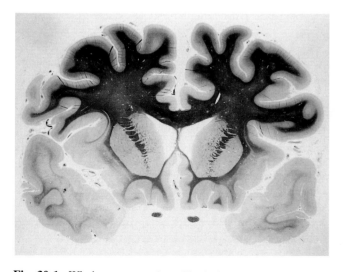

Fig. 30-1. Whole-mount section of brain from a patient who died from acute encephalopathy following exposure to multiple toxins. (Hematoxylin and eosin/Luxol fast blue, ×1.)

edema in toxic encephalopathies, some of its complications may produce "false-localizing" signs; e.g., transtentorial herniation may lead to occlusion of the posterior cerebral artery, compression of the third cranial nerve, or compression of the cerebral peduncle. On cut section, the edematous brain is soft, there may be blurring of the gray-white junction, and the lateral ventricles are compressed. The brain stem, particularly the pons, may show slender hemorrhages, another complication of transtentorial herniation. Cerebral edema secondary to vascular damage, as in lead encephalopathy, or direct damage to CNS myelin, as in triethyltin encephalopathy, is largely confined to the white matter. In contrast, edema resulting from diffuse cytotoxic damage, as in thallium intoxication, affects both gray and white matters and has been observed to impart a "moth-eaten" appearance to the cortical ribbon. Disappointingly, the histological manifestations of cerebral edema can be slight: myelin pallor and mild gliosis. Other commonly encountered macroscopic findings that are often coincident with edema are small hemorrhages about vessels, usually scattered throughout the white matter; however, they may have a characteristic distribution, such as about the third ventricle, aqueduct of Sylvius, and floor of the fourth ventricle, as in methanol intoxication.

Neuronal degeneration following exposure of the human CNS to toxicants may be diffuse or localized. For example, high-dose thallium or carbon disulfide (CS_2) intoxication has been reported to yield neuronal degradation in a wide array of CNS structures. Macroscopically, changes of generalized atrophy may be observed. In contrast, a number of central neurotoxicants demonstrate remarkable specificity in the population of neurons affected, e.g., chronic ethanol abuse and degeneration of neurons in the internal granular cell layer of the anterosuperior cerebellum, methyl mercury–induced degeneration of the calcarine cortex, and neuronal degeneration in the pallidoluysian system (globus pallidus and subthalamic nucleus of Luys) following manganese intoxication. Whether the primary lesion is focal or generalized, secondary degeneration of fiber pathways may be observed. Histologically, at low magnification, a greater than one-third decrease in the normal neuron density must occur before neuronal degradation can be recognized easily. At higher magnification, the cytological features of neuronal degradation vary with etiology. Central chromatolysis is a common finding in disease processes that are intrinsic to neurons or that produce proximal axonal damage. Neuron enlargement, rounding of the cytoplasmic membrane with loss of normal concavity, eccentric displacement of the nucleus, and hyalinization of the cytoplasm with loss of stainable Nissl substance are all characteristic. A morphologically related but pathophysiologically distinct change, neuronal swelling with vacuolization of the cytoplasm (hydropic degeneration) has also been observed following neurotoxicant exposure (e.g., thallium). Another common form of response to injury in neurons is coagulative necrosis, or "red neuron" formation as assessed by hematoxylin and eosin staining. This is an early defining feature of hypoxic/ischemic damage. In this instance, there is contraction of the neuron soma, deeply eosinophilic discoloration of the cytoplasm, and karyolysis. This is in sharp contrast to cytoplasmic condensation with basophilia that is characteristic of autolysis (postmortem change). Lastly, although intraneuronal inclusions are common to primary degenerative disease of brain (e.g., Lewy bodies in idiopathic Parkinson's disease), they are uncommon in neurotoxic disease of the CNS. Abnormal intraneuronal inclusions, however, have been reported in neurons following intoxication with heavy metals.[26]

Under normal circumstances, an astrocyte's soma is not apparent by light microscopy, but rather its fine cytoplasmic processes blend imperceptibly with the surrounding neuropil. Response to recent injury produces primarily a hypertrophy of astrocytes with development of prominent, eosinophilic cell bodies that are strongly immunoreactive for glial fibrillary acidic protein (GFAP). These reactive, hypertrophied astrocytes also are known as protoplasmic astrocytes or gemistocytes. As astrocytic reaction to injury enters a chronic phase, the morphological features become more subtle. Now there are a few gemistocytes, but there is a slight increase in the density of astrocyte nuclei and a coarsening of astrocytic processes that can be difficult to appreciate by hematoxylin and eosin staining but that is more apparent with immunohistochemical staining for GFAP. These morphological changes have been substantiated by the immunoblotting studies of O'Callaghan and co-workers who have shown early but transient elevation in GFAP immunoreactivity following exposure to different neurotoxicants.[132,133] Another morphological feature of chronicity is the formation of Rosenthal fibers: glassy, eosinophilic, corkscrew-shaped cytoplasmic bodies that are immunoreactive for GFAP, ubiquitin, and alpha-B-crystallin. Lastly a more specific type of astrocyte response to injury that does not involve cytoplasmic changes is the formation of Alzheimer type II astrocytes. Hyperammonemic states, resulting from hepatic failure of a variety of causes, may produce an encephalopathy that, by light microscopy, is characterized by enlarged astrocyte nuclei with cleared chromatin, prominent nucleoli, and convoluted nuclear membranes.

Microglia, or rod cells, are inconspicuous elements of the uninjured CNS but can assume prominence following tissue damage. There are two basic patterns of microglial response to injury: microglial nodules (focal) and microgliomatosis. Microglial nodules are a radial arrangement of microglia and astrocytes, usually surrounding a virally infected or degenerating neuron. Microgliomatosis, in contrast, is a diffuse prominence of rod cells that is present in some CNS infections, e.g., general paresis, and has been reported following neurotoxicant exposure. Although microglia can phagocytize devitalized tissue, blood-derived monocytes appear to be the primary scavengers of destroyed parenchyma.

Histopathological changes in CNS myelin are most easily approached from the initial observation of myelin pallor, or a decreased density in stainable myelin. Myelin pallor results from three general processes: dysmyelination (abnormal production), demyelination (abnormal degradation), or decreased white matter tissue density secondary to an infiltrating process, such as edema or astrogliosis. The term "demyelination" should be reserved for those lesions characterized by selective loss of myelin with relative sparing of axons and other tissue elements as well as an influx of phagocytic cells that imbibe the myelin debris. Examples of diseases that produce such lesions are multiple sclerosis, central pontine myelinolysis, Marchiafava-Bignami disease, and progressive multifocal leukoencephalopathy. Demyelination can also follow the intramyelinic edema induced by triethyltin or hexachlorophene intoxication. Myelin pallor secondary to neurotoxicant exposure, however, is more commonly due to a combination of edema and astrogliosis.

Peripheral nervous system. Pathological examination of the human peripheral nervous system is, for all practical purposes, limited to evaluation of nerve biopsy specimens, and the vast majority of these are of the sural nerve, a pure sensory nerve. Peripheral nervous system lesions are most easily conceptualized as either axonal degeneration with or without regeneration or demyelination with remyelination. It should be stressed that these processes rarely exist in pure forms.

Axonal degeneration is the more common finding in toxicant-induced peripheral neuropathies. Seen in cross section, it is revealed microscopically by a decreased number of myelinated axons and by the presence of degenerating axons. An optimal technique for viewing axons along several internodes is teased fiber preparations that show linear collections of phagocytic cells that are digesting myelin and axonal debris; an appearance generally referred to as "dying-back" axonopathy. As originally proposed, this process describes a specific pathogenetic sequence, such as toxic injury to the neuronal soma, that results in "dying back" of the distal axon, circumstances not appropriate for many neurotoxicants. Indeed, careful studies have suggested that multifocal "chemical transection" of the axon followed by wallerian-type degeneration of the distal segment is a common consequence of toxicant injury. The morphological presentation of both of these pathogenetic processes is similar, and a meaningful distinction between them in a nerve biopsy specimen usually is not possible.

Axonal regeneration, as evidenced by axonal sprouting, may occur in a pure axonopathy because the neuron soma has remained intact. Axonal sprouting is manifested as multiple, small, thinly myelinated neurites within a single Schwann cell basement membrane. Of course, if the neu-

ronal soma has been destroyed, the axon degenerates and axonal sprouting cannot occur.

A final feature of axonopathies that is characteristic of some neurotoxicant-induced diseases is the distal giant axonal swelling (Fig. 30-2). These large eosinophilic collections within axons have been shown to be composed of massive accumulations of neurofilaments. Identical neurofilament-filled axonal swellings also are seen in a rare familial neuropathy termed giant axonal neuropathy. This is in sharp distinction to the morphologically similar axonal spheroids that have been observed in characteristic locations in neurologically intact older people as well as in patients with neuraxonal dystrophies. Although under experimental conditions neurofilamentous axonal swellings may be produced anywhere along the axon, in neurotoxicant-induced diseases in humans (e.g., *n*-hexane or CS_2), they have been reported only in the distal portion of long axons of both the central and the peripheral nervous systems and were accompanied by degeneration of the distal axonal segment.

Segmental demyelination is the other major class of pathological lesions in the peripheral nervous system. Inappropriately thin myelin sheaths, shortening of internodal distances, and variation of myelin thickness among inter-

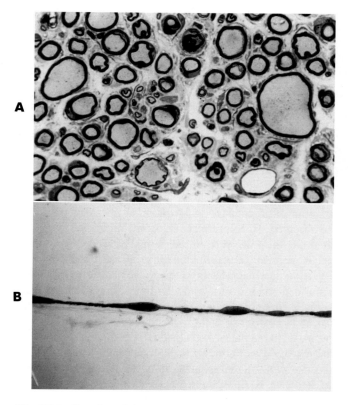

Fig. 30-2. Samples of the muscular branch of the posterior tibial nerve from rats exposed by inhalation to 800 ppm carbon disulfide (CS_2), 5 days/wk for 90 days. **A,** Plastic-embedded 5 μm section. (Toluidine blue, ×52.) **B,** Teased-fiber preparation. (Osmium tetroxide, x10.)

nodal segments of the same axon are all observed during the remyelination that follows demyelination. Recurrent episodes of demyelination with remyelination may lead to hypertrophic neuropathy that is characterized by "onion bulb" formation, a feature produced by redundant basement membrane material around a thinly myelinated axon.

Catalog of neurotoxic lesions in humans

The vast majority of information on human neurotoxicants has come from the study of intoxicated humans (Table 30-1). Typically, knowledge of a neurotoxicant initiates with a cluster of neurological symptoms in a group of patients that share some activity. After much investigation, the suspect neurotoxicants are removed from the environment, the population of patients is followed by physicians, and laboratory scientists investigate the compounds. For example, following reports from Japan of n-hexane–induced axonopathy,[193] three factory workers[86] and habitual glue sniffers[6,102,178] in the United States were reported to have developed distal sensorimotor polyneuropathy from n-hexane exposure. A few years later, an industrial outbreak of distal sensorimotor polyneuropathy in Ohio was traced to methyl n-butyl ketone (2-hexanone) exposure.[4] As discussed further in a later section, both compounds have been shown to share a common chemical pathogenetic mechanism that involves covalent cross-linking of neurofilament proteins. Analogous events have occurred with methyl mercury, hexachlorophene, chlordecone, triethyltin, manganese, leptophos, MPTP, and many other neurotoxicants. Table 30-1 contains a compilation of pathological data for human neurotoxicant-induced disease obtained from such case series. The majority of this information stems from acute and subacute exposures, when causal relationships are easier to establish, although studies have begun to address chronic low-dose exposures.

BIOCHEMICAL MECHANISMS OF SELECTED NEUROTOXIC LESIONS

Viewed from the perspective of neurotoxicology, the two most intriguing regions of the nervous system are the basal ganglia and hippocampus of the CNS and the distal extent of the longest axons of both the central and the peripheral nervous systems. Both of these structures commonly are damaged after neurotoxic insult, and, as described subsequently, groups of apparently unrelated compounds can produce similar-appearing lesions at each site. In the following sections, the biochemical mechanisms that are thought to underlie these lesions with shared topographical and morphological features are discussed.

Basal ganglia and hippocampus

Historical background. The selective vulnerability of the deep cerebral gray matter to a variety of pathological processes has been recognized for decades. For example, the globus pallidus and striatum may be injured following

ischemia, hypoglycemia, hypoxemia, or anemia as well as following exposure to endogenous toxins (e.g., bilirubin in neonates) or exogenous toxicants.[93,94] In an attempt to explain the heightened sensitivity of this region to injurious processes, Vogt and Vogt advanced the "pathoclisis" theory that proposed unspecified chemical and physiological properties peculiar to this region were responsible. Alternatively, it was hypothesized that idiosyncrasies of this region's vascular supply were the culpable factor. Over the past decade, the explosion of data indicating a role for glutamate and other excitatory amino acids (EAAs) in neurodegeneration and the remarkable investigations of MPTP-induced parkinsonism have led to a sophisticated modification of Vogt and Vogt's original theory: that selective vulnerability of certain neuron populations may be due to a heightened sensitivity to endogenous EAAs[17,45] Before discussing specific neurotoxicants that can damage this region of the brain, a synopsis of EAAs in neurological diseases is in order.

Excitatory amino acids in neurological disease

EAAs and their cell surface receptors (EAARs) have been proposed to participate in a wide array of neurological diseases—primarily ischemia, hypoglycemia, and epilepsy, but also chronic neurodegeneration, trauma, human immunodeficiency virus (HIV) dementia, and neuropathic pain.[113,120,121] Although a bewildering number of experiments and experimental systems have provided indirect support for a role of EAARs in neurological diseases, relatively few observations have directly linked EAAs with neurodegeneration. Among these, the most compelling have been "experiments of nature," in which animals or humans were exposed to high doses of EAAR agonists and subsequently developed neurological disease.[171] Although a few rare, geographically circumscribed neurological diseases have been linked to chronic dietary consumption of foods containing EAAR agonists, the identity of the responsible agents has not yet been fully resolved.[54,171] The domic acid intoxications that occurred in the maritime provinces of Canada in late 1987 are an exception.[138,171] A total of 107 patients were identified who suffered an acute illness that most commonly presented as gastrointestinal disturbance, severe headache, and short-term memory loss within 24 to 48 hours of ingesting mussels. Of these, 12 patients required intensive care because of seizures and myoclonus, coma, or cardiorespiratory complications. A subset of the more severely afflicted patients was subsequently shown to have chronic memory deficits, motor neuropathy, and decreased medial temporal lobe glucose metabolism by positron-emission tomography (PET). Neuropathological investigation of four patients who died within 4 months of intoxication disclosed neuronal loss with reactive gliosis that was most prominent in the hippocampus and amygdala but also affected regions of the thalamus and cerebral cortex. The responsible agent was identified as domic acid, a

Table 30-1. Catalog of occupational and environmental neurotoxicants in humans

Neurotoxicant	Neurological findings	Neuropathological and imaging findings
Acrylamide	Encephalopathy* Truncal ataxia† SMPN‡	Not documented. Not documented. Axonal degeneration predominantly affecting large myelinated axons.[69,90]
Aluminum	Dementia, myoclonus, epilepsy, and focal neurological signs have been observed in patients undergoing chronic renal dialysis.[3] Rapidly progressive encephalopathy was reported after occupational exposure.	Spongiosis in cerebral midcortical layers, mild reactive astrocytosis, and microgliomatosis have been observed.[33,148] Diffuse brain edema only was observed at autopsy.[118] The role of aluminum in the pathogenesis of Alzheimer's disease and other rare neurodegenerative diseases is controversial.[185,186]
Arsenic inorganic	SMPN, often with pain as a primary feature,*/§,‡ is most common. Acute intoxication may mimic Guillain-Barré syndrome[53]	Axonal degeneration with regeneration was reported in acute exposure, and demyelination with remyelination was observed in chronic exposure.[39,76,95,134]
Arsenic organic	Encephalopathy	Petechial hemorrhages with perivascular demyelination and hemorrhagic necrosis were observed in the cerebral white matter and brain stem.[92]
Carbon disulfide	Psychotic symptoms,† encephalopathy,† and parkinsonism§[140] Distal SMPN‡	Few autopsy studies have been reported (reviewed in ref. 5). These showed diffuse edema of brain with swollen endothelial cells and perivascular hemorrhages, loss of large neurons in the cerebral cortex and cornu Ammonis as well as slight changes in the striatum and cerebellum and scattered areas of myelin degeneration and gliosis in the brain and spinal cord. The peripheral nervous system was unremarkable. More recent studies of disulfiram neuropathy have documented a distal axonopathy that in one instance showed neurofilament accumulation.[20,125,126,131]
Carbon monoxide	Encephalopathy and parkinsonism*/§	Generalized edema was observed. Hypoxic/ischemic damage to cerebrum, bilateral necrosis of globus pallidus, and perivascular demyelination have been reported in survivors of acute poisonings.[40,74,75,101,142,147,168]
Chlordecone (kepone)	Tremor, opsoclonus, and encephalopathy†	Sural nerve biopsies revealed decreased number of unmyelinated fibers and endoneural fibrosis.[117]
Cocaine	Cocaine abuse has been associated with an increased risk of cerebrovascular disease, cerebral perfusion defects, and cerebral atrophy.[65,67,99]	Nonspecific
Cyanide	Encephalopathy and parkinsonism*/§	Generalized edema was reported following fatal acute exposure. Delayed changes of global hypoxic/ischemic damage have been observed: bilateral necrosis of the globus pallidus and striatum, laminar necrosis of the cerebral cortex, and loss of cerebellar Purkinje cells.[61,80,154,180,183]
Dimethyamino-propionitrile	Flaccid neurogenic bladder, male sexual dysfunction, sensory loss in sacral dermatomes and distal SMPN†	Sural nerve biopsy from a severely intoxicated patient showed mildly decreased density of myelinated and unmyelinated axons with axonal swellings containing neurofilaments.[139]
Domic acid	Headache, seizures, hemiparesis, opthalmoplegia, and coma* Anterograde memory deficits and SMPN§	Neuronal loss was seen primarily in the hippocampus and amygdala.[138,176]

Table 30-1. Catalog of occupational and environmental neurotoxicants in humans—cont'd.

Neurotoxicant	Neurological findings	Neuropathological and imaging findings
Ethanol¶	Fetal alcohol syndrome†	Abnormalities of brain development that most commonly include microcephaly, neuroglial heterotopias, brain stem and cerebellum malformations with hydrocephalus, and agenesis of the corpus callosum.[44,136,190]
	Wernicke-Korsakoff syndrome‡	Petechial hemorrhages, neuronal loss, gliosis, and capillary proliferation are present in the mamillary bodies and periventricular gray matter of the midbrain and hindbrain. Older lesions may cavitate.[92]
	Slowly progressive truncal ataxia‡	Atrophy of superior cerebellar vermis and cerebellar hemispheres that is characterized by loss of internal granular neurons and Purkinje cells with Bergmann gliosis.[92]
	Distal SMPN‡	Primarily distal axonal degeneration.[92]
	Marchifava-Bignami disease‡	Partial demyelination and necrosis of the corpus callosum have been observed.[92]
	Increased risk for cerebrovascular accidents	Nonspecific.[65,67,73]
Ethylene glycol	Acute encephalopathy	Generalized edema with scattered petechial hemorrhages throughout the brain and meningitis have been observed. Oxalate crystal deposition in meninges and brain is characteristic.[19,68,153,169]
Ethylene oxide	Acute encephalopathy[83]	Nonspecific
	Cognitive impairment‡[46]	Not documented
	SMPN†	Axonal degeneration with regeneration.[83,105,163]
n-Hexane and 2-Hexanone (methyl-n-butyl ketone)	Euphoria, narcosis*	Not documented
	Distal SMPN†,‡	Axonal swelling with thinned myelin sheaths and axonal degeneration was present in the distal portion of long axons of the spinal cord and PNS. Axonal regeneration was observed in the PNS.[4,6,23,60,86,97,102,150,170,172,178,193] Autopsy of a patient with a 12-year history of glue sniffing also showed diffuse cerebral and cerebellar atrophy.[60]
Lead inorganic	Encephalopathy†,‡ (more common in children)	Generalized edema with scattered petechial hemorrhages occurred; however, herniation was unusual. Microscopically a protein-rich perivascular exudate, endothelial necrosis, and thrombosis were observed throughout the neuraxis. Microglial nodules have been reported. Focal degeneration of cerebellar Purkinje and internal granule cells with reactive gliosis has been demonstrated.[87,104]
	Children with signs of plumbism but no encephalopathy may develop neurobehavioral deficits or delays.[179]	Not documented
	Asymptomatic children may be at increased risk for neurobehavioral deficits or delays.[179]	Not documented
	Motor neuropathy primarily of upper extremities†,‡ (more common in adults)	Axonal degeneration with regeneration.[87,104]
	Asymptomatic adults may be at increased risk for cerebrovascular accidents.‡[179]	Nonspecific
Lead organic	Acute encephalopathy	Atrophy of cerebellar vermis and adjacent hemispheres was observed in patients who habitually inhaled leaded gasoline.[98,184] Microscopic sections showed Purkinje cell loss, internal granular cell atrophy, and Bergmann gliosis. One report documented other changes that suggest global hypoxia as a contributing factor.[184]
	Asymptomatic adults may be at increased risk for cerebrovascular accidents.‡	Nonspecific

Continued.

Table 30-1. Catalog of occupational and environmental neurotoxicants in humans—cont'd.

Neurotoxicant	Neurological findings	Neuropathological and imaging findings
Leptophos	Rigidity and spasticity as well as numerous other central and peripheral CNS findings[161]	Not documented.
Manganese	Extrapyramidal movement disorder‡ Emotional and psychiatric disturbances†	Bilateral atrophy of the pallidum and/or putamen with neuron loss, gliosis, and sometimes pigment deposition have been observed (reviewed in refs. [15,16,175,192]).
Mercury inorganic	Dementia and emotional lability	Degeneration of cerebellar granule cells and deposition of mercury granules in the inferior olive, dentate nucleus, and choroid plexus have been reported.[49]
Mercury organic	Gait ataxia Concentric visual field deficit	Degeneration of the calcarine and cerebellar cortices, particularly at the depths of sulci, is characteristic. Less severely affected structures commonly include the precentral, postcentral, and temporal cortices. The atrophic cerebral cortex shows neuronal degeneration and reactive astrocytosis. The cerebellum has selective loss of the internal granular cells. Secondary, symmetrical degeneration of the pyramidal tracts has been noted.[36,165]
	Perioral and extremity paresthesias	Findings in the peripheral nervous system have been variable; ranging from no abnormality to degeneration of dorsal root ganglion cells and posterior columns.[36,165]
Methanol	Blindness*,† Parkinsonism§	Retinal ganglion cell degeneration[18] Bilateral putaminal necrosis with or without hemorrhage and widespread hypoxic/ischemic damage is characteristic.[119,141]
Methyl bromide	Acute encephalopathy with seizures* SMPN, weakness, coordination defects, extrapyramidal movement disorders, and psychosis†,‡[127,194]	Cerebral edema with petechial and subarachnoid hemorrhages was reported.[127,145] One patient who was maintained artificially for 30 days following acute exposure had, at autopsy, symmetrical lesions in the mamillary bodies and inferior colliculi that resembled the changes of Wernicke's encephalopathy.[173]
MPTP	Parkinsonism	No human autopsy studies have been reported. Clinical and neuroimaging studies in humans have localized the lesion to the substantia nigra.[14,189]
Polychlorinated biphenyls and polychlorodibenzofurans	Sensory neuropathy. Neurobehavioral deficits or delays**[38,100]	Not documented.
Thallium	Acute encephalopathy	Generalized edema of both gray and white matter with petechial hemorrhages, chromatolysis of ganglion cells in the brain and spinal cord, and microgliomatosis with minimal astrogliosis have been reported.[146]
	SMPN	Axonal degeneration with secondary myelin loss.[48,112]
Triethyltin and Hexachlorophene‖	Encephalopathy*,†	Generalized edema of the white matter characterized by intramyelinic vacuoles.[115,116,128,166,167]
Trimethyltin	Limbic-cerebellar syndrome*[22,159]	Central chromatolysis, membrane-bound neuronal cytoplasmic inclusions, neuronophagia, and neuron loss most concentrated in limbic structures were the results of the single reported autopsy.[22]

Table 30-1. Catalog of occupational and environmental neurotoxicants in humans—cont'd.

Neurotoxicant	Neurological findings	Neuropathological and imaging findings
Tri-*o*-cresyl phosphate	Cholinergic crisis* Distal SMPN§	None reported Axonal degeneration of central and peripheral long axons with axonal regeneration in the PNS.
Trichloroethylene	Sensorimotor neuropathy primarily restricted to cranial nerve V	Symmetrical demyelination and axonal degeneration of the entire length of cranial nerve V as well as associated ganglion cell degeneration was observed.[34,62]
Toluene	Euphoria* Amnesia, dementia, cerebellar ataxia, pyramidal tract and oculomotor dysfunction, tremor, and deafness[25,64,78,123,158]	Not documented. A single autopsy showed diffuse cerebral myelin pallor, but not demyelination.[158]

MPTP, 1-Methyl-4-phenyl-1,2,3,6-tetrahydropyridine; *SMPN*, Sensorimotor distal neuropathy; *PNS*, peripheral nervous system.
*Acute (less than one month).
†Subacute (less than one year).
‡Chronic (greater than one year).
§Delayed.
‖Infants and children.
¶In combination with nutritional deficiencies.
**Prenatal exposure.

potent structural analog of glutamate that had been concentrated in cultivated mussels.

It seems that a variety of neurodegenerative processes can involve secondarily the overstimulation of EAARs; however, the pathogenesis is not fully understood. Experimental studies have outlined a cascade of events through which EAAR stimulation may lead to neurodegeneration. Initially the effective synaptic concentration of EAAs is increased. Rapid degeneration, the form that occurs in the presence of agonist, is thought to be mediated by a depolarization-dependent increase in sodium and chloride permeability that is followed by osmotic swelling and neuronal lysis. Delayed toxicity, which develops after the agonist has been removed, appears to operate through disruption of intraneuronal calcium levels with subsequent inappropriate activation of calcium-dependent enzymes, mitochondrial damage, or increased generation of partially reduced oxygen species.[45,160] The characteristic tissue manifestation of EAAR overstimulation, produced by local injection of an EAAR agonist into rodent striatum, is selective neuronal degeneration and slight gliosis but with preservation of glia and axons. This is often referred to as an "excitotoxic lesion" in experimental animals and is essentially identical to the hippocampal lesions in patients who died following domic acid poisoning.

Many experimental studies have supported this sequence of events in acute insults, such as ischemia, in which there is a dramatic increase in extracellular glutamate and in which it has been shown that EAAR antagonists can diminish the ultimate amount of tissue damage. Some investigators have proposed that chronic neurodegeneration, as seen in amyotrophic lateral sclerosis, Huntington's disease, and

Parkinson's disease, also may result from increased sensitivity to endogenous glutamate toxicity.[17] The scientific basis for this proposal comes largely from the study of MPTP.

The history of MPTP-induced parkinsonism in young adults who inadvertently injected themselves with this compound is well-known.[107] MPTP has been shown to act as a protoxicant that, after entering the brain, is metabolized by glial monoamine oxidase (MAO-B) to the toxic metabolite 1-methyl-4-phenylpyridinium cation (MPP+), which is then selectively transported into nigral neurons via a dopamine transporter. Once inside these neurons, MPP+ acts as a mitochondrial toxin by inhibiting the formation of complex I of the electron transport chain. Other pyridinium metabolites also may contribute to cytotoxicity by producing partially reduced oxygen species.[96] It has been demonstrated in rats that neuronal degeneration following MPTP exposure can be diminished by an EAAR antagonist. Before this, it had been observed that impairment of energy metabolism in tissue culture facilitated the transition of glutamate from neurotransmitter to excitotoxin.[130] Building on these observations, other laboratories have demonstrated selective neuronal degeneration with sparing of other tissue elements ("excitotoxic lesions") in rat striatum following local injection of cellular respiration inhibitors other than MPP+.[17,81] These experimental findings have been synthesized into an hypothesis proposing that defective mitochondrial respiration may secondarily increase the sensitivity of neurons to endogenous glutamate and thus culminate in chronic neurodegeneration.

Pathological findings with basal ganglia and hippocampal neurotoxicants. The basal ganglia are a varyingly defined group of subcortical gray matter that, for our purposes, include the claustrum, striatum (caudate and putamen), pallidum (pars interna and externa of the globus pallidus), subthalamic nucleus of Luys, and substantia nigra. Exact clinicopathological mapping of these structures is still under investigation, and it is simplest to state that damage to this region produces some combination of bradykinesia, rigidity, tremor, involuntary movements (extrapyramidal movement disorders), and psychiatric manifestations.[152] The amygdala is commonly grouped anatomically with the basal ganglia; functionally, however, it is related more closely to the hippocampus and limbic system, structures that are thought to subserve motor function, complex behavior, and memory.

Toxicants that can have a major effect on these structures are carbon monoxide (CO), cyanide (CN), methanol, carbon disulfide (CS_2), manganese (Mn), trimethyltin (TMT), domic acid, and MPTP. Intoxication by each of these compounds has been demonstrated to produce disease in humans with tissue lesions confirmed by either autopsy or neuroimaging studies. When considering the tissue lesions produced by these neurotoxicants in the basal ganglia and hippocampus, one can divide them into those that are histotoxic, ultimately manifesting as cystic necrosis with destruction of all tissue elements, and those that are selectively cytotoxic to neurons but sparing of other tissue elements.

Histotoxicants. CO, CN, and methanol compose the histotoxic group of basal ganglia and hippocampal neurotoxicants. It must be stressed that all three agents are systemic toxicants with profound effects on the cardiorespiratory system. Patients who survive acute intoxication often develop delayed neurological sequelae. In these cases, pathological examination reveals lesions in the basal ganglia and hippocampus as well as other sites of the CNS that follow the typical temporal, topographical, and morphological patterns of global hypoxic/ischemic injury.[75,142]

Carbon monoxide. Delayed encephalopathy from acute CO exposure is relatively common in intoxicated patients requiring hospitalization (reviewed in Choi[40] and Ginsberg[74]). The clinical picture in encephalopathic patients is often broad, including motor, cognitive, and psychiatric dysfunction in addition to parkinsonism. The older medical literature contains several reports of post mortem examination of patients who survived the initial intoxication but later succumbed. Gray matter lesions consist of bilateral cystic necrosis of the globus pallidus that frequently extends into the adjacent internal capsule, laminar necrosis of the cerebral cortex, neuronal loss in the cornu Ammonis of the hippocampus, granular atrophy of the arterial border zones, and focal necrosis of the cerebellum. Several patterns of white matter necrosis also have been identified as sequelae of acute CO intoxication in humans.[74] The central importance of pallidal lesions to parkinsonian symptoms was underscored by a case report that described bilateral lucencies of the globus pallidus by computed tomog-

raphy (CT) in a survivor of CO intoxication who had a pure parkinsonian syndrome.[101] Other case reports describing patients with more complex neurological dysfunction also have demonstrated lesions in the basal ganglia by CT or magnetic resonance imaging (MRI).[40,147,168] Data from carefully controlled studies on rats, cats, and monkeys have generally indicated that systemic hypotension is the best predictor of CNS damage following carbon monoxide intoxication, although direct cytotoxic action of CO may contribute to the leukoencephalopathy.[137] One laboratory demonstrated that, at least in part, neurodegeneration induced by systemic CO exposure could be impeded by EAAR antagonists.[91]

Despite numerous epidemiological studies of cigarette smokers and workers in various industrial settings, no specific neurological deficits can be attributed to chronic low-level exposure to CO.

Cyanide. Three autopsy studies document the pathological changes in the brains of patients who died more than 24 hours after acute CN intoxication.[85,180] In one case, the patient remained comatose for 36 hours before death, and although the globus pallidi were reported grossly as soft, no histological examination was made. The second patient survived 16 days following intoxication but did not demonstrate an extrapyramidal movement disorder. Pathological changes were limited to laminar necrosis of the cerebral cortex and marked cerebellar Purkinje cell degradation. The most recent case concerns a man who survived 19 months after attempting suicide with potassium cyanide (KCN). Within 4 months, he had developed generalized rigidity, bradykinesia, and resting tremor of the arms. At autopsy, the putamen and globus pallidus were shrunken and spongy, the subthalamic nucleus showed neuronal loss and gliosis, the occipital lobes contained laminar necrosis in the arterial border zone, there was neuronal loss in the zona compacta of the substantia nigra, and marked loss of Purkinje cells was seen in the cerebellar hemispheres. The hippocampi were noted specifically to be unremarkable.[180] These autopsies have been corroborated by more recent neuroimaging studies.[61,80,154,183] Elegant experiments that were conducted in rats and monkeys[29,30] led to the conclusion that hypoxic-ischemic damage, rather than direct histotoxicity, is the major cause of delayed CNS damage after CN exposure.

Chronic exposure to CN has been linked to "cassavism," a spastic paraparesis of the lower extremities that has been observed in indigent populations that consume large amounts of cassava roots in their diets.[171] Although some investigators have proposed that hydrolysis of cyanogenic glycosides with release of CN is the mechanism of toxicity,[135] others have proposed alternative agents, also contained within these roots, that may play a central role in the development of this disease. Chronic occupational exposure to CN has been associated with a variety of nonspecific neurological signs and symptoms; however, these examples are complicated by exposure to multiple agents, and no pathological data are available.

Methanol. Methanol-induced damage to the basal ganglia, in contrast to CO, is directed principally at the putamen rather than the globus pallidus. Patients surviving methanol intoxication have been observed to develop cystic necrosis of the putamen that commonly involves adjacent structures, ischemic cell change in the hippocampus, laminar necrosis of the cerebral cortex, and cystic necrosis of cerebral white matter.[119,141] Although retinal ganglion cell degeneration appears to be mediated through formate, a metabolite of methanol, it is not clear what direct role methanol or its metabolites play in other CNS lesions. The striking similarity between the pathological changes produced by methanol, CO, and CN exposure promotes the reasonable assumption that all share similar pathogenetic mechanisms. There are examples of methanol-intoxicated patients, however, who lacked clinical evidence of marked hypoxia or hypotension but who later developed CNS lesions.[119] Furthermore, there is clearly preferential involvement of the putamen following methanol exposure, whereas other causes of global hypoxia/ischemia tend to involve the globus pallidus. It seems likely that methanol and its metabolites, in addition to global hypoxia/ischemia, contribute directly to the development of CNS lesions other than retinal degeneration.

Neuronal cytotoxicants. The second group of basal ganglia and hippocampal neurotoxicants are those that produce selective neuronal loss, resulting in cytotoxic lesions that are quite different from the histotoxic lesions already described. These agents include MPTP, domic acid, Mn, and TMT. Although MPTP and domic acid serve as scientific paradigms for this type of CNS lesion, Mn and TMT are examples of occupational neurotoxicants that produce selective neuronal loss. In contrast to the histotoxicants discussed previously, Mn and TMT are not significant systemic toxicants, and the signs and symptoms that accompany exposure are largely limited to the CNS. The pathological lesions that result from Mn or TMT intoxication are restricted to gray matter and do not overlap with the temporal or morphological features of hypoxic-ischemic damage.

Manganese. There have been many case series and individual reports from all over the world concerning occupational exposure to Mn dust (reviewed in references 63, 129, and 164) as well as a few accounts of apparent iatrogenic exposure to Mn.[55,124] In one of the more exhaustive studies, a cohort of 13 symptomatic patients employed as manganese miners was identified.[122] The range of time exposed to manganese dust was 8 months to 20 years. Consistently observed signs and symptoms were psychomotor disturbances or locura manganica (manganic madness) in the early phases of disease that was followed by generalized muscle weakness, gait abnormalities, and impaired speech. Other commonly reported features were clumsi-

ness, tremor, impotence, memory dysfunction, and sleep disturbances. Some years later, a separate group of investigators reexamined most of these patients and concluded that bradykinesia and dystonia were the major clinical findings.[15,16]

A separate cohort of six workers from a ferromanganese factory displayed bradykinesia, rigidity, clumsiness, and gait abnormalities, but not neuropsychiatric disturbances, as the most common signs and symptoms.[88] All six had been exposed to elevated manganese concentrations for more than 2 years and had elevated blood and hair manganese levels. Repeat neurological examination 4 years later demonstrated slow progression of symptoms, despite cessation of manganese exposure, and limited response to levodopa therapy.[89] This same group of investigators performed PET studies on four patients with early parkinsonism secondary to chronic manganese exposure.[191] Their results suggested that the early effects of manganism are directed at cerebral structures that are postsynaptic to the nigrostriatal system, including the striatum and pallidum. Furthermore, diffusely decreased cerebral glucose metabolism was observed in patients demonstrating extrapyramidal movement disorders but who did not manifest neuropsychiatric impairment.

Despite the relatively large population of clinically evaluated patients, only a few autopsy studies of patients who suffered from manganism have been performed (reviewed in references 15, 16, and 192). The consistent pathological finding is atrophy of the basal ganglia, characterized by neuronal loss and mild gliosis. The lesion tends to focus in the pallidoluysian system, but the striatum and even the thalamus may be equally affected.[35] Involvement of the substantia nigra is unusual, but neuronal degeneration and even occasional Lewy bodies have been reported.[21] In one patient, frontal atrophy was described grossly,[35] and in another diffuse cortical gliosis was noted.[21] Uncharacterized pigment deposition was identified in the striatum of one patient.[35]

Manganism was initially thought to mimic closely idiopathic Parkinson's disease. It was soon realized, however, that the clinical and pathological manifestations of these two diseases are different. Some investigators have proposed that the pathological changes in patients with manganism more closely parallel those seen in striatonigral degeneration,[51,106] a process that primarily results in tissue damage to the putamen and substantia nigra.[1] Rather, it is our opinion that Mn-induced neurodegeneration should be considered a form of pallidoluysian atrophy.[15,93]

Experiments in monkeys have detailed the pathophysiological events that occur following Mn intoxication.[56,57,59] Following 5 months of repetitive subcutaneous injection of manganese oxide, the animals developed the typical extrapyramidal movement disorder of manganism. Pathological examination revealed bilateral severe neuron loss and gliosis in the globus pallidus but no other significant changes in the remainder of the brain. Neurochemical analysis demonstrated Mn levels that were greatest in the globus pallidus and putamen, reaching concentrations in excess of tenfold greater than control animals, and marked depletion of dopamine and dihydroxyphenylalanine acetic acid (dopac) in these same brain structures. Furthermore, Mn had the greatest toxic effect on dopaminergic systems in this region and only minor effects on the serotoninergic and cholinergic systems, a finding that was later corroborated by PET studies.[58] Another group of investigators failed to produce neurological abnormalities in monkeys following 2 years of exposure to inhaled Mn; however, these animals did show significant reduction in caudate and pallidal dopamine concentrations as well as small increases in basal ganglia Mn levels.[24]

Many experiments directed at understanding the mechanisms of Mn-induced neurotoxicity have been performed in other mammals and in vitro. Although results have varied depending on the system used, method of administration, and age of animal, the results are broadly consonant with those described earlier (reviewed in references 15, 16, and 51). Experimental evidence has been presented to support the following possible mechanisms: (1) Mn^{3+}-accelerated dopamine or dopac oxidation with generation of cytotoxic quinones and partially reduced oxygen species[11,52,79,188] that may be augmented by increased dopamine turnover[15]; (2) inhibition of cellular protective mechanisms by Mn[110,187]; (3) enhancement of mitochondrial P-450 activity[111]; and (4) disruption of mitochondrial calcium levels and inhibition of oxidative phosphorylation.[70,71] This last potential mechanism is particularly interesting in light of the observation that neurodegeneration following direct injection of Mn into rat striatum could be partially blocked by an EAAR antagonist or interruption of corticostriatal glutaminergic efferents.[31] These investigators also observed a reduction in tissue adenosine triphosphate (ATP) levels, and they proposed that Mn-induced neurodegeneration was mediated by EAAR stimulation secondary to impaired cellular respiration. The relative importance of these potential mechanisms and their possible interrelations are not known.

Trimethyltin. Clinical experience with the consequences of TMT exposure is more limited than with Mn. We are aware of three case series that report on workers who became symptomatic following exposure to high levels of TMT.[22,66,159] In one report, two chemists who were exposed chronically to TMT developed memory loss, disorientation, and tonic-clonic seizures from which they recovered.[66] Acute exposure of another group of six workers to TMT resulted in disorientation, complex partial and tonic-clonic seizures, limbic system dysfunction, nystagmus, ataxia, and mild sensory neuropathy. Two patients remained seriously disabled by the limbic-cerebellar syndrome, and one patient died. At autopsy, the neuropathological findings included central chromatolysis, membrane-bound neuronal cytoplasmic inclusions, neuronophagia,

and neuron loss. These findings were most concentrated in the amygdala but were also found in other limbic system structures (the hippocampi were not mentioned specifically), basal ganglia, temporal cortex, and pontine nuclei. Severe Purkinje cell loss was observed in the cerebellar cortex.[22] No white matter abnormality was identified.

High-dose exposure of rats to TMT has been shown to produce widespread neuronal degeneration in the CNS that is most prominent in the hippocampus (small neurons of the fascia dentata and pyramidal cells of cornu Ammonis), pyriform cortex, and amygdala.[13,27,28,32] As with many other pathological processes that involve hippocampal pyramidal cells, sparing of CA2 neurons has been observed.[32] Also, preferential involvement of hippocampal pyramidal cells, relative to the neurons of the fascia dentata, has been reported following chronic, low-dose exposure.[26] One study noted increased GFAP immunoreactivity in affected structures following exposure.[13] Ultrastructurally, initial neuronal cytoplasmic changes included multifocal collections of dense-cored vesicles and tubules as well as membrane-bound vacuoles. This was followed by the accumulation of autophagic vacuoles and polymorphic electron-dense bodies in the cytoplasm. Importantly, ultrastructural alterations in mitochondria were not observed in the initial stages of neuron degeneration.[26]

The biochemical mechanism of TMT-mediated neuronal degeneration is unclear but may involve a protein named stannin that is present in TMT-sensitive neurons[177] or stimulated release of excitatory amino acids. Structure-function analysis in rats showed that one or more methyl groups was required for trialkyltin-mediated neuron cytotoxicity, whereas one or more ethyl groups was required for the development of intramyelinic edema as observed following triethyltin exposure. The severity of neuron injury or edema increased with increasing number of methyl or ethyl substituents, respectively.[2]

Other neurotoxicants and lesions of the basal ganglia. CS_2 commonly is included in the litany of agents that selectively produce lesions in the basal ganglia. Although chronic exposure to CS_2 clearly can produce a central and peripheral distal axonopathy (see below) and has been related to extrapyramidal movement disorders in humans,[37,140] data are sparse and conflicting about what lesions are produced in the CNS by CS_2. There have been few autopsy studies of humans chronically exposed to CS_2, and these have yielded inconsistent pathological patterns.[5] A more recent report described MRI studies of four patients with extrapyramidal movement disorders who were repeatedly exposed to grain fumigants that contained CS_2. These imaging studies showed lesions that were consistent with demyelination in the cerebral white matter of two patients. No mention was made of the basal ganglia.[140] Results from experiments using monkeys exposed to CS_2 over many months did show cystic degeneration of the basal ganglia; however, each monkey was accidentally exposed to near lethal concentrations, resulting in respiratory arrest at least once during the course of this investigation.[149] Therefore, as described previously, the observed pathological changes may have been delayed consequences of systemic toxicity. Subacute exposure of dogs to uncontrolled, high concentrations of CS_2 similarly was noted to produce neuron degradation primarily in the cerebral cortex and striatum in addition to axonopathy.[5] This last study is particularly intriguing in light of several case reports of extrapyramidal movement disorders in patients who took massive doses of disulfiram, of which CS_2 is a major metabolite, and who later were shown by CT or MRI to harbor lesions in the putamen and pallidum.[103,108] A single report of an autopsy of a patient who developed an extrapyramidal movement disorder following disulfiram therapy showed bilateral, cavitated lesions of the pars externa of the globus pallidus and surrounding gliosis[84] (as reviewed in Krauss and co-workers[103]). As noted with some of the experimental studies, however, this patient developed extrapyramidal movement disorder after documented cardiorespiratory collapse, and so a firm conclusion about the neuronal cytotoxicity of CS_2 remains elusive.

Before concluding our discussion of neurotoxicants that damage the basal ganglia, attention should be drawn to the potential role of neurotoxicants in idiopathic Parkinson's disease. Of the primary neurodegenerative diseases, Parkinson's disease has been thought to be heavily influenced by environmental factors, although this issue has been reopened.[143,162] Although MPTP and Mn provide sufficient clinical, pathological, and experimental data to conclude that parkinsonism may result from toxicant exposure, there is no consensus on the contribution of toxicants to idiopathic Parkinson's disease. General conclusions from several epidemiological studies are that the cause of Parkinson's disease is likely to be multifactorial and that one of the factors may be environmental toxicants, especially agrochemicals (reviewed in references 96 and 175). The identity of specific toxicants and their relative effects on different subsets of parkinsonian patients, however, remains to be elucidated.

Summary. In this section we have tried to draw stark distinction between two classes of neurotoxicants that damage the basal ganglia and hippocampus. The first group, including CO, CN, and methanol, produces CNS damage as a delayed consequence of acute, life-threatening exposure. These agents produce histotoxic lesions in several sites of the CNS, and these most likely are the result of global hypoxic-ischemic injury. With the exception of methanol, this group of neurotoxicants exerts little direct toxicity in the CNS. The second group are the neuron cytotoxicants; Mn and TMT are the clearest examples of occupational neurotoxicants belonging to this class. In this instance, chronic exposure yields little systemic toxicity but over the course of years results in slowly progressive neurological dysfunction. Tissue damage is restricted to neuronal loss and rea-

tive gliosis. The mechanisms of Mn or TMT neurotoxicity are unclear.

Axonopathy

Distal sensorimotor polyneuropathy is probably the most common manifestation of neurotoxicant exposure in humans. A variety of toxicants, including n-hexane, methy-n-butyl ketone (2-hexanone), CS_2, acrylamide, and organophosphorus esters, results in degeneration of the distal portions of the longest, largest myelinated axons in the peripheral and central nervous systems, an observation encapsulated in the term central-peripheral distal axonopathy. The increased susceptibility of these axons may be the product of the great distances over which vital molecules and organelles must be transported, the volume of cytoplasm that must be maintained, and the increased number of axonal targets for neurotoxicants. A morphologically striking subset of the central-peripheral distal axonopathies is those characterized by neurofilamentous axonal swellings. Investigations have detailed the biochemical steps through which two chemically dissimilar compounds, CS_2 and n-hexane, may produce clinically and morphologically identical lesions.

Distal axonopathies: n-hexane and carbon disulfide. As with many environmental neurotoxicants, the neurotoxicity of n-hexane and CS_2 was first recognized in humans and then verified in experimental animals. Hexane is a versatile nonpolar solvent used commercially for laminating and as a glue solvent in furniture and shoe production, where exposure may occur through inhalation and skin absorption. Cases of neuropathy from industrial exposure date to the mid-1960s and have been reported in the United States, France, Japan, and Morocco.[86,193] Inhalant abuse of n-hexane–containing mixtures has also been an important source of exposure and is responsible for some of the most severe cases of n-hexane–induced neuropathy.[6] CS_2 represents one of the earliest known industrial toxicants. Its toxicity was recognized more than a century ago in Europe, where it was used for the cold vulcanization of rubber.[47] Today the major uses of CS_2 are as a solvent in the laboratory and as a reactant in the production of cellophane and rayon from cellulose. The acute toxicity of CS_2 resulting from high-level exposure is manifested as narcosis and psychosis. Reduction of ambient levels of CS_2 in the workplace diminished the occurrence of these overt, acute signs but also provided an appropriate environment for chronic, low-dose exposure and its major complication, distal axonopathy.

Despite the different chemical structures, chronic exposure to either n-hexane or CS_2 can produce identical pathological changes. The primary lesion produced by both n-hexane and CS_2 develops in the distal axon of the longest and largest sensory and motor nerves of the central and peripheral tracts. Initially, multifocal fusiform axonal swellings develop at the proximal side of nodes of Ranvier at distal but preterminal sites (Fig. 30-2, *A*). Ultrastructural changes at the swellings include massive accumulations of disorganized 10 nm neurofilaments, decreased numbers of microtubules, thin myelin, and segregation of axoplasmic organelles and cytoskeletal components.[77] As axonal swellings enlarge, thinning and retraction of myelin becomes increasingly apparent (Fig. 30-2, *B*). Demyelination may occur partially through mechanical retraction at associated swellings, but evidence suggests that a direct action on Schwann cells also is possible.[144] Schwann cells develop increased cytoplasmic contents and proliferate around swollen and demyelinated axons with intrusion of their cell processes into the axoplasm. Distal to swellings, axons may become shrunken and then degenerate. With continued exposure, more proximal swellings occur with subsequent degeneration. Investigations on *n*-hexane and CS$_2$ have detailed their fate within biological systems and have provided insight into their mechanisms of action. The key to their shared clinical and pathological profiles appears to be the ability of each compound to generate protein-bound electrophilic species that can covalently cross-link neurofilament proteins.

Hexane is successively metabolized by hepatic ω-1 oxidation to its toxic metabolite 2,5-hexanedione (Fig. 30-3).[50] Intermediates in this oxidative pathway are also potentially neurotoxic and one, methyl *n*-butyl ketone (2-hexanone), also has been associated with distal axonopathies in humans exposed occupationally.[4,23] The neurotoxicity of each intermediate is proportional to the level of 2,5-hexanedione produced, and compounds such as methyl ethyl ketone that enhance ω-1 oxidation also potentiate the toxicity of 2,5-hexanedione precursors.[7,151] Neurotoxicity

of diketones requires an irreversible reaction of diketone with protein amine groups to form a pyrrole (Fig. 30-4). Diketones with other than γ spacing are incapable of forming pyrroles and are not neurotoxic. Although pyrrole formation is a necessary step for neurotoxicity, it is not sufficient. There is a requirement for pyrrole oxidation to a reactive intermediate that is then followed by protein cross-linking. That pyrrole formation, oxidation, and protein cross-linking are requisite for neurotoxicity of γ-diketones is evident from the following: (1) γ-diketones such as 3,4-diacetyl-2,5-hexanedione that rapidly form pyrroles but do not oxidize or result in protein cross-linking are not neurotoxic[174]; (2) when rates of pyrrole oxidation are increased either by inductive effects (e.g., meso-3,4-dimethyl-2,5-hexanedione, that forms pyrroles at the same rate as 2,5-hexanedione[72]) or hyperbaric oxygen,[155] the neurotoxic endpoint is reached more rapidly; and (3) diketones that undergo pyrrole formation and oxidation more rapidly than 2,5-hexanedione are more potent neurotoxicants and produce swellings at more proximal locations; *d,l*-3,4-dimethyl-2,5-hexanedione is more than 30 times more potent than 2,5-hexanedione.[10,156] Although the exact protein

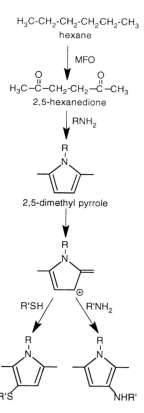

Fig. 30-4. Covalent cross-linking of proteins by hexane. Activation of hexane to 2,5-hexanedione occurs through ω-1 oxidation. Once formed, 2,5-hexanedione combines with the first protein amine to generate a 2,5-dimethyl pyrrole derivative. The pyrrolyl derivative then undergoes oxidation to an electrophilic intermediate that is followed by addition of a second protein nucleophile.

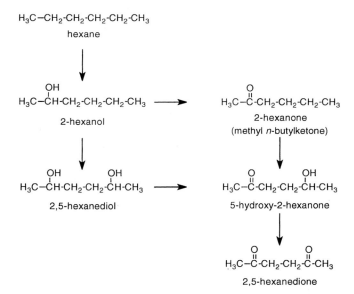

Fig. 30-3. Metabolism of hexane. Successive hepatic ω-1 oxidations of hexane produce 2,5-hexanedione, the neurotoxic species.

cross-linking structures have not been determined, addition of sulfhydryls and amines has been shown to occur at the 3 position of 2,5-dimethyl pyrrole in the presence of oxygen.[8]

The ability of CS_2 to cross-link proteins covalently also has been investigated in an attempt to explain how these chemically dissimilar compounds produce identical changes in the axon. Using Carbon-13 nuclear magnetic resonance (NMR) and specific isotopic labeling, a mechanism was demonstrated through which CS_2 can cross-link proteins covalently under physiological conditions (Fig. 30-5).[181] The cross-linking sequence initiates with CS_2 adding to a protein amine group forming a monoalkyl dithiocarbamate. The next step requires generation of isothiocyanate either through loss of sulfhydryl ion from dithiocarbamate or oxidation of dithiocarbamate through bis-thiocarbamoyl disulfide to isothiocyanate. Once formed, isothiocyanate adducts can undergo nucleophilic addition with sulfhydryl or amine groups to produce dithiocarbamate ester and thiourea cross-linking structures. Because dithiocarbamate esters form reversibly under physiological conditions, they too may serve as a source of isothiocyanate. The relative stability of thiourea and the greater abundance of amine groups in biological systems suggest that thiourea may be the more biologically relevant cross-linking structure.

Considerable similarity exists, therefore, between the sequence of events leading to cross-linking by 2,5-hexanedione and CS_2. Both compounds initially react with protein amine groups to form an adduct. The initial adducts then oxidize (pyrrole) or decompose (dithiocarbamate) generating a reactive electrophilic intermediate that undergoes nucleophilic addition. Although the specific cross-linking structures have been determined for CS_2, they are still under investigation for 2,5-hexanedione.[8]

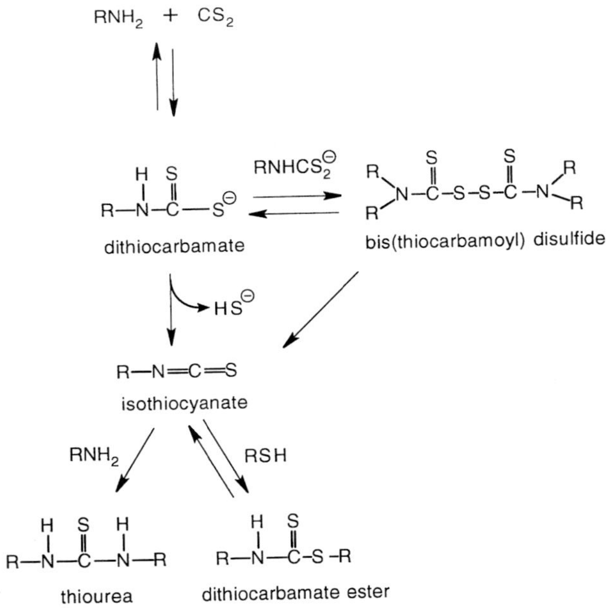

The massive accumulation of disorganized intermediate filaments within axonal swellings and the correlation between protein cross-linking and neurotoxicity suggest that neurofilament protein cross-linking may be the neurotoxic mechanism of 2,5-hexanedione and CS_2. Indeed, cross-linking of neurofilaments by 2,5-hexanedione has been demonstrated in vivo.[72,109,174] Although protein derivatization and cross-linking are expected to occur in proteins both within and outside the nervous system, neurofilament proteins may be more susceptible to progressive derivatization and cross-linking owing to their considerable stability and slow rate of transport down the axon. Additionally the prolonged juxtaposition of neurofilament subunits within neurofilaments may favor the formation of intermolecular cross-linking structures. The demonstration of spectrin dimers produced by CS_2 in vivo[182] suggests that cross-linking by CS_2 may also occur in other cytoskeletal proteins. If CS_2 also cross-links neurofilament proteins, it may provide a link to explain how these two agents produce identical neuropathological changes.

Proximal axonopathies. Proximal axonal swellings occur in motor neuron diseases of humans (e.g., amyotrophic lateral sclerosis and Werdnig-Hoffmann disease), but they have not been reported in humans following environmental toxicant exposure. Proximal axonal swellings, however, have been produced experimentally in laboratory animals by the administration of 3,3'-iminodipropionitrile (IDPN) or 3,4-dimethyl-2,5-hexanedione.[9] IDPN is not a naturally occurring compound, and knowledge of its biological effects was derived from investigations on the role of nitriles in the production of lathyrism associated with consumption of *Lathyrus* spp. Following a single 1 to 2 g/kg dose of IDPN in the rat, a peculiar behavioral change consisting of excitability, circling, and choreiform movements was observed.[41] Within 48 hours, proximal axonal swellings consisting of disorganized neurofilaments could be detected immediately distal to the initial segment and progressed in size over 3 to 4 weeks.[42] Demyelination with remyelination resulting in onion bulb formation occurred with extended exposures. Surprisingly, axonal loss or wallerian degeneration does not typically occur, and the most striking pathological change distal to the swelling is reduced axonal caliber.[43] Interruption of the slow component of axonal transport has been suggested as a mechanism for IDPN toxicity,[82] but relatively little is known regarding the molecular mechanism of this compound. Experimental studies done in rats using IDPN or crotonitrile demonstrated a specific lesion occurring in the hair cells of the vestibular apparatus as a

Fig. 30-5. Covalent cross-linking of proteins by carbon disulfide (CS_2). Addition of CS_2 to the first protein amine yields a monoalkyl dithiocarbamate. Isothiocyanate is then generated either from successive oxidation through disulfide formation or directly from the dithiocarbamate by elimination of the sulfhydryl ion. Once formed, the isothiocyanate undergoes nucleophilic addition with a second protein amine or sulfhydryl to produce thiourea or dithiocarbamate ester cross-linking structures.

potential target to account for the behavioral changes induced by these compounds.[114] Because crotonitrile produces behavioral changes identical to IDPN but does not produce proximal axonal swellings, the possibility exists that two separate mechanisms are responsible for these effects.

Summary. There is considerable evidence indicating a role for neurofilament cross-linking in CS_2-induced and 2,5-hexanedione–induced neuropathy; however, the mechanism through which cross-linking produces neurofilament-filled axonal swellings has not been elaborated. Several hypotheses have been presented, including physical blockage of neurofilament transport at nodes of Ranvier or interference with posttranslational modification of neurofilament proteins required for transport of neurofilaments. This question is complicated by the fact that the normal functional role of neurofilaments in the axon is still undetermined. Additionally the relationship between neurofilamentous axonal swellings and degeneration of the axon remains to be established. The IDPN model has demonstrated that axonal swellings alone are not sufficient to produce degeneration,[43] and is contrasted by acrylamide toxicity that results in axonal degeneration with much less neurofilament accumulation than CS_2 or 2,5-hexanedione.[12] Clearly, these questions need to be addressed in future investigations to obtain a better understanding of the underlying mechanisms of distal axonopathies.

CONCLUSION

Recurring "epidemics" of large-scale, acute exposures unequivocally demonstrate that humans are being exposed frequently to neurotoxicants. Once a compound is recognized as a neurotoxicant, contemporary regulations limit high-dose exposures; however, chronic low-dose exposure usually continues. The major problem that lies before clinicians and researchers is to discover those neurotoxicants that are biologically active following chronic exposure and to discern which of these is contributing to the progression of chronic neurological diseases. Clear answers to these questions await elucidation of the toxic mechanism of the injurious compounds.

REFERENCES

1. Adams RD, Salam-Adams M: *Striatonigral degeneration.* In Vinken PJ, Bruyn G, Klawans HL, editors: *Handbook of clinical neurology,* New York, 1986, Elsevier Science Publishers.
2. Aldridge WN et al: The toxicity and neuropathology of dimethylethyltin and methyldiethyltin in rats, *Neuropathol Appl Neurobiol* 13:55-69, 1987.
3. Alfrey AC, LeGendre GR, Kaehny WD: The dialysis encephalopathy syndrome, *N Engl J Med* 294:184-188, 1976.
4. Allen N, et al: Toxic polyneuropathy due to methyl *n*-butyl ketone. An industrial outbreak, *Arch Neurol* 32:209-218, 1975.
5. Alpers BJ, Lewy FH: Changes in the nervous system following carbon disulfide poisoning in animals and in man, *Arch Neurol Psychiatry* 44:725-739, 1940.
6. Altenkirch H, Mager J, Stoltenburg G, Helmbrecht J: Toxic poly-neuropathies after sniffing a glue thinner, *J Neurol* 214:137-152, 1977.
7. Altenkirch H, Stoltenburg G, Wagner HM: Experimental studies on hydrocarbon neuropathies, *J Neurol* 219:159, 1978.
8. Amarnath V et al: The mechanism of nucleophilic substitution of alkylpyrroles in the presence of oxygen, *Chem Res Toxicol* 7:56-61, 1994.
9. Anthony DC et al: The effect of 3,4-dimethyl substitution on the neurotoxicity of 2,5-hexanedione. II. Dimethyl substitution accelerates pyrrole formation and protein crosslinking, *Toxicol Appl Pharmacol* 71:372-382, 1983.
10. Anthony DC Boekelheide K, Graham DG: The effect of 3,4 dimethyl substitution on the neurotoxicity of 2,5-hexanedione. I. Accelerated clinical neuropathy is accompanied by more proximal swellings, *Toxicol Appl Pharmacol* 71:362-371, 1983.
11. Archibald FS, Tyree C: Manganese poisoning and the attack of trivalent manganese upon catecholamines, *Arch Biochem Biophys* 256:638-650, 1987.
12. Asbury AK, Brown MJ: *The evolution of structural changes in distal axonopathies.* In Spencer PS, Schaumburg HH, editors: *Experimental and clinical neurotoxicology,* Baltimore, 1980, Williams & Wilkins.
13. Balaban CD, O'Callaghan JP, Billingsley ML: Trimethyltin-induced neuronal damage in the rat brain: comparative studies using silver degeneration stains, immunocytochemistry and immunoassay for neuronotypic and gliotypic proteins, *Science* 26:337-361, 1988.
14. Ballard PA, Tetrud JW, Langston JW: Permanent human parkinsonism due to 1-methyl-4-phenyl-1,2,3,6-tetrahydropyridine (MPTP): Seven cases, *Neurology* 35:949-956, 1985.
15. Barbeau A: Manganese and extrapyramidal disorders. A critical review and tribute to Dr. George C. Cotzias, *Neurotoxicology* 5:13-36, 1984.
16. Barbeau A, Inoue N, Cloutier T: Role of manganese in dystonia, *Adv Neurol* 14:339-351, 1976.
17. Beal MF: Does impairment of energy metabolism result in excito-toxic neuronal death in neurodegenerative illness. *Ann Neurol* 31:119-130, 1992.
18. Benton Jr CD, and Calhoun Jr FP: The ocular effects of methyl alcohol poisoning. Report of a catastrophe involving 320 persons, *Am J Ophthalmol* 36:1677-1685, 1952.
19. Berger JR, Ayyar R: Neurological complications of ethylene glycol intoxication. Report of a case, *Arch Neurol* 38: 724-726,
20. Bergouignan FX et al: Disulfiram neuropathy, *J Neurol* 235:382-383, 1988.
21. Bernheimer H et al: Brain dopamine and the syndromes of Parkinson and Huntington. Clinical, morphological and neurochemical correlations, *J Neurol Sci* 20:415-455, 1973.
22. Besser R, et al: Acute trimethyltin limbic-cerebellar syndrome, *Neurology* 37:945-950, 1987.
23. Billmaier D et al: Peripheral neuropathy in a coated fabrics plant, *J Occup Med* 16:655-671, 1974.
24. Bird ED, Anton AH, Bullock B: The effect of manganese inhalation on basal ganglia dopamine concentrations in *Rhesus* monkey, *Neurotoxicology* 5:59-66, 1984.
25. Boor JW, Hurtig HI: Persistent cerebellar ataxia after exposure to toluene, *Ann Neurol* 2:440-442, 1977.
26. Bouldin TW et al: Pathogenesis of trimethyltin neuronal toxicity. Ultrastructural and cytochemical observations, *Am J Pathol* 104:237-249, 1981.
27. Bouldin TW, Goines ND, Krigman MR: Trimethyltin retinopathy. Relationship of subcellular response to neuronal subspecialization, *J Neuropathol Exp Neurol* 43: 162-174, 1984.
28. Bouldin TW et al: Differential vulnerability of mixed and cutaneous nerves in lead neuropathy, *J Neuropathol Exp Neurol* 44:384-396, 1985.

29. Brierley JB, Brown AW, Calverley J: Cyanide intoxication in the rat-physiological and neuropathological aspects, *J Neurol Neurosurg Psychiatry* :39:129-140, 1976.
30. Brierley JB et al: Cyanide intoxication in *Macaca mulatta, J Neurol Sci* 31:133-157, 1977.
31. Brouillet EP et al: Manganese injection into the rat striatum produces excitotoxic lesions by impairing energy metabolism, *Exp Neurol* 120:889-894, 1993.
32. Brown AW et al: The behavioral and neuropathologic sequelae of intoxication by trimethyltin compounds in the rat, *Am J Pathol* 97: 59-82, 1979.
33. Burks JS et al: A fatal encephalopathy in chronic haemodialysis patients, *Lancet* 1:764-768, 1976.
34. Buxton PH, Hayward M: Polyneuritis cranialis associated with industrial trichloroethylene poisoning, *Neurol Neurosurg Psychiatry* 30:511-517, 1967.
35. Canavan MM, Cobb S, Drinker CK: Chronic manganese poisoning. Report of a case, with autopsy, *Arch Neurol Psychiatry* 32:501-513, 1934.
36. Chang LW: *Mercury.* In Spencer PS, Schaumburg HH, editors: *Experimental and clinical neurotoxicology,* Baltimore, 1980, Williams & Wilkins.
37. Chapman LJ et al: Finger tremor after carbon disulfide-based pesticide exposures, *Arch Neurol* 48:866-870, 1991.
38. Chen YCJ, et al: Cognitive development of Yu-Cheng (oil disease) children prenatally exposed to heat-degraded PCBs, *JAMA* 268:3213-3218, 1992.
39. Chhuttani PN, Chopra JS: *Arsenic poisoning.* In Vinken PJ, Bruyn GW, editors: *Handbook of clinical neurology,* Amsterdam, 1979, Elsevier Science Publishers.
40. Choi IS: Delayed neurologic sequelae in carbon monoxide intoxication, *Arch Neurol* 40:433-435, 1983.
41. Chou SM, Hartmann HA: Axonal lesions and waltzing syndrome after IDPN administration in rats: with a concept "axostasis," *Acta Neuropathol* 3:428-450, 1964.
42. Chou SM, Hartman HA: Electron microscopy of focal neuroaxonal lesions produced by β-β′ iminodipropionitrile (IDPN) in rats, *Acta Neuropathol* 4:590-603, 1965.
43. Clark A, Griffin JW, Price DL: The axonal pathology in chronic β,β′-iminodipropionitrile intoxication, *J Neuropathol Exp Neurol* 39:42-55, 1980.
44. Clarren SK et al: Brain malformations related to prenatal exposure to ethanol, *J Pediatr* 92:64-67, 1978.
45. Coyle JT, Puttfarcken P: Oxidative stress, glutamate, and neurodegenerative disorders, *Science* 262:689-695, 1993.
46. Crystal HA et al: Cognitive impairment and sensory loss associated with chronic low-level ethylene oxide exposure, *Neurology* 38:567-569, 1988.
47. Davidson M, Feinlab M: Carbon disulfide poisoning: a review, *Am Heart J* 83:100-114, 1972.
48. Davis LE et al: Acute thallium poisoning: toxicological and morphological studies of the nervous system, *Ann Neurol* 10:38-44, 1981.
49. Davis LE et al: Central nervous system intoxication from mercurous chloride laxatives, *Arch Neurol* 30:428-431, 1974.
50. Di Vincenzo GD, Kaplan CJ, Dedinas J: Characterization of the metabolites of methyl *n*-butyl ketone, methyl iso-butyl ketone, and methyl ethyl ketone in guinea pig serum and their clearance, *Toxicol Appl Pharmacol* 36:311, 1976.
51. Donaldson J: The physiopathologic significance of manganese in brain: its relation to schizophrenia and neurodegenerative disorders, *Neurotoxicology* 8:451-462, 1987.
52. Donaldson J, McGregor D, Labella F: Manganese neurotoxicity: a model for free radical mediated neurodegeneration? *Can J Physiol Pharmacol* 60:1398-1405, 1982.
53. Donofrio PD et al: Acute arsenic intoxication presenting as Guillain-Barre-like syndrome, *Muscle Nerve* 10:114-120, 1987.
54. Duncan MW: β-*Methylamino-L-Alanine (BMAA) and amyotrophic lateral sclerosis-Parkinsonism dementia of the western Pacific.* In Langston JW, Young A, editors: *Neurotoxins and neurodegenerative disease,* New York, 1992, NY Academy of Science.
55. Ejima A et al: Manganese intoxication during total parenteral nutrition, *Lancet* 339:426, 1992.
56. Eriksson H, Lenngren S, Heilbronn E: Effect of long-term administration of manganese on biogenic amine levels in discrete striatal regions of rat brain, *Arch Toxicol* 59:426-431, 1987.
57. Eriksson H, et al: Effects of manganese oxide on monkeys as revealed by a combined neurochemical, histological and neurophysiological evaluation, *Arch Toxicol* 61:46-52, 1987.
58. Eriksson H et al: Manganese induced brain lesions in *Macca fasicularis* as revealed by positron emission tomography and magnetic resonance imaging, *Arch Toxicol* 66:403-407, 1992.
59. Eriksson H et al: Receptor alterations in manganese intoxicated monkeys, *Arch Toxicol* 66:359-364, 1992.
60. Escobar A, Aruffo C: Chronic thinner intoxication: clinico-pathologic report of a human case, *J Neurol Neurosurg Psychiatry* 43:986-994, 1980.
61. Feldman JM, Feldman MD: Sequelae of attempted suicide by cyanide ingestion: a case report, *Int J Psychiat Med* 20:173-179, 1990.
62. Feldman RG: *Trichlorethylene.* In Vinken PJ, Bruyn GW, editors: *Handbook of clinical neurology,* Amsterdam, 1979, Elsevier Science Publishers.
63. Feldman RG: *Manganese as possible ecoetiologic factor in Parkinson's disease.* In Langston JW, Young A, editors: *Neurotoxins and neurodegenerative disease,* New York, 1992, NY Academy of Sciences.
64. Filley CM, Heaton RK, Rosenberg NL: White matter dementia in chronic toluene abuse, *Neurology* 40:532-534, 1990.
65. Filley CM, Kelly JP: Alcohol- and drug-related neurotoxicity, *Curr Opin Neurol Neurosurg* 6:443-447, 1993.
66. Fortemps E et al: Trimethyltin poisoning: a report of two cases, *Int Arch Occupat Environ Health* 6:1-5, 1978.
67. Freilich RJ, Byrne E: Alcohol and drug abuse, *Curr Opin Neurol Neurosurg* 5:391-395, 1992.
68. Friedman et al: Consequences of ethylene glycol poisoning, *Am J Med* 32:891-902, 1962.
69. Fullerton PM: Electrophysiological and histological observations on peripheral nerves in acrylamide poisoning in man, *J Neurol Neurosurg Psychiatry* 32:186-192, 1969.
70. Gavin CE, Gunter KK, Gunter TE: Manganese and calcium efflux kinetics in brain mitochondria. Relevance to manganese toxicity, *Biochem J* 266:329-334, 1990.
71. Gavin CE, Gunter KK, Gunter TE: Mn^{2+} sequestration by mitochondria and inhibition of oxidative phosphorylation, *Toxicol Appl Pharmacol* 115:1-5, 1992.
72. Genter MB et al: Evidence that pyrrole formation is a pathogenetic step in γ-diketone neuropathy, *Toxicol Appl Pharmacol* 87:351-362, 1987.
73. Gill JS et al: Alcohol consumption—a risk factor for hemorrhagic and non-hemorrhagic stroke, *Am J Med* 90:489-496, 1991.
74. Ginsberg MD: *Carbon monoxide.* In Spencer PS, Schaumburg HH, editors: *Experimental and clinical neurotoxicology,* Baltimore, 1980, Williams & Wilkins.
75. Ginsberg MD, Hedley-Whyte ET, Richardson Jr EP: Hypoxic-ischemic leukoencephalopathy in man, *Arch Neurol* 33:5-14, 1976.
76. Goebel HH et al: Polyneuropathy due to acute arsenic intoxication: biopsy studies, *J Neuropathol Exp Neurol* 49:137-149, 1990.
77. Gottfried MR et al: The morphology of carbon disulfide neurotoxicity, *Neurotoxicology* 6:89-96, 1985.

78. Grabski DA: Toluene sniffing producing cerebellar degeneration, *Am J Psychiatry* 118:461-462, 1961.
79. Graham DG: Catecholamine toxicity: a proposal for the molecular pathogenesis of manganese neurotoxicity and Parkinson's disease, *Neurotoxicology* 5:83-96, 1984.
80. Grandas F, Artieda J, Obeso JA: Clinical and CT scan findings in a case of cyanide intoxication, *Movement Dis* 4:188-193, 1989.
81. Greene JG et al: Inhibition of succinate dehydrogenase by malonic acid produces an excitotoxic lesion in rat striatum, *J neurochem* 61:1151-1154, 1993.
82. Griffin JW et al: Slow axonal transport of neurofilament proteins: impairment by β,β′-iminodiporpionitrile, *Science* 202:633, 1978.
83. Gross JA, Haas ML, Swift TR: Ethylene oxide neurotoxicity: report of fourt cases and review of the literature, *Neurology* 29:978-983, 1979.
84. Hanawa S, Matsushita M: An autopsy case of disulfiram induced psychosis with parkinsonian syndrome, *Seishin Shinkeigaku Zasshi* 84:503-512, 1982.
85. Haymaker W, Ginzler AM, Ferguson RL: Residual neuropathological effects of cyanide poisoning. A study of the central nervous system of 23 dogs exposed to cyanide compounds, *Milit Surg* 11:231-245, 1952.
86. Herskowitz A, Ishii N, Schamburg H: n-Hexane neuropathy: a syndrome occurring as a result of industrial exposure, *N Engl J Med* 285: 82, 1971.
87. Hirano A, Iwata M: *neuropathology of lead intoxication*. In Vinken PJ, Bruyn GW, editors: *Handbook of clinical neurology*, Amsterdam, 1979, Elsevier Science Publishers.
88. Huang C-C et al: Chronic manganese intoxication, *Arch Neurol* 46:1104-1106, 1989.
89. Huang C-C et al: Progression after chronic manganese exposure, *Neurology* 43:1479-1483, 1993.
90. Igisu H et al: Acrylamide encephaloneuropathy due to well water pollution, *J Neurol Neurosurg Psychiatry* 38:581-584, 1975.
91. Ishimaru H, et al: Effects of N-methyl-D-aspartate receptor antagonists on carbon monoxide-induced brain damage in mice, *J Pharmacol Exp Ther* 261:349-352, 1992.
92. Jacobs JM, Le Quesne PM: *Toxic disorders*. In Vinken PJ, Bruyn GW, Klawans JL, editors: *Handbook of clinical neurology*, Amsterdam, 1986, Elsevier Science Publishers.
93. Jellinger K: *Exogenous lesions of the pallidum*. In Vinken PJ, Bruyn GW, Klawans HL, editors: *Handbook of clinical neurology*, Amsterdam, 1986, Elsevier Science Publishers.
94. Jellinger K: *(Exogenous) striatal necrosis*. In Vinken PJ, Bruyn GW, Klawans HL, editors: *Handbook of clinical neurology, Amsterdam, 1986, Elsevier Science Publishers.*
95. Jenkins RB: Inorganic arsenic and the nervous system, *Brain* 89:479-497, 1966.
96. Jenner P, Schapira AHV, Marsden CD: New insights into the cause of Parkinson's disease, *Neurology* 42:2241-2250, 1992.
97. Joong S, Kim JM: Giant axonal swelling in "Huffer's" neuropathy, *Arch Neurol* 33:583-586, 1976.
98. Kaelan C, Harper C, Vieira BI: Acute encephalopathy and death due to petrol sniffing: neuropathological findings, *Aust NZ J Med* 16:804-807, 1986.
99. Kaku DA, Lowenstein DH: Emergence of recreational drug abuse as a major risk factor for stroke in young adults, *Ann Intern Med* 113:821-827, 1990.
100. Kimbrough RD: Human health effects of polychlorinated biphenyls (PCBs) and polybrominated biphenyls (PBBs), *Ann Rev Pharmacol Toxicol* 27:87-111, 1987.
101. Klawans HL et al: A pure parkinsonian syndrome following acute carbon monoxide intoxication, *Arch Neurol* 39:302-304, 1982.
102. Korobkin R et al: Glue-sniffing neuropathy, *Arch Neurol* 32:158-162, 1975.
103. Krauss JK et al: Dystonia and akinesia due to pallidoputaminal lesions after disulfiram intoxication, *Movement Dis* 6:166-170, 1991.
104. Krigman MR, Bouldin TW, Mushak P: *Lead*. In Spencer PS, Schaumburg HH editors: *Experimental and clincal neurotoxicology*, Baltimore, 1980, Williams & Wilkins.
105. Kuzuhara S et al: Ethylene oxide polyneuropathy, *Neurology* 33:377-380, 1983.
106. Langston JW, Irwin I, Ricaurte GA: Neurotoxins, parkinsonism and Parkinson's disease, *Pharmacol Ther* 32:19-49, 1987.
107. Langston JW, Langston EB, Irwin I: MPTP-induced parkinsonism in human and non-human primates—clinical and experimental aspects, *Acta Neurol Scand* 70:49-54, 1984.
108. Laplane D et al: Lesions of basal ganglia due to disulfiram, *J Neurol Neurosurg Psychiatry* 55:925-929, 1992.
109. Lapodula DM et al: Cross-linking of neurofilament proteins of rat spinal cord in vivo after administration of 2,5-hexanedione, *J Neurochem* 46:1843-1850, 1986.
110. Liccione JJ, Maines MD: Selective vulnerability of glutathione metabolism and cellular defense mechanisns in rat striaum to manganese, *J Pharmacol Exp Ther* 247:156-161, 1988.
111. Liccione JJ, Maines MD: Manganese-mediated increase in the rat brain mitochondrial cytochrome P-450 and drug metabolism activity: susceptibility of the striatum, *J Pharmacol Exp Ther* 248:222-227, 1989.
112. Limos LC et al: Axonal degeneration and focal muscle fiber necrosis in human thallotoxicosis: histopathological studies of nerve and muscle, *Muscle Nerve* 5:698-706, 1982.
113. Lipton SA, Rosenberg PA: Excitatory amino acids as a final common pathway for neurological disorders, *N Engl J Med* 330:613-622, 1994.
114. Llorens J et al: The behavioral syndrome caused by a 3,3′-iminodipropionitrile and related nitriles in the rat is associated with degeneration of the vestibular sensory hair cells, *Toxicol Appl Pharmacol* 123:199-210, 1993.
115. Martin-Bouyer G et al: Outbreak of accidental hexachlorophene poisoning in France, *Lancet* 1:91-95, 1982.
116. Martinez AJ, Boehm R, Hadfield MG: Acute hexachlorophene encephalopathy: clinico-neuropathological correlation, *Acta Neuropathol (Berl)* 28:93-103, 1974.
117. Martinez AJ et al: Chlordecone intoxication in man. II. Ultrastructure of peripheral nerves and skeletal muscle, *Neurology*, 28:631-635, 1978.
118. McLaughlin AIG et al: Pulmonary fibrosis and encephalopathy associated with the inhalation of aluminum dust, *Br J Industr Med* 19:253-263, 1962.
119. McLean DR, Jacobs H, Mielke BW: Methanol poisoning: a clinical and pathological study, *Ann Neurol* 8:161-167, 1980.
120. Meldrum BS: Excitatory amino acid receptors and disease, *Curr Opin Neurol Neurosurg* 5:508-513, 1992.
121. Meldrum B, Garthwaite J: Excitatory amino acid neurotoxicity and neurodegenerative disease, *TIPS* 11:379-387, 1990.
122. Mena I et al: Chronic manganese poisoning. Clinical picture and manganese turnover, *Neurology* 17:128-136, 1967.
123. Meulenbelt J, de Groot G, Savelkoul TJF: Two cases of acute toluene intoxication, *Br J Industr Med* 47:417-420, 1990.
124. Mirowitz SA, Westrich TJ, Hirsch JD: Hyperintense basal ganglia on T1-weighted MR images in patients receiving parenteral nutrition, *Radiology* 181:117-120, 1991.
125. Moddel G et al: Disulfiram neuropathy, *Arch Neurol* 35:658-660, 1978.
126. Mokri B, Ohnishi A, Dyck PJ: Disulfiram neuropathy, *Neurology* 31:730-735, 1981.
127. Moses H, Klawans HL: *Bromide intoxication*. In Vinken PJ, Bruyn GW, editors: *Handbook of clinical neurology*, Amsterdam, 1979, Elsevier Science Publishers.

128. Mullick FG: Hexachlorophene toxicity—human experience at the Armed Forces Institute of Pathology, *Pediatrics* 51:395-399, 1973.

129. Nelson K et al: Manganese encephalopathy: utility of early magnetic resonance imaging, *Br J Industr Med* 50:510-513, 1993.

130. Novelli A et al: Glutamate becomes neurotoxic via the *N*-methyl-D-aspartate receptor when intracellular energy levels are reduced, *Brain Res* 451:205-212, 1988.

131. Nukada H, Pollock M: Disulfiram neuropathy. A morphometric study of sural nerve, *J Neurol Sci* 51:51-67, 1981.

132. O'Callaghan JP: *Assessment of neurotoxicity using assays of neuron and glial-localized proteins: chronology and critique.* In Tilson H, Mitchell C, editors: *Neurotoxicology,* New York, 1992, Raven Press.

133. O'Callaghan JP: Quantitative features of reactive gliosis following toxicant-induced damage of the CNS, *Ann NY Acad Sci* 679:195-211, 1992.

134. Ohta M: Ultrastructure of sural nerve in a case of arsenical neuropathy; *Acta Neuropathol (Berl)* 16:233-242, 1970.

135. Osuntokun BO: An ataxic neuropathy in Nigeria. A clinical, biochemical and electrophysiological study, *Brain* 91:215-247, 1968.

136. Peiffer J et al: Alcohol embryo- and fetopathy, *J Neurol Sci* 41:125-137, 1979.

137. Penney DG: Acute carbon monoxide poisoning: animal models: a review, *Toxicology* 62:123-160, 1990.

138. Perl TM et al: An outbreak of toxic encephalopathy caused by eating mussels contaminated with domoic acid, *N Engl J Med* 322:1775-1780, 1990.

139. Pestronk A, Keogh JP, Griffin JW: *Dimethylaminopropionitrile.* In Spencer PS, Schaumburg HH, editors: Baltimore, 1980, Williams & Wilkins.

140. Peters HA et al: Extrapyramidal and other neurologic manifestations associated with carbon disulfide fumigant exposure, *Arch Neurol* 45:537-540, 1988.

141. Phang PT et al: Brain hemorrhage associated with methanol poisoning, *Crit Care Med* 16:137-140, 1988.

142. Plum F, Posner JB, Hain RF: Delayed neurological deterioration after anoxia, *Arch Int Med* 110:56-63, 1962.

143. Poirier J, Kogan S, Gauthier S: Environment, genetics and idiopathic Parkinson's disease, *Can J Neurol Sci* 18:70-76, 1991.

144. Powell HC et al: Schwann cell abnormalities in 2,5-hexanedione neuropathy, *J Neurocytol* 7:517, 1978.

145. Prain JH, Smith GH: A clinical-pathological report of eight cases of methyl bromide poisoning, *Br J Industr Med* 9:44-49, 1952.

146. Prick JJG: *Thallium poisoning.* In Vinken PJ, Bruyn GW, editors: *Handbook of clinical neurology, Amsterdam, 1979, Elsevier Science Publishers.*

147. Pulst S-M, Walshe TM, Romero JA: Carbon monoxide poisoning with features of Gilles de la Tourette's syndrome, *Arch Neurol* 40:443-444, 1983.

148. Reusche E, Seydel U: Dialysis-associated encephalopathy: light and electron microscopic morphology and topography with evidence of aluminum by laser microprobe mass analysis, *Acta Neuropathol* 86:249-258, 1992.

149. Richter R: Degeneration of the basal ganglia in monkeys from chronic carbon disulfide poisoning, *J Neuropathol Exp Neurol* 4:324-353, 1945.

150. Rizzuto N, Terzian H, Galiazzo-Rizzuto S: Toxic polyneuropathies in Italy due to leather cement poisoning in shoe industries, *J Neurol Sci* 31:343-354, 1977.

151. Robertson PJ, White EL, Bus JS: Effects of methyl ethyl ketone pretreatment on hepatic mixed-function oxidase activity and on in vivo metabolism of *n*-hexane, *Xenobiotica* 19:721-729, 1989.

152. Rogers D: Psychiatric consequences of basal ganglia disease, *Semin Neurol* 10:262-266, 1990.

153. Roscher AA: A new histochemical method for the demonstration of calcium oxalate in tissues following ethylene glycol poisoning, *Am J Clin Pathol* 55:99-104, 1971.

154. Rosenberg NL, Myers JA, Martin WRW: Cyanide-induced parkinsonism: clinical, MRI, and 6-fluorodopa PET studies, *Neurology* 39:142-144, 1989.

155. Rosenberg CK et al: Hyperbaric oxygen accelerates the neurotoxicity of 2,5-hexanedione, *Toxicol Appl Pharmacol* 87:374-379, 1987.

156. Rosenberg CK et al: dl-versus meso-3,4-dimethyl-2,5-hexanedione: a morphometric study of the proximodistal distribution of axonal swellings in the anterior root of the rat, *Toxicol Appl Pharmacol* 87:363-373, 1987.

157. Rosenberg NL et al: Central nervous system effects of chronic toluene abuse—clinical, brainstem evoked response and magnetic resonance imaging studies, *Neurotoxicol Teratol* 10:489-495, 1988.

158. Rosenberg NL et al: Toluene abuse causes diffuse central nervous system white matter changes, *Ann Neurol* 23:611-614, 1988.

159. Ross WD et al: Neurotoxic effects of occupational exposure to organotins, *Am J Psychiatry* 138:1092-1095, 1981.

160. Rothman SM, Olney JW: Glutamate and the pathophysiology of hypoxicischemic brain damage, *Ann Neurol* 19:105-111, 1986.

161. Schaumburg HH, Spencer PS: *Selected outbreaks of neurotoxic disease.* In Spencer PS, Schaumburg HH, editors: *Experimental and clinical neurotoxicology,* Baltimore, 1980, Williams & Wilkins.

162. Schoenberg BS: Environmental risk factors for Parkinson's disease: the epidemiologic evidence, *Can J Neurol Sci* 14:407-413, 1987.

163. Schroder et al: Ethylene oxide polyneuropathy: clinical follow-up study with morphometric and electron microscopic findings in a sural nerve biopsy, *Neurology* 232:83-90, 1985.

164. Seppalainen AM, Haltia M: *Carbon disulfide.* In Spencer PS, Schaumburg HH, editors: *Experimental and clinical neurotoxicology,* Baltimore, 1980, Williams & Wilkins.

165. Shiraki H: *Neuropatholigic aspects of organic mercury intoxication, including Minamata disease.* In Vinken PJ, Bruyn GW, editors: *Handbook of clinical neurology,* Amsterdam, 1979, Elsevier Science Publishers.

166. Shuman RM et al: Neurotoxicity of hexachlorophene in the human: I. A clinicopathologic study of 248 children, *Pediatrics* 54:689-695, 1974.

167. Shuman RM, Leech RW, Alvord Jr EC: Neurotoxicity of hexachlorophene in humans. II. A clinicopathological study of 46 premature infants, *Arch Neurol* 32:320-325, 1975.

168. Silverman CS, Brenner J, Murtagh FR: Hemorrhagic necrosis and vascular injury in carbon monoxide poisoning: MR demonstration, *AJNR Am J Neuroradiol* 14:168-170, 1993.

169. Smith DE: Morphological lesions due to acute and subacute poisoning with antifreeze (ethylene glycol), *Arch Pathol* 51:423-433, 1951.

170. Spencer PS, Couri D, Schaumburg HH: *n-Hexane and methyl n-butyl ketone.* In Spencer PS, Schaumburg HH, editors: *Experimental and clinical neurotoxicology,* Baltimore, 1980, Williams & Wilkins.

171. Spencer PS, Ludolph AC, Kisby GE: *Are human neurodegenerative disorders linked to environmental chemicals with excitotoxic properties?* In Langston JW, Young A, editors: *Neurotoxins and neurodegenerative disease,* New York, 1992, NY Academy of Sciences.

172. Spencer PS et al: Nervous system degeneration produced by the industrial solvent methyl *n*-butyl ketone, *Arch Neurol* 32:219-222, 1975.

173. Squier MV, Thompson J, Rajgopalan B: Case report: neuropathology of methyl bromide intoxication, *Neuropathol Appl Neurobiol* 18:579-584, 1992.

174. St. Clair MBG et al: Pyrrole oxidation and protein cross-linking as necessary steps in the development of γ-diketone neuropathy, *Chem Res Toxicol* 1:179-185, 1988.

175. Tanner CM, Langston JW: Do environmental toxins cause Parkinson's disease? A critical review, *Neurology* 3:17-30, 1990.

176. Teitelbaum JS et al: Neurologic sequelae of domoic acid intoxication due to the ingestion of contaminated mussels, *N Engl J Med* 322:1781-1787, 1990.

177. Toggas SM et al: Molecular mechanisms of selective neurotoxicants: studies on organotin compounds, *Ann NY Acad Sci* 679:157-177, 1992.

178. Towfighi J et al: Glue sniffer's neuropathy, *Neurology* 26:238-243, 1976.

179. *Toxicological profile for lead 1993*, US Department of Health and Human Services, 1993, Washington, DC.

180. Uitti RJ et al: Cyanide-induced parkinsonism: a clinicopathologic report, *Neurology* 35:921-925, 1985.

181. Valentine WM et al: Covalent cross-linking of proteins by carbon disulfide, *Chem Res Toxicol* 5:254-262, 1992.

182. Valentine WM, Graham DG, Anthony DC: Covalent cross-linking of erythrocyte spectrin by carbon disulfide in vivo, *Toxicol Appl Pharmacol* 121:71-77, 1993.

183. Valenzuela R, Court J, Godoy J: Delayed cyanide induced dystonia, *J Neurol Neurosurg Psychiatry,* 55:198-199, 1992.

184. Valpey R et al: Acute and chronic progressive encephalopathy due to gasoline sniffing, *Neurology* 28:507-510, 1978.

185. Verity MA: Neurotoxins and environmental poisons, *Curr Opin Neurol Neurosurg* 5:401-405, 1992.

186. Verity MA: Environmental neurotoxicity of chemicals and radiation, *Curr Opin Neurol Neurosurg* 6:437-442, 1993.

187. Vescovi A et al: Interactions of manganese with human brain glutathione-*S*-transferase, *Toxicology* 57:183-191, 1989.

188. Vescovi A et al: Dopamine metabolism alterations in a manganese-treated pheochromocytoma cell line (PC12), *Toxicology* 67:129-142, 1991.

189. Winder H et al: Bilateral fetal mesencephalic grafting in two patients with parkinsonism induced by 1-methyl-4-phenyl-1,2,3,6-tetra-hydropyridine (MPTP), *N Engl J Med* 327:1556-1563, 1992.

190. Wisniewski K et al: A clinical neuropathological study of the fetal alcohol syndrome, *Neuropediatrics* 14:197-201, 1983.

191. Wolters EC et al: Positron emission tomography in manganese intoxication, *Ann Neurol* 26:647-651, 1989.

192. Yamada, M et al: Chronic manganese poisoning: a neuropathological study with determination of manganese distribution in the brain, *Acta Neuropathol* 70:273-278, 1986.

193. Yamada S: An occurrence of polyneuritis by *n*-hexane in the polyethylene laminating plants, *Jap J Industr Health* 6:192, 1964.

194. Zatuchni J, Hong K: Methyl bromide poisoning seen initially as psychosis, *Arch Neurol* 38:529-530, 1981.

Chapter 31

SKELETAL SYSTEM

H. Clarke Anderson

This chapter is dedicated to the memory of Dame Janet Vaughan, 1899-1993, pioneer radiobiologist and pathologist who was among the first to study the biological hazards of bone-seeking radioisotopes. Dame Janet founded the MRC Bone Research Laboratory at the Nuffield Orthopaedic Center, Oxford, which initially was solely devoted to studies of the biological effects of bone-seeking radioisotopes. She was trained as a physician, and after medical school, she practiced hematology. In the late 1920s while on staff at Hammersmith Hospital, she pioneered the use of minced liver to treat pernicious anemia. During World War II, she directed the entire blood supply service for North-West London. From 1945 to 1967, she was the renowned Principal of Somerville College, Oxford. Her whole life and her singular scientific achievements were characterized by a relentless concern for excellence.

BONE DEVELOPMENT, GROWTH, AND MECHANISMS OF MINERALIZATION

Bones develop and grow by means of two major mechanisms: (1) "endochondral" growth within preexisting cartilage, as characterized by elongation at cartilaginous growth plates (epiphyseal plates) situated at the ends of the long bones, and (2) "intramembranous" appositional growth of bone as characterized by cortical bone growth under the periosteum and by osteoblasts on surfaces of medullary bone trabeculae.

Endochondral bone growth is a symmetrical and polarized process in which chondrocytes multiply in the proliferative zone of the growth plate and their daughter cells accumulate as stacked cell columns in single file (Fig. 31-1). The daughter cells progress through a life cycle that includes maturational hypertrophy, synthesis and secretion of cartilage matrix containing matrix vesicles, senescence, and finally programmed cell death and disruption, which occurs near the base of the growth plate.[36] The entire life cycle takes only about 2 to 3 days to complete in a growing animal.[60] In synchrony with chondrocyte hypertrophy and then senesence, predetermined areas of matrix calcify to form longitudinally oriented bars of calcified matrix (Fig. 31-1). Calcification of cartilage begins in matrix rather than in cells and is initiated by extracellular matrix vesicles.[2,3] Once initiated, calcification extends by a process of epitaxial crystal proliferation, infiltrating the adjacent collagenous matrix.[2] Calcium phosphate in the form of crystalline hydroxyapatite is the predominant form of mineral in growth plate cartilage matrix and also in the matrix of newly formed bone.

Ultimately the calcified regions of the growth plate are converted to bone (Fig. 31-1) in a process that involves: (1) chondroclast resorption in the metaphysis of deceased

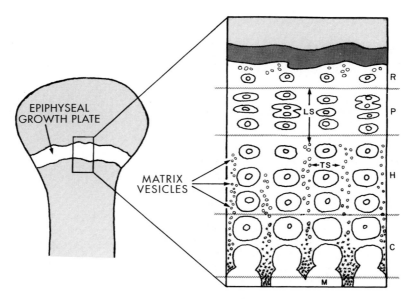

Fig. 31-1. Diagram of the epiphyseal growth plate of a long bone, the site at which growth in length occurs. The growth plate is subdivided into the following anatomical regions: The reserve zone *(R),* at the top of the growth plate, contains apparently inactive chondrocytes. The proliferative zone *(P)* is a zone of active cell division where cell columns first appear, thus allowing the matrix to be anatomically subdivided into transverse matrix septa *(TS),* separating cells within a column, and longitudinal septa *(LS),* separating adjacent cell columns. The hypertrophic zone *(H)* contains enlarging chondrocytes and many matrix vesicles, found in clusters in the longitudinal septa. The first mineral crystals arise within matrix vesicles of the hypertrophic zone (see Fig. 31-3). The calcifying zone *(C)* contains degenerating chondrocytes. This is the level at which proliferating mineral spreads from matrix vesicles radially outward to infiltrate the interstices of the longitudinal septal matrix. At the base of the growth plate lies the bony metaphysis *(M)* with small vessels that invade the uncalcified transverse matrix septa and degenerative cells, leaving calcified longitudinal septa on which osteoblasts from the marrow deposit new bone (the primary spongiosa). (From Anderson HC: *Calcium in biological systems,* New York, 1985, Plenum Press; with permission.)

cartilage cells and uncalcified cartilage matrix, which persists mainly as transverse bars between the cells; (2) capillary ingrowth into the spaces created by resorption of disrupted chondrocytes and uncalcified matrix; and (3) preosteoblast migration from the underlying marrow. These cells line up along the projecting calcified cartilage septa, where they deposit bone matrix beneath their basilar surfaces in a polarized manner. Bone matrix contains more collagen and less proteoglycan than does cartilage matrix. Mineralization is also initiated in bone by matrix vesicles.[3,6] Bone matrix vesicles are derived from the basolateral surfaces of osteoblasts, apparently by a "pinching-off" process. Hydroxyapatite mineral proliferates to involve the entire matrix except for an unmineralized zone beneath the osteoblast. The advancing border of mineral is referred to as the "calcification front" (Fig. 31-2). The calcification front moves toward the osteoblast by appositional mineral accumulation, but at sites of active osteoblastic bone growth, the calcification front does not keep up and usually is separated from the basal surface of the osteoblast by a layer of uncalcified "osteoid" matrix.

Membrane bone formation shares many similarities with endochondral bone formation. In this instance, however, osteoblasts arise by maturation of osteoprogenitor cells, either from the periosteum, a fibrous layer covering the bone cortex, or from endosteal osteoprogenitor cells of the marrow stroma. Osteoblasts begin the polarized deposition of a layer of new osteoid matrix on preexisting bony surfaces with cartilage being absent. As before, matrix vesicles of osteoid initiate calcification, which then is self-propagating by a process of epitaxial crystal growth. For a suggestion of the mechanism by which matrix vesicles initiate calcification, see Figs. 31-3 and 31-4.

FLOURIDE

When apatite mineral forms in an extracellular fluid containing fluoride, fluoroapatite is formed with fluorine atoms incorporated into the crystal lattice of calcium phosphate apatite. The substitution of fluorine into the apatite crystal structure causes an increase in hardness and a decrease in solubility of apatite.[8,28]

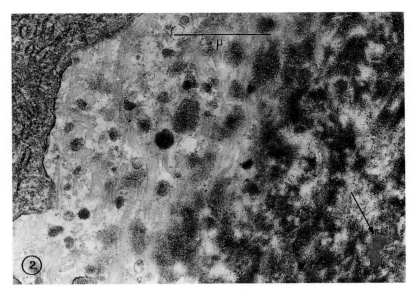

Fig. 31-2. The mineralization front of a developing bone is seen as a diagonal boundary zone lying at the edge of densely mineralized bone matrix *(right two fifths of field)* at its junction with unmineralized osteoid matrix *(midleft)*. Numerous matrix vesicles are also present in the unmineralized osteoid between the mineralized matrix and an osteoblast *(upper left)*. This electron micrograph is from the cortical surface of a developing femur in an 8-day-old chick embryo. The arrow indicates a homogeneous density within dense mineral, which may represent a residual matrix vesicle. (×35,000.) (From Anderson HC, Reynolds JJ: Pyrophosphate stimulation of calcium uptake into cultured embryonic bones. Fine structure of matrix vesicles and their role in calcification, *Dev Biol* 34:211, 1973; with permission.)

Fluoride metabolism

Most fluoride enters the body by ingestion in water and food. The normal dietary intake of fluoride is between 1 and 3 mg daily, and an intake of up to 4 mg is considered to be safe.[15] The rate of absorption of fluoride from the intestine varies with the form of fluoride ingestion. Sodium fluoride and monofluorophosphate are readily absorbed, whereas fluoride compounds containing aluminum, calcium, magnesium, or chloride are less readily absorbed.

After fluoride enters the blood stream, it is distributed into two metabolic compartments, one with a turnover time of only a few hours (located in the blood and soft tissues) and one with a half-life of up to several years (located in the mineral of bones and teeth). The body burden of fluoride is best reflected by the concentration of fluoride in bone. Fluoride deposition into bone mineral is not homogeneous but is mainly localized in regions that were undergoing active bone formation and matrix mineralization at the time of exposure to fluoride. During mineralization, fluoride ions are fixed to the surfaces of apatite crystals or are exchanged into the apatite crystal lattice by substitution with hydroxyl ions.

Although fluoride is released slowly from bone, having a half-life of 8 to 9 years,[37] there is a considerable local reutilization of fluoride as the element is released by resorption of bone mineral but then recaptured "on site" in adjacent areas of new bone formation.[49] Because of its slow release from bone, the measurement of fluoride in bone samples constitutes the best indication of the fluoride exposure history of a patient.

Effect of fluoride on bone cells

Osteoblasts and osteoblast-derived cells, cultured in vitro in the presence of fluoride, demonstrate both an increase in proliferative activity and an increase in alkaline phosphatase expression,[35] the latter being an indication of differentiation. There has been considerable debate as to whether fluoride is capable of causing genetic mutations of the sort that might precede cancer development. Jones and co-workers[59] and Tsutsui and co-workers[112] reported an increase in broken chromosomes and sister chromatid exchanges in cultures exposed to fluoride. Li,[69] who has carried out similar studies, questions whether fluoride is truly genotoxic.

The predominant in vivo effect of fluoride on bone cells appears to be a promotion of bone formation. In patients treated with fluoride, there is an increase in osteoblast-covered, bone-forming surfaces.[16] The relative area of bone-resorbing surfaces may be unchanged or moderately increased. Thus, the coupling of bone formation and bone resorption appears to be unbalanced by fluoride in favor of bone formation,[16] at least in the endosteum. The overall effect of fluoride on cortical bone, however, may be just the reverse; i.e., in the cortex of the femoral neck, fluoride ap-

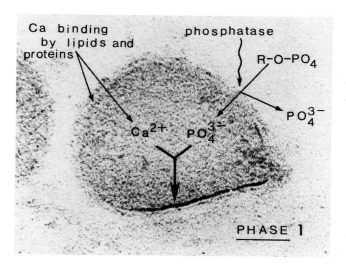

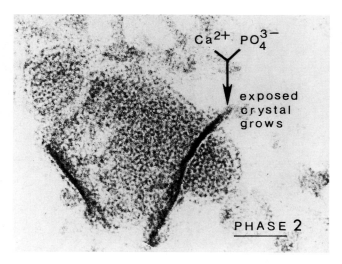

Fig. 31-3. Scheme for mineralization in matrix vesicles. During *phase 1,* intravesicular calcium concentration is increased by its affinity for lipids and calcium *(Ca)*-binding proteins of the vesicle membrane interior. Phosphatase (e.g., alkaline phosphatase, pyrophosphatase, or adenosine triphosphatase) at the vesicle membrane acts on ester phosphate of matrix or vesicle fluid to produce a local increase in phosphate/(PO_4) in the vicinity of the vesicle membrane. The intravesicular ionic product of $[Ca^{2+}] \times [PO_4^{3-}]$ is thereby raised, resulting in initial deposition of $CaPO_4$ near the membrane. (From Anderson HC: Introduction to the second conference on matrix vesicle calcification, *Metab Bone Dis Rel Res* 1:83. Copyright 1978, with kind permission from Elsevier Science Ltd, The Boulevard, Langford Lane, Kidlington OX5 1GB, UK.)

Fig. 31-4. With accumulation and growth, intravesicular crystals are exposed to the extravesicular environment. *Phase 2* begins with exposure of preformed apatite crystals to extravesicular fluid, which in normal animals is supersaturated with respect to apatite, enabling further crystal proliferation. Matrix vesicles pictured are in rat growth plate cartilage. (From Anderson HC: Introduction to the second conference on matrix vesicle calcification, *Metab Bone Dis Rel Res* 1:83. Copyright 1978, with kind permission from Elsevier Science Ltd, The Boulevard, Langford Lane, Kidlington OX5 1GB, UK.)

pears to cause a decrease in percent mineralized bone and an increase in bone fragility.[63,103] Inhibition of bone mineralization has also been reported frequently in fluorosis[66] and is characterized by the deposition of poorly mineralized "mottled" osteoid in halos of matrix surrounding osteocytes.[16] Although fluorotic bone may appear on x-ray film to be more dense than normal, the resultant irregularities of mineralization actually lead to brittleness with reduced bone strength.[103]

Epidemiology, clinical features, and pathology of skeletal fluorosis

Skeletal fluorosis most commonly results from years of exposure to elevated fluoride in drinking water. Soil and water fluoride are endemically elevated in certain geographical areas, including India,[34,66] Africa,[25] and mainland China (Li, personal communication, 1993). Cases of fluorosis also have resulted from prolonged consumption of fluoride-rich mineral waters from certain European spas.[16] Wine fluorosis has been described in Spain owing to ingestion of large amounts of local wine to which fluoride was added to stop fermentation.[106] Industrial fluorosis has resulted from inhalation of fluorinated gases produced by the processing of cryolite asbestos[47] or of released fluorinated dust. Iatrogenic fluorosis may be caused by prolonged ingestion of fluoridated antiinflammatory agents,[9] and the

current therapeutic use of large doses of fluoride to treat osteoporosis constitutes a potential cause of iatrogenic fluorosis.

In recent years, many soft drinks and other beverages have been manufactured using fluoridated water.[21,68] The sometimes quite high consumption of these beverages, particularly by young individuals, can as much as double the daily intake of fluoride. Because the fluoride content of processed beverages is quite variable from brand to brand, this new environmental source of fluoride renders the epidemiological prediction of fluoride intake less reliable.

Clinical findings in children exposed to high levels of systemic fluoride include mottled tooth enamel, enamel dysplasia, caries, and gingivitis.[68] In adults, there is often generalized bone and joint pain with stiffness of the spine and other joints. The most severe effects include deformities of the spine[96] and limbs (Fig. 31-5), with knock knees,[66] and, ultimately, crippling resulting in a bedridden state.[25] X-ray films show predominantly osteosclerosis of the spine, pelvis, and ribs with a pattern of increased trabecular markings.[106,111] There also may be irregular periosteal new bone formation with osteophytes and exostoses. The urine fluoride content is usually at least five times normal.[31,34] Although the medullary bone formed in fluorosis is usually more dense, there is an increased incidence of fracture,[15,57] suggesting that fluorotic bone is abnormally brittle and less able to withstand mechanical force.

The pathological picture resulting from prolonged expo-

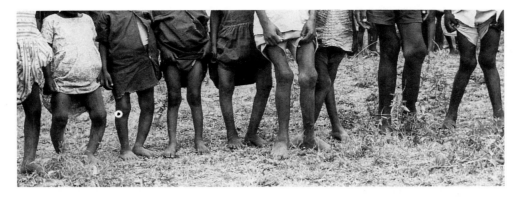

Fig. 31-5. Crippling form of skeletal fluorosis—endemic genu valgum. (From Christie DP: The spectrum of radiographic bone changes in children with fluorosis, *Radiol* 136:85, 1980; with permission.)

sure to high levels of fluoride is characterized by osteosclerosis of bone (Fig. 31-6).[15] Histological changes, which are usually evaluated in biopsies of non–weight-bearing iliac crest bone, include an increase in the volume of bone trabeculae, and increased bone formation rate as indicated by an increase in osteoid surfaces, the thickness of osteoid seams, tetracycline-labeled bone surfaces, and "active," osteoblast-covered bone trabecular surfaces. Often, there is a lag in osteoid mineralization rate, which probably accounts for the increase in osteoid volume that has been described, and there is a zone of poorly mineralized "mottled" osteoid in the matrix around osteocytes.[15] Although the bone resorption rate may be normal or increased, usually the rate of bone formation exceeds that of resorption, thus leading to osteosclerosis. An exception to this rule has been reported in the cortices of long bones, in which a negative balance of resorption over formation apparently exists.[92] Also, increased cortical resorption associated with fluoride has been noted in the fracture-prone femoral neck.[103]

Therapeutic uses of fluoride

Most of the literature suggests that exposure to low doses of fluoride in drinking water can prevent dental caries.[48] The effect is presumed to be due to an increase in hardness and durability of the hydroxyapatite of tooth enamel by substitution of fluoride ion into the crystalline structure of apatite. In the original studies, the reduction in cavities in communities with fluoridated water was on the order of 50%.[102] More recent studies set the number in the range of 10% to 30%.[48] The fluoridation of water supplies to prevent dental caries has proved to be relatively innocuous. One frequently encountered complication of exposure of preerupted teeth during the first few years of life, however, is the development of mottled tooth enamel, i.e., mild fluorosis. Since the initiation of fluoridation in the 1940s, the prevalence of mottled enamel has increased in North America to the current level of approximately 20% to 25% in U.S. school children.[21] Milder forms of enamel fluorosis

are not regarded by the U.S. Environmental Protection Agency (EPA) as a significant public health problem but rather as a cosmetic effect. The increased prevalence of mild dental fluorosis in recent years is almost certainly due to a nationwide increase in the exposure of infants and children to environmental sources of fluoride such as supplemental fluoride in infant formula, food, soft drinks, and swallowed toothpaste. The debate continues regarding the efficacy and advisability of involuntary water fluoridation to combat caries.[21,26,57]

A second major therapeutic use of fluoride has been in the treatment of osteoporosis in an attempt to reduce the fracture rate.[44] A decade ago, oral fluoride in relatively high doses was advocated to promote increased vertebral bone density in postmenopausal osteoporosis and to forestall vertebral crush fractures. However, the evidence obtained from clinical trials supporting the hypothesis that fluoride can prevent fractures is weak.[63,98] Therefore, the trend is away from the use of fluoride therapy in osteoporosis.

Relation, if any, between fluoride exposure and osteosarcoma

Since artificial fluoridation of a water supply was begun in Grand Rapids, Michigan, in 1945 as an anticaries measure, there has been continued questioning and concern about a possible carcinogenic effect from involuntary fluoride exposure.[52] Partly to allay these concerns, a series of epidemiological and animal studies have been conducted. To date, none have demonstrated a statistically convincing relationship between environmental fluoride exposure and the genesis of any form of cancer.[118]

In 1990, the results of a federally sponsored animal study were released that showed a slight increase in osteosarcomas in rats treated with extremely high doses of fluoride in their drinking water.[82] In this study by the U.S. National Institutes of Environmental Health Sciences (NIEHS), one out of 50 male rats receiving 100 ppm and 3 out of 80 male rats receiving 175 ppm of fluoride in drinking water developed osteosarcoma. This was above the incidence of os-

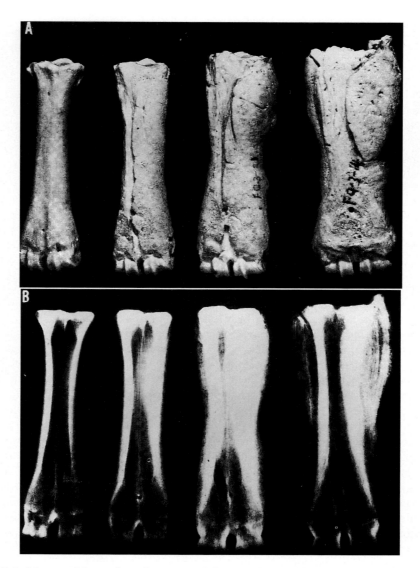

Fig. 31-6. Metatarsal bones from four cows of the same breed, size, and age depicting various degrees of fluoride-induced periosteal hyperostosis. *Left to right,* normal to excessive osteofluorosis. Note that the articular surfaces appear normal. **A,** Gross appearance. **B,** Radiographic appearance. (From Shupe JL: *Disease of Cattle,* ed 2, Santa Barbara, Calif, American Veterinary Publications, p. 740; with permission.)

teosarcoma in the control group of 0.5 per 100 rats. It was concluded that the increase in osteosarcomas observed in the treated group was "equivocal," meaning that there was "a marginal increase in neoplasms that may be chemically related."

A Canadian epidemiological study found no significant difference in osteosarcoma incidence in Edmonton, a city where water is fluoridated, versus Calgary, where it is not.[56] An updated analysis of cancer deaths by the U.S. National Cancer Institute's (NCI) Surveillance Epidemiology and End Results (SEER) program of cancer registries showed an increase in osteosarcoma in young males under age 20 from 3.6 to 5.5 cases per million, counterbal-

anced by a decrease in incidence in young females to 3.7 cases per million from 3.8 per million, and concluded, as before, that there is no discernible trend relating fluoride to osteosarcoma[118] or any other malignancy.[55] Thus, present epidemiological and toxicological data do not confirm a relationship between fluoride exposure and the development of osteosarcoma. It is reasonable to conclude that exposure to fluoride at levels currently considered safe does not cause any notable increase in osteosarcoma risk. If a small risk of osteosarcoma has escaped detection by epidemiological studies, it is not likely to be an important factor in the prevalence of human osteosarcoma.

LEAD (see Chapter 4)

Environmental lead is one of the most important toxic agents in modern civilization. This soft metal, known from ancient times, is used in a wide variety of industrial processes and products, including paint, battery-making and burning, welding and foundry work, lead smelting, mining, and, until recently, as an additive to gasoline. Geochemical analysis of lead in the Arctic and Antarctic ice caps indicates that within the last 100 years there has been a 400-fold increase in the natural prevalence and concentration of lead.[81] The increasing concentration of lead in the polar ice caps reflects a growing lead contamination of the atmosphere and water worldwide.

Environmental lead most often gains access to the blood stream by inhalation. An important alternate route of lead uptake in children, however, is through ingestion, particularly of paint chips from older houses (see Chapter 3). Lead toxicity may be manifested in adults as kidney disease[12,108] or impaired hematopoeisis.[51] In children, lead has been the cause of considerable public health concern because exposure during fetal life or in early childhood has been related to mental incapacitation, including low intelligence quotient (IQ), a poor attention span, and learning disabilities[71,84,85] (see Chapter 4). Furthermore, unacceptably high blood lead levels were detected in 12.2% of black children, usually living in older, lead-painted, peeling housing in city centers, as compared with only 2.0% of white children, usually living in middle-class circumstances.[73]

Once it enters the body, lead is bone-seeking. The calcified tissues accumulate approximately 90% of the body burden of lead,[86] and its release rate from bone is slow, with a half-life of approximately 8 years.[86] Thus, the lead level in bone is a good indication of an individual's lead exposure over a period of years. The release of high levels of stored lead from bone as a result of bone resorption constitutes a cause of sustained damaging effects on other tissue, such as brain, kidneys, and bone marrow. Postmenopausal women experiencing rapid bone loss owing to osteoporosis are believed to be particularly at risk for the development of systemic lead toxicity.[105]

Metabolism of lead and cellular effects

After being absorbed in the respiratory tract or intestine, lead enters the blood stream and thence the bone. The half-life of lead in the blood stream is short, of the order of 1 to 2 days, whereas lead incorporated into bone turns over slowly with a half-life of approximately 8 years.[86] Molecular lead is incorporated into the crystal lattice of hydroxyapatite of bones and teeth, where it is substituted for calcium.[104] Lead also substitutes for calcium in several biological reactions: In the plasma membrane, lead replacement of Ca^{2+} interferes with Ca^{2+}-dependent signal transduction as mediated through calmodulin and protein kinase C.[19] Lead affects Ca^{2+}-related ion pumps at the cell surface, interfering with the normal exclusion of Ca^{2+} from the cytosol and thus producing abnormally high cytosolic and mitrochondrial Ca^{2+} levels. Lead also poisons enzymes by binding to disulfide groups. In the bone marrow, lead inhibits aminolevulinic acid dehydratase and ferroketolase, both being enzymes involved in heme synthesis. As a consequence, iron is displaced from heme. The synthesis of a zinc-substituted protoporphyrin results, which blocks red cell synthesis and leads to a microcytic, hypochromic, mildly hemolytic anemia.

Lead-containing acid-fast inclusion bodies accumulate in the nucleus and, to a lesser extent, in the cytoplasm of osteoclasts (but not osteoblasts) in 95% of cases,[17,114] renal tubular cells in 68% of cases, and liver cells in 37% of cases. These inclusion droplets (Fig. 31-7) are comprised mostly of alpha$_2$ microglobulin, a lead-binding protein that apparently mediates the transport of lead into nuclei of the respective cells.[42] These inclusions are considered pathognomonic for lead intoxication. Biochemical studies of the lead-binding protein of these inclusions suggest that it may function in a protective fashion by binding lead that otherwise might react with and inhibit the enzyme alphalevulinic acid dehydratase (ALAD), which functions in the second stage of heme synthesis.[42] In osteoclasts, lead inhibition of resorption may be linked to an inhibition of carbonic anhydrase II, which is known to be sensitive to lead. Carbonic anhydrase II is concentrated at the resorption pole of the osteoclasts; i.e., at the "ruffled border," where this enzyme appears to function in the secretion of hydrogen ions that promote local mineral dissolution.[40,113]

Pathological and clinical features of human plumbism

Exposure to lead in utero is associated with low birth weight and prolonged gestation, resulting in infants who are small for gestational age.[11] Lead readily crosses the placental barrier[45] and is associated with developmental skeletal abnormalities, including the fusion of two or more vertebrae, delayed ossification, and delayed deciduous tooth development. Although bone is a "sink" for lead coming from the bloodstream, the pathological changes owing to lead toxicity observed in the skeleton are less severe than those seen in the central nervous system, bone marrow, or kidney. Lead tends to accumulate at sites where mineral is being actively deposited, i.e., within the bony epiphyses and metaphyses. These deposits are visualized as "lead lines" on x-ray film; i.e., increased density at the ends of long bones (Fig. 31-8) or in the cranial vault on the x-ray film.[19] The lead-line of bone appears to be due to a failure of resorption and remodeling by chrondroclasts and osteoclasts of the metaphysis, allowing a local buildup of radiodense, lead-containing calcified cartilage matrix.[32]

In bone, the main pathological effect of lead seems to be to slow skeletal growth.[94] Human congenital lead poisoning is associated with delayed skeletal and dental development at birth.[89] There may be increased bone density of the cranial vault and delayed tooth eruption. Postnatal

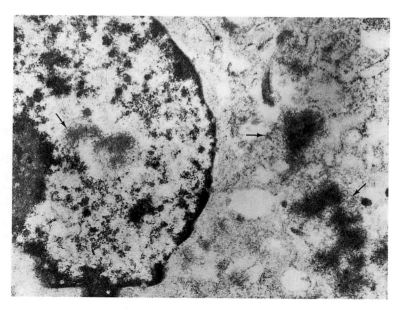

Fig. 31-7. Intranuclear and intracytoplasmic lead-containing inclusion droplets in an osteoclast from the proximal metaphysis of a rat tibia, 7 days after injection of a single 4 mg/kg dose of lead acetate. Electron micrograph stained with uranium. (×15,000.) (From Van Mullem PJ, Stadhouders AM: Bone marking and lead intoxication. Early pathological changes in osteoclasts. *Virchows Arch [B]* 15:345, 1974. Copyright Springer-Verlag; with permission.)

skeletal growth is also slower in children with low-level lead intoxication.[67] At the tissue level, there is a decreased rate of bone formation, prolonged closure of the epiphyses, and a slower bone turnover rate.[5] As indicated previously, cellular toxicity is evidenced by the appearance of intranuclear and intracytoplasmic lead-containing inclusions in osteoclasts.[17,114] There is an overall decrease in the rate of formation of bone matrix (osteoid) and retarded formation of new bone at the growth plates.[51]

Children are particularly vulnerable to the damaging effects of lead on the central nervous system. Acute lead toxicity in neonates and children may cause edema of the brain, demyelination of the white matter, death of cortical neurons, and astrocytic and capillary proliferation in areas of damage. Even low levels of lead have been shown in epidemiological studies to cause irreversible mental impairment in infants and children as manifested by a slight reduction in IQ, poor reading scores, learning disabilities, and retarded psychomotor development.[84] In adults, lead toxicity is associated with muscle weakness and, at times, paralysis, which may be due to a direct toxic effect of lead on muscle[51] or, perhaps, to peripheral neuropathy.

The toxic effect of lead on bone marrow hematopoeisis is typically manifested by a hypochromic, microcytic anemia. As mentioned previously, lead inhibits the activity of delta aminolevulinic dehydratase, an enzyme required for iron incorporation into heme. The result is a disproportionate increase in zinc-containing protoporphyrin and a decrease in circulating erythrocyte protoporphyrin. Lead-

intoxicated red cells typically demonstrate a fine basophilic stippling.[51]

The kidney is a major target organ for lead toxicity in adults.[27] The characteristic pathological change of renal lead toxicity is chronic nephritis, predominantly of tubules and interstitial connective tissue, i.e., "tubulointerstitial" nephritis, with interstitial fibrosis, chronic inflammation, and the appearance of eosinophilic droplets in tubular epithelial cells. These pathological changes are associated with the clinical picture of Fanconi's syndrome, characterized by glycosuria, aminoaciduria, phosphaturia, and, in late stages, hyperuricemia (see Chapter 32).

The diagnosis of lead toxicity is often difficult to make: in children vague central nervous system symptoms reflective of intellectual, behavioral, or motor impairment are easily overlooked. In adults there are often gastrointestinal disturbances characterized by colic with acute crampy abdominal pains. In children, there may be a "lead line" of dark discoloration of the gums at the base of teeth. The presence of hypochromic microcytic anemia with basophilic stippling of red cells is often diagnostic. To confirm the diagnosis of lead toxicity, it is necessary to demonstrate an elevated blood level of lead, above 50 μg/dl. Although it is possible to lower blood levels of lead significantly by chelation therapy,[24] if the bone lead level is very high, then chelation therapy may not permanently bring blood lead levels to normal. Often it is necessary to assess the body stores of lead by measuring bone or tooth lead levels. This can be done noninvasively by x-ray fluorescence techniques using iodine-125 or cadmium-109 as an x-ray source to bombard and excite K- or L-x-ray backscatter from either deep or superficial bone mineral,[86] or from the enamel surface of teeth.[104]

RADIATION AND BONE-SEEKING RADIONUCLIDES
Skeletal effects of external beam radiation

External beam electromagnetic radiation comes usually in the form of gamma rays or x-rays, either therapeutically administered or accidentally received, as may occur with occupational exposure. These types of radiation can penetrate tissues deeply, however, they engage in relatively few molecular interactions passage through tissue. Thus it is said that these types of radiation exhibit a low linear energy transfer (LET) and a low relative biological effectiveness (RBE). As discussed in Chapter 11, the dose of absorbed radiation is usually stated in rads (r), or the more recent term, grays (gy), with 1 gy equaling 100 r. Radiation of any type produces damaging effects at the cellular level by one or more of several mechanisms, including (1) direct damage to DNA molecules, producing mutations with genetic or cancerous potential, and (2) the intracellular induction of highly reactive free radicals by ionizing H_2O to hydrogen and hydroxyl ions that then enter into damaging interactions with enzymes and membranes as well as DNA (see Chapter 21).

Growth retardation is a frequently observed effect of external radiation. This is most notable in children and adolescents who are irradiated while undergoing growth at the epiphyseal plates in bones and/or active periosteal and endosteal new bone formation.[95] Although mature bone and cartilage is relatively insensitive to radiation, the actively dividing chondrocytes of the growth plate and actively dividing osteoblasts of growing bones are easily damaged and stop dividing as a result of only modest doses of external radiation.[101] A frequently encountered clinical example of this is the shortening of stature resulting from therapeutic irradiation of the spine in children treated for neoplastic processes that infiltrate the spinal canal.[95] As little as 6 Gy (600 rad) can cause a reduction of cell division in growth plate chondrocytes.[78,101] Furthermore, in utero exposure to external ionizing radiation may result in microcephaly, presumably owing to an interference of skull growth, and is associated with mental retardation.[79,80] In Hiroshima and Nagasaki, the incidence of microcephaly and mental retardation in offspring was greatest after exposure of mothers at 8 to 15 weeks of gestation.[79] In children exposed to the atom bomb blasts, doses of less than 10 Gy caused arrested growth of tooth buds and resulted in failure of permanent teeth to develop.[78] Fractionated doses of external radiation in excess of 25 Gy to the ends of the long bones in growing children also have been shown to cause slipped capital epiphyses,[116] an effect that probably results from

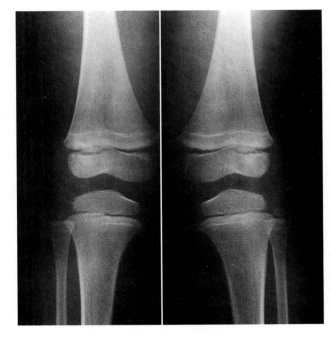

Fig. 31-8. "Lead lines" of increased radiodensity in epiphyses of a child suffering from lead poisoning. (Courtesy of Marilyn Pearl, M.D.)

damage to proliferating osteoblasts and capillary endothelium at the growing metaphysis and epiphyseal plate.

Adults exposed to bone radiation often show poor resistance to infection and increased susceptibility to fracture in the irradiated bones.[10,97] Exposure to both therapeutic and atom bomb–generated external radiation is associated with a significant increase in the incidence of hyperparathyroidism.[38] The radiation-induced form of hyperparathyroidism is associated mostly with parathyroid adenomas, although it is also associated with diffuse parathyroid gland hyperplasia, in about the same ratio of adenomas to hyperplasias as is seen in the nonradiated population. Clinical indications of hyperparathyroidism include high serum calcium, low serum phosphate (PO_4), and elevated alkaline phosphatase, all indicative of the metabolic effect of excessive circulating parathyroid hormone (PTH) and reflecting an increased rate of bone loss owing to PTH-driven bone resorption.

Bone-seeking radionuclides

Radionuclides that are bone-seeking, i.e., metabolically concentrated in bone (Fig. 31-9), include isotopes of calcium, phosphorus, strontium, radium, and alkaline earth elements, all of which tend to accumulate diffusely throughout mineralized bone matrix (the "volume seekers"), plus plutonium and thorium, which tend to be concentrated at the periosteal and endosteal surfaces of bone.[107] Bone-seeking radionuclides in general liberate subatomic particles. That is, they release either alpha or beta particles of

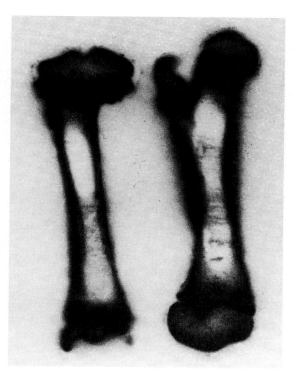

Fig. 31-9. Autoradiograph of animal bones after Strontium-90 ingestion. Dark areas represent strontium deposition, which is most marked near the epiphyseal plates, with substantial deposition in all visualized osseous cortex. (Case courtesy of Marvin C. Bell. From Mettler FA, Mosely RD: *Direct effects of radiation.* In Mettler FA, Mosby RD, editors: *Medical effects of ionizing radiation,* Orlando, 1985, Grune & Stratton; with permission.)

lower intrinsic energy that do not penetrate tissues deeply (usually only a few microns in depth), but that exhibit high LET and thus cause more numerous molecular interactions in the tissues penetrated.

In the early 1900s, radium-containing patent medicines were given as a tonic to promote general health and well-being. The dramatic event that brought the practice of radium therapy to a halt in the United States was a report in *The New York Times* in 1932 describing the extensive radiation damage that occurred in a wealthy and prominent Long Island socialite who had been chronically dosing himself with one such radium-containing patent medicine called "Radithor."[72] The patient's health deteriorated severely after about 2 years of *ad libitum* ingestion of Radithor. His teeth began falling out, and radiological examination revealed mandibular necrosis similar to that seen in radium watch dial painters, discussed in the next section.[7,76,93] Pathological and degenerative changes seen in radionuclide-irradiated bone include aseptic necrosis and fibrous thickening of the walls of small marrow arteries and arterioles, plus the appearance of a layer of fibroblastic cells covering the bone surfaces of the endosteum.[107]

Carcinogenesis by radiation

The carcinogenic effects of bone-seeking radionuclides and external beam radiation are well-known. The history of radiation-induced cancer begins with radium dial painters in the early 1900s who painted luminous numbers on watch faces. The dial painters used isotopes of radium, Radium-226 and Radium-228, which have relatively long half-lives of 5.8 years and 1600 years, respectively. They kept their fine paint brushes in a relatively pointed configuration by intermittently licking the bristles. This group of workers acquired a massive exposure to radium over a period of years, which was metabolically concentrated in bones and associated with a roughly 100-fold increase in the incidence of bone tumors, mainly osteosarcomas (Fig. 31-10).[7,76,93]

Intravenous administration of radium-226 or plutonium-239 has been used to induce osteosarcomas in beagle dogs.[20] Similarly, $32PO_4$ and strontium-90 (Sr-90), when given systemically, caused significant increases in osteosarcoma incidence in animals.[13,41,75,87] However, there are no epidemiological data indicating an increase of osteosarcoma or any other bone tumor in those working on the atomic bomb at Los Alamos, New Mexico, who were accidentally exposed to a large dose of plutonium.[115] Nor is there any epidemiological evidence of increased bone cancer in individuals exposed to external radiation or radioactive fallout in the Hiroshima and Nagasaki nuclear bomb blasts,[78,80] nor among exposed individuals at Three Mile Island or Chernobyl nuclear reactor accidents.[100] Theoretically, Sr-90 and plutonium-239 must continue to be regarded as potential causes of bone cancer in individuals exposed to fallout. In actuality, however, external exposure to these radionuclides in air or water leads to little uptake into the blood stream or bone because of poor absorption from the gastrointestinal tract, and most of the radioisotope taken up by inhalation is deposited in pulmonary lymph nodes. A cohort of 26 Manhattan Project workers who were heavily exposed to plutonium has been carefully followed.[78,115] At the 32-year observation point, there was no increase in mortality above expected rates and no evidence of an increase in the frequency of bone cancer or any other form of cancer in the exposed group.

External beam radiation therapy, as used for a variety of neoplasms and other conditions, is known to predispose to the development of bone tumors, particularly osteosarcomas.[61] Children and young adults are especially susceptible to the development of bone tumors, and there has been a striking increase in the incidence of secondary bone sarcomas in children who are treated with radiation for retinoblastoma. These children may be especially predisposed to the development of radiation-induced tumors because many have an inherited genomic mutation in the retinoblastoma (Rb) gene. The mutated Rb gene is believed no longer to function as a tumor suppressor gene. Also, homozygosity of the Rb gene locus is known to be associated with a predilection for osteosarcoma, even in the absence of retinoblastoma development.[29]

ALUMINUM

This element is one of the commonest in the earth's crust. On ingestion or inhalation, aluminum enters the blood stream and is deposited in bone, where its turnover and release are slow. Aluminum's fate in the body somewhat parallels the pattern of uptake and release of lead.

Environmental sources of aluminum

Aluminum is present to a variable degree worldwide in drinking water. The most frequent overt form of aluminum toxicity seen in recent years has been described in patients with chronic renal disease who were being dialyzed. In some instances, the water used in the dialysis bath was relatively high in aluminum content. Thus, aluminum was essentially dialyzed into the patients' systemic circulation during hemodialysis to remove nitrogenous wastes from the blood. Also, in these dialysis patients, aluminum-containing antacids were and still are being given by mouth to block phosphate absorption through the gut, and hence to lower the often elevated serum phosphate levels. Aluminum hydroxide phosphate blockers probably constitute the current major source of absorbed aluminum in dialysis patients.

Toxic effects of aluminum on bone

Aluminum is deposited at the mineralization front in areas of active bone formation and growth (Fig. 31-11). Nondecalcified bone sections stained for aluminum[74,99] show a dense deposition line of aluminum, which is precipitated in this particular stratum of the bone matrix because this was a mineralizing surface at the time that the patient was exposed to a significant dose of aluminum.

Aluminum exposure in renal dialysis patients is associated with two separate abnormalities of bone: an excessive accumulation of unmineralized osteoid (dialysis osteomalacia) and an inhibition of osteoblastic activity and bone turnover. Generally the amount of aluminum accumulated correlates well with the histological severity of one or the other of these two abnormalities. The normal aluminum content of bone is approximately 5 to 7 mg/kg of dry weight, whereas in aluminum-related bone disease, levels often exceed 80 to 100 mg/kg. Potentially toxic levels of aluminum also have been observed in solutions used for total parenteral nutrition (TPN). In this case, the aluminum was contained in the casein hydrolysate component, which is prepared by hydrolysis using an aluminum catalyst. Characteristic aluminum-associated osteomalacia and encephalopathy were observed in patients receiving TPN.[64]

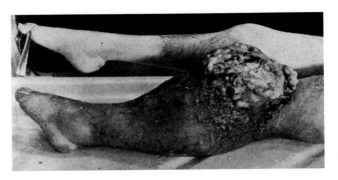

Fig. 31-10. Osteosarcoma arising in the tibia of a radium watch dial painter who was heavily exposed to Radon-226 and Radium-228. (From Aub JC et al: The late effects of internally-deposited radioactive materials in man, *Medicine* 31:221-329, 1952; with permission.)

Effects of aluminum on bone

The presence of toxic levels of aluminum in bone results in inhibition in the number of functional osteoblasts, thus leading to low bone formation rate, low bone turnover, and low bone and serum alkaline phosphatase (the characteristic enzyme expressed by functioning osteoblasts) so-called aplastic osteodystrophy.[30,43,83] Aluminum inhibits bone formation by reducing the surface area of trabecular bone, where osteoblasts are actively secreting bone matrix, but it does not reduce the thickness of osteoid deposits in areas where active bone formation persists.

Aluminum can inhibit the rate of mineral deposition at the "calcification front" in bone trabeculae.[43,117] Aluminum may inhibit the mineralization process by inhibiting alkaline phosphatase at the site of initial mineralization[70] or by inhibiting the physicochemical process of apatite crystal growth, as has been demonstrated in in vitro models of apatite formation.[14] Retardation of bone mineralization by parenteral aluminum, resulting in osteomalacia, has been convincingly demonstrated in animals,[33,110] and there is a strong correlation in dialysis patients between the bone content of aluminum and the presence of osteomalacia in biopsy specimens.[53,77]

Clinical and pathologic features of aluminum-induced bone disease

Aluminum-induced bone disease most often presents a picture of osteomalacia with characteristic attendant symptoms of bone pain; frequent spontaneous fractures of ribs, vertebrae, and hips; and muscle weakness.[109,117] Diagnostic signs include the presence of diffuse osteopenia on bone x-ray film and in bone absorptiometry, pseudofractures (Looser's zones) on x-ray film, and increased osteoid seam thickness in the undecalcified bone biopsy specimen (Fig. 31-11). The clinical picture is often complicated by a superimposed element of secondary hyperparathyroidism, which is seen in patients with chronic renal disease and typ-

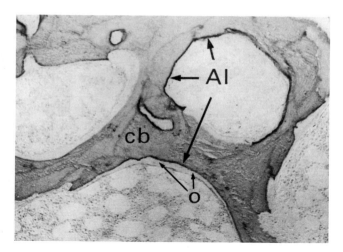

Fig. 31-11. Section of undecalcified transiliac bone biopsy in a patient with chronic renal disease on hemodialysis, stained by the aluminon procedure. Aluminum *(Al)* appears as dark-staining linear deposits at several mineralization fronts, which are covered by excessive osteoid *(O)*. *cb,* Niobium. (From Charon SA et al: Case report: high bone turnover associated with an aluminum-induced impairment of bone mineralization, *Bone* 7:319. Copyright 1986, with kind permission from Elsevier Science Ltd., The Boulevard, Langford Lane, Kidlington OX5 1GB, UK.)

ified by bone changes that include increased osteoclast numbers, increased resorptive surfaces with Howship's erosion "lacuna" of bone, and fibroblast proliferation of marrow (i.e., osteitis fibrosa). Because of a frequently superimposed hyperparathyroid bone disease, the clinical laboratory findings in dialysis-induced osteomalacia are often not typical of pure osteomalacia. For example, the serum calcium level is often near normal, the phosphate level is elevated instead of being reduced as is often the case in osteomalacia, and the alkaline phosphatase is only modestly elevated if at all because of the direct inhibition of osteoblast expression of alkaline phosphatase by aluminum.[43,83]

The diagnosis of aluminum-induced osteomalacia is best confirmed by a nondecalcified bone biopsy specimen. This is the only method by which the presence of increased osteoid can be proved conclusively. The histomorphometric analysis of amount and distribution of aluminum in bone is more sensitive than is evaluation by direct chemical analysis.[74,99] As alluded to previously, the characteristic histopathological features of aluminum-induced osteomalacia include increased osteoid seam thickness, decreased osteoblast-covered "active" surfaces of bone spicules, decreased surface area occupied by the mineralization front, ATA-staining or ASA-staining aluminum deposits[99] at the junction of surface osteoid and underlying bone mineralization fronts (Fig. 31-11), decreased tetracycline-measured bone formation rate, and the presence of "clouds" of small foci of patchy calcification in nonmineralized osteoid surrounding osteocytes.[18] The significance of these areas of patchy calcification is unknown, but they could represent

foci of arrested initial calcification arising in matrix vesicles[4] with punctate mineral foci enlarging and spreading incompletely into the surrounding collagenous matrix.[58] These patchy foci of calcification around osteocytes are known to contain deposits of aluminum. The coating of mineral by aluminum may temporarily inhibit the progress of mineral propagation.

Nonosseous toxic effects of aluminum

Aluminum is a well-known cause of encephalopathy in dialysis patients.[39,88] "Dialysis dementia" or "dialysis encephalopathy" is characterized clinically by dementia, dysarthria-apraxia of speech, asterixis, myoclonus, focal seizures, and an abnormal electroencephalogram pattern. This form of severe encephalopathy was considered to be the most frequent cause of death in a series of dialysis patients studied by Alfrey and colleagues[1] when the condition was first described. Aluminum has been shown experimentally to be toxic to the central nervous system, causing seizures and progressive encephalopathy.[62,65] Aluminum has also been localized in the brains of dialysis patients with encephalopathy and was concentrated in neurons of the cerebral cortex, the red nucleus, and the olivary nuclei.[39] Electron microscopy showed electron-dense small acicular crystalline deposits in the lysosomes of these cells, which contained aluminum and phosphate. Thus the ability of aluminum to cause encephalopathy in dialysis patients appears to be well established.

A role for environmental aluminum in the pathogenesis of dementia in Alzheimer's disease (AD) and the typical pathological changes seen in the brain in AD remains controversial. Perl and colleagues[90,91] put forward the hypothesis that aluminum causes AD, based on (1) the clinical similarity between AD and a type of dementia and encephalopathy attributed to environmental aluminum exposure that occurred in natives of the island of Guam and (2) the finding of trace amounts of aluminum in the olfactory tracts and hippocampal lesions of AD patients. The finding of trace amounts of aluminum in AD brain tissue has been confirmed[91] and denied[22]; one can only conclude that the aluminum hypothesis of AD pathogenesis is unproved at present.

Localized massive pathological soft tissue calcification, designated "tumoral calcinosis," is well-known to be associated with aluminum toxicity in hemodialysis patients.[119] These distinctive calcium phosphate deposits are often found in a periarticular location and are not a usual concomitant of the typical lung, stomach, and kidney pathological calcifications often seen in dialysis patients who are suffering from secondary hyperparathyroidism. The mechanism by which aluminum toxicity can lead to periarticular calcium phosphate deposits (while inhibiting mineralization in bone) is not clear at all. The only common factor in a series of such patients was the finding of elevated serum phosphate levels.[119]

REFERENCES

1. Alfrey AC, LeGendre GR, Kaehny WD: The dialysis encephalopathy syndrome. Possible aluminum intoxication, *N Engl J Med* 294:184, 1976.
2. Anderson C, Path MRC, Danylchuk KD: The effect of chronic low level lead intoxication on the haversian remodeling system in dogs, *Lab Invest* 37:466, 1977.
3. Anderson HC: Vesicles associated with calcification in the matrix of epiphyseal cartilage, *J Cell Biol* 41:59, 1969.
4. Anderson HC: Mechanism of mineral formation in bone, *Lab Invest* 60:320, 1989.
5. Anderson HC, Johnson TF, Avramides A: Matrix vesicles in osteomalacic bone, *Metab Bone Dis* 2S:79, 1980.
6. Anderson HC, Reynolds JJ: Pyrophosphate stimulation of calcium uptake into cultured embryonic bones. Fine structure of matrix vesicles and their role in calcification, *Dev Biol* 34:211, 1973.
7. Aub JC et al: The late effects of internally-deposited radioactive materials in man, *Medicine* 31:221, 1952.
8. Baud CA: Biophysical study of bone mineral in biopsies of osteoporotic patients before and after long term treatment with fluoride, *Bone* 9:361, 1988.
9. Baud CA, Boivin G, Demeurisse O: Drug induced skeletal fluorosis, *Fluoride* 15:54, 1982.
10. Bell RS et al: Fractures following limb salvage surgery and adjuvant radiation for soft tissue sarcoma, *Clin Orthop* 271:265, 1991.
11. Bellinger D et al: Weight gain and maturity in fetuses exposed to low levels of lead, *Environ Res* 54:151, 1991.
12. Bennett WM: Lead nephropathy, *Kidney Int* 28:212, 1985.
13. Bensted JPM, Blackett NM, Cameron DA: Histological and dosimetric considerations of bone tumour production with radioactive phosphorous, *Br J Radiol* 34:160, 1961.
14. Blumenthal NC, Posner AS: In vitro model of aluminum-induced osteomalacia: inhibition of hydroxyapatite formation and growth, *Calcif Tissue Int* 36:439, 1984.
15. Boivin G, Meunier PJ: *Fluoride and bone: toxicological and therapeutic aspects.* In Cohen RD, Lewis B, Alberti KGMM, Denman AM, editors: *The molecular basis of acquired disease,* London, 1990, Bailliere & Tindall.
16. Boivin G et al: Skeletal fluorosis: histomorphometric analysis of bone changes and bone fluoride content in 29 patients, *Bone* 10:89, 1989.
17. Bonucci E et al: Osteoclast changes induced by lead poisoning (Saturnism), *Appl Pathol* 1:241, 1983.
18. Boyce BF et al: Histological and electron microprobe studies of mineralization in aluminum-related osteomalacia, *J Clin Pathol* 45:502, 1992.
19. Bressler JP, Goldstein GW: Mechanisms of lead neurotoxicity, *Biochem Pharmacol* 41:479, 1991.
20. Bruenger FW, Lloyd RD, Miller SC: The influence of age at time of exposure to ^{226}Ra or ^{239}Pu on distribution, retention, postinjection, survival and tumor induction in Beagle dogs, *Radiat Res* 125:248, 1991.
21. Burt BA: The changing patterns of systemic fluoride intake, *J Dent Res* 71:1228, 1992.
22. Chafi AH et al: Absence of aluminum in Alzheimer's disease brain tissue: electron microprobe and ion microprobe studies, *Neurosci Lett* 123:61, 1991.
23. Charon SA et al: Case report: high bone turnover associated with an aluminum-induced impairment of bone mineralization, *Bone* 7:319, 1986.
24. Chisolm JJ Jr: Evaluation of the potential role of chelation therapy in treatment of low to moderate lead exposures, *Env Health Perspect* 89:67, 1990.
25. Christie DP: The spectrum of radiographic bone changes in children with fluorosis, *Radiology* 136:85, 1980.
26. Colquhoun J: Flawed foundation: a re-examination of the scientific basis for a dental benefit from fluoridation, *Commun Health Stud* 14:288, 1990.
27. Cramer K et al: Renal ultrastructure, renal function, and parameters of lead toxicity in workers with different periods of lead exposure, *Br J Ind Med* 31:113, 1974.
28. DenBesten PK, Thariani H: Biological mechanisms of fluorosis and level and timing of systemic exposure to fluoride with respect to fluorosis, *J Dent Res* 71:1238, 1992.
29. Dryja TP et al: Chromosome 13 homozygosity in osteosarcoma without retinoblastoma, *Am J Hum Genet* 38:59, 1986.
30. Dunstan CR et al: Effect of aluminum and parathyroid hormone on osteoblasts and bone mineralization in chronic renal failure, *Calcif Tissue Int* 36:133, 1984.
31. Ehrnebo M, Ekstrand J: Occupational fluoride exposure and plasma fluoride levels in man, *Int Arch Occup Env Health* 58:179, 1986.
32. Eisenstein R, Kawanoue S: The lead line in bone—a lesion apparently due to chondroclastic indigestion, *Am J Pathol* 80:309, 1975.
33. Ellis HA, McCarthy JH, Herrington J: Bone aluminum in haemodialysed patients and in rats injected with aluminum chloride: relation to impaired bone mineralization, *J Clin Pathol* 32:832, 1979.
34. Faccini JM, Teotia SPS: Histopathologic assessment of endemic skeletal fluorosis, *Calcif Tissue Res* 16:45, 1974.
35. Farley JR, Wergedal JE, Baylink DJ: Fluoride directly stimulates proliferation and alkaline phosphatase activity of bone-forming cells, *Science* 222:330, 1983.
36. Farnum CE, Wilsman NJ: Cellular turnover at the chondro-osseous junction of growth plate cartilage: analysis by serial sections at the light microscopic level, *J Orthop Res* 7:654, 1989.
37. Forbes GB et al: Bone mineral turnover in a patient with osteogenesis imperfecta estimated by fluoride excretion, *Calcif Tissue Res* 25:283, 1978.
38. Fujiwara S et al: Hyperparathyroidism among atomic bomb survivors in Hiroshima, *Radiat Res* 130:372, 1992.
39. Galle P et al: Progressive myoclonic encephalopathy in dialysis patients, *Nouv Presse Med* 8:4091, 1979.
40. Gay CV et al: Current studies on the location and function of carbonic anhydrase in ocleoclasts, *Ann NY Acad Sci* 429:473, 1984.
41. Giddes-Dwyer V et al: Transplantation and tissue culture studies of radiation-induced osteosarcoma in the rat, *Pathology* 6:71, 1974.
42. Goering PL, Fowler BA: Mechanisms of renal lead binding protein protection against lead-inhibition of delta-aminolevulinic dehydratase, *J Pharm Exp Ther* 234:365, 1985.
43. Goodman WG, Duarte MEL: Aluminum: effects on bone and role in the pathogenesis of renal osteodystrophy, *Min Electrolyte Metab* 17:221, 1991.
44. Gordon SL, Corbin SB: Summary of workshop on drinking water fluoride influence on hip fracture in bone health. (National Institutes of Health, 10 April, 1991.) *Osteoporosis Int* 2:109, 1992.
45. Goyer RA: Transplacental transport of lead. *Envir Health Perspect* 89:101, 1990.
46. Grandjean P: Classical syndromes in occupational medicine: occupational fluorosis through 50 years: clinical and epidemiological experiences, *Am J Ind Med* 3:227, 1992.
47. Grandjean P, Juel K, Jensen OM: Mortality and cancer morbidity after heavy occupational fluoride exposure, *Am J Epidemiol* 121:57, 1985.
48. Grembowski D, Fiset L, Spadafora RDH: How fluoridation affects adult dental caries, *J Am Dent Assoc* 123:49, 1992.
49. Guo MK et al: Retention of skeletal fluoride during bone turnover in rats, *J Nutr* 118:362, 1988.
50. Hass GM et al: Relations between lead poisoning in rabbit and man, *Am J Pathol* 45:691, 1964.
51. Hass GM, Landerholm W, Hemmens A: Inhibition of intercellular

matrix synthesis during ingestion of inorganic lead, *Am J Pathol* 50:815, 1967.

52. Hileman B: Fluoridation of water. Questions about health risks and benefits remain after more than 40 years, *Chem Eng News* pp 26-42, Aug 1, 1988.

53. Hodsman AB et al: Bone aluminum and histomorphometric features of renal osteodystrophy, *J Clin Endocrinol* 54:539, 1982.

54. Hodsman AB et al: Do serum aluminum levels reflect underlying skeletal aluminum accumulation and bone histology before or after chelation by deferoxamine, *J Lab Clin Med* 106:674, 1985.

55. Hoover RN et al: Fluoridation of drinking water and subsequent cancer incidence and mortality. In *Report of the Ad Hoc Subcommittee on Fluoride of the Committee to Coordinate Environmental Health and Related Programs,* Washington, DC, 1991, US Public Health Service.

56. Hrudey S et al: Drinking water fluoridation and osteosarcoma, *Can J Public Health* 81:415, 1990.

57. Inkovaara JA: Is fluoride treatment justified today? *Calcif Tissue Int* 49(suppl):568, 1991.

58. Johnson TF, Morris DC, Anderson HC: Matrix vesicles and calcification of rachitic rat osteoid, *J Exp Pathol* 4:123, 1989.

59. Jones CA, Callahan MF, Huberman E: Sodium fluoride promotes morphological transformation of syrian hamster embryo cells, *Carcinogenesis* 9:2279, 1988.

60. Kember NF: Cell population kinetics of bone growth: the first 10 years of autoradiographic studies with tritiated thymidine, *Clin Invest* 76:213, 1971.

61. Kim JH, Chu SC, Woodard HQ: Radiation induced soft tissue and bone sarcoma, *Radiology* 129:501, 1978.

62. Klatzo I, Wisniewski H, Streicher E: Experimental production of neurofibrillary degeneration: I. light microscopic observations, *Neuropathol Exp Neurol* 24:187, 1965.

63. Kleerekoper M, Balena R: Fluorides and osteoporosis, *Ann Rev Nutr* 11:309, 1991.

64. Klein GL et al: Aluminum as a factor in the bone disease of long-term parenteral nutrition, *Trans Assoc Am Phy* 95:155, 1982.

65. Kopelhoff LM, Barrera SE, Kopelhoff N: Recurrent convulsive seizures in animals produced by immunologic and chemical means, *Am J Psychiatry* 98:881, 1942.

66. Krishnamachari KAVR: Skeletal fluorosis in humans: a review of recent progress in the understanding of the disease, *Prog Food Nutr Sci* 10:279, 1986.

67. Lauwers MC et al: Comparison of biometric data of children with high and low levels of lead in the blood, *Am J Phys Anthropol* 69:107, 1986.

68. Leverett DH: Fluorides and the changing prevalence of dental caries, *Science* 217:26, 1982.

69. Li YM: Genotoxic effects of fluoride: a controversial issue, *Mutat Res* 195:127, 1998.

70. Lieberherr M et al: In vitro effects of aluminum on bone phosphatases: a possible interaction with bPTH and vitamin D3 metabolites, *Calcif Tissue Int* 34:280, 1982.

71. Lippman M: Lead and human health: background and recent findings, *Env Res* 51:1, 1990.

72. Macklis RM: Radithor and the era of mild radium therapy, *JAMA* 264:615, 1990.

73. Mahaffey KR et al: National estimates of blood lead levels: United States 1976-1980, *N Engl J Med* 307:573, 1982.

74. Maloney NA et al: Histological quantitation of aluminum in iliac bone from patients with renal failure, *J Clin Lab Med* 99(2):206, 1982.

75. Martin TJ: Parathyroid hormone-responsive adenylate cyclase in induced transplantable osteogenic rat sarcoma, *Nature* 260:436, 1976.

76. Martland HS: The occurrence of malignancy in radioactive persons, *Am J Cancer* 15:2435, 1931.

77. McClure J et al: Bone histoquantitative findings and histochemical staining reactions for aluminum in chronic renal failure patients treated with haemodialysis fluids containing high and low concentrations of aluminum, *J Clin Pathol* 36:1281, 1983.

78. Mettler FA, Mosely RD: *Medical effects in ionizing radation.* In Mettler FA, Mosely RD, editors: *Medical effects of ionizing radiation,* Orlando, 1985, Grune & Stratton.

79. Miller RW: Delayed radiation effects in atomic bomb survivors. *Science* 166:569, 1969.

80. Morgan C: Hiroshima, Nagasaki and the RERF, *Am J Pathol* 98:843, 1980.

81. Muorozumi M, Chow TJ, Peterson C: Chemical concentrations of pollutant lead in aerosols, terrestrial dusts and sea salts in Greenland and Antarctic snow strata, *Geochim Cosmochim Acta* 33:1247, 1969.

82. National Toxicology Program: *Toxicology and carcinogenesis studies of sodium fluoride (CAS No. 7681-49-4) in F344/N rats and B6C3F1 mice.* (Drinking water studies.) Publication No. 91-2848, Technical Report 393, Washington, DC, 1991, US Department of Health and Human Services.

83. Nebeker HG, Coburn JW: Aluminum and renal osteodystrophy (review), *Ann R Med* 37:79, 1986.

84. Needleman HL et al: Deficits in psychological and classroom performance of children with elevated dentine lead concentration in the general population, *N Engl J Med* 300:689, 1979.

85. Needleman HL et al: Long term effects of low doses of lead in childhood, *N Engl J Med* 11:83,1990.

86. Nordberg GF, Mahaffey KR, Fowler BA: Introduction and summary. International workshop on lead in bone: implications for dosimetry and toxicology, *Env Health Perspect* 91:3, 1991.

87. Owen M, Sessions HA, Vaughan JM: The effect of a single injection of high dose ^{90}Sr (500-100 MCi/kg) in rabbits, *Br J Cancer* 11:229, 1957.

88. Parkinson IS et al: Fracturing dialysis osteodystrophy and dialysis encephalopathy: an epidemiologic survey, *Lancet* 1:406, 1979.

89. Pearl M, Boxt LM: Radiographic findings in congenital lead poisoning, *Radiology* 136:83, 1980.

90. Perl DP, Brody AR: Alzheimer's disease: x-ray spectrometric evidence of aluminum accumulation in neurofibrillary tangle-bearing neurons, *Science* 208:297, 1980.

91. Perl DP, Good PF: Aluminum, Alzheimer's disease, and the olfactory system, Ann NY Acad Sci 640:8, 1991.

92. Phipps KR, Burt BA: Water-borne fluoride and cortical bone mass: a comparison of two communities, *J Dent Res* 69:1256, 1990.

93. Polednak AP, Stehney AF, Roland RE: Mortality among women first employed before 1930 in the U.S. radium dial painting industry, *Am J Epidemiol* 107:179, 1978.

94. Pounds JG, Long GJ, Rosen JF: Cellular and molecular toxicity of lead in bone, *Env Health Perspect* 91:17, 1991.

95. Probert JC, Parker BR: Effects of radiation therapy on bone growth, *Radiology* 114:155, 1975.

96. Rao BS, Taraknath VR, Sista VN: Ossification of the posterior longitudinal ligament and fluorosis, *J Bone Joint Surg [Br]* 74:469, 1992.

97. Regen EM, Wilkins WE: The influence of roentgen irradiation on the rate of healing of fractures and phosphatase activity of the callus of adult bone, *J Bone Joint Surg* 18:69, 1936.

98. Riggs BL: Treatment of osteoporosis with sodium fluoride or parathyroid hormone, *Am J Med* 91(S5B):S37, 1991.

99. Romanski SA et al: Detection of subtle aluminum-related renal osteodystrophy, *Mayo Clin Proc* 68:419, 1993.

100. Royal HD: *Three Mile Island and Chernobyl.* In Metler FA, editor: *Medical management of radiation accidents,* Boca Raton, Fla, 1990, CRC Press.

101. Rubin P et al: Radiation induced dyplasia of bone, *AJR Am J Roentgenol* 82:206, 1959.

102. Russell AL, Elvolve E: Domestic water and dental caries relationship in an adult population, *Public Health Rep* 66:1389, 1951.

103. Schnitzler CM et al: Bone fragility of the peripheral skeleton during fluoride therapy for osteoporosis, *Clin Orthop* 261:268, 1990.

104. Shapiro IM et al: X-ray fluorescence analysis of lead in teeth of urban children in situ: correlation between tooth lead level and the concentration of blood lead and free erythroporphyrins, *Environ Res* 17:46, 1978.

105. Silbergeld EK, Schwartz J, Maheffy K: Lead and osteoporosis: mobilization of lead from bone in post menopausal women, *Environ Res* 47:79, 1988.

106. Soriano M, Manchon F: Radiological aspects of a new type of bone fluorosis, periostitis deformans, *Radiology* 87:1089, 1966.

107. Spiers FW, Vaughn J: The toxicity of bone-seeking radionuclides, *Leukemia Res* 13:347, 1989.

108. Staessen JA et al: Impairment of renal function with increasing blood lead concentration in the general population, *N Engl J Med* 327:151, 1992.

109. Sundaram M, Dessner D, Ballal S: Solitary, spontaneous cervical and large bone fractures in aluminum osteodystrophy, *Skel Radiol* 20:91, 1991.

110. Talwar HS et al: Influence of aluminum on mineralization during matrix induced bone development, *Kidney Int* 29:1038, 1986.

111. Teotia SPS, Teotia M, Teotia NPS: Skeletal fluorosis: roentgenological and histopathological study, *Fluoride* 9:91, 1976.

112. Tsutsui T, Suzuki N, Ohmori M: Sodium fluoride–induced morphological and neoplastic transformation chromosome aberrations, sister chromatid exchanges, and unscheduled DNA synthesis in cultured Syrian hamster embryo cells, *Cancer Res* 44:938, 1984.

113. Vaananen HK, Parvinen EK: High active isoenzyme of carbonic anhydrase in rat calvaria osteoclasts—immuno-histochemical study, *Histochemistry* 78:481, 1983.

114. Van Mullen PJ, Stadhouders AM: Bone marking and lead intoxication. Early pathological changes in osteoclasts, *Virchows Arch [B]* 15:345, 1974.

115. Voelz GL et al: A 32 year medical follow-up on Manhattan project plutonium workers, *Health Phys* 37:445, 1979.

116. Walker SJ et al: Slipped capital femoral epiphysis following radiation and chemotherapy, *Clin Orthop* 159:186, 1981.

117. Ward MK et al: Osteomalacic dialysis osteodystrophy: evidence for a water-borne etiological agent, probably aluminum, *Lancet* 1:841, 1978.

118. Young FE: Public Health Service report on fluoride benefits and risks, *JAMA* 266(8):1061, 1991.

119. Zins B et al: Tumoral calcifications in hemodialysis patients: possible role of aluminum toxicity, *Nephron* 60:260, 1992.

Chapter 32

URINARY SYSTEM

Michael Kashgarian

The kidney is the principal excretory organ of the body and is a major route for excretion of toxins absorbed by any route. The kidney and urinary tract are particularly vulnerable to toxin exposure because the kidney receives 25% of the cardiac output and filters 160 to 180 L of glomerular ultrafiltrate per day. Furthermore, the contents of that filtrate are concentrated nearly 200-fold to produce urine in the range of 500 to 2000 ml per day. This process of filtration and concentration of soluble toxins makes the kidney the organ with the highest likelihood of significant exposure to xenobiotics.

The kidney itself is not a single homogeneous organ but rather a collection of a million individual organ units or nephrons (for detailed review of renal structure and function see Seldin and Giebisch[79]). The nephron is the basic functional unit of the kidney and consists of the glomerulus, the primary semipermeable filter for blood, and a complex tubule system, which functions as both a reabsorptive and a secretory system to modify the primary filtrate further (Fig. 32-1). The tubule has several functional units, each with specific transport characteristics

and different susceptibility to injury. The proximal tubule is responsible for the absorption of approximately 50% to 60% of the solutes and water filtered at the glomerulus. In addition, salts, sugars, amino acids, and metabolites are also reabsorbed in this segment. It also contains a well-developed endocytic lysosomal apparatus that is involved in the reabsorption and degradation of macromolecules from the ultrafiltrate. Peroxisomes or microbodies are present, and the proximal tubule is a major source of the enzyme cytochrome P-450 in the kidney. It is likely that this is the site where protein-bound toxins are dissociated and metabolized and detoxified by lysosomal mechanisms and the action of mixed function oxidases. It is the site for secretion of organic acids and toxins that have been conjugated to glucuronide after reabsorption. The loop of Henle is responsible for generating the medullary concentration gradient by virtue of its countercurrent anatomy. Final modification of the urine is made in the collecting ducts before excretion into the collecting system. Although there are differences in susceptibility of the various tubular segments to different toxins, the proximal tubule appears to be the major target for a wide variety of toxins. Toxins that are concentrated within the urine, however, are associated with distal nephron damage and injury of the collecting system urothelium.

Tubular-vascular relationships are also an important morphological feature of the kidney. The relationship of the macula densa of the distal tubule, the renin-secreting cells of the juxtaglomerular apparatus, and the afferent and efferent arterioles of the glomerulus is of particular importance. Feedback regulation of glomerular function to maintain glomerular tubular balance is mediated through this anatomical relationship. The renin-angiotensin system not only functions as a regulator of renal function, but also plays a major role in the pathogenesis of systemic hyper-

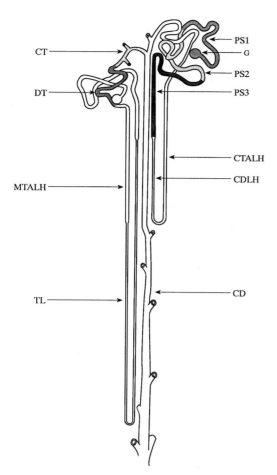

Fig. 32-1. Diagram of cortical and juxtamedullary nephrons demonstrating nephron segments. *G,* Glomerulus; *PS1,* S1 segment of proximal tubule; *PS2,* S2 segment of proximal tubule; *PS3,* S3 segment of proximal tubule; *CDLH, CTALH,* cortical descending and ascending limbs of the loop of Henle; *MTALH,* medullary loop of Henle; *TL,* thin limbs of Henle; *DT,* distal tubule; *CT,* connecting and collecting tubule; *CD,* collecting duct.

tension. Damage of these relationships, either structural or functional, may manifest not as renal dysfunction but rather as systemic hypertension. Another special vascular configuration of importance is the formation of vasa recta, which extend into the medulla. This configuration forms a countercurrent multiplier system involved in urinary concentration as well as in specialized postglomerular diversion of blood flow in the juxtamedullary nephrons. Destruction of the countercurrent system results in a loss of the ability of the kidney to concentrate urine, as is manifested by renal diabetes insipidus. Even the interstitial tissue has a specific function because medullary interstitium contains lipid-rich interstitial cells, which synthesize prostaglandins. The kidney is also an endocrine organ and is the site of production of the hormone erythropoietin, responsible for regulating hematopoiesis.

MECHANISMS OF INJURY

The mechanisms by which xenobiotics can mediate renal injury can be either direct through cytotoxicity or indirect by the induction of a systemic inflammatory or immunological reaction. Direct cytotoxic mechanisms depend on dose and exposure duration. Indirect reactions are often idiosyncratic and are more frequently dependent on the route of entry. Furthermore, the clinical manifestations of toxin-induced renal injury may be related directly to the renal injury itself or to secondary systemic effects of renal injury as manifested by hypertension and renal insufficiency. The nature of the injury may be determined to some extent by factors unrelated to the toxin, such as preexisting renal disease, or extrarenal factors that can affect renal dosage, such as abnormal liver function. In addition, the differences of susceptibility of different nephron segments can modify the renal response to toxins. Genetic toxicity with the development of neoplasia may be a delayed effect of the toxin or its metabolite with occurrence of disease at a time distant from the occurrence of exposure.

The most dramatic form of renal toxicity is acute tubular necrosis.[42,84,94] It has been long recognized that poisoning with heavy metals and organic solvents can lead to dose-dependent acute tubular epithelial cell necrosis manifested clinically by acute renal failure. The route of exposure to the toxin is generally irrelevant and can be through ingestion, inhalation, or cutaneous absorption. Although most instances of nephrotoxic acute tubular necrosis are the result of industrial accidents or accidental or intentional ingestion, it must be recognized that numerous therapeutic agents, such as aminoglycoside antibiotics[28] and the antineoplastic agent cisplatin, are known causes of toxic renal damage.[75,84]

Heavy metal–induced acute cell injury is largely the result of metal binding to the sulfhydryl groups of cell membrane proteins and enzymes. Binding to cell membrane proteins results in increased membrane permeability and inhibition of ATPase-dependent transport functions.[23,32,36] The most vivid example of heavy metal toxicity is that of mercuric chloride poisoning, in which widespread necrosis of proximal tubules occurs.[24] Binding of heavy metals to disulfide groups of enzymes and other proteins alters tertiary structure, resulting in denaturation, and thereby interferes with numerous metabolic functions, including uncoupling of mitochondrial oxidative phosphorylation. The effects sometimes may not be as dramatic and may present as chronic, functional tubular disturbances, such as Fanconi syndrome with aminoaciduria rather than cell necrosis with acute renal failure.[32,33] Acute lead nephropathy is perhaps the best example. The severity of heavy metal toxicity is modulated by the presence of metal binding proteins, metallothioneins, in the liver and kidney. Although these proteins are abundant and readily inducible, excessive dosage or exposure can overwhelm the ability to bind and deactivate the toxic effects of heavy metals.[14,15] This mechanism

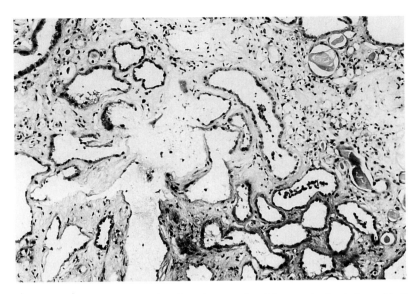

Fig. 32-2. Toxic acute tubular necrosis. There is necrosis of the proximal tubular epithelium with denudation of the basement membrane and rupture of luminal contents into the interstitium. There is marked interstitial edema and a leukocytic interstitial infiltrate. Some tubules show sloughing of cells into the lumen. (Hematoxylin and eosin ×350.)

has been shown to be important in the development of cadmium nephropathy. Organic solvents induce acute cellular cytotoxicity through the production of free radicals when they are metabolized by cytochrome P-450 and mixed function oxidases. Generation of free radicals results in lipid peroxidation and plasma membrane damage.[78,79]

Toxic acute tubular necrosis is most obvious in the proximal convoluted tubules (Fig. 32-2).[9,35,42] Although the necrosis is generally nonspecific, in some cases, distinctive morphological changes can be identified. For example, with mercuric chloride sublethally injured cells may contain large acidophillic inclusions, whereas carbon tetrachloride poisoning is characterized by the accumulation of lipids.[84]

Clinically, acute tubular necrosis is manifested in most instances by the presence of oliguric acute renal failure. The mechanisms that have been invoked to induce the oliguria range from alterations of glomerular tubular feedback secondary to inhibition of tubular transport function, arteriolar vasoconstriction, back leak of tubular fluid in areas of tubular damage, and obstruction from necrotic debris.[9,35,42,84] A good example of toxin-related tubular obstructive nephropathy is the case of ethylene glycol toxicity, in which obstruction with calcium oxalate crystals gives a characteristic histological picture.[25,84] A significant number of patients with toxic acute renal failure may not have oliguria and may, in fact, be polyuric. Such patients tend to follow a more benign clinical course, and this may be related to the dose to which the individual has been exposed.

Direct cytotoxic damage to the glomeruli is unusual and is not usually considered as a potential mechanism of renal

toxicity. Nevertheless, some examples of this mechanism have been used to develop experimental models of glomerular injury. Puromycin aminonucleoside (a cytotoxic agent) causes glomerular podocyte detachment, swelling, and foot process effacement, resulting in nephrotic range proteinuria.[22,26] Similar functional consequences result when the polyanionic sites of the proteoglycans incorporated into the basement membrane are blocked by the heparin antagonist protamine.[22] It is also possible that the glomerular sclerosis that accompanies chronic nephrotoxicity is the result of such a mechanism involving direct cytotoxic effects on the mesangial cell. This would result in mesangiolysis followed by matrix deposition and glomerular obsolescence (Fig. 32-3). This lesion is seen in humans as an acute response to certain snake venoms.[57]

Chronic nephrotoxicity is more insidious in its onset and clinical manifestations. It can mimic other primary renal diseases and may manifest itself by minor functional abnormalities or by systemic effects of renal damage, such as hypertension or progressive renal failure. Low molecular weight proteinuria such as an increased excretion of β_2 microglobulin has been used as an indicator of mild tubular damage[90] and is frequently used to screen individuals for the nephrotoxic effects of occupational exposures. It is often difficult to identify the specific nephrotoxic agent, and epidemiological studies that show an association of a particular agent with chronic renal failure or hypertension does not necessarily imply a cause-and-effect relationship. Indeed, even the identification of increased tissue levels of the suspect toxin may not be sufficient to identify a causal relationship. Increased levels could be due to lack of ex-

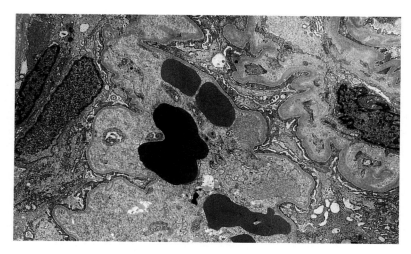

Fig. 32-3. Electron micrograph of a glomerulus with mesangiolysis. There is loss of the normal architecture of the glomerulus with loss of the entire mesangial structure. The glomerular basement membrane forms a belt around the merged capillaries, which contain red cells and fragments of denuded endothelium and mesangial cells. ($\times 10,500$.)

cretion in a patient who has renal insufficiency for other causes.[16] Nonetheless, there are several studies that have found an association of impaired renal function with increased blood lead concentrations in the general population and evidence of renal impairment and hypertension with chronic hydrocarbon exposure.* Chronic interstitial nephritis, the lesion best correlated with chronic nephrotoxicity, is often idiopathic, and a direct causal agent cannot be specifically identified.[19] Although epidemiological studies do raise suspicions, the effects of prolonged exposure to low levels of potential nephrotoxins often cannot be firmly established. Mild and subtle metabolic effects of nephrotoxins have been shown to increase apoptosis in experimental and in vitro situations;[48] it is not clear that this direct effect is mimicked in human disease. Chronic low-level exposure may enhance the susceptibility to injury by substances that are generally not considered to be nephrotoxic.

Even more difficult to assess are immunological complications associated with toxin exposure. Most glomerular disease is immune complex mediated, and in the vast majority of cases, it is classified as idiopathic and the immunogen is unknown. Although it is likely that in most instances an infectious antigen or autoantigen is the likely inciting factor, the possibility does exist that environmental toxins may contribute to the pool of immune complex–mediated glomerular disease of unknown cause.† Environmental toxins, particularly natural toxins, may function as haptens and therefore as immunogens after they have become protein bound. One reasonably well-recognized example of this mechanism is the occurrence of minimal change disease following allergic reactions to the bite of venomous insects.

Environmental exposure to toxins has also been implicated in the pathogenesis of autoimmune disease (see Chapter 25). Experimental studies have demonstrated that subcutaneous injection of mercuric chloride or inhalation of mercury vapor can induce an autoimmune glomerulonephritis that involves both circulating immune complexes and antibodies directed against basement membrane antigens.[10,17,38,64] It has been demonstrated that this disease is the result of a T-cell–dependent polyclonal B cell activation, which results in the production of antibodies against self-antigens and non–self-antigens. Well-controlled and well-designed epidemiological and occupational studies, however, have not demonstrated a mercury-induced effect on the immune system.[49,67] There has been considerable interest and concern raised about the potential deleterious effects on the immune system by mercury in dental amalgams.[51] This is a potential source for low-level exposure over a long period of time, and there have been some sporadic individual case reports suggesting an association with autoimmune diseases. A careful review of the literature and of the few well-conducted studies of the general population and dental workers fails to reveal any evidence of an effect on the immune system induced by mercury in dental amalgam.[18,51] Similar studies of occupational exposure to inorganic mercury have also been negative. Chronic hydrocarbon exposure has also been suggested potentially to mediate immunological alterations. There are numerous reports of antiglomerular basement membrane–mediated disease associated with hydrocarbon exposure.[5,92,93] In addition, several population studies suggest an increased incidence of primary glomerular disease and hypertension in individuals with chronic exposure. Although the evidence is somewhat more convincing than that for mercury,[17,44] it is still nevertheless a speculative association.[49]

*References 4, 13, 33, 37, 64, 86, 97.
†References 5, 10, 11, 17, 38, 44, 63, 77, 92, 93.

One definite area in which immunology plays a role in relationship to environmental agents is the development of allergic interstitial nephritis after exposure to a variety of therapeutic agents. Agents implicated include antibiotics, diuretics, anticonvulsants, and most recently nonsteroidal antiinflammatory drugs (NSAIDs).[15] These reactions definitely appear to be idiosyncratic and not dose related, and the incidence appears to be relatively low. This has been borne out with the experience of having NSAIDs sold as over-the-counter medications. Despite widespread use of these analgesics, there has been no truly significant increase in the incidence or prevalence of allergic interstitial nephritis.

SPECIFIC NEPHROTOXIC AGENTS
Heavy metals

It has already been stated that heavy metals exert their toxicity by binding to disulfide groups of enzymes and other proteins and thereby interfere with metabolic function[23,32,36,58,78] (see Chapter 4). Among the heavy metals, those that are recognized as being most important as nephrotoxins following environmental or occupational exposure are lead, mercury, cadmium, and arsenic. Gold and platinum have been implicated after therapeutic use, and other metals, including antimony, chromium, cobalt, copper, nickel, and uranium, have been implicated after massive exposure.

Lead. Although nephrotoxicity associated with chronic occupational exposure to lead has been well described, the potential of chronic low-level environmental exposure to cause chronic renal disease is less well defined.[7,20,33,95] Occupations in which lead exposure is known to be a hazard include those that relate to lead smelting, mining, plumbing, battery-making, or the use of lead paints or lead glazes.[29,95] The form of environmental exposure that has received the greatest public attention is the exposure to paint dust and flakes from older buildings where lead base paints had been used extensively.[33,39] As the primary excretory organ, a rapid accumulation of lead occurs in the kidneys, where specific lead-binding proteins have been identified. Lead is concentrated in the nuclei, and characteristic dark intranuclear inclusions are seen in both acute and chronic lead nephrotoxicity. In acute lead nephropathy, there is evidence of tubular necrosis with nuclear dropout and the presence of the intranuclear inclusions in the sublethally injured cells.[32,33] The inclusions are noted to be persistent for many years even after removal from lead exposure. Although acute tubular necrosis can occur, acute lead nephropathy is more likely to present itself as a tubular reabsorptive defect characterized by the Fanconi syndrome with aminoaciduria, phosphaturia, and glycosuria.

Chronic lead nephropathy was recognized as early as the late nineteenth century, in which contraction and granularity of the kidneys was a regular feature of individuals with occupational chronic lead exposure.[20] The question as to whether environmental exposure at levels lower than those of lead industry workers can cause chronic lead nephropathy is a matter of significant debate. A quoted study from Australia described cases of renal insufficiency occurring many years after childhood lead exposure.[37] The renal findings in these patients were essentially relatively nonspecific and consisted of contracted kidneys with a chronic interstitial nephritis.[56] There are reports that suggest that the association of lead exposure with chronic renal disease may be coincidental and that individuals with hypertensive nephrosclerosis and moderate renal insufficiency have a decreased ability to excrete lead.[16,29,62] One study presents further evidence to suggest that exposure to lead may impair renal function in the general population.[18] The authors found that creatinine clearance rates were inversely correlated with blood lead and zinc protoporphyrin levels. A tenfold increase in blood lead concentration was associated with a reduction of creatinine clearance by 10 to 13 ml/min. They also found a positive correlation between serum β_2 microglobulin and blood levels. Although these data can be accepted as demonstrating that chronic low-level lead exposure can be associated with progressive renal disease, the authors recognize that renal impairment owing to other causes may also lead to an increase in blood lead concentrations because of decreased excretion. These findings are similar to a previous study, which showed that elevated blood lead concentrations were correlated with hypertension.[3,4,64] Although extremely difficult to assign a cause-and-effect relationship between environmental lead exposure and chronic renal disease, the possibility does exist that they may be causally related.

Mercury. The effects of mercury on the kidney are more protean than those of lead. Mercury can exhibit its effect both directly as a cellular toxin[24] and indirectly by inducing autoimmune mechanisms.[10,17] The effects are similar whether the mercury is in an organic or a metallic form. The form of mercury may influence, however, the relative dosage to the kidney and therefore modulate the severity of the toxic reactions. As with other heavy metals, mercury reacts with free sulfhydryl groups, but it has also been demonstrated to inhibit oxidative phosphorylation in mitochondria. This mechanism probably explains the predilection of the hypoxia-sensitive S3 (latter third) segment of the proximal tubule to mercury-induced necrosis.[9]

Acute mercury poisoning represents a classic cause of acute tubular necrosis and was once relatively common because of the wide use of mercuric compounds therapeutically as diuretics and more generally as disinfectants.[24,27] Exposure to as little as 0.5 g of mercuric salts can produce tubular necrosis. There is necrosis of the S3 segment of the proximal tubule, but larger doses have been demonstrated to affect other tubular segments as well.

Although it has been suggested that chronic exposure to mercury may result in chronic interstitial nephritis, chronic

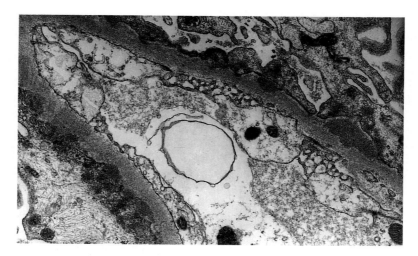

Fig. 32-4. Membranous glomerulopathy associated with heavy metal exposure. There are electron dense deposits on the epithelial side of the glomerular basement membrane. These correspond to immune complexes seen by immunoflourescence microscopy. (×22,500.)

exposure has been more consistently associated with the indirect effects of mercury exposure on the immune system.* Membranous glomerulonephropathy has been reported in a variety of instances, including both industrial exposure and therapeutic exposure (Fig. 32-4).[44] Although the mechanism has not been clearly identified, it is thought by some that tubular damage caused by mercury may release tubular brush border antigens and lead to the formation of autoantibodies, which then result in a membranous nephropathy similar to that seen in experimental Heymann's nephritis. An alternate hypothesis, and one that is more likely, is that mercury induces T cell–mediated polyclonal B cell activation with the production of a wide variety of autoantibodies.[10] In support of this is that antiglomerular basement membrane disease has also been identified in humans with occupational exposure and in animals injected with mercuric chloride.[77] This hypothesis is best supported by demonstrations of autoimmune glomerulonephritis with both a linear and a membranous pattern in rats exposed to mercury either as a salt injected subcutaneously or through inhalation of mercury vapor.[38,67] It is of interest, however, that a number of studies of chronic low-level occupational exposure have not shown any adverse effects on renal function.[67] The results of these studies argue strongly against the hypothesis presented by some that dental amalgam may be a sufficient source of mercury to induce autoimmune disease in humans.[51,72]

Cadmium. Cadmium acting as an important nephrotoxin became clear in reports from Japan, where villagers eating food grown in soil heavily contaminated by industrial cadmium developed bone disease and renal failure.[59,76] A prominent feature of cadmium nephrotoxicity is hypercalciuria with the development of renal stones associated

*References 10, 17, 32, 44, 75, 77.

with osteoporosis and osteomalacia. Nephrolithiasis is also a common occurrence in cadmium workers. Cadmium becomes bound to metallothioneins[14,15] and therefore has a predilection for accumulation in proximal tubular epithelium and may explain the tubular dysfunction that results in hypercalciuria. Histologically the lesion is one of chronic interstitial fibrosis with tubular atrophy and nephrocalcinosis, which is essentially nonspecific in its pattern and distribution. Although it has been suggested that chronic cadmium exposure can be associated with increased incidence of hypertension, the problem of interpreting these data is similar to that seen with lead exposure.[16,59]

Other metals. Tubular necrosis has been reported with massive exposure to a variety of other metals, including chromium, bismuth, copper, and antimony.[74] Arsenicals have been widely used in the agricultural industry, where excessive exposure has also been implicated in the pathogenesis of acute tubular necrosis.[31] Uranium workers have been shown to have an increase in urinary β_2 microglobulin excretion as compared with control individuals, but it is not known whether this can contribute to the development of hypertension or chronic renal failure.[74] As mentioned previously, the use of gold compounds therapeutically in patients with rheumatic diseases has been associated with the development of a membranous nephropathy.

Organic chemicals

Organic chemicals are ubiquitous and are used not only in industry, but also in everyday household activities. Although some organic compounds such as halogenated hydrocarbons are extremely toxic, others such as gasoline are less toxic. The nephrotoxicity of all organic compounds is directly dose-dependent. Because of their ubiquitous nature, organic solvents are probably responsible for more cases of nephrotoxic tubular necrosis than are heavy met-

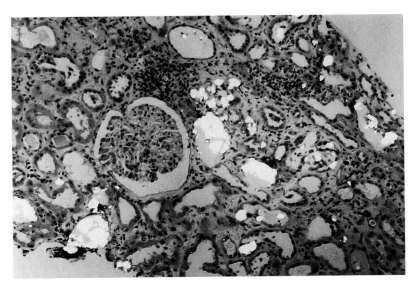

Fig. 32-5. Oxalate nephropathy following chronic ingestion of massive doses of vitamin C. Oxalate crystals are seen occluding tubules and are associated with interstitial edema and leukocytic infiltration. A similar picture is seen with ingestion of glycols. (Hematoxylin and eosin ×350.)

als. In addition, there appears to be synergistic effects of different organic compounds. Alcoholics appear to be more susceptible to the toxic effect of organic solvents. It is theorized that the effect of organic compounds is amplified by the presence of alcohol, and doses normally not expected to be toxic become so.

Of particular concern are the halogenated hydrocarbons, which are frequently used as dry cleaners and include trichloroethylene, ethylene dichloride, and the now obsolete dry cleaning compounds chloroform and carbon tetrachloride.[34] These are extremely toxic compounds, and exposure by inhalation or ingestion to even modest amounts can be lethal. Although symptoms referable to other organ systems, particularly the liver, may predominate, acute tubular necrosis does contribute to a death in these individuals.[96]

The question of chronic effects of hydrocarbon exposure is, as with other nephrotoxins, difficult to assess. Some epidemiological studies suggest that occupational hydrocarbon exposure is associated with renal dysfunction.[37,97] A large number of case reports have suggested that hydrocarbons can be associated with immunological alterations, and they have been implicated in the development of idiopathic membranous glomerulonephropathy and antiglomerular basement membrane antibody–mediated disease.[50,89,93] Again, although these sporadic reports do suggest a potential relationship, good experimental models are not available, and a definite causal relationship in humans has been difficult to establish.

Another group of compounds that are a major source of nephrotoxic tubular injury are the glycols.[25] A variety of glycols are toxic to the kidney. Ethylene glycol is widely

used as antifreeze, and its availability has resulted in numerous cases of ingestion as a substitute for alcohol. Ethylene glycol is oxidized by alcohol dehydrogenase to oxalic acid, which is secreted by the renal tubules. Glycol poisoning thus produces vacuolar degeneration of the proximal tubules with precipitation of oxalate crystals in the tubule lumina.[83] This is a characteristic histological picture and is similar to oxalate nephrosis seen with ingestion of large amounts of vitamin C (Fig. 32-5).

Other organic compounds that have been associated with toxic tubular necrosis include methanol, phenol, and petroleum products. All of these require either ingestion or heavy inhalation exposure. Until recently, evaluation of toxicity related to exposure to gasolines was complicated by the presence of lead additives, and renal lesions were often attributed to lead toxicity rather than to the hydrocarbon itself. Phenols, in addition to producing tubular necrosis, have been associated with bilateral cortical necrosis.

Silica and berylliosis

Silica as an occupational toxin is primarily recognized for the development of pulmonary lesions, which are generally considered to be the major adverse effect (see Chapter 28). In one study of patients with severe silicosis, however, 40% had renal insufficiency, 20% had proteinuria, and 45% had urinary concentration defects.[63] Autopsy studies have suggested that there may be an increased incidence of glomerulonephritis or vasculitis in patients with silicosis.[11,45] It is not clear whether these associations are circumstantial or whether indeed silicosis also can affect systemic immunity and thereby initiate immune-mediated renal disease. The kidneys can also be involved as a secondary manifestation in patients with berylliosis. The granulomatous pulmonary disease is often associated with hypercalcemia and hypercalciuria, which can lead to an increased incidence of renal stones and nephrocalcinosis.

GENETIC TOXICITY AND NEOPLASIA

Just as the kidney is particularly susceptible to the cytotoxic effects of xenobiotics because it is an excretory organ, the epithelia of the kidney and collecting system are also vulnerable to genetic toxicity and the development of neoplasia. Indeed, one of the earliest recognized occupational diseases was carcinoma of the bladder in aniline dye workers.[68] The strong association of bladder cancer with a variety of occupations and other environmental hazards has generated considerable interest in the urinary tract as a target for the potential carcinogenic effects of substances commonly encountered in the environment. Although a definite relationship has been established for transitional cell carcinoma of the collecting system to certain occupational exposures, we do not know what proportion of sporadic transitional cell carcinoma of the urinary tract in the general population can be attributed to environmental exposure to lower levels of related carcinogens. The matter is further complicated by the fact that pathogenesis of cancer is a multistep process involving a number of different genetic alterations that can occur over a period of time. Furthermore, environmental agents can function either directly as initiating carcinogens or indirectly as promoters unmasking a previous genetic injury (see Chapter 26).

Carcinogenic environmental agents act either directly or by producing intermediate metabolites that act as the offending agent. For example, heavy metals, which are important nephrotoxins from a cytotoxic point of view, also bind to purine and pyrimidine bases, thereby adversely affecting the normal process of DNA repair. The prime example of intermediate metabolites being carcinogenic is derived from analysis of the carcinogenic affect of aniline dyes. Aniline dyes are metabolized by oxidation in the liver, conjugation with glucuronic acid, and excretion in the urine. Further hydrolysis by the urothelium results in the production of hydroxylamine, which acts as the direct carcinogen. Because of these complexities, environmental agents that have been implicated in the cause of renal cell or bladder cancer are classified into three categories, those in which there is an established relationship, those in which the relationship is strongly associated or suspicious, and those which are theorized and yet unproven.

The molecular biology and genetics of renal cell carcinoma has received considerable attention because one of the known predisposing factors has been an association with von Hippel-Lindau disease, and this has led to genetic investigation of both familial and sporadic cases.[69] The most prominent finding has been cytogenetic changes associated with the short arm of chromosome 3, including deletions, insertions, and translocations. In one study, a putative re-

nal cell carcinoma gene was located on 3p.[19,21] This is of particular interest because the gene of von Hippel-Lindau disease is localized to that same region. This study found the renal cell carcinoma gene was expressed in all normal kidney samples examined, but gene expression was 20% or less in the majority of renal cell carcinomas.[69] Alterations of chromosome 3p were found in clear nonpapillary renal cell carcinomas, whereas papillary carcinomas demonstrated other genetic abnormalities, including trisomy involving chromosomes 7, 12, and 17. The genetic defect seen in oncocytic lesions was a translocation of 5 and 11. The alterations of chromosome 17 are of particular interest because lesions of 17p have been reported in many tumors, and it is of note that the tumor suppressor gene p53 is assigned to that region. The potential role of tumor suppressor genes suggests that pathogenesis of renal cell carcinoma involves a two-hit mechanism in which sporadic initiation is followed by deletion of specific tumor suppressor genes. The multistep process is an indication that it is likely that environmental factors contribute significantly to renal carcinogenesis.

A number of case-control studies of renal cancer have demonstrated an increased incidence in certain industries, including the chemical, petroleum, and metal processing industries.* Of particular interest is that in some studies white collar workers in those same industries also appear to have an increased risk for renal cell cancer even though they have had no direct exposure to the putative agent. Similarly, architects have been identified as being at increased risk for renal cell carcinoma.[50,54] Thus, although it is recognized that obvious occupational exposure is associated with an increased incidence, the realization that even casual exposure may function as a potential etiological factor is not generally considered. Minimal, casual, or "harmless" exposure is often not asked about when taking a patient's medical history because it is believed that such exposure is too ubiquitous to have any direct or specific affect on the patient's disease. The finding of an increased incidence of renal cell cancer in architects and in white collar workers of selected industries suggests that even casual exposure may be a contributing factor. Another study that did not target specific industries and that adjusted for obesity, smoking, and coffee consumption found that there was an increased risk for men in a mixed category of various white collar occupations.[65] There was no clustering of cases into particular subcategories of industry or occupation, and no other specific risk factors were identified. It is of interest to compare these findings with those of studies that have found a decreased risk in male farmers. One could possibly conclude that the recirculated air of offices is likely to be more carcinogenic than the open fresh air of farm fields.

The one environmental toxin that has been associated with both renal and urothelial cancer is tobacco smok-

*References 8, 18, 34, 43, 52, 68, 80, 82.

ing.[47,53] This association holds not only in the general population, but also in studies of occupational exposure. As an example, one case-control study of fishermen in Japan, who have exposure to aniline dyes through the use of dyed maggots as bait, found no significant risk related to dye exposure but rather demonstrated a definite relationship to cigarette smoking.[85] Similarly, another study has demonstrated that there is a greater risk of renal cell carcinoma in cadmium workers who smoke as compared with nonsmoking workers, whereas both smoking and nonsmoking workers are at greater risk than the general population. The role of smoking in renal cell cancer, although recognized, has been relatively difficult to evaluate because there has been considerable heterogeneity in the published estimates of the relative risk. A case-control study from Italy has more clearly established this relationship. A significant positive relationship was demonstrated between dose, i.e., amount and duration of smoking history, and the risk of renal cell cancer. The relative risk was roughly double that of nonsmokers.[47]

The case for environmental exposure in the pathogenesis of urothelial cancer is well established. A case for a positive correlation has been demonstrated for contact with arylamines, excess phenacetin consumption, and cigarette smoking.* A wide variety of substances have been implicated as etiological agents, but roles have not been completely established, and a number of therapeutic reagents are included, including cyclophosphamide. Other substances that have close structural relationships to proven carcinogens have also been suggested as playing a potential role and include such commonly used substances as coffee, saccharin, cyclamates, and nitrates and nitrosamine from smoked foods. Also of particular interest is the potential role of tryptophan as a promoter but not necessarily an initiator of urothelial cancer. Urothelial cancers can involve any part of the collecting system, including the renal pelvis ureters as well as the bladder. Although transitional cell tumors of the bladder are more common, there appears to be an increasing incidence of upper tract tumors, particularly in cigarette smokers.[81] One special instance that deserves mention is the unusually frequent occurrence of transitional cell carcinoma of the bladder of the inhabitants of a few villages in the vicinity of the Danube River and its tributaries.[70] This is the same population that is afflicted with a chronic tubulointerstitial nephritis commonly called Balkan endemic nephropathy.[31] Although the pathogenesis is still obscure, the similarity to the picture seen with phenacetin ingestion strongly suggests that an environmental agent is responsible for Balkan nephritis and carcinoma of the urinary tract.

Another potential environmental effect that deserves discussion is the relationship between parental occupation and congenital renal disease in offspring. One study has demonstrated a possible relationship between Wilms tumor and parental occupation, suggesting that the fetus may be a particularly susceptible target for gene toxicity. The Wilms tumor susceptibility gene WT1 maps to the chromosome 11p 13 site.[12,21,66] The gene encodes a zinc finger protein that acts as a tumor suppressor.[71] Small deletions or mutations can alter gene function, and because the WT1 gene product is associated with epithelial differentiation,[46] mutation is associated with inhibition of differentiation and initiation of congenital neoplasia. Thus, 11p 13 WT1 appears to play a crucial role in regulating the proliferation and differentiation of nephroblasts and thus is important in embryonic development. In the case-control study conducted to examine the relationship between Wilms tumor and parental occupation exposure, no consistent pattern of increased risk was found for parental exposure to hydrocarbons or lead.[61] There was strong suggestive evidence, however, that the offspring of vehicle mechanics, auto body repairmen, and welders did indeed have an increased risk. Although chance could not be excluded because of the nature of the population studied, a potential role of environmental exposure with fetal genitourinary abnormalities cannot be dismissed. Another study that examined the association of congenital anomalies with parental occupation found a positive correlation of urinary tract anomalies to parental occupation in the printing industry.[61]

CONCLUDING REMARKS

Environmental and occupational exposure constitutes an important part of the etiology of renal disease. It appears to contribute to the pool of patients with end-stage renal disease of unknown cause as well as to those instances of renal disease and renal and urothelial neoplasia in which a specific association has been defined. With our advancing knowledge of the molecular biology of cell injury, immunity, and neoplasia, we may be able to narrow further the gap between epidemiological studies that suggest a potential association with the actual demonstration of a direct relationship of a specific toxin with a specific renal disease.

REFERENCES

1. Abralman PA, Keane WF: Glomerular and interstitial disease induced by non steroidal anti-inflammatory drugs, *Am J Nephrol* 4:1, 1984.
2. Atanassov N, Donovski L, Kumanov H: *Tumours of the urinary passages in endemic nephropathy.* In Puchlev A et al, editors: *Proc. Second International Symposium on Endemic Nephropathy,* Sofia, 1974, Bulgarian Academy of Sciences.
3. Batuman V: Lead Nephropathy, gout, and hypertension, *Am J Med Sci* 305:241, 1993.
4. Beevers DG et al: Blood lead and hypertension, *Lancet* 2:1, 1976.
5. Beirne G: Glomerulonephritis associated with hydrocarbon solvents, *Environ Res* 23:422, 1980.
6. Bengtsson T et al: Transitional cell tumours of the renal pelvis in analgesic abusers, *Scand J Urol Nephrol* 2:145, 1968.
7. Bennett MW: Lead nephropathy, *Kidney Int* 28:212, 1985.
8. Bertazzi PA et al: Mortality study of cancer risk among oil refinery workers, *Int Arch Occup Environ Health* 61:261, 1989.

*References 6, 40, 44, 55, 80, 81.

9. Biber TUL et al: A study of micropuncture and microdissection of acute renal damage in rats, *Am J Med* 44:664, 1962.

10. Bigazzi PE: Lessons from animal models: the scope of mercury-induced autoimmunity, *Clin Immunol Immunopathol* 65:81, 1992 (editorial).

11. Bonnin A et al: Silicosis associated with crescentic IgA mesangial nephropathy, *Nephron* 47:229, 1987.

12. Brown KW et al: Inactivation of the remaining allele of the WT1 gene in a Wilms' tumour from a WAGR patient, *Oncogene* 7:763, 1992.

13. Carmignani M et al: Renal mechanisms in the cardiovascular effects of chronic exposure to inorganic mercury in rats, *Br J Ind Med* 49:226, 1992.

14. Chan HM et al: Exogenous metallothionein and renal toxicity of cadmium and mercury in rats, *Toxicology* 76:15, 1992.

15. Cherian MG, Goyer RA, Delaquerriere-Richardson L: Cadmium-metallothionein-induced nephropathy, *Toxicol Appl Pharmacol* 38:399, 1976.

16. Cory-Slechta DA: Lead exposure during advanced age: alterations in kinetics and biochemical effects, *Toxicol Appl Pharmacol* 104:67, 1990.

17. Druet P et al: Immunologically mediated glomerulonephritis induced by heavy metals, *Arch Toxicol* 50:187, 1982.

18. Eklund G, Izikowitz L, Molin C: Malignant tumours in Swedish dental personnel: a comparative study with the total population as well as with some specific occupational groups, *Swed Dent J* 14:249, 1990.

19. Eknoyan G, Schrier RW, Gottschalk CW: *Diseases of the kidney,* ed 5, Boston, 1993, Little, Brown.

20. Emmerson BT: Chronic lead nephropathy, *Kidney Int* 4:1, 1973.

21. Erlandsson R et al: A gene near the D3F15S2 site on 3p is expressed in normal human kidney but not or only at a severely reduced level in 11 of 15 primary renal cell carcinomas (RCC), *Oncogene* 5:1207, 1990.

22. Fishman JA, Karnovsky MJ: Effects of aminonucleoside of puromycin on glomerular epithelial cells, *Am J Pathol* 118:398, 1985.

23. Fowler BA, DuVal G: Effects of lead on the kidney: roles of high-affinity lead-binding proteins, *Environ Health Perspect* 91:77, 1991.

24. Freeman RB et al: Renal tubular necrosis due to nephrotoxicity of organic mercurial diuretics, *Ann Intern Med* 57:34, 1962.

25. Friedman EA et al: Consequences of ethylene glycol poisoning. Report of four cases and review of the literature, *Am J Med* 32:891, 1962.

26. Fujiwara Y: Ultrastructural study of the effect of steroids on amino-nuclesive nephrosis in the rat, *Vircows Arch* 405:11, 1984.

27. Galle P, Morel-Maroger L: Les lesions renales du saturnisme humain et experimental, *Nephron* 2:273, 1965.

28. Gary NE et al: Gentamycin associated acute renal failure, *Arch Intern Med* 136:1101, 1976.

29. Gerhardsson L et al: Kidney effects in long term exposed lead smelter workers, *Br J Ind Med* 49:186, 1992.

30. Gerhardt RE, Crecelius EA, Hudson JB: Moonshine-related arsenic poisoning, *Arch Intern Med* 140:221, 1980.

31. Gloor FJ: Changing concepts in pathogenesis and morphology of analgesic nephropathy as seen in Europe, *Kidney Int* 13:27, 1978.

32. Goyer RA: The renal tubule in lead poisoning. I. Mitochondrial swelling and aminoaciduria, *Lab Invest* 19:71, 1968.

33. Goyer RA: Lead toxicity: from overt to subclinical to subtle health effects, *Environ Health Perspect* 86:177, 1990.

34. Harrington JM et al: Renal disease and occupational exposure to organic solvents: a case referent approach, *Br J Ind Med* 46:643, 1989.

35. Henry LN, Lane CE, Kashgarian M: Studies of the pathophysiology of acute renal failure, *Lab Invest* 19:309, 1968.

36. Hitzfeld B, Planas-Bohne F, Taylor D: The effect of lead on protein and DNA metabolism of normal and lead-adapted rat kidney cells in culture, *Biol Trace El Res* 21:87, 1989.

37. Hotz P et al: Hydrocarbon exposure, hypertension and kidney function tests, *Int Arch Occup Environ Health* 62:501, 1990.

38. Hua J et al: Autoimmune glomerulonephritis induced by mercury vapour exposure in the Brown Norway rat, *Toxicology* 79:119, 1993.

39. Inglis JA, Henderson DA, Emmerson BT: The pathology and pathogenesis of chronic lead nephropathy occurring in Queensland, *J Pathol* 124:65, 1978.

40. Jensen OM et al: The Copenhagen case-control study of renal pelvis and ureter cancer: role of analgesics, *Int J Cancer* 44:965, 1989.

41. Johansson S, Wahlqvist L: Tumours of urinary bladder and ureter associated with abuse of phenacetin-containing analgesics, *Acta Pathol Microbiol Scand [A]* 85:768, 1977.

42. Kadamani S, Asal NR, Nelson RY: Occupational hydrocarbon exposure and risk of renal cell carcinoma, *Am J Ind Med* 15:131, 1989.

43. Kashgarian M: Acute renal failure. *Pathol Ann* 15:335, 1980.

44. Kibukamusoke JW, Davies DR, Hutt MSR: Membranous nephropathy due to skin-lightening cream, *Br Med J* 2:646, 1974.

45. Kolev K, Doitschiniv D, Todorov D: Morphologic alterations in the kidneys by silicosis, *Medicina del Lavora* 61:205, 1970.

46. Kreidberg JA et al: WT-1 is required for early kidney development, *Cell* 74:679, 1993.

47. LaVecchia C et al: Smoking and renal cell carcinoma, *Cancer Res* 50:5231, 1990.

48. Ledda-Columbano GM et al: Cell deletion by apoptosis during regression of renal hyperplasia, *Am J Pathol* 135:657, 1989.

49. Longworth S et al: Renal and immunological effects of occupational exposure to inorganic mercury, *Br J Ind Med* 49:394, 1992.

50. Lowery JT et al: Renal cell carcinoma among architects, *Am J Ind Med* 20:123, 1991.

51. Mandel ID: Amalgam hazards. An assessment of research *J Am Dent Assoc* 122(9):62, 1991; published erratum appears in *J Am Dent Assoc* 122:10, 1991.

52. McCredie M, Stewart JH: Risk factors for kidney cancer in New South Wales. IV. occupation, *Br J Ind Med* 50:349, 1993.

53. McCredie M, Stewart JH, Ford JM: Analgesics and tobacco as risk factors for cancer of the ureter and renal pelvis in man, *J Urol* 130:28, 1983.

54. McLaughlin JK et al: Renal cell cancer among architects and allied professionals in Sweden, *Am J Ind Med* 21:873, 1992.

55. Mihatsch MJ et al: Phenacetinabusus. III, *Schweiz Med Wochenschr* 110:255, 1980.

56. Morgan JM, Hartley MW, Miller RE: Nephropathy in chronic lead poisoning, *Arch Intern Med* 118:17, 1966.

57. Morita T et al: Mesangiolysis: sequential ultrastructural study of HABO snake venom induced glomerular lesions, *Lab Invest* 38:94, 1978.

58. Nolan CV, Shaikh ZA: Lead nephrotoxicity and associated disorders: biochemical mechanisms, *Toxicology* 73:127, 1992.

59. Nomiyama K: Recent progress and perspectives in cadmium health effects studies, *Sci Total Environ* 14:199, 1980.

60. Olshan AF, Teschke K, Baird PA: Paternal occupation and congenital anomalies in offspring, *Am J Ind Med* 20:447, 1991.

61. Olshan AF et al: Wilms' tumor and paternal occupation, *Cancer Res* 50:3212, 1990.

62. Omae K et al: No adverse effects of lead on renal function in lead-exposed workers, *Ind Health* 28:77, 1990.

63. Osorio AM et al: Silica and glomerulonephritis: case report and review of the literature, *Am J Kidney Dis* 9:224, 1987.

64. Osterloh JD et al: Body burdens of lead in hypertensive nephropathy, *Arch Environ Health* 44:304, 1989.

65. Partanen T et al: Renal cell cancer and occupational exposure to chemical agents, *Scand J Work Environ Health* 17:231, 1991.

66. Pelletier J et al: Germline mutations in the Wilms' tumor suppressor gene are associated with abnormal urogenital development in Denys-Drash syndrome, *Cell* 67:437, 1991.

67. Piikivi L, Ruokonen A: Renal function and long-term low mercury vapor exposure, *Arch Environ Health* 44:146, 1989.

68. Poole-Wilson DS: Occupational tumours of the renal pelvis and ureter arising in the dye-making industry, *Proc R Soc Med* 62:93, 1969.

69. Presti JC Jr et al: Histopathological, cytogenetic, and molecular characterization of renal cortical tumors, *Cancer Res* 51:1544, 1991.

70. Radovanovic Z et al: Papillary transitional cell tumours, Balkan nephropathy, and β_2-microglobulin, *Lancet* 2:689, 1981 (letter).

71. Rauscher FJ et al: Binding of the Wilms' tumor locus zinc finger protein to the EGR-1 consensus sequence, *Science* 250:1259, 1990.

72. Reinhardt JW: Side-effects: mercury contribution to body burden from dental amalgam, *Adv Dent Res* 6:110, 1992.

73. Roberts RS et al: A study of mortality in workers engaged in the mining, smelting, and refining of nickel. II: mortality from cancer of the respiratory tract and kidney, *Toxicol Ind Health* 5:975, 1989.

74. Roels HA et al: Urinary kallikrein activity in workers exposed to cadmium, lead or mercury vapour, *Br J Ind Med* 47:331, 1990.

75. Safirstein R et al: Cisplatin nephrotixicity, *Am J Kid Dis* 8:356, 1986.

76. Saito H et al: Chronic cadmium poisoning induced by environmental cadmium pollution. Renal lesions (multiple proximal tubular dysfunctions) identified in residents of cadmium-polluted Hosogoe, Kosaka town, Akita prefecture, Japan, *Jpn J Med* 16:2, 1977.

77. Sapin C, Druet E, Druet P: Induction of antiglomerular basement membrane antibodies in the Brown-Norway rat by mercuric chloride, *Clin Exp Immunol* 28:173, 1977.

78. Schreiner GE, Maher JF: Toxic nephropathy, *Am J Med* 38:409, 1965.

79. Seldin DW, Giebisch G: *The kidney, physiology and pathophysiology,* ed 2, New York, 1993, Raven Press.

80. Shinka T et al: Clinical study on urothelial tumors of dye workers in Wakayama City, *J Urol* 146:1504, 1991.

81. Silverman DT et al: Bladder cancer and occupation among Swedish women, *Am J Ind Med* 16:239, 1989 (letter).

82. Sinks T et al: Renal cell cancer among paperboard printing workers, *Epidemiology* 3:483, 1992.

83. Smith DE: Morphologic lesions due to acute and subacute poisoning with antifreeze (ethylene glycol), *Arch Pathol* 51:423, 1951.

84. Solez K, Heptinstall RH: *Pathology of the kidney,* ed 4, Boston 1992, Little, Brown.

85. Sorahan T, Sole G: Coarse fishing and urothelial cancer: a regional case-control study, *Br J Cancer* 62:138, 1990.

86. Staessen JA et al: Impairment of renal function with increasing blood lead concentrations in the general population. The Cadmibel Study Group, *N Engl J Med* 327:151, 1992.

87. Stoeckle JD, Hardy HL, Weber AL: Chronic beryllium disease. Long-term follow-up of sixty cases and selective review of the literature, *Am J Med* 46:545, 1969.

88. Sullivan JB Jr: Immunological alterations and chemical exposure, *J Toxicol Clin Toxicol* 27:311, 1989 (review).

89. Sumpio B, Hayslett JP: Renal handling of proteins in normal and diseased states, *Quart J Med* 57:611, 1985.

90. Thun MJ, Baker DB, Smith AB: *Uranium and nephrotoxicity.* NIOSH health hazard evaluation report, Canon City, Co, 1981, Cotter Corp, HETA.

91. Tubbs RR et al: Membranous glomerulonephritis associated with industrial mercury exposure, *Am J Clin Pathol* 77:409, 1982.

92. Van der Laan G: Chronic glomerulonephritis and organic solvents. A case control study, *Int Arch Occup Environ Health* 47:1, 1980.

93. VanWhy SK et al: Induction and intracellular localization of HSP-72 after renal ischemia, *Am J Physiol* 263:F769, 1992.

94. Wedeen RP et al: Occupational lead nephropathy, *Am J Med* 59:630, 1975.

95. Woods WW: The changes in the kidneys in carbon tetrachloride poisoning, and their resemblance to those in the "crush syndrome," *J Pathol Bacteriol* 58:767, 1946.

96. Yaqoob M: Renal impairment with chronic hydrocarbon exposure, *Q J Med* 86:165, 1993.

Chapter 33

REPRODUCTIVE SYSTEM

Donald R. Mattison
John E. Craighead

Reproduction by the individual male and female, as well as the couple, is a complex interdependent process. Over the past two decades, increasing attention has been devoted to the vulnerability of reproduction to interruption by exposures to chemical, physical, and biologic agents.[3,12,26] This increased interest by the scientific and medical public is the result of several factors including epidemiologic data suggesting human vulnerability to reproductive toxicity, changes in demographics and life-style factors, increasing numbers of female employees in occupations traditionally filled by males, and the increasing age of workers.

Not all attempts at reproduction are successful (Table 33-1). Among 1000 couples attempting pregnancy, approximately 60% conceive during each cycle of unprotected intercourse. Preimplantation loss is thought to be high, with as many as half of the conceptions succumbing before implantation. Between 30% and 70% of pregnancies detectable by a sensitive and specific hCG immunoassay survive.

Between 15% and 60% of these are lost subsequently, leaving clinically recognized pregnancy occurring in about 20% to 30% of conceptions. It is estimated that about 10% to 30% of unprotected cycles of intercourse result in the birth of a living child at the end of pregnancy (Fig. 33-1).

Given the complex series of events needed for successful reproduction, it is not surprising that reproductive or developmental failure should occur as a result of physiologic, infectious, and environmental causes (Table 33-2). In order to appreciate the potential impact of toxicants on reproduction, it is necessary to explore the factors influencing reproductive success and failure.

At present, the incidence and etiology of reproductive failure within and across various human populations are uncertain. This is because it is necessary for pregnancy to have been attempted in order to recognize reproductive failure. It has been estimated that between 10% and 20% of couples have impaired fertility (Table 33-3). Moreover, surgical sterilization increases from about 4% at age 15 to 24 to almost 50% at age 35 to 44.[23,24] Between the years 1965 and 1982, the percent of infertile married women in the age range of 15 to 24 years increased, but there was no change in the prevalence of infertility among those older than 25 (Table 33-4). The origin of increased infertility among these younger women is poorly defined. Infectious diseases are thought to play a substantial role, but the impact of environmental factors is unknown.[24] There has been little attempt to explore the impact of other potential causes of infertility among these young women. Because fertility is highest among younger couples,[6] this change is of concern.

Factors that influence fertility include age, frequency of intercourse, and the cycle day(s) on which intercourse occurs. As women pass through puberty and enter adulthood, their ability to conceive increases (Fig. 33-2). In a study of

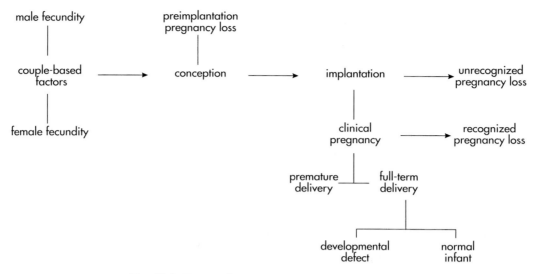

Fig. 33-1. Range of outcomes of attempts at pregnancy.

Table 33-1. Life table of reproductive and developmental success

Reproductive or developmental event	Outcome*
Couples attempting pregnancy	1000
Conception (occurs at mid-cycle 14 days before menses)	600-1000
Pre-implantation loss (30% to 50% loss between conception and implantation)	(300-500)
Chemical pregnancy (+hCG, from 7 days before missed menses until 7 weeks)	300-700
Unrecognized pregnancy loss (15% to 60% up to 7 weeks)	(45-420)
Clinical pregnancy (clinically recognized)	200-300
Clinically recognized spontaneous abortion (15% to 25%)	(30-75)
Continuing pregnancy (beyond 28 weeks)	170-300
Stillbirth (beyond 28 weeks, <3%)	(10-15)
Premature, postmature, growth retardation (about 10%)	(20-30)
Term births	110-300
Developmental abnormality	
(3 to 5% identified at birth)	(3-12)
(5 - 15% identified over first year of life)	(6-35)

*The numbers in parentheses represent reproductive or developmental loss or failure.

Data adapted from Mattison DR, Jelovsek FR: *Environmental and occupational exposure.* In Evans MI, editor: *Reproductive risks and prenatal diagnosis,* Norwalk, Conn, 1992, Appleton and Lange; Kline J, Stein Z, Susser M: *Conception to birth: epidemiology of prenatal development,* New York, 1989 Oxford University Press.

the effect of age of the wife at marriage on fertility rate and delays in conception, it was observed that the fertility rate increased from 93 per 1000 at age 16 to 276 per 1000 at age 24. A comparable decrease in conception delay from 11.7 months to 5.3 months was also found. Age at the end of the reproductive life span alters female fecundity (although it appears to have little or no effect on male fecundity).

Frequency of intercourse also impacts on fertility. Barrett and Marshall evaluated its effect on the number of conceptions occurring within 6 months of the time contraception was stopped.[4,5] Frequency of intercourse appears to impact on fertility and on the cycle-specific fertility rate. Among couples who had intercourse less than once per week, there were 17% pregnancies over a period of 6 months, whereas among those engaging in intercourse more often than four times per week, the cumulative conception rate was 83% (Fig. 33-3).[6] Data from Barrett and Marshall[5] can be used to calculate the cycle-specific fertility rate, which is the probability of becoming pregnant per cycle of unprotected intercourse (Table 33-5). With all other things being equal, couples that have unprotected intercourse daily have a high probability of conceiving. The likelihood of conception also varies with the day of the cycle on which intercourse occurs, as does the risk for early pregnancy loss (Fig. 33-4). Highest fecundity occurs during the several days before ovulation and falls rapidly thereafter. The rate of early pregnancy loss appears to decline when intercourse occurs near the time of ovulation but increases rapidly thereafter.

In general, the causes of infertility are thought to be roughly one third male attributable, one third female, and one third couple.[6,23,24,35] The defined causes of infertility depend on the individual or couple. Data from medical clinics may misrepresent the actual causes of infertility, but it is the best estimate of the etiology of infertility available (Table 33-6). Although sperm count, motility, and morphology as well as semen composition might be expected to impact on male fecundity,[22,30,41-45] only sperm count has been clearly demonstrated to have an effect.[20] Female fecundity is influenced by age, with declining fecundity beyond age 35[21,33] (Table 33-4). Age and prior reproductive history have a strong influence on the risk for spontaneous abortion.[10,23,34]

Reproductive toxicity is defined as a delay in pregnancy, an increase in early pregnancy loss, or subfertility or absolute infertility, resulting from an exposure to a physical, biologic or chemical agent that alters the reproductive performance of either partner or of the couple. *Developmental toxicity* is defined as an alteration in the structure or function of a developing embryo, fetus, infant, child, or adult resulting from an exposure to the male or female either before or after conception or during development. Developmental alterations include death (in utero or after birth), alterations in growth or body weight (or both), and either structural or functional abnormalities of the offspring (see Chapter 34). Given these definitions, it is clear that there are multiple adverse reproductive outcomes that could result from exposure to toxicants in the environment or work place. Unfortunately, the role of environmental and occupational factors in the etiology of most reproductive disease remains incompletely defined.

REPRODUCTIVE TOXICANTS

Information on the impact of many common drugs and chemicals on reproduction is lacking. When adequate human data are not available, the results of animal studies must be relied upon. Unfortunately, the quality and quantity of animal data vary considerably and information is often nonexistent or insufficient to evaluate potential human reproductive toxicity. A recent National Research Council report estimated that sufficient information exists on only 34% of pesticides and inerts, 22% of cosmetics, 45% of drugs, and 20% of food additives to permit critical evaluation of reproductive or developmental toxicity.[25] A recent survey by the Organization for Economic Cooperation and Development found that only 367 of 948 (39%) organic and 148 of 390 (38%) inorganic, high-production-volume chemicals had been satisfactorily evaluated for reproductive or developmental hazard.

To examine the information available to physicians and other health professionals, a survey of the 1993 *Physicians Desk Reference* (PDR) on reproductive effects of commonly prescribed medications was conducted. In this review, special attention was given to the sections of the PDR labeled *contraindications, warnings,* and *precautions.* If reproductive effects were not noted, it was assumed that data were not available. If only one gender was noted, it was assumed that only that gender was used for determining an effect (Table 33-7). It is important to note that these 50 prescription drugs account for about one third of all prescription medications used in the United States during 1992. Studies had been conducted to define reproductive toxicity in only 31 of these 50 medications and most (20 of 31) were not

Table 33-2. Individual and couple dependent factors that influence reproductive success

Reproductive endpoint factor	Impact on Endpoint
Male Fecundity	
Mumps	Decrease sperm production
Fever	Decrease sperm production
Varicocele	Decrease sperm production
Diabetes	Decrease libido, increase impotence
Hypertension	Decrease libido, increase impotence
Prescription drugs	Decrease libido, impair spermatogenesis, increase impotence
Smoking	Decrease libido, impair spermatogenesis, alter impotence
Alcohol	Decrease testicular function, alter libido and impotence
Substances of abuse	Impair testicular function, alter libido and impotence
Female Fecundity	
Contraception	Decrease fecundity and fertility
Tubal ligation	Decrease fecundity and fertility
Infection	Decrease fecundity, impair tubal function
Prescription drugs	Impair ovulation, fecundity, and libido
Smoking	Impair fecundity, alter libido
Alcohol	Impair fecundity, alter libido
Substances of abuse	Impair fecundity, alter libido
Age	Decrease fecundity
Couple-specific factors	
Infections	Decrease fecundity and fertility
Prescription drugs	Decrease fecundity and fertility
Alcohol	Decrease fecundity and fertility
Substances of abuse	Decrease fecundity and fertility
Early pregnancy loss	
Maternal age	Increase abortion
Smoking	Increase abortion, decrease fecundity and libido
Alcohol	Increase abortion, decrease fecundity and libido
Substances of abuse	May have effect; difficult to separate from lifestyle factors
Infection	Increase abortion and ectopic pregnancy
History	Increase abortion

identified as reproductive toxicants. Reproductive effects were noted: four altered female fecundity, six altered male fecundity—but in two reports, the gender was not noted.

MALE REPRODUCTIVE TOXICITY

Historically, most attention to the role of occupational and environmental exposures has focused on adverse

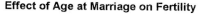

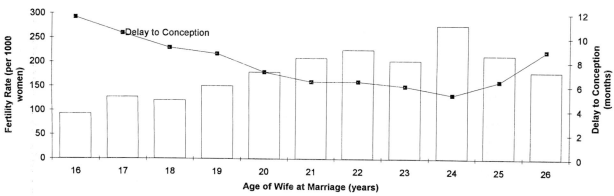

Fig. 33-2. Effect of age at marriage on fertility rate and time to conception. (Adapted from Belsey MA: *Infertility: prevalence, etiology and natural history.* In Bracken, MB, editor: *Perinatal epidemiology,* New York, 1984, Oxford University Press, pp 255-282.)

Table 33-3. Distribution of reproductive status among married couples

Fertility Status	Age of Wife		
	15-24(%)	25-34 (%)	35-44
Surgically Sterile			
Contraceptive	4	19	28
Noncontraceptive	0.4	7	19
Impaired fertility	11	16	19
Fertile	85	59	34

Adapted from Mosher WD, Pratt WF: *Fecundity and infertility in the United States,* 1965–1982 NCHS advance data 104, publication PHS 85-1250, 1985, pp 1-8.

Table 33-4. Percent of married women who are infertile (excluding surgical sterilization)

Age	1965	1976	1982
15-19	0.6	2	2
20-24	4	7	11
25-29	7	11	9
30-34	14	16	14
35-39	18	23	24
40-44	28	31	27

Adapted from Mosher WD, Pratt WF: Fecundity and infertility in the United States, 1965–1982 NCHS advance data 104, PHS 85-1250, 1985, pp 1-8.

reproductive outcome in the male and adverse developmental outcome in the female. This may, in part, result from the ready access to biological markers of male reproductive function. For example, semen can be readily obtained and provides material for biochemical and morphological analysis. As a result, it has generally been possible to evaluate the impact of environmental or occupational exposures on male reproductive function. The prototypical example of a compound that stimulated this interest is dibromochloropropane (DBCP). In the mid-1970s, workers who were exposed to DBCP became concerned about infertility. Clinical evaluation revealed a very high rate of infertility, which was subsequently shown to result from exposure to DBCP. This chemical is also instructive in another regard, that is, the use of toxicologic data gathered in animals to protect human health. It was tested for reproductive toxicity in the early 1960s and shown to produce testicular toxicity in all species tested.[38] For reasons that are unclear, this information was not used to protect workers exposed to DBCP, and an evaluation of the effect of DBCP on humans was not carried out. This delay in recognition of the potential

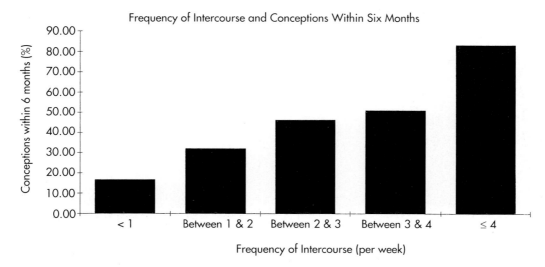

Fig. 33-3. Effect of frequency of intercourse and resulting conception within a 6-month period.

Table 33-5. Effect of frequency of intercourse on cycle-specific fertility rate

Frequency of intercourse	Cycle-specific fertility
Daily	0.68
Every other	0.43
Every third	0.31
Every fourth	0.24
Every fifth	0.20
Every sixth	0.17
Every seventh	0.14

Adapted from Barrett JC, Marshall J: The risk of conception on different days of the menstrual cycle, *Popul Studies* 23:455, 1969.

vulnerability of the human male reproductive system demonstrates the importance of animal studies in assessing toxicity. This section briefly summarizes the sites of vulnerability in the male reproductive system.

Four specific aspects of male fecundity are vulnerable to interruption: neuroendocrine function, testicular function, the function of accessory structures, and reproductive behavior. In the male, neuroendocrine interactions link the hypothalamus and pituitary with the testis. The testis is a site of production of steroid hormones, including androgens and the peptide hormone inhibin. The accessory structures (epididymis, vas deferens, prostate, and seminal vesicles) provide routes for egress of sperm and products that support ejaculation and fertilization.

The hypothalamus and pituitary interact with other organs by means of hormonal and neuronal signals, integrating data influencing reproduction. In the normal sexually mature male, the hypothalamus synthesizes and releases gonadotropin stimulating hormone (GnRH) into the hypothalamic-hypophyseal portal system, which flows to the pituitary. The pituitary responds to the pulsatile stimu-

Table 33-6. Causes of infertility in couples evaluated in infertility clinics

Etiology	Range reported (%)
Male	20-50
Azospermia	5-15
Oligospermia	15-40
Female	25-85
Tubal	5-85
Ovulation	5-50
Cervix/uterus	5-50
Multiple causes	10-25
Unexplained	0-20

Adapted from data in Belsey MA: Infertility: prevalence, etiology and natural history. In *Bracken MB, editor:* Perinatal *epidemiology,* New York, 1984, Oxford University Press, pp 255-282; Mosher WD, Pratt WF: Reproductive impairment among married couples: United States vital and health statistics, National Survey of Family Growth Series 23 #11, PHS 83-1987, 1982; Mosher WD, Pratt WF: Fecundity and infertility in the United States, 1965–1982, NCHS advance data 104, PHS 85-1250, pp 1-8, 1985; PHS 85-1250; Speroff Glass RH, Kase NG: *Clinical gynecologic endocrinology and infertility,* Baltimore, MD, 1983. Williams & Wilkins.

lus of GnRH with the release of luteinizing hormone (LH) and follicle stimulating hormone (FSH). The LH targets the Leydig cells within the testis to stimulate the synthesis and release of testosterone, which acts at many different sites throughout the body, including the hypothalamus and pituitary, where it provides negative feedback. The FSH acts on both the Sertoli cell and the seminiferous tubules. A polypeptide product of the Sertoli cells, inhibin, acts to enhance spermatogonia maturation and exerts feedback control on the pituitary. Toxic damage to the seminiferous tubules can increase inhibin blood concentrations and, as a result, reduce FSH production.

Under the influence of testosterone and FSH, Sertoli

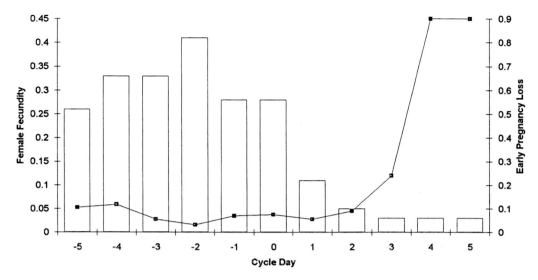

Fig. 33-4. Female fecundity and early pregnancy loss in relation to time of intercourse during the mid-menstrual cycle.

cells act to initiate spermatogenesis within the seminiferous tubules, a process that requires over 70 days from spermatogonia to spermatid. In experimental animals, the careful delineation of these stages has allowed definition of the specific stages that are vulnerable to a toxicant. Maturation continues, even after the spermatid leaves the testis and enters the epididymis, where it acquires mobility and undergoes a morphologic and functional transformation, resulting in fertilization capability.

Based on animal studies and human data (including epidemiologic and clinical studies), a number of compounds have been identified as hazards for male reproduction. They include metals, pesticides, organic solvents, pharmaceuticals, and physical agents (Table 33-8). Obviously, the actual impact on human male reproductive function requires exposure to sufficient quantities of the chemical at the appropriate time during reproduction.

EXAMPLES OF HUMAN MALE REPRODUCTIVE TOXINS
Dibromochloropropane

Epidemiological studies conducted in occupational settings have now conclusively established the toxic effects of 1,2-dibromo-3-chloropropane (DBCP) on spermatogenesis in seemingly otherwise healthy workers in the pesticide industry. Prior to the recognition of its toxicity, this chemical was widely used as a fumigant for soil nematodes because it had little toxicity for the root systems of plants.

In the initial studies, some, but not all, workers exposed to DBCP in a chemical factory for periods of 3 or more years had sperm counts of less than 1×10^6/ml associated with elevated concentrations of blood FSH and

LH.[41] Workers with relatively short exposures (less than 3 months) were not affected. Among men who had been exposed but were not azospermic, sperm motility was often reduced, and abnormal sperm forms were increased in number. Unfortunately, in this study and those discussed next, well-documented data on ambient air concentrations of DCBP are not available. Nonetheless, the initial observations have been confirmed in studies of workers in several different factories (Table 33-9). Systematic attempts have been made to document the long-term toxic effects.[8,9] Among those most severely affected, the outcome has been variable (Table 33-10), but evidence of permanent damage to the seminiferous tubules proved to be common. The mechanism of the toxic effects of DBCP on spermatogenesis appears to involve the metabolic generation of an epoxide, which produces testicular damage. It is of interest that affected male workers have not experienced systemic disease, and females apparently have not developed fertility problems. In addition, teratogenic effects have not been recognized among the offspring of exposed men and women.

Ethylene dibromide

Ethylene dibromide (EDB; dibromoethane) is a highly reactive alkylating agent that is widely used as a fumigant of soil, grains, fruit, and timber. It is also employed in the petroleum refining industry as a scavenger. The possibility of effects of EDB on human spermatogenesis was suggested by its chemical similarity to DBCP and the results of studies in animals. In this work, EDB was found to alter spermatid morphology in bulls and rams and reduced spermatogenesis in rats.[3] However, the dosages used in these experimental studies and the toxicity exhibited by

Table 33-7. Reported reproductive and developmental effects of commonly used drugs

Drug	Use or indication	Gender preference for indication	Reproductive effects noted
Premarin (Wyeth-Ayerst)	Estrogen replacement	Female	Yes, gender not defined
Amoxil (SmithKline Beecham)	Antibiotic, broad spectrum	None	No data noted
Zantac (Glaxo)	Histamine H2 receptor antagonist used to treat duodenal ulcer disease	None	Yes, male
Lanoxin (Burroughs Wellcome)	Cardiac glycoside, cardiac disease	None	Studies not conducted
Synthroid (Boots)	Synthetic levothyroxin, thyroid hormone replacement	None	Studies not conducted
Xanax (Upjohn)	Benzodiazepine, antianxiety agent	None	No data noted
Procardia XL (Pfizer)	Calcium channel blocker, antianginal	None	Reduced fertility, gender not noted
Vasotec (Merck Sharp & Dohme)	Angiotensin converting enzyme inhibitor, antihypertensive	None	No data noted
Ceclor (Lilly)	Antibiotic	None	Studies conducted, no effects noted
Seldane (Marion Merrell Dow)	Histamine H1 Receptor antagonist	None	Studies conducted, no effects noted
Naprosyn (Syntex)	Nonsteroidal antiinflammatory	None	Studies conducted, no effects noted
Calan SR (Searle)	Calcium channel blocker, angina, hypertension	None	Female fertility studied, no effect
Capoten (Squibb)	Angiotensin converting enzyme inhibitor, antihypertensive	None	No data noted
Mevacor (Merck Sharp & Dohme)	Cholesterol lowering agent,	None	Yes, male, no data noted for female
Augmentin (SmithKline Beecham)	Antibiotic, infections	None	Studies conducted, no effects noted
Tagamet (SmithKline Beecham)	Histamine H2 receptor antagonist, ulcer	None	Studies conducted, no effects noted, male impotence at high dose
Prozac (Dista)	Serotonin uptake inhibitor, depression	None	Studies conducted, no effects noted
Proventil Aerosol (Schering)	Beta adrenergic bronchodilator, asthma	None	Studies conducted, no effects noted
Trimox (Apothecon)	Antibiotic, infection	None	No data found
Dyazide (SmithKline Beecham)	Diuretic, hypertension		No studies conducted
Provera (Upjohn)	Progestin, hormone treatment	Female	Yes, male and female
Lopressor (Geigy)	Beta-adrenergic blocking agent, hypertension	None	Studies conducted, no effects noted
Ortho-Novum 7/7/7-28 (Ortho)	Oral contraceptive	Female	Yes, male and female
Micronase (Upjohn)	Sulfonurea, diabetes	None	Studies conducted, no effects noted
Tenormin (ICI Pharma)	Beta-adrenergic blocking agent, hypertension	None	Studies conducted, no effects noted
Ventolin Aerosol (Allen & Hanburys)	Beta-adrenergic, bronchodilator	None	Studies conducted, no effects noted
Dilantin (Parke-Davis)	Antiepileptic, seizure disorders	None	No data noted
Cipro (Miles)	Antibiotic, infections	None	Studies conducted, no effects noted

Continued.

Table 33-7. Reported reproductive and developmental effects of commonly used drugs—cont'd.

Drug	Use or indication	Gender preference for indication	Reproductive effects noted
Coumadin Sodium (Du Pont)	Anticoagulant, clotting disorders	None	Studies not conducted
Cardizem (Marion Merrell Dow)	Calcium channel blocker, angina	None	Studies conducted, no effects noted
Humulin (Lilly)	Human insulin, diabetes	None	No data noted
Lasix Oral (Hoechst-Roussel)	Diuretic, hypertension	None	Studies conducted, no effects noted
Ibuprofen (Boots)	Nonsteroidal antiinflammatory	None	No data noted
Lopid (Parke-Davis)	Lipid regulating agent	None	Yes, male and female
Voltaren (Geigy)	Nonsteroidal anti-inflammatory	None	Studies conducted, no effects noted
DiaBeta (Hoechst-Roussel)	Sulfonurea, diabetes	None	Studies conducted, no effects noted
Amoxicillin Trihydrate (Warner Chilcott)	Antibiotic	None	No data noted
Glucotrol (Roenig)	Sulfonurea, diabetes	None	Studies conducted, no effects noted
Zestril (Stuart)	Angiotensin converting enzyme inhibitor, hypertension	None	Studies conducted, no effects noted
Amoxicillin Trihydrate (Biocraft)	Antibiotic	None	No data noted
Triphasil-28 (Wyeth-Ayerst)	Oral contraceptive	Female	Yes, female
Darvocet-N 100 (Lilly)	Narcotic analgesic	None	No data noted
Pepcid Merck Sharp & Dohme	Histamine H2 receptor antagonist, ulcer	None	Studies conducted, no effects noted
Theo-Dur (Key)	Bronchodilator	None	No data noted
Cardizem SR (Marion Merrell Dow)	Calcium channel blocker, angina	None	No data noted
Polymox (Apothecon)	Antibiotic	None	No data noted
Acetaminophen/Codeine (Puropac)	Analgesic, narcotic analgesic	None	No data noted
Tylenol/Codeine (McNeil)	Analgesic, narcotic analgesic	None	No data noted
Hismanal (Janssen)	Histamine H1 receptor antagonist, antiallergy	None	Studies conducted, no effects noted
Triamterine and hydrochlorothiazide (Rugby)	Diuretics	None	No data noted

the rodents precluded a predictive assessment of the chemical's potential effects of humans. Possible answers to this question were provided by a study of workers in a Hawaii fruit-processing plant who were chronically exposed to EDB.[28] Among these men, a significant decrease in sperm count per ejaculate and an increase in abnormal spermatids was found (Table 33-11). The number of men with oligospermia also increased. As with so many studies of this type, the effects of EDB on reproductive outcome were not assessed. Although poor semen quality impairs fertility, pregnancies do occur when sperm counts are reduced and a relatively high proportion of morphologically abnormal spermatids are found.

Additional halogenated compounds

A number of different halogenated hydrocarbons having estrogenic properties contaminate the environment as a result of indiscriminate or uninformed use in the past (see Chapters 8 and 26). These lipotropic chemicals tend to accumulate in human adipose tossie and persist indefinitely in tissues because of their extended half-lives. Accordingly, concern has focused on the effects of these compounds on reproduction, in part, supported by the experimental observations summarized in Table 33-12. Studies thus far have failed to demonstrate effects on the human reproductive system.

Scattered, poorly documented reports allege effects of

Table 33-8. Examples of factors and toxicants that may impair male and female fecundity

Male fecundity		Female fecundity	
Factors	**Toxicants**	**Factors**	**Toxicants**
Vasectomy	DBCP	Contraception	DDT and metabolites
Mumps	EDB	Tubal ligation	Carbaryl
Fever	Lead	Infection	Kepone
Varicocele	Carbon disulfide	Prescription drugs	Lead
Diabetes	Kepone	Smoking	PAH
Hypertension	Boron	Alcohol	Ionizing radiation
Prescription drugs	Carbaryl	Age	DES
Smoking	Cadmium	Abused substances	2-Ethoxy acetic
Alcohol	Methylmercury		Anesthetic gases
Abused substances	Ionizing radiation		Aniline
	DES		Benzene
	Chloroprene		Carbon disulfide
	Ethylene oxide		Chloroprene
	Glycol ethers		Glycol ethers
	Hexane		Formaldehyde
	Vinyl chloride		Methylmercury
			Pesticides
			Phthalic acid ester
			PCBs
			Styrene
			Toluene
			Vinyl chloride

DBCP, Dibromochloropropane; *DDT*, dichlorodiphenyltrichloroethane; *DES*, diethylstilbestrol; *EDB*, ethylene dibromide; *PAH*, p-aminohippuric acid; *PCBs*, polychlorinated biphenyls.

the polychlorinated biphenyls on fertility and the development of the conceptus.[14,15,32,37] These reports are difficult to assess from the limited amount of published information available.

Ethylene glycol ethers

Glycol ethers are widely used in the chemical industry and have numerous commercial applications. At high levels of environmental exposure, the various chemicals in this family of compounds manifest systemic toxic effects in humans. In animal experimentation, testicular toxicity has been found, however, little information exists on the effects of glycol ethers on human reproduction. In a study of painters chronically exposed to varying concentrations of 2-ethoxyethanol and 2-methoxyethanol, an increase in the number of men with azospermia and oligospermia was found. The mean sperm counts (per ml of semen) and the total counts (per ejaculate) were reduced, but the decreases for the group as a whole were not found to be statistically significant when compared to controls.[40] This elaborate, carefully conducted study requires confirmation before conclusions can be drawn.

Lead

Information linking lead exposure to reproductive failure in the male is limited. In the past, various lead-containing compounds found applications as spermatocides.

Table 33-9. Dibromochloropropane effects on spermatogenesis as assessed by sperm counts of manufacturers

	Exposed*	Not exposed
Azospermia	13	3
Oligospermia (<20 × 10⁶/ml)	17	0
Normospermia	70	97
Median (× 10⁶/ml)	46	79

*Quantitative information documenting exposure is not available.
Adapted from Milby TH, Whorton D: Epidemiological assessment of occupationally related, chemically induced sperm count suppression, *J Occup Med* 22:77, 1980.

However, only a few studies have been carried out in men with lead blood concentrations now considered to be toxic.[16] Cullen and colleagues[7] evaluated seven symptomatic young men with long-term occupational or avocational lead exposures who had blood lead concentrations greater than 60 μg/dl. The evidence accumulated in detailed clinical and pathologic investigations strongly suggested an effect both on the hypothalamic-pituitary axis and on the testes. Measures of thyroid function and glucocorticoid production demonstrated depressed tropic hormone activity. Sperm counts were evaluated in six of the men. Two exhibited oligospermia, and two had azospermia. Biopsies

Table 33-10. Long-term outcome of exposure to dibromochloropropane

Case no	Sperm Cessation of exposure	Concentration (10⁶/ml) 12-24 months	5-17 years	Motility (%) 4-7 years	Follicle-stimulating hormone, (ImU/ml) Cessation of exposure	4-7 years
1	0	25	74	49	28	—
2	0	0	0.04	33	13	—
3	0	30	12	—	—	—
4	24	9	45	30	10	19
Normal	≥20			≥40	1.5-13ImU/ml	

Adapted from Eaton M, et al: Seven year follow-up of workers exposed to 1,2-dibromo-e-chloropropane, *J Occup Med* 28:1145, 1986.

Table 33-11. Ethylene dibromide effects on spermatogenesis as assessed by sperm counts on fruit processors

	Exposed	Not Exposed
Azospermia and Oligospermia	22	5
Sperm counts (mean)	81	140
Abnormal forms (% mean)		
Macrocephalic heads	1.4	1.7
Tapered heads	4.2	2.5
Absent heads	2.1	1.4
Abnormal tails	6.5	5.7

Adapted from Ratcliffe JM, et al: Semen quality in papaya workers with long-term exposure to ethylene dibromide, *Br J Ind Med* 44:317, 1987.

Table 33-12. Summary of experimental effects of halogenated hydrocarbons in male rats and mice

	Dosage	Route	Effect
Dibromochloropropane	>3 ppm	Inhalation, subcutaneous	Seminiferous tubule atrophy
Hexachlorocyclohexane	>25 ppm	Diet	Seminiferous tubule atrophy
Chloroprene (Kepone)	≥50 ppm	Diet	Testicular atrophy
Polychlorinated biphenyls (PCBs)	about 50-100 ppm	Diet	Decreased spermatogenic infertility

Adapted from Zenick H: *Mechanisms of environmental agents by class associated with adverse male reproductive outcomes.* In: *Reproduction: the new frontiers in occupational and environmental health research,* New York, 1984, Alan R Liss, pp 335-361.

of the testicle of the latter two men demonstrated prominent pathologic alteration in the seminiferous tubules, with a significant reduction in spermatogenesis (Figs. 33-5 and 33-6).

FEMALE REPRODUCTIVE TOXICITY

Although considerable attention has focused on the female with respect to developmental toxicology, less has been directed to the vulnerability of the female reproductive system. In part, this is because assessment of most biological markers of female reproductive performance requires invasive measures. One of the unique features of the female reproductive system is the continuous change in hormonal and structural characteristics during the menstrual cycle. Thus, in evaluating female fecundity, it is necessary to conduct assessments throughout the cycle (a more stringent requirement than is needed for the male reproductive system).

Normal female fecundity requires a functionally intact neuroendocrine system, ovary, uterus, and normal sexual behavior. The neuroendocrine system is centered in the hypothalamus and pituitary. The functional unit of the ovary is the follicle, consisting of oocyte and the investing layers of granulosa and thecal cells. After release from the ovary, the oocyte is transported through the fallopian tube (where fertilization usually occurs) into the uterus (where it normally implants). Anatomic abnormalities of these structures are common causes of reproductive failure.

Periodic release of GnRH by the hypothalamus into the portal system exerts control over the female reproductive system. It is necessary, but not sufficient, for normal function and stimulates the release of FSH and LH from the pituitary into the bloodstream. The FSH acts on the ovary to support the growth of follicles. In the absence of

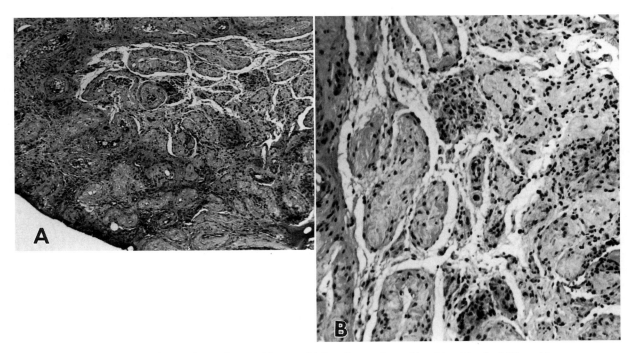

Fig. 33-5. Testicular biopsy from a 42-year-old foundry worker with a blood lead of 55 mg/dl. He was azospermic and had elevated blood concentrations of follicle stimulating hormone and lutinizing hormone. The testosterone levels were at the lower margin of the normal range. (Courtesy of Mark Cullen. Case reported in Cullen MR, Kayne RD, Robins JM: Endocrine and reproductive dysfunction in men associated with occupational inorganic lead intoxication, *Arch Environ Health* 39:431, 1984.)

FSH, follicles mature and then undergo apoptosis. Under the continued influence of FSH, follicle growth continues and estrogen production increases until the negative feedback mechanisms reverse, stimulating the release of LH from the pituitary. Sustained high levels of LH result in the disruption of the ovulatory follicle with the release of the oocyte and the subsequent development of the corpus luteum.

This brief overview of reproductive physiology emphasizes the complexities inherent in conducting definitive epidemiological and clinical studies of reproductive toxicology in women. Indeed, a critical analysis of the contemporary literature yields little conclusive information regarding the effects of environmental agents on reproductive efficiency. Summarized next and in Table 33-8 is information on a select few environmental toxicants that have been associated with female reproductive failure.

EXAMPLES OF HUMAN FEMALE REPRODUCTIVE TOXINS
Cigarette smoking

The adverse influences of smoking on female reproduction and fetal development have long been recognized.[18,19,30] Smoking accelerates the onset of menopause and may be associated with the osteoporosis that so frequently follows. An analysis of the impact of ciga-

rette smoking is invariably complex because smoking appears to have a diversity of effects on the reproductive system. Moreover, epidemiological studies are difficult to conduct because the exposures to mainstream and side stream smoke are so variable among members of the general population. Cigarette smoke, nicotine, or both have demonstrable effects in the experimental animal. Nicotine delays the prolactin response in the nursing mother and blunts the proestrus surge of luteinizing hormone and prolactin in a dose-dependent fashion. Exposure of rats to cigarette smoke frequently inhibits ovulation. A direct action on the development of the corpus luteum has also been demonstrated in experimental animals.[18]

In humans, female fertility is clearly affected by smoking (Fig. 33-7).[36] Smokers experience a higher frequency of secondary amenorrhea and abnormal vaginal bleeding.[11] Endocrinologic studies[17] have demonstrated decreases in urinary excretion of estrogen during the luteal phase of the menstrual cycle in female smokers. Cycle-specific fertility has been evaluated by at least two groups of workers.[1,2,13] In the study of Howe and colleagues,[13] 59% of nonsmoking women had delivered by 12 months after termination of contraception, whereas only 49% of those who smoked more than one pack each day were pregnant.

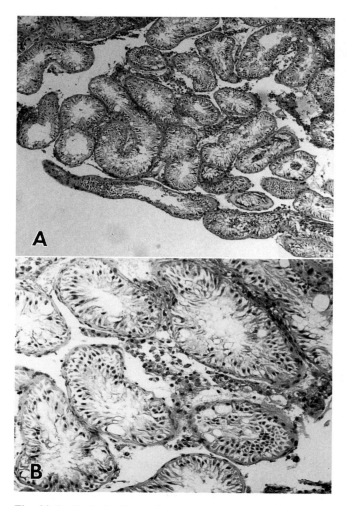

Fig. 33-6. Testicular biopsy from a battery worker with a history of blood lead concentrations ranging from 60 to 80 mg/dl and complaints of arthralgia and intermittent abdominal pain. The biopsy was obtained 16 months after exposure ceased. At the time he was azospermic and had an increased blood follicle stimulating hormone level, but a normal blood testosterone level. (Courtesy of Mark Cullen. Case reported in Cullen MR, Kayne RD, Robins JM: Endocrine and reproductive dysfunction in men associated with occupational inorganic lead intoxication *Arch Environ Health* 39:431, 1984.)

Studies undertaken to explore the effects of smoking on the timing of menopause have consistently shown that menopause occurs 1 to 4 years earlier in smokers than in nonsmokers (Fig. 33-8). The effects appear to be dosage-dependent. The mechanisms involved in this phenomenon are unknown. In experimental animals, polycyclic aromatic hydrocarbons have been found to destroy oocytes in a dosage-dependent manner, but the effects are variably influenced by the age, strain, and species of animal. In addition, the amounts of the agent required to induce a response may have little relevance to the human experience. Thus, the results of these animal experiments are difficult to interpret.

Nitrous oxide

During the administration of anesthesia, anesthetists can be exposed to concentrations of nitrous oxide (N_2O) ranging from 100 to 400 ppm with documented peak levels several times higher. This agent is widely used in human and veterinary surgery and in both obstetric and dental anesthesia. The equipment, as well as the operative procedure and duration, obviously has profound effects on exposure, but personnel often experience exposures repeatedly and usually on a daily basis. In recent years, the use of waste gas scavengers has significantly reduced exposure to operating room personnel.

Retrospective studies have documented increased rates of spontaneous abortion among women working in this setting. An increase in the incidence of congenital abnormalities in offspring of nurse anesthetists has also been claimed. Because of the inevitable variables and confounding factors, as well as the difficulties inherent in identifying appropriate control groups for retrospective studies, however, this work has been subject to question.

Recently, Rowland and colleagues[31] reported the results of a study of the reproductive histories of 7000 female dental assistants who were regularly exposed to N_2O. Women exposed to high concentrations (i.e., unscavengered N_2O) for 5 or more hours per week were found to be significantly less fertile than those who experienced substantially lesser amounts of exposure. Indeed, each hour of N_2O exposure resulted in a 6% reduction in the likelihood of conception during each menstrual cycle. Only 11% of the women exposed repeatedly to unscavengered N_2O became pregnant during the first cycle of unprotected intercourse, whereas 27% of unexposed women conceived. Over 40% of the heavily exposed women required more than 1 year to become pregnant. Unfortunately, this study failed to assess whether women were rendered infertile as a result of their work with N_2O.

Inorganic and organic lead

An adverse effect of lead upon pregnancy outcome has long been recognized. Lead has a direct effect on the ovary and can cause follicular atresia in rodents and in nonhuman primates.[27,29,39] In the past, it was employed as an abortifacient. The risk of premature termination of pregnancy has been found to increase substantially in women with elevated (above 14 µg/dl) blood lead concentrations. Lead absorption from the digestive tract is increased during pregnancy, and with calcium deprivation it is mobilized from bone. Lead crosses the placenta, resulting in fetal tissue concentrations equivalent to those of the mother. As discussed in Chapters 4 and 30, lead toxicity is often manifested as neurobehavioral and developmental abnormalities in infants and children.

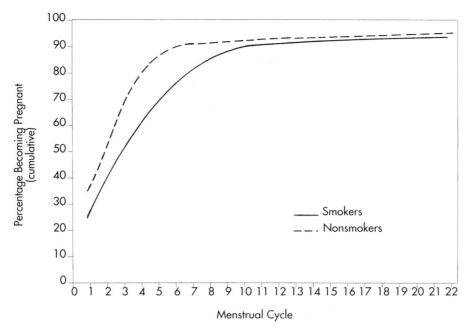

Fig. 33-7. Effect of smoking on the time of conception. (Adapted from Tokuhata GM: Smoking in relation to infertility and fetal loss, *Arch Environ Health* 17:353, 1968.)

CONCLUDING REMARKS

Few areas of environmental and occupational health science are more resistant to critical inquiry than the study of reproductive toxicology. The complexities of human reproduction and the difficulties in scientifically evaluating it are compounded by variability in exposures to specific toxic substances with a background of confounding factors.

Outcome measures are also confounded by the difficulties inherent in assessing the fecundity of both the male and female and their union as a pair. In addition, the teratogenic effects of various toxic substances (resulting in early, unrecognized spontaneous abortions) require definition. When attempting to characterize the potential hazard of a drug or chemical exposure, it is necessary to evaluate a hierarchy of information. In only a few cases are sufficient human data available to accomplish this task. More often, it is necessary to rely on the outcome of animal investigations. These studies appear to identify correctly many human reproductive toxicants, but they also have brought to our attention many additional chemicals that do not appear to be toxic for human reproduction. After a chemical has been identified as a potential hazard, it is necessary to characterize the dose-response relationship, as well as the site and mechanism of action. These steps are required in order to appropriately extrapolate animal data to humans for estimating qualitatively and quantitatively the risk to reproduction. The next step is to characterize the exposure. What

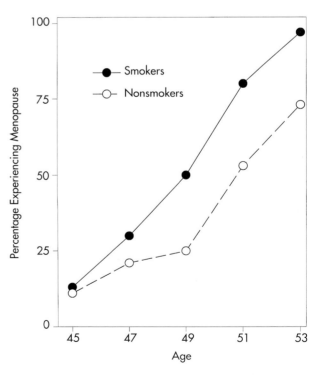

Fig. 33-8. Effect of smoking on the time of onset of menopause. (Adapted from Tokuhata GM: Smoking in relation to infertility and fetal loss, *Arch Environ Health* 17:353, 1968.)

concentration, duration, and relationship of the exposure to the critical milestones of reproduction exist? Most chemical reproductive toxicants have "biologic windows" in which they produce their adverse effects. Exposure outside these windows is associated with a substantially reduced risk to the reproductive process.

REFERENCES

 1. Baird DD, Wilcox AJ: Cigarette smoking associated with conception delay, *JAMA* 253:2679, 1985.
 2. Baird DD, Wilcox AJ: Future fertility after prenatal exposure to cigarette smoke, *Fertil Steril* 46:368, 1986.
 3. Barlow SM, Sullivan FM: *Reproductive hazards of industrial chemicals: an evaluation of animal and human data,* London, 1982, Academic Press.
 4. Barrett JC: Fecundability and coital frequency, *Popul Studies* 25:309, 1971.
 5. Barrett JC, Marshall J: The risk of conception on different days of the menstrual cycle, *Popul Studies* 23:455, 1969.
 6. Belsey MA: *Infertility: prevalence, etiology and natural history.* In Bracken MB, editor: *Perinatal epidemiology,* New York, 1984, Oxford University Press, pp 255-282.
 7. Cullen MR, Kayne RD, Robins JM: Endocrine and reproductive dysfunction in men associated with occupational inorganic lead intoxication, *Arch Environ Health* 39:431, 1984.
 8. Eaton M, et al: Seven year follow-up of workers exposed to 1,2-dibromo-3-chloropropane, *J Occup Med* 28:1145, 1986.
 9. Goldsmith JR, Potashnik G, Israeli R: Reproductive outcomes in families of DBCP-exposed men, *Arch Environ Health* 39:85, 1984.
10. Gurrero VR, Rojas OI: Spontaneous abortion and aging of human ova and spermatozoa, *N Engl J Med* 293:573, 1975.
11. Hammond EC: Smoking in relation to physical complaints, *Arch Environ Health* 3:28, 1961.
12. Hemminki K, Sorsa M, Vainio H, editors: *Occupational hazards and reproduction,* Washington, DC, 1985, Hemisphere.
13. Howe G, et al: Effects of age, cigarette smoking and other factors on fertility: findings in a large prospective study, *Br Med J* 290:1697, 1985.
14. Jacobson JL, Jacobson SW, Humphrey HEB. Effects of *in utero* exposure to polychlorinated-biphenyls and related contaminants on cognitive-functioning in young children. *J Pediatr* 116:38, 1990.
15. Jacobson SW, et al: The effect of intrauterine PCB exposure on visual recognition memory, *Child Dev* 56:856, 1985.
16. Lancranjan I, et al: Reproductive ability of workmen occupationally exposed to lead, *Arch Environ Health* 30:396, 1975.
17. MacMahon B, et al: Cigarette smoking and urinary estrogens, *N Engl J Med* 307:1062, 1982.
18. Mattison DR: The effects of smoking on reproduction from gametogenesis to implantation, *Environ Res* 28:410, 1982.
19. Mattison DR, et al: The effect of smoking on oogenesis, fertilization, and implantation, *Semin Reprod Endocrinol* 7:291, 1989.
20. Meistrich ML, Brown CC: Estimation of the increased risk of human infertility from alterations in semen characteristics, *Fertil Steril* 40:220, 1983.
21. Menker J, Trussell, J, Larsen U. (1987) Age and infertility, *Science* 233:1389,1987.
22. Milby TH, Whorton D: Epidemiological assessment of occupationally related, chemically induced sperm count suppression, *J Occup Med* 22:77, 1980.
23. Mosher WD, Pratt WF: Reproductive impairment among married couples: United States vital and health statistics, National Survey of Family Growth Series 23 #11 1982 (PHS 83-1987), 1982.
24. Mosher WD, Pratt WF: Fecundity and infertility in the United States, 1965–1982 NCHS advance data 104 (PHS 85-1250), 1985.
25. National Research Council: Biomarkers in reproductive and developmental toxicology; *Environ Health Perspect* 74:1, 1987.
26. Paul M, editor: *Occupational and environmental reproductive hazards: a guide for clinicians,* Baltimore, 1993, Williams & Wilkins.
27. Petrusz P, et al: Lead poisoning and reproduction: effects on pituitary and serum gonadotropins in neonatal rats, *Environ Res* 19:383, 1979.
28. Ratcliffe JM, et al: Semen quality in papaya workers with long-term exposure to ethylene dibromide, *Br J Ind Med* 44:317, 1987.
29. Rom WN: Effects of lead on the female and reproduction: a review, *Mt Sinai J Med* 43:542, 1976.
30. Rosenberg MJ, et al: Sperm as an indicator of reproductive risk among petroleum refinery workers, *Br J Ind Med* 42:123, 1985.
31. Rowland AS, et al. Reduced fertility among women employed as dental assistants exposed to high levels of nitrous oxide, *N Engl J Med* 327:993, 1992.
32. Saxena MC, et al: Role of chlorinated hydrocarbon pesticides in abortions and premature labor, *Toxicology* 17:323, 1980.
33. Schwartz D, Magauz MJ: Female fecundity as a function of age: results of artificial insemination in 2193 nulliparous women with azospermic husbands, *N Engl J Med* 306:404, 1982.
34. Simpson JL: In editors: *Obstetrics: normal and problem pregnancies,* Gabbe SG, Niebyl JR, Simpson JL, New York, 1986, Churchill Livingstone, p 1148.
35. Speroff L, Glass RH, Kase NG: *Clinical gynecologic endocrinology and infertility,* Baltimore, 1983, Williams & Wilkins.
36. Tokuhata GM: Smoking in relation to infertility and fetal loss, *Arch Environ Health* 17:353, 1968.
37. Tomczak S, Baumann K, Lehnert G: Occupational exposure to hexachlorocyclohexane: IV, sex hormone alterations in HCH-exposed workers, *Int Arch Occup Environ Health* 48:283, 1981.
38. Torkelson TR, Toxicologic investigations of 1,2-dibromo-3-chloropropane, *Toxicol Appl Pharmacol* 3:545, 1961.
39. Vermande-VanEck GJ, Meigs JW: Changes in the overy of the Rhesus monkey after chronic lead intoxication, *Fertil Steril* 11:223, 1960.
40. Welch LS, et al: Effects of exposure to ethylene glycol ethers in shipyard painters: II, male reproduction, *Am J Med* 14:509, 1988.
41. Whorton MD, et al: Infertility in male pesticide workers, *Lancet* 2, 1259, 1977.
42. Whorton, M.D., et al: Testicular functions among carbaryl-exposed employees, *J Toxicol Environ Health* 5:929, 1979.
43. Wyrobek AJ, et al: Sperm studies in anesthesiologists, *Anesthesiology* 55:527, 1981.
44. Wyrobek AJ, et al: Sperm shape abnormalities in carbaryl-exposed employees, *Environ Health Perspect* 40:255,1986.
45. Wyrobek, AJ, et al: An evaluation of human sperm as indicators of chemically induced alterations of spermatogenic function, *Mutat Res* 115:73, 1983.
46. Zenick H: Mechanisms of environmental agents by class associated with adverse male reproductive outcomes. In: Reproduction: the new frontiers in occupational and environmental health research, New York, 1984, Alan R Liss, pp 335-361.

Chapter 34

TERATOLOGY

Anthony R. Scialli

MANIFESTATIONS OF DEVELOPMENTAL TOXICITY

During the 1960s, the imagination of the general public was captured by thalidomide. To this day, images of babies with limb reduction defects represent for many people the potential adverse effects of medication exposure during pregnancy. Added to normal parental concerns about the physical development of their offspring is a fear that toxicants in the environment and at work are prevalent and that exposure of pregnant women to these agents imposes a substantial risk of abnormal embryonic development.

The fears of prospective parents and their physicians may exceed the actual risk involved in most occupational and environmental exposures. Although the magnitude of risk associated with an exposure is an important consideration, it is necessary also to consider the range of responses of the conceptus to toxicants. As discussed in this chapter, not all malformations are due to developmental toxicants, and not all developmental toxicity is manifested as malformation. There are, in fact, four categories of adverse developmental outcome considered under the rubric of developmental toxicity: malformation, growth impairment, death, and functional impairment.

Malformation

The incidence of structural abnormalities in human offspring is usually cited at between 3% and 8%, although some estimates are higher. The range represents differences in incidence based on what kind of malformations are considered and when in the life of the individual malformations are sought. For example, at birth, 2% or 3% of infants are diagnosed with a major malformation. Minor malformations occur in about 1.5% of newborns; these defects are variably included when overall malformation rates are cited. Thus, about 5% of infants at birth have an anomaly diagnosed.[16] Another 6% of children have anomalies ascertained over the first year of life. There is evidence that follow-up of children to age 10 can identify a cumulative congenital anomaly rate as high as 15%.[24] Malformation rates are higher among conceptuses that do not survive to birth: spontaneous abortuses have a malformation rate of

Table 34-1. Rates for specific abnormalities, 1974-1988*

Malformation	Rate (per 10,000 infants)
Anencephaly	0.8-18.4
Spina bifida	1.8-17.5
Encephalocele	0.3-3.2
Hydrocephaly	2.1-8.5
Microtia	0.1-6.4
Transposition of the great vessels	0-5.4
Hypoplastic left heart syndrome	0-3.4
Cleft palate	2.6-10.1
Cleft lip	5.2-16.3
Esophageal atresia	0.4-3.6
Anorectal atresia	1.4-5.5
Renal agenesis/dysgenesis	0.2-4.1
Hypospadias	2.3-29.7
Epispadias	0-0.7
Bladder exstrophy	0-0.8
Limb reduction defects	3.1-8.0
Diaphragmatic hernia	0.3-4.4
Abdominal wall defects	1.9-6.8
Omphalocele	0.8-3.9
Gastroschisis	0.4-2.3
Conjoined twins	0-0.3
Down syndrome	5.2-15.3

Compiled by the author from data presented in International Clearinghouse for Birth Defects Monitoring Systems: *Congenital malformations worldwide,* Amsterdam, 1991, Elsevier.

*Rates give the range of the lowest to highest geographical regions (mean rates for the reporting interval).

Table 34-2. Causes of birth defects

Type of cause	Percentage of total
Unknown	65
Genetic (e.g., single gene defects)	20
Chromosomal	5
Maternal illness, including alcoholism	4
Infection	3
Mechanical	2
Toxicants	1

Adapted from Brent RL, Beckman DA: Principles of teratology. In Evans MI, editor, *Reproductive risks and prenatal diagnosis,* Norwalk, CT, 1992, Appleton & Lange.

20%.[72] The excess of malformations among pregnancy losses is not surprising given the adverse effects of many structural derangements on viability of the conceptus.

Rates of specific malformations vary with geographical location and with time. Table 34-1 shows the rates of selected malformations reported from the International Clearinghouse for Birth Defects Monitoring Systems. Surveillance systems such as this can be used to evaluate possible associations of malformations with exposures or other factors.[57] It is apparent from Table 34-1 that specific malformations are relatively common in some areas and unusual in others. For example, spina bifida was reported from New Zealand at a rate of 17.5 per 10,000 infants but at a rate only one tenth as high from Finland. For defects that are detectable by antenatal diagnosis, such as spina bifida, reported rates reflect not only the rate of occurrence, but also the reporting region's use of screening technologies and pregnancy interruption for abnormal fetuses. Note, however that there is prominent geographical variability for abnormalities for which effective screening does not exist; for example, the nearly tenfold difference in rates for esophageal atresia reflects the relative rarity of the defect in Sichuan, People's Republic of China, compared with a high rate in Italy.

Most malformations are not believed to be caused by exposure to toxicants. Pharmaceutical agents, for which exposure information is often most accessible, are believed to play a role in only about 1% of congenital anomalies.[4,17] Exposure to other xenobiotic chemicals, such as those encountered in the workplace and industry, probably account for relatively few additional malformations. Table 34-2 details the distribution of causes of birth defects by type. Although authors may disagree by a few percent for some of these categories, the observation that most birth defects do not have a specific identifiable cause is well accepted. It is possible that some of these malformations represent ignorance about developmentally toxic exposures that have yet to be described; however, a convincing case can be made that the unknown category includes multifactorial interactions of genetic predisposition and environmental influence as well as spontaneous errors of development.[6] In fact, when studying embryology, it is a wonder that it ever goes right, let alone that it sometimes goes wrong.

Growth impairment

Infants with congenital anomalies tend to be smaller than average, regardless of the cause of the anomaly. About 25% of fetuses with severe early-onset intrauterine growth retardation are chromosomally abnormal.[85] Toxicants that have been associated with fetal growth impairment are listed in the box on the next page. Decreased fetal growth may be a consequence of alterations in uterine perfusion or of placental toxicity; however, the association of growth impairment with birth defects is also consistent with abnormal cell death in the conceptus, one of the major postulated mechanisms of developmental toxicity. This mechanism is discussed more fully later.

Of special note is the fetal growth deficit associated with ethanol, a cause of structural malformations and mental impairment as well as of growth impairment. The small stature and head circumference of offspring affected by ethanol developmental toxicity appears to persist into adolescence and adulthood, associated with persistent impairment of intellect and behavior.[77,98] The smallness of infants with

Examples of toxicants associated with impairment of fetal growth

Drugs of abuse

Cigarette smoking
Ethanol
Heroin

Pharmaceutical agents

Glucocorticoids
Propranolol
Phenytoin
Warfarin

Infectious agents

Herpes simplex
Cytomegalovirus
Rubella
Toxoplasmosis

fetal alcohol syndrome is, then, a harbinger of continued smallness and neurological impairment yet to come (see Chapter 14).

Death

Death of the conceptus before 20 weeks is defined as spontaneous abortion (miscarriage); thereafter, fetal death is called stillbirth. Spontaneous abortion is a common event, the incidence of which depends on the sensitivity of the test used to diagnose pregnancy. Because most spontaneous abortions occur early, with low maternal serum levels of human chorionic gonadotropin (hCG), many pregnancy losses are not recognized as such and are considered to be menstrual periods. If a sensitive hCG assay is used on serial urine samples collected by noncontracepting women, about 30% of pregnancies are found to abort.[86] Fewer than half of the abortions occur in clinically recognized pregnancies. Of the clinical pregnancies that abort, at least half are karyotypically abnormal.[3] These aneuploid conceptuses are considered to represent meiotic errors in germ cells or mitotic errors shortly after fertilization.

There are few data on toxicants as a cause of early human pregnancy loss; however, experience in experimental animals suggests that embryo death is a common manifestation of xenobiotic toxicity. In addition to direct destruction of the embryo as a mechanism of embryolethality, alterations in the uterine environment from hormonally active agents might interfere with normal implantation and produce early embryo loss.[15]

Stillbirth occurs in about 8 per 1000 pregnancies. About half of these deaths are classified as asphyxial or associated with maternal illnesses such as hypertension, and a quarter of stillbirths have no identifiable cause.[38] Birth de-

fects are found in about 20% of stillborn fetuses. Infection is responsible for perhaps 5% of stillbirths and is the only cause of late fetal death that can be reliably associated with environmental exposures. Parvovirus B19, for example, can be occupationally acquired by health or child care workers. This infection is a cause of fetal anemia, hydrops, and death.[22]

Functional impairment

Congenital organ-system dysfunction is difficult to assess: the presentation may not occur for years after birth, and postnatal causes may be possible contributors. Cerebral palsy, for example, is a congenital motor disorder that initially presents during childhood. Although there is a perception among lay people and even among some physicians that cerebral palsy is due to birth injury, in fact, it is not.[37,48] In most instances in which the timing of the neurological damage can be determined, the disease is found to have its origins in the antepartum period. Some postnatal insults, however, can give rise to cerebral palsy–like motor disorders. For example, excessively high neonatal serum concentrations of bilirubin can result in damage to the basal ganglia as part of a syndrome called kernicterus.

Developmental toxicants can also produce functional disorders in anatomically normal children. One example is Minamata disease, an instance of methylmercury poisoning reported first in Japan in 1952 and again in 1964. The abnormalities in affected children included ataxia; mental retardation; and disturbances of gait, vision, and speech. The disease was named for Minimata Bay, an area of the island of Kyūshū. The 1952 epidemic was associated with organic mercurials discharged by a chemical plant into the Minimata River. The chemicals entered the food chain and were ultimately consumed in fish caught from the bay. The 1964 poisonings occurred in the Niigata prefecture on the main island of Honshū, and were associated with effluent from another factory at that site.[45] Another episode of human methylmercury exposure occurred in Turkey in 1971. Treated grain that was intended for planting was mistakenly diverted to the making of bread and thousands of people, including pregnant women, were poisoned (see Chapter 4).

The brain abnormality in Minimata disease is characterized by abnormal neuronal migration and orientation. Thus, on a histological level, affected individuals can be said to have a structural abnormality. The fact remains, however, that this and other disorders of function may be observed in children who do not appear malformed by physical examination. There has been considerable discussion as a result about what kind of disorders are subsumed under the heading "birth defect." This is largely a semantic issue: it matters little in human and economic cost whether a disability is based primarily on a gross structural defect, a histologically identifiable abnormality, or a biochemical disorder.

MECHANISMS OF TOXICITY

There is a perception that embryos and fetuses are uniquely at risk for injury from environmental and occupational exposures; however, conceptal tissue is subject to the same mechanisms of toxicity as other tissues.

Cell death

Perhaps the most widely seen response to toxicant exposure is cell death. Because of the importance of cell populations in developmental events, cell death may have widespread ramifications in the embryo or fetus. Cells not only provide the architectural framework for the conceptus, but also interact with other cells, both through anatomic cell-cell connections and through the production of biochemical mediators. For example, neuronal migration in parts of the brain involves cells following paths established by previously migrated neurons or glial cells. If excessive death occurs among cells responsible for laying down migratory guideposts, subsequent migration among living cells might be impaired.

A model of cell death as a mediator of developmental toxicity is provided by x-irradiation. In experimental animals, irradiation during pregnancy results in decreased fetal size, brain weight, and thickness of the cerebral cortex as well as abnormalities in neurological function.[30,51] The animal experiments are consistent with the developmental toxicity of ionizing radiation noted after the atomic bombings of Japan at the end of World War II. Adverse effects consisted predominantly of microcephaly and mental retardation, and fetuses were most susceptible during the late first and early second trimesters, at the time of maximal neuronal proliferation in the fetal brain (see Chapter 11).[54]

The belief that cell death is responsible for a substantial proportion of the adverse effects seen after toxicant exposure led to the popularization of the "all-or-none" principle. This concept predicts that exposure of the conceptus from fertilization up to about a week after implantation is likely to result in either pregnancy loss or in survival of a normal embryo, with survival of a malformed embryo less likely. The all-or-none principle is based on the observation that cells in the early embryo lack commitment to the formation of specific tissues and maintain a degree of totipotency. Thus, if toxicant exposure of a blastocyst around the time of implantation destroys a small population of cells, neighboring cells can proliferate to fill in the gap. If, however, a large number of cells are killed, there will be insufficient surviving cells to reconstitute the embryo, and the pregnancy will be lost. Experimental support exists for this idea. For example, exposure of preimplantation mouse embryos to methylmethanesulfonate, a DNA strand breaker, results in loss of embryos or birth of normally formed, although small, pups.[21]

Later in development, as cells become committed to specific developmental pathways, death of key populations is more likely to leave irreparable damage in a living embryo

or fetus. For example, hydroxyurea is an inhibitor of DNA synthesis but can also produce rapid cell death through the production of free radicals in tissue. When pregnant rabbits are treated with hydroxyurea, cell death is detectable within hours in the limb bud mesenchyme of the fetus, and pups surviving to term bear several kinds of birth defects, including limb reduction defects. Administration of free radical scavengers with hydroxyurea results in a decrease in histological evidence of cell death in the limb bud and a decrease in the incidence of limb reduction defects at term (see Chapter 21).[19]

It should be noted that some cell death within the developing embryo is a normal event. Tissue modeling requires the disappearance of certain cells according to a predetermined schedule. Limb outgrowth, for example, is limited by zones of programmed cell death in the apical ectodermal ridge, a collection of specialized cells at the distal margin of the limb bud. Failure of cell death to occur when appropriate may produce abnormalities; for example, aspirin induces polydactyly in rats in association with alterations in programmed cell death in the limb bud.[36,69]

Genotoxicity

Because genetic material determines so much of the structure and function of organisms, it is sometimes assumed that congenital abnormalities are usually due to genetic abnormalities. In Table 34-2, however, genetic and chromosomal abnormalities are considered to explain perhaps one quarter of birth defects. When toxicant-induced defects are considered, the proportion owing to genetic damage is believed to be even smaller, as discussed subsequently.

Genes are segments of DNA coding ultimately for protein products. If the DNA sequence is altered, as in sickle cell anemia, the protein product may be altered and the function of the organism impaired. This view of genetic abnormality is overly simple: turning a segment of DNA into protein is a complex process involving DNA-associated histones that must be removed from the DNA section to be transcribed, RNA and regulatory proteins that interact with DNA, splicing molecules that modify the transcription product, and three-dimensional modifications of the polypeptide that results from RNA translation. There are many opportunities in this scheme for abnormalities to be introduced; geneticists have identified large numbers of spontaneously occurring or hereditary disorders that arise through different errors in these processes.

An important question is whether and how often exposures to chemical or physical agents can result in genetic damage that produces an abnormality in the offspring. One aspect of this question is whether genotoxicity owing to a chemical or physical agent can be specific enough to alter a single base pair, as in sickle cell anemia, and leave the rest of the genome intact. This degree of targeting appears unlikely; however, isolated base pair change is only one kind of genetic abnormality. Other genotoxicity may occur through destruction of genes, a much less targeted event. For example, when cancer is induced by a mutagenic agent, one possible mechanism is the disabling of repressor genes, permitting unrestricted clonal growth of a cell. The mutagenic agent need not hit the right target in every cell with which it comes in contact: transformation of a single cell may be sufficient to produce a malignancy.

By contrast, transformation of a single cell in a developing embryo would not be expected to have an impact on the development or function of the organism. If, for example, a single limb bud cell were to be genetically altered, the thousands of neighboring limb bud cells would be expected to compensate for the aberrant cell. The induction of cancer by a mutagenic agent is sometimes described as a stochastic event, from the Greek *stokastikos*, meaning skillful in aiming. Stochastic events are probablistic; that is, if a specified number of x-ray photons are directed at a tissue, there is a probability that one of them will alter the genome in exactly the way required for a malignancy to be produced. Nonstochastic toxicity depends on an effect being produced by the cumulative action of the toxicant. The cell death mechanism, discussed earlier, is an example of a nonstochastic mechanism of toxicity. If toxicant exposure produces sufficient cell death, an adverse outcome is manifested. If the amount of cell death is insufficient, there is repair and normal development. Such nonstochastic mechanisms show thresholds; that is, there are doses below which toxicity is not seen. Stochastic phenomena do not show thresholds because exposure to even a single photon or molecule is associated with a finite probability of the transforming event.

What is the experimental evidence regarding the role of genotoxicity in abnormal embryonic development? In fact, nearly all mutagenic agents can produce birth defects when given to pregnant animals, but this finding may be explained by the cytotoxicity of mutagens; in other words, cell death is readily produced by agents that damage the genome. Experimental teratologists have noted for decades that agents producing birth defects characteristically show a threshold dose below which no abnormalities are produced, suggesting a nonstochastic phenomenon. Classic work using x-irradiation in mice, for example, demonstrated the kind of all-or-nothing effect that would be expected from a cell death mechanism.[62]

There are, however, animal data that indicate a genotoxicity mechanism for some developmental toxicants. The production of heritable alterations in phenotype, for example, is a strong argument that the genome has been altered by an experimental exposure. Mutagen treatment of the germ cells of male or female mice has been shown to produce an increase in anomalies in the F_3 generation; that is, the grandchildren arising from the treated gametes show phenotypic alterations.[49] The experimental induction of dominant mutations in mammals, chiefly rodents, has

been an area of active research since the 1960s, and there are several examples of chemical agents as well as ionizing radiation that can produce this sort of genotoxicity (reviewed by Selby[70]). Adverse effects on pregnancy outcome can also be mediated by premating treatment of male rodents (reviewed by Olshan and Faustman[52]). In these experiments, the usual adverse outcome is early pregnancy loss; however, a small increase in the incidence of abnormal live pups has been noted. Such paternally mediated developmental toxicity is most likely to occur with treatment during spermatid development, after meiosis has been completed. During this phase, the germ cell chromatin undergoes special packaging, with replacement of DNA-associated histones by protamines. There is evidence that gamete damage with alkylating agents during this period is due to alkylation of the associated protamines rather than alkylation of DNA. Such damage to the protein constituents of chromatin might interfere with faithful replication or transcription of the genome. Because this sort of damage leaves the DNA code intact, it is sometimes called "epigenetic" rather than genetic. Treatment of male rodents with toxicants also can produce germ cell chromosome abnormalities associated with phenotypic abnormalities in viable offspring (see Chapter 20).[63]

Other evidence for genetic or epigenetic damage as a cause of developmental toxicity comes from experiments in which treatment during the so-called all-or-none period resulted in an increase in abnormal live fetuses near term. Among the first agents shown capable of producing such effects was ethylene oxide, an alkylating agent used as a sterilant. Treatment of female mice within hours of mating caused early pregnancy loss but also later fetal death and malformation.[23,64] The production of fetal effects with this treatment at the zygote stage is consistent with genetic or epigenetic damage that is perpetuated throughout generations of embryonic cells.

Evaluation of genotoxicity as a mechanism of adverse human pregnancy outcome has not resolved the question of how often genetic or epigenetic damage from toxicants is responsible for congenital anomalies. Birth defect syndromes can certainly be transmitted through generations; however, the production of such syndromes by xenobiotics has not been demonstrated. Much effort has been put into characterizing paternal exposures that are associated with adverse pregnancy outcome in the offspring; such an effect would be evidence of a genetic or epigenetic mechanism of developmental toxicity. The epidemiology literature (reviewed by Colie[13] and by Olshan and Faustman[53]) includes suggestive associations between paternal exposures (such as solvents) or occupations (such as automobile mechanics) and adverse outcome, particularly miscarriage and childhood cancers. These data, however, lack consistency and in instances of childhood cancer cannot exclude postnatal exposure to carcinogens.

Data from survivors of cancer therapy, including ionizing radiation and genotoxic drug treatment, have not shown an increase in congenital anomalies in subsequently conceived offspring.[20,27,28,44] This lack of association is in agreement with follow-up of atomic bomb survivors, in whom subsequently conceived pregnancies showed no increase in adverse pregnancy outcome attributable to genetic damage.[66] The lack of an effect in these populations may be due to the inability to detect a small but significant increase in an isolated abnormality because such an increase may not significantly increase the overall birth defect rate. In addition, subjects in these studies conceived at varying times after the genotoxic exposure. It is conceivable that with time, germ cell injury may have been repaired or affected germ cells eliminated in some individuals, thus obscuring an effect.

Impaired cell function

If cell death can disrupt embryogenesis by depriving the conceptus of important cellular participants in future developmental events, it follows that sublethal interference with cell function could have similar results. For example, an agent that inhibits protein synthesis might prevent a cell from synthesizing important mediators of development, even without killing the cell. Important enzymes, such as dihydrofolate reductase, thymidilate synthetase, and DNA polymerase, may be inhibited by xenobiotics that interfere with cell division at doses lower than those lethal to the cell. Such xenobiotics have been associated with birth defects in animals and in some instances in humans. Carbonic anhydrase, which is important in the regulation of blood pH, is inhibited by acetazolamide, a cause of limb reduction defects in rodents. 6-Aminonicotinamide, a niacin antagonist, increases palatal clefting and limb defects in experimental animals.

It should also be remembered that nonmalforming developmental toxicity may occur by mechanisms similar to those responsible for toxicity in children and adults. For example, women receiving drugs with anticholinergic activity may give birth to nenonates with meconium ileus. Withdrawal syndromes are seen in newborns whose mothers have used opioid drugs late in pregnancy, and renal impairment, intestinal injury, and premature ductal closure are sometimes encountered in fetuses exposed to the prostaglandin synthetase inhibitor indomethacin.[50]

Hormones and hormonally active agents are particularly relevant in this regard: androgenic agents, for example, can masculinize the external genitalia of female fetuses by inducing abnormal differentiation in tissues that normally respond to endogenous androgens in male fetuses. Although examples of such exposures in humans are confined to pharmacological agents, environmental and occupational exposures to estrogenic pesticides have raised concerns; some of these agents have been shown to alter genital development in rodents (see Chapter 8).[79]

Maternal toxicity

In mammals, the pregnant organism meets the nutrient, respiratory, and osmoregulatory and thermoregulatory needs of the conceptus. It is not surprising, then, that illness in the mother may have adverse effects on the embryo or fetus. Severe or prolonged maternal hypotension, for example, can result in reductions in uterine perfusion that are damaging to an otherwise normal conceptus.

It is not always a simple matter to determine if adverse developmental effects are due entirely or in part to maternal toxicity. Animal studies characteristically test agents at doses up to those producing some maternal toxicity, to be sure that the doses used have a biological effect in the species under investigation. If developmental toxicity appears only at a maternally toxic dose and not at lower doses, the question arises whether the mother and conceptus are demonstrating sensitivity to the same dose or whether the adverse effects in the conceptus are merely due to impairments in maternal physiology.

Diflunisal, for example, produces skeletal abnormalities in the offspring of treated rabbits. This agent also produces hemolytic anemia in the pregnant does, and the fetal abnormalities have been shown to be due to the maternal anemia rather than to a direct effect of the drug on the fetal skeleton.[11]

Some teratologists believe that there are characteristic malformations in experimental animals that suggest maternal toxicity (Table 34-3).[34,35] These abnormalities may be defects to which a given species or strain is genetically prone, with maternal illness providing the insult necessary to cross a developmental threshold, producing the adverse effects in the offspring. Other teratologists have not been able to confirm a pattern of abnormalities associated with maternal toxicity in experimental animals; in fact, only extra ribs in the mouse have been found reliably to be a common associate of maternal illness.[33]

It is clear, however, that maternal conditions such as malnutrition, electrolyte disturbance, or hypercapnea may be associated in experimental animals with adverse effects on the offspring, either by themselves or as potentiators of the toxicity of xenobiotics (reviewed by Chernoff et al[10]). There is little information on how often xenobiotic-induced maternal illness is a mediator of human developmental toxicity.

Placental toxicity

Besides providing an interface for maternal-fetal gas and nutrient exchange, the placenta is metabolically active, producing a number of hormones (see box on next page). In addition to these substances, a number of placental peptides have been identified, the functions of which have not been completely characterized. Thus, toxicants that interfere with placental function may produce adverse effects by impairing oxygenation or nutrition of the conceptus or by altering placental biosynthetic and secretory function.

Table 34-3. Fetal abnormalities associated with maternal toxicity in animal teratology studies

Species	Abnormalities
Mouse	Exencephaly
	Open eye
	Hemivertebrae
	Fused vertebral arches or centra
	Fused, missing, or extra ribs
	Fused or scrambled sternebrae
Rat/rabbit	Fused, retarded, missing, or split vertebrae
	Fused, extra, missing, or wavy ribs
	Missing, fused, or nonaligned sternebrae
	Exophthalmia, anophthalmia, or micophthalmia
	Cleft palate
	Umbilical hernia
	Ectrodactyly or syndactyly
	Bent or shortened long bones
	Crooked, short, or absent tail
Hamster	Fused ribs
	Exencephaly
	Encephalocele
	Microphthalmia or anophthalmia
	Omphalocele
	Shortened or crooked tail
	Cleft lip
	Ectrodactyly or syndactyly

From Scialli AR: *A clinical guide to reproductive and developmental toxicology*, Boca Raton, Fla, 1992, copyright CRC Press. Adapted from Khera 1984, 1985.[34,35]

In humans, placental dysfunction may be seen in hypertensive disorders in which vascular disease compromises transfer of nutrients. The resultant adverse effect is growth restriction of the fetus. An analogous toxic effect occurs with cigarette smoking, in which vascular effects of nicotine or gas-exchange effects of carbon monoxide or a combination of factors result in a reduction in fetal growth.

Cadmium, which is concentrated in the placentae of smokers,[59] has been shown to produce substantial developmental toxicity in rats via a placental mechanism. When administered to pregnant dams after embryogenesis is complete, cadmium results in fetal death and premature birth. This toxicity occurs despite very small amounts of cadmium reaching the fetus[74]; in fact, direct injection of the fetus produces less toxicity than treatment of the mother.[40] Cadmium toxicity in this model appears to be mediated by metal-associated reductions in uteroplacental blood flow and nutrient transport.[18,40] There is no direct evidence that cadmium toxicity is an important factor in the human developmental toxicity of cigarette smoke; however, the possibility remains that metal damage to the placenta is a contributing factor to this toxicity.

CONCEPTUS SELECTIVITY

Although developmental toxicity can occur through mechanisms that affect tissues in general, the toxicants that

Placental hormones

Chorionic gonadotropin
Placental lactogen
Chorionic adrenocorticotropin
Chorionic thyrotropin
Parathyroid hormone–related protein
Gonadotropin-releasing hormone
Corticotropin-releasing hormone
Thyrotropin-releasing hormone
Growth hormone–releasing hormone
Neuropeptide Y
Inhibin
Activin
Progesterone
Estrogens (chiefly estriol and estradiol)

selectively target the conceptus are of greatest concern. To understand this concern, it is helpful to use the historical perspective of one of the best-known episodes in teratology.

Thalidomide

The modern era of birth defect research dates from the work of Hale in the 1930s. This investigator worked in animal husbandry and was interested in factors that affect the reproductive success of commercially important animals. The experiment for which he is best known involved the feeding of vitamin A–deficient diets to pregnant sows, resulting in the birth of piglets with anophthalmia.[25]

It had been known since the eighteenth century that avian embryo development could be disrupted by environmental manipulations, chiefly incubation at nonphysiological temperatures. Mammalian development, however, was considered to be privileged because of maternal homeostatic mechanisms. In addition, the placenta was believed to be an effective screen that protected the conceptus from noxious agents and ensured the transport of necessary nutrients and gases.

The question asked by Hale was how the placenta would transport a necessary nutrient, in this case vitamin A, if the nutrient were withheld from the mother. The finding that nutrient deprivation could be associated with congenital anomalies was an important turning point in thinking about the protected status of mammalian reproduction. The Hale study prompted other investigators to explore the potential developmental effects of other nutrient deficiencies.[84]

It is not easy, however, to create diets selectively deficient in specific nutrients. For example, if the effects of a deficiency of the amino acid serine were to be evaluated, a serine-free diet probably would also be deficient in other amino acids and in protein in general. One approach to this problem was to synthesize analogues of nutrients, compounds that would enter metabolic pathways in competition with the targeted nutrient. Azaserine, for example, can be used to simulate a serine-deficient diet and has been shown to cause birth defects in the offspring of treated rats.[46]

Among the most clinically successful of the nutrient analogues were the folic acid antagonists, aminopterin and methotrexate, which were used in cancer therapy and the latter of which is used currently in the treatment of arthritis and psoriasis as well as some malignancies. Folic acid is a required factor for thymidilate synthetase, which catalyzes a rate-limiting step in DNA synthesis. Aminopterin, the older of the two folic acid antagonists, was known in 1950 to interfere with normal pregnancy, as might be expected from inhibition of DNA synthesis.[82] Because of this property, aminopterin was used as an abortifacient in unwanted pregnancies in humans, a practice that led to the birth of malformed infants among those that failed to abort.[43,81,83]

In 1957, thalidomide was marketed as a sedative/hypnotic in Europe, and over the next 4 years it became one of the most widely prescribed drugs for this indication in many parts of the world. In late 1959 and 1960, German and Australian clinicians became aware of an epidemic of phocomelia, an unusual kind of limb reduction defect. By the end of 1961, thalidomide had been removed from commerce in England and Germany. The phocomelia epidemic ended 9 months later.

The unique feature of the thalidomide episode was the safety of the drug for adults. Part of the commercial success of this agent was due to this lack of toxicity, even when taken in overdosage. Yet normal sedative use of the agent, even for short periods of time, had dramatic toxic effects on the embryo. Other agents that had been shown to damage the embryo, such as aminopterin, also produced considerable toxicity in the adult. Thus, thalidomide became the first widely known example of an agent with *selective* toxicity for the conceptus.

The importance of selective toxicity is in the estimation of risk attendant on human exposure. It is not farfetched, for example, to be concerned about the developmental effects of lead because lead has known hematological, neurological, and other organ-system toxicity in experimental animals and humans. The embryotoxicity of the anticonvulsant valproic acid was not suspected for many years, partly because the drug does not have prominent general toxicity (see Chapter 4).

A/D ratio

It is considered axiomatic that any compound produces toxicity in an organism if a sufficient dose is administered; therefore, agents are not categorized as toxic and nontoxic or as teratogenic and nonteratogenic. Rather the concept of selective conceptus toxicity has led to efforts to compare doses of a compound at which developmental toxicity occurs with doses at which more generalized toxicity occurs. Such a comparison can be expressed as the so-called A/D ratio, a ratio between the dose at which *A*dult toxicity oc-

curs and the dose at which *D*evelopmental toxicity occurs. If an agent has a high A/D ratio, the dose at which developmental toxicity occurs is much lower than the dose at which adult toxicity occurs, and the agent is considered a potential hazard. If the A/D ratio is near 1, the conceptus and the adult show similar susceptibility to the toxic effects of the agent.

One attraction of the A/D ratio is the ability to evaluate the relative sensitivity of developing and adult tissues in nonhuman animals and even, perhaps, in in vitro systems. There has been interest, for example, in the use of an artificial embryo made by dissociating cells of the coelenterate *Hydra* and permitting them to reassociate. The differentiation of cells in the artificial embryo into tentacles can be monitored as a developmental event, and different concentrations of a test compound can be used to try to inhibit the event. The developmentally toxic concentration can be compared to the concentration necessary to produce toxicity in mature *Hydra*. The resulting A/D ratio has been found by the assay's developers to be reasonably predictive of A/D ratios obtained with the same compounds in rodent studies.[31]

The utility of the A/D ratio as a predictor of human developmental hazard has not gained universal acceptance. Not all investigators have found A/D ratios in one species to be predictive of those in other species. This is likely due in part to differences in maternal handling of the administered compound, which determines how much if any of the active toxicant reaches the conceptus. Mice, for example, are not sensitive to the developmental toxicity of 13-*cis*-retinoic acid (isotretinoin, the acne medication marketed as Accutane) because they biotransform it only slowly to all-*trans*-retinoic acid, which is the proximate toxicant. In addition, use of the A/D ratio to identify hazards can work only with agents to which human exposure produces no adult toxicity. Many agents that are developmentally toxic in humans are encountered at adult toxic doses. An example is ethanol, which gives rise to reproducible developmental effects at doses that are also toxic to women with chronic ethanol ingestion. Thus, the A/D ratio for ethanol is about 1, and a fetus would not be protected by a decision to not worry about ethanol based on this ratio.

In standard developmental toxicity studies, the potential relationship between adult and conceptus toxicity is used in the choice of doses when the experiments are designed. It is assumed that if an agent is developmentally toxic, such toxicity will be manifested at doses similar to those producing maternal toxicity. In other words, compounds are not considered to have A/D ratios much less than 1. By selecting test doses to include one at which maternal toxicity (usually a small impairment of weight gain) occurs, it is believed that developmental toxicity would be uncovered. Maternal toxicity then is used as a biological indicator that an adequate dose has been selected to produce an effect in that species. If there is no developmental toxicity present despite exposure that produces maternal toxicity, it is assumed that the potential for adverse effects in the conceptus is negligible. Note that the converse does not follow: if a compound produces toxicity in the conceptus at maternally toxic doses, it is not clear that the compound is directly toxic to the embryo or fetus because maternal toxicity may have been a mediator of the adverse effect. In such instances, the kind and degree of toxicity in mother and conceptus may be relevant. For example, if an exposure produces decreased food intake and weight loss in the dam, and the developmental toxicity consists of a modest decrease in fetal weight, a relationship between developmental and maternal toxicity is plausible.

PRINCIPLES OF TERATOGENICITY

With the preceding discussion as background, we can review general principles of developmental toxicology that were popularized in 1977 by Wilson.[88] Although the production of birth defects is only one of the manifestations of developmental toxicity, Wilson's principles, which were developed from classic animal teratology experiments, can be applied to all manifestations. Five of the six principles were first articulated in 1959, even before thalidomide toxicity was recognized[87]; it is interesting that these principles have required little modification in the intervening decades.

Genetic-environment interaction

Susceptibility to teratogenesis depends on the genotype of the conceptus and the manner in which this interacts with environmental factors.

As a general rule, the sensitivity of individuals to toxicants varies, and at least part of this variability is genetically determined. Thus, a dose of medication that is therapeutic in one person may produce unacceptable side effects in another. The sensitivity of conceptuses also differs from one individual to another. Within a population of pregnant animals given the same dose of test agent, some litters have many affected members, and other litters are normal. Even within litters, there are pups showing different responses to the same toxicant.

There has been considerable interest in whether toxicant response is most influenced by the genotype of the mother or of the conceptus, but it appears that both mother and conceptus may play a role in determining toxicity, depending on the agent. An example of these dual determinants is in the intrauterine response of mice to polycyclic aromatic hydrocarbons (PAHs). PAHs are ubiquitous environmental pollutants found, for example, in cigarette smoke. PAH toxicity is in large measure produced by biotransformation products of the hydrocarbons; therefore, organisms with substantial biotransformation capabilities experience more toxicity. Biotransformation enzymes can be induced by exposure to PAHs, and the degree of inducibility is determined at a genetic locus called the "Ah locus." Thus, Ah

reactive mice experience more PAH toxicity than nonreactive mice. The presence of the kinds of inducible enzymes that can biotransform PAHs has been demonstrated in early murine embryos.[22] By mating mice of different zygosity for the Ah locus, experiments can be performed in which Ah-reactive or Ah-nonreactive dams bear pups of mixed Ah status.[73] Such studies show that when an Ah-nonreactive dam is treated with PAHs, only the Ah-reactive pups in her litter manifest toxicity. If, however, an Ah-reactive dam is treated, all pups show toxicity, suggesting that the mother's ability to biotransform PAHs into more toxic compounds is sufficient to damage all her young, regardless of their individual status (see Chapters 5 and 26).

In humans, a role for the conceptus in determining toxicant susceptibility has been demonstrated with regard to phenytoin. This anticonvulsant appears to produce toxicity through a reactive intermediate that is the product of biotransformation by a ubiquitous microsomal enzyme system. All humans appear to produce this reactive intermediate, regardless of genotype. Detoxification of the intermediate, however, proceeds at different rates depending on the genetic endowment of an enzyme called epoxide hydrolase. The genotype of the conceptus is an important determinant of phenytoin toxicity: offspring with low epoxide hydrolase activity appear to be at substantially greater risk of suffering adverse phenytoin developmental effects than are offspring with high detoxification activity.[8]

Stage dependency

Susceptibility to teratogenic agents varies with the developmental stage at the time of exposure.

It makes sense that to produce limb defects in an embryo, a toxicant needs to be applied at the time of limb development. This sample of conventional wisdom appears too simple to warrant much discussion; however, considerable bad advice has been given as a result of misinterpretation of this principle. Because most organ systems assume a recognizable form in the first trimester of human pregnancy, the assumption is made that this is the stage at which susceptibility to birth defects is greatest. As a result, some clinicians have counseled avoidance of all exposures during the first trimester and avoidance of none thereafter.

In fact, it should be recognized that important developmental events occur throughout gestation as well as during early childhood and that exposure to a toxicant after the first trimester may have serious consequences. Minamata disease, discussed earlier, is produced with late-pregnancy exposures to methylmercury. Ionizing radiation is more effective at producing mental retardation at 16 weeks than at 6 weeks. Warfarin, although it produces an embryopathy with first-trimester usage.also can cause central nervous system damage with later trimester usage.[26,55] Angiotensin converting enzyme inhibitors can cause oligohydramnios, fetal skull defects, and death; they appear to produce developmental toxicity only when administered *after* the first

---

Mechanisms of developmental toxicity

Mutation
Chromosomal damage
Mitotic interference
Altered nucleic acid integrity/function
Lack of normal precursors
Altered energy sources
Changes in membrane characteristics
Osmolar imbalance
Enzyme inhibition

From Wilson JG: *Current status of teratology.* In Wilson JG, Fraser FC, editors: *Handbook of teratology,* New York, 1977, Plenum Press.

trimester,[5] as do agents that cause premature constriction of the ductus arterious, fetal growth impairment, and preterm labor.

The stage dependency of toxicity then is not meant to imply that some stages are susceptible and others are not, only that toxicity at each stage may result in different kinds of damage and that some agents may be more damaging at one period than another.

Mechanisms

Teratogenic agents act in specific ways (mechanisms) on developing cells and tissues to initiate abnormal embryogenesis (pathogenesis).

It has been observed that different agents can produce similar kinds of abnormalities. The facial features of the fetal alcohol and fetal hydantoin syndromes, for example, are similar. One explanation for similar abnormalities arising from different agents is the presence of final common pathways of abnormal embryogenesis. When Wilson wrote this principle, he envisioned nine diverse mechanisms of developmental toxicity (see box above). Each of these mechanisms was presumed capable of producing one of five abnormal pathogenetic states. These states included excessive (or reduced) cell death, failed cell interactions, reduced biosynthesis of cell products, impeded cell movement, or mechanical disruption of tissues. According to Wilson, the five pathogenetic states could result in one of two general final common pathways: a deficiency of cells or cell products or abnormal tissue growth or differentiation.

As an example, ionizing radiation exposure at adequate doses and at sensitive times in gestation damages nucleic acids (the second and fourth mechanisms in the box above), thereby producing excessive cell death in the brain (the first of the pathogenetic states), leading to a deficiency of neurons (the first of the final common pathways) in the cortex. If a different agent produced the same degree of excessive cell death in the same population of cells, even through a different mechanism, it would not be surprising if the resulting impairment were similar to radiation-induced microcephaly and mental retardation.

Manifestations of abnormal development

The final manifestations of abnormal development are death, malformation, growth retardation, and functional disorder.

The four manifestations of developmental toxicity were discussed in detail at the beginning of this chapter. Wilson, in his formulation of this principle, indicated that these four manifestations may not be entirely independent of one another. For example, a toxicant might produce death by inducing abnormalities of structure or function incompatible with survival. Structural and functional changes might induce one another, much as the defects of tetralogy of Fallot arise from the abnormal hemodynamic consequences of pulmonic stenosis.

The four endpoints of developmental toxicity are not discrete; there is a continuum of response for many toxicants. The continuum may extend over a dose range, so a small dose of a toxicant may have no effect, whereas larger doses successively may produce growth impairment, malformation, and then death. The continuum may extend over time; that is, a dose of an agent during the preimplantation period may produce death, with the same dose during the embryonic and fetal period producing malformation and functional damage. Finally the continuum may extend over a population, with some members being sensitive to malforming effects and other members being sensitive to functional or growth effects of the same exposure.

Access of agents to the conceptus

The access of adverse environmental influences to developing tissues depends on the nature of the influences (agent).

Wilson developed this principle to distinguish between agents such as ionizing radiation that gain direct access to the conceptus and agents that are handled by the mother's body before getting to the offspring. Although such a difference appears self-evident, it is worth emphasizing here that maternal handling of xenobiotics appears to be one of the most important determinants of access to the conceptus of toxicants. Many otherwise toxic substances are biotransformed to nontoxic products by the mother and pose no developmental risk as a result. Other compounds may be bioactivated to more toxicant agents by the pregnant animal, as in the Ah-responsive mouse dam exposed to PAHs. Agents that are extensively protein bound by the pregnant adult may not reach the conceptus as a result. Other toxicants, such as ethanol, may attain ready equilibrium between mother and conceptus.

Toxicokinetics, the study of how xenobiotic agents are handled by the organism, has become an important aspect of developmental toxicology research.[47] Special attention has been given to the development of models, often computer simulated, by which toxicokinetic parameters are predicted. Modeling has been used, for example, to characterize the disposition of 2-methoxyethanol in pregnant mice.[12]

This compound is of particular interest because it is a commonly encountered occupational exposure and because developmental toxicity from 2-methoxyethanol appears to be due to one of its metabolites, 2-methoxyacetic acid. The development of a predictive model can be expected to assist in applying the results of animal testing to an estimation of human risk from an exposure.

Dose-response relationship

Manifestations of deviant development increase in degree as dosage increases from the no-effect level to the totally lethal level.

As discussed earlier, most developmental toxicologists believe that threshold exposures exist below which toxicity does not occur. This concept is important in counseling exposed individuals because an exposure should not be viewed as simply safe or unsafe. Rather an exposure can be thought of as entailing a risk of developmental toxicity that might range from 0 to 100% (although no agents in humans have produced a 100% risk of developmental toxicity). Although the agent is a central determinant of how much risk exists, the dose of the agent is also important. It is assumed that there is a dose of thalidomide, for example, at which developmental toxicity would not be seen.

The fact that developmental toxicologists believe in the concept of a threshold dose does not mean that the threshold is necessarily easy to identify. Ethanol is one agent for which threshold questions commonly arise. Consumption by a pregnant woman of more than 2 oz/day of absolute ethanol is associated with a 30% to 40% risk of fetal alcohol syndrome.[14,76-78] Consumption of 1 oz/day is less commonly associated with fetal alcohol syndrome but may produce modest growth impairment in the fetus.[42] It has not been possible to demonstrate an increase in adverse pregnancy outcome with lower doses of ethanol; however, the question arises whether ethanol is safe at lower doses or whether the abnormalities are so infrequent or subtle that they simply have escaped detection (see Chapter 14).

The probabilistic approach of the dose-response paradigm assumes that members of a population differ in sensitivity to a toxicant. At low doses, all members are resistant. As the dose is raised, an increasing proportion of the population becomes affected. In some instances, particularly susceptible subsets of a population may be identifiable. It is believed, for instance, that young children are more sensitive to the adverse cognitive effects of lead. The possible sensitivity of the fetus to lead neurotoxicity led to concerns that women who work with this metal might impose such toxicity on their intrauterine offspring at exposure levels much lower than those producing adult toxicity. These concerns resulted in discriminatory employment practices that were subsequently overturned by the Supreme Court in the Johnson Controls case (reviewed by Scialli[68]).

LACTATION

Breastfeeding is the most complete source of infant nutrition and can provide the total fluid and food needs of the baby for at least 6 months after birth. It is unfortunate that many health care providers discourage nursing in the face of exposures to xenobiotics without evidence that the exposure provides risk to the infant.

Milk formation

The unit of milk production is the saclike alveolus, a ball of cells within a network of maternal blood vessels. Much of the milk is derived from maternal plasma, the constituents of which are either processed by the alveolar cells or enter the milk space through aqueous pores between the cells. Milk is a complex mixture of water, proteins, fats, carbohydrates, and cells. The relative contribution of different milk constituents changes with gestational age at delivery, time of day, time during a feeding, and time since delivery. For example, preterm milk has relatively more protein than milk produced at term, a difference that may persist for 2 months.[9] Colostrum, produced for the first days after birth, is high in immunoglobulins. Over the next 2 weeks, a transitional milk higher in lipid and lactose is produced, leading to mature milk. Within a feeding the first milk, called foremilk, is lower in fat than the creamier hindmilk.

Most xenobiotics enter milk by diffusion from maternal plasma. Pharmaceutical agents are generally small molecules, and few of them have difficulty gaining access to milk. The presence of an agent in the milk is sometimes interpreted as a contraindication to breastfeeding; however, despite nearly all agents gaining access to milk, there are few agents that make nursing inadvisable.

Distribution of xenobiotics in milk

At equilibrium, agents are distributed between maternal plasma and milk by principles of diffusion as modified by factors such as degree of ionization, lipid solubility, and protein binding. Because ionized species do not diffuse well, agents that acquire a charge in milk tend to accumulate in that compartment. Milk is usually somewhat more acidic than plasma, and weak bases are more ionized in milk than in plasma. As the nonpolar molecules diffuse into milk and ionize, diffusion reequalizes the concentrations of the nonpolar species, driving more of the compound into the milk. Examples of agents concentrated in milk by this mechanism are atenolol, metoprolol, metoclopramide, and terbutaline. Acidic drugs are relatively excluded from milk by a similar mechanism: they are more ionized in plasma and diffuse out of milk more readily than they diffuse into milk.

Xenobiotics that are lipid soluble are present in milk, which contains about 4% fat. If there are extensive stores of a compound in maternal lipid stores, breast milk may be the most effective means of excreting the compound. This

Table 34-4. Breast milk exposures contraindicated by the American Academy of Pediatrics

Drug	Comment
Amphetamine	Case reports of irritable infants
Bromocriptine	Suppresses lactation: no documented adverse effect on nursing infant
Cocaine	Case reports of intoxicated infants
Cyclophosphamide	Case reports of neutropenia in infants
Cyclosporine	Unknown effects on infant; contraindication appears to be based on undocumented fears of immune suppression
Doxorubicin	Unknown effects; concentrated in milk
Ergotamine	Case report of vomiting, diarrhea, convulsions
Heroin	May appear in milk at higher concentrations than other opioids
Lithium	Infant plasma levels reported to be ⅓ to ½ those of mother; case reports of symptomatic infants
Marijuana	No known adverse effect; appears to be contraindicated under the general principle that people who care for infants should not use recreational drugs
Methotrexate	Undocumented concerns about immune suppression and carcinogenesis; milk levels are known to be low
Nicotine	Case reports of cardiovascular and gastrointestinal toxicity in infants
Phencyclidine	Concentrated in milk in mice; considered inappropriate for use by the caretakers of young children
Phenindione	Anticoagulant toxicity documented in a single case report; it does not appear that such toxicity is shared by warfarin
Radionuclides	Gallium-67, indium-111, iodine-125 and iodine-131, technetium-99m, and nuclides of sodium are considered to require temporary cessation of nursing because of the presence of radioactivity in milk. Of these agents, the iodine nuclides impose a plausible risk of thyroid toxicity

List adapted from American Academy of Pediatrics Committee on Drugs: The transfer of drugs and other chemicals into human milk, *Pediatrics* 93:137, 1994. Comments are those of the author, not the American Academy of Pediatrics.

route of excretion, for example, is a quantitatively important way of decreasing the maternal body burden of polychlorinated biphenyls and of some organochlorine insecticides.[60] It should be noted that despite the presence of these environmental contaminants in milk, adverse effects on the offspring are difficult to document and do not appear to outweigh the benefits of breastfeeding for the child.[61]

Protein binding in maternal blood is an effective way to prevent a xenobiotic from being free to diffuse into milk. Most opioids are so extensively bound in maternal blood that they are present in only trace amounts in the milk and are not an important exposure for the nursing infant.

Determinants of effect on the infant

As is the case for toxicants in general, dose is an important determinant of the effect of breast milk contaminants on the nursling. Even when the concentration in milk is similar to that in maternal plasma, the dose ingested by the infant is typically small. Ethanol, for example, is present in milk at a concentration of 1 mg/ml if a woman is intoxicated (i.e., a plasma concentration of 0.1 g/dl). An ounce of such milk contains 30 mg of ethanol, or about 0.2% of a mixed drink. Corrected for a term infant's weight, ingestion of this amount of ethanol produces a plasma concentration of 0.002 g/dl, 50 times lower than the mother's plasma concentration.

There are instances in which even small amounts of a toxicant can produce symptoms in a newborn. Caffeine, for example, is biotransformed slowly by infants at term and even more slowly by preterm infants. Ingestion of large

Table 34-5. References to assist clinicians with developmental toxicology questions

Reference	Comments
Bennett (1988)[2]	Contains the conclusions of a World Health Organization working group on drugs and lactation
Briggs, Freeman, Yaffe (1990)[7]	A compendium of nearly exclusively pharmaceutical agents; animal data are generally not considered in this source
Paul (1993)[56]	Written expressly to address environmental and occupational exposures, although most of the discussions have general applicability
Schardein (1993)[65]	Concentrates on teratogenic effects, that is, structural malformations
Scialli (1992)[67]	A general guide for clinicians; does not contain entries for individual agents
Shepard (1992)[71]	An encyclopedic listing of short summaries for each of 2243 agents; also available by computer and CD-ROM (see text)

amounts of caffeine by nursing women results in small exposures of the child but can result in bioaccumulation of the alkaloid because of the slowness with which the compound is handled.

The potential toxicity of a xenobiotic in breast milk may be attenuated by poor oral absorption of the compound. Aminoglycoside antibiotics, for example, are not absorbed from the gastrointestinal tract of the infant despite being present in the milk. Tetracycline is poorly absorbed in the

---

North American Teratology Information Services

Arizona Teratogen Information Program
(602) 795-5674, (800) 362-0101 (Arizona only)

California Teratogen Information Service
(619) 294-6084, (800) 532-3749 (California only)

Teratogen Information and Education Service (Denver, Colo)
(303) 861-6395, (800) 332-2082 (Colorado only), (800) 525-4871 (Wyoming only)

Connecticut Pregnancy Exposure Information Service
(203) 679-1502, (800) 325-5391 (Connecticut only)

Teratogen Information Service (Gainesville, Fla)
(904) 392-3050

Teratogen Information Service (Tampa, Fla)
(813) 974-2262

Centers for Disease Control and Prevention (Atlanta, Ga)
(404) 488-4967

Illinois Teratogen Information Service
(312) 908-7441, (800) 252-4847 (Illinois only)

Indiana Teratogen Information Service
(317) 274-1071

University of Iowa Teratogen Information Service
(319) 356-2674

Prenatal Diagnostic and Genetic Clinic (Wichita, Kan)
(316) 688-2362

Massachusetts Teratogen Information Service
(617) 787-4957, (800) 322-5104 (Massachusetts only)

Embryology Teratology Unit, Massachusetts General Hospital (Boston, Mass)
(617) 726-1742

TERAS, Brigham and Women's Hospital (Boston, Mass)
(617) 732-6507

Occupational and Environmental Reproductive Hazards Center,
University of Massachusetts Medical Center (Worcester, Mass)
(508) 856-2818

Nebraska Teratogen Project
(402) 559-5071

New Jersey Pregnancy Risk Information Service
(908) 745-6659, (800) 287-3015 (New Jersey only)

Perinatal Environmental and Drug Consultation Service (Rochester, NY)
(716) 275-3638

Teratogen Information Service (West Seneca, NY)
(716) 674-6300, extension 4812

Division of Medical Genetics (Grand Forks, ND)
(701) 777-4277

Pregnancy Healthline (Philadelphia, Pa)
(215) 829-3601

Pregnancy Safety Hotline (Pittsburgh, Pa)
(412) 687-7233

Department of Reproductive Genetics (Pittsburgh, Pa)
(412) 647-4168

Pregnancy Riskline (Salt Lake City, Utah)
(801) 583-2229

Vermont Pregnancy Risk Information Service
(802) 658-4310

Central Laboratory for Human Embryology, University of Washington (Seattle, Wash)
(206) 543-3373

Wisconsin Teratogen Project
(608) 262-4716, (800) 442-6692

Great Lakes Genetics (Milwaukee, Wis)
(414) 475-7400, (414) 475-7223

Eastern Wisconsin Teratogen Service (Milwaukee, Wis)
(414) 357-6555

Poison and Drug Information Service (Calgary, Alberta, Canada)
(403) 670-1059

Department of Genetics, Children's Hospital of Eastern Ontario
(613) 737-2275

Safe Start Program (Hamilton, Ontario, Canada)
(416) 521-2100, extension 6788

Fetal Risk Assessment from Maternal Exposure Program (London, Ontario)
(519) 685-8293

Motherisk Program (Toronto, Ontario, Canada)
(416) 813-6780

Department of Medical Genetics, University of British Columbia (Vancouver, British Columbia, Canada)
(604) 875-2157

British Columbia Drug and Poison Information Centre (Vancouver, British Columbia, Canada)
(604) 682-2344, extension 2126

---

presence of milk, and infants exposed through nursing are, of course, taking this medication with milk.

The American Academy of Pediatrics (AAP) publishes recommendations on drugs and breastfeeding.[1] Table 34-4 lists those agents considered contraindicated by the AAP. It should be noted that many contraindications are based on only a few case reports or on concerns about the mechanism of action of the agents even without reports of exposure.

Most agents for which recommendations are made are pharmaceuticals; considerably fewer data exist for environmental and occupational exposures. As discussed earlier, many pesticides and polychlorinated biphenyls are found in breast milk, but their presence is not considered to outweigh the benefits of nursing. Because much of the food chain has become contaminated with these compounds, infants will be exposed to them throughout their lives; nursing represents an enriched source of lipid-soluble contaminants but not the only source.

Heavy metals, particularly lead, have also been investigated as breast milk contaminants. When lactating monkeys were given lead at highly toxic doses, achieving blood lead concentrations of 116 μg/dl, milk concentrations were 222 μg/dl, and the offspring had blood lead concentrations of 30 μg/dl.[80] By contrast, a survey of normal lactating women showed mean blood lead concentrations of 12 μg/dl with corresponding milk concentrations of 0.3 μg/dl.[58] Another survey found milk lead concentrations to be about 1 μg/dl; infant daily lead intake from this source was estimated to be 0.9 to 2.3 μg/kg/day.[75] This can be compared with a permissible daily intake of lead of 5 μg/kg/day. Other investigators have concluded that lead concentrations in breast milk do not correlate well with concentrations in maternal blood.[53]

In industrialized countries where environmental controls have not been enforced, heavy contamination of the population with pesticides and metals has occurred. Data from such areas suggest that although breast milk contamination also occurs under these conditions, the economic and health benefits of nursing continue to be greater than documented risks from using breast milk as the infant's nutrition source.[39]

SOURCES OF INFORMATION

Health care providers are often asked to give advice on the potential developmental toxicity of therapeutic, occupational, and environmental exposures. It is not sufficient simply to counsel avoidance of all exposures; such advice is impractical and may impose undue economic hardship. In addition, employment discrimination for fetal protection is illegal in the United States.[68] Clinicians can go to the original literature for information, but access to a medical library and sufficient time for research may be limiting factors. There are a number of information sources that can be used to assist in providing information based on data.

Books

A number of books have been written specifically to help clinicians understand developmental toxicology and to give information about specific agents (Table 34-5). It should be understood that book publishing results in a product that is many months old at the time it first appears on the market. The rapidity with which biomedical information ages should be kept in mind when books are consulted.

Computerized databases

There are two computerized databases in North America, access to which is available by modem or by other electronic access, including compact disk (CD-ROM). REPROTOX®, based in Washington, DC, can be contacted at (202) 293-5137. TERIS, based in Seattle, Washington, and Vancouver, British Columbia, can be contacted at (206)

543-2465. REPROTOX provides summaries of the literature on several thousand agents, including occupational and environmental exposures, and will research agents on request if they are not already in the database. TERIS provides interpretive summaries based on the deliberations of a panel of teratologists. A CD-ROM subscription that includes both services and the computer version of Shepard (see Table 34-5) is available from Micromedex, (800) 525-9083.

Teratology information services

A number of centers are available in North America to handle telephone inquiries from professional and laypeople with developmental toxicology questions (see box on previous page). Although these centers are operated independently, an Organization of Teratology Information Services has been set up to foster common approaches to the training of counselors and quality assurance of services.

The large number of reference sources and the increasing quantity and quality of developmental toxicology information should permit an informed discussion on most occupational and environmental exposures. The goal of counseling should be to avoid exposures that are likely to produce toxicity, to provide information about possible adverse outcomes of such exposures, to decrease anxiety about low-risk exposures, and to prevent the unnecessary abortion of wanted pregnancies.

REFERENCES

1. American Academy of Pediatrics Committee on Drugs: The transfer of drugs and other chemicals into human milk, *Pediatrics* 91:137, 1994.
2. Bennett PN: *Drugs and human lactation,* Amsterdam, 1988, Elsevier.
3. Boué J, Boué A, Lazar P: Retrospective and prospective epidemiological studies of 1500 karyotped spontaneous human abortions, *Teratology* 12:11, 1975.
4. Brent RL: The complexities of solving the problems of human malformations, *Clin Perinatol* 24:491, 1986.
5. Brent RL, Beckman DA: Angiotensin-converting enzyme inhibitors, an embryopathic class of drugs with unique properties: information for clinical teratology counselors, *Teratology* 43:543, 1991.
6. Brent RL, Beckman DA: *Principles of teratology.* In Evans MI, editor: *Reproductive risks and prenatal diagnosis,* Norwalk, Conn, 1992, Appleton & Lange.
7. Briggs GG, Freeman RK, Yaffe SJ: *Drugs in pregnancy and lactation,* 3rd ed, Baltimore, 1990, Williams & Wilkins.
8. Buehler BA, et al: Prenatal prediction of risk of the fetal hydantoin syndrome, *N Engl J Med* 322:1567, 1990.
9. Butte NF, et al: Longitudinal changes in milk composition of mothers delivering preterm and term infants, *Early Hum Devel* 9:153, 1984.
10. Chernoff N, Rogers JM, Kavlock RJ: An overview of maternal toxicity and prenatal development: considerations for developmental toxicity hazard assessments, *Toxicology* 59:111, 1989.
11. Clark RL, et al: Diflunisal-induced maternal anemia as a cause of teratogenicity in rabbits, *Teratology* 30:319, 1984.
12. Clarke DO, et al: Pharmacokinetics of 2-methoxyethanol and 2-methoxyacetic acid in the pregnant mouse: a physiologically based mathematical model, *Toxicol Appl Pharmacol* 121:239, 1993.
13. Colie CF: Male mediated teratogenesis, *Reprod Toxicol* 7:3, 1993.

14. Committee on Scientific Affairs, American Medical Association: Fetal affects of maternal alcohol use, *JAMA* 249:2517, 1983.
15. Cummings AM, Laskey J: Effect of methoxychlor on ovarian steroidogenesis: role in early pregnancy loss, *Reprod Toxicol* 7:17, 1993.
16. Czeizel A: *Epidemiological studies of congenital abnormalities in Hungary.* In Kalter H, editor: *Issues and reviews in teratology,* vol 6, New York, 1993, Plenum Press.
17. Czeizel A, Racz J: Evaluation of drug intake during pregnancy in the Hungarian case-control surveillance of congenital anomalies, *Teratology* 42:505, 1990.
18. Daneilsson BR, Dencker L: Effects of cadmium on the placental uptake and transport to the fetus of nutrients, *Biol Res Preg Perinatol* 5:93, 1984.
19. DeSesso JM, Goeringer GC: Ethoxyquin and nordihydroguaiaretic acid reduce hydroxyurea developmental toxicity, *Reprod Toxicol* 4:267, 1990.
20. Dodds L, et al: Case-control study of congenital anomalies in children of cancer patients, *BMJ* 307:164, 1993.
21. Fabro S, McLachlan JA, Dames NM: Chemical exposure of embryos during the preimplantation stages of pregnancy: mortality rate and intrauterine development, *Am J Obstet Gynecol* 148:929, 1984.
22. Filler R, Lew KJ: Developmental onset of mixed-function oxidase activity in preimplantation mouse embryos, *Proc Natl Acad Sci USA* 78:6991, 1981.
23. Generoso WM, et al: Exposure of female mice to ethylene oxide within hours after mating leads to fetal malformation and death, *Mutat Res* 176:269, 1987.
24. Hakosalo JK: Cumulative detection rates of congenital malformations in a ten-year follow-up study, *Acta Pathol Microbiol Scand* 242(suppl A):1, 1973.
25. Hale F: The relation of vitamin A to anophthalmos in pigs, *Am J Ophthalmol* 18:1087, 1935.
26. Hall JG, Pauli RM, Wilson KM: Maternal and fetal sequelae of anticoagulation during pregnancy, *Am J Med* 68:122, 1980.
27. Hawkins MM: Is there evidence of a therapy-related increase in germ cell mutation among childhood cancer survivors? *J Natl Cancer Inst* 83:1643, 1991.
28. Hawkins MM, Smith RA: Pregnancy outcomes in childhood cancer survivors: probably effects of abdominal radiation, *Int J Cancer* 43:399, 1989.
29. International Clearinghouse for Birth Defects Monitoring Systems: *Congenital malformations worldwide,* Amsterdam, 1991, Elsevier.
30. Jensh RP, Brent RL: Effects of prenatal X-irradiation on the 14th-18th days of gestation on postnatal growth and development in the rat, *Teratology* 38:431, 1988.
31. Johnson EM, Gabel BE: An artificial "embryo" for detection of abnormal developmental biology, *Fundam Appl Toxicol* 3:243, 1983.
32. Jordan EK, Sever JL: Fetal damage caused by parvovirus infections, *Reprod Toxicol* 8:161, 1994.
33. Kavlock RJ, Chernoff N, Rogers EH: The effect of acute maternal toxicity on fetal development in the mouse, *Teratogenesis Carcinog Mutagen* 5:3, 1985.
34. Khera KS: Maternal toxicity—a possible factor in fetal malformation in mice, *Teratology* 29:411, 1984.
35. Khera KS: Maternal toxicity: a possible etiological factor in embryofetal deaths and fetal malformations in rodent-rabbit species, *Teratology* 31:129, 1985.
36. Klein KL, Scott WJ, Wilson JG: Aspirin induced teratogenesis: a unique pattern of cell death and subsequent polydactyly in the rat, *J Exp Zool* 216:107, 1981.
37. Kuban KCK, Leviton A: Cerebral palsy, *N Engl J Med* 330:188, 1994.
38. Lammer EJ, et al: Classification and analysis of fetal deaths in Massachusetts, *JAMA* 261:1757, 1989.
39. Lederman SA: *Environmental contaminants and their significance for breastfeeding in the central Asian republics,* New York, 1993, Wellstart International.
40. Levin AA, Miller RK: Fetal toxicity of cadmium in the rat: maternal vs. fetal injections, *Teratology* 22:1, 1980.
41. Levin AA, Miller RK: Fetal toxicity of cadmium in the rat: decreased uteroplacental blood flow, *Toxicol Appl Pharmacol* 58:297, 1981.
42. Little RE, et al: Fetal growth and moderate drinking in early pregnancy, *Am J Epidemiol* 123:270, 1986.
43. Meltzer HG: Congenital abnormalities due to attempted abortion with 4-aminopterylglutamic acid, *JAMA* 161:1253, 1956.
44. Mulvihill JJ, et al: Pregnancy outcomes in cancer patients. Experience in a large cooperative group, *Cancer* 60:1143, 1987.
45. Murakami U: Organic mercury problem affecting intrauterine life, *Adv Exp Biol Med* 27:301, 1972.
46. Murphy ML, Karnofsky DA: Effect of azaserine and other growth-inhibiting agents on fetal development in the rat, *Cancer* 9:955, 1956.
47. Nau H, Scott WJ Jr: *Pharmacokinetics in teratogenesis,* Boca Raton, Fla, 1992, CRC Press.
48. Newton ER: The relationship between intrapartum obstetric care and chronic neurodevelopmental handicaps in children, *Reprod Toxicol* 4:85, 1990.
49. Nomura T: X-ray- and chemically induced germ-line mutation causing phenotypic anomalies in mice, *Mutat Res* 198:309, 1988.
50. Norton S, Kimler BR: Correlation of behavior with brain damage after in utero exposure to toxic agents, *Neurotoxicol Teratol* 9:145, 1987.
51. Norton ME, et al: Neonatal complications after the administration of indomethacin for preterm labor, *N Engl J Med* 329:1602, 1993.
52. Olshan AF, Faustman EM: Male-mediated developmental toxicity, *Annu Rev Public Health* 14:159, 1993.
53. Ong CN, et al: Concentrations of lead in maternal blood, cord blood, and breast milk, *Arch Dis Child* 60:756, 1985.
54. Otake M, Schull WJ: In utero exposure to A-bomb radiation and mental retardation: a reassessment, *Br J Radiol* 57:409, 1984.
55. Pati S, Helmbrecht GD: Congenital schizencephaly associated with warfarin exposure, *Reprod Toxicol* 8:115, 1994.
56. Paul M: *Occupational and environmental reproductive hazards,* Baltimore, 1993, Williams & Wilkins.
57. Robert E: Handling surveillance types of data on birth defects and exposures during pregnancy, *Reprod Toxicol* 6:205, 1992.
58. Rockway SW, et al: Lead concentration in milk, blood, and hair in lactating women, *Int Arch Occup Environ Health* 53:181, 1984.
59. Roels HA, et al: Placental transfer of lead, mercury, cadmium and carbon monoxide in women. III. Factors influencing the accumulation of heavy metals in the placenta and the relationship between metal concentrations in the placenta and in maternal and cord blood, *Environ Res* 16:236, 1978.
60. Rogan WJ, et al: Polychlorinated biphenyls (PCBs) and dichlorodiphenyl dichloroethane (DDE) in human milk: effects of maternal factors and previous lactation, *Am J Public Health* 76:172, 1986.
61. Rogan WJ, et al: Polychlorinated biphenyls (PCBs) and dichlorodiphenyl dichloroethane (DDE) in human milk: effects on growth, morbidity, and duration of lactation, *Am J Public Health* 77:1294, 1987.
62. Russell LB: X-ray induced developmental abnormalities in the mouse and their use in the analysis of embryological patterns, *J Exp Zool* 114:545, 1950.
63. Rutledge JC, et al: Increased incidence of developmental anomalies among descendants of carriers of methylenebisacrylmaide-induced balanced reciprocal translocations, *Mutat Res* 229:161, 1990.
64. Rutledge JC, Generoso WM: Fetal pathology produced by ethylene oxide treatment of the murine zygote, *Teratology* 39:563, 1989.
65. Schardein JL: *Chemically induced birth defects,* 2nd ed, New York, 1993, Marcel Dekker.

66. Schull WJ, Otake M, Neel JV: Genetic effects of the atomic bombs: a reappraisal, *Science* 213:1220, 1981.

67. Scialli AR: *A clinical guide to reproductive and developmental toxicology,* Boca Raton, Fla, 1992, CRC Press.

68. Scialli AR: Fetal protection policies in the United States, *Semin Perinatol* 17:50, 1993.

69. Scott WJ, Klein KL, Wise LD: Review: pathogenesis of preaxial polydactyly, *Congen Anom* 21:441, 1981.

70. Selby PB: Experimental induction of dominant mutations in mammals by ionizing radiations and chemicals, *Iss Rev Teratol* 5:181, 1990.

71. Shepard TH: *Catalog of teratogenic agents,* 7th ed, Baltimore, 1992, Johns Hopkins University Press.

72. Shepard TH, Fantel AG, Fitzsimmon J: Congenital defect rates among spontaneous abortuses: twenty years of monitoring, *Teratology* 39:325, 1989.

73. Shum S, Jensen NM, Nebert DW: The murine Ah locus: in utero toxicity and teratogenesis associated with genetic differences in benzo[a]pyrene metabolism, *Teratology* 20:365, 1979.

74. Sonawane BR, et al: Placental transfer of cadmium in rats: influence of dose and gestational age, *Environ Health Perspect* 12:97, 1975.

75. Sternowsky HJ, Wessolowski R: Lead and cadmium in breast milk. Higher levels in urban vs rural mothers during the first 3 months of lactation, *Arch Toxicol* 57:41, 1985.

76. Streissguth AP, Barr HM, Martin DC: Alcohol exposure in utero and functional defects in children during the first four years of life. In *Mechanisms of alcohol damage in utero,* CIBA Foundation Symposium 105, London, 1984, Pittman.

77. Streissguth AP, Clarren SK, Jones KL: Natural history of the fetal alcohol syndrome: a 10-year follow-up of eleven patients, *Lancet* 2:85, 1985.

78. Streissguth AP, et al: Fetal alcohol syndrome in adolescents and adults, *JAMA* 265:1961, 1991.

79. Swartz WJ, Corkern M: Effects of methoxychlor treatment of pregnant mice on female offspring of the treated and subsequent pregnancies, *Reprod Toxicol* 6:431, 1992.

80. Tachon P, et al: Lead poisoning in monkeys during pregnancy and lactation, *Sci Tot Environ* 30:221, 1983.

81. Thiersch JB: Therapeutic abortions with folic acid antagonist 4-aminopteroylglutamic acid (4-amino P.G.A.) administered by oral route, *Am J Obstet Gynecol* 63:1298, 1952.

82. Thiersch JB, Phillips FS: Effect of 4-amino pteroylglutamic acid (aminopterin) on early pregnancy, *Proc Soc Exp Biol Med* 74:204, 1950.

83. Warkany J, Beaudry PH, Hornstein S: Attempted abortion with aminopterin (4-aminopterylglutamic acid), *Am J Dis Child* 97:274, 1959.

84. Warkany J, Nelson RC: Appearance of skeletal abnormalities in the offspring of rats reared on a deficient diet, *Science* 92:383, 1940.

85. Weiner CP, Williamson RA: Evaluation of severe retardation using cordocentesis—hematologic and metabolic alterations by etiology, *Obstet Gynecol* 73:225, 1989.

86. Wilcox AJ, et al: Incidence of early pregnancy loss, *N Engl J Med* 31:189, 1988.

87. Wilson JG: Experimental studies on congenital malformations, *J Chron Dis* 10:111, 1959.

88. Wilson JG: Current status of teratology. In Wilson JG, Fraser FC, editors, *Handbook of teratology,* New York, 1977, Plenum Press.

Chapter 35

PHONATION

Robert Thayer Sataloff

Environmental and occupational pollution is ubiquitous. Pollution is encountered in the home, the workplace, the air we breathe, the food chain, and even in the medical treatment room. For centuries physicians have tried to understand and control toxic substances to prevent bodily injury. Many substances are toxic to the voice, but few are understood fully. Although anecdotal experience is extensive, little research has been done to determine the vocal effects of various pollutants. Nevertheless, it appears that injury to the vocal tract caused by environmental or occupational pollution is not rare. Various kinds of pollution must be considered.

ANATOMY, PHYSIOLOGY, AND VOICE ASSESSMENT

Vocal anatomy and function are extremely complex, and we have begun to understand them only in the last two decades. Details of anatomy and physiology of phonation are beyond the scope of this chapter but should be reviewed in other literature.[13,26-28,30]

The larynx is essential to normal voice production, but the anatomy of the voice is not limited to the larynx. The vocal mechanism includes the abdominal and back musculature, rib cage, lungs, the pharynx, oral cavity, and nose. Each component performs an important function in voice production, although it is possible to produce voice even without a larynx, for example, in patients who have undergone laryngectomy. In addition, virtually all parts of the body play some role in voice production and may be responsible for voice dysfunction. Even something as remote as a sprained ankle may alter posture, thereby impairing abdominal, back, and thoracic muscle function and resulting in vocal inefficiency, weakness, and hoarseness.

The larynx is composed of four basic anatomical units: (1) skeleton, (2) intrinsic muscles, (3) extrinsic muscles, and (4) mucosa. The mucosa is of particular interest. It consists of five layers (Fig. 35-1).[13] The thin, lubricated epithelium covering the vocal folds forms the area of contact between the vibrating vocal folds and acts somewhat like a capsule, helping to maintain vocal fold shape. The epithelium lining most of the vocal tract is pseudostratified, ciliated columnar epithelium, typical respiratory epithelium involved in handling mucous secretions. The vibratory margin of the vocal fold is covered with stratified squamous epithelium, better suited to withstand the trauma of vocal fold contact. The superficial layer of the lamina propria, also known as Reinke's space, is made up of loose fibrous components and matrix. It contains few fibroblasts. The intermediate layer of the lamina propria contains more fibroblasts and consists primarily of elastic fibers. The deep layer of the lamina propria is composed primarily of collagenous fibers and is rich in fibroblasts. The thyroarytenoid or vocalis muscle makes up the body of the vocal fold and is one of the intrinsic laryngeal muscles. The region of the intermediate and deep layers of the lamina propria is called the vocal ligament and lies immediately below Reinke's space. Functionally, the various layers have different mechanical properties and act somewhat like ball bearings of different sizes in allowing the smooth shearing action necessary for proper vocal fold vibration. The posterior one

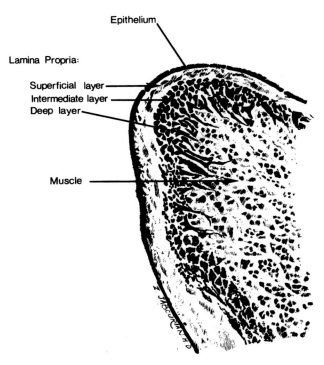

Fig. 35-1. Cross-section through the midportion of the vocal fold, in the coronal plane. The vocal fold consists of epithelium; superficial; intermediate, and deep layers of lamina propria; and vocalis muscle. There is also a complex basement membrane that connects the epithelium to the superficial layer of the lamina propria.

third (approximately) of the vocal fold is cartilaginous, and the anterior two thirds are membranous (from the vocal process forward) in adults. Most of the vibratory function critical to sound quality occurs in the membranous portion.

Mechanically the vocal fold structures actually act more like three layers consisting of the cover (epithelium and Reinke's space), transition (intermediate and deep layers of the lamina propria), and body (the vocalis muscle). Understanding this anatomy is important because different pathological entities occur in different layers. Moreover, fibroblasts are responsible for scar formation.

The physiology of voice production is exceedingly complex, beginning with volition in the cerebral cortex. The new science of neurolaryngology is only beginning to clarify the many important neurological and neuromuscular pathways and interactions. Peripherally the vocal folds act as the oscillator of the vocal tract, creating a sound like the buzz of a trumpet mouthpiece. This sound passes through the supraglottic vocal tract (e.g., pharynx, oral cavity, nasal cavity), which acts like a series of interconnected resonators and is responsible, in large measure, for voice quality. The power source of the voice is infraglottic and consists of the thorax and its contents, the abdominal muscles, and the back muscles. They generate a force that propels

air between the vocal folds. Defects anywhere in the system may produce voice dysfunction. For example, if the support mechanism (power source) is impaired, attempts at compensation usually involve hyperfunction of neck and larynx muscles, which are not designed for power source functions. This commonly produces vocal injuries, such as nodules, hemorrhages, and cysts.

Technological advances in the 1980s now allow comprehensive voice evaluation using strobovideolaryngoscopy for slow-motion assessment of the vibratory margin and voice laboratory equipment to quantify voice function (acoustic, aerodynamic, phonatory, electromyographic). These advances are recent, however, and state-of-the-art evaluation is still only available in relatively few medical centers. Nevertheless, it is essential when evaluating environmental and occupational voice disorders.

ATMOSPHERIC POLLUTION
Inhaled pollutants

Vocal tract injury caused by inhaled pollution is most obvious. In extreme cases, the vocal effects of inhaled substances are self-evident. Such problems are usually seen following fires or industrial accidents in which hydrocarbons or other substances are inhaled, and pulmonary and laryngeal dysfunction ensue. More subtle voice dysfunction may result from chronic inhalation of atmospheric pollutants. Some such substances injure the airway topically. Other inhaled pollutants are absorbed into the body and may remain there for prolonged periods of time. In both scenarios, the consequent voice dysfunction may be more severe and prolonged than one would expect, even when there is no secondary gain (such as litigation) that might confuse the clinical presentation. The mechanisms of these problems remain obscure. Certainly, substances that directly injure the mucosa of the vocal folds and the rest of the respiratory tract can interfere with the mechanics of vibration. When irritants result in coughing, this physiological response may also cause substantial vocal fold injury, including mucosal disruption and vocal fold hemorrhage. It is equally clear that pollutants that alter pulmonary function may have adverse effects on the voice. The lungs act as the power source for phonation. It has been well established that impairment in power source function can result in compensatory muscular tension dysphonia, voice fatigue, hoarseness and other quality changes, and even structural lesions such as vocal nodules. Such power source alterations may be caused by any agent that produces obstructive or restrictive lung disease or that alters abdominal and thoracic muscle function and coordination. Clinically, however, it appears that voice dysfunction may also occur following exposure to toxic pollutants that do not produce obvious or measurable topical or pulmonary alterations. Allergy is often involved as an explanation, but the mechanism in many of these cases is not understood. Indeed, it is unclear even whether such conditions result in injury to nerves, control mechanisms, surface integrity, other factors, or combinations of such mechanisms. To prevent, diagnose, and treat such problems and predict their long-term courses, we need a much better understanding of the effects of inhaled toxins on the vocal tract, including not only upper and lower airway structures, but also neurological components.

A general review of environmental and occupational pollutants is beyond the scope of this chapter (see Chapters 2 and 3). A few particularly important substances, however, have been identified by the U.S. Environmental Protection Agency (EPA), recognized by the federal government,[9] and listed in the Indoor Air Quality Act of 1990. Many of these pollutants have known consequences that strongly suggest concomitant voice effects, although specific voice studies have not been conducted in most instances. A review of some of the pollutants listed by the EPA provides a useful overview of the problem and potential for adverse vocal consequences.

Radon found in soil, well water, and some building materials is known to cause lung cancer. An association with laryngeal cancer has not been firmly established. Environmental tobacco smoke causes irritation to mucous membranes, pulmonary effects, and cancer, all of which are known to affect the vocal folds and voice adversely. Biological contaminants from humans and animals can cause allergic reactions, infectious diseases, and other toxic effects that may involve laryngeal function. Although this subject has not been well studied, it is intuitively obvious, for example, to anyone who is allergic to cats and has tried to speak or sing following acute exposure to feline dander.

Volatile organic compounds in paints, adhesives, solvents, office machinery, and other substances can also cause irritation, cancer, and neurotoxic effects. Formaldehyde, which is present in plywood, particle board, upholstery, and other substances, has also been associated with mucosal irritation, allergy, and cancer. Polycyclic aromatic hydrocarbons from kerosene heaters and woodstoves are associated not only with irritation and cancer, but also with decreased immune function. Conceivably, this might be associated with more frequent upper respiratory tract infection and concomitant voice dysfunction. Pesticides may cause neurotoxicity, although specific involvement of the voice pathway has not been studied.

Asbestos present in building material and other substances has been causally related to cancer and asbestosis. Asbestosis causes decreased pulmonary function, which affects the voice.

Carbon monoxide from combustion causes a variety of problems, including exacerbation of cardiopulmonary dysfunction in compromised patients. This suggests that chronic carbon monoxide exposure may cause voice dysfunction through power source compromise, especially in the elderly. Nitrogen dioxide from combustion is known to cause decreased pulmonary function in asthmatics, changes in anatomy and function of the lungs, increased susceptibility to infection in animals, and other compromises of function essential for normal, healthy voice production. It also appears to be synergistic with other pollutants. Similar effects may be seen with exposure to sulfur dioxide from combustion of sulfur-containing fuels. Combustion particles (such as soot) may also cause irritation to respiratory tissues and decrease lung function. Various household sprays and aerosols may also cause adverse effects.

Clinical experience and our current understanding of vocal anatomy and physiology have taught us that the voice is exquisitely sensitive to even subtle changes in health or environment. These changes are particularly obvious in professional singers whose vocal function may be impaired substantially by influences as minor as dust in a theater or decreased humidity on an airplane.[27] Consequently, one is compelled to suspect that pollutants such as those reviewed here cause voice dysfunction, despite the paucity of scientific proof.

Although relatively few studies have been done to investigate the effects of inhaled pollutants on the voice, review of some of those available in the literature provides helpful insights. In 1968, Klayman[17] reported on the otolaryngological effects of insecticide exposure. He reported on several patients with epidermoid carcinoma of the larynx who had been exposed to insecticides. All of the insecticides were nonarsenicals and highly absorbable through skin, lungs, and gastrointestinal tract, producing irritation to the eyes, nose, and throat.[17] Also in 1968, Becker and coworkers[4] reviewed the effect on health of the 1966 Eastern Seaboard air pollution episode. They found that there was a definite relationship between air pollution levels and symptoms of irritative phenomena, including hoarseness; increased cough; shortness of breath; chest constriction; nausea; vomiting; and irritation of the mucous membranes of the eyes, nasal passages, pharynx, and bronchial tree. They also reported that individuals with chronic obstructive pulmonary disease were affected most adversely by increasing air pollution levels.[4]

Snow[29] investigated the effects of carbon black inhalation on the larynx and trachea. His 1970 study used golden hamsters exposed for varied periods of time to air containing various quantities of carbon black, a substance used in the manufacture of the majority of black objects, including tires, paints, and ink. Snow found that prolonged inhalation of sufficient quantities of carbon black produced subepithelial changes in the thyroarytenoid fold, including edema, and retention of amorphous eosinophilic material in subglottic and tracheal glands. No tumor formation or pathological changes in the epithelium were noted. Snow concluded that inhalation of this inert dust "cannot be considered innocuous" and that further study was needed.[29]

In 1971, Amdur[1] reviewed the toxicology of aerosols formed by oxidation of sulfur dioxide. She reported that the particulate oxidation product, sulfuric acid, has an increased irritant potency in comparison with sulfur dioxide.

Furthermore, particulate size is important in predicting irritant potency and response, suggesting that analysis of mass concentration alone was not sufficient. She observed that the particulate size of greatest importance was at the submicron level. She reported that sulfuric acid mist promotes laryngeal spasms and spasmodic bronchostenosis, which can cause death. It can also produce parenchymal lung damage. She noted that "an equivalent amount of sulfur produces a less irritant response if it is present as sulfur dioxide gas than if it is present as particulate sulfate or sulfuric acid." Laryngeal changes (other than spasm) were not studied specifically, but substantial impairment of pulmonary function was documented. This phenomenon, along with direct irritation, is likely to affect the voice.[1]

In 1972, Baskevill[3] reported on the effects of atmospheric toxic agents on the larynges of children. He attempted to correlate air pollution with dysphonia in children. He quoted previous literature and presented anecdotal observations suggesting that an association exists, but a causal relationship was not established clearly. He also highlighted the importance of respiratory dysfunction and repeated upper respiratory infections on the voice, observing that these conditions may be caused by pollution and thereby exert at least secondary effects on the voice.[27]

In 1975, Kruysse and co-workers[21] investigated the consequences of acetaldehyde vapor on Syrian golden hamsters. They noted severe histopathological changes in the respiratory tract, including necrosis, inflammatory changes, hyperplasia, and metaplasia; the upper segments of the respiratory tract were much more severely affected than the lower parts.[21] They looked at tissue from various areas, including the nose and larynx. Nasal findings included necrotizing rhinitis. Laryngeal studies showed that areas normally lined by respiratory epithelium appeared to be covered with stratified squamous epithelium, often keratinized. The vocal fold edge, which is normally lined by stratified squamous epithelium, was covered with a thick layer of keratin. Substantial damage to tracheal epithelium was also noted.

Wehner and associates[36] studied the effects of chronic inhalation of asbestos and cigarette smoke in hamsters in 1975. They found that animals exposed to asbestos developed lung lesions earlier and more severely than controls exposed to sham or smoke. Laryngeal lesions in the asbestos plus smoke–exposed group were essentially the same as those in the asbestos plus sham smoke–exposed group. Interestingly, there was a significantly lower incidence of laryngeal lesions and of malignant tumors in the asbestos plus smoke–exposed group than in the smoke-exposed controls. The authors believed that this was due to earlier death from asbestosis.[36]

In 1976, Wehner and coworkers[35] at the National Cancer Institute used Syrian hamsters to investigate the effects of diethylnitrosamine and cigarette smoke. They found that diethylnitrosamine caused a significant increase in epithelial lesions of the larynx, including papillomas, and that cigarette smoke inhalation had a significant potentiating effect on the incidence of these lesions.[35]

In 1983, Matsuo and associates[23] reviewed 191 patients with polypoid vocal folds seen over a 10-year period. They found that long-lasting hoarseness was the most common symptom; that most patients were smokers; and that "vocal abuse, alcohol drinking, and air pollution did not prove to be etiologic factors."[25] The study used examinations, questionnaires, and retrospective review. Exposure to air pollution was recorded as "present" or "absent," and air analysis was not performed.

Of course, the deleterious effects of tobacco smoke have been reported extensively (see Chapter 13). They include deleterious effects throughout the upper and lower respiratory tract, including the larynx, and both active and passive smoke exposure have been implicated. The literature on tobacco is too extensive to cite meaningfully in this paper, but its adverse consequences have been well established.[31-33] In addition to pulmonary disease that can impair voice function and lead to cancer, cigarette smoke has been associated with a variety of vocal fold lesions, including polypoid chorditis (Reinke's edema). Matsuo and co-workers[23] found smoking to be the most common associated factor in 191 patients with this condition reported in 1983. Interestingly, they noted specifically that air pollution did not appear to be an etiological factor.

Numerous authors have looked at the association between laryngeal disease and various occupations associated with exposure to environmental pollution. Most such studies have suggested a relationship between occupational exposure to environmental toxins and laryngeal disease, although the causal relationship has not been proved conclusively in most cases. Chovil[6] suggests, for example, that the apparent association of laryngeal cancer with asbestos and possibly other occupational exposures can be accounted for by the hypothesis that chronic vocal abuse peculiar to certain working conditions acts as a promoting factor for active carcinogens found mainly in tobacco smoke. This notion is speculative, however, and extensive further study is needed.

In a more recent report, Leonard and colleagues[22] studied the effects of ambient inhaled ozone on vocal fold mucosa in Bonnet monkeys. They noted differences in vocal fold mucosa, including increases in the thickness of epithelial and connective tissues and inflammatory changes with associated disruptions in glands and blood vessels. Ozone is a major component of smog and is a common environmental pollutant in many metropolitan areas. Ozone also has been associated with alterations in pulmonary function, including reduced forced vital capacity and forced expiratory volume,[5,15] biochemical changes, cellular injury, and structural alterations in the lower respiratory tract[11,12,16,37]; and nasal mucosal changes and ciliary damage.[14] Although these abnormal consequences of ozone exposure secondary to pollution throughout the vocal tract might affect the voice, in and of themselves, the investigation by Leonard and colleagues[22] appears to be the first to recognize potentially serious voice implications of ozone exposure. In particular, they noted that, after 7 days of ozone exposure, epithelium that appeared to be normal clinically was markedly abnormal histologically, suggesting that ozone-induced changes may be difficult to detect using routine clinical methods. The long-term effects of chronic ozone exposure remain unknown, but in the lungs, ozone has been shown to produce metaplasia, resulting in replacement of one type of epithelium by another that is more resistant to toxic irritation.[2] The consequences of these and other vocal fold changes on vocal fold function and voice quality remain unknown. Clearly, available preliminary evidence dictates a need for additional research into the effects of this especially common environmental pollutant.

Ingested pollutants

In addition to inhaled pollutants, physicians are commonly confronted with ingested substances that may affect voice function adversely through toxicity. Those that cause alteration of neurological function are of particular interest. Such substances include not only widely recognized neurotoxins, such as lead, but also more common substances, including alcohol, caffeine, various drugs (prescribed and recreational), and possibly chemicals such as preservatives and insecticides. Optimal vocal health depends on fine motor control. Little is known about the effects of many commonly ingested chemicals on the neurological components of the vocal tract. Naturally, toxic environmental and occupational pollutants can be absorbed in other ways, such as through the skin. Moreover, the effects of such pollutants need not be neurolaryngological. They may simply produce mucosal drying, irritation, or other topical symptoms. Some pollutants are also capable of provoking respiratory response that alters voice at least temporarily, especially in people particularly sensitive or allergic to the pollutant. Monosodium glutamate may be an example. It is reasonable to speculate, however, that substances that affect neurological control mechanisms or function may affect the voice adversely, and these possibilities warrant research.

Other pollutants

Pollutants need not be ingested or inhaled to affect the voice adversely. For example, noise intense enough to interfere with auditory feedback used ordinarily for voice control may be considered a pollutant with voice effects. The question of causal relationship between noise and dysphonia has been investigated by several authors.* Most suggested an association between voice dysfunction and high

*References 8, 10, 18-20, 24, 25, 34.

noise levels, attributing vocal fold abnormalities to voice abuse associated with the need to speak over loud noise. These studies were primarily anecdotal, however, and not controlled. Although the hypothesis is intuitively attractive, it is unproven. Interestingly, Van Dijk and co-workers[34] performed a rather extensive evaluation of 539 workers from seven industries, finding no correlation between hoarseness and noise exposure in their study of the nonauditory effects of noise in industry. Review of the available literature confirms that the effects of noise pollution on the voice remain unknown and that this subject is also greatly in need of thorough investigation.

FUTURE RESEARCH

Recognizing the substantial body of research on the effects of pollution on other bodily functions, it is reasonable to wonder why there is so little information about the vocal effects. The paucity of information is due neither to lack of interest nor to lack of clinical indications that pollution-related voice problems exist. Rather, it is a consequence of technological development. Until recently, accepted, practical methods for quantifying voice function were not available. Although histological study of the vocal folds and other components of the vocal tract in animals is possible, the human voice is unique. This is true not only in terms of anatomy (humans are the only species with a vocal ligament), but also, even more importantly, in terms of function. Consequently, assessment of the effects of pollutants on voice quality requires human study. There are still few clinical voice laboratories for such research,[7] and most of those have been active for less than 5 years. Although reasonably good research is possible today, even now, standards for most objective voice measures and for reporting have not been established. As these problems are addressed and as technology for voice measurement improves, we are likely to see substantial progress toward answering many questions about vocal effects of environmental and occupational pollution.

REFERENCES

1. Amdur MO: Aerosols formed by oxidation of sulfur dioxide, *Arch Environ Health* 23:459, 1971.
2. Barr B, et al: Distal airway remodeling in rats chronically exposed to ozone, *Am Rev Respir Dis* 137:924, 1988.
3. Baskervill RD: Internal laryngeal injury in children due to ingestion of atmospherical toxic agents, *J School Health* 42:377, 1972.
4. Becker WH, Schilling FJ, Verma MP: The effect on health of the 1966 eastern seaboard air pollution episode, *Arch Environ Health* 16:414, 1968.
5. Bedi J, Horvath S, Drechsler-Parks D: Adaptation by older individuals repeatedly exposed to 045 parts per million ozone for two hours, *J Air Poll Control Assoc* 39:194, 1989.
6. Chovil A: Laryngeal cancer: an explanation for the apparent occupational association, *Med Hypotheses* 7:951, 1981.
7. Colton RH: The inner voice, *J Voice* 4:91, 1990.
8. Drasoveanu C, Asgian B, Mulfay G: Influenta zgomotului industrial asupra fonatiei, *Rev Chir [Chir]* 28:175, 1983.

9. Environmental Protection Agency Report No. EPA/400/1-89/001C, vol 2, Washington, DC, 1989, Environmental Protection Agency.

10. Feder RJ: The professional voice and airline flight, *Otolaryngol Head Neck Surg* 92:251, 1984 (editorial).

11. Folinsbee L, McDonnell W, Horstman D: Pulmonary function and symptom responses after 66-hour exposure to 012 ppm ozone with moderate exposure, *J Air Poll Control Assoc* 38:28, 1988.

12. Fujinaka L, et al: Respiratory bronchiolitis following long-term ozone exposure in bonnet monkeys: a morphometric study, *Exp Lung Res* 8:167, 1985.

13. Gould WJ, Sataloff RT, Spiegel JR: *Voice surgery,* St. Louis, 1993, Mosby-Year Book.

14. Harkema J, et al: Response of the macaque nasal epithelium to ambient levels of ozone, *Am J Pathol* 128:29, 1987.

15. Horstman D, et al: *Changes in pulmonary function and airway reactivity due to prolonged exposure to typical ambient ozone (O₃) levels.* In Schneider T, Lee S, Walters G, Grant L, editors: *Atmospheric ozone research and its policy implications,* Amsterdam, 1989, Elsevier.

16. Hyde D, et al: *Ozone induced structural changes in monkey respiratory system.* In Schneider T, et al, editors: *Atmospheric ozone research and its policy implications,* Amsterdam, 1989, Elsevier.

17. Klayman MB: Exposure to insecticides, *Arch Otolaryngol* 88:142, 1968 (letter to the editor).

18. Klingholz F: Effect of noise on phonation. Einfluss von Larm auf die Stimmgebung, *MMW* 124:1005, 1982.

19. Klingholz F: Voice and noise, *Stimme und Larm Z Gesamte Hyg* 20:571, 1974.

20. Krajcovic I: Hlasove poruchy zamestnancov hlucnych pracovisk svermovych zeleziarni Podbrezova, *Cesk Otolaryngol* 37:33, 1988.

21. Kruysse A, Feron VJ, Til HP: Repeated exposure to acetaldehyde vapor, studies in Syrian golden hamsters, *Arch Environ Health* 30:449, 1975.

22. Leonard RJ, George LC, Faddis B: Effects of ambient inhaled ozone on vocal fold mucosa in bonnet monkeys, *J Voice* 5(4):304, 1993.

23. Matsuo K, Kamimura M, Hirano M: Polypoid vocal folds. A 10-year review of 191 patients, *Auris Nasus Larynx* 10(suppl):37S, 1983.

24. Otto B, et al: An analysis of the relation between dysphonia in shipyard workers and working in noise, *Bull Inst Marit Trop Med Gdynia* 31:185, 1980.

25. Rontal E, et al: Vocal cord dysfunction—an industrial health hazard, *Ann Otol Rhinol Laryngol* 88:818, 1979.

26. Sataloff RT: The human voice, *Sci Am* 267:108, 1992.

27. Sataloff RT: *Professional voice: the science and art of clinical care,* New York, 1993, Raven Press.

28. Scherer RS: *Physiology of phonation: a review of basic mechanics.* In Ford CN, Bless DM, editors: *Phonosurgery: assessment and surgical management of voice disorders,* New York, 1991, Raven Press.

29. Snow JB: Carbon black Inhalation into the larynx and trachea, *Laryngoscope* 80:267, 1970.

30. Sundberg J: *Science of the singing voice,* DeKalb, Ill, 1987, Northern Illinois University Press.

31. Surgeon General's Report: *The health consequences of smoking: nicotine addiction,* Rockville, Md, 1988, U.S. Department of Health and Human Services.

32. Surgeon General's Report: *Reducing the health consequences of smoking: 25 years of progress,* Rockville, Md, 1989, U.S. Department of Health and Human Services.

33. Surgeon General's Report: *The health benefits of smoking cessation: executive summary,* Rockville, Md, 1990, U.S. Department of Health and Human Services.

34. van Dijk FJ, Souman AM, de Vries FF: Non auditory effects of noise in industry. VI. A final field study in industry, *Int Arch Occup Environ Health* 59:133, 1987.

35. Wehner AP, Busch RH, Olson RJ: Effects of diethylnitrosamine and cigarette smoke on hamsters, *J Natl Cancer Inst* 56:749, 1976.

36. Wehner AP, et al: Chronic inhalation of asbestos and cigarette smoke by hamsters, *Environ Res* 10:368, 1975.

37. Wilson D, Plopper C, Dungworth D: The response of the macaque traceobronchial epithelium to acute ozone injury, *Am J Pathol* 116:193, 1984.

Chapter 36

AUDITORY FUNCTION

Robert Thayer Sataloff
Joseph Sataloff

Diagnosing occupational hearing loss
Cochlear biology: current concepts
Sensorineural hearing loss
The 4000-Hz audiometric dip
Histopathology of noise-induced hearing loss
Exposure to hazardous noise

Noise-induced hearing loss has been recognized since the industrial revolution. There are now approximately 8 million people with occupational hearing loss (OHL) in American industry, rendering OHL our most prevalent industrial "disease." Similar problems exist in most countries with noisy industries. Although classified as a disease, OHL is actually the cumulative result of repetitive injury to the cochlear hair cells. Society's neglect of hearing loss, especially OHL, has produced human and economic consequences that affect nearly every household in industrialized countries. This is particularly regrettable because noise-induced hearing loss is almost completely preventable at little cost.

Occupational physicians, otolaryngologists, and otologists are called on with increasing frequency to assess hearing problems purportedly related to the workplace. Unfortunately, few residency training programs or otology fellowships provide the special training necessary for expert management of this complex subspecialty. Many unique factors must be taken into account when considering a diagnosis of OHL and when providing advice to employees, management, and the legal professions. These factors have been discussed in detail in other publications,[14] and only a few areas are summarized in this chapter. Although pathol-

ogists rarely have the opportunity to review histological materials from living patients with OHL, basic knowledge of current concepts in cochlear biology and OHL is valuable for any pathologist concerned with prevalent problems in occupational and environmental medicine.

DIAGNOSING OCCUPATIONAL HEARING LOSS

The American College of Occupational Medicine Noise and Hearing Conservation Committee promulgated a position statement on the distinguishing features of occupational noise-induced hearing loss.[9] This statement summarizes the currently accepted opinions of the medical community regarding diagnosis of OHL. The American Occupational Medicine Association (AOMA) Committee defined occupational noise-induced hearing loss as a slowly developing hearing loss over a long period (several years) as the result of exposure to continuous or intermittent loud noise. The committee stated that the diagnosis of noise-induced hearing loss is made clinically by a physician and should include a study of the noise exposure history. It also distinguishes OHL from acoustic trauma, a sudden change in hearing resulting from a single exposure to a sudden burst of sound, such as an explosive blast. The committee recognized that the principal characteristics of occupational noise-induced hearing loss are as follows:

1. It is always sensorineural, affecting the hair cells in the inner ear.
2. It is almost always bilateral. Audiometric patterns are usually similar bilaterally.
3. It almost never produces a profound hearing loss. Usually, low-frequency limits are about 40 dB and high-frequency limits about 75 dB.
4. Once the exposure to noise is discontinued, there is

no substantial further progression of hearing loss as a result of the noise exposure.

5. Previous noise-induced hearing loss does not make the ear more sensitive to future noise exposure. As the hearing threshold increases, the rate of loss decreases.

6. The earliest damage to the inner ears reflects a loss at 3000, 4000, and 6000 Hz. There is always far more loss at 3000, 4000, and 6000 Hz than at 500, 1000, and 2000 Hz. The greatest loss usually occurs at 4000 Hz. The higher and lower frequencies take longer to be affected than the 3000 to 6000 Hz range.

7. Given stable exposure conditions, losses at 3000, 4000, and 6000 Hz usually reach a maximal level in about 10 to 15 years.

8. Continuous noise exposure over the years is more damaging than interrupted exposure to noise, which permits the ear to have a rest period.

COCHLEAR BIOLOGY: CURRENT CONCEPTS

The organ of Corti in the inner ear contains approximately 15,000 hair cells resting on a basilar membrane. These hair cells are arranged in long rows conforming to the spiral shape of the organ of Corti. There are approximately 4000 inner hair cells arranged in a single row and almost three to four times as many outer hair cells, which run in three to five parallel rows. There is a tunnel between the inner and outer hair cells (Fig. 36-1). There are also various types of supporting cells in the inner ear that relate to the nerve fibers as well as to the inner ear. About 95% of the auditory nerve fibers terminate on the inner hair cells and only 5% on the many outer hair cells.[19] As long as there are adequate supporting cells in the inner ear, the nerve fibers do not seem to show much degeneration. If the hair cells and the supporting cells are damaged, however, the nerve fibers supplying them degenerate, so that many cases of sensory hearing loss progress to the sensorineural type.

The hair cells change mechanical vibrations into electrochemical impulses that can be interpreted by the nervous system. As the hairs or cilia covering the tops of the inner and outer hair cells are deflected, an electrical current flows across the top of the cell, leading to a nerve impulse. Outer hair cells are in contact with the tectorial membrane, a gel-like structure that appears to assist in ciliary deflection and restoration of position. Contact between the cilia of the inner hair cells and the tectorial membrane is slight, or possibly nonexistent.[8] The hair cells are contained in the organ of Corti, which rests on the basilar membrane in the cochlear partition. The partition itself also moves because of complex fluid phenomena. Acoustic vibrations result in a wave that travels through the cochlea.[1] Motion of the cochlear partition is important to hearing, and impairment of motion may be responsible for some kinds of hearing loss, including presbycusis. At present, it is believed that the frequency-selective properties of the auditory system are due to mechanical processes within the cochlea, rather than to complex peripheral neural interactions as previously believed. Many of the mysteries of auditory physiology, however, remain unsolved. For example, there is a suggestion that an active, energy-producing system exists in the cochlear partition and is responsible for the sharp mechanical tuning abilities of the ear.[6] This structure, however, has not really been identified or explained. In fact, even the roles of the inner and outer hair cells are not well understood. Several histological peculiarities of the outer hair cells remain unexplained. For example, there are many subsurface layers in the outer hair cells that appear to be specialized for calcium storage, and the cylindrical external surface is surrounded by the fluid of the organ of Corti (in contrast to inner hair cells, which are closely juxtaposed to supporting cells). These outer hair cell findings are not commonly associated with sensory receptor cells, and they suggest that the outer hair cells may be serving functions as yet undiscovered. Interestingly the outer hair cells appear to contain the ingredients associated with active nonmuscle contraction. Nevertheless, it is clear that when outer hair cells are damaged, hearing loss occurs, and the frequency of the hearing loss is directly related to the area of outer hair cell damage. Outer hair cell loss also damages or eliminates fine-tuning capabilities. In addition, absence of the outer hair cells changes markedly the neural output from the cochlea, even though this outflow originates primarily from the inner hair cells.

Despite the many unanswered questions of cochlear physiology, it is clear that, despite the small neural distributions to the outer hair cells, they are extremely important to hearing. They are also fragile. Damage to the auditory system usually is first seen as outer hair cell injury, with noise and direct head trauma typically destroying the outer row of outer hair cells first. Many ototoxic drugs tend to injure initially the inner row of outer hair cells. The maximum hearing loss (threshold shift) that occurs when the outer hair cells are lost is about 50 dB. The hearing loss exceeds 60 dB only when the inner hair cells also become damaged. When all the hair cells are lost, no stimuli are available to excite the nerve endings, and consequently there is no sensation of hearing, although the nerve itself may be intact. Considerably more research is necessary to clarify the functions of even the hair cells, let alone the entire auditory system. The reader is encouraged to consult an excellent summary by Dallos[2] for a review of other concepts in cochlear physiology as well as other sources.

In addition to the afferent bundles from the ear to the brain, there is also an efferent bundle of Rasmussen that carries impulses to the ear from the brain. This efferent tract appears to have a role in the inhibition of impulses, and its fibers appear to stimulate the outer hair cells, causing a change in the mechanical properties of the organ of Corti and cochlear partition.

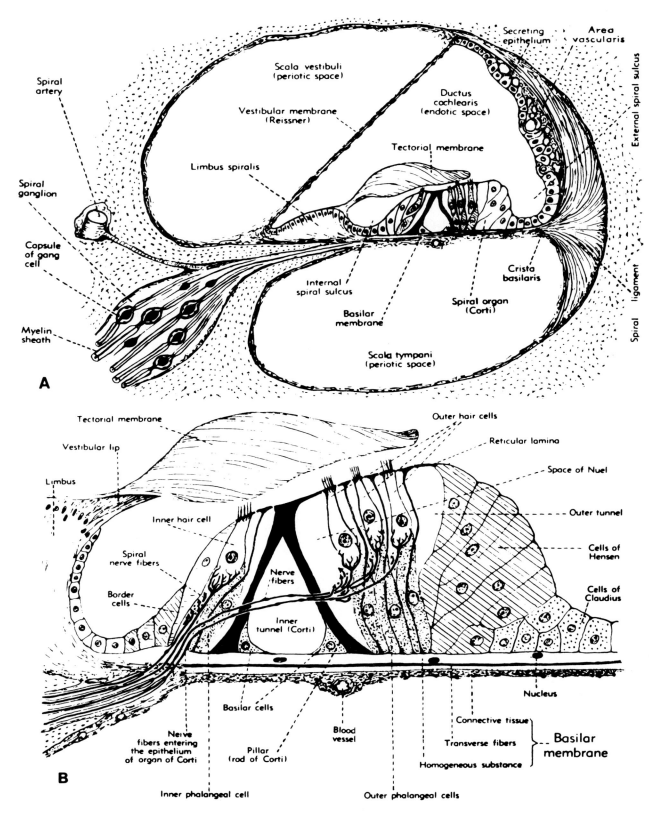

Fig. 36-1. A cross-section of the organ of Corti. **A,** Low magnification. **B,** Higher magnification. (From Sataloff J, Sataloff RT: *Occupational hearing loss,* 2nd ed, New York, 1993, Marcel Dekker, Inc., NY; with permission.)

The relation of the hair cells to the nerve is the basis for explaining the phenomenon of recruitment, which is most evident in endolymphatic hydrops (Ménière's syndrome). It is found also in patients whose hearing has been damaged by certain drugs. The precise explanation for recruitment of loudness in its varying forms still is not clear. The essential element for recruitment is damage to the hair cells that is disproportionately large compared with the nerve fiber supply. The mechanism seems to be that enough hair cells are damaged to reduce the threshold, but enough remain so that when the sounds gets loud enough, a normal number of nerve fibers are excited as if all the hair cells were present. Although this explains most types of recruitment, it does not provide a satisfactory explanation for the phenomenon of hyperrecruitment, in which the sound in the damaged ear is not merely as loud as that in the normal ear but actually is perceived by the patient as even louder. This suggests that the number of nerve impulses ascending the auditory nerve is even greater per unit of time than the normal ear. Patients with hyperrecruitment are those who complain habitually that noises are bothersome and exceptionally loud.

Some patients with damage to the inner ear and marked recruitment can detect small changes in sound intensity, smaller than those that even the normal ear can detect. The ear seems to become ultrasensitive to loudness. This phenomenon technically is called reduced intensity difference-limen or, briefly, reduced difference-limen. Its occurrence has a logical explanation similar to that of recruitment of loudness.

Certain facts should be clarified about the ability of present-day hearing tests to detect damage to the sensorineural pathway. Although an audiogram may show a 0 dB hearing level, which is considered to be normal, it does not necessarily indicate that the sensorineural mechanism is undamaged. Many nerve fibers can be destroyed without affecting threshold hearing for pure tones. As many as 75% of the auditory nerve fibers supplying a certain cochlear area can be sectioned without creating a substantial change in hearing threshold level. This must be considered in the interpretation of hearing tests and in visualizing auditory pathway damage. It also should be borne in mind that when octave bands are measured, acuity in the many frequencies between the octave points measured is unknown (especially in the large area between 4000 and 8000 Hz).

SENSORINEURAL HEARING LOSS

Habitual exposure to occupational noise damages the hair cells in the cochlea, causing a sensory hearing loss. No damage to the outer or middle ear (conductive loss) is caused by routine daily exposure to loud industrial noise. Ultimately, some of the nerve fibers supplying the damaged hair cells may also become damaged from many causes and result in a neural loss of hearing as well.

THE 4000-HZ AUDIOMETRIC DIP

Figure 36-2 shows a composite audiogram of the classic progress of many cases of OHL. This pattern is seen in hearing loss caused by gunfire as well as exposure to continuous noise, such as in weaving mills and some metal plants. The earliest damage occurs between 2000 and 8000 Hz. Some noise sources, such as paper-making machines, can damage the 2000 Hz frequency somewhat before the higher frequencies, whereas noise exposure such as chipping and jackhammers characteristically damages the higher frequencies severely before affecting the lower ones. In general, however, the frequencies below 3000 Hz are almost never damaged by occupational noise without earlier damage to the higher frequencies.

It has been known for many years that prolonged exposure to high-intensity noise results in a classic audiogram showing a 4000 cycle dip in which hearing is better at 2000 and 8000 Hz. Unfortunately the fact that noise produces this 4000-Hz dip has led some physicians to assume that any comparable dip is produced by noise. This error can lead to misdiagnosis and can result in undesirable medical and legal consequences. Although there are numerous hypotheses that attempt to explain the 4000-Hz dip in noise-induced hearing loss,[5,7,17,18] its pathogenesis remains uncertain. It is known, however, that in most cases this loss initially affects hearing between 4000 and 6000 Hz and then spreads to other frequencies.[3,16] Frequencies higher than those usually measured clinically may be tested on special audiometers and are helpful in diagnosing noise-induced hearing loss in selected cases.[11] This hearing loss may re-

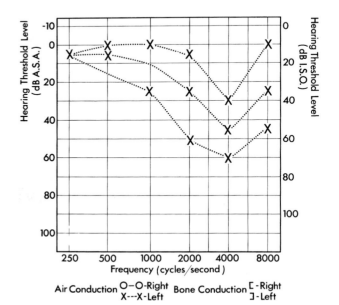

Fig. 36-2. Series of audiometric curves showing a "classic" progressive loss that may be found in employees with excessive noise exposure. (From Sataloff J, Sataloff RT: *Occupational hearing loss,* 2nd ed, New York, 1993, Marcel Dekker, Inc., NY; with permission.)

sult from steady-state or interrupted noise, although the intensities required to produce comparable hearing losses differ,[12] and controversy exists as to the nature of the actual cochlear damage.[4,10,12,23] Noise-induced hearing loss may be temporary or permanent. The 4000-Hz dip is generally bilateral and symmetrical. One common exception is the hearing loss seen in rifle fire: the ear closest to the barrel is worse (left ear in a right-handed shooter) because it is closest to the explosion, and the other ear is protected by the "head shadow." This asymmetry may disappear over time with extensive additional gunfire, particularly from louder weapons. Other types of acoustic trauma, such as that from blast injuries, may result in other audiometric patterns or in a 4000-Hz dip, but they are not considered in this discussion.

It is important to recall that sound of a given frequency spectrum and intensity requires a certain amount of time to produce hearing loss in most subjects. Although the necessary exposure varies from person to person, a diagnosis of noise-induced hearing loss requires a history of sufficient noise exposure. Guidelines for estimating how much noise is necessary to cause hearing loss in most people have been established by the scientific community and the federal government.[15]

HISTOPATHOLOGY OF NOISE-INDUCED HEARING LOSS

Histological studies of human inner ears damaged by noise reveal diffuse degeneration of hair cells and nerves

in the second quadrant of the basal turn of the cochlea, the area sensitive to 3000 to 6000-Hz sounds (Figs. 36-3, 36-4, and 36-5). Similar findings have been demonstrated in cochlear hair cells in first-order neurons in experimental animals exposed to loud noise. The histopathology of noise-induced hearing loss remains a controversial subject, and

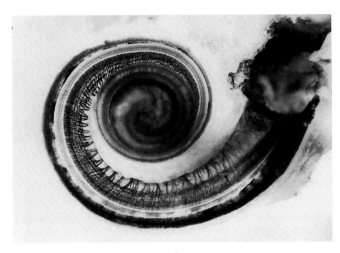

Fig. 36-4. The left cochlea of a 76-year-old male cancer patient with hypertension and generalized arteriosclerosis. Note the patchy degeneration of the organ of Corti in the lower basal turn and the nerve degeneration. This is typical of presbycusis. Paraformaldehyde 11 hours postmortem, Osmium Tetroxide (OsO₄). (Courtesy of Lars-Goran Johnsson; from Sataloff J, Sataloff RT: *Occupational hearing loss,* 2nd ed, New York, 1993, Marcel Dekker, Inc., NY; with permission.)

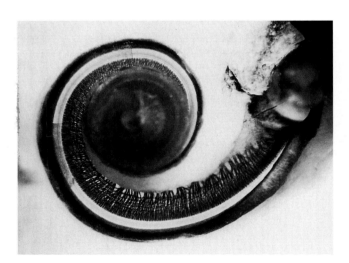

Fig. 36-3. Anterolateral view of the left cochlea from a 17-year-old female car accident victim. Most of the vestibular portion of the membranous wall of the cochlea, Reissner's membrane, and the tectorial membrane have been removed for surface preparations. At 12 o'clock a part of Reissner's membrane is still in situ, and at 9 o'clock, a portion of the spiral ligament is arching over the scala vestibuli. (Courtesy of Lars-Goran Johnsson; from Sataloff J, Sataloff RT: *Occupational hearing loss,* 2nd ed, New York, 1993, Marcel Dekker, Inc., NY; with permission.)

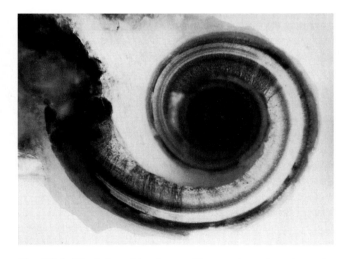

Fig. 36-5. The left cochlea from a 59-year-old male patient who had worked in noisy surroundings and had been an enthusiastic hunter. There is a total loss of hair cells and nerve fibers in the middle of the basal turn. Note in the upper basal turn the presence of nerve fibers in an area where no organ of Corti remains. This appearance is typical of advanced noise-induced hearing loss. Paraformaldehyde 8 hours postmortem, OsO₄. (Courtesy of Lars-Goran Johnsson.)

many questions are still unanswered.[15,20-22] In particular, it is interesting to note that initial damage occurs in the hair cells. Secondary neural degeneration in the area of hair cell damage usually does not occur when only outer hair cells have been destroyed but appears to require damage to inner hair cells as well as supporting cells. No significant neural degeneration has been noted in adjacent areas. In addition, maximal damage to the cochlea secondary to noise exposure is essentially never total.

EXPOSURE TO HAZARDOUS NOISE

Comprehensive understanding of the nature of OHL and the risks of specific noise exposures has been hindered by the difficulties associated with scientific studies in an industrial setting. Sataloff and Sataloff[15] have provided a brief review of the old literature and an in-depth discussion of the most comprehensive recent study highlighting the complexity of the problem and the clinical and scientific findings that form the basis for the guidelines set forth in this chapter. This information is extremely important to anyone attempting to understand this subject and especially to any professional attempting to render judgments regarding causation of a hearing impairment.

Patients who have actually worked for many years on weaving looms, paper-making machines, boilers, sheet metal, riveters, jackhammers, chippers, and the like nearly always have some degree of OHL, especially if they have not worn effective ear protection. Many other patients, however, have marked hearing losses that could not possibly have been caused by their minimal exposures to noise. Almost all patients working in industry can claim that they have been exposed to a great deal of noise. It is essential to get more accurate information by obtaining, if possible, a written work history and time-weighted average of noise exposure from the employer. If a physician does not have firsthand knowledge of the noise exposure in a patient's job, a definitive diagnosis should be delayed until such information is made available.

Many publications have perpetuated the idea that exposures below 90 dBA can produce handicapping hearing losses in the speech frequencies. A critical review of the most quoted publications reveals that all these reports contain serious shortcomings, casting considerable doubt on their conclusions.[15] The Inter-Industry Noise Studies[13,24,25] are the best conducted and monitored research projects relating hearing loss and noise exposure, but even these authors emphasize the need for additional valid and reliable research. The 85 and 90 dB noise exposure levels designated by the Occupational Safety and Health Administration are the levels at which initiation of hearing conservation programs is recommended. They are not necessarily the levels at which hearing becomes impaired in the speech frequencies even after years of exposure. Individuals who have handicapping hearing loss in their speech frequencies and are habitually exposed to less than 90 dBA probably

have hearing losses from other causes. These losses have developed regardless of their jobs. It is important to find the specific causes for their hearing losses rather than to make misleading, unjustified, and hasty diagnoses of OHL.

OHL is a complex problem. Accurate diagnosis requires an understanding of current concepts in cochlear biology, meticulous clinical evaluation, and an accurate assessment of noise exposure. Additional research is needed to answer the many remaining questions regarding pathogenesis and prevention of OHL.

REFERENCES

1. Bekesy G: *Experiments in hearing,* New York, 1960, McGraw-Hill.
2. Dallos P: Cochlear neurobiology: revolutionary developments, American Speech and Hearing Association (ASHA), June/July:50 1988.
3. Gallo R, Glorig A: Permanent threshold shift changes produced by noise exposure and aging, *Am Ind Hyg Assoc J* 25:237, 1964.
4. Johnsson L-G, Hawkins JE: Degeneration patterns in human ears exposed to noise, *Ann Otol Rhinol Laryngol* 85:725, 1976.
5. Kellerhals B: Pathogenesis of inner ear lesions in acute acoustic trauma, *Acta Otolaryngol* 73:249, 1972.
6. Kim DO: Active and nonlinear cochlear biomechanics and the role of outer-hair-cell subsystem in the mammalian auditory system, *Hearing Res* 22:105, 1986.
7. Lawrence M: Current concepts of the mechanism of occupational hearing loss, *Am Ind Hyg Assoc J* 25:269, 1964.
8. Lim DJ: Functional structure of the organ of Corti: a review, *Hearing Res* 22:117, 1986.
9. Orgler GK, et al: American Occupational Medicine Association Noise and Hearing Conservation Committee guidelines for the conduct of an occupational hearing conservation program, *J Occup Med* 29:981, 1987.
10. Salmivalli A: Acoustic trauma in regular Army personnel: clinical audiologic study, *Acta Otolaryngol* 22(suppl):1, 1967.
11. Sataloff J, Vassallo L, Menduke H: Occupational hearing loss and high frequency thresholds, *Arch Environ Health* 14:832, 1967.
12. Sataloff J, Vassallo L, Menduke H: Hearing loss from exposure to interrupted noise, *Arch Environ Health* 18:972, 1969.
13. Sataloff J et al: Intermittent exposure to noise: effects on hearing, *Ann Otol Rhinol Laryngol* 92:623, 1983.
14. Sataloff RT: The 4,000-Hz. audiometric dip: not always noise, *Ear Nose Throat J* 59:251, 1980.
15. Sataloff RT, Sataloff J: *Occupational hearing loss,* 2nd ed, New York, 1993, Marcel Dekker.
16. Schneider EJ, et al: The progression of hearing loss from industrial noise exposure, *Am Ind Hyg Assoc J* 31:368, 1970.
17. Schuknecht HF: *Pathology of the ear,* Cambridge, Mass, 1974, Harvard University Press.
18. Schuknecht HF, Tonndort J: Acoustic trauma of the cochlea from ear surgery, *Laryngoscope* 70:479, 1960.
19. Spoendlin H: *The organization of the cochlear receptor,* Basel, 1966, S. Karger.
20. Spoendlin H: Primary structural changes in the organ of Corti after acoustic over-stimulation, *Acta Otolaryngol* 1:166, 1971.
21. Spoendlin H: Histopathology of nerve deafness, *J Otolaryngol* 14:282, 1985.
22. Spoendlin H, Brun JP: Relation of structural damage to exposure time and intensity in acoustic trauma, *Acta Otolaryngol* 75:220, 1973.
23. Ward D, Fleer RE, Glorig A: Characteristics of hearing losses produced by gunfire and steady noise, *J Audiol Res* 1:325, 1961.
24. Ward WD, Glorig A: Protocol of inter-industry noise study, *J Occup Med* 17:760, 1975.
25. Yerg RA, et al: Inter-industry noise study, *J Occup Med* 20:351, 1978.

Chapter 37

THE EYE

Gordon K. Klintworth
Michael G. Hitchcock

Nutritional deficiencies
    Vitamin A
    Vitamin B complex
    Vitamin C (ascorbic acid)
    Vitamin D (calciferol)
    The vitamin E family (tocopherols)
Nutritional excesses
    Vitamin excesses
    Excessive calcium or vitamin D

As a light receptor, the eye's delicate and sensitive structure is at variance with its exposed location on the face. The eye is protected by the common sense of its owner, natural reflexes, its bony orbit, and thin eyelids. The eye's environment is dictated by nature, especially climate, and human actions, both intentional and unintentional.

Environmental factors may be the primary cause of an eye disease or accentuate a preexisting disorder. For example, photophobia and lacrimation are precipitated in thyroid eye disease by strong light, smoke, wind, or a dry atmosphere.

We have applied an etiologic classification for the different forms of environmental eye injury. Although inevitably there is overlap in the pathogenesis of different injuries, we have attempted to avoid repetition.

ORGANISMS

Countless pathogenic organisms reach the eye and invade the ocular tissues via several routes. They may be inoculated directly onto the conjunctiva by aerosol from the cough of an infected person or contaminated water or be deposited on the eye by flies, unsterile eyedrops, contaminated fingers, a shared towel, or an unsterilized instrument in a physician's office. Accidental or surgical trauma may open the conjunctiva to organisms. Circulating blood brings organisms from distant sites.

Many bacteria, viruses, fungi, chlamydia, protozoa, helminths, and insects may cause ocular disease (see Figs. 37-1 and 37-2). Most bacteria and fungi that grow on the surface of the conjunctiva and eyelids are nonpathogenic and do not invade the underlying tissues unless the ocular mucous membrane is breached. Patients undergoing surgical procedures in the hospital are prone to nosocomial infections.

Parasitic diseases have distinct geographical distributions. For example, those that involve ocular tissues in southeast Asia include gnathostomiasis, dracunculiasis, and sparganosis.

Organisms affecting the eye are discussed first by type; then organisms with specific environmental predisposing factors are discussed.

Types of organisms

Bacteria. Conditions predisposing to bacterial ulcerative keratitis include contact lenses, topical corticosteroids, accidental trauma, dry eyes, trichiasis, and a poor blink reflex. Causes of acute bacterial conjunctivitis include *Neisseria gonorrhoeae, N. meningitidis, Hemophilus influenzae,* staphylococci, and streptococci. Bacterial endophthalmitis most often follows intraocular surgery, accidental penetrating trauma, or bacterial keratitis or scleritis. Although bacterial endophthalmitis is an uncommon complication of cataract extraction (0.09% to 0.5%), the frequency of this procedure produces numerous cases. A considerable number of cases of postsurgical endophthalmitis represent nosocomial infections caused by bacteria on the eyelids and conjunctiva being inadvertently implanted during surgery. Examples include *Staphylococcus epidermidis,* but also *S. aureus, Streptococcus sp., Proteus sp.,* and *Propionibacterium acnes* (the most frequently recovered anerobic microorganism).

The possibility of bacterial endophthalmitis is a major concern in many operations of the eye. For example, the created fistula in individuals undergoing trabeculectomy for glaucoma is a potential path for microorganisms to enter the eye, and infected filtering blebs spread directly and rapidly into the eye.

Viruses. Molluscum contagiosum, which often affects the eyelids, is spread by direct contact with infected cells in showers, swimming baths, sharing of towels, and sexual contact. Papillomavirus probably causes warts and papillomas of the eyelids and conjunctiva as well as squamous dysplasias and carcinomas of the conjunctiva and eyelid.[110,123] Papillomavirus common antigen has been identified in conjunctival papillomas by immunohistochemical methods and in situ hybridization. Human papillomavirus type 16 (HPV 16) has been demonstrated in a recurrent squamous cell carcinoma of the lower eyelid by using the polymerase chain reaction.

A strong causal relationship exists with the Epstein-Barr virus and Burkitt's lymphoma, which often involves the orbit and is the most common cause of proptosis among children in parts of Africa.

Rubella virus infection during the first trimester of pregnancy can cause cataracts, deafness, and mental retardation.[77] Later in pregnancy, the effects are less frequent and less severe.[127]

Cytomegalovirus is the most common opportunistic infection of the retina, and systemic immune suppression predisposes to it. One percent of infants are infected in utero; many others become infected during the first 6 months of life, mostly from breast milk.

Several serotypes of adenovirus (types 8, 10, 19, 37) are responsible for conjunctivitis or keratoconjunctivitis. Sometimes uveitis is associated. This self-limiting infection often occurs in epidemics and can be spread by rubbing the eyes with contaminated hands, by ophthalmologic instruments, and by inadequately chlorinated swimming pools.

Recurrent bouts of herpes simplex keratitis are thought to be triggered by environmental factors that include sunlight and physical trauma.

Chlamydia. Trachoma, the leading cause of blindness

in many developing countries is produced by *Chlamydia trachomatis* serovars A, B, Ba, and C. The disease is most prevalent in dry regions where poor personal hygiene, filth, inadequate public sanitation, and countless flies are features of the environment.[61,94] Infection is spread by several routes, including direct contact, fomites, flies, and contaminated fingers or water. After reproducing within the conjunctival epithelium, *C. trachomatis* elicits a mixed acute and chronic inflammatory cell infiltrate. Lymphoid aggregates and macrophages accumulate in the conjunctival stroma. This chronic infection causes progressive scarring of the conjunctiva and cornea. The eyelids become distorted, and the eyelashes abrade the cornea. The cornea becomes vascularized and opaque, and fibrovascular tissue extends into the cornea between the epithelium and Bowman's layer (pannus). Involved eyes are prone to secondary bacterial infections, and eventually blindness ensues.

Fungi. Factors predisposing to ocular fungal infection include penetrating ocular trauma (especially with plant, wood, and vegetable matter), iatrogenic instrumentation, intravenous catherization, intravenous drug abuse, contaminated irrigating solutions or prosthetic devices (such as contact lenses, punctal occlusive plugs, aqueous shunt tubing, and intraocular lenses), scleral buckling materials, defective operating room air control, topical or systemic corticosteroids and other immunosuppressive agents, treatment of local corneal diseases with topical antibiotics and corticosteroids, cataract extraction with excessive instrumentation, and keratoplasty with contaminated donor storage media.[138]

Some fungi affecting the eye and orbital tissue have characteristic geographic distributions based on the environmental living conditions of the pathogen. Aspergillosis, which may involve the orbit, for example, occurs more commonly in areas with a hot, humid climate. *Coccidioides immitis* is endemic in the southwestern United States, northwestern and central Mexico, Venezuela, and the Gran Chaco Plain of South America. *Blastomyces dermatitidis (Ajellomyces dermatitidis),* the causative agent of North American blastomycosis, is found most frequently in the southeastern United States but also occurs in other areas of the United States, Canada, and Africa. *Histoplasma capsulatum (Emmonsiella capsulata)* is endemic to the Ohio River and Mississippi River valleys and the Appalachian Mountains in the United States and causes a characteristic ocular syndrome (ocular histoplasmosis syndrome) in regions where it is endemic. *Histoplasma duboisii* is found in Nigeria.

A warm, moist climate and an agricultural environment may influence the exposure of healthy eyes to fungi, and the pathogens causing fungal keratitis differ strikingly within geographical areas. Fungal keratitis is infrequent in northern latitudes. In the United States, *Aspergillus, Candida, Cephalosporium,* and *Fusarium* are the most frequently isolated genera. Many fungi are ubiquitous in air, soil, and organic waste, and *Fusarium* is the predominant

cause of fungal keratitis in the southern United States.[95]

The airborne fungi belonging to the Zygomycetes, settle in the paranasal sinuses, and readily enter the orbital tissues, causing severe disease in susceptible hosts such as poorly controlled diabetics.

The conjunctiva, eyelid, or intraocular tissues may become locally infected by *Sporothrix schenckii,* a saprophyte found on plants, green vegetables, and grass. Ocular sporotrichosis has generally been a localized infection, and this fungus rarely causes systemic disease after entering the body at a site of injury. Cryptococcosis that may be acquired from pigeon droppings and unpasteurized cow's milk can affect the eye.

Rhinosporidiosis, caused by the enigmatic *Rhinosporidium seeberi* most often involves the nasal mucosa, producing vascularized polyps. The conjunctiva may also be affected. The disease has been detected in most countries except Australia and New Zealand; it is most prevalent in India and Sri Lanka. The mode of transmission of the etiologic agent, which has been neither grown in culture nor transmitted experimentally, remains unknown, but handling infected horses, cattle, pets, and other animals has been implicated. Water and dust are also suspected of spreading this noncontagious disease. A recent provocative review suggests that the disease is not due to fungus, but is a storage disease due to the defective degradation of ingested tapioca.[3]

Protozoa. Aside from acquiring toxoplasmosis by the accidental ingestion of *Toxoplasma* oocysts from exposure to fecal material from cats, humans may develop the disease by ingesting undercooked beef, pork, or mutton contaminated by *Toxoplasma* cysts. Although cases of this nature can occur in isolation, a major epidemic of ocular toxoplasmosis in Brazil is believed to have been due to the ingestion of contaminated meat.[71] Ocular toxoplasmosis complicates acquired immunodeficiency disorder (AIDS),[79] but this usually results from a reactivation of dormant infection.

Toxoplasma, the most commonly identified cause of retinochoroiditis has two separate developmental cycles. An enteroepithelial cycle comprising asexual and sexual stages of reproduction occurs within the feline ileum. It gives rise to oocysts, which are shed in large numbers in the feces of the cat after a brief infective illness. The oocysts remain viable in soil and dirt for many months, depending upon climatic conditions. An extraintestinal cycle also takes place in the cat and other warm-blooded animals, including humans.

Approximately 10% of children born to mothers infected by *Toxoplasma* during pregnancy (evidenced by seroconversion) manifest congenital toxoplasmosis. The risk of congenital toxoplasmosis relates to when maternal infection occurs. The protozoon is particularly likely to be transmitted to the fetus when the mother acquires toxoplasmosis during the final month of pregnancy. The infection, however, will be subclinical in infancy. Earlier maternal infec-

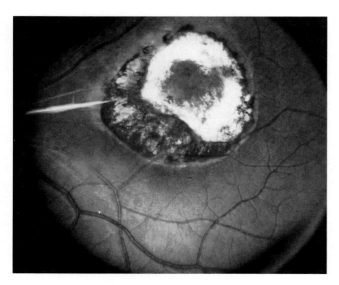

Fig. 37-1. Toxoplasmosis of the macula has produced a large atrophic scar surrounded by a rim of pigment epithelium hyperplasia. (From Klintworth GK, Landers MB III: *The eye: structure and function in disease*, Baltimore, 1976, Williams & Wilkins; with permission.)

tion less often involves the fetus but commonly causes severe disease. Most frequently they develop retinochoroiditis during childhood. Many patients with toxoplasmic retinochoroiditis present for the first time as young adults.

The typical retinochoroidal lesion is a granuloma (Fig. 37-1) with central coagulative necrosis surrounded by lymphocytes, plasma cells, epithelioid cells, and occasional giant cells. *Toxoplasma* may be evident within the central and surrounding areas. Retinal necrosis is usually striking, and the subjacent choroid is necrotic or is replaced by epithelioid cells. Lymphocytes and plasma cells frequently infiltrate the surrounding choroid. Free-living *Acanthamoeba* can cause serious keratitis, live mainly in stagnant water, and are present in many water supplies. These worldwide facultative parasites can withstand the heat of a bath tub as well as near-freezing swimming water.[33] *Acanthamoeba castellani* and *A. polyphaga* account for most cases of amoebic keratitis.[19,31,33,160] Initial reports of acanthamoeba keratitis followed trauma, but far more cases are linked with wearing contact lenses.

The microsporidial protozoan *Nosema* most frequently parasitizes fish and arthropods. *Nosema cuniculi* differs in normally residing in mammals, especially rodents, and rarely it has been identified in humans. Exceptional examples of nosemal keratitis have been reported from Sri Lanka, Botswana, and the southern United States.[18,146] One of these cases was a boy who developed a necrotizing stromal keratitis 6 years after being gored by a goat.[18] Ocular nosematosis has been reported in the absence of antecedent trauma in several mammalian species including the cat and blue fox.[14,18] Microsporidia may also infect the cornea in

persons with AIDS.[116] The lesions consist of an acute inflammatory reaction with stromal vascularization, and reparative scarring *Nosema* are present within macrophages and lying free.

The bite of tsetse flies transmits trypanosomes to humans, causing trypanosomiasis. African trypanosomiasis caused by *Trypanosoma brucei* sometimes produces pronounced urticaria of the eyelids, often with preauricular lymphadenopathy and uveitis, as well as inflammation of the corneal stroma. Trypanosomes may even be observed in the aqueous. In parts of Central and South America, bites of tsetse flies infected with *T. cruzi* cause South American trypanosomiasis (Chagas' disease). Pronounced unilateral eyelid swelling and periorbital edema and conjunctivitis (Romaña's sign) commonly ensue. In contrast to African trypanosomiasis, intraocular lesions have not been documented.

Ocular complications are not usual in leishmaniasis, although bilateral anterior uveitis, sometimes complicated by angle-closure glaucoma, may follow visceral leishmaniasis (kala azar). These abnormalities probably result from allergic phenomena and not from a direct infection by *Leishmania donovani*. The ulcers or elevated nodules of granulomatous inflammation of cutaneous leishmaniasis caused by the inoculation of *L. mexicana* and *L. braziliensis* during bites of the sandfly (usually *Phlebotomus* spp.) predominate on exposed skin surfaces including the eyelids. Conjunctival and corneal lesions are rare.

Helminths

Tapeworms. Patients with cysticercosis, the parasitic disease caused by the ingestion of eggs from the pig tapeworm *(Taenia solium),* frequently have an intraocular cyst.[100] Although persons with the tapeworm can develop cysticercosis, especially by poor personal hygiene, a major source of this condition is food contaminated by affected unhealthy food attendants.

Hydatid cysts derived from the ingestion of the eggs of *Echinococcus granulosus (Taenia echinococcus)* usually form in the liver and other tissue sites. On rare occasions, the orbit is involved,[75] but, unlike cysticercosis, an intraocular location is not a feature.

Retrobulbar neuropathy occasionally complicates the vitamin B_{12} deficiency caused by the fish tapeworm *(Diphyllobothrium latum).*[25]

Sparganosis caused by the plerocercoid larvae of *Spirometra* is often acquired in southeast Asia from the eating of raw or inadequately cooked meat of infected frogs, snakes, and mammals.[100] It may also be acquired from infected frog flesh applied to open wounds and inflamed eyes as a poultice. This amphibian is an intermediate host in the life cycle of diphyllobothriid tapeworms of the genus *Spirometra,* and the larva may leave the amphibian tissue to enter those of humans, producing sparganosis. Sparganosis may also be acquired by ingesting contaminated water or the meat of infected animals. After initial conjunctival edema, a nodule may form on the eyelids and orbit.[54,133,178]

Nematodes. Onchocerciasis, the most significant parasitic disease affecting the eye, is caused by the nematode *Onchocerca volvulus,* which produces keratitis, pannus formation, anterior uveitis, chorioretinitis, and secondary glaucoma. *Onchocerca volvulus* is transmitted by bites of infected black simulian flies (*Simulium* sp.), which breed in certain swift-running rivers in parts of tropical west Africa, South America, Guatemala, and Mexico. Following the death of intracorneal microfilariae, an inflammatory response causes corneal opacification, secondary glaucoma, and visual impairment ("river blindness").

The ingestion of raw or inadequately cooked infected meat from several wild and domesticated animals, but especially pork, infested with *Trichinella spiralis* causes trichinosis. The eating of infected mollusks can also cause trichinosis. The myositis produced by larvae of this roundworm involves the striated skeletal muscle, including the extraocular muscles.

Loiasis, caused by the filarial nematode *Loa loa,* occurs in the rainforests of central and west Africa. It is transmitted by the bite of mango flies. The threadlike migrating adult worm often crosses the globe within the subconjunctival tissues, hence the connotation African "eyeworm." Migrating worms do not elicit an inflammatory reaction, but static worms become surrounded by neutrophils, eosinophils, plasma cells lymphocytes, and foreign body granulomatous reaction with multinucleated giant cells. The eyelids may become swollen and itchy.

The nematodes *Toxocara canis* and *T. cati* (*T. mystax*) live in the intestine of dogs and cats, respectively. The parasites affect humans if they ingest the embryonated ova. After hatching, the other larvae invade the intestinal wall and travel to the liver and then to other tissues via the systemic circulation. Sometimes the *Toxocara* settle in retinal and other ocular vessels and produce small granulomas that may cause a unilateral loss of vision, and the lesions may simulate a retinoblastoma clinically.

Of the several species of *Baylisascaris,* one associated with raccoons (*B. procyonis*) has caused a fatal illness in humans and may cause ocular disease.[98,99]

Thelaziasis, which affects only the eye in humans, is caused by *Thelazia callipaeda* (oriental eye worm) or *T. californiensis.* Humans are incidental hosts of this helminthic disease that is probably transmitted by flies, but the mode of transmission remains unknown.[100]

A possible association has been noted between malignant Mooren's corneal ulcer in African males with *Ascaris lumbricoides* and *Ancylostoma.*[101,161]

Insects. Lesions in the eye may be of the foreign body type, as in ophthalmia nodosa (see the section on Foreign Bodies); venomous, as in bee and wasp stings (see the section on Animal Venoms); or because of the direct invasion of the ocular tissues, as in ophthalmomyiasis. In ophthalmomyiasis, the nature of the botfly depends on the inter-

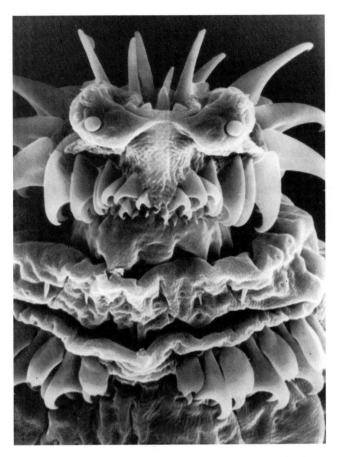

Fig. 37-2. Scanning electron micrograph of a horse botfly larva, *Gasterophilus intestinalis.*

mediate host—cattle (cattle botfly, *Hypoderma bovis*), horse (horse botfly, *Gasterophilus* spp.) (Fig. 37-2), sheep (sheep botfly, *Oestrus ovis*), or rodents (*Cuterebra*)—and the prevalence varies with the geographical area. The ocular lesions vary with the botfly species. Some botfly larvae, such as *O. ovis,* remain within the conjunctival sac, causing an external ophthalmomyiasis, but the larva of other botflies, such as *Cuterebra,* can penetrate the globe and burrow through the sclera and into the eye, where that may cause pain, visual symptoms, and a characteristic linear destruction of the retinal pigment epithelium (internal ophthalmomyiasis).[44] The life cycle of botflies normally involves an intermediate animal host, and the human eye is usually involved only accidently after a botfly egg reaches the moist conjunctival sac and hatches, liberating the first instar larva.

Modes of spread

Contaminated food. Diseases affecting the eye that are spread by the eating of inadequately cooked meat that contains the living parasite include angiostrongylosis, cysticercosis, hydatid cysts, sparganosis, toxoplasmosis, paragonimiasis, gnathostomiasis, and trichinosis (see the previous section on Helminths). Angiostrongylosis results from eating infected raw mollusks, prawns, crabs or planarians or vegetables contaminated with mucus from infected mollusks. Paragonimiasis is acquired by eating infected raw or undercooked crustaceans such as crabs and crayfish. Gnathostomiasis is transmitted by eating raw and infected fish, chicken, pork, frogs, or snakes.

During times of food shortage in the Middle Ages, many devastating epidemics resulted from ergotism caused by the eating of rye contaminated with the ergot fungus *(Claviceps purpurea)*.[20] During acute ergotism, retinal vessels undergo a temporary vasoconstriction, and retinal edema is accompanied by an amblyopia with a central scotoma and contracted peripheral visual field.[97]

Airborne organisms. The eye is constantly exposed to a wide variety of bacteria, fungi, and viruses that reach the ocular surface from the air. Most bacteria and fungi that grow on the surface of the conjunctiva and eyelids are nonpathogenic. Certain highly virulent bacteria such as *Neisseria gonorrhoeae, N. meningitidis,* and *Corynebacterium diphtheriae* are capable of directly invading the cornea, but most bacteria cannot penetrate intact corneal epithelium.

Contaminated water. Many microorganisms survive in inadequately chlorinated swimming pools. Adenovirus is spread in this way and causes swimming pool conjunctivitis.[184] Molluscum contagiosum, which often produces nodular lesions of the eyelid and chronic keratoconjunctivitis, may also be transmitted in swimming pools.[55]

Acanthamoeba survive in solutions for storing contact lenses. The earlier widespread use of salt tablets dissolved in tap water appeared to be a source of some of these infections. *Pseudomonas* is another organism known to live in solutions for storing contact lenses.

Parasitic diseases affecting the eye that are transmitted by drinking water include dracunculiasis and cysticercosis. Entering water that contains *Schistosoma* leads to schistosomiasis.

Insects. Several parasitic diseases affecting the ocular tissues are inoculated into humans by the bites of insects: *onchocerciasis* (black flies), loiasis (mango flies), African trypanosomiasis (tsetse flies), leishmaniasis (sandfly), malaria, dirofilariasis, bancroftian and Brugian filariasis (mosquitoes), South American trypanosomiasis (reduviid bugs). Another disease affecting the eye is spread by the bites of deer ticks; Lyme disease is caused by *Borrelia burgdorferi.*[193] Rickettsial diseases are transmitted by ticks (Rocky Mountain spotted fever, boutonneuse fever, Queensland tick fever, Siberian tick fever), fleas (murine endemic typhus), human body lice (epidemic typhus, trench fever), rat louse (endemic typhus), mites (rickettsial pox, scrub typhus), and other blood-sucking arthropods. Flies *(Musca domestica)* also contribute to the spread of trachoma, and they are suspected of transmitting thelaziasis.

Exposure to animals. Animals that spread diseases to the ocular tissues include cats (toxoplasmosis, cat scratch fever, toxocariasis), fowl (Newcastle disease), sheep *(Oestrus ovis),* dogs (toxocariasis), raccoons *(Baylisascaris),* pigeons (cryptococcosis), bats (histoplasmosis), rodents *(Cuterebra),* caterpillars (ophthalmia nodosa), frogs (gnathostomiasis, sparganosis), fish (gnathostomiasis), pigs (trichinosis, gnathostomiasis), chicken (gnathostomiasis), crabs (angiostrongylosis, paragonimiasis), crayfish (paragonimiasis), crustaceans (paragonimiasis), mollusks (angiostrongylosis), prawns (angiostrongyliasis), and snakes (gnathostomiasis).

The cat scratch bacillus *(Rochalimaea hensalae)* is the most common cause of Parinaud's oculoglandular syndrome, a suppurative granulomatous conjunctivitis with preauricular necrotizing granulomatous lymphadenitis with stellate abscesses.[188] Infection follows inoculation, especially by the claws of cats, but sometimes the conjunctiva is contaminated by close contact with a cat, perhaps by licking around the eye.

Newcastle disease virus induces a fatal pneumonitis in fowl and can cause severe unilateral follicular conjunctivitis in humans.

Filth. Filth predisposes to trachoma where the disease is endemic. *Baylisascaris* and toxocariasis are spread by the oral ingestion of food or other materials contaminated with the parasitic ova.

Unknown. The mode of transmission of some diseases affecting the eye, such as rhinosporidiosis and thelaziasis, is unknown.

Microorganisms are a common cause of diarrhea, and individuals with severe diarrhea are at risk for cataracts, according to a case-control study of 300 patients with cataracts and 609 age-matched controls in Oxfordshire, England.[185] Other studies, such as one in southern India, do not support the hypothesis that individuals with a positive history of severe diarrhea are at increased risk of developing visually disabling cataracts.[23]

ATMOSPHERE

Oxygen can form unstable free radicals, especially superoxide and hydroxyl ions, which are lethal to cells in high concentration. Defense mechanisms against oxygen radicals include superoxide dismutase, catalase, and glutathione peroxidase. Other naturally occurring antioxidants are vitamin E (tocopherol) and vitamin C (see Chapter 21).

If defenses are insufficient, the radicals are reduced by electrons from lipids within intracellular membranes. This lipoperoxidation damages mitochondria and other organelles. Enzyme systems involving sulfhydryl groups and oxidation of glutathione are inhibited.

Oxidative stress is believed to be important in age-related cataractogenesis. Oxygen species cause proteins such as the lens crystallins to aggregate and precipitate.[24,170] Exogenous photooxidation and endogenous reduction of oxygen may occur. The antioxidant status of people as measured by serum levels of vitamin E, vitamin C, and carotenoids at different ages, with and without cataracts, support this view. However, data linking blood levels to lens concentrations of these substances are lacking, (see Chapter 9).

Numerous microorganisms within the atmosphere are disseminated to the surface of the eye via the air (see the section on Organisms).

Exposure to oxygen

Hyperbaric oxygen. Hyperbaric oxygen chambers are used to treat a variety of diseases, including radionecrosis. Oxygen at elevated atmospheric pressure causes myopia, mainly in individuals at least 50 years old. It seems to result from a change in the refractive power of the crystalline lens.[8,9] This usually resolves completely after exposure is discontinued.

The lenses of several species can be damaged by excessive oxygen. The lens epithelium of guinea pigs is damaged by elevated oxygen tensions[137] and cataracts have been created in mice with oxygen.[162]

Hypoxia. Retinal hemorrhages, which may be asymptomatic, and edema of the optic nerve head occur at high altitudes in acute mountain illness and high-altitude edema.[37]

Ambient oxygen. The crystalline lens is continually exposed to light and ambient oxygen; even at normal oxygen levels, oxidative stress is believed to affect the lens and to be important in age-related cataractogenesis. The lens contains defense mechanisms against toxic products of oxygen and can readily detoxify exogenous hydrogen peroxide. However, a possible association between some human cataracts and elevated levels of aqueous hydrogen peroxide has generated considerable interest in the role of the glutathione redox cycle and the pentose phosphate pathway in protecting the lens from hydrogen peroxide toxicity. Photooxidative damage hence is suspected of being an important high-risk factor in age-related and other forms of cataractogenesis. Comparative studies of the incidence of cataracts in different countries support the notion that some cataracts are related to the intensity and duration of sunlight, particularly ultraviolet light (see Chapters 10 and 21).

The retinopathy of prematurity (ROP, or retrolental fibroplasia) occurs in the retina of premature infants (Fig. 37-3). It is characterized by the formation of proliferating fibrovascular tissue at the junction of the vascularized and yet to be vascularized portions of the retina. By spreading onto the retinal surface, this abnormal fibrovascular tissue frequently causes tractional retinal detachment, which in a small percentage of cases results in a retrolental mass.

Although the clinical aspects of this entity were initially defined by Terry in 1942,[182] a decade passed before the link with oxygen therapy was established. Epidemiologic data implicated the oxygen-enriched incubators used for nursing premature newborn babies. The relationship to oxygen was later established in a controlled clinical trial[144] and in experimental animal studies.[16,17,143]

There are five clinical stages, beginning at the margin of the developing vasculature: stage 1, demarcation line;

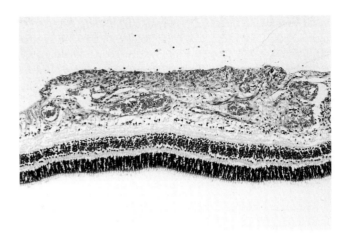

Fig. 37-3. Pronounced vascularization is evident in the inner portion of this retina following the cessation of oxygen administration to a new premature infant. (Hematoxylin and eosin ×74.) (From Klintworth GK, Landers MB III: *The eye: structure and function in disease*, Baltimore, 1976, Williams & Wilkins; with permission.)

stage 2, ridge; stage 3, ridge with extraretinal fibrovascular proliferation; stage 4, subtotal retinal detachment; and stage 5, total retinal detachment. The condition may arrest spontaneously, particularly in the early stages.

Microscopic correlates of these stages are as follows: A thin rim of tissue consisting of spindle-shaped cells and differentiating endothelium is normally located anterior to the developing retinal vasculature. In early ROP, both cell types undergo hyperplasia, and the normally inapparent border between the vascularized and avascular retina becomes clinically visible. With further proliferation, the surface forms a ridge. Developing blood vessels and glial tissue within the ridge may penetrate the retinal inner limiting lamina to emerge on the retinal surface. Further proliferation of the extraretinal tissue leads to vascular invasion of the vitreal cavity and, depending on the severity of the vitreoretinal proliferation, variable degrees of retinal detachment ensue. With total retinal detachment, the retina and extraretinal fibrovascular tissue may then be pulled anteriorly toward the back of the lens in the final cicatricial phase that evoked the name *retrolental fibroplasia*.

Only blood vessels at the retinal periphery are affected in older, near-term babies. The circulation on the temporal side of the retina is the last to be established, being farthest from the optic nerve head, and the effects of oxygen toxicity at this stage are prone to provoke neovascularization in this region alone.

The vasoproliferative disease is presumably preceded by retinal ischemia as retinal vessels initially undergo an autoregulatory vasoconstriction in response to high levels of inspired oxygen, according to animal studies. Eventually endothelial cells degenerate, starting with the most recently differentiated cells.

Despite usually increased activity with hyperoxia, superoxide dismutase decreases in neonatal kittens exposed to high levels of oxygen. Low levels of vitamin E in premature infants may leave the premature retina inadequately prepared to cope with slight increases in oxygen. Retinal metabolism in utero is predominantly anerobic. The retinal capillaries of some extremely small babies may not tolerate normal atmospheric oxygen concentrations. In some instances, arterial blood oxygen levels are within normal limits, but their carbon dioxide values are strikingly elevated. Hypercapnia may prevent the arteriolar constriction response to hyperoxia and increase oxygen delivery to the retina.

Through rigorous monitoring of the oxygen content in incubators and the blood oxygen of neonates, the incidence of ROP has diminished, but it remains a problem because of difficulties in balancing the prevention of ROP with adequate cerebral oxygenation in the newborn.

Airborne allergens and pollutants

Pollens and other airborne allergens can lead to hay fever, as well as vernal and other forms of allergic conjunctivitis (see Chapters 6 and 25). Some allergens can settle on contact lens and precede allergic reactions, such as giant follicular conjunctivitis. Severe air pollution by chemicals, as in smog, can irritate the eye and produce an acute keratoconjunctivitis (see Chapter 2).

Atmospheric pollutants and other potentially toxic substances are detoxified in the lens by glutathione S-transferases, a group of enzymes that catalyze the conjugation of a diverse group of foreign chemicals to glutathione. Some forms of glutathione S-transferase express selenium-independent glutathione peroxidase II activity toward lipid hydroperoxides.

Evaporation

Environmental factors, such as arid air, that predispose to evaporation can also adversely effect the eye. Evaporation from the cornea may lead to supersaturation and precipitation of calcium ions in the superficial cornea, particularly in the interpalpebral region. The importance of evaporation in the genesis of corneal calcification is underscored by experimental studies in which calcific band keratopathy is accentuated by open eyes and prevented by eyelid closure. The precipitation of the calcium in the superficial cornea may follow a reduced solubility of calcium caused by the rise in pH produced by the loss of carbon dioxide.[42]

Excessive evaporation of the secretions on the surface of the eye exposes the cornea to desiccation, resulting in a distinct disorder of the ocular mucous membrane (keratoconjunctivitis sicca). Other causes of this dry eye syndrome include the Stevens-Johnson syndrome, toxic epidermal necrolysis, avitaminosis A, trachoma, chemical burns, and irradiation of the eyelids. The corneal epithelium may desquamate as filamentous threads (filamentous keratopathy), and secondary infection often ensues.

TOXIC AGENTS

Numerous chemicals, detergents, cosmetics, and animal toxins are deleterious to the eye and its adjacent structures. Some medicines also have toxic side effects, and an extensive literature on ocular toxicology exists.[59,65,76,147] As a group, toxic injuries only account for a minor proportion of human blindness. Some toxins affecting the ocular tissues follow occupational exposure in industry (such as carbon disulfide, toluene diisocyanate, silver, platinum, organic solvents, hydroquinones, or quinones), agriculture (pesticides), health care (ethylene gas), domestic situations (lead, cosmetics, polychlorobiphenyl, detergents, drain cleaners), and war (nerve gas). Children suffer a disproportionate number of domestic chemical injuries.

These toxic chemicals may be inorganic, such as battery hydrochloric acid, or organic, such as hydrocarbons. Some are refined or made by humans; others exist free in nature within living plants or animals. Most toxic chemicals affecting the eye reach it in a gaseous, liquid, or solid state by direct contamination. Other toxins reach the ocular tissues via the bloodstream after their ingestion or inhalation.

Adverse corneal responses to toxins may occur immediately but frequently become manifest only after chronic exposure.[65]

Evidence for an oncogenic role of chemicals in ocular tumors is weak, but the prevalence of choroidal melanoma was greater than expected in a population of current and former workers at a chemical plant that produced a variety of suspected carcinogens.[4]

The severity of chemical injury from direct ocular exposure depends on the concentration of the substance, its chemical and physical properties, and the duration of contact. The last is influenced by the victim's speed of blink and avoidance of exposure, as well as the rapidity with which the substance is diluted, either by lacrimation or irrigation. Solubility and the ability of the chemical to penetrate the ocular tissue are of prime importance. Materials such as lime that adhere to the conjunctiva and dissolve slowly are particularly dangerous. The corneal epithelium and corneal endothelium, as well as the conjunctival epithelium, present barriers to ionized substances that otherwise pass with ease through the outer coat; the reverse situation applies to lipids. A substance with dual properties can achieve the greatest and most rapid penetration. Enzymes and/or structural proteins are damaged reversibly or irreversibly by a wide variety of substances, and cell death may then result. Because of space restrictions, only a few of the common classes of chemicals that are hazardous to the eye are discussed here.

Following exposure to one of numerous chemical agents, the ocular surface membrane may develop a nonspecific conjunctivitis, keratoconjunctivitis or another toxic reaction.

In many countries, consumer products are required to be

tested for ocular toxicity in animal models. Debates focus on the validity of different test protocols, such as the concentration of product to apply, and the most appropriate animal subject, if any, to use.[152]

Acids

An inadvertent splash of acid, such as that from an automobile battery, in the eye is capable of causing serious damage. Because acid substances denature and coagulate proteins, the corneal and conjunctival epithelia are destroyed on contact with acid and may later slough. However, the insoluble acid proteinates that form become barriers to deeper penetration of the acid and although external injury may be severe, the inner eye usually remains intact. If the acid is concentrated, however, the entire cornea and its cellular elements can be completely devastated. In contrast to alkalis, lipoidal barriers are not destroyed, and the tendency toward symblepharon and corneal vascularization is usually less following acid burns than after alkali burns. Corneal thinning and necrosis may be followed by adherence of the conjunctiva to the cornea (pseudopterygium) and an accumulation of abundant polymorphonuclear leukocytes in the ocular anterior chamber (hypopyon). Hydrofluoric acid penetrates the corneal stroma and leads to endothelial damage, iridocyclitis, trabecular meshwork destruction, and secondary glaucoma.

Alkalis. Dishwashing detergents in both solid and liquid form typically have an alkaline pH. Sodium hydroxide is used as a drain cleaner because of its effectiveness in denaturing the proteins present in hair, which often block drains. Similar potency is evident in eye contact. Ocular burns from alkali may be willfully inflicted.

Cell death is immediate when alkali reaches the cornea. Unlike acids, alkalis saponify the lipids, resulting in the disintegration of cell membranes. The bulbar surface epithelium may slough. Keratocytes and the corneal endothelium may be destroyed; if the alkali penetrates deeper, the lens, iris, and ciliary body may also be damaged. A pronounced acute inflammatory reaction ensues. The corneal stroma that first becomes devitalized and edematous may appear to melt away and eventually becomes thinned, vascularized, and scarred. With destruction of the epithelial stem cells at the corneoscleral limbus, corneal ulceration and sometimes perforation result from inadequate epithelial regeneration. In the absence of surviving corneal or corneoscleral limbal epithelium, conjunctival epithelium may slowly migrate over the corneal surface. Damage to the epithelial basement membrane retards healing further, and degradation of the components of the extracellular matrix in the basement membrane may result in a poorly adherent epithelium. Destruction of the trabecular meshwork, together with an associated iridocyclitis, can lead to peripheral anterior synechiae and a secondary closed-angle glaucoma. Corneal clouding follows corneal endothelial destruction, and the lens almost invariably becomes cataractous. Collagenase,

which is elaborated by the injured ingrowing epithelium and by polymorphonuclear leukocytes, enters the devitalized tissue and accounts for the "corneal melting" observed clinically and experimentally.[32] The action of collagenase is facilitated by a reduction in extracellular matrix that is consistently found in alkali-burned corneas, or possibly by a partial denaturation of stromal collagen.

Methanol

Methanol may contaminate ethanol preparations. It is also used as a solvent, as an antifreeze solution, and as a fuel. Human methanol poisoning is characterized by formic acidemia. Aside from causing death and central nervous system dysfunction, methanol ingestion can lead to serious visual impairment and blindness. The effects of methanol intoxication include blurred vision, loss of central vision, and complete blindness some 18 to 48 hours after ingestion. Hyperemia and edema of the optic nerve head and surrounding retina occur in some individuals, whose vision later becomes permanently impaired.[22] Following methanol intoxication, persons with marked metabolic acidosis develop optic atrophy, which is sometimes followed by severe retinal edema. One catastrophe involved 320 persons who ingested a mixture containing 35% methanol and 15% ethanol.[22]

Species differences in methanol metabolism have made it difficult to study its ocular toxicity. Methanol toxicity is ordinarily restricted to humans and nonhuman primates. In the rhesus monkey, methanol intoxication conspicuously affects the optic nerve instead of the retina and produces edema of the optic disc as well as mydriasis and a poor pupillary response to light.[21]

Retinal edema and photoreceptor degradation occur in animal models. It has been suggested that stasis in the flow of materials along optic nerve axons is the critical injury in methanol poisoning. Other species are resistant to the accumulation of formate and the associated metabolic and visual toxicity. An understanding of the ocular effect of methanol has been aided by the development of a rodent model of methanol-induced visual toxicity.[58,134] The oxidation of methanol's toxic metabolite, formic acid, is inhibited in rats treated with subanesthetic concentrations of nitrous oxide, and these animals develop formic acidemia, metabolic acidosis, and visual toxic reactions after methanol intoxication analogous to human methanol poisoning[134] Electroretinographic and morphologic abnormalities in the retina occur; generalized retinal edema, vacuolation in the photoreceptors, and retinal pigment epithelium follow methanol administration, as well as swollen and disrupted mitochondria in the photoreceptor inner segments, optic nerve, and the retinal pigment epithelium.[134] Visual dysfunction as reflected by reductions in the flash-evoked cortical potential and electroretinogram (ERG) occurs coincident with blood formate accumulation. Alterations in the ERG take place at formate concentrations lower than those associated with other visual alterations and supply a functional indication of direct retinal toxicity in the toxicity of methanol.[58]

Metals

After prolonged exposure to heavy metals, such as silver, gold, and mercury, the conjunctiva, cornea, and other ocular tissues may become pigmented from the tissue deposition of the metal (see Chapter 4).

Silver. Silver solutions have traditionally been instilled into neonatal eyes as sterilizing agents to prevent gonococcal ophthalmitis. A long-term side effect of this medication is corneal and conjunctival argyrosis. Similar pigmentary changes in the cornea have been noted in the silver industry in persons producing silver nitrate, silver oxide, and silver solder.[132,164,171] Silver pigmentation of the lacrimal sac may also occur.[171]

Copper. Copper and its alloys incite suppuration, with hypopyon, and a vitreous abscess leading to retinal detachment and ultimately phthisis bulbi. A less pronounced reaction may lead to a slow retinal degeneration. With a slow diffusion of copper from an intraocular foreign body composed of a copper alloy, a green-blue ring may appear in the peripheral cornea at the level of Descemet's membrane, and the iris, zonular fibrils, and vitreous framework may become discolored (chalcosis). The deposition of copper in the deeper layers of the anterior lens capsule produces a cataract characterized by colorful powdery opacities arranged as a central disk with radiating petal-like spokes (sunflower cataract), and tiny metallic flecks often form on the retina.

Iron. An iron-containing foreign body may severely damage and discolor ocular structures. The retina is particularly sensitive to iron and is injured early, but staining is late and not in areas where the retina is most damaged. As the ocular structures become discolored, the foreign body may diminish in size and even disappear completely. Iron diffuses throughout the eye to be taken up by cells of the iris, ciliary body, choroid, and cornea. Retinal detachment or chorioretinal adhesions may also occur. Frequently, as a late event, injury to the trabecular meshwork and an infiltration of iron-laden macrophages in the anterior chamber angle cause glaucoma. Clinical and experimentally produced siderosis bulbi secondary to intraocular blood can damage the outer retina and discolor the ocular tissues similarly.

Iron overload, as in South African Bantu consumption of large amounts of iron-rich beer and food cooked in iron pots, may develop a gold-brown ring at the corneoscleral limbus[69] (see Chapter 9).

Platinum. Platinum and its salts are allergens and produce marked irritation of mucous membranes as well as the skin.[155] Soluble compounds are more toxic than the insoluble metallic forms.

Lead. Lead poisoning is a concern around older houses with flaking paint. Low- to moderate-level exposure to lead causes chronic damage to the retinal rods.[63,132,164] Optic disc edema may also occur.[78]

Other metals. Optic neuritis may accompany arsenic poisoning,[172] and papilledema occurs with gold, mercury, and thallium toxicity.[78] Mercurial vapors and phenylmercuric nitrate can cause calcific band keratopathy.[192]

Other organic compounds

Pesticides. Workers with pesticides are exposed to organophosphates, organochlorines (including dichlorodiphenyltrichloroethane [DDT]), and other chemicals. Fenthion is associated with altered pigmentation about the fovea of the retina, which reduces vision in many subjects. Abnormal ocular movements evoked by pesticides include an abnormal spontaneous and rapid conjugate movement of the eyes in the vertical plane with a slow return to the midposition (atypical ocular bobbing) as documented in acute poisoning with organophosphate pesticides.[84]

Dioxin. Chloracne, an acneform eruption, often follows the ingestion of chlorinated phenolic agents such as dioxins[27,153] (see Chapter 27; Color Plate 7). It may also follow many years after a chemical industrial explosion liberating tetrachlorodibenzo-p-dioxin.[153] The eyelids are often involved and conjunctivitis may also be present. Chloracne may persist for years and differs from acne vulgaris in the distribution and appearance of the lesions. Sometimes xerotic skin, pigmentation, and follicular hyperkeratosis are associated. The primary lesion is a follicular plug containing keratinous material.[197] Chemical workers exposed to chlorinated dioxins are at risk of developing chloracne, with the incidence noted as highest among the youngest workers and among those who worked in the production of chlorinated phenols rather than with products derived from those materials.[27]

Aldehydes. Solutions of formaldehyde used as a tissue fixative in pathology release a vapor that is irritating to the eyes and respiratory system but does not appear to have long-term effects in humans.[186] The eyes of nurses and technicians are exposed to the irritant chemical glutaraldehyde when they disinfect endoscopes used for examination of the bowel in patients.[136]

Polychlorobiphenyl. The accidental addition of polychlorobiphenyl (PCB), with components of polychlorodibenzofuran and polychloroquaterphenyl, to rice oil used for food caused serious intoxication in an area of Japan in the late 1960s (called Yusho).[15] There were severe cutaneous and mucous membrane eruptions resembling acne. A separate series of cases in Taiwan in the early 1980s showed swelling and abnormal pigmentation of the conjunctiva, hypersecretion, and swelling of the meibomian glands.[66] The higher the blood levels of PCB, the more severe the ocular disease. Most of the changes appeared reversible.

Carbon disulfide. Workers exposed to carbon disulfide

in viscose rayon factories develop an increased incidence of microaneurysms of the small retinal blood vessels and degenerative changes of the pigmentary epithelium. These abnormalities correlate with the degree of carbon disulfide exposure.[96]

Toluene diisocyanate. Toluene diisocyanates used in the manufacture of foam rubber have been associated with painless corneal epithelial edema in exposed workers.[117]

Hydroquinones and quinones. After prolonged ocular exposure, pigmentation of the cornea and conjunctiva develops as an occupational hazard in workers employed in the manufacture of hydroquinones or quinones, an oxidation product of aniline.[7]

Miscellaneous causes of pigmentation. Hyperpigmentation of the eyelids may follow industrial exposure to mercury and other compounds, including tars, hydrocarbon-rich oils, and phenols.[192] Conjunctival pigmentation can follow the use of mascara or other eyeliners.[192]

Gaseous toxins

Chlorine. Chlorine is used to disinfect swimming pools or as a constituent of other disinfection reagents. Aside from pulmonary disease, laryngitis, bronchitis, and rhinitis, swimmers sometimes develop conjunctivitis, which may be a result of repeated exposure to chlorine in swimming pools.[198]

Ethylene gas. Ethylene oxide is used to sterilize heat-sensitive objects, especially in the medical field. Individuals exposed to massive doses of this gas suffer lens opacification, probably as a result of its alkylating properties.[51] People working with ethylene oxide must protect themselves, as chronic exposure carries similar risks of developing subcapsular cataracts.[50]

Nerve gas. Organophosphates are used as a "nerve gas." Sarin, a potent cholinesterase inhibitor and nerve gas, causes intense miosis, which may take months to cure in survivors.[150] Mustard gas is a potent irritant of the skin, eyes, and respiratory tract. Death follows within minutes of significant exposure, but chronic eye, skin, and lung disease affects survivors.

Animal venoms

Aside from the direct injury caused by their bites, snakes and numerous insects may injure the eye and surrounding tissue by the inoculation of venoms. The bite of the brown recluse spider is capable of producing a necrotic skin lesion, and extensive local life-threatening complications may involve the eyelids.[57] A bee sting may be responsible for unilateral optic neuritis leading to loss of vision.[168] Linear keratitis responsive to corticosteroids may follow a wasp sting.[129]

A Chesapeake Bay sea nettle is capable of producing a severe iritis and raised intraocular pressure.[73] Conventional medical treatment can control the iritis and raised intraoc-

ular pressure, but residual signs may persist for years.

Certain snakes including the spitting cobra *(Naja nigricollis)* and the ringhals cobra *(Hemachatus haemachatus)* have evolved the ability to cast oculotoxic venom spray from their mouths toward prey or threat. The venom can be ejected in a fine jet for a distance of 6 or more feet into the eyes and can cause intense ocular pain with conjunctival edema, corneal opacification, and photophobia.[91]

SUBSTANCE ABUSE
Tobacco (see Chapter 13)

Tobacco-alcohol amblyopia. In adults, cigarette smoking in combination with alcohol abuse may cause altered vision with symmetric scotomata, altered color vision, diminished visual acuity, and loss of discrimination between red and green light. Folate deficiency is common in patients with the so-called tobacco-alcohol amblyopia. The possible role of cyanide from tobacco smoke, folate, and other dietary deficiencies in tobacco-alcohol amblyopia is reviewed by Dang.[46] With cessation of ethanol abuse and the use of vitamins, improvement is possible, but complete recovery is exceptional.

Several independent studies have indicated that cigarette smoking increases the risk of cataract, especially the nuclear sclerotic type.* Some investigations have drawn attention to an increased incidence of posterior subcapsular cataracts[40] or cataract extraction in cigarette smokers.[82]

In confined spaces, particulate and gaseous components of tobacco smoke are capable of causing eye irritation. Individuals with thyroid ophthalmopathy have a greater frequency of smoking than healthy individuals with Graves' disease without severe ophthalmopathy.[166]

Ethanol (see Chapter 14). The vast majority of children born with the fetal alcohol syndrome have one or more eye abnormalities. The ocular teratogenic effect of ethanol, one of the most widespread teratogenetic disorders, spans from early pregnancy through late gestation. Short palpebral fissures, poor vision, ptosis, esotropia, and epicanthal folds are features of the fetal alcohol syndrome, and microphthalmia, myopia, coloboma, blepharophimosis, hypoplasia of the optic nerve, and tortuous retinal veins are occasionally found.[86,173-175]

In the fetal alcohol syndrome, the corneas are often opaque at birth due to variations in thickness in Bowman's layer and deterioration of the anterior zone of Descemet's membrane.[56] This opacification is frequently restricted to the central cornea (Peters' anomaly), and the corneal endothelium is also altered. A hypoplastic optic nerve head and tortuosity of retinal vessels are frequently found.

An alcoholic with pancreatitis can develop a retinopathy with superficial cotton wool spots and hemorrhages,[90] prob-

---

*References 40, 82, 102, 148, 156, 159, 191.

ably by fat embolism. Alcoholics are prone to bacterial keratitis and numerous other infections.[121]

Illicit drugs (see Chapter 15)

Damage to the eye following drug abuse may result from the illicit substances themselves, contaminants mixed with the drugs, the method of administration, or injury sustained during an altered state of consciousness.[125] Intravenously administered illicit drugs are often contaminated with talc, cornstarch, or other foreign particles that occasionally accumulate in choroidal and other ocular blood vessels, sometimes eliciting granulomas.[111] Other ocular manifestations of illicit drug use include blepharospasm (marijuana),[125] ptosis (opiates),[125] defective ocular accommodation (cocaine, opiates, marijuana, and amphetamines),[125] conjunctival edema (marijuana),[125] corneal epithelial toxicity (cocaine),[36] and retraction of the upper eyelids (amphetamines and cocaine).[65,76] Visual illusions thought to be due to lesions in the parietooccipital or temporoparietal lobes of the cerebrum also occur in illicit drug users.[115]

Drug abusers are vulnerable to a variety of infections, including tuberculosis and AIDS, that may involve the ocular tissue. Retinal and other ophthalmic lesions are common in AIDS and may be the presenting manifestation of this contemporary plague, usually as a consequence of opportunistic infection by cytomegalovirus, herpes simplex, herpes zoster, atypical mycobacteria, *Cryptococcus neoformans,* or *Toxoplasma gondii.* Fungal and bacterial endophthalmitis may follow intravenous injections with contaminated needles.[125,177] Metastatic *Bacillus cereus* endophthalmitis associated with illicit intravenous drug use is a newly emerging intraocular infection and the absence of an apparent primary site of infection is the rule in these patients.[85]

Drug abuse has not been clearly established as a cause of ocular developmental anomalies, but several women have given birth to offspring with malformations of the eye after abusing amphetamines, marijuana, and/or LSD,[26,122] as well as quinine used to "cut" heroin.[35,124]

Self-removal of the eyes has been reported in drug abusers, especially those preoccupied with religious thoughts, including Matthew 5:29: "if your right eye causes you to sin, pluck it out and throw it away; it is better that you lose one of your members than that your whole body be thrown into hell."[154,183]

PHYSICAL TRAUMA

Like other environmentally induced disorders physical trauma is a significant preventable cause of blindness.[47,48] Ocular injuries occur in industry, farming, sports, travel, explosions, assaults, gunshots, self-mutilation, and even excessive eye rubbing. More than 80% of patients presenting to emergency rooms in western hospitals with penetrating ocular trauma are males.[140] Most of these injuries take place at work (25% to 50%) and during sporting and rec-

reational activities (up to 25%), but many also take place at home (about 25%), and children are particularly prone to ocular injury. Automobile accidents, assault, and other situations account for the minority of ocular injuries due to physical trauma. Rare penetrating injuries to the eye have been recorded from dog, rat, and human bites. Aside from the effects of physical trauma, such bites predispose to infection largely as a result of flora in the saliva. People who frequently handle venomous animals such as in zoos are particularly at risk of bites.

Protective eyewear is available for many activities with significant risk of eye injury and is increasingly being mandated. Unlike the usual glass or CR39 allyl resin spectacles worn for visual acuity, such glasses do not shatter on impact to cause ocular injury.

Direct injury

The eye may be injured by a direct blow from a blunt object, a fall (Fig. 37-4), a collision, or a high-pressure shock wave of air or water, as from an explosion or even a bullet passing through the orbit but without actually touching the globe. The concussing force may lacerate the ocular tissues, causing hemorrhage, tissue loss, and cell disruption.

The entrance of a blunt object, such as a stick, into the orbit may force the eye against an orbital wall, rupturing the globe. The pressure wave generated by a bullet rapidly traversing the orbit may severely damage the orbital contents and even rupture the ocular wall contralateral to the site of impact. The optic nerve may also be avulsed. A missile passing through the orbit may cause retinal and choroidal tears and/or hemorrhage, even if the globe is not ruptured.

Complications of a ruptured globe include loss of intraocular contents, cataract, glaucoma, vitreous hemorrhage, hyphema, uveitis, and autoimmune reactions (pha-

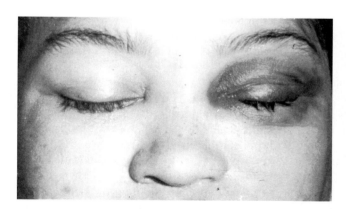

Fig. 37-4. This hemorrhage of the upper and lower lids of the left eye followed a fall onto the back of the head. A fracture of the base of the skull typically causes such a circumscribed hemorrhage. (From Klintworth GK, Landers MB III: *The eye: structure and function in disease*, Baltimore, 1976, Williams & Wilkins; with permission.)

coanaphylaxis, and sympathetic ophthalmia). Vitreous and retina may extend to or extrude through a corneal or scleral wound.

Following any penetrating injury of the globe, intraocular cysts may form, presumably from the implantation of nonkeratinizing or keratinizing epithelium (derived from conjunctiva or skin). Penetrating and perforating injuries of the eye predispose to infection. Especially if incorporated in a wound through the outer ocular wall, damage to the uvea of one eye may elicit an autoimmune reaction (sympathetic ophthalmia) that destroys vision in the other eye previously spared the direct effects of the trauma.

Indirect injury

Major nonocular trauma can produce clinically significant retinal disease known as "traumatic retinopathy of Purtscher." Several days after compression or crush injuries of the abdomen or chest, long bone fractures, or head trauma, cotton wool spots and hemorrhages may appear in the retina. Should the patient recover from the original trauma, such lesions usually resolve over time and seldom produce a permanent defect. This retinopathy probably results from different mechanisms, with fat embolism sometimes occluding the retinal and choroidal arterioles producing retinal areas of nonperfusion. Particularly in crush injuries, arterial spasm and venous reflux may also play a role.

Autoimmune reaction

Injuries to the uvea of one eye may elicit an autoimmune reaction (sympathetic ophthalmia) that destroys vision in the other eye. Similarly, lens damage may be followed by an autoimmune lens-induced uveitis (phacoanaphylactic uveitis).

Foreign bodies

In a survey of almost 3000 penetrating eye injuries in the workplace, one third had an intraocular foreign body.[47] Foreign material may enter the eye during its perforation by sharp objects such as twigs, thorns, fragments of glass, metal, or rock. When propelled at a considerable velocity, a foreign particle may traverse the eye completely. More often it remains in the wall of the globe or ends up in the vitreous or another part of the eye (Fig. 37-5). A small inert foreign body may remain intraocularly for a prolonged time without eliciting a detectable reaction.

Significant visual impairment may even follow chemically inert foreign bodies, such as those that produce intraocular hemorrhage as they enter the eye. The track of a foreign body through the globe may later be a site of fibroblastic proliferation from the point of the perforation, and the formation of collagenous bands can lead to retinal and/or choroidal detachment.

Some ocular tissues react more violently than others to a specific foreign body. An extraneous object in the vascu-

lar uvea is more likely to provoke an inflammatory response than one lodged in the avascular lens or vitreous. The shape and sharpness of a foreign material can also influence its damaging effects, especially if it remains mobile within the eye. Particularly animal and vegetable foreign matter can provoke a marked granulomatous response, whereas metals such as gold, silver, and platinum may merely become encapsulated by fibrous tissue. Relatively inert substances, such as carbon, clay, glass, rock, stone, and certain plastics, can damage the eye during entry and by migration when within the ocular tissue. Glass in the anterior chamber angle can cause recurrent iridocyclitis and corneal edema. In the retina, it may be encapsulated by glial proliferation. Certain metals may be sterilized by heat during propulsion, but still damage ocular tissues. Aluminum, lead, mercury, nickel, and zinc can elicit inflammation, particularly when lodged in the posterior segment. Copper- and iron-containing foreign bodies are particularly toxic (see the section on Toxin Agents).

Cotton, wood, and other extraneous vegetable material commonly elicit granulomatous inflammation as well as fibrous or glial proliferation. Sometimes, especially following an explosion, relatively inert bone or skin enters the globe. Rarely, eyelashes enter the globe and remain within the anterior chamber or at least partially in apposition to or incarcerated in adjacent iris, cornea, or lens. The hair usually excites little or no response, but an early or late inflammatory reaction can be sufficiently severe to destroy the globe. A granuloma can form, and occasionally epithelial implantation cysts may accompany the cilia; their origin may be from the follicle at its base.

The sharply pointed hairs of caterpillars can enter the conjunctival sac after accidentally falling there or being blown or rubbed into the eye.[43,80,187] Aside from causing a conjunctivitis, the hairs can burrow into the eye and produce a severe intraocular inflammatory reaction. Sharply pointed caterpillar hairs, which are brittle and easily broken, burrow into the tissue and migrate by passive move-

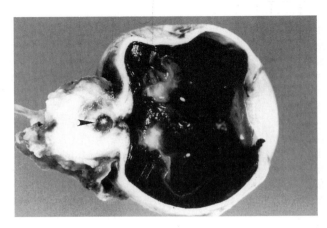

Fig. 37-5. BB pellet in optic nerve of child who was accidentally shot by this "toy."

ment that may be related to blinking, extraocular movements, pulse, and perhaps to the movement of the ciliary musculature and continued rubbing. In addition to causing direct mechanical injury, the hairs apparently contain noxious substances rather than a secreted venom. A keratoconjunctivitis is common, and following the intraocular entry of the caterpillar hairs iridocyclitis may develop. Nodules later appear in the conjunctiva and occasionally the iris. Choroiditis, retinal perivasculitis, and vitritis are sometimes associated, and endophthalmitis may culminate in a blind, painful eye. The hairs of a cocoon can even enter the eye while one dries the face with a towel containing a cocoon.[80,187]

Hairs or spines of plants may enter the conjunctiva and cornea and cause a severe reaction similar to that of ophthalmia nodosa. They may fall into the conjunctival sac, be blown in, or be accidentally rubbed into the ocular tissues. Filamentous foreign material derived from blankets, sweaters, or stuffed animals may cause granulomatous conjunctivitis.[189]

Manners of injury

Occupational trauma. The vast majority of individuals injuring a eye at work are adult men, mostly in construction, manufacturing and agricultural activities.[147] Hammering is probably the most frequent single task producing a penetrating wound.[139,142] Engineering and mechanical tasks, such as drilling and grinding, are frequently implicated. Being below structures from which materials can drop down into the eye also commonly predisposes to ocular injury.[5,119] In order of decreasing frequency, projectiles, sharp objects, blunt objects, and blasts cause eye injury at work by the mechanisms described earlier. Metallic fragments are the most common work-related foreign bodies, followed in frequency by wood, brick dust, paint, and nonspecific dust and grit.[126]

Protective goggles do not prevent all eye injuries. For example, metal dust may fall from the forehead into the eye after eye wear is removed. Workers may resist using eye shielding because of discomfort, fogging, and scratching of the lenses or screens. More than 90% of injured workers in the National Eye Trauma System Registry were not wearing safety eyewear.[47] Even when compliance is good among machinery operators, bystanders may be unexpectedly hit by flying particles, even several feet from the source of the projectile.[139]

In 1992, the National Eye Trauma System Registry published data on 635 penetrating eye injuries that occurred in the workplace.[47] One third had hyphema and one third had traumatic cataract. In two thirds, the posterior segment of the eye was damaged, with almost one half having a vitreous hemorrhage and one third of each having incarcerated tissue, a foreign body, scleral laceration or rupture, or retinal tear. Retinal detachment occurred in 10%.

Another important, but fortunately infrequent, occupa-

tional cause of ocular injury is machines that pump liquids under high pressure, often reaching 2000 to 10,000 lbs/in^2 (140 to 170 bar). In construction, farm, industrial, and oil field equipment, streams of liquids that may be fine and almost invisible are sometimes released under high pressure from hydraulic lines or fuel injectors during use or malfunction. The ejected liquids can cause serious ocular injuries, even if the liquids do not contain noxious substances, and the reaction created by the injection of foreign material into the orbit may be difficult to treat.[87]

Recreational trauma. Recreational injuries are common in contact sports and in ball or projectile games. Circumstances of the injury vary widely, depending on culture, climate, and human imagination in devising new pastimes.

The number of injuries may be moderated by education and enforcement of rules concerning the style of play and use of ocular safeguards. Since the early 1980s, laws in the United States have mandated the use of eye protection in ice hockey and racquet sports. Protective eyewear has successfully reduced ocular injury, particularly in some professional sports. The Canadian Standards Association has set an example in the study and prevention of eye injury in sport.[141]

Boxers risk severe eye injury in addition to the increasingly documented chronic brain damage. In a study of 74 boxers applying for a new or renewed license in New York in the late 1980s, two thirds had had at least one ocular injury.[70] The mean age of the boxers was 25 years. Cutaneous scarring was included in this overall number. About one fifth had abnormalities of the anterior chamber angle of the eye (tears in the ciliary body, synechiae, and increased angle pigmentation) or cataracts (mostly posterior subcapsular). One quarter of the boxers had retinal tears. The more bouts a boxer had fought, and the more he had lost, the more likely the presence of a retinal tear. The devastating wounds suffered by the eye and the brain in boxing have led numerous national medical associations to recommend that boxing be banned.

In American football, the faceguard and rules against holding reduce blunt ocular trauma and eye gouging. A thin polycarbonate screen in the faceguard can protect players from opponents' fingers and foreign material such as dust and mud. Other forms of football including soccer, rugby union, and rugby-league have a risk of eye injury by elbows, fingers, and impact with the ground.

In a study of 163 competitive squash players in Australia, one quarter had experienced ocular trauma, and approximately one tenth had more than one wound.[67] Males were more frequently affected. About 17 injuries occurred per 100,000 playing hours, with more being caused by a squash racquet than the ball. One third of the lesions were "black eyes"; another third were eyelid or periorbital lacerations. Hyphema or subconjunctival or retinal hemorrhage was present in approximately one quarter. Corneal abrasions were infrequent. When squash balls travel at approximately 40 miles per hour, they can penetrate the open-frame style of eye guards. In contrast, solid polycarbonate lenses resist speeds in excess of 90 miles per hour. In this investigation only about one tenth of the players voluntarily used protective eyewear, often after previous injury. Medical advice provided insufficient incentive for the remainder of the group. Perceived discomfort, inconvenience, or even increased chance of injury from wearing eye protection was common. Despite this, most players in the study supported compulsory use of protective eyewear.

The emphasis on eye protection in the racquet sports, where the risk of injury is obvious, has left badminton as a leading cause of eye injury in Canada.[141] The lighter shuttlecock and racquet still transfer enough energy to damage the eye. Since the early 1980s, Canada has mandated eye protection for racquet sports.

Ice hockey has many instruments for injuring the eye, with possible player speeds exceeding 30 miles per hour.[45] The puck travels at more than 100 miles per hour in professional hockey. Yet, the hockey stick produces more eye injuries than the puck. Periorbital trauma is more frequent than hyphema and other internal ocular injuries. Despite regulations, hockey players who are not wearing certified face protectors or visors continue to suffer from hyphema, corneal abrasions and lacerations, occasional orbital fractures, and devastating ruptured globes.[45] The use of helmets, with mandatory face masks since 1976, has decreased eye injuries markedly in North American amateur leagues.

In golf, the ocular tissues can be injured from a direct blow from a club or golf ball and also from the expulsion of material maintained under extremely high pressure in the liquid center of some golf balls. Individuals cutting or unwinding the rubber band beneath the outer shell of such a golf ball can be struck with this central material, which is usually a mixture of zinc and barium sulfates. After being ejected with explosive force, the liquid can penetrate the conjunctiva or skin and produce a white lesion with black birefringent particles, mainly within macrophages.[93]

In the early 1980s, "war games" using a carbon dioxide–pressurized gun firing dye-containing plastic pellets became popular in several countries.[120] Eye injuries have been frequent, even though players are issued protective eyewear. Fogging of the eyewear from heat and humidity encourages players to remove eye protection intermittently, making the eye a potential target for the pellet, which usually bursts on contact. The most frequent injuries are soft tissue hemorrhage, corneal lacerations, hyphema, and retinal damage.

In indoor cricket, either a polyurethane ball or a tennis ball is bowled from one end of a pitch toward a batter protecting three wickets, behind which is the wicket keeper or backstop. Eye injuries are not as frequent as soft tissue sprains and fractures, but wicket keepers are at eye level with the oncoming ball and have their vision obstructed by the batter.[62] They are at greatest risk for periorbital lacerations, corneal abrasion, hyphema, lens dislocation, vitreous hemorrhage, commotio retinae, and other eye injuries and benefit most from protective glasses.

An obviously dangerous weapon called an *aerial dart* or *flechette* was a popular backyard projectile until the late 1980s, when it was banned in the United States.[169] Its effectiveness in causing death when dropped from French aircraft in World War I was repeated when it was sold as a toy in the United States. Penetrating injuries of the eye and scalp caused infections, blindness, and death.

Eye injuries can follow such diverse activities as shooting, baseball, snow skiing, volleyball, snowmobiling, and lacrosse.[83,109,128] In Kuwait, the commonest cause of eye injury in children is a catapulted missile.[6]

Domestic trauma. Concussion forces are usually responsible for domestic ocular traumatic injuries. Penetrating and perforating wounds caused by sharp instruments such as broken glass, needles, scissors, knives, and even houseplants, occur more often than gunshot wounds, but gunshots are more likely to cause blindness. The popping of champagne corks is hazardous to the eye.

Accidents involving riding and pushing lawnmowers affect the limbs, but the eyes are not always spared the force of the high-velocity blades and the material that is thrown by the shielding built into the mower. Weed whackers are a further potential source of ocular injuries if adequate protective eye shields are not worn.

Fireworks are regulated in many countries because of the high incidence of injuries, with most occurring in adolescents and children. In the United States, two thirds of these injuries occur in the few weeks prior to and following Independence Day; in other countries, injuries from fireworks are also linked to festivals. Direct heat causes more damage than hits by the flying fireworks, or smaller fragments of foreign material. The hands and fingers suffer twice as often as the eyes.[131]

Injury from therapeutic procedures and devices

Ocular surgery. Many complications may follow cataract surgery, drainage operations for glaucoma, keratoplasty, and other surgical procedures on the eye. These include infections, hemorrhage, detached retina, vitreous loss, and cystoid macular edema. Corneal transplantation may also be complicated by immunogenic graft rejection, especially if the cornea is vascularized, and corneal edema may develop if the endothelium of the donor tissue is compromised. Whereas AIDS has apparently not been transmitted by way of a corneal transplant, bacterial and fungal endophthalmitis and keratitis as well as hepatitis, Creutzfeldt-Jakob disease, and rabies have occurred in recipients.*

Contact lenses. Most wearers of contact lenses have no adverse effects; some develop problems from oxygen deprivation, adherent antigens, or infections. Infections are dis-

*References 10, 11, 53, 74, 176.

cussed elsewhere in this chapter. Direct trauma of a contact lens rubbing against the cornea can cause epithelial abrasions that stain with fluorescein. With hard lenses, this has a predilection for the 3 and 9 o'clock positions, apparently occurring where the tear film breaks at those sites. Overwear of a contact lens, especially one made of polymethyl methacrylate, can lead to severe, extremely painful epithelial breakdown. A small proportion of soft and rigid contact lens wearers develop clinically significant contact lens-induced corneal warpage. Epithelial breakdown and corneal ulceration predispose to infection. Loss of vision results from corneal scarring or destruction of the eye if endophthalmitis ensues. Common causes of these ulcers include *Pseudomonas aeruginosa, Streptococcus pneumoniae,* and *Serratia marcescens. Acanthamoeba,* a ubiquitous, free-living, nonparasitic protozoan, is responsible for a severe infection in contact lens wearers (see the section on Protozoa). The incidence of ulcerative keratitis in contact lens wearers is low, but the vast number of individuals using contact lenses makes ulcerative keratitis an important complication of lens wearers. Infections tend to be more common in soft lens wearers (both day wear and extended wear) than in hard or gas-permeable lenses.

Contact lenses impair normal corneal metabolism and oxygenation. Placement of the lens on the cornea increases the risk of a minor abrasion, thereby allowing bacteria to gain access to the stroma. Poor hygiene and the improper handling and cleaning of lenses result in bacterial contamination. Contaminated lenses inoculate the tear film with abnormally high concentrations of bacteria.

The ocular surface membrane may be adversely affected by certain chemical contaminants of contact lenses. For example, chlorobutanol and chlorhexidine, which are used as preservatives in some contact lens cleaning solutions, may cause a mild conjunctivitis when the contact lens is placed on the eye.

For further information on contact lenses, the reader should consult the excellent review written by Bruce and Brennan.[34]

Prosthetic intraocular lenses. A wide variety of complications may follow the implantation of intraocular lenses. Common problems include dislocation, iris erosion, endothelial cell loss, trabecular meshwork damage, cystoid macular edema, glaucoma, and corneal edema.

Epidemics of endophthalmitis have occurred from bacterial[68] or fungal[145] contaminated prosthetic lenses in persons undergoing cataract extraction and the implantation of intraocular lens. Faulty sterilization techniques have resulted in endophthalmitis, sometimes in multiple patients implanted with lenses from the same batch. Endophthalmitis may also follow the introduction of soiled intraocular lenses, as occurred in the epidemic that followed contamination by *Paecilomyces lilacius* in the manufacturer's sterilizing solution.[145]

The residual polishing compound fused to the surface of dry-sterilized intraocular lenses can produce a sterile iritis and endophthalmitis. The alkaline caustic storage fluid used to sterilize the surface of prosthetic lenses may result in the leaching of small barium-containing crystals from the glass storage vials.[106]

Amniocentesis. Thrusting a needle into the gravid uterus during amniocentesis, particularly without the benefit of real-time ultrasound guidance, puts the fetal eye at risk for injury. Rarely, ocular trauma may occur.[157]

Self-inflicted injuries. Most patients with keratoconus, a common disorder in which the cornea becomes cone shaped as its stroma becomes thin, rub their eyes excessively. Eye rubbing is a feature of several conditions associated with keratoconus including atopic disease, the wearing of contact lenses, Down's syndrome and other causes of mental retardation, and it may play a role in the pathogenesis of keratoconus.[104] Mentally disturbed individuals sometimes willfully injure their ocular tissues by inserting or injecting noxious substances or by plucking their own eye from the orbit.[154,183]

Battered baby syndrome. Since Caffey[38] first described children with intracranial hemorrhages and fractures of bones without external evidence of abuse, pronounced shaking of the infants as a form of punishment has become recognized as the cause of such injuries. Ocular injuries are common in this battered baby syndrome and include eyelid lacerations, subluxed and dislocated lenses, cataracts (which may be bilateral), periorbital and intraocular hemorrhage, glaucoma (sometimes suspected of being congenital in type), anterior chamber angle recession, iridodialysis, iris neovascularization, retinal dialysis, optic atrophy, and edema of the optic nerve head. These infants frequently have injured brains, and an intracranial subdural hemorrhage may extend toward the eye along the optic nerve sheath. Retinal and vitreous hemorrhage may also accompany intracranial hemorrhage. Approximately 20% of individuals suffering from traumatic subarachnoid or subdural hemorrhages develop intraocular hemorrhages, mostly confined to the juxtapapillary and macular areas. Blood may also accumulate beneath the internal limiting membrane of the retina. In a study of 20 infants injured solely by being shaken without other evidence of abuse, retinal hemorrhages were noted in 12 of the 18 cases examined by ophthalmoscopy.[118] The acceleration-deceleration forces associated with shaking are thought to account for the high incidence of retinal hemorrhages. Other findings included subdural hemorrhage (10 cases), cerebral contusion (8 cases), and subarachnoid hemorrhage (5 cases). Ten of the 17 survivors were significantly disabled, with abnormalities that included motor impairment, seizures, developmental delay, and also blindness and visual impairment. The relatively large head size and weight, weak neck musculature, and delicate, friable vasculature, together with the incomplete myelination of the brain are suspected of making young infants particularly vulnerable to shaking.

Birth injury. Hemorrhages at different depths in the retina are common, especially in birth injury, and sometimes spread to the subhyaloid space and vitreous. Edema, often involving much of the retina, can form at the posterior pole of the eye and the site of injury following trauma. Clinically apparent whitish areas resolve completely over several days, but at the macula the edema may persist as a cystoid maculopathy that leads to degenerative and/or proliferative alterations in the adjacent retinal pigment epithelium or to lamellar holes in the macula. Following the resorption of the retinal hemorrhages, the involved area may remain destroyed and be evident as cystoid spaces or as atrophic areas within the retina; sometimes associated with gliosis.

RADIATION

The superficial location of the eye exposes the ocular tissues to many types of radiation.[147] The eyes are exposed throughout life to solar radiation and light from various other sources. Major contributors of radiation from natural sources include radon, cosmic rays, and radionuclides within the earth, as well as radioactive isotopes within the body. Additional exposure to radiation occurs in such diverse situations as defective microwave ovens in the home and radiotherapy of neoplasms within and near the eye. Certain occupations, such as some forms of mining and aerospace work, may also lead to ocular radiation exposure.

Nonionizing radiation that can damage the ocular tissue includes ultraviolet (UV) light, visible light, infrared light, and microwaves. The ionizing radiation of high-frequency electromagnetic waves of relatively short wavelength (gamma rays and x rays) is a major cause of ocular damage.

Solar-induced lesions (see Chapter 10)

Radiation from the sun spans a wide range of the electromagnetic spectrum that includes visible, UV, and infrared light. Solar radiation is suspected of playing an important role in the pathogenesis of several disorders of the eye and eyelids. In some conditions, the adverse effects of solar radiation result from radiation of a specific wavelength. In most entities, unequivocal evidence to implicate a precise wavelength remains lacking, hence the justification for the designation "actinic rays."

Largely because of difficulties in quantitating the cumulative effect of chronic low-dosage UV light and other solar exposure, evidence to implicate solar irradiation in the pathogenesis of ocular disease has been indirect. Evidence for solar irradiation has largely been derived from apparent increases in the prevalence of the condition with outdoor activities, with increasing age, and in populations living at latitudes closer to the equator. Even in regions with high ambient UV light, large individual variations in personal exposure vary throughout life and depend on such variables as wearing appropriate glasses and hats when outdoors, and

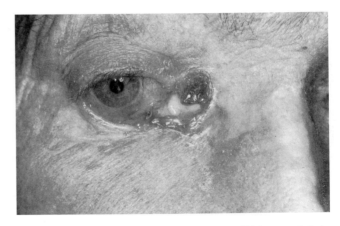

Fig. 37-6. A basal cell carcinoma of the eyelid has eroded the tissue of the medial canthus. (From Klintworth GK, Landers MB III: *The eye: structure and function in disease*, Baltimore, 1976, Williams & Wilkins; with permission.)

this makes it difficult to specifically implicate solar radiation.

Eyelid. The cumulative effect of chronic solar irradiation contributes to numerous pathologic conditions of the eyelids, including actinic keratosis, solar (senile) keratosis, basal cell carcinoma, and squamous cell carcinoma. Basal cell carcinoma forms mainly on the lower eyelid in fair-skinned adults and is commonly preceded by prolonged exposure to sunlight (Fig. 37-6). In the Western Hemisphere, squamous cell carcinoma of the eyelid is uncommon and composes 9% of all eyelid malignancies.[149] In Japan, squamous cell carcinoma is the most frequent malignancy of the eyelid. When the eyelid contains sun-induced cutaneous tumors, the skin in other sun-exposed areas of the body often has precancerous lesions and other malignant cutaneous tumors. Persons with oculocutaneous albinism are predisposed to sun-induced neoplasms, lentigines, solar keratoses, and squamous cell carcinoma, but the incidence of melanoma is low.[194]

Solar radiation potentiates the toxic effects of isotretinoin, sulfonamides, barbiturates, phenothiazines, and dimethylchlortetracycline, and phototoxic reactions with these agents may result in blepharitis.[60,64,192]

Retina. Sungazing under the influence of drugs or purposely for secondary gain, as has been detected in military personnel, or watching a solar eclipse can cause a macular lesion with loss of central vision. This "solar retinitis" or "eclipse retinopathy," which is sometimes bilateral, begins as macular edema with loss of the foveal reflex. The underlying retinal pigment epithelium may be lost and surrounded by hyperpigmentation, and the maculopathy may progress to a macular hole or cyst.

Conjunctiva and cornea

Pingueculae. Localized yellowish conjunctival nodules adjacent to the corneoscleral limbus in the interpalpebral fissure (pingueculae) can appear before the end of the sec-

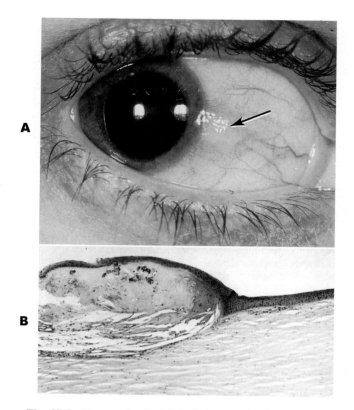

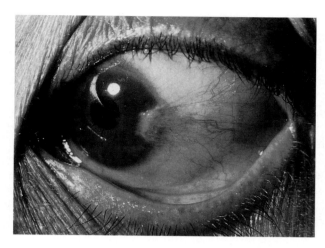

Fig. 37-8. Pterygium. (From Klintworth GK, Landers MB III: *The eye: structure and function in disease*, Baltimore, 1976, Williams & Wilkins; with permission.)

Fig. 37-7. Pinguecula. **A,** Clinical photograph of a pinguecula at the nasal limbus. **B,** Light micrograph of pinguecula with histological features equivalent to dermal actinic elastosis. (**A,** From Klintworth GK, Landers MB III: *The eye: structure and function in disease*, Baltimore, 1976, Williams & Wilkins; **B,** from Klintworth GK: *Degenerations, depositions, and miscellaneous reactions of the ocular anterior segment.* In Garner A, Klintworth, GK editors: *Pathobiology of ocular disease: a dynamic approach*, ed 2, Marcel Dekker, Inc., NY, 1994; with permission.)

ond decade, but occurs predominantly in middle and late life (Fig. 37-7). The incidence of these frequently bilateral lesions increases with age.

Pingueculae are common in tropical and subtropical countries, less frequent in places of greater latitude, and rare in England, Finland, and other countries. The incidence of pingueculae correlates with outdoor work. Histopathologically, pingueculae are identical to actinic elastosis of the skin but have more non–fiber-forming aggregates. They frequently contain focal calcifications and autofluorescent spheroidal bodies (see the section on Chronic Actinic Keratopathy).

Pingueculae commonly coexist with pterygia, but the association of UV radiation exposure with pinguecula is weaker than with pterygia and chronic actinic keratopathy.

Pterygia. Chronic ocular exposure to solar UV light is suspected of causing epibulbar pterygia. Pterygia, which consist of a fold of vascularized bulbar conjunctiva encroaching onto the cornea in the horizontal meridian (Fig. 37-8), usually first appear in the dominant eye, perhaps be-

cause persons facing the sun keep the dominant eye open while closing the nondominant eye.

Although varying in different countries, pterygia are most prevalent in tropical and subtropical countries and less common in regions located further from the equator. They are common in Australia, Greenland, Hawaii, Jordan, Peru, and parts of continental United States, but are uncommon in Japan and rare in Britain, Finland, and elsewhere. Pterygia are common in fishermen and in other workers exposed to excessive UV radiation from the sun. The prevalence of pterygia correlates positively with lower latitudes and high UV levels. Differences in lifestyle explain discrepancies in the prevalences in the racial groups and between males and females. The incidence of pterygia increases with age, and there is a predilection for men and outdoor workers. Welders exposed to excess UV radiation have a significantly high incidence of pterygia, and the incidence is closely related to the length of employment. In regions where pterygia are endemic, such as the Sahara Desert, their presence correlates with the severity and the duration of exposure to predisposing factors.

Pterygia are frequently associated with other putative sun-induced ocular lesions, such as conjunctival spheroidal degeneration and pingueculae. The vast majority of pterygia are associated with conjunctival actinic elastosis, but some can apparently develop in the absence of pingueculae, as in India.

Solar radiation has long been suspected as causing pterygia, as their prevalence, like solar radiation, diminishes with increasing latitude. Ample circumstantial evidence implicates chronic UV light in the pathogenesis of pterygia. Pterygia are associated with a broad band of UV radiation exposure (290 to 400 nm), and their frequency correlates positively with the degree of exposure to UV radiation. Because pterygia are not an occupational disease of furnace workers, stokers, and other individuals exposed to heat, infrared radiation is probably not a cause.

It is noteworthy, however, that the correlation between pterygia and other ocular lesions thought to result from chronic UV radiation, such as pingueculae, conjunctival spheroidal degeneration, and chronic actinic keratopathy, is weak. Also, although pterygia are uncommon in Japan, conjunctival spheroidal degeneration and pingueculae are common in that country.

Despite evidence implicating UV light in the causation of pterygia, other environmental factors probably also play a role. For example, a survey of ocular disease among Punjabi Indians who immigrated to British Columbia, Canada (an area with less solar irradiation than India), suggests that sawmill workers may be prone to pterygia. The prevalence of pterygia in Punjabi Indian workers in sawmills (an indoor occupation) in both British Columbia and New Delhi is higher than Punjabi farmers (an outdoor occupation) in India. In Canada pterygia are commoner in Indian (12%) than other sawmill workers (2%). Moreover, the likelihood of pterygia increases with duration of employment in the mill. A higher prevalence rate in sawmill workers than in controls has also been found in Taiwan and Thailand.

Repeated conjunctival microtrauma and, to a lesser degree, other causal factors are also suspected of causing pterygia. In some, but not all, geographic regions where pterygia are prevalent, dust, wind and excessive desiccation coexist with the sun glare. Desiccation is not essential because a high incidence of pterygia occurs in certain areas of high humidity.

An inherited susceptibility to ptergyia seems likely. Unilateral or bilateral pterygia have occurred in two or more generations of several families. Blood relatives of persons with ptergygia are more vulnerable than the general population. Some pedigrees are consistent with an autosomal dominant mode of transmission, and some familial cases lack a history of unusual exposure to the elements.

Racial differences in the incidence of pterygia, which may reflect a genetic predisposition, occur in some geographic areas such as Aruba, an island off the coast of Venezuela, and Canada.

Chronic actinic keratopathy (climatic droplet keratopathy). In an entity notorious for its many names, white, grayish, or yellow opacities appear in the conjunctiva, on either side of the peripheral cornea, and in the horizontal meridian, where they commonly resemble oil droplets. A popular connotation for the condition is *climatic droplet keratopathy,* but this designation, like many of its other names, has serious semantic shortcomings. First, the climate of a region designates the long-term manifestastions of weather. It reflects different atmospheric phenomena, such as temperature, wind, moisture, and various air pollutants. Solar radiation, the most likely causal culprit, is not part of the climate according to the traditional use of the word, but rather a factor influencing it. Also, *droplet,*

although descriptive of a solitary clinical feature, lacks precision and ignores many established aspects of the disorder. We prefer the designation *chronic actinic keratopathy (CAK).*

With time, the deposits become more numerous, increase in size, and sometimes form a band across the cornea as they extend centrally. In what appears to be an earlier and less severe manifestion of the less common CAK, numerous discrete yellowish globules occasionally gather in the interpalpebral portion of the conjunctiva adjacent to a clinically normal cornea (conjunctival spheroidal degeneration). Such globules may be present in the cornea and conjunctiva.

Many of the globules manifest autofluorescence when examined by slit-lamp biomicroscopy. Like pingueculae and pterygia, the nasal conjunctiva is affected more often than the temporal conjunctiva, which is rarely involved in Eskimos perhaps because of their eye shape and narrow palpebral fissure.

The prevalence of conjunctival spheroidal degeneration varies in different populations; it is high in Jordan, low in Denmark, and rises with increasing age.

Individuals affected with conjunctival spheroidal degeneration and CAK are predominantly men who are or have been fishermen, divers, trappers, stockworkers, or other outdoor workers. In Labrador the only affected women have spent a considerable amount of time outdoors. In Australian aborigines, the prevalence in men who have worked as stockmen for more than 20 years is 41%, but only 8% for women aged 45 years or more.

Chronic actinic keratopathy is caused by exposure to some environmental factor related to the proportion of time spent outdoors. In some regions with a high prevalence of severe CAK, eyes become exposed to climatic extremes, evaporation, and the traumatic aftermath of wind-blown sand or ice. For example, in the Dahlak Islands in the Red Sea, shade is nonexistent. Possible causal factors include evaporation in areas of low humidity, microtrauma from wind-blown minute particles like snow and ice (in snowbound regions such as Labrador and Newfoundland), or dust and sand (as in the deserts of North Africa and the Middle East), as well as solar irradiation. The climate varies considerably in geographical areas where CAK is recognized, and injurious environmental factors in some regions are absent in other locations with the keratopathy, indicating that they are not essential to its development. For instance, CAK can develop where the atmosphere lacks excessive particulate matter. Evaporation could predispose to the precipitation of the proteins in the superficial cornea, as it does in calcific band keratopathy, but excessive evaporation from the cornea does not seem to be important. It occurs in some arid areas and in regions like Labrador, where the air contains negligible water vapor, but it is also found in regions where the humidity is not low. Also, similar stromal deposits are not features of the dry eye syndrome or in exposure keratopathy, where excessive evaporation takes place.

It appears worldwide, but it is most prevalent and severe in certain geographic areas, such as Labrador, the Dahlak Islands in the Red Sea, northern Cameroon, Australia, and Saudi Arabia, where UV light exposure is high. Ultraviolet light is reflected by snow, desert, and water, which are prominent in some areas where CAK is severe. The incidence and severity of CAK are less in the northern than in the southern parts of the Arctic region.

Extracellular, variably sized proteinaceous granules and concretions are identified in unstained tissue sections. They manifest an intense yellow autofluorescence under fluorescence microscopy. Similar bodies occur in pingueculae and in conjunctival spheroidal degeneration. The identity of the protein that makes up the bulk of concretions remains unknown. Although not always evident clinically, actinic elastosis (the histopathologic counterpart of pingueculae) is common in tissue sections, and these lesions contain identical concretions. However, UV light probably produces CAK at energy levels too low to cause acute keratoconjunctivitis because a history of repeated episodes of AKC is usually lacking in individuals with CAK.

The prevalence and gravity of CAK appear to be directly related to levels of sunlight exposure, and UV light from solar irradiation is the prime suspect for the fundamental causal factor. The potential for excessive exposure to radiant energy from the sun is common to all geographic areas where CAK is prevalent, and UV light seems to be the most probable form of energy to implicate. The high incidence of CAK in places where sand, snow, and surf predominate is readily accounted for by the fact that most UV-B light that strikes the ocular surface is indirect, scattered, or reflected radiation (albedo). Chronic actinic keratopathy is not a disorder of extreme northern latitudes, where adverse weather exists and probably the sun fails to rise high above the horizon, causing less pronounced effects of UV light than in more southern areas.

In Britain, where the population is to some extent protected from UV irradiation by a blanket of clouds, CAK is less common than in countries with higher levels of sunlight. Absorption of solar radiant energy can account for the predisposition for the exposed interpalpebral part of the eye, the usual bilaterality of the condition, the preponderance of outdoor occupations that also reflects the gender difference, and the increased incidence with advancing years due to an increased time of solar exposure. Additional observations support the hypothesis that CAK follows the cumulative effect of chronic solar irradiation. Advanced CAK was found in a 30-year-old black subject with xeroderma pigmentosum, an inherited disease in which individuals are sensitive to light with a wavelength of 280 to 310 nm. Morphologically, CAK is associated with conjunctival elastosis in the same eye and has concretions indistinguishable from those found in pingueculae and cutaneous actinic elastosis (solar elastosis).

Abundant evidence implicates prolonged sunlight exposure in dermal actinic elastosis. It is restricted to skin that is exposed to solar irradiation, it is most severe in areas receiving the most intense and prolonged solar exposure, it is less evident in heavily pigmented skin that is protected from UV light, it can be produced experimentally with UV light, and in whites sun-induced cutaneous tumors, such as basal cell carcinomas and melanomas, are associated with it.

Sclera. Discrete slate gray areas immediately in front of medial and lateral rectus muscle insertions are common in the elderly[163] (Fig. 37-9). Although often referred to as *plaques,* these lesions are not flattened elevations but part of the sclera. Although rare prior to the seventh decade, scleral plaques increase in incidence with age thereafter. The discolored areas have an increased translucency to light, and the dark color results from an enhanced visibility of the underlying ciliary body.

The scleral thickness at the site of the "plaque" is either normal or slightly increased. A spectrum of histopathologic abnormalities in the affected sclera includes an increased hematoxylinophilia of the collagen, decreased cellularity, and the presence of corkscrew-shaped fibers. Extensive plaques calcify.

Pingueculae may hide the "plaque" from view. Although this relationship has received little attention, it has also been found in a histologic study of eyes obtained postmortem. Of the various hypotheses for the pathogenesis of senile plaques, the one implicating a culmination of chronic UV light irradiation is the most attractive in view of the putative actinically induced histopathologic connective tissue abnormalities.

Lens. Another puzzling disease for which an environmental cause has been suspected in the pseudoexfoliation syndrome (PSX). This condition is characterized by the ap-

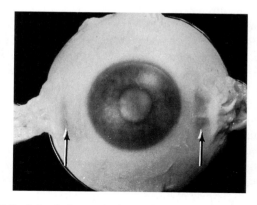

Fig. 37-9. Scleral plaques in front of the medial and lateral rectus muscles *(arrows).* (From Klintworth GK: *Degenerations, depositions, and miscellaneous reactions of the ocular anterior segment.* In Garner A, Klintworth GK, editors: *Pathobiology of ocular disease: a dynamic approach,* ed 2, New York, 1994, Marcel Dekker, Inc., NY; with permission.)

pearance of a basement membrane–like material on the lens capsule and other tissues. The prevalence of PSX in northern Finland, Lapland, Iceland, northern Russia, and Saudi Arabia and among Navajo Indians in the United States and Australian aborigines is high, and the frequency rises with increasing age in all populations. Only the Eskimo population is virtually free of PSX. The prevalence of PSX varies considerably, both within and between countries. In three areas—Birmingham (Britain), Bonn (Germany), and Bergen (Norway)—on the same latitude and receiving similar exposure to UV light, the number of patients with PSX is more or less the same in geriatric homes, with some 3% affected in the seventh decade, increasing to 11% in the tenth decade.[1]

A significant relation to UV light—the only seriously investigated environmental factor—has been reported in Australian aborigines[180] and in Pakistan.[130] Data about an association with pingueculae, pterygia, and chronic actinic keratopathy are conflicting. In one study, PSX was six times more frequent in patients with CAK than in controls.[151]

Specific nonionizing electromagnetic radiation (see Chapters 10 and 12)

Microwaves. Most applications of microwave (1 mm to 30 cm; 1000 to 300,000 megacycles/sec) as used in radar, communications, heating in homes and industry, and scientific endeavors are safe and do not injure the eye. Prolonged exposure to microwaves, as from household appliances, has been associated with the formation of cataracts.[105]

Visible light. Sources of light that may potentially damage the eye include the sun, directly viewed fluorescent light, fluorescent or mercury-vapor streetlights, tungsten-halogen automotive headlights of oncoming cars, and photographic flashes. The adverse effects of light are more severe in infants and children, whose ocular media transmit more blue and UV light, than in adults.[114] The yellow carotenoid pigments of the human macula that normally block blue light from the retina display considerably less absorbance in the UV-A range.[81] Carotenoid pigments have a photoprotective antioxidant property. Because the retinal carotenoid levels are three to four times lower in infants than in adults,[28] the effect of light on the retina of infants is enhanced.

Excessive visible light (380 to 760 nm), as well as light of specific colors such as violet (397 to 424 nm), blue (455 to 492 nm), or red (647 to 723 nm) can injure the retina, especially the photoreceptors and the retinal pigment epithelium. Threshold lesions are associated with rises in temperature of only 2.5° C to 3° C, and heating the animal to 42.5° C in the dark does not result in retinal damage. The effect of light may be potentiated by heat, and the susceptibility of these tissues to noxious effects of intense light is probably determined by their rate of metabolism, which in turn is related to their temperature. Retinal edema and degeneration of photoreceptor outer segments ensues, but later the photoreceptor cells and retinal pigment epithelium become repaired and regenerate. Similar irradiation under conditions of hypothermia produces less damage.

An accumulation of lipofuscin within the retinal pigment epithelium, especially at the macula, may reflect retinal light damage. The most rapid accumulation of this pigment takes place during infancy and childhood.[190]

Numerous experimental and clinical studies have documented iatrogenic retinal injury by light. The damage principally involves the external retina and retinal pigment epithelium. Light damage may be a complication of using the indirect ophthalmoscope, the slit lamp, an overhead surgical lamp, or a fiberoptic endoscopic illuminator during vitreoretinal operations, such as during the surgical removal of preretinal membranes.[108,196] An operating microscope as used in cataract extraction, epikeratophakia, combined anterior segment procedures, glaucoma procedures, and other operations may also injure the retina. The nature and extent of the retinal damage is influenced by the power, exposure time, and wavelenth of the light. Even ophthalmologists who use lasers or operating microscopes are prone to their adverse effects. They can develop subtle but definite changes in color vision after chronic exposure to argon blue light and develop a decreased discrimination for colors in a tritan color confusion axis.[12]

First described more than a century ago, age-related macular degeneration usually begins after the age of 50 years and progressively impairs central vision with increasing age. The connotations *age-related macular degeneration* (AMD) and *age-related maculopathy* are preferable to the earlier term, *senile macular degeneration*. This condition is the most common cause of blindness in the Western world, and high levels of exposure to blue or visible light may be related to its development.[181] It is associated with a variety of pigmentary and atrophic alterations in the region of the macula, including deposits on Bruch's membrane (hard and soft drusen), basal laminar deposits beneath the macula, an organization of hemorrhage beneath the retinal pigment epithelium, retinal pigment epithelial degeneration, increased retinal pigmentation in the macular region, subretinal scarring or exudates (serous or hemorrhagic), subretinal lipid deposits, and serous or hemorrhagic detachment of the retinal pigment epithelium. Late forms of the disease have been designated the *nonexudative* (dry or atrophic) or *exudative* (neovascular) varieties of age-related maculopathy.

In the United States this maculopathy has a prevalence rate of 1.5% to 1.8%.[30,103,112] This prevalence varies at different ages; it is 8.5% in those 43 to 54 years old, and it rises to 36.8% in persons at least 75 years old.[113] Aside from age, other risk factors include exposure to sunlight, dermal actinic elastosis, race, iris color, zinc, and smoking. In an analysis of watermen on the Chesapeake Bay, affected patients had significantly higher exposure to blue or visible light over the preceding 20 years than age-matched controls.[181] There was no difference in respect to UV-A or UV-B. Some risk factors may also reflect an effect of sunlight. Smoking elevates the risk of neovascular and/or exudative AMD, whereas carotenoids decrease the risk of it.[88]

Retinopathy of prematurity. Retinopathy of prematurity (ROP) is clearly related to the oxygen exposure (see the section on atmosphere), but light is also suspected of being a contributing factor. The incidence of ROP is reduced if premature infants are protected from light with a neutral density filter over the incubators.[72] This effect may relate to reduced oxygen consumption relative to free oxygen radical formation.

Ultraviolet light. As discussed previously, solar UV radiation has been implicated in many ocular lesions (see Chapter 10). Ultraviolet light having a wavelength of 200 to 290 nm (UV-C) is damaging to DNA and amino acids but is blocked by the stratospheric ozone layer; UV-B (290 to 320 nm), which is partially blocked by the ozone layer, is the least dangerous; UV-A (320 to 400 nm) is particularly hazardous for individuals taking photosensitizing medications. Solar UV light is reflected, especially from water, snowfields, and deserts. Aside from sunlight, other sources of UV light are sunlamps, arc welding, UV lamps used to sterilize rooms, and other industrial sources. Almost all UV light below 295 nm is absorbed by the cornea and especially its epithelium. Ultraviolet light of longer wavelengths (295 to 400 nm) and great intensity is absorbed by the lens and affects its anterior cortex and subcapsular region. In the eye with a crystalline lens, little or no UV light reaches the retina.

Overabundant ocular exposure to UV light over short periods produces acute keratoconjunctivitis. Symptoms from a superficial punctate keratopathy follow after a latent period of several hours. Mitosis is inhibited, and the damaged epithelium sloughs after loosening from its basement membrane. Severe exposure leads to corneal edema and ulceration, conjunctivitis, and iritis.

Chronic exposure to solar UV radiation has been implicated as the major causal factor in the development of squamous cell carcinoma of the conjunctiva (Fig. 37-10).[41] In many parts of the world, this neoplasm is one of the least malignant forms of squamous cell carcinoma, especially if treated early, but in some countries such as Saudi Arabia it behaves aggressively and metastasizes widely.

Epithelial dysplasia of the conjunctiva is analogous to actinic (senile) keratosis of the eyelid and, like the latter disorder, it is usually associated with elastosis of the underlying connective tissue (pinguecula) and a pterygium is also occasionally present.

Several investigations point to an association between human cataractogenesis and UV radiation or sunlight (see box on next page and Fig. 37-11). Sunlight has been impli-

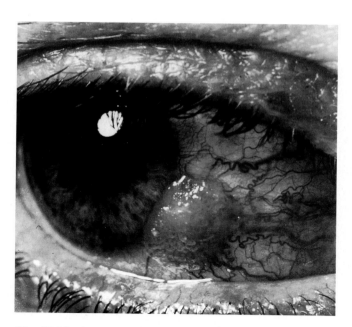

Fig. 37-10. A squamous cell carcinoma of the conjunctiva is located at the corneoscleral limbus. (From Klintworth GK, Landers MB III: *The eye: structure and function in disease*, Baltimore, 1976, Williams & Wilkins; with permission.)

cated as a major causative factor in brown nuclear cataracts, and many arguments support and refute this hypothesis. A prevailing view is that the generation of singlet oxygen and/or free radicals, directly or indirectly, by UV radiation is a major factor in cataractogenesis. Following UV irradiation, singlet oxygen, superoxide anion (O_2^-), hydroxyl radical (OH^-), hydrogen peroxide and other reactive oxygen free radicals are produced in the lens (see Chapter 22).

The lens is especially prone to photochemical stress because of the continuous entry of electromagnetic radiation. Potentially damaging photosensitization and photooxidative changes occur in the human lens throughout life. Photochemical and photooxidative reactions play important roles in normal lens biochemistry, pigment formation, and cataractogenesis. The interactions between UV light and various biomolecules has been extensively studied in the lens, and excellent reviews on the photochemistry and photobiology of the lens are available.[52,195] The photooxidation of free or protein-bound tryptophan within the lens by near-UV radiation leads to brown discoloration. Major absorbers of near-UV light are free or bound aromatic amino acids (tryptophan, tyrosine, and phenylalanine), numerous pigments, and fluorescent chromophores. Among the amino acids, tryptophan absorbs 95% or more of the radiant energy. Other endogenous light-absorbing biomolecules in the lens are 3-hydroxykynurenine and its fluorescent glucoside. Sunlight in the presence of air causes the oxidative cleavage of tryptophan to *N*-formylkynurenine.

Oxygen increases the rate of photolysis, and substances such as glutathione, ascorbic acid, and vita-

Some environmental causes of cataracts

Physical agents
Electric current
Heat
Lightning
Trauma
Ultrasound

Radiation
x rays
Beta rays
Fast neutrons
Microwaves
Infrared light
Ultraviolet light

Hemodialysis (hyperosmolar cataract)

Drugs and toxins
Thallium
Psolaren (with ultraviolet light)

Metallic foreign bodies
Iron
Copper

Bacteria
Treponema pallidum

Viruses
Cytomegalovirus
Herpes simplex
Rubella

Protozoa
Toxoplasma gondii

Nematodes
Onchocerca volvulus

Deficiency states
Certain amino acids
Riboflavin
Rickets
Tryptophan
Severe protein deficiency

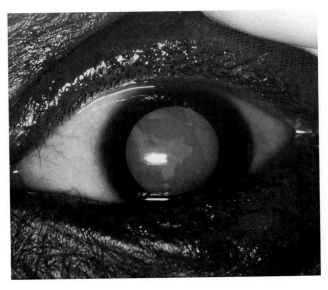

Fig. 37-11. A mature cataract completely fills the pupil of this eye. (From Klintworth GK, Landers MB III: *The eye: structure and function in disease*, Baltimore, 1976, Williams & Wilkins; with permission.)

oxide generated by near-UV radiation is mainly responsible for the hexokinase inactivation.

They are caused by the interaction of light with endogenous photosensitizers, resulting in the generation of singlet oxygen, free radicals, and other active species such as hydrogen peroxide. Active oxygen species such as hydrogen peroxide could also accumulate in the lens by light-independent mechanisms, that is, by uptake from ocular fluids surrounding the tissue or through the metabolically generated univalent reduction of oxygen intracellularly. Photochemically generated hydrogen peroxide would seem to represent the major source, and under normal conditions hydrogen peroxide is detoxified by protective mechanisms.

A population-based, case-control study of 838 Chesapeake Bay watermen revealed a significant association between total cumulative UV-B exposure and the risk of developing cortical cataracts.[179] Ultraviolet-B exposure was approximately 21% higher in watermen with cortical opacities than in those without opacities; however, nuclear cataracts and UV-B exposure were not associated. Another case-control study on a rural population in eastern Maryland disclosed a significant association between UV-B exposure and increased risk of posterior subcapsular cataracts.[2] A good correlation exists between cataracts and UV exposure in experimental animals. In lens proteins, tryptophan residues are the main absorbers of UV-B radiation, and the exposure leads to the production of photosensitizers, such as N-formylkynurenine and its derivatives. In the presence of oxygen, fluorescent products arise, and additional photochemicals lead to the cross-linking and aggregation of lens proteins.

Because of the profound sensitivity of skin, including

min E can under certain conditions act as quenchers.

Indirect evidence indicates that this pigmentation results from the generation of free radicals and other reactive species produced after exposure of photosensitizers to near-UV radiation.

Several lens enzymes are inactivated by near-UV light in the presence of tryptophan or some of its oxidation products. Some studies raise the possibility that hydrogen per-

that of the eyelid, to light in individuals with xeroderma pigmentosum, the skin of individuals with this disorder becomes acutely erythematous in early childhood on exposure to sunlight, and increased pigmentation, telangiectasia, and actinic keratoses (solar keratoses) subsequently develop. As a consequence of the deficient ultraviolet endonuclease, the impaired repair of UV damaged DNA in affected individuals predisposes them profoundly to several types of malignant sun-induced cutaneous tumors, including basal and squamous cell carcinoma and malignant melanoma,[138] as well as conjunctival squamous cell carcinoma.

Ultraviolet light is suspected of reactivating ocular herpes simplex in humans, and it has been shown to do so in mice treated with immunosuppressive drugs.[165]

Infrared irradiation

Intense infrared (400 to 723 nm) irradiation, to which thermal glassworkers, blast furnace operators, steelworkers, and smelter workers are exposed, affects the lens capsule, causing it to exfoliate, and this rare lesion is more or less restricted to individuals with these occupations. Anterior and posterior subcapsular opacities, iridoschisis, and acute blepharitis may also follow infrared irradiation.

Lens capsular exfoliation is typically bilateral, and the superficial lamellae of the anterior capsule separate from the deeper layers and peel away more or less concentrically. Sometimes a posterior polar cataract accompanies exfoliation of the lens capsule. A heat cataract may also occur without the lens capsular exfoliation.

Lasers

A laser (*l*ight *a*mplification by *s*timulated *e*mission of *r*adiation) can emit light at any specific wavelength. Aside from their deleterious effects on the eye, lasers have important therapeutic applications in the treatment of ocular diseases.[114,147,167] The armamentarium of ophthalmologists includes several different lasers: argon (mainly 488 and 514.5 nm), krypton (530.8, 568.2, and 647.1 nm), carbon dioxide (10,600 nm), eximer (*e*xcited *dimer*)(argon fluoride 193 nm, krypton chloride 222 nm, krypton fluoride 249 nm, xenon chloride 308 nm, xenon fluoride 351 nm), dye (360 to 960 nm, depending on the organic dye used), ruby (694.3 nm), and neodymium:yttrium aluminum garnet (Nd:Yag)(532 nm) lasers. For example, lasers can seal peripheral retinal holes and tears. They are also used in the treatment of narrow-angle glaucoma by producing iridotomy and laser trabeculoplasty is a method of treatment for open-angle glaucoma. Laser energy is also used to destroy the ciliary processes (cyclophotocoagulation) in the treatment of glaucoma. Excimer cyclophotocoagulation lasers are used to remove scars or other anterior corneal lesions. The Nd:YAG laser is used most frequently to produce an opening in the posterior capsule, which may opacify following extracapsular cataract surgery.

The effect of the laser can be divided into thermal, photochemical, and ionizing modes. Photons, the smallest units of light energy, are absorbed by ocular pigments, and thermal energy is produced; this causes a local heating of the tissue with coagulation of the tissue protein, inflammation, and scarring. Photochemical effects are due to a chemical reaction in the tissue caused by absorption of high- or low-energy waves. The ionizing effects are the result of plasma production in the tissues by high energy and very short exposure times. Accidental laser exposure, as in the military, can damage the eye.

The increase in pigment density in the macular pigment epithelium (as compared with the retinal periphery) results in a high absorption of laser energy in the macular region for a given exposure. The changes following xenon-arc photocoagulation can be more pronounced, with destruction of the entire retinal architecture. Excimer lasers are used to remove scars or other anterior corneal lesions.

Laser burns have sharply defined margins and cause the sensory retina to adhere to the retinal pigment epithelium (Fig. 37-12). The inner retinal layers are spared, but the retinal pigment epithelium becomes irregularly clumped. Rods and cones are degenerate, and nuclei in the outer nuclear layer become pyknotic and dispersed.

Complications of laser photocoagulation include retinal hemorrhages, visual field defects, lens opacities, transient myopia, ischemic papillitis, cystoid macular edema, traction, and exudative retinal detachment.

Ionizing radiation

Severe ocular damage may follow embryonic or fetal exposure to high levels of x-radiation (see Chapter 11). Radiation damage to the ocular anlagen produces anophthal-

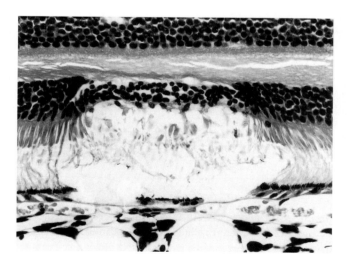

Fig. 37-12. An acute chorioretinal lesion was produced by a gallium arsenide laser. (Hematoxylin and eosin ×360.) (From Klintworth GK, Landers MB III: *The eye: structure and function in disease*, Baltimore, 1976, Williams & Wilkins; with permission.)

mia, microphthalmia, cataracts, coloboma, eyelid anomalies, and retinal pigmentary changes.[29,49] After the eleventh week, little damage is produced in the eye except for cataracts or a predisposition to early cataracts.

Cataracts form in the region of the lens receiving radiation. The epithelium of the germinative zone of the lens is most sensitive to x-irradiation, and an initial inhibition of mitotic activity begins within an hour and continues for several days. This is followed by more mitoses than normal, these reaching a peak 2 to 3 weeks after exposure. After several months, the lens epithelium becomes disorganized, and the lens fibers opacify. After a single dose of x-irradiation, the epithelial cells of the rat lens become markedly vacuolated and swollen. Eventually the entire lens epithelium shrinks, but the lens capsule is not conspicuously affected. The time lag between the radiation and the onset of morphologic abnormalities varies with the radiation dose and the species. Posterior cell migration precedes radiation-induced posterior subcapsular cataracts. X-irradiation interferes with the normal differentiation of lens epithelium into lens fibers. The lens bow nuclei becomes displaced posteriorly, and abnormal nucleated fibers accumulate in the posterior lens cortex.

Of the ocular tissues, the lens appears to be most susceptible to ionizing radiation. The damage of alpha, beta, and gamma rays becomes apparent proportional to the dose of the ionizing particles and the energy delivered to the tissue. Proliferating cells at the lens equator are most vulnerable, and after a latent period these cells may degenerate and opacify. The rapidly growing lenses of young individuals are more vulnerable than lenses of the elderly and may become completely opaque. In most experimental animals, irradiation at various wavelengths across the electromagnetic spectrum induces cataracts that appear to result from oxidative changes and/or the generation of free radicals in the lens. Survivors of the atomic bombing of Hiroshima and Nagasaki developed more extensive axial opacities and polychromatic changes in the posterior subcapsule than control populations not exposed to ionizing radiation.[135] Neutrons ionize by interacting with atomic nuclei in the tissues. Fast neutrons can cause cataracts.[107]

Intravenous methotrexate, cytosine arabinoside, lomustine, and 5-fluorouracil may all potentiate radiation-induced optic neuropathy.[89]

A mild, acute blepharitis sometimes follows irradiation to the orbit, globe, or eyelids; chronic radiation dermatitis develops months to years after treatment. A dose of 4000 rad produces severe atrophy, vascular occlusion, and fibrosis. Squamous or basal cell carcinomas may emerge in these areas after many years.

Squamous cell carcinoma. Aside from fair skin, excessive UV radiation, and xeroderma pigmentosa, x-ray irradiation predisposes to squamous cell carcinoma of the eyelid. The skin, including the hair follicles of the eyelids, may

atrophy, resulting in loss of hair. Skin may also ulcerate and heal poorly. Epithelial cells may become hyperplastic and morphologically abnormal. Telangiectatic vessels commonly emerge, and eventually basal or squamous cell carcinomas can appear.

Initially, the conjunctiva becomes acutely inflamed, but later it atrophies as telangiectatic vessels become prominent. In severe cases a loss of mucus glands and lacrimal secretions leads to the "dry eye syndrome." Closure of the puncta, symblepharon, conjunctival and corneal keratinization, and eventual carcinoma are possible sequelae. Corneal involvement may be secondary to the loss of conjunctival and lacrimal secretions. The cornea may develop hypoesthesia followed by a punctate or filamentary keratopathy and ulceration. Late corneal manifestations include stromal vascularization and scarring, aseptic necrosis, and perforation.

Particularly when cobalt plaques emitting high doses of ionizing radiation are applied to the eye in the therapy of intraocular malignant tumors, scleral necrosis may develop.

Following high doses of ionizing radiation, retinal degeneration with an infiltration of retinal pigment epithelium, retinal neovascularization with vitreous hemorrhages, iris neovascularization, and glaucoma may also develop.

In experimental animals, high doses of gamma radiation rapidly cause a degenerative retinopathy characterized by edema, nuclear pyknosis, and photoreceptor disintegration. Retinas of young animals are more sensitive than those of older animals.

Iridocyclitis, followed by atrophy of the iris and ciliary body and pigment dispersion in the anterior chamber angle leading to glaucoma, may also occur.

Particularly osteogenic sarcoma, but also fibrosarcoma, other sarcomas and epithelial neoplasms may follow radiotherapy for retinoblastoma.[158]

Astronauts are exposed to cosmic rays consisting of protons, alpha particles, and other particles, despite the protective covering of their spaceships. Although significant visual abnormalities have not been detected in any of the numerous astronauts who have been exposed to radiation in space, individuals involved in space travel have reported minute visual images thought to be due to the impact of cosmic rays on the retina. Galactic and solar cosmic rays are a serious radiation hazard for space exploration, especially for anticipated long-duration missions such as those designed for lunar habitat or a Mars transfer vehicle.

ULTRASOUND

Ultrasonography using sound having a frequency of greater than 30,000 Hz is used by ophthalmologists to evaluate certain ocular abnormalities, especially when the ocular contents are opaque. Although these brief examinations do not cause adverse effects, the frequency of the ultrasonic waves and the intensity and duration of the stimulus produce thermal, mechanical, and chemical effects that may

engaged in manufacture of hydroquinone, *Arch Ophthalmol* 38:812, 1947.

8. Anderson B Jr, Farmer JC Jr: Hyperoxic myopia, *Trans Am Ophthalmol Soc* 76:116, 1978.

9. Anderson B Jr, Shelton DL: Axial length in hyperoxic myopia. In: Bone AA, Bachrach AJ, Greenbaum Jr LJ, editors: *Proceedings, 9th International Symposium on Underwater and Hyperbaric Physiology,* Undersea and Hyperbaric Medical Society, Bethesda, Maryland, 1987, pp 607-611.

10. Anderson LJ, et al; Nosocomial rabies: investigation of contacts of human rabies cases associated with a corneal transplant, *Am J Public Health* 74:370, 1984.

11. Antonios SR, et al: Contamination of donor cornea: postpenetrating keratoplasty endophthalmitis, *Cornea* 10:217, 1991.

12. Arden GB, et al: A survey of color discrimination in German ophthalmologists. Changes associated with the use of lasers and operating microscopes, *Ophthalmology* 98:567, 1991.

13. Armstrong RC, Monie IWL: Congenital eye defects on rats following maternal folic-acid deficiency during pregnancy, *J Embryol Exper Morphol* 16:531, 1966.

14. Arnesen K, and Nordstoga K: Ocular encephalitozoonosis (nosematosis) in blue foxes. Polyarteritis nodosa and cataract, *Acta Ophthalmol (Copenh)* 55:641, 1977.

15. Asahi M: Clinical features and pathogenesis of Yusho (PCB poisoning) (Review). (In Japanese), *Sangyo Ika Daigaku Zasshi* 15:1, 1993.

16. Ashton N, Ward B, Serpell G: Role of oxygen in the genesis of retrolental fibroplasia: preliminary report, *Br J Ophthalmol* 37:513, 1953.

17. Ashton N, Ward B, Serpell G: Effect of oxygen on developing retinal vessels with particular reference to the problem of retrolental fibroplasia *Br J Ophthalmol* 38:397, 1954.

18. Ashton N, Wirasinha PA: Encephalitozoonosis (nosematosis) of the cornea, *Br J Ophthalmol* 57:669, 1973.

19. Auran JD, Starr MB, Jakobiec FA: Acanthamoeba keratitis. A review of the literature, *Cornea* 6:2, 1987.

20. Barger G: *Ergot and ergotism,* London, 1931, Oxford Medical Publisher.

21. Baumbach GL, et al: Methyl alcohol poisoning. IV. Alterations of the morphological findings of the retina and optic nerve, *Arch Ophthalmol* 95:1859, 1977.

22. Benton CD, Calhoun FP Jr: The ocular effects of methyl alcohol poisoning: report of a catastrophe involving 320 persons, *Am J Ophthalmol* 36:1677, 1953.

23. Bhatnagar R, et al: Risk of cataract and history of severe diarrheal disease in southern India, *Arch Ophthalmol* 109:696, 1991.

24. Bhuyan KC, Bhuyan DK: Superoxide dismutase of the eye: relative functions of superoxide dismutase and catalase in protecting the ocular lens from oxidative damage, *Biochim Biophys Acta* 542:28, 1978.

25. Bjorkenheim B: Optic neuropathy caused by vitamin-B_{12} deficiency in carriers of the fish tapeworm, *Diphyllobothrium latum, Lancet* 1:688, 1966.

26. Bogdanoff B, et al: Brain and eye abnormalities. Possible sequelae to prenatal use of multiple drugs including LSD, *Am J Dis Child* 123:145, 1972.

27. Bond GG, et al: Incidence of chloracne among chemical workers potentially exposed to chlorinated dioxins, *J Occup Med* 31:771, 1989.

28. Bone RA, et al: Analysis of the macular pigment by HPLC: retinal distribution and age study, *Invest Ophthalmol Vis Sci* 29:843, 1988.

29. Brent RL: *Radiations and other physical agents.* In: Fraser, F.C. and Wilson, J.G. editors: *Handbook of Teratology,* New York, 1977, Plenum Press, pp 153-201.

30. Bressler NM, et al: The grading and prevalence of macular degeneration in Chesapeake Bay watermen, *Arch Ophthalmol* 107:847, 1989.

31. Brincker P, Gregersen E, Prause JU: Acanthamoeba keratitis, clinico-pathological report of 2 cases, *Acta Ophthalmol (Copenh)* 66:210, 1988.

32. Brown SI, Weller CA, Akiya S: Pathogenesis of ulcers of the alkaliburned cornea, *Arch Ophthalmol* 83:205, 1970.

33. Brown TJ, Cursons RT: Pathogenic free-living amebae (PFLA) from frozen swimming areas in Oslo, Norway, *Scand J Infect Dis* 9:237, 1977.

34. Bruce AS, Brennan NA: Corneal pathophysiology with contact lens wear, *Surv Ophthalmol* 35:25, 1990.

35. Burns RP, Steele A: *Ocular changes in drug abusers: symposium on ocular therapy* ed 6, St Louis, 1973, Mosby–Year Book.

36. Burstein, N.L: Corneal cytotoxicity of topically applied drugs, vehicles and preservatives, *Surv Ophthalmol* 25:15, 1980.

37. Butler FK, Harris DJ Jr, Reynolds RD: Altitude retinopathy on Mount Everest, 1989, *Ophthalmology* 99:739, 1992.

38. Caffey J: The whiplash shaken infant syndrome: manual shaking by the extremities with whiplash-induced intracranial and intraocular bleedings, linked with residual permanent brain damage and mental retardation, *Pediatrics* 54:396, 1974.

39. Cashwell LF Jr., et al: Idiopathic true exfoliation of the lens capsule, *Ophthalmology* 96:348, 1989.

40. Christen WG, et al: A prospective study of cigarette smoking and risk of cataract in men, *JAMA* 268:989, 1992.

41. Clear AS, Chirambo MC, Hutt MS: Solar keratosis, pterygium, and squamous cell carcinoma of the conjunctiva in Malawi, *Br J Ophthalmol* 63:102, 1979.

42. Cogan DG, Albright F, Bartter FC: Hypercalcemia and band keratopathy: report of nineteen cases, *Arch Ophthalmol* 40:624, 1948.

43. Corkey JA: Ophthalmia nodosa due to caterpillar hairs, *Br J Ophthalmol* 39:301, 1955.

44. Custis PH, et al: Posterior internal ophthalmomyiasis. Identification of a surgically removed Cuterebra larva by scanning electron microscopy, *Ophthalmology* 90:1583, 1983.

45. Daly PJ, Sim FH, Simonet WT: Ice hockey injuries. A review, *Sports Med* 10:122, 1990.

46. Dang CV: Tobacco-alcohol amblyopia: a proposed biochemical basis for pathogenesis, *Med Hypotheses* 7:1317, 1981.

47. Dannenberg AL, et al: Penetration eye injuries in the workplace. The National Eye Trauma System Registry, *Arch Ophthalmol* 110:843, 1992.

48. Dannenberg AL, Parver LM, Fowler CJ: Penetrating eye injuries related to assault. The National Eye Trauma System Registry, *Arch Ophthalmol* 110:849, 1992.

49. Dekaban AS: Abnormalities in children exposed to x-radiation during various stages of gestation: tentative timetable of radiation injury to the human fetus. I, *J Nuclear Med* 9:471, 1968.

50. Deschamps D, et al: Etude en milieu professionnel de la toxicité de l'oxyde d'éthylène sur le cristallin. Difficulté des enquêtes épidémiologiques sur la cataracte. *J Fr Ophtalmol* 13:189, 1990.

51. Deschamps D, et al: Toxicity of ethylene oxide on the lens and on leukocytes: an epidemiological study in hospital sterilisation installations, *Br J Ind Med* 47:308, 1990.

52. Dillon J: *Photochemical mechanisms in the lens.* In Maisel H, editor: *The ocular lens, structure, function and pathology,* New York, 1985, Marcel Dekker, pp 349-366.

52A. Doughman D, Ingram JJ, Bourne WM: Experimental band keratopathy: electron microscope x-ray analysis of aqueous and corneal calcium concentrations, *Invest Ophthalmol* 9:471, 1970.

53. Duffy P, et al: Possible person-to-person transmission of Creutzfeldt-Jakob disease, *N Engl J Med* 290:692, 1974 (letter).

54. Duke-Elder S: *Diseases of the outer eye.* In Duke-Elder S, editor: *System of ophthalmology,* vol 8, London, 1965, Henry Kimpton, pp 420-421.

55. Easty DL, Williams C: *Viral and rickettsial disease.* In Garner A,

Klintworth GK, editors: *Pathobiology of ocular disease,* New York, 1994, Marcel Dekker, pp 227-262.

56. Edward DP, et al: Diffuse corneal clouding in siblings with fetal alcohol syndrome, *Am J Ophthalmol* 115:484, 1993.

57. Edwards JJ, Anderson RL, Wood JR: Loxoscelism of the eyelids, *Arch Ophthalmol* 98:1997, 1980.

58. Eells JT: Methanol-induced visual toxicity in the rat, *J Pharmacol Exp Ther* 257:56, 1991.

59. Ellis PP: *Ocular therapeutics and pharmacology,* ed 7, St Louis, 1985, Mosby–Year Book.

60. Ferguson J, Johnson BE: Photosensitivity due to retinoids: clinical and laboratory studies, *Br J Dermatol* 115:275, 1986.

61. Forsey T, Darougar S: Transmission of chlamydiae by the housefly, *Br J Ophthalmol* 65:147, 1981.

62. Forward GR: Indoor cricket injuries, *Med J Aust* 148:560, 1988.

63. Fox DA, Katz LM, Farber DB: Low level developmental lead exposure decreases the sensitivity, amplitude and temporal resolution of rods, *Neurotoxicology* 12:641, 1991.

64. Fraunfelder FT, LaBraico JM, Meyer SM: Adverse ocular reactions possibly associated with isotretinoin, *Am J Ophthalmol* 100:534, 1985.

65. Fraunfelder FT, Meyer SM: *Drug-induced ocular side effects and drug interactions,* Philadelphia, 1989, Lea & Febiger.

66. Fu YA: Ocular manifestation of polychlorinated biphenyls intoxication, *Prog Clin Biol Res* 137:127, 1984.

67. Genovese MT, et al: Eye injuries among pennant squash players and their attitudes towards protective eyewear, *Med J Aust* 153:655, 1990.

68. Gerding DN, et al: Treatment of *Pseudomonas endophthalmitis* associated with prosthetic intraocular lens implantation, *Am J Ophthalmol* 88:902, 1979.

69. Gillman T: Nutrition, liver disease and some aspects of ageing in Africans, *Ciba Found Colloq Ageing* 3:104, 1957.

70. Giovinazzo VJ, et al: The ocular complications of boxing, *Ophthalmology* 94:587, 1987.

71. Glasner PD, et al: An unusually high prevalence of ocular toxoplasmosis in southern Brazil, *Am J Ophthalmol* 114:136, 1992.

72. Glass P: Light and the developing retina, *Doc Ophthalmol* 74:195, 1990.

73. Glasser DB, et al: Ocular jellyfish stings, *Ophthalmology* 99:1414, 1992.

74. Gode GR, Bhide NK: Two rabies deaths after corneal grafts from one donor, *Lancet* 2:791, 1988 (letter).

75. Gomez Morales A, et al: Hydatid cysts of the orbit. A review of 35 cases, *Ophthalmology* 95:1027, 1988.

76. Grant WM: *Toxicology of the eye,* ed 2, Springfield, Ill, 1974, Charles C Thomas.

77. Gregg NM: Congenital cataract following German measles in the mother, *Trans Ophthalmol Soc Aust* 3:35, 1941.

78. Griffin JD, Garnick MB: Eye toxicity of cancer chemotherapy: a review of the literature, *Cancer* 48:1539, 1981.

79. Grossniklaus HE, et al: Toxoplasma gondii retinochoroiditis and optic neuritis in acquired immune deficiency syndrome. Report of a case, *Ophthalmology* 97:1342, 1990.

80. Gunderson T, Heath P, Garron LK: Ophthalmia nodosa, *Trans Am Ophthalmol Soc* 48:151, 1950.

81. Handelman GJ, et al: Biological control of primate macular pigment. Biochemical and densitometric studies, *Invest Ophthalmol Vis Sci* 32:257, 1991.

82. Hankinson SE, et al: A prospective study of cigarette smoking and risk of cataract surgery in women, *JAMA* 268:994, 1992.

83. Harada T, et al: Bilan sur 164 cas de traumatismes oculaires dus à certain sports, *J Fr Ophtalmol* 8:455, 1985.

84. Hata S, Bernstein E, Davis LE: Atypical ocular bobbing in acute organophosphate poisoning, *Arch Neurol* 43:185, 1986.

85. Hatem G, Merritt JC, Cowan CL Jr: Bacillus cereus panophthalmitis after intravenous heroin, *Ann Ophthalmol* 11:431, 1979.

86. Hinzpeter EN, Renz S, Löser H: Augenveränderungen bev Alkoholembryopathie, *Klin Monatsbl Augenheilkd* 200:33, 1992.

87. Holds JB, et al: Hydraulic orbital injection injuries, *Ophthalmology* 100:1475, 1993.

88. Hyman LG, et al: Risk factors for age-related maculopathy, *Invest Ophthalmol Vis Sci* 33(suppl):801, 1992.

89. Imperia PS, Lazarus HM, Lass JH: Ocular complications of systemic cancer chemotherapy, *Surv Ophthalmol* 34:209, 1989.

90. Inkeles DM, Walsh JB: Retinal fat emboli as sequela to acute pancreatitis, *Am J Ophthalmol* 80:935, 1975.

91. Ismail M, et al: The ocular effects of spitting cobras: I. the ringhals cobra *(Hemachatus haemachatus)* venom-induced corneal opacification syndrome, *J Toxicol Clin Toxicol* 31:31, 1993.

92. Jacques PF, et al: Antioxidant status in persons with and without senile cataract, *Arch Ophthalmol* 106:337, 1988.

93. Johnson FB, Zimmerman LE: Barium sulfate and zinc sulfate deposits resulting golf-ball injury to the conjunctiva and eyelid, *Am J Clin Pathol* 44:533, 1965.

94. Jones BR: Changing concepts of trachoma and its control, *Trans Ophthalmol Soc UK* 100:25, 1980.

95. Jones DB, Forster FK, Rebell G: Fusarium solani keratitis treated with natamycin (pimaricin): eighteen consecutive cases, *Arch Ophthalmol* 88:147, 1972.

96. Karai I, Sugimoto K, Goto S: A fluorescein angiographic study on carbon disulfide retinopathy among workers in viscose rayon factories, *Int Arch Occup Environ Health* 53:91, 1983.

97. Kaunitz J: Chronic endemic ergotism and its relation to thromboangiitis, *Arch Surg* 25:1135, 1932.

98. Kazacos KR, Vestre WA, Kazacos EA: Raccoon ascarid larvae *(Baylisascaris procyonis)* as a cause of ocular larva migrans, *Invest Ophthalmol Vis Sci* 25:1177, 1984.

99. Kazacos KR, et al: Diffuse unilateral subacute neuroretinitis syndrome: probable cause, *Arch Ophthalmol* 102:967, 1984.

100. Kean BH, Sun T, Elsworth RM: *Color atlas/text on ophthalmic parasitology,* New York, 1991, Igaku-Shoin.

101. Kietzman B: Mooren's ulcer in Nigeria, *Am J Ophthalmol* 65:679, 1968.

102. Klein BE, et al: Cigarette smoking and lens opacities: the Beaver Dam eye study, *Am J Prev Med* 9:27, 1993.

103. Klein R, Klein BE, Linton KL: Prevalence of age-related maculopathy. The Beaver Dam eye study, *Ophthalmology* 99:933, 1992.

104. Klintworth GK: *Degenerations, depositions, and miscellaneous reactions of the ocular anterior segment. In Garner A, Klintworth GK, editors: Pathobiology of ocular disease,* ed 2. New York, 1994, Marcel Dekker, pp 743-797.

105. Klintworth GK, Garner A: *The causes, types, and morphology of cataracts. In Garner A, Klintworth GK, editors: Pathobiology of ocular disease, ed 2, New York, 1994, Marcel Dekker, pp 481-532.*

106. Klintworth GK, Streeten BW, Eagle RC Jr: *Applications of energy dispersive microprobe analysis in ophthalmic pathology. In Ingram P, Shelburne JD, Roggli VI, editors: Microprobe analysis in medicine,* New York, 1989, Hemisphere, pp 253-290.

107. Konishi N: Electron microscopic study of rabbit lenses irradiated with fast electrons, *Acta Soc Ophthalmol Jpn* 70:1367, 1966.

108. Kuhn F, Morris R, Massey M: Photic retinal injury from endoillumination during vitrectomy, *Am J Ophthalmol* 111:42, 1991.

109. Lapidus CS, et al: Eye injuries in lacrosse: women need their vision less than men? *J Trauma* 32:555, 1992.

110. Lauer SA, Malter JS, Meier JR: Human papillomavirus type 18 in conjunctival intraepithelial neoplasia, *Am J Ophthalmol* 110:23, 1990.

111. Lederer CM Jr, Sabates FN: Ocular findings in the intravenous drug abuser, *Ann Ophthalmol* 14:436, 1982.

112. Leibowitz HM, et al: The Framingham Eye Study monograph: an ophthalmological and epidemiological study of cataract, glaucoma, diabetic retinopathy, macular degeneration, and visual acuity in a

general population of 2631 adults, 1973-1975, *Surv Ophthalmol* 24:335, 1980.

113. Lerman S: Biophysical aspects of corneal and lenticular transparency, *Curr Eye Res* 3:3, 1984.

114. L'Esperance FA Jr: *Ophthalmic Laser,* ed 3, 2 vol, St Louis, 1989, Mosby–Year Book.

115. Levi L, Miller NR: Visual illusions associated with previous drug abuse, *J Clin Neuro Ophthalmol* 10:103, 1990.

116. Lowder CY, et al: Microsporidia infection of the cornea in a man seropositive for human immunodeficiency virus, *Am J Ophthalmol* 109:242, 1990.

117. Luckenbach M, Kielar R: Toxic corneal epithelial edema from exposure to high atmospheric concentration of toluene diisocyanates, *Am J Ophthalmol* 90:682, 1980.

118. Ludwig S, Warman M: Shaken baby syndrome: a review of 20 cases, *Ann Emerg Med* 13:104, 1984.

119. Macewen CJ: Eye injuries: a prospective survey of 5671 cases, *Br J Ophthalmol* 73:888, 1989.

120. Mamalis N, et al: Blunt ocular trauma secondary to "war games," *Ann Ophthalmol* 22:416, 1990.

121. Margo CE: *Ocular disease due to bacteria.* In Garner A, Klintworth GK, editors: *Pathobiology of ocular disease,* New York, 1994, Marcel Dekker, pp 275-297.

122. Margolis S, Martin L: Anophthalmia in an infant of parents using LSD, *Ann Ophthalmol* 12:1378, 1980.

123. McDonnell JM, Mayr AJ, Martin WJ: DNA of human papillomavirus type 16 in dysplastic and malignant lesions of the conjunctiva and cornea *N Engl J Med* 320:1442, 1989. Erratum, 321:63.

124. McKinna AJ: Quinine induced hypoplasia of the optic nerve, *Canad J Ophthalmol* 1:261, 1966.

125. McLane NJ, Carroll DM: Ocular manifestations of drug abuse, *Surv Ophthalmol* 30:298, 1986.

126. Mencia-Gutierrez E, et al: Perforating ocular wounds in occupational accidents, *Ophthalmologica* 197:97, 1988.

127. Menser MA, Dods L, and Harley JD: A twenty-five-year follow-up of congenital rubella, *Lancet* 2:1347, 1967.

128. Missliwetz J, Lindermann A: Gunshot wounds caused by Fiocchi anticrime cartridges (plastic bullets), *Am J Forensic Med Pathol* 12:209, 1991.

129. Miyashita K: Wasp sting–induced linear keratitis, *Ann Ophthalmol* 24:143, 1992.

130. Mohammed S, Kazmi H: Subluxation of the lens and ocular hypertension in exfoliative syndrome, *Pakistan J Ophthalmol* 2:77, 1980.

131. Morell T, Lohmann M, Basse PN: Injuries due to fireworks. (In Danish), *Ugeskr Laeger* 154:3736, 1992.

132. Moss AP, et al: The ocular manifestations and functional effects of occupational argyrosis. *Arch Ophthalmol* 97:906, 1979.

133. Muller R: *Worms and disease: a manual of medical helminthology,* London, 1975, Heinemann.

134. Murray TG, et al: Methanol poisoning. A rodent model with structural and functional evidence for retinal involvement, *Arch Ophthalmol* 109:1012, 1991.

135. Nefzger MD, Miller RJ, Fujino T: Eye findings in atomic bomb survivors of Hiroshima and Nagasaki: 1963-1964, *Am J Epidemiol* 89:129, 1969.

136. Newman MA, Kachuba JB: Glutaraldehyde: a potential health risk to nurses, *Gastroenterol Nurs* 14:296, 1992.

137. Nichols CW, et al: Histologic alterations produced in the eye by oxygen at high pressure, *Arch Ophthalmol* 87:417, 1972.

138. O'Brien TP, Green WR: *Fungus infections of the eye and periocular tissues.* In Garner A, Klintworth GK, editors: *Pathobiology of ocular disease,* New York, 1994, Marcel Dekker, pp 299-333.

139. Owen P, Keightley SJ, Elkington AR: The hazards of hammers, *Injury* 18:61, 1987.

140. Parver LM, et al, editors: Characteristics and causes of penetrating eye injuries reported to the National Eye Trauma System Registry, 1985-91, *Public Health Rep* 108:625, 1993.

141. Pashby TJ: Eye injuries in Canadian sports and recreational activities, *Can J Ophthalmol* 27:226, 1992.

142. Patel BC, Morgan LH: Work-related penetrating eye injuries, *Acta Ophthalmol (Copenh)* 69:377, 1991.

143. Patz A, et al: Oxygen studies in retrolental fibroplasia. II. The production of the microscopic changes of retrolental fibroplasia in experimental animals, *Am J Ophthalmol* 36:1511, 1953.

144. Patz A, Hoeck LE, de la Cruz E: Studies on the effect of high oxygen administration in retrolental fibroplasia. I, Nursery observations, *Am J Ophthalmol* 35:1248, 1952.

145. Pettit TH, et al: Fungal endophthalmitis following intraocular lens implantation. A surgical epidemic, *Arch Ophthalmol* 98:1025, 1980.

146. Pinnolis M, et al: Nosematosis of the cornea. Case report, including electron microscopic studies, *Arch Ophthalmol* 99:1044, 1981.

147. Pitts D, Kleinstein RN: *Environmental vision: interactions of the eye, vision and the environment,* Boston, 1993, Butterworth-Heinemann.

148. Ravenholt RT: Cigarette smoking and risk of cataracts, *JAMA* 269:747, 1993 (letter).

149. Reifler DM, Hornblass A: Squamous cell carcinoma of the eyelid, *Surv Ophthalmol* 30:349, 1986. Erratum, 31:77.

150. Rengstorff RH: Accidental exposure to sarin: vision effects, *Arch Toxicol* 56:201, 1985.

151. Resnikoff S, Filliard G, Dell'Aquila B: Climatic droplet keratopathy, exfoliation syndrome, and cataract, *Br J Ophthalmol* 75:734, 1991.

152. Rhodes C, et al: A balanced approach to the detection, characterisation and mechanism of the toxicity of industrial chemicals, *J Toxicol Sci* 12:243, 1987.

153. Rodriguez-Pichardo A, Camacho F: Chloracne as a consequence of a family accident with chlorinated dioxins, *J Am Acad Dermatol* 22:1121, 1990 (letter and comment).

154. Rosen DH, Hoffman AM: Focal suicide: self-enucleation by two young psychotic individuals, *Am J Psychiatry* 128:1009, 1972.

155. Roshchin AV, Veselov VG, and Panova AI: Industrial toxicology of metals of the platinum group, *J Hyg Epidemiol Microbiol Immunol* 28:17, 1984.

156. Roy H: Cigarette smoking and risk of cataracts, *JAMA* 269:748, 1993 (letter).

157. Rummelt V, Rummelt C, Naumann GO: Congenital nonpigmented epithelial iris cyst after amniocentesis. Clinicopathologic report on two children, *Ophthalmology* 100:776, 1993.

158. Sahel JA, Albert DM: *Tumors of the retina.* In Garner A, Klintworth GK, editors: *Pathobiology of ocular disease, New York, 1994, Marcel Dekker, pp 1471-1514.*

159. Salchert JJ: Cigarette smoking and risk of cataracts, *JAMA* 269:747, 1993 (letter).

160. Samples JR, et al: Acanthamoeba keratitis possibly acquired from a hot tub, *Arch Ophthalmol* 102:707, 1984.

161. Schanzlin DJ: *Scientific foundations and clinical practice.* In Smolin G, Thoft R, editors: *The cornea,* Boston, 1987, Little Brown, pp 321-327.

162. Schocket SS, et al: Induction of cataracts in mice by exposure to oxygen, *Isr J Med Sci* 8:1596, 1972.

163. Scroggs MW, Klintworth GK: Senile scleral plaques: a histopathologic study using energy-dispersive x-ray microanalysis, *Hum Pathol* 22:557, 1991.

164. Scroggs MW, Lewis JS, Proia AD: Corneal argyrosis associated with silver soldering, *Cornea* 11:264, 1992.

165. Shimeld C, et al: Reactivation of latent infection and induction of recurrent herpetic eye disease in mice, *J Gen Virol* 71:397, 1990.

166. Shine B, et al: Association between Graves' ophthalmopathy and smoking, *Lancet* 335:1261, 1990.

167. Sliney D, Wolbarsht M: *Safety with lasers and other optical sources: a comprehensive handbook,* New York, 1980, Plenum Press.

168. Song HS, Wray SH: Bee sting optic neuritis. A case report with visual evoked potentials, *J Clin Neuro Ophthalmol* 11:45, 1991.

169. Sotiropoulos SV, et al: Childhood lawn dart injuries. Summary of 75 patients and patient report, *Am J Dis Child* 144:980, 1990.

170. Spector A, Garner WH: Hydrogen peroxide and human cataract, *Exp Eye Res* 33:673, 1981.

171. Spencer WH, et al: Endogenous and exogenous ocular and systemic silver deposition, *Trans Ophthalmol Soc UK* 100:171, 1980.

172. Spiteri MA, James DG: Adverse ocular reactions to drugs, *Postgrad Med J* 59:343, 1983.

173. Stromland K: Ocular involvement in the fetal alcohol syndrome, *Surv Ophthalmol* 31:277, 1987.

174. Stromland K: Alcohol during pregnancy damages eye and vision development (Review). (In Swedish), *Nord Med* 107:313, 1992.

175. Stromland K, Miller M, and Cook C: Ocular teratology, *Surv Ophthalmol* 35:429, 1991.

176. Stuart JC, Linn JG Jr: *Candida albicans* transmission by penetrating keratoplasty, *Cornea* 3:285, 1984.

177. Sugar HS, Mandell GH, Shalev J: Metastatic endophthalmitis associated with injection of addictive drugs, *Am J Ophthalmol* 71:1055, 1971.

178. Tansurat P: *Sparganosis.* In Marcial-Rojas RA, editor: *Pathology of protozoal and helminthic diseases with clinical correlation,* Baltimore, 1971, Williams & Wilkins, pp 585-591.

179. Taylor HR: Ultraviolet radiation and the eye: an epidemiologic study, *Trans Am Ophthalmol Soc* 87:802, 1990.

180. Taylor HR, Hollows FC, Moran D: Pseudoexfoliation of the lens in Australian Aborigines, *Br J Ophthalmol* 61:473, 1977.

181. Taylor HR, et al: Visible light and risk of age-related macular degeneration, *Trans Am Ophthalmol Soc* 88:163, 1990.

182. Terry TL: Extreme prematurity and fibroblastic overgrowth of persistent vascular sheath behind each crystallin lens. I. Preliminary report, *Am J Ophthalmol* 25:203, 1942.

183. Thomas RB, Fuller DH: Self-inflicted ocular injury associated with drug use, *J S C Med Assoc* 68:202, 1972.

184. Turner M, et al: Community outbreak of adenovirus type 7a infections associated with a swimming pool, *South Med J* 80:712, 1987.

185. Van Heyningen R, Harding JJ: A case-control study of cataract in Oxfordshire: some risk factors, *Br J Ophthalmol* 72:804, 1988.

186. Wartew GA: The health hazards of formaldehyde, *J Appl Toxicol* 3:121, 1983.

187. Watson PG, Sevel D: Ophthalmia nodosa, *Br J Ophthalmol* 50:209, 1966.

188. Wear DJ, et al: Cat scratch disease bacilli in the conjunctiva of patients with Parinaud's oculoglandular syndrome, *Ophthalmology* 92:1282, 1985.

189. Weinberg JC, et al: Conjunctival synthetic fiber granuloma. A lesion that resembles conjunctivitis nodosa, *Ophthalmology* 91:867, 1984.

190. Weiter JJ, et al: Retinal pigment epithelial lipofuscin and melanin and choroidal melanin in human eyes, *Invest Ophthalmol Vis Sci* 27:145, 1986.

191. West S: Does smoke get in your eyes? *JAMA* 268:1025, 1992 (editorial).

192. Wilson FM: Adverse external ocular effects of topical ophthalmic medications, *Surv Ophthalmol* 24:57, 1979.

193. Winterkorn JM: Lyme disease: neurologic and ophthalmic manifestations, *Surv Ophthalmol* 35:191, 1990.

194. Witkop CJ Jr, et al: *Albinism.* In Scriver CR, et al, editors: *Metabolic basis for inherited diseases,* New York, 1989, McGraw-Hill, pp 2905-2947.

195. Zigman S: *Photobiology of the lens.* In Maisel H, editor: *The ocular lens, structure, function and pathology,* New York, 1985, Marcel Dekker, pp 301-347.

196. Zilis JD, Machemer R: Light damage in detached retina, *Am J Ophthalmol* 111:47, 1991.

197. Zugerman C: Chloracne. Clinical manifestations and etiology, *Dermatol Clin* 8:209, 1990.

198. Zwick H, et al: Increased sensitization to aeroallergens in competitive swimmers, *Lung* 168:111, 1990.

The letter f following page numbers indicates
figures; t indicates tables.